Principles and Practice of Neurocritical Care

Hemanshu Prabhakar
Vasudha Singhal • Kapil G Zirpe
Harsh Sapra
Editors

Principles and Practice of Neurocritical Care

Springer

Editors
Hemanshu Prabhakar
Department of Neuroanaesthesiology and Critical Care
All India Institute of Medical Sciences
New Delhi, Delhi, India

Vasudha Singhal
Department of Neuroanesthesiology and Neurocritical Care
Medanta The Medicity
Gurugram, Haryana, India

Kapil G Zirpe
Department of Neuro Trauma Unit
Ruby Hall Clinic
Pune, Maharashtra, India

Harsh Sapra
Department of Neuroanesthesia and Neurocritical care
Medanta The Medicity
Gurgaon, Haryana, India

ISBN 978-981-99-8058-1 ISBN 978-981-99-8059-8 (eBook)
https://doi.org/10.1007/978-981-99-8059-8

This Springer imprint is published by the registered company Springer Nature Singapore Pte Ltd.
The registered company address is: 152 Beach Road, #21-01/04 Gateway East, Singapore 189721, Singapore

To our patients, who taught us more than books.

Foreword

I am delighted to introduce the Society of Neurocritical Care of India's *Principles and Practice of Neurocritical Care* which represents a collaborative effort from esteemed authors across the world.

This volume showcases the collective wisdom and expertise of its international authorship. It offers up-to-date knowledge on a wide range of topics presented from a variety of perspectives. There are chapters dedicated to basic principles, monitoring, and neuropharmacology. In other chapters, authors address extracranial impacts of neurological disease and integrate them in chapters focusing on supportive care. The series of chapters written in a case-based format are particularly useful for early career neurointensivists. This comprehensive volume finishes with discussions of ethics and brain death.

Each chapter reflects the authors' commitment to the field of neurocritical care. Drawing from experiences in diverse healthcare systems, the authors offer valuable clinical insights and recommendations. This book serves as both a guide for aspiring neurocritical care professionals and a companion for experienced practitioners.

Collaboration and global cooperation have become essential in advancing medical knowledge, and this book exemplifies that spirit. By bringing together international authorship, it symbolizes the unity of the medical community in its pursuit of excellence and improved patient care worldwide and explores practice in limited resource settings.

I extend my gratitude to the authors for their dedication and contributions to this important endeavor. Their commitment to sharing knowledge will undoubtedly inspire practitioners to provide the highest level of care for critically ill neurological patients.

To the readers, I encourage you to embrace this volume with an open mind and a thirst for learning. May it enable your journey toward mastery of the practice of neurocritical care, and may the patients entrusted to your care benefit from this knowledge.

Michael Diringer
Professor of Neurology
Washington University School of Medicine
St Louis, MO, USA
July 26, 2023

Preface

Neurocritical Care is the intensive care management of patients with neurological problems. The field of neurocritical care has changed considerably over the recent years. The change has been brought about primarily with the advances in imaging and monitoring of the brain and the spinal cord. We now understand the functions of the brain better than what we did until a decade or so ago.

The Editors of this volume are very excited to present the first edition of the *Principles and Practice of Neurocritical Care*. The book tries to cover all the essential concepts of neurocritical care. Divided into many sections, the book covers from topics related to the basics of neurocritical care, neuromonitoring, neuropharmacology, systemic and supportive neurocritical care, and case-based discussions. It also includes important topics such as management of pediatric, geriatric, and pregnant patients with neurologic problems. The book will describe some of the commonly performed procedures in the neuro-intensive care unit as well. This book will serve as a quick reference guide to all intensivists managing neurosurgical patients. It would be useful for general intensivists who occasionally have to manage neurologic patients and trainees and fellows. The book has a straightforward and systematic approach to various clinical problems encountered during intensive care management of neurologic patients.

We thank the contributors for doing an outstanding job of producing such authoritative chapters. On behalf of SNCC, we feel privileged to have prepared this first edition of the book for the society. We learned a lot in editing this book, and I sincerely hope you will find it a valuable source of education.

New Delhi, Delhi, India — Hemanshu Prabhakar
Gurugram, Haryana, India — Vasudha Singhal
Pune, Maharashtra, India — Kapil G Zirpe
Gurugram, Haryana, India — Harsh Sapra

The original version of this book has been revised. A foreword by Michael Diringer has been included in the book.

Acknowledgments

We wish to acknowledge the support from the administrations of All India Institute of Medical Sciences (AIIMS), New Delhi (India), Medanta—The Medicity, Gurugram and Ruby Hall Clinic, Pune, for allowing us to carry out this academic task.

Very special thanks to Dr. Charu Mahajan and Dr. Indu Kapoor, for their constructive criticism and inputs in this academic endeavor.

Special thanks are due to the team of Springer—Dr. Naren Aggrawal, Jagjeet Kaur Saini, Sinchu Mohan, Sukanya Kumar, and all involved in this project.

New Delhi, Delhi, India — Hemanshu Prabhakar
Gurugram, Haryana, India — Vasudha Singhal
Pune, Maharashtra, India — Kapil G Zirpe
Gurugram, Haryana, India — Harsh Sapra

Contents

Part V Systemic Neurocritical Care

Part VI Supportive Neurocritical Care

Part I

History of Neurocritical Care

1 Introduction to Neurocritical Care

Indu Kapoor and Hemanshu Prabhakar

Neurocritical care is a super-specialized zone where intensive care is provided to patients with neurological and neurosurgical diagnosis. It provides both medical and surgical treatments to life-threatening conditions in such patients [1]. The first neurocritical care unit (NCCU) was established in 1932 at the Johns Hopkins University by a neurosurgeon named Walter Dandy and was solely dedicated to postoperative monitoring of neurosurgical patients under the guidance of anesthesiologists [2]. The earliest involvement of neurologists was in the 1950s in Europe during the poliomyelitis epidemic when neurosurgical patients required ventilator support due to bulbar and neuromuscular weakness [3, 4]. Neurosurgical conditions, including both non-traumatic (brain tumors, subarachnoid hemorrhage (SAH), intracranial aneurysms, spinal cord tumors, multiple spinal instrumentation) and traumatic (traumatic brain injury, spinal cord injury) mechanisms, might require intensive care support. In neurological conditions like myasthenia gravis, status epilepticus, and Guillian–Barré syndrome, acute ischemic stroke often requires intensive care intervention. A focused history and comprehensive neurological examination is the key to any treatment strategy for patients admitted to the NCCU. The important components of medical history include information from relatives, time since the symptoms first appeared, past psychiatric treatment, drug abuse, or any other significant medical details. The examination comprises higher mental function assessment followed by motor examination, sensory evaluation, cranial nerve examination, and testing of coordination, gait, and reflexes. The level of consciousness assessment is prudent in any neurological or neurosurgical patient. Apart from assessing arousal, which includes spontaneous eye opening, fixed gaze, and purposeful voluntary movements, various scores are used in the NCCU to monitor the level of consciousness, including the Glasgow Coma Scale (GCS), the GCS-Pupil (GCS-P), and the Full Outline of Unresponsiveness (FOUR) score. The main difference between the GCS score and GCS-P score is that the latter assesses brain stem function, i.e., the pupillary reflex. In the GCS-P score, the pupillary reactivity score is subtracted by the GCS score. The pupillary reactivity score is summarized as follows: both pupils are nonreactive to light: 2; single pupil is reactive to light: 1; and both pupils are reactive to light: 0 [5]. The minimum value in the GCS score is 3, whereas for the GCS-P score, it is 1. The FOUR score, apart from the level of consciousness assessment, also provides additional information on brain stem function, breathing pattern, visual tracking, and respiratory drive [6]. Delirium is a fluctuating

I. Kapoor · H. Prabhakar (✉)
Department of Neuroanaesthesiology and Critical Care, All India Institute of Medical Sciences (AIIMS), New Delhi, India

H. Prabhakar et al. (eds.), *Principles and Practice of Neurocritical Care*,
https://doi.org/10.1007/978-981-99-8059-8_1

state characterized by altered attention, spatiotemporal disorientation, disorganized thinking, and alteration of awareness. Delirious patients can be hypoactive, hyperactive, or, alternatively, both. Tools like the Confusion Assessment Method for the Intensive Care Unit (ICU) (CAM-ICU) [7] or the ICU Delirium Screening Checklist (ICU DSC) [8] can be used to assess the presence and degree of delirium. In these patients, neuroimaging plays multiple roles both during the acute phase and at the time of follow-up or the monitoring phase. In the acute phase, most of the time, computed tomography (non-contrast) of the head suffices, which helps in differentiating structural causes from non-structural ones. Magnetic resonance imaging (MRI) may be indicated in some patients to identify smaller ischemic lesions. During monitoring or the follow-up phase, imaging modalities are helpful in identifying secondary brain injuries. More advanced neuroimaging modalities like MR spectroscopy, positron imaging tomography, etc. can help in predicting the outcome in patients with traumatic brain injury [9]. Neuromonitoring is a robust tool for neurointensivists who manage patients in the NCCU. The aims of neuromonitoring are to diagnose worsening neurological function, identify secondary brain injuries, improve the pathophysiological understanding of cerebral disease in critical illness, provide clear physiological data to guide and individualize therapy, and assist in prognostication [10]. Introduction of advanced monitoring modalities to the management of neurocritically ill patients has been shown to improve the overall outcome [11]. Various monitoring methods that can be used in the NCCU include intracranial pressure (ICP), cerebral oximetry, jugular venous oximetry ($SjvO_2$), brain tissue oxygen tension ($PbtO_2$), transcranial Doppler (TCD), cerebral microdialysis, electroencephalography (EEG), and somatosensory evoked potential (SSEP) [10]. Neurological biomarkers are quantitative indicators of brain dysfunction following neurological injuries. These include s-100β, neuron-specific enolase (NSE), amyloid-β and tau, glial fibrillary acidic protein, etc. An emerging body of evidence suggests that multi-marker panels may enhance sensitivity and specificity for acute neurological injury [12, 13].

The impact of neurointensive care on outcomes in terms of mortality and length of stay in patients with life-threatening neurological and neurosurgical illnesses has been reported by various studies [14–19]. Particularly in patients with subarachnoid hemorrhage (SAH), neurointensivist-managed ICUs have reported positive efficacy and outcomes pertaining to their length of intensive care unit stay [18, 20] and hospital discharge status (home, rehabilitation facility, nursing home, and death) [21]. Mirski et al. compared patients with intracranial hemorrhage treated in the NCCU with those treated in the general ICU and observed a lower hospital mortality rate in the former [14]. According to a survey conducted by [22] patients admitted to the NCCU had higher rates of invasive monitoring and ICP monitoring and more nutritional support compared to those in medical or surgical ICUs [22]. However, the mechanical ventilation rate and intravenous sedation were found to be lower in patients admitted to the NCCU. There are numerous similar studies demonstrating improvement in hospital stay, ICU stay, mortality, and overall expenditure when patients were treated in the NCCU. Varelas et al., in their observational study, analyzed 1087 patients before and 1279 after the neurointensivist appointment and observed an independent positive impact on patient outcomes, including lower ICU mortality, length of stay, and discharge to a skilled nursing facility and a higher discharge home [23]. In their review, combining their study's data with those of the older literature, Kramer et al. revealed that more than 40,000 patients were assessed in observational studies that compared their stay in neurological versus general ICUs. [24] Although their results were heterogeneous, admission to the NCCU was found to be associated with lower mortality and a greater chance of favorable recovery. Markandaya et al. conducted a survey among intensivists in North America, in which 70% of the respondents acknowledged that admittance to the NCCU with neurointensivists would improve the quality of care of neurocritically ill patients [25]. Neurocritical care in adults with a life-threatening neurological disease is a distinct discipline that has developed from critical care medicine and neurology. Pediatric neurocritical care is a new frontier of pediatric critical care medicine and pediatric neurology; however, it does not have the equivalent parallels with neurocritical care in adults and the track record in health-care research [26]. The most effective strategies across the field of implementation science that can facilitate deployment of neurocritical care pathways in the pediatric NCCU include planning, educating, restructuring, financing, managing quality, and attending to the policy context [27]. Using a combination of these strategies, several institutions have improved patient morbidity and mortality. Emerging evidence supports the implementation of evidence-based care pathways, which has been shown to improve outcomes, for critically ill children with two common neurological diagnoses, namely, status epilepticus and traumatic brain injury. [27] According to a survey on the current perception and practice in pediatric neurocritical care, 20% of the respondents had a pediatric NCCU at their institution [28]. In all, 46% of the respondents believed that a specialized, clinical, pediatric neurocritical care service improves the quality of care of critically ill children [28]. The authors also found that pediatric neurocritical care programs are not uncommon; however, there is no clear agreement on the optimal role or benefit of this area of practice subspecialization. The literature still lacks data on the impact of NCCU care on the long-term outcome and quality of life of both adult and pediatric patients.

References

1. Kuroda Y. Neurocritical care update. J Intensive Care. 2016;4:36.
2. Wijdicks EFM, Kramer AH. Critical care neurology part I: neurocritical care. Oxford: Elsevier Science; 2017.
3. Prabhakar H, Ali Z. Textbook of neuroanesthesia and neurocritical care. 1st ed. Singapore: Springer; 2019.
4. Prabhakar H. Neurointensive care. 1st ed. New Delhi: Oxford University Press; 2019.
5. Brennan PM, Murray GD, Teasdale GM. Simplifying the use of prognostic information in traumatic brain injury. Part 1: the GCS-pupils score: an extended index of clinical severity. J Neurosurg. 2018;128:1612–20.
6. Wijdicks EF, Bamlet WR, Maramattom BV, Manno EM, McClelland RL. Validation of a new coma scale: the FOUR score. Ann Neurol. 2005;58:585–93.
7. Ely EW, Margolin R, Francis J, May L, Truman B, Dittus R, et al. Evaluation of delirium in critically ill patients: validation of the confusion assessment method for the intensive care unit (CAM-ICU). Crit Care Med. 2001;29:1370–9.
8. Bergeron N, Dubois MJ, Dumont M, Dial S, Skrobik Y. Intensive care delirium screening checklist: evaluation of a new screening tool. Intensive Care Med. 2001;27:859–64.
9. Vespa PM. Imaging and decision-making in neurocritical care. Neurol Clin. 2014;32:211–24.
10. Stocchetti N, Le Roux P, Vespa P, Oddo M, Citerio G, Andrews PJ, et al. Clinical review: neuromonitoring—an update. Crit Care. 2013;17:201.
11. Prabhakar H. Neuromonitoring techniques. 1st ed. Elsevier; 2017.
12. Laskowitz DT, Kasner SE, Saver J, Remmel KS, Jauch EC. Clinical usefulness of a biomarker-based diagnostic test for acute stroke: the biomarker rapid assessment in ischemic injury (BRAIN) study. Stroke. 2009;40:77–85.
13. Turck N, Vutskits L, Sanchez-Pena P, Robin X, Hainard A, Gex-Fabry M, Fouda C, Bassem H, Mueller M, Lisacek F, Puybasset L, Sanchez JC. A multiparameter panel method for outcome prediction following aneurysmal subarachnoid hemorrhage. Intensive Care Med. 2010;36:107–15.
14. Mirski MA, Chang CW, Cowan R. Impact of a neuroscience intensive care unit on neurosurgical patient outcomes and cost of care: evidence-based support for an intensivist-directed specialty ICU model of care. J Neurosurg Anesthesiol. 2001;13:83–92.
15. Diringer MN, Edwards DF. Admission to a neurologic/neurosurgical intensive care unit is associated with reduced mortality rate after intracerebral hemorrhage. Crit Care Med. 2001;29:635–40.
16. Suarez JI, Zaidat OO, Suri MF, Feen ES, Lynch G, Hickman J, et al. Length of stay and mortality in neurocritically ill patients: impact of a specialized neurocritical care team. Crit Care Med. 2004;32:2311–7.
17. Varelas PN, Eastwood D, Yun HJ, Spanaki MV, Hacein Bey L, Kessaris C, et al. Impact of a neurointensivist on outcomes in patients with head trauma treated in a neurosciences intensive care unit. J Neurosurg. 2006;104:713–9.
18. Varelas PN, Schultz L, Conti M, Spanaki M, Genarrelli T, Hacein-Bey L. The impact of a neuro-intensivist on patients with stroke admitted to a neurosciences intensive care unit. Neurocrit Care. 2008;9:293–9.
19. Burns JD, Green DM, Lau H, Winter M, Koyfman F, DeFusco CM, et al. The effect of a neurocritical care service without a dedicated neuro-ICU on uality of care in intracerebral hemorrhage. Neurocrit Care. 2013;18:305–12.

20. Josephson SA, Douglas VC, Lawton MT, English JD, Smith WS, Ko NU. Improvement in intensive care unit outcomes in patients with subarachnoid hemorrhage after initiation of neurointensivist co-management. J Neurosurg. 2010;112:626–30.
21. Samuels O, Webb A, Culler S, Martin K, Barrow D. Impact of a dedicated neurocritical care team in treating patients with aneurysmal subarachnoid hemorrhage. Neurocrit Care. 2011;14:334–40.
22. Kurtz P, Fitts V, Sumer Z, Jalon H, Cooke J, Kvetan V, et al. How does care differ for neurological patients admitted to a neurocritical care unit versus a general ICU? Neurocrit Care. 2011;15:477–80.
23. Varelas PN, Conti MM, Spanaki MV, Potts E, Bradford D, Sunstrom C, et al. The impact of a neurointensivist-led team on a semiclosed neurosciences intensive care unit. Crit Care Med. 2004;32:2191–8.
24. Kramer AH, Zygun DA. Neurocritical care: why does it make a difference? Curr Opin Crit Care. 2014;20:174–81.
25. Markandaya M, Thomas KP, Jahromi B, Koenig M, Lockwood AH, Nyquist PA, et al. The role of neurocritical care: a brief report on the survey results of neurosciences and critical care specialists. Neurocrit Care. 2012;16:72–81.
26. Tasker RC. Pediatric neurocritical care: is it time to come of age? Curr Opin Pediatr. 2009;21:724–30.
27. Markham C, Proctor EK, Pineda JA. Implementation strategies in pediatric neurocritical care. Curr Opin Pediatr. 2017;29:266–71.
28. Murphy SA, Bell MJ, Clark ME, Whalen MJ, Noviski N. Pediatric neurocritical care: a short survey of current perceptions and practices. Neurocrit Care. 2015;23:149–58.

Part II

Basic Principles of Neurocritical Care

Neurological Examination in Neurocritical Care

2

Ravindra Ghawat and Jayram Navade

2.1 Introduction

Every patient in the intensive care unit (ICU) must undergo a neurological examination in some form for a good clinical evaluation (fever, shock, multiorgan failure). Patients with neurological conditions require a detailed neurological examination in the ICU (an altered mental status (AMS), seizures, unconsciousness, neurodeficit). Neuroexamination, assessment, and diagnosis in the neurocritical unit are all quite challenging for the clinicians as history is inadequate, most of the time from the attendants; the symptoms and signs are not forthcoming; the patients are drowsy with altered sensorium and sometimes sedated; and systemic diseases may show neurological signs. Some presentations are clear (e.g., postictal state after a seizure or a diabetic with hypoglycemia), whereas some are subtle (an unresponsive patient). The differential diagnoses are enormous. To obtain data from multiple sources, a structured and systematic approach with a high index of suspicion is necessary to detect and address the potentially catastrophic events. In this chapter, we will discuss how to maximize the output of our examination.

A patient can get admitted to a neurocritical ICU with either (1) a primary neurological problem (e.g., stroke, traumatic brain injury, brain tumor, epilepsy, meningitis) or (2) a secondary neurological problem (e.g., encephalopathy, hyponatremia, hypoglycemia, drugs, sepsis, etc.).

There is no consensus on the optimal order of a neurological examination. The examination may differ depending on the patient's level of consciousness, which can range from alert and oriented to comatose. In this context, we will discuss the differences between the neurological examination of a conscious patient, a patient with an altered sensorium, and a patient in a coma.

Box 2.1 Indications for neuro-ICU admissions:

- Impaired level of consciousness; coma.
- Impaired mental function.
- Impaired airway protection.
- Progressive respiratory impairment or the need for mechanical ventilation (Box 2.1).
- Seizures and status epilepticus management.
- Determination of brain death.
- Prevention of further damage to the central nervous system.
- Clinical or computed tomographic evidence of raised intracranial pressure (ICP) caused by a space-occupying lesion, a cerebral edema, or hemorrhagic conversion of a cerebral infarct.

R. Ghawat (✉) · J. Navade
Critical Care Medicine, Jupiter Hospital, Thane, Maharashtra, India

H. Prabhakar et al. (eds.), *Principles and Practice of Neurocritical Care*, https://doi.org/10.1007/978-981-99-8059-8_2

- General medical complications that develop in the course of a neurological illness (e.g., hyper/hypotension, aspiration pneumonia, sepsis, cardiac arrhythmias, pulmonary emboli).
- Monitoring (e.g., level of consciousness, respiratory function, ICP, continuous electroencephalography (EEG)).
- Specific treatments (e.g., neurosurgical intervention, intravenous or arterial thrombolysis).
- Evaluation of a neurological disease that occurs in the course of a severe medical disease.

Box 2.2 Neurological Indications for Mechanical Ventilation

- Failure of central regulation of respiration (apnea, ataxic or cluster breathing).
- Inability to protect the airway.
- Brain swelling with a depressed level of consciousness (Glasgow Coma Scale <9).
- Impending neuromuscular respiratory failure (forced vital capacity <20 mL/kg, tachypnea, dyspnea at rest, use of accessory muscles, staccato speech).

Respiratory failure must be anticipated before the emergence of hypoxia and/or hypercapnia. Thus, the threshold for intubation is lower in the context of rapidly progressive neuromuscular weakness [1].

2.2 The ABCDE (Airway, Breathing, Circulation, Disability, Exposure) Approach and the ABCGS (Airway, Breathing, Circulation, Glucose, or Seizures) Approach

2.2.1 Initial Assessment

For any patient with an altered level of consciousness, identifying and promptly treating alterations using the ABCGS (Airway, Breathing, Circulation, Glucose, or Seizures) approach is a priority. This has to be followed by a detailed neurological assessment to check for the presence of any focal neurodeficit, suggesting a structural abnormality (e.g., stroke), or for the absence of one, suggesting generalized neurological depression (e.g., sedation or septic encephalopathy). The examination should attempt to determine whether the neurological change is immediately reversible (e.g., hypoglycemia) or irreversible (e.g., stroke). A quick "ABCDE approach" not only helps in patient stabilization but also aids in excluding and treating many reversible causes of a decreased sensorium.

The Airway: The airway should be assessed for patency, the presence of foreign bodies, and for their ability to clear out secretion and prevent aspiration by assessing the level of consciousness and cough, gag, and swallowing reflexes. The aim is to correct and prevent hypoxia and hypercarbia, both of which have a causative and additive association with a decline in the sensorium. The decision regarding endotracheal intubation is, however, ambiguous and tricky and needs to be individualized to suit the patient. Although a Glasgow Coma Scale (GCS) of <8 is considered an indication, one need not rush toward intubation, keeping in mind certain reversible causes of the altered sensorium, such as hypoglycemia, seizure, benzodiazepine overdose, syncope, and Transient ischemic attack (TIAs). However, some patients with a structural lesion, such as an intracranial hemorrhage, a tumor, traumatic brain injury, and status epilepticus, showing an acute decline in the sensorium from a GCS of 15 to 8, would warrant an immediate endotracheal intubation and mechanical ventilation. Endotracheal intubation also prevents aspiration in the lungs. Concurrently, care should be taken to immobilize the cervical spine in patients with a head injury and a suspected spine injury. Airway adjuvants like the nasal and oral airways may be used in appropriate indications.

Breathing: Maintaining the patency of the airways, in most of the cases, would address the breathing trouble. Patients with raised intracranial pressure, sedation, persistent drowsiness, and status epilepticus need to be mechanically ventilated. Mechanical ventilation prevents and treats atelectasis, hypoxia, and hypercarbia. Oxygen supplementation will be required in some patients.

Circulation: It is important to rectify both hypotension and hypertension and look for arrhythmias. The presence of hypertension with bradycardia may point toward the possibility of severe intracranial hypertension and an impending herniation and should be treated immediately. Hypotension may worsen the neurological status and cause further brain damage and needs to be treated with fluid resuscitation and vasopressors and inotropes. The patient should be kept isovolumic. Invasive hemodynamic monitoring is required, and, in patients with raised intracranial pressure, ICP monitoring is also warranted. Arrythmias, as a cause of hypotension and hypoperfusion with a subsequent decline in the sensorium (syncope in most cases), should be looked for.

Disability: This is one of the most important steps in the evaluation of patients with an altered sensorium. It includes assessment of the level of consciousness (GCS or AVPU (Alert, Verbal, Pain, Unresponsive) score), pupillary size and reaction with eye examination (to rule out space-occupying lesions in the brain), facial deviation and/or motor power in the limbs (hemiparesis in a stroke), involuntary movements (seizures), and brainstem reflexes.

Exposure: A quick head-to-toe examination should be performed to look for signs of trauma, petechiae, infectious sources such as indwelling catheters, needle pricks in intravenous drug abusers, or transdermal drug patches [2].

2.2.2 History and General Examination

A good probe into the history is a must to know the patient's concurrent medical illnesses (such as diabetes, hypertension, seizures, renal failure, hypothyroidism, psychiatric issues), any history of trauma, fever, headaches, drug history, possible toxic ingestion, etc. Simultaneously, vital signs should be checked, including pulse oximetry, heart rate and rhythm, blood pressure, respiratory rate, breathing patterns, and temperature. A focused examination and vital signs may provide significant leads to the cause of the altered sensorium.

Heart rate: Bradycardia is associated with raised intracranial pressure (ICP), medication overdose with sympatholytic drugs (e.g., clonidine) or sedative hypnotics (e.g., barbiturates), organophosphorus poisoning, and hypothermia. Tachycardia is seen in patients with sepsis (presenting with hypotension), intracranial hemorrhage (due to sympathetic overactivity), psychotropic drug poisoning, and ketamine overdose.

Blood pressure: Hypotension is a common presenting feature of patients with sepsis. It can also be a feature of drug overdosage (e.g., antihypertensives, tricyclic antidepressants, sedative hypnotics, clonidine). Hypertension may be seen as a part of the Cushing reflex in patients with raised ICP or in patients with posterior reversible hypertensive encephalopathy (PRES). It is also common in ketamine and phencyclidine intoxication.

Respiratory rate and breathing patterns: Bradypnea is seen in opioid and sedative hypnotic overdose. In the setting of a structural neurological disease, bradypnea is an ominous sign and points toward a medullary involvement. Tachypnea is a feature of patients presenting with metabolic acidosis due to any cause—diabetic ketoacidosis, uremia, alcoholism, drug overdose, sepsis, and so on. Different kinds of breathing patterns can be observed and may help in localizing the lesions and in identifying the source of the altered sensorium. Cheyne–Stokes breathing (alternating hyperpnea and periods of apnea) may be observed with bilateral cortical and forebrain lesions, upper brainstem dysfunction, raised intracranial pressure, toxic encephalopathy, central medullary lesions, Cardiovascular system (CVS) and respiratory system (RS) (carbon monoxide poisoning), and chronic hypoxia at altitude; a similar pattern is seen in normal people during deep sleep. Central neurogenic hyperventilation (sustained rapid breathing) may be seen in upper pontine and midbrain lesions, whereas irregular shallow and halting breathing patterns (apneustic or ataxic breathing) are observed in the mid-lower pons and dorsomedial medulla, respectively. Acidotic (Kussmaul) respiration is sustained, and deep sighing hyperventilation is seen in diabetic ketoacidosis and uremia.

Temperature: Hyperthermia may be reflective of a septic etiology for the altered sensorium. Fever may also be seen in patients with traumatic brain injury, pontine hemorrhage, subarachnoid hemorrhage (SAH), meningoencephalitis, hypothalamic injury, salicylate poisoning, or environmental exposure. Hypothermia is usually caused by an environmental factor. Other causes include severe sepsis, hypoglycemia, hypothyroidism, sedative hypnotic overdose, acute spinal cord transaction, or brain death. For each degree increase in temperature, the normal metabolic demand is increased by 10%. This may increase cerebral edema and infarction.

Other useful physical findings in an unconscious patient [3]

Examination site	Physical findings	Probable diagnosis
Head	Contusion; postauricular ecchymosis (Battle's sign) Ventriculoperitoneal shunt	Trauma Hydrocephalus; shunt malfunction
Face	Facial deviation Sallow, puffy appearance	Stroke Hypopituitarism
Eyes	Periorbital ecchymosis (raccoon eyes) Papilledema Icterus	Trauma Increased intracranial pressure Hepatic dysfunction, hepatic encephalopathy, hemolytic anemia
Ears	Hemotympanum/bleeding	Trauma
Nose	Excessive discharge/bleeding	Trauma, cerebrospinal fluid (CSF) rhinorrhea
Neck	Stiffness Enlarged thyroid	Subarachnoid hemorrhage, meningitis, infection Thyroid disorders
Heart	Arrhythmias	Hypoxic/ischemic encephalopathy
Abdomen	Small hard liver/shrunken/nodular	Hepatic encephalopathy
Skin	Petechiae, splinter hemorrhage, ecchymosis Telangiectasia Vesicular rash Needle pricks Cyanosis Cherry red spots Grayish blue cyanosis Localized cyanosis Hypermelanosis (increased pigment)	Coagulopathy; subacute bacterial endocarditis, fat embolism syndrome, meningococcemia, Disseminated intravascular coagulation (DIC), Thrombotic thrombocytopenic purpura (TTP), drugs Chronic alcoholism, vascular malformations of the brain Herpes simplex, varicella, Behcet disease, or drugs Drug overdose or withdrawal Carbon dioxide (CO_2) narcosis, hypoxia Carbon monoxide poisoning Methemoglobinemia Arterial emboli, vasculitis Porphyria, Addison's disease, chronic nutritional deficiency
Lymph nodes	Adenopathy	Infections, tuberculosis, immunocompromised hosts
Miscellaneous	Acetone, alcohol breath Fever Tongue laceration; incontinence, fall, dislocation, fracture Asterixis/flapping tremors	Ketoacidosis; alcohol intoxication Infection Postictal state Metabolic encephalopathies

Immediate Management (Box)

1. Establish a quick intravenous access and start fluids (correct hypotension) while managing the airway, breathing, and circulation.
2. Send blood (serum chemistries, basic hematology, arterial blood gas (ABG), ammonia, toxicology screens).
3. Check bedside blood glucose.
4. Administer 50 mL of 50% dextrose intravenous (IV) if the blood sugar is <70 mg/dL.
5. Administer IV thiamine 100 mg.
6. Administer IV naloxone 0.4–2 mg, repeat up to 4 mg if necessary (opioid toxicity).

7. Administer IV flumazenil 0.1 mg, not >3 mg/h (benzodiazepine overdose).
8. Administer IV lorazepam 4 mg slowly over 2–3 min or fosphenytoin 20 mg/kg at 50 mg/min (for suspected seizure).
9. Administer IV mannitol 1–1.5 mg/kg bolus (for raised ICP).
10. Draw blood cultures and initiate broad-spectrum antibiotics (for sepsis).

Hypoglycemia is a quickly reversible, potentially life-threatening cause of an altered mental status. Thiamine prevents the precipitation of acute Wernicke's encephalopathy (especially in patients with nutritional deficiency, in chronic alcoholics, and in malnourished patients). A clinical suspicion of opioid toxicity is raised if there is a history of illicit drug use, apnea or bradypnea, or pinpoint pupils. Benzodiazepine overdose is suspected if there is a history of drowsiness, ataxia, slurred speech, or respiratory depression. Signs of raised ICP like hypertension, bradycardia, unequal pupils, drowsiness, etc. must be looked for. Drowsiness, muscle twitching, and tongue bite may indicate a seizure. Clinical signs and symptoms of sepsis should be assessed. Functional (hysteria) acute decline in the sensorium should always be taken into account. A reasonably sensitive and specific sign of functional unresponsiveness is the presence of firm resistance to eye opening. Another sign is the eye gaze sign, in which the patient tends to look at the ground when turned on one side. Moreover, when the patient's arm that is suspended over his/her face is released, it tends to move away and does not fall over the face. The presence of nystagmus with caloric stimulation in an apparently comatose patient supports a diagnosis of psychogenic unresponsiveness, though not perfectly specific.

2.2.3 Neurological Examination of a Conscious Patient

In a conscious patient, a neurological examination typically involves evaluating various domains, including mental status, cranial nerves (CNs), motor system, sensory system, reflexes, and coordination. Mental status is evaluated by assessing orientation to place, person, and time, attention, mood and affect coherence, comprehension, memory, recall, language, and executive function. Cranial nerves are examined for signs of abnormalities, such as smell, vision and visual fields, eye movements, facial weakness, vision changes, hearing loss, and balance problems. The motor system is assessed for strength, tone, and coordination. The sensory system is evaluated for the presence of sensory deficits, such as numbness, tingling, or loss of sensation. Reflexes are checked for their amplitude and symmetry, and coordination is assessed by testing finger-to-nose, heel-to-shin, and rapid alternating movements.

Neurological Examination of a Patient with an Altered Sensorium

In a patient with an altered sensorium, the neurological examination requires modifications, as the patient may be confused, drowsy, or obtunded. The focus of the examination is on assessing the level of consciousness, the presence of focal neurological deficits, and signs of brainstem dysfunction. The level of consciousness is evaluated using a standardized scale, such as the Glasgow Coma Scale (GCS), which assesses eye opening, verbal response, and motor response. Focal neurological deficits, such as weakness or numbness on one side of the body or face, may suggest a stroke or other neurological disorders. Signs of brainstem dysfunction, such as pupillary abnormalities, abnormal eye movements, and altered respiratory patterns, may indicate a more severe neurological condition. A patient with an altered mental status should be assessed for their response to normal voice, loud voice, light touch, and central pain and for their ability to differentiate between a higher function of "awareness" (e.g., purposeful movement, recognition of family) and arousability (grimacing to only pain). This is followed by determination of the Glasgow Coma Scale (GCS).

Five point assessment

1. Mental status: An altered mental status (AMS) is not a disease; it is a symptom. The com-

monly used assessment tool for mental status is the Mini-Mental State Examination (MMSE) or the Montreal Cognitive Assessment (MoCA) [4].
2. Cranial nerves: This includes evaluating the functions of 12 cranial nerves that are involved in the patient's ability to follow visual fields, move their eyes, sense smells, taste, hear, and perform facial movements [5].
3. Motor function: The patient should be examined for muscle strength, tone, and coordination. This includes evaluating muscle groups throughout the body, checking for muscle atrophy or fasciculations, and testing for pronator drift. The commonly used assessment tool for motor function is the Medical Research Council (MRC) grading system [6].
4. Sensory functions: Assessment of sensory functions includes the ability to sense touch, pain, and temperature. This includes testing for dermatome patterns and peripheral nerve function. The commonly used assessment tool for sensory function is the American Spinal Injury Association (ASIA) sensory examination [7].
5. Reflexes: The examiner should assess deep tendon reflexes, including the biceps, triceps, brachioradialis, patellar, and Achilles reflexes. The commonly used assessment tool for reflexes is the four-point scale.

2.2.4 Neurological Examination of a Patient in a Coma

Clinical levels of altered consciousness [3] (modified from Halls)

Terminology	Eye response	Wakefullness	Sensorium	Remarks
Lethargy	Closed	Arousable	Mildly impaired	
Stupor	Closed	Arousable with effort	Markedly impaired	
Coma	Closed	Unarousable	Not applicable	
Akinetic mutism (abulic state, coma vigil)	Open	Wakeful	Impaired	Secondary to bilateral frontal/basal forebrain dysfunction
Locked-in syndrome	Open	Wakeful	Normal	Secondary to basis pontis dysfunction; voluntary blinking and vertical eye movements remain intact
Psychogenic unresponsiveness	Closed	Wakeful, arousable with effort, voluntary closure of eyes	Normal	Prolonged, motionless, dissociative attack, catatonia

For a patient in a coma, the neurological examination is focused on assessing the level of coma, the presence of brainstem reflexes, and the absence of voluntary movements. The examination also includes assessing the pupillary response, motor function, reflexes, and cranial nerves. The presence of focal neurological deficits can suggest a specific underlying cause of coma, such as a stroke or traumatic brain injury.

Brainstem reflexes, such as the pupillary light reflex, corneal reflex, and oculocephalic reflex, are assessed to determine the integrity of the brainstem. The absence of voluntary movements suggests a more severe neurological injury and may indicate the need for further testing, such as imaging studies or electroencephalography (EEG).

The most used scale for assessing the level of consciousness is the Glasgow Coma Scale (GCS). It assesses three components of consciousness: eye opening, verbal response, and motor response. Depending upon their performance on these components, patients are assigned a score of 3 (minimum) out of 15 (maximum) (see table). A patient is considered more alert and responsive if the score is higher. However, it does not take into account alteration in the brainstem functions, hemiparesis, or aphasia; also, it becomes a bit tricky to assign scores based on verbal response in intubated patients. In addition to the GCS, depending on the clinical situation, other scales may be used to assess the level of consciousness: Full Outline of Unresponsiveness (FOUR) score and the Alert, Verbal, Pain, Unresponsive (AVPU) scale. The Full Outline of Unresponsiveness (FOUR) score (see table) evaluates four categories of neurological function: eye response, motor response, brainstem reflexes, and respiration. Each category is scored on a scale of 0–4, with the maximum score of 16 indicating a normal neurological function (see table). The main difference between the GCS and the FOUR score is that the FOUR score incorporates an assessment of brainstem function and respiratory pattern (instead of the verbal score), can be reliably used even in intubated patients in the ICU, and can thus provide additional information about the severity of brain injury. The AVPU scale (see table) is a simple, easy to use and remember, and quick assessment tool, often used in the prehospital setting and in the emergency department by paramedical or nonmedical personnel. However, it is not as detailed as the GCS or the FOUR score and does not provide as much information about the patient's neurological function. The AVPU scale consists of four categories: alertness, verbal response, response to pain, and unresponsiveness.

The Glasgow coma scale [8]

Eye opening	Best verbal response	Best motor response	Score
No response	No response	No response	1
To speech	Incomprehensible sounds	Abnormal extension (decerebrate)	2
To pain	Inappropriate words	Abnormal flexion (decorticate)	3
Spontaneously	Confused	Flexion withdrawal from pain	4
	Oriented toward time, place, and person	Localizes pain	5
		Obeys commands	6

The AVPU scale [9]

A	The patient is awake
V	The patient responds to verbal stimulation
P	The patient responds to painful stimulation
U	The patient is completely unresponsive

The FOUR score [10]

Eye response	Motor response	Brainstem reflexes	Respiration	Score
Eyelids open, blinking to command	Makes sign (thumbs up, fist or peace sign)	Pupil and corneal reflexes present	Not intubated, regular breathing pattern	4
Eyelids open but not tracking	Localizes pain	One pupil wide and fixed	Not intubated, Cheyne–stokes breathing pattern	3
Eyelids closed but open to loud voice	Flexion response to pain	Pupil or corneal reflexes absent	Not intubated, irregular breathing	2
Eyelids closed but open to pain	Extension response to pain	Pupil and corneal reflexes absent	Breathes above ventilator rate	1
Eyelids closed with pain	No response to pain	Absent pupil, corneal and cough reflexes	Breathes at ventilator rate or apnea	0

2.3 Examination of Cranial Nerves (CNs) [5, 11]

The cranial nerves are arranged in pairs along the brainstem in descending order. There are five motor nerves (CNs III, IV, VI, XI, and XII), three sensory nerves (CNs I, II, and VIII), and four mixed motor and sensory nerves (CNs V, VII, IX, and X). A dysfunction of the cranial nerves produces effects on the same side (ipsilateral). In a conscious and alert patient, who can participate in the examination, all cranial nerves can be tested. However, in an unconscious patient, only some of the cranial nerves can be tested. These are tested by stimulating a sensory nerve and looking for a reflex motor response. In brainstem herniation syndromes, cranial nerve function can be lost in descending order (if the origin of the injury is above the tentorium). CNs I and II are located above the brainstem. CNs III–XII are located along the brainstem. CN XI (accessory) has its origin in the spine, rising to give the appearance of a CN located between X and XII. CN III is situated at the level of the tentorium. Sudden loss of CN III function (decreased reactivity and dilation of the pupil) indicates herniation at the top of the brainstem. This is the most important CN to test in critical care. Asymmetrical loss of any CN function indicates unilateral compression.

Most of the brainstem reflex tests involve testing cranial nerve function for accuracy because of their arrangement along the brainstem. CN IV (the only cranial nerve that arises from the posterior cord) provides contralateral function. Symptoms remain ipsilateral, with the reason being its length and point of crossing wherein compression typically occurs after crossing. However, this is rarely a significant CN to test in the critical care population.

Examination of cranial nerves

CN	Name	Main function	Testing in the ICU	Clinical significance/ remark
I	Olfactory (sensory)	Smell	Block one nostril and test the ability to smell from the contralateral nostril (peppermint, coffee)	Dysfunction causes loss of taste to food. May be injured with the anterior basal skull fracture. Testing omitted in most critical care assessments
II	Optic (sensory)	Sight information from each of the four visual fields of each eye travels via a unique pathway between the retina and the brain. Homonymous hemianopia is a visual field defect that involves either the two right or the two left halves of the visual fields of both eyes	Each eye must be tested separately. Recognition of objects or people. Ability to see objects in all eight fields. Acuity of vision, eye chart, reading. Light reflex tests CNs II and III remember to test with glasses on. Fundoscopy. Detailed testing post-ICU discharge	Occipital lobe damage causes loss of vision to the opposite visual field of one or both eyes (hemianopia) Optic chiasma lesion causes bitemporal hemianopia Homonymous hemianopia—Cerebral infarction, intracranial hemorrhage, multiple sclerosis, epilepsy, dementia, Alzheimer's disease Traumatic brain injury Both pupils should constrict to light shone in either eye

CN	Name	Main function	Testing in the ICU	Clinical significance/ remark
III	Oculomotor (motor)	Pupillary constriction. Opening of the eyelids. Eye movement (all directions, except those of CNs IV and VI; CNs III, IV, and VI are tested together)	Light reflex. Eye opening. Ability to follow an object upward, horizontally toward the nose, straight down, and downward/laterally	Deconjugate gaze causes diplopia, mydriasis Trauma, herniation syndromes, aneurysm compression due to aneurysm/tumor True CN III compression should cause decreased responsiveness to both direct and consensual testing
IV	Trochlear (motor)	Downward and nasal rotation of the eye. Enables movement of the superior oblique muscle	Ability to follow an object in the downward, nasal field of vision	Vertical diplopia (double vision vertically). Tortional diplopia (image tilted or rotated). Head injury. Congenital cranial dysinnervation syndrome
V	Trigeminal (sensory and motor)	Primarily sensory: Feeling to the face in three branches: V1: Ophthalmic (forehead, cornea, nose), V2: Maxillary (cheeks), V3: Mandibular (jaw) motor: Chewing Largest of the cranial nerves	Light touch and pin sensation to the forehead, cheek, and jaw region Ability to raise cheeks (chew), corneal reflex tests the V1 branch of CN V (sensation) and CN VII (blink)	Trauma, post-surgery pain
VI	Abducens (motor)	Horizontal and lateral movement of the eye innervates the lateral rectus muscle	Ability to follow an object in the horizontal/ temporal gaze	Horizontal diplopia, inability to abduct the eye Atherosclerosis, meningitis, encephalitis, cavernous sinus thrombosis, Diabetes mellitus (DM), Hypertension (HT), temporal arteritis
VII	Facial (motor and sensory)	Primarily motor: Face movement, eyelid closure, tearing of the eye, salivation, sensation/taste to the front two-third of the tongue	Eye closure, face movement (smile, assess nasolabial fold, show teeth), inability to wrinkle the forehead on the side of facial weakness indicates CN VII dysfunction; forehead wrinkle preserved in stroke	Cerebral stroke, space-occupying lesion Bell's palsy Trauma

CN	Name	Main function	Testing in the ICU	Clinical significance/ remark
VIII	Auditory or vestibulocochlear (sensory)	Hearing, balance, vestibular system sends information about head movement to the pons; makes CN III/VI move the eyes together for horizontal eye movement	Response to voice or sound, tuning fork, balance during mobilization, detailed testing post-ICU discharge, doll's eyes, and cold caloric test	Determination of brain death Horizontal nystagmus Vertigo with upright positioning or impaired horizontal eye movement may indicate CN VIII disorders
IX	Glossopharyngeal (sensory, motor, and parasympathetic)	Sensation to the back of the tongue/tonsils, parotid secretion, contraction stylopharyngeus muscle	CNs IX and X collectively tested by touching each side of the back of the throat and observing for gag response	Ability to clear out throat secretions, difficulty in swallowing, taste impairment over post one-third of the tongue, palate, and pharynx determination of brain death
X	Vagal (sensory and motor, parasympathetic)	Contraction larynx/pharynx, parasympathetic fibers of the thoracoabdominal viscera, coughing, sneezing, swallowing, vomiting	CNs IX and X collectively tested by touching each side of the back of the throat and observing for gag response	Vasovagal syncope overreaction of the vagus nerve to extreme heat, hunger, pain, anxiety, etc. DM viral infections, abdominal surgeries, scleroderma
XI	Accessory/spinal (motor)	Shoulder shrug, head rotation, sternocleidomastoid, and trapezius	Ability to shrug the shoulder or turn the head against resistance	Posterior and lateral cervical triangle surgeries, neck trauma, motor neuron disease, poliomyelitis, brachial neuritis, syringomyelia
XII	Hypoglossal (motor)	Tongue movement	Ability to move the tongue side to side. Can test against resistance by pressing the tongue against the cheek, thus providing resistance with a finger outside the cheek	Bilateral damage (radiation) tumor, infections, trauma, stroke, internal carotid artery dissection Dysarthria (CNs IX, X, and XII)

2.3.1 Motor Functions and Assessment

A motor function refers to the ability of the body's muscles to perform voluntary movements and maintain posture. Symmetrical spontaneous/localized movements and response to painful stimuli should be observed. If the patient can obey commands, then the motor response can be described using the 0–5/5 Motor Scoring Scale. The components of motor function that are evaluated during a neurological examination include muscle strength, tone, and coordination. The following tests may be performed to assess these components:

Muscle strength and grading: The patient should be asked to perform specific movements against resistance. Alternatively, the patient may be asked to push against their hand or a resistance band. One hand should be placed above the joint being examined to stabilize the joint and isolate the specific movement. In the upper extremities, shoulder and wrist abduction and extension and flexion at the elbow, wrist, and finger should be tested. In the lower extremities, flexion and extension at the hip, knee, and ankle (dorsiflexion and plantar flexion) should be tested. The commonly used scale for grading muscle strength is the 0–5 Medical Research Council scale (MRC), where

0 = no contraction;
1 = visible muscle twitch but no movement of the joint;
2 = weak contraction insufficient to overcome gravity;
3 = weak contraction that is able to overcome gravity but no additional resistance;
4 = weak contraction that is able to overcome some resistance but not full resistance; and
5 = normal; able to overcome full resistance.

The main feature of the MRC scale is its reproducibility, and the major limitation of the scale is its insensitivity to subtle differences in strength. Clinicians try to compensate for this using intermediate grades, such as 3+ or 5-; however, there is no consensus on how these intermediate grades are to be defined. The muscles should also be inspected and palpated for evidence of atrophy and fasciculations (random, involuntary muscle twitches).

Muscle tone: Muscle tone is the degree of tension in a muscle at rest. Abnormal muscle tone indicates a neurological or musculoskeletal disorder. Evaluation is conducted by passively moving the patient's limbs and assessing the resistance encountered. Tone is qualitatively assessed by asking the patient to relax and then passively manipulating their limbs. Several forms of increased tone (hypertonia) are distinguished, including spasticity, rigidity, and paratonia. Decreased tone (hypotonia) also occurs. *Spasticity* results in a "*clasp-knife phenomenon*," in which the limb moves freely for some distance and then there is a "*catch*" and more force is required to move the limb until at a certain point; then, again, there is a sudden release and the limb moves freely. Spasticity is mostly seen in the flexors of the upper extremity and in the extensors of the lower extremity. *Rigidity* is characterized by increased resistance throughout the movement. When the resistance is uniform, it is lead-pipe rigidity, whereas rhythmic interruption of the resistance, producing a "ratchet-like effect," is cogwheel rigidity. Rigidity can be accentuated by distracting the patient. *Paratonia* (also called Gegenhalten) is increased resistance that becomes less prominent with distraction and is commonly seen in anxious or demented patients.

Coordination: Coordination refers to the ability of the body to perform smooth and accurate movements and usually reflects cerebellar function. Limb weaknesses and encephalopathy may be confounding factors. Commonly used tests to assess coordination are as follows:

Finger-to-nose test: The patient is asked to touch his/her nose with his/her finger and then touch the physician's finger held in front of him while alternating between the two. Observations are made for both accuracy and tremor.

Heel-to-shin test: The patient is asked to run their heel down the front of the opposite shin, from the knee to ankle, while maintaining a straight line. Observations are made for both accuracy and tremor.

Rapid alternating movements: The patient is asked to rapidly pronate and supinate their hand against a stable surface (e.g., a table, patient's own thigh), observing for speed, accuracy, and rhythm rapidly and alternately. Impaired ability is known as *dysdiadochokinesis*.

Finger tapping: The patient is asked to make a fist with their hand and then to extend their thumb and index finger and tap the tip of their index finger on the tip of their thumb as quickly as possible, observing for speed, accuracy, and regularity of rhythm.

Pronator drift: The patient is asked to stretch out both their arms at a level, fully extended with their palms facing straight up (90° to his/her body/modify position as tolerated), and then close their eyes. Observations are made for 5–10 s to check whether either of the arms tend to pronate (so that the palm turns inward) and drift downward. A unilateral pronator drift in one arm points toward an upper motor neuron lesion affecting that arm. If one palm rotates toward the floor, then it is more sensitive than waiting for the arm to drift downward.

Involuntary movements: The patient is observed throughout the history and physical examination for the following:

Tremors: Shaking movements in one or more parts of the body.
Chorea: Rapid, jerky twitches, similar to myoclonus but more random in location and more likely to blend into one another.
Flaps/asterixis: Sudden lapses of sustained posture from involuntary interruption in muscle contraction.
Athetosis: Slow, writhing movements of the limbs.
Ballismus: Large-amplitude, flinging limb movements.
Myoclonus: Rapid, shock-like muscle jerks.
Tics: Abrupt, stereotyped, coordinated movements or vocalizations.
Dystonia: Maintenance of an abnormal posture or repetitive twisting movements.
Clonus: More than five sustained involuntary contractions following muscle stretching.
Fasciculations: Spontaneous muscle twitching.
Gait assessment: When the patient is unaware, their casual gait should be observed. The patient is asked to walk a short distance toward or away on tiptoes or in tandem like walking on a tightrope; their balance, stride, festination (an involuntary tendency to accelerate and become smaller), and overall gait are all assessed.
The Romberg test: The Romberg test is often used in conjunction with other neurological exams, such as the finger-to-nose test or heel-to-toe walk, to assess the patient's overall coordination and motor function. It is also commonly used to evaluate patients with conditions that affect balance and coordination, such as Parkinson's disease, multiple sclerosis, or peripheral neuropathy. The Romberg test evaluates a person's balance and proprioception, which is the ability to perceive the position and movement of one's body. The test is commonly used to assess the functioning of the sensory and vestibular systems.

The patient is asked to stand with their feet together, arms at their sides, and eyes closed for up to 60 s. The patient is observed for any swaying or loss of balance. If the patient sways significantly or loses balance, then this may indicate a problem with their proprioception or vestibular system. Care should be taken as loss of balance can result in falls or injury.

2.3.2 Reflex Examination

Reflex testing can help assess the integrity of the motor and sensory pathways and may be used to diagnose neurological conditions such as spinal cord injury, multiple sclerosis, or stroke. Reflex testing is a common part of a neurological examination and involves testing the patient's deep tendon reflexes, which are mediated by the spinal cord and lower motor neurons. It is important to note that abnormal reflexes are not always indicative of a specific diagnosis and may require further evaluation and testing. Relaxation is most important during the reflex examination; hence, patients should be distracted by engaging them in conversation while testing their reflexes.

Tendon reflexes: The commonly tested reflexes are the biceps, triceps, brachioradialis, knee (patellar), and ankle (Achilles). The joint to be examined should be kept at about 90° and fully relaxed. The joint should be supported by the person conducting the test. With the other arm, the end of the hammer should be held; the head of the hammer should be allowed to drop like a pendulum to strike the tendon while looking for the contraction of the muscle and tendon under consideration. Anatomical positions for various reflex testing include the following:

Biceps (C5–6 roots): Just anterior to the elbow.
Triceps (C6–7 roots (mainly C7)): Just posterior to the elbow.
Brachioradialis (C5–6 roots): About 10 cm above the wrist on the radial aspect of the forearm.
Knee (L3–4 roots, mainly L4): Just below the patella.
Ankle (S1 root): Just behind the ankle.

Difficult-to-elicit reflexes can be amplified using reinforcement procedures like clenching the teeth or hooking the flexed fingers of both hands together and pulling (the Jendrassik maneuver) when testing lower extremity reflexes. Clonus is a rhythmic sustained contraction of muscle induced by stretching the tendon. Usually, it is tested at the ankle and is elicited by suddenly dorsiflexing the patient's foot and maintaining light upward pressure on the sole. It becomes difficult to detect slight asymmetry, when the reflexes are brisk. For the most sensitive and best comparison, the stimulus should be reduced until it is just barely above the threshold for eliciting the reflex.

Grading reflexes: The most common convention for grading deep tendon reflexes is simple but not precise: absent (0), reduced, hypoactive (1), normal (2), increased hyperactive (3), clonus (4), and sustained clonus (5). Comparison between reflexes in one part of the body and another, as well as corresponding reflexes on the right and left, where even subtle asymmetry may be significant, is much more important than the absolute reflex grade.

The Babinski reflex test: This test evaluates the plantar reflex, which is the reflex response of the toes to stimulation on the sole of the foot. During this test, a pointed object, such as a hammer, a key, or a pen, is used to stroke the sole of the foot in an upward motion, starting from the heel and moving toward the toes. In a normal response, the toes will flex or curl downward (flexor plantar response). However, in an abnormal response, the big toe will extend upward (dorsiflexion), whereas the other toes fan out, which is known as the extensor plantar response or the "Babinski sign." The presence of the Babinski sign can indicate a damage to the brain or the spinal cord. The Babinski sign may be present in infants up to the age of 2 years, as their nervous system is still developing.

Upper Motor vs. Lower Motor Neuron Disease

During assessment of motor function, symmetry is one of the most important considerations. Once asymmetrical weakness is noted, this weakness is evaluated to determine whether the cause is likely due to a problem in the upper or lower motor neuron pathway. The upper motor neuron pathway begins in the motor strip of the contralateral cerebral hemisphere and terminates in the spinal cord. Following impulse transmission to the end of the upper motor neuron pathway, the impulse synapses with the lower motor neuron (the spinal nerve root) to activate the muscle. Motor weakness can occur as a result of upper motor neuron damage (such as a stroke or cord injury) or a lower motor neuron injury (e.g., injury to the brachial plexus or disc protrusion against a spinal nerve).

Features	Upper motor neuron disease (UMND)	Lower motor neuron disease (LMND)
Site of the lesion	In the motor cortex, corticospinal tracts, or brainstem	In the anterior horn cells of the spinal cord or the cranial nerve nuclei
Signs and symptoms	Muscle weakness, stiffness, spasticity, exaggerated reflexes, and abnormal Babinski sign, presence of clonus	Muscle weakness, atrophy, fasciculations, decreased reflexes and muscle tone (hypotonia)
Muscle tone	Increased (spasticity)	Decreased (flaccidity)
Reflexes (2+ is normal reflex, 3+ or 4+ is increased)	Increased/brisk	Decreased
Distribution	Bilateral or unilateral	Mostly unilateral
Examples of diseases	Stroke, cerebral palsy, multiple sclerosis	Spinal muscular atrophy, amyotrophic lateral sclerosis

During the early spinal shock phase of an acute spinal cord injury, the temporary loss of reflexes can cause a paralysis-like lower motor neuron injury. While upper motor neuron causes for hemiplegia are more common, lower motor neuron injury can also be seen in critical care. Examples include:

1. Brachial plexus injury: Motor nerves from the cervical spine (C5–8 and T1), which join to form a plexus that passes below the collar bone, are collectively responsible for all arm and hand movements. Flaccid paralysis of the arm with decreased upper extremity deep tendon reflexes, associated with a shoulder injury, may indicate brachial plexus injury.
2. The cranial nerves are lower motor neurons (CNVII). Injury to CN VII causes ipsilateral facial paralysis with an inability to close the eyelid or wrinkle the forehead. Stroke or brain injury causes contralateral facial paralysis due to the inability to stimulate the contralateral CN VII. At least some ability to close the eye is preserved if the facial weakness is due to a stroke as the upper branches of both CN VIIs (responsible for forehead wrinkling) are simultaneously activated by messages from either side of the brain and forehead wrinkling. A basal skull (middle fossa) fracture may be suspected if there is bleeding or drainage from the ear canal. A lower motor neuron injury (CN VII) is believed to be a cause of associated facial weakness. An inability to close the eye or wrinkle the forehead on the side of the facial paralysis in this condition is likely due to CN VII damage rather than stroke.
3. Any spinal cord injury that causes disc protrusion may cause a lower motor neuron weakness.

2.3.3 Motor Examination in an Unconscious Patient

Asymmetries of movements, muscle tone, and reflexes often indicate a hemiplegia of the nonmoving side, suggesting involvement of the opposite cerebral hemisphere or upper brainstem. The patient needs to be checked for purposeful movements like crossing the midline, approaching the stimulus, actively withdrawing from the stimulus, or pushing the examiner's hand away. Acute structural disease also causes decreased muscle tone or flaccidity. Flexion and extension movements are representative of reflex responses arising from subcortical structures. *Decorticate posturing* consists of upper extremity adduction and flexion at the elbows, wrists, and fingers, with lower extremity extensions like extension and adduction at the hip, extension at the knee, and plantar flexion and inversion at the ankle. This occurs with dysfunction at the cerebral cortical level or below and may reflect a "release" of other spinal pathways. *Decerebrate posturing* consists of extension adduction and pronation of the upper extremity, together with extension of the lower extremity, and indicates dysfunction below the red nucleus, allowing the vestibulospinal tract to predominate. Patients with decorticate posturing in response to pain have a relatively better prognosis than do those with decerebrate posturing. *Reflex posturing* is also seen in deep metabolic coma (e.g., hypoglycemia) without affection of the muscle tone. *Bilateral rigidity* has been described in neuroleptic malignant syndrome, malignant hyperthermia, and hepatic coma.

Multifocal myoclonus strongly suggests a metabolic or toxic etiology. Tremor and asterixis are suggestive of a metabolic encephalopathy. These occur with the limbs held in a posture against gravity. A tremor is usually rapid and is often present when the limb is actively moved (postural action tremor). Myoclonic twitches of the facial muscles or fingers, more synchronous or rhythmic movements, or spontaneous nystagmus point toward the possibility of nonconvulsive status epilepticus (NCSE). *Opisthotonos* is extreme hyperextension and spasticity of the head, neck, and back. The causes include tetanus, rabies, meningoencephalitis, malaria, syphilis, traumatic brain injury, hydrocephalous, strychnine poisoning, and drowning.

2.3.4 Sensory Testing

Assessment of sensory function is an important aspect of a neurological examination. It involves evaluating a patient's ability to perceive different types of sensory stimuli (i.e., light touch, pain and temperature, vibration, joint position sense) and then the discriminative sensory functions (i.e., point localization, two-point discrimination, stereognosis, graphesthesia, and extinction). The former accounts for the integrity of the afferent sensory pathways, whereas the latter tests the ability of sensory and association cortices to analyze and interpret sensory inputs. Following are the tests for assessment of sensory functions:

Light touch testing: This test involves using a soft brush or cotton swab to touch different parts of the patient's skin. The patient is asked to tell the examiner where they feel the touch and whether it feels the same or different from other parts of their body.

Pinprick testing: This test involves using a sharp object, such as a pin, to prick the patient's skin. The patient is asked to report any pain or discomfort they feel and to identify the location of the prick.

Temperature testing: This test involves using hot and cold stimuli to test the patient's ability to perceive changes in temperature. The examiner can use hot or cold water, ice packs, or thermal stimulators to apply the stimuli to the patient's skin. The patient is asked to report whether the stimuli feel hot or cold and to identify the location of the stimuli.

Vibration testing: This test involves using a tuning fork to test the patient's ability to sense vibrations. The examiner places the tuning fork on the patient's skin and asks the patient to report whether they feel any vibration and to identify the location of the vibration.

Proprioception testing: This test involves testing the patient's ability to sense joint position by asking the patient to identify the position of a limb without looking at it. The examiner moves the patient's limb and asks the patient to report where they think their limb is located.

Stereognosis testing: This test involves placing an object in the patient's hand and asking the patient to identify it without looking at it. The patient may be asked to identify the shape, texture, or size of the object.

Graphesthesia: The examiner draws a number from 0 to 9 on the patient's index finger using a ballpoint pen, and, with closed eyes, the patient is asked to identify these numbers. This is repeated with several other numbers and compared with the other hand. Graphesthesia in the feet need not be tested.

Two-point discrimination testing: This test involves touching the patient's skin with two points of a caliper and asking the patient to identify whether they feel one or two points. The distance between the two points is gradually increased until the patient can no longer discriminate between one or two points.

Eye moments and positions [12] (Gaze)

Brain structure	Type of eye movement affected	Direction of eye movement	Abnormality
Pons	Horizontal gaze	Lateral gaze	Paralysis of lateral gaze toward the side of the lesion
Medulla	Horizontal and vertical gaze	All directions	Complete paralysis of eye movements or nystagmus
Midbrain	Vertical gaze	Upward or downward gaze	Paralysis or limited range of vertical gaze
Cerebellum	Gaze holding	All directions	Inability to maintain fixation on a moving target

The eye muscles are controlled by three sets of cranial nerves, namely, CN III, CN IV (trochlear), and CN VI (abducens), with their nuclei being in the upper midbrain, lower midbrain, and pontomedullary junction, respectively. Proper eye movement control requires a network of interconnections between these nuclei so that the eyes move conjugatively. This interconnection is the medial longitudinal fasciculus (MLF), which is also integrated with the vestibular nuclei and is responsible for reflex conjugate eye movement due to positional head changes. An MLF lesion manifests as impaired adduction on the affected side with nystagmus in the other abducting eye ("Internuclear ophthalmoplegia or INO"). Horizontal nystagmus suggests alcoholics and antiepileptic drug intoxication, whereas vertical nystagmus is seen in brainstem dysfunction. *Opsoclonus* (also known as the dancing eye, dancing feet syndrome) is characterized by rapid involuntary movements of the eyes in all directions. It is commonly seen in children and is associated with ataxia and myoclonus. Common causes are neuroblastoma, viral encephalitis, meningitis, malaria. In adults, it is observed in paraneoplastic syndromes, breast and lung cancers, and rarely in falciparum malaria [13].

Gaze palsy is characterized by an abnormal eye movement wherein the two eyes have limited movement in one direction but can move conjugately. *Gaze centers* are the cortical and brainstem regions responsible for conjugate gaze. Gaze palsy occurs due to malfunction of gaze centers or interruption of the pathways leading from them. In *supranuclear gaze palsy*, only voluntary gaze is impaired. The reflexes can still activate the brainstem neurons responsible for gaze as the lesion is in a cortical gaze center. In *nuclear gaze palsy*, the neurons cannot be activated either voluntarily or by reflexes like the oculocephalic (doll's eye) reflex as the lesion is in the brainstem gaze center. Gaze deviation is a feature of ipsilateral hemispheric lesions, contralateral pontine lesions, or a seizure focus.

Inspection of the fundi may yield important diagnostic clues. A subhyaloid hemorrhage is virtually pathognomonic for aneurysmal subarachnoid hemorrhage in a comatose patient. Papilledema indicates raised intracranial pressure (ICP) or malignant hypertension. Roth spots (white-centered hemorrhages) are usually associated with bacterial endocarditis but can also be seen in leukemia, vasculitides, and diabetic retinopathy.

2.3.5 Pupillary Size and Reflex

The most important cranial nerve reflexes regarding coma are the pupillary, corneal, and vestibulocochlear reflexes. Pupils are tested for size, symmetry, and reactivity (response to light). The normal pupillary size is 3–7 mm and is bilaterally equal. In trans-tentorial herniation, the pupils become reduced in size (4–5 mm) after the initial dilatation and remain unreactive to light and are called mid-position, fixed pupils. Pinpoint pupils (meiosis) are seen in pontine lesions and opioid overdose, whereas dilated pupils (mydriasis) are seen in tricyclic antidepressants and drug intoxication. For pupillary reflex testing, a four-point assessment should be conducted:

(a) Direct light response in the left eye.
(b) Direct light response in the right eye.
(c) Consensual light response in the left eye.
(d) Consensual light response in the right eye.

When assessing for possible brain death, a detailed review of cranial nerve function is required.

Pupillary size/changes in coma

	Size	Reactivity	Comments
Bilateral			
	Normal or small	Normal	Toxic metabolic disturbance
	Mid-position (3–5 mm)	Poor	Midbrain dysfunction; drugs (glutethimide (Doriden))
	Small (pinpoint)	Poor	Pontine dysfunction; drugs (narcotics)
	Large	Poor	Toxic metabolic disturbance (anoxia); drugs(anticholinergics) brain death, deep coma, barbiturate intoxication, and hypothermia
Unilateral			
	Large	Unreactive	Ipsilateral midbrain pathology or compression of ipsilateral CN III: Uncal herniation, posterior communicating artery aneurysm/potential neurosurgical emergency (e.g., extradural hematoma)
	Small	Minimal	Ipsilateral sympathetic dysfunction, Horner's syndrome, hypothalamic damage

2.3.6 Brainstem Reflexes

A careful assessment of brainstem reflexes provides information about the functioning of the various components of the brainstem. Some of the brainstem reflexes are pupillary reflex (size, reaction to light, symmetry), corneal reflex, gag and cough reflexes, oculocephalic reflex, vestibulo-ocular reflex, visual threat response, etc. Their assessment and testing help in the diagnosis of brainstem death and posterior circulation such as basilar occlusion syndromes.

Testing of various reflexes and their clinical significance

Reflex	Location (brain)	Clinical significance	Examples of diseases
Pupillary light reflex	Midbrain	Tests the integrity of CN II and CN III	Optic neuritis, anisocoria
Corneal reflex	Pons and medulla	Tests the integrity of CN V and CN VII	Brainstem lesions, trigeminal neuralgia
Vestibulo-ocular reflex (VOR), caloric reflex	Pons and medulla	Tests the integrity of CN VIII and the vestibular nuclei	Acoustic neuroma, labyrinthitis
Gag reflex/pharyngeal reflex	Medulla	Tests the integrity of CN IX and CN X	Bulbar paralysis, brainstem tumors, myasthenia gravis, Guillain–Barré syndrome
Jaw jerk reflex	Pons and medulla	Tests the integrity of CN V	Trigeminal neuralgia, masseter weakness
Oculocardiac reflex (doll's eye)	Pons and medulla	Decreased heart rate with pressure on the eye	Trigeminal neuralgia, ocular tumors
Cough reflex	Medulla	Tests the integrity of CN X	Bulbar paralysis, neurodegenerative diseases
Breathing pattern	Midbrain, pons, and medulla	Abnormalities suggest dysfunction of brainstem respiratory centers	Traumatic brain injury, brainstem stroke

2.3.7 Neuroexamination in Pediatrics

A great deal of information can be obtained from simple observation, such as the overall muscle tone, symmetric movement of all extremities, strength of cry, and the child's level of interaction with parents. A neurological assessment includes clinical history, a detailed neurological examination, and an additional general physical examination relevant to child neurology.

History: This includes the chief complaint or reason for visit, pattern of symptoms like static, progressive, or episodic, any localizing symptom, and duration. Birth history includes gestational age, birth weight, and complications during pregnancy and delivery. Prenatal history includes exposure to any drugs, radiations, gestational infections, age at the time of exposure, maternal age, and weight gain during pregnancy. Perinatal history includes type of delivery (spontaneous induced or cesarean section), length of labor, fetal presentation, Apgar score, need for resuscitation, or intensive care admission at the time of birth. Postnatal history includes occurrence of seizure, any sign of encephalopathy, and use of therapeutic hypothermia.

Developmental history (milestones, delays, regression): A detail probe into the social and motor milestones, medical history (previous illnesses, surgeries, hospitalizations), family history of neurological disorders, and genetic conditions is warranted. The health status of first-degree relatives should be asked as many of neurological disorders are inherited. Any current and past medications and the history and nature of allergies should also be examined.

A detailed general physical examination relevant to child neurology, including height, weight, head circumference, dysmorphic features, fontanels, sutures, skin rashes or birth marks, and external genitalia, should be assessed.

Detailed neurological examination: This should start during child visit, and the inspection should be conducted while the child is seated on the parent's lap. Mental status examination, including the level of consciousness, behavior, and speech, should be assessed. Cranial nerves, including visual acuity, pupillary reactions, facial movements, and hearing, should be examined. All cranial nerves should be examined for motor or sensory test, by observation for specific movements and responses, but the examination is less reliable in pediatric patients. Motor system examination assessment includes strength, tone, and coordination. Posture and involuntary movements like chorea, athetosis, myoclonus, tremors, tics, stereotype, and handwriting moment should be looked for. The sensory system, including touch, pain, temperature, vibration, and position sense, should be examined. Sensory examination in a child below 5–6 years can be unreliable and may need to be repeated for confirmation. Deep tendon reflex assessment is the same as in adults. Superficial reflexes, including plantar reflex (S1), conjunctival reflex, superficial abdominal reflexes, and cremasteric reflex (L1–2), should be examined. Gait and balance can be assessed by seeing the child while walking on the floor, with barefooted and exposed legs and feet. Cerebellar function, including coordination, and the finger–nose–finger test should be assessed. The entire length of the spine should be examined to rule out congenital spinal cord anomaly such as spina bifida and tethered cord syndrome. Any gross lesion like meningocele and myelomeningocele should be assesses. Assessment of abnormal movements, including seizures, tremors, dystonia, chorea, and tics, should be performed. Systemic examination relevant to the clinical scenario should be performed, for example, ophthalmological examination (strabismus, nystagmus, optic disc abnormalities), cardiovascular examination (heart murmur, cyanosis), respiratory examination (breathing sound, respiratory distress), abdominal examination (organomegaly), and musculoskeletal examination (joint abnormalities, scoliosis).

In conclusion, a neurological examination in a neurocritical care unit is quite challenging. It requires a thorough and systematic approach, including a detailed probe into the history. In the pediatric population, it becomes even more difficult. In a comatose patient, various scales are useful for functional assessment. Early and prompt clinical evaluation and diagnosis allows for immediate and proper management.

References

1. Howard RS, Kullmann DM, Hirsch NP. Admission to neurological intensive care: who, when, and why? J Neurol Neurosurg Psychiatry. 2003;74(suppl 3):iii2–9.
2. Singhal V. Clinical approach to acute decline in sensorium. Indian J Crit Care Med. 2019;23(Suppl 2):S120.
3. Schmidt GA, Wood LD, Hall JB. Principles of critical care. Third Edition -Coma,persistent vegetative state and brain death by Alex J. Rosengart,Roberta L.Novakovic Jeffrey I. Frank Chapter 67 page 1038 (1037-1051)McGraw-Hill Professional; 2005.
4. Folstein MF, Folstein SE, McHugh PR. "Mini-mental state": a practical method for grading the cognitive state of patients for the clinician. J Psychiatr Res. 1975;12(3):189–98.
5. Masdeu JC, Biller J. Localization in clinical neurology. Lippincott Williams & Wilkins; 2011.
6. Bohannon RW. Manual muscle testing: does it meet the standards of an adequate screening test? Clin Rehabil. 2005;19(6):662–7.
7. Marino RJ, Barros T, Biering-Sorensen F, Burns SP, Donovan WH, Graves DE, Haak M, Hudson LM, Priebe M. International standards for neurological classification of spinal cord injury. J Spinal Cord Med. 2003;26(sup1):S50–6.
8. Teasdale G, Jennett B. Assessment of coma and impaired consciousness: a practical scale. Lancet. 1974;304(7872):81–4.
9. Wijdicks EF, Bamlet WR, Maramattom BV, Manno EM, McClelland RL. Validation of a new coma scale: the FOUR score. Ann Neurol. 2005;58(4):585–93.
10. Yang YC, Lin PC, Liu CY, Tzeng I, Lee SJ, Hou YT, Chen YL, Chien DS, Yiang GT, Wu MY. Prehospital shock index multiplied by AVPU scale as a predictor of clinical outcomes in traumatic injury. Shock. 2022;58(6):524–33.
11. https://www.lhsc.on.ca/media/2014/download.
12. Ramat S, Leigh RJ, Zee DS, Optican LM. What clinical disorders tell us about the neural control of saccadic eye movements. Brain. 2007;130(1):10–35.
13. Poungvarin NI, Praditsuwan RU. Opsoclonus in malaria: the first report in the literature. J Med Assoc Thai. 1990;73(8):462–6.

3 Cerebrospinal Fluid Dynamics

Dona Saha and Priyank Tapuria

3.1 Introduction

Comprehensive knowledge of the cerebrospinal fluid (CSF) system is essential for our understanding of health and disease state within the central nervous system (CNS). CSF is a protective fluid for the brain and spinal cord and is valuable for maintaining stable intracranial pressure (ICP). It helps provide mechanical protection and facilitates the transport of nutrients and hormones from one area to another and also plays a crucial role in protein and waste clearance within the CNS. It further helps in communication between the CNS, the peripheral nervous system (PNS), the lymphatic system, the vascular system, and thus immune system and thus aids in maintaining CNS homeostasis [1–3]. This chapter aims to explain the existing knowledge and new theories underlying the CSF system, its secretion, flow, and reabsorption, which are much debated. The most controversial topics regarding the glymphatic system and CNS lymphatics have been specially mentioned to try and bridge these theories. The second section reviews how the dynamics of CSF change in different neurological diseases and the relationship between CSF and ICP.

3.2 CSF-Containing Spaces [4]

CSF is generated within the brain and occupies two spaces, namely, the macroscopic space (the ventricular system and the subarachnoid space) and the narrow extracellular space (ECS) in between the neurons and glia. These two spaces are in continuity around the perivascular space (PVS). The total volume of the macroscopic space can range from 50 mL in newborns to 140–150 mL in adults, in which the ventricular spaces make up approximately 16%–17% of the total CSF volume. The ECS, on the other hand, has an estimated volume of 300–350 mL in adults. In humans, the formation rate is estimated to be 0.35–0.40 mL/min or 500–600 mL per day. This means that approximately 0.25% of the total CSF volume in adults is replenished with newly formed fluid each minute. The entire volume of the CSF is replaced approximately four times a day, with a turnover time of 5–7 h (Tables 3.1 and 3.2).

D. Saha (✉)
Department of Neuro-Anaesthesia and Critical Care, Kalinga Institute of Medical Sciences, Bhubaneswar, Odisha, India

P. Tapuria
Department of Cardiac Anaesthesia, Care Hospital, Bhubaneswar, Odisha, India

H. Prabhakar et al. (eds.), *Principles and Practice of Neurocritical Care*,
https://doi.org/10.1007/978-981-99-8059-8_3

Table 3.1 Distribution of CSF in different spaces by volume [5]

Space	CSF volume (mL)
Cranial subarachnoid space	100
Spinal subarachnoid space	25
Lateral ventricular horns	25–30
Third ventricle	2–3
Fourth ventricle	2–3

Table 3.2 CSF volume and pressure values according to age [6]

Age group	CSF volume (mL)	CSF pressure (mmHg)
Infants	40–60	1.5–6.0
Younger children	60–100	3.0–7.0
Older children	80–120	10–15
Adults	100–160	10–15

3.3 CSF Production

3.3.1 From the Choroid Plexus (CP)

The classical theory states that CSF in the ventricles is produced from the choroid plexus (CP) capillaries and circulates through the ventricles and in the subarachnoid space. It accounts for 80–90% of total CSF production [1, 5–7]. The remaining 10–20% is extra-choroidal production. The choroid plexuses are numerous villi that project into the lateral, third, and fourth ventricles of the brain. These are highly vascularized structures. Those located within the lateral ventricles stretch from the lower horn to the central region of the ventricle. The blood supply to the choroid plexuses in the main body of the lateral and third ventricles is provided by the posterior and anterior choroidal arteries, respectively. Meanwhile, the choroid plexuses in the temporal horns and the fourth ventricle are nourished by the superior and posterior inferior cerebellar arteries, respectively [8].

The choroid plexuses originate from the ependymal cells that protrude from the pia mater into the ventricles. They consist of a single layer of epithelial cells that are supported by a basement membrane, CP stroma or the interstitial space, and capillaries with fenestrations (Fig. 3.1a). The epithelial cells are closely interconnected through tight junctions, which makes the layer relatively impermeable and forms the blood–CSF barrier (BCSFB) [9]. Meanwhile, the underlying capillaries, which are perforated, are relatively permeable, allowing for the passage of substances from the bloodstream to the stroma. The choroid plexus epithelium is not only equipped with a barrier function but is also explicitly designed for secretion. An electron microscopic examination of rat choroidal epithelial cells displays a highly developed brush border on the apical membrane that faces the ventricle. The basolateral membrane, which is on the side of the epithelium facing the blood, also has numerous infoldings that expand its surface area. The epithelial cells also have abundant mitochondria and an exceptionally developed endoplasmic reticulum, which are common characteristics of cells that secrete substances [10].

The Role of Ion Channels in CSF Secretion from the CP

The capillary endothelium lining the CP is different from those lining other cerebral vessels, as the former does not have tight junctions between its cells and is leaky [11]. As blood enters the CP, fluid is filtered through the endothelial fenestrations and has a composition similar to that of interstitial fluid (ISF) in other parts of the body, which is rich in proteins [1]. This fluid is present within the CP stroma or the interstitial space. From here, selected constituents are transported across the relatively impermeable CP epithelium into the ventricular CSF through specialized, tightly regulated ion channels and water transport. Therefore, CSF is not simply an ultrafiltrate of blood but an actively secreted product [12].

Ion Transport

CSF secretion is dependent upon the unidirectional transport of ions because of the polarity of the epithelial cells, i.e., the ion channels in the basolateral membrane are different from those in the apical membrane. Various techniques are used to determine the expression of these channels (isotope flux study, reverse transcription-

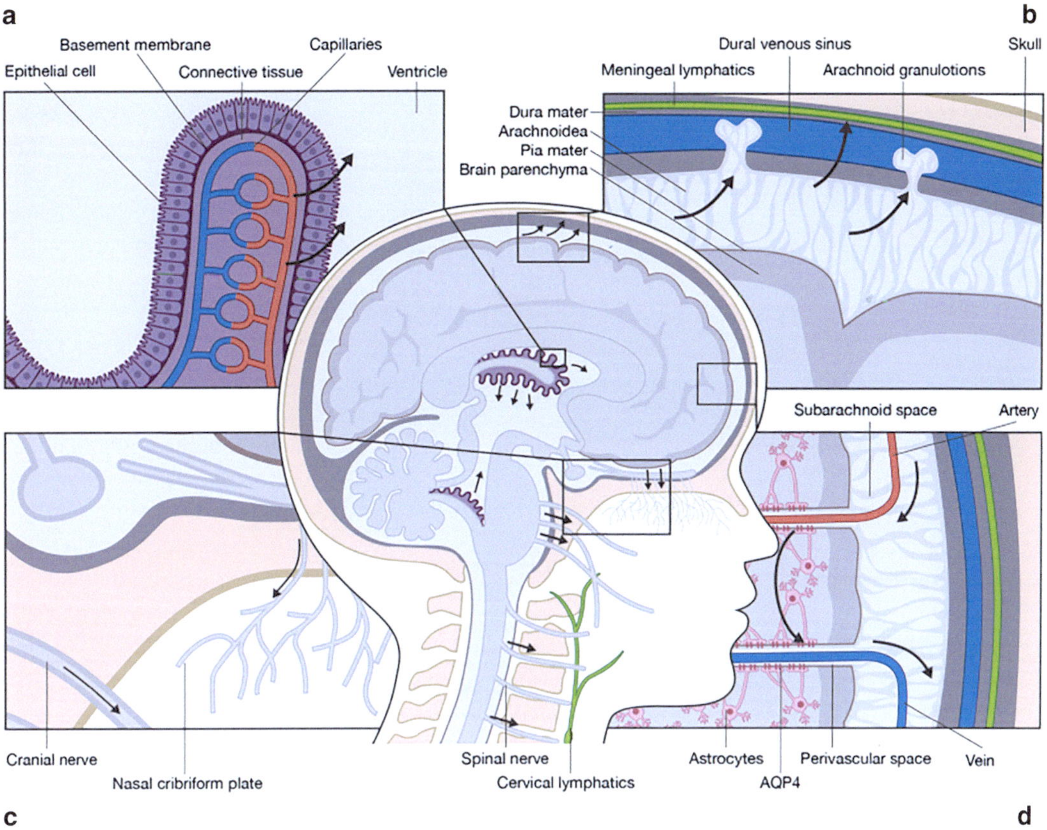

Fig. 3.1 A schematic overview of the cerebrospinal fluid system. The primary site of CSF production is the choroid plexuses located within the lateral, third, and fourth ventricles of the brain. (**a**) The choroid plexuses consist of leaky epithelial cells, a basement membrane, a connective tissue, and fenestrated capillaries. CSF production is mediated by ionic transport that generates osmotic gradients and water transport from the blood system to the ventricular system. (**b**) Several anatomical sites are responsible for CSF absorption, e.g., arachnoid granulations, meningeal lymphatics, (**c**) cranial nerve sheaths, and the nasal cribriform plate to the cervical lymphatics. (**d**) One essential function of CSF is the delivery of nutrients and the removal of waste products. The most recently proposed mechanism for waste removal has been the glymphatic system. The CSF enters from the perivascular spaces surrounding the arteries into the brain parenchyma via mechanisms that include AQP4 water channels located at the astrocytic end feet. Within the brain parenchyma, CSF disperses and intermixes with the interstitial fluid (ISF) and waste products. The mixture of CSF, ISF, and waste products enters the perivascular spaces surrounding veins by unknown mechanisms, e.g., AQP4 water channels. From the perivascular spaces, the mixture leaves the brain parenchyma. (Reproduced with permission from Wichmann et al. [9])

polymerase chain reaction (RT-PCR), in situ hybridization) [10].

The main mechanisms are Na^+, Cl^-, and HCO^{3-} secretion into the CSF and thus net water following the concentration gradient and K reabsorption from CSF (Fig. 3.2a).

Na^+ secretion: The choroid epithelium is highly unusual in that the Na^+–K^+–ATPase is located on the apical membrane rather than on the basolateral membrane in most other cells. This pump drives Na^+ into the CSF space.

K^+ absorption: The Na^+–K^+–ATPase removes K^+ from the CSF. More K^+ may be absorbed by the apical Na^+–K^+–$2Cl^-$ cotransporter using the energy of the Na^+ gradient.

HCO_3^- secretion: This is generated inside the epithelial cells by the action of carbonic anhydrase by combining carbon dioxide and water.

$$CO_2 + H_2O = H_2CO_3 = H^+ + HCO_3^-$$

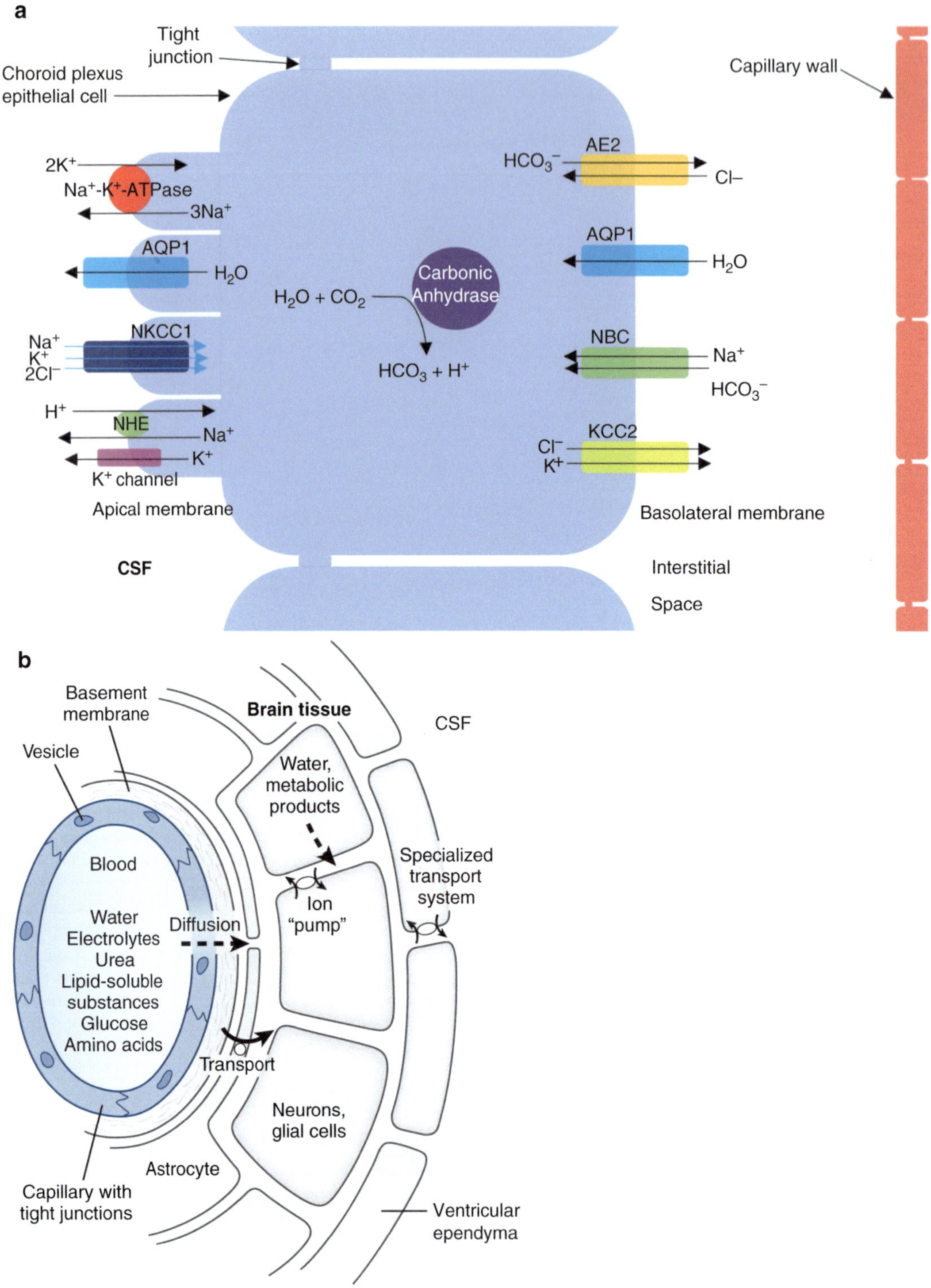

Fig. 3.2 (**a**) Transepithelial ion transport at the choroid plexus. Reproduced with permission from Bothwell et al. [13]. (**b**) Water and other constituents of plasma cross the blood–brain barrier (capillary endothelial cells, basement membrane, and astrocyte foot processes) into the brain ECS space by diffusion or transport. This fluid diffuses toward the macroscopic CSF space and subarachnoid space. Water and other cellular metabolites are added to the ECS from neurons and glial cells. (Reproduced with permission from Artru [4])

H^+ is released to the CP stroma via a Na^+–H^+ exchanger, and HCO_3^- is secreted into the CSF via the Cl^- channel and the Na^+–HCO_3^- cotransporter.

Cl^- secretion: Cl^- is concentrated within the epithelial cell by the $Cl^-HCO_3^-$ anion exchanger in the basolateral membrane and then flows across the apical membrane via the Cl^- channel.

Water secretion: Water follows an osmotic gradient generated by the secretion of Na^+, HCO_3^-, and Cl^- toward the CSF. Aquaporin channels have the ability to transport water bidirectionally across cell membranes in response to changes in the osmotic pressure gradient. They have a narrow pathway, which is an extremely tight fit for water and helps water molecules to pass rapidly with no resistance. Aquaporin 1 (AQP1) is highly expressed on the apical membrane [14, 15]. However, its role in CSF secretion is undetermined due to its low expression on the basolateral membrane. The other water transport methods are along with cotransporters like glucose transporter GLUT1, independent of the osmotic gradient [16].

3.3.2 Extra-Choroidal CSF Formation

The blood–brain barrier (BBB), which is composed of endothelial cells that line the cerebral capillaries and are connected by tight junctions, acts as the regulated gateway for the exchange of ions, molecules, and cells between the blood and the brain [17]. Approximately 10–20% of CSF secretion is attributed to fluid transport across the BBB [18]. The interstitial fluid (ISF) is thus produced as a result of fluid secretion through the BBB, filling the narrow extracellular space between the neurons and glia in the brain tissue. Meanwhile, the cerebrospinal fluid occupies the brain's ventricles and subarachnoid space [19].

About 60% of the extra-choroidal cerebrospinal fluid is produced by the oxidation of glucose by the neurons and glial cells in the brain tissue and freely enters the brain's extracellular fluid. The other 40% is derived from ultrafiltration from the cerebral capillaries [4]. In most cases, the passage of large and polar molecules across the blood–brain interface is restricted by the tight junctions of the capillaries. However, substances such as water, electrolytes, glucose, amino acids, urea, lipid-soluble materials, and a number of small nonelectrolytes can pass more easily through this interface [20]. Some of these substances may be actively transported by the astrocyte layer that surrounds the capillary endothelium, whereas others may simply diffuse into the brain's extracellular fluid. The movement of water appears to be largely influenced by osmotic forces [21] (Fig. 3.2b).

Movement of Glucose

The concentration of glucose in the CSF at the choroid plexus or in mixed samples is about 60% of that in the blood. This proportion remains unchanged unless the blood glucose level rises above 15–20 mM (270–360 mg/dL). The entry of glucose into the CSF occurs through facilitated transport, which enables glucose to cross the blood–CSF barrier more rapidly than expected based on its lipid solubility [22]. The transport process follows saturable kinetics, and the rate is directly related to glucose concentration in the serum. It is independent of the glucose concentration gradient between the serum and CSF [23].

Movement of Proteins

The entry of proteins from the blood into the CSF at the choroid plexus and extra-choroidal sites is limited, resulting in lower protein content in the CSF (0.03 g/dL) compared to the plasma (7 g/dL), with a CSF/plasma ratio of 0.004 [13]. The permeability of the blood–CSF barrier to albumin increases with age and is similar between males and females [24]. If there is no structural barrier separating the brain's ECS and the macroscopic CSF space, then the proteins that enter the brain's ECS will drain into the macroscopic CSF space by bulk flow. Once in the CSF, the proteins are transported along with it through the macroscopic pathways and are cleared from the CSF space into the dural venous sinuses. This "sink effect" of flowing CSF helps maintain a low protein concentration in both the CSF and the brain, far from equilibrium with the blood [4].

3.4 CSF Composition

From the discussion till now, it is clear that CSF is a clear aqueous solution that has a different composition compared to plasma, with higher concentrations of sodium, chloride, and magnesium and lower concentrations of glucose, proteins, amino acids, uric acid, potassium, bicarbonate, calcium, and phosphate. The differences in composition between the CSF and an ultrafiltrate of plasma suggest that active secretion occurs during the formation of the CSF. The concentrations of these substances in the macroscopic spaces can vary depending on the location of the sample, as diffusion between the CSF and the brain's ECS occurs as it flows through the ventricles and subarachnoid spaces. The concentrations of the CSF constituents are significantly affected during neuroendoscopy [25] (Table 3.3).

Table 3.3 Composition of CSF and plasma in humans [4]

Feature/component	Mean CSF value/concentration	Mean plasma value/concentration
Specific gravity	1.007	1.025
Osmolality (mOsm/kg H_2O)	289	289
pH	7.31	7.41
PCO_2 (mmHg)	50.5	41.1
Sodium (mEq/L)	141	140
Potassium (mEq/L)	2.9	4.6
Calcium (mEq/L)	2.5	5.0
Magnesium (mEq/L)	2.4	1.7
Chloride (mEq/L)	124	101
Bicarbonate (mEq/L)	21	23
Glucose (mg/100 ml)	61	92
Protein (mg/100 mL)	28	7000
→ Albumin	→ 23	→ 4430
→ Globulin	→ 5	→ 2270
→ Fibrinogen	→ 0	→ 300

3.5 Continuity between the Ventricular CSF and the Brain ECS

The exchange of CSF and interstitial fluid is believed to occur in the perivascular spaces or the Virchow–Robin spaces (VRSs) [26], which are low-resistance pathways surrounding the blood vessels supplying the brain parenchyma. These histologically defined spaces are located around the perforating arteries and veins as they penetrate deep with their pial layer from the subarachnoid space into the brain tissue (Fig. 3.3a). Here, the interaction between the CSF and ISF allows for the bidirectional flow of fluid between the brain's extracellular space and the subarachnoid space. This exchange is believed to serve the purpose of distributing compounds from one region of the brain to another, such as melatonin, as well as from the systemic circulation, such as vitamin C and folate, into the central nervous system through the choroid plexus. More details of the VRSs and perivascular spaces can be found in Brinker et al. [26].

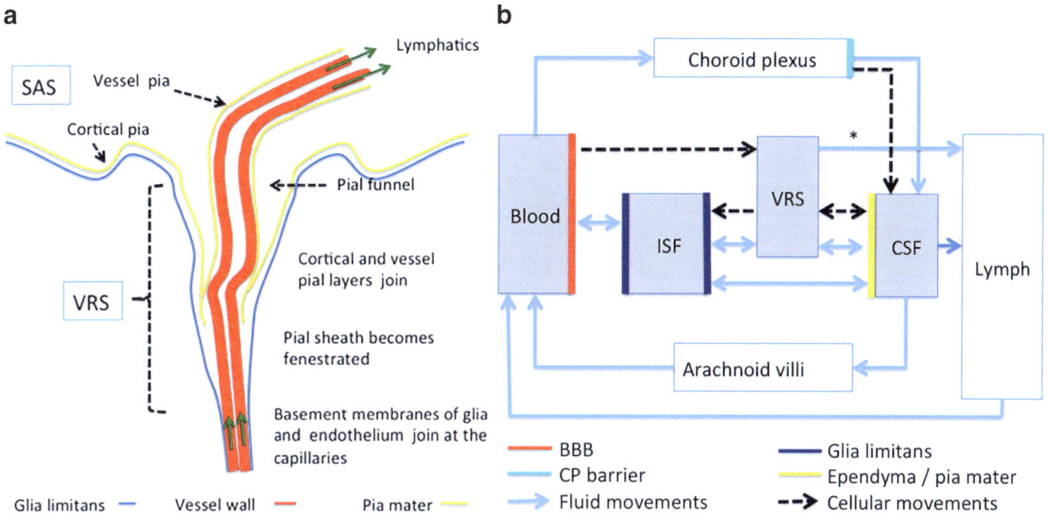

Fig. 3.3 (**a**) The morphology of Virchow–Robin and perivascular spaces. Delineated by basal membranes of the glia, pia, and endothelium, the Virchow–Robin space (VRS) depicts the space surrounding the vessels penetrating into the parenchyma. Reproduced with permission from Brinker et al. [26]. (**b**) A diagram of CSF "circulation." This diagram summarizes fluid and cellular movements across the different barriers of the brain compartments (blood, interstitial fluid, Virchow–Robin space, cerebrospinal fluid space comprising the cerebral ventricles, basal cisterns, and cortical subarachnoid space). (Reproduced with permission from Brinker et al. [26])

3.6 The Role of the Glymphatic System

The CNS requires a means of removing waste products generated by its highly active metabolic regions. This function is performed by the CSF system, including the recently proposed glymphatic system [27]. Despite being the focus of much research, the exact mechanisms of the glymphatic system remain unclear and much debated. The glymphatic system is believed to be a fluid exchange system between CSF and interstitial ISF in the brain, facilitated by astrocytes [27, 28]. CSF is believed to be conveyed from the subarachnoid space into the periarterial spaces surrounding the penetrating arteries and then into the brain parenchyma, with the help of the water channel protein aquaporin 4 (AQP4). AQP4 is expressed on the vascular end feet of astrocytes [29]. However, the role of AQP4 remains a point of contention in the study of the glymphatic system (Fig. 3.1d). Within the brain, CSF and ISF mix with waste products and leave the brain via the perivenous spaces, which are poorly understood [27]. The mixture then returns to the subarachnoid space and potentially exits the CNS through the meningeal lymphatic vessels, nerve sheaths, or nasal cribriform plate into the deep cervical lymph nodes [30].

In cases of neurological injury such as traumatic brain injury (TBI), subarachnoid hemorrhage (SAH), and ischemic stroke, the glymphatic function—a mechanism responsible for the clearance of extracellular proteins in the brain—appears to decrease [31–33]. This impaired function can harm patients as the clearance of proteins becomes disrupted. Research has shown that amyloid-β clearance is reduced when the glymphatic function is impaired in mice without the *AQP4* gene [27]. Similarly, tau clearance is also impaired following TBI when the glymphatic function is reduced [32]. The attenuation of glymphatic function and protein clearance is associated with AQP4 distribution, which is altered after TBI. A reduction in protein clearance can have significant implications, such as the development or early onset of dementia or Alzheimer's disease, in which the aggregation of these proteins is reported [34].

3.7 CSF Flow

There are two primary types of movements involved in CSF flow dynamics in the ventricular system and subarachnoid spaces: convective flow and pulsatile flow [35]. The unidirectional motion from the lateral ventricles' choroidal plexuses through the left and right foramina of Monro into the third ventricle, passing through the cerebral aqueduct into the fourth ventricle, is referred to as convective flow (Fig. 3.4). The CSF then exits the ventricular system through three apertures (two lateral foramina of Luschka and one median foramen of Magendie). It enters the cerebral subarachnoid space, the spinal subarachnoid space, and the central canal of the spinal cord. Convective flow is believed to be driven by the hydrostatic pressure gradients that exist between the choroid plexuses, where pressure is high (15 mmHg), and arachnoid granulations, where pressure is low (9 mmHg). Ependymal cell cilia create currents that move the CSF toward the fourth ventricle and its foramina, leading to subarachnoid spaces.

Having said that, convective flow is unidirectional. Recent studies have shown constant CSF movement without a net unidirectional displacement of CSF, indicating the presence of pulsatile flow [18]. Unlike convective flow, which moves in a single direction, pulsatile flow involves bidirectional movement, with the CSF moving in both upward (cranial) and downward (caudal) directions along the spinal cord and in varying directions toward the brain. Earlier theories suggested that the choroid plexuses were responsible for generating pulsatile CSF motion [36]. However, two main theories have emerged, namely, the cardiac-driven theory and the respiratory-driven theory, to explain the origin of pulsatile CSF motion. According to the cardiac-driven theory, changes in blood volume are

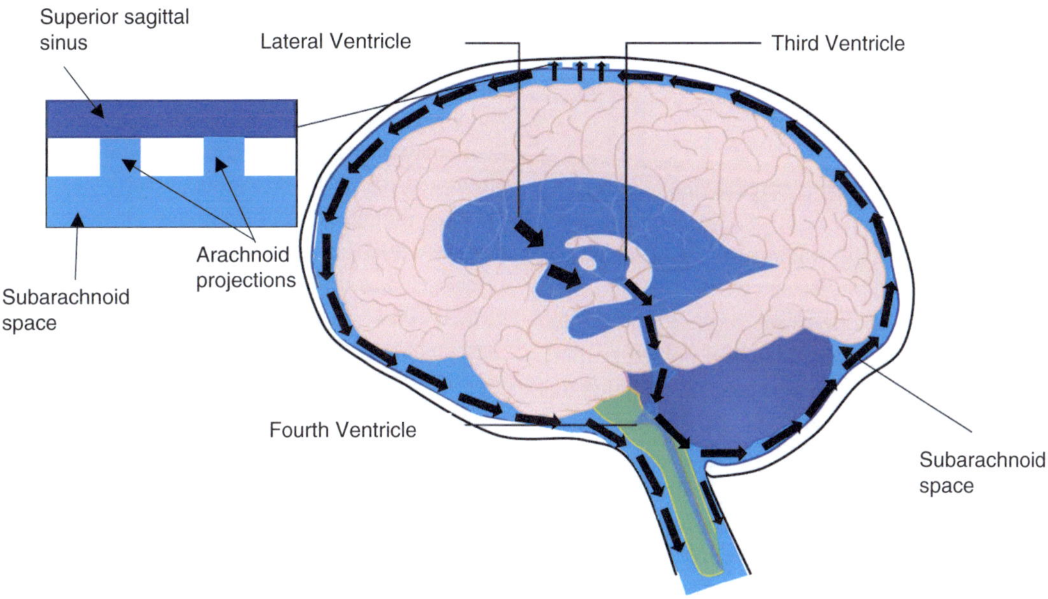

Fig. 3.4 The conventional view of CSF flow. CSF is produced in the ventricles, beginning in the lateral ventricles and flows toward the subarachnoid space. CSF circulates in the subarachnoid space and drains into the subarachnoid space (via arachnoid projections) and the spinal cord. The arrows depict the flow of CSF from the lateral ventricle origin. (Reproduced with permission from Bothwell et al. [13])

directly and indirectly transmitted to the CSF. This theory proposes that the pulsations of blood vessels are transmitted to the CSF both directly and indirectly through other tissues [37, 38]. On the other hand, the respiratory-driven theory suggests that changes in intrathoracic pressure are transmitted through the venous system into the CSF [38]. Although natural respiration may not generate as much force as forced respiration, this theory proposes that changes in intrathoracic pressure during respiration cause the movement of CSF. It is commonly believed that inspiration causes cranial movement of CSF, whereas expiration results in caudal movement [39]. The cardiac-driven force is believed to be responsible for the basic pulsatile CSF flow, whereas the respiratory-driven force is responsible for the larger pulsatile CSF flow.

Radioisotope studies have demonstrated that within a few minutes, labeled CSF moves from the ventricles to the basal cisterns and begins to accumulate along the area of the superior sagittal sinus over the course of 12–24 h. The labeled CSF is observed to enter the low cervical-high thoracic region at 10–20 min, the thoracolumbar area at 30–40 min, the lumbosacral cul de sac at 60–90 min, and the basal cisterns at 2–2.5 h. Approximately 20–33% of the labeled CSF is able to reach the intracranial cavity within 12 h [18, 40].

3.8 CSF Reabsorption

CSF passes from the subarachnoid space into venous blood through arachnoid villi and macroscopic arachnoid granulations. Intracranial arachnoid villi are located within the dural wall bordering the superior sagittal sinus and venous lacunae, and the spinal arachnoid villi are located within the dural wall bordering the dural sinusoids on the dorsal nerve roots. Traditional estimates were that, under usual conditions, 85–90% of CSF is reabsorbed at intracranial sites and 10–15% at spinal sites [4].

There are several theories of CSF absorption; apart from the classical theory described above, the other theories suggest other sites for CSF reabsorption: first, via cranial meningeal lymphatics embedded in the dura mater alongside the arterial and venous vessels, and second, via the cribriform plate and cranial nerve sheaths into the cervical lymphatics [13]. Refer to Fig. 3.1b, c.

3.8.1 Meningeal Lymphatics

In 1787, the Italian anatomist Paolo Mascagni initially reported the presence of a lymphatic network in the meninges of the brain, a finding that has been recently translated and published [41]. The rediscovery of this network has revealed that meningeal lymphatic vessels are located within the dura mater, alongside the arteries, veins, and cranial nerves [2, 28]. The lymphatic network in the meninges helps clear waste from the brain and provides a direct connection between the CNS and the PNS [42]. It is suggested that specific entry points along the vessels facilitate the entry of solutes and immune cells from the CSF into the meningeal lymphatics. Although the brain and spinal cord have significant anatomical differences, it is reasonable to assume that the spinal cord has a similar waste clearance and lymphatic system as proposed for the brain.

3.8.2 Continuous Fluid Exchange [13]

A contemporary and contentious theory about CSF dynamics drifts away from the notion of CSF production, flow, and drainage at specific locations within the cranial compartment. Instead, it suggests that there is a consistent exchange of fluid among the CSF from the choroid plexus, interstitial fluid (ISF) in ECS, blood, and parenchyma throughout the entire system, driven by osmotic and hydrostatic forces. This hypothesis opposes the "classical" and lymphatic CSF hypotheses, which are supported by a considerable amount of evidence demonstrating CSF production at the choroid plexus and CSF drainage via the arachnoid villi or extracranial lymphatics. The main issue with this new hypothesis is that water exchange between the CSF, ISF, and parenchyma does not necessarily indicate overall CSF movement, as water can move independently of the ions comprising CSF. Therefore, water exchange and CSF exchange should be investigated separately. Some researchers have attempted to merge this modern model with the existing model of CSF drainage. However, this perspective is far from being embraced by most scientists, and more evidence is required to integrate this concept into our current understanding.

3.9 CSF Dynamics and ICP Elevation

Alterations in CSF can affect ICP because the intracranial compartment, consisting of the brain, blood, and CSF within the rigid skull, is a closed system. The balance between cerebral blood inflow and outflow is crucial for maintaining normal ICP. The Monro–Kellie hypothesis states that a change in one of the brain, blood, or CSF volume will result in a reciprocal change in one or both of the other two. If this is not possible, then an increase in volume will lead to increased ICP [43]. A sudden increase in ICP can reduce cerebral perfusion pressure (CPP), which is determined by subtracting ICP from the mean arterial pressure (MAP) and can predispose the brain to ischemia, particularly when autoregulation of cerebral blood vessels is impaired, as in the case of stroke. Chronic elevation of ICP can lead to papillary edema, vision loss, and death. The normal range of ICP in healthy adults is approximately 5–15 mmHg, and increases to 30 mmHg are considered pathological, whereas 40 mmHg is life-threatening [44].

Before we deal with different diseases and their effect on CSF dynamics, we have to understand a few physiological concepts. The rate of CSF formation (V_f) is generally not influenced by changes in ICP within certain limits. V_f remains constant, regardless of whether ICP is 2-cm H_2O or 20-cm H_2O, and only when ICP rises significantly enough to decrease CPP to below

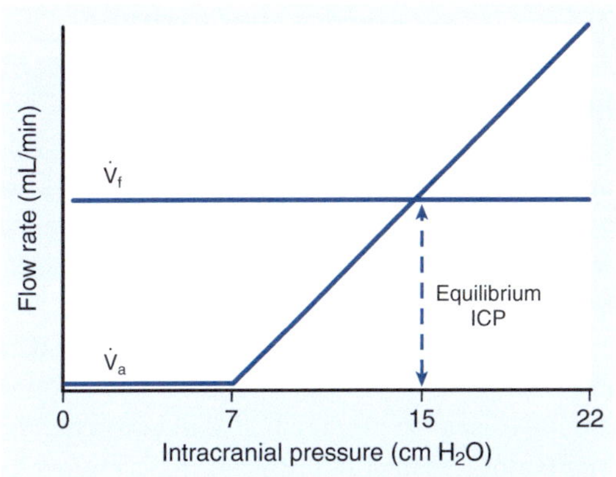

Fig. 3.5 Rates of CSF formation (V'_f) and reabsorption (V'_a) are plotted as functions of ICP. (Reproduced with permission from Artru [4])

~70 mmHg, will V_f decrease. Conversely, the rate of CSF reabsorption (V_a) is highly sensitive to changes in ICP. At ICP levels below 7-cm H_2O, minimal reabsorption occurs, whereas V_a increases proportionally to ICP at levels above 7-cm H_2O [45]. The relationship between ICP and V_a is linear up to 30-cm H_2O because, in this range, the resistance to reabsorption (R_a) is relatively constant. The point of intersection between the plots of V_f/ICP and V_a/ICP is known as the equilibrium pressure [4]. At this pressure, the rates of CSF formation and reabsorption are equal, resulting in no net change in the CSF volume (Fig. 3.5). Various drugs, e.g., anesthetic drugs (both intravenous (IV) and inhalational), opioids, steroids, diuretics, vasopressin, digoxin, and theophylline variables, affect production and reabsorption and affect the ICP, whereas muscle relaxants like succinylcholine and vecuronium produce no change in V_f or R_a [4].

Other neurogenic and metabolic factors can also affect both V_f and R_a, as summarized in Table 3.4 [4].

CNS disorders, such as hydrocephalus, intracerebral hemorrhage (ICH), subarachnoid hemorrhage (SAH), and ischemic stroke, can cause increased intracranial pressure. A detailed review of altered CSF dynamics in each of these CNS disorders is discussed below.

Table 3.4 Neurogenic and metabolic factors affecting Vf and Ra

Factors	Effects
Adrenergic nerves • Sympathectomy • Stimulation	• Increases V_f by 33% (increases carbonic anhydrase activity by 150%) • Decreases V_f by 32%
Cholinergic nerves • Agonists (acetylcholine, carbachol) • Antagonists	• Reduces V_f by 25–55% • Increases V_f
Hypothermia • For every 1 °C decrease	Decreases V_f (by reducing the activity of the active secretory and transport processes and by decreasing CBF) • V_f is decreased by 11%
pH • Metabolic acidosis • Metabolic alkalosis • Hypocapnia – Prolonged – Acute	• No change in V_f • Decreases V_f • No change • Decreases V_f

3.10 Hydrocephalus

This is a condition in which there is an accumulation of fluid in the brain and dilated ventricles due to disruptions in CSF secretion, flow, or drainage, resulting in increased ICP [46]. Most cases (about 95%) are caused by disruptions in CSF flow, often due to tumors within the ventricular system or transient obstructive hydrocephalus resulting from intraventricular hemorrhage. Nonobstructive hydrocephalus can also occur when there is decreased absorption within the ventricular system, and increased CSF secretion due to tumors of the choroid plexus can also lead to hydrocephalus if not compensated for by increased outflow.

3.11 Idiopathic Intracranial Hypertension (IIH)

IIH refers to elevated ICP in the absence of lesions or disruptions in CSF. It has a global incidence of 0.03–2.2 per 100,000, and obesity is a major risk factor [47]. The primary treatment is acetazolamide, which inhibits carbonic anhydrase to reduce CSF secretion. However, this approach targets the symptom rather than the cause. A ventricular or lumbar CSF shunt is often required. The use of acetazolamide in IIH management may negatively impact other aspects of CNS health since CSF has roles in protein and metabolite clearance.

3.12 Traumatic Brain Injury

Aquaporins have been implicated in developing edema in TBI, and upregulation of AQP4 and AQP9 has been observed in animal models of TBI [48]. This upregulation is associated with hypoxia-inducible factor-1α (HIF-1α), indicating that hypoxia plays a role in aquaporin upregulation in TBI and other CNS injuries, such as ischemic stroke.

A condition in which there is disruption of the BBB, e.g., vasogenic edema, leads to the leakage of proteins and fluid into the brain ECS, resulting in multiple complications like increased intracranial pressure, acute posttraumatic seizures, immune response, and limitations in treatment options with hyperosmolar therapy. On the other hand, cytotoxic edema, which can occur shortly after an injury, leads to cellular swelling due to changes in the osmotic balance between the intracellular compartment and ECS [49]. As a result of this, there is an alteration in the ionic milieu of the ECS that drives water from the intravascular compartment through the damaged BBB and increases ICP further. This secondary edema is also known as ionic edema.

3.13 Intracerebral Hemorrhage

In instances of intracerebral hemorrhage (ICH), the rise in ICP occurs due to an increase in volume that enters the intracranial compartment via a lesion and is independent of CSF. To determine whether targeting CSF secretion with acetazolamide could counter this elevation in ICP, a few researchers investigated using a rat model of ICH [50]. They discovered that while acetazolamide did not lessen the average ICP, it did decrease the number of transient ICP spikes, characterized by a 1-min peak with an increase of more than 20 mmHg. Moreover, ICP was more stable in the treated rats, which is an indication of enhanced intracranial compliance. This example demonstrates that even though CSF was not the primary cause of the elevated pressure, targeting CSF was still beneficial in reducing the effects of ICH [48]. If CSF can be targeted in this manner for ICP conditions that do not directly stem from CSF abnormalities, then it can certainly be applied to those in which CSF imbalance is the primary cause.

3.14 Subarachnoid Hemorrhage

SAH is a type of stroke that occurs when there is a rupture of blood vessels into the subarachnoid space, accounting for approximately 5% of all strokes [51]. A neurological injury following SAH is characterized as biphasic, with the initial brain injury caused by global ischemia and toxicity of subarachnoid blood. Delayed brain injury occurs in around 30% of patients, which refers to delayed neurological deterioration resulting from delayed cerebral ischemia and typically presents up to 2 weeks post-stroke. Vessel rupture in SAH can also cause hydrocephalus, vasospasm, and increased ICP [50]. Studies have revealed that 81% of SAH patients experience at least one episode of elevated ICP (defined as ICP > 20 mmHg for 5 min), and 36% had the "highest mean ICP" of >20 mmHg. The rise in ICP observed in patients is associated with poor clinical outcomes [52], making it necessary to investigate therapies to target this ICP elevation.

Although the role of CSF in elevated ICP following SAH is not fully understood, some clinical observations have reported disruptions to CSF flow associated with SAH, and studies of animal SAH models support these observations. Disruption of CSF flow along the "glymphatic" pathway has been observed following SAH, and this disruption was sustained for at least 4 days with improved distribution at 30 days [33]. Increased ICP following SAH presents patients with additional risks and may contribute to delayed brain injury. Reports of impaired CSF flow following SAH provide insight into the mechanisms underlying this ICP rise and create new pathways for exploring therapeutic tactics to reduce this ICP in the hope of preventing secondary degeneration. A study has already examined the use of tissue plasminogen activator (tPA) in preserving CSF flow post-SAH and found that an intracisternal injection of recombinant tPA was able to lower ICP, increase cortical blood volume, and partially restore CSF flow 24 h after SAH [53].

3.15 Ischemic Stroke [13]

Elevation of ICP has been observed in animals and humans following an ischemic stroke, which can lead to reduced cerebral blood flow, blood–brain barrier disruption, and altered fluid movement. Although edema development has long been associated with ICP elevation, recent studies have suggested that alterations in CSF volume may also contribute to increased ICP, particularly in smaller strokes where edema volume could not be correlated with the out-of-proportion increase in ICP [13]. The choroid plexus, a major site of CSF secretion, may be impacted by an ischemic stroke, leading to changes in CSF secretion and subsequent ICP elevation. Studies in rat models have shown reduced blood supply to the lateral ventricle choroid plexus and increased BCSFB permeability following a stroke. Morphological studies have also identified swelling of the choroid plexus epithelium and markers of proliferation following stroke occlusion [54]. Understanding how fluid exchange at the choroid plexus is altered following an ischemic stroke may be significant for exploring therapeutic strategies to reduce ICP and prevent secondary damage.

Exploring the expression and activity of transient receptor potential vanilloid 4 (TRPV4, a mechano- and osmotic-sensitive channel) in the choroid plexus following an ischemic stroke would be an interesting path of investigation [55]. TRPV4 channels have been shown to be involved in regulating CSF and are highly expressed in choroid plexus epithelial cells. Upregulation of TRPV4 channels following ischemia has been associated with greater neuronal injury [56], and targeting these channels has been shown to alleviate cardiac ischemia/reperfusion injury in mice [57]. Therefore, investigating these receptors in the choroid plexus after an ischemic stroke can potentially lead to new therapeutic strategies for managing ICP elevation and reducing secondary brain injury.

Aquaporins play a crucial role in CSF secretion, and overexpression of AQP4 has been associated with increased CSF secretion and subsequent cognitive decline in aged mice with hypoxia-induced hydrocephalus [58]. After an ischemic stroke, AQP4 expression is temporarily reduced or lost around 24 h post-stroke, possibly as a mechanism to limit water influx via the water channels and reduce brain edema. However, AQP4 expression partially recovers by 72 h post-stroke to support the absorption of excess fluid. Although there have been attempts to develop pharmacological inhibitors of AQP4 to reduce brain edema following ischemia, they have not been successful so far [59, 60].

3.16 Conclusions

This chapter presents an overview of our current knowledge of CSF dynamics, with a particular emphasis on how these dynamics affect ICP during neurological diseases. Additionally, it points out some of the discrepancies within the field. The clinical implications of these findings are highly relevant to understanding and treating neurological diseases that involve impaired brain fluid homeostasis. Although our understanding of the CSF system has improved significantly, many processes still need clarification. Notably, most research has been focused on the brain, leaving a significant knowledge gap regarding the spinal cord. The anatomical and physiological differences between the two systems make it challenging to transfer the findings from the brain to the spinal cord, which is why more research is necessary to investigate the mechanisms in the spinal cord.

References

1. Damkier HH, Brown PD, Praetorius J. Cerebrospinal fluid secretion by the choroid plexus. Physiol Rev. 2013;93(4):1847–92.
2. Aspelund A, Antila S, Proulx ST, Karlsen TV, Karaman S, Detmar M, et al. A dural lymphatic vascular system that drains brain interstitial fluid and macromolecules. J Exp Med. 2015;212(7):991–9.
3. Louveau A, Smirnov I, Keyes TJ, Eccles JD, Rouhani SJ, Peske JD, et al. Structural and functional features of central nervous system lymphatic vessels. Nature. 2015;523(7560):337–41.
4. Artru AA. Cerebrospinal fluid. In: Cottrell and Patel's Neuroanesthesia. 6th ed. Elsevier; 2017. p. 59–73.
5. Wood JH. Physiology, pharmacology, and dynamics of cerebrospinal fluid. In: Wood JH, editor. Neurobiology of cerebrospinal fluid 1. Boston, MA: Springer US; 1980. p. 1–16. https://doi.org/10.1007/978-1-4684-1039-6_1.
6. Majumdar A, Jana A, Jana A, Biswas S, Bhatacharyya S, Bannerjee S. Importance of Normal values of CSF parameters in term versus preterm neonates. J Clin Neonatol. 2013;2(4):166.
7. Hladky SB, Barrand MA. Mechanisms of fluid movement into, through and out of the brain: evaluation of the evidence. Fluids Barriers CNS. 2014;11(1):26.
8. Javed K, Reddy V, Lui F. Neuroanatomy, choroid plexus. StatPearls: StatPearls Publishing; 2022. https://www.ncbi.nlm.nih.gov/books/NBK538156/.
9. Wichmann TO, Damkier HH, Pedersen M. A brief overview of the cerebrospinal fluid system and its implications for brain and spinal cord diseases. Front Hum Neurosci. 2022;15:15. https://doi.org/10.3389/fnhum.2021.737217.
10. Brown PD, Davies SL, Speake T, Millar ID. Molecular mechanisms of cerebrospinal fluid production. Neuroscience. 2004;129(4):957–70.
11. Mortazavi MM, Griessenauer CJ, Adeeb N, Deep A, Bavarsad Shahripour R, Loukas M, et al. The choroid plexus: a comprehensive review of its history, anatomy, function, histology, embryology, and surgical considerations. Childs Nerv Syst ChNS Off J Int Soc Pediatr Neurosurg. 2014;30(2):205–14.
12. Christensen HL, Nguyen AT, Pedersen FD, Damkier HH. Na(+) dependent acid-base transporters in the choroid plexus; insights from slc4 and slc9 gene deletion studies. Front Physiol. 2013;4:304.
13. Bothwell SW, Janigro D, Patabendige A. Cerebrospinal fluid dynamics and intracranial pressure elevation in neurological diseases. Fluids Barriers CNS. 2019;16(1):9.
14. Kozono D, Yasui M, King LS, Agre P. Aquaporin water channels: atomic structure molecular dynamics meet clinical medicine. J Clin Invest. 2002;109(11):1395–9.
15. Agre P. The aquaporin water channels. Proc Am Thorac Soc. 2006;3(1):5–13.
16. MacAulay N, Zeuthen T. Water transport between CNS compartments: contributions of aquaporins and cotransporters. Neuroscience. 2010;168(4):941–56.
17. Abbott NJ, Patabendige AAK, Dolman DEM, Yusof SR, Begley DJ. Structure and function of the blood-brain barrier. Neurobiol Dis. 2010;37(1):13–25.
18. Orešković D, Klarica M. The formation of cerebrospinal fluid: nearly a hundred years of interpretations and misinterpretations. Brain Res Rev. 2010;64(2):241–62.
19. Abbott NJ, Pizzo ME, Preston JE, Janigro D, Thorne RG. The role of brain barriers in fluid movement in the CNS: is there a "glymphatic" system? Acta Neuropathol (Berl). 2018;135(3):387–407.
20. Chikly B, Quaghebeur J. Reassessing cerebrospinal fluid (CSF) hydrodynamics: a literature review presenting a novel hypothesis for CSF physiology. J Bodyw Mov Ther. 2013;17(3):344–54.
21. Buishas J, Gould IG, Linninger AA. A computational model of cerebrospinal fluid production and reabsorption driven by Starling forces. Croat Med J. 2014;55(5):481–97.
22. Hochwald GM, Gandhi M, Goldman S. Net transport of glucose from blood to cerebrospinal fluid in the cat. Neuroscience. 1983;10(3):1035–40.
23. Hochwald GM, Magee J, Ferguson V. Cerebrospinal fluid glucose: turnover and metabolism. J Neurochem. 1985;44(6):1832–7.
24. Pakulski C, Drobnik L, Millo B. Age and sex as factors modifying the function of the blood-cerebrospinal fluid barrier. Med Sci Monit Int Med J Exp Clin Res. 2000;6(2):314–8.

25. Salvador L, Valero R, Carrero E, Caral L, Fernández S, Marín JL, et al. Cerebrospinal fluid composition modifications after neuroendoscopic procedures. Minim Invasive Neurosurg MIN. 2007;50(1):51–5.
26. Brinker T, Stopa E, Morrison J, Klinge P. A new look at cerebrospinal fluid circulation. Fluids Barriers CNS. 2014;11(1):10.
27. Iliff JJ, Wang M, Liao Y, Plogg BA, Peng W, Gundersen GA, et al. A paravascular pathway facilitates CSF flow through the brain parenchyma and the clearance of interstitial solutes, including amyloid β. Sci Transl Med. 2012;4(147):147ra111.
28. Jessen NA, Munk ASF, Lundgaard I, Nedergaard M. The glymphatic system: a Beginner's guide. Neurochem Res. 2015;40(12):2583–99.
29. Trillo-Contreras JL, Toledo-Aral JJ, Echevarría M, Villadiego J. AQP1 and AQP4 contribution to cerebrospinal fluid homeostasis. Cell. 2019;8(2):197.
30. Mestre H, Mori Y, Nedergaard M. The Brain's Glymphatic system: current controversies. Trends Neurosci. 2020;43(7):458–66.
31. Gaberel T, Gakuba C, Goulay R, Martinez De Lizarrondo S, Hanouz JL, Emery E, et al. Impaired glymphatic perfusion after strokes revealed by contrast-enhanced MRI: a new target for fibrinolysis? Stroke. 2014;45(10):3092–6.
32. Iliff JJ, Chen MJ, Plog BA, Zeppenfeld DM, Soltero M, Yang L, et al. Impairment of glymphatic pathway function promotes tau pathology after traumatic brain injury. J Neurosci. 2014;34(49):16180–93.
33. Golanov EV, Bovshik EI, Wong KK, Pautler RG, Foster CH, Federley RG, et al. Subarachnoid hemorrhage—induced block of cerebrospinal fluid flow: role of brain coagulation factor III (tissue factor). J Cereb Blood Flow Metab. 2018;38(5):793–808.
34. Apostolova LG. Alzheimer Disease. Contin Minneap Minn. 2016;22(2 Dementia):419–34.
35. Yildiz S, Thyagaraj S, Jin N, Zhong X, Heidari Pahlavian S, Martin BA, et al. Quantifying the influence of respiration and cardiac pulsations on cerebrospinal fluid dynamics using real-time phase-contrast MRI. J Magn Reson Imaging JMRI. 2017;46(2):431–9.
36. Takizawa K, Matsumae M, Hayashi N, Hirayama A, Sano F, Yatsushiro S, et al. The choroid plexus of the lateral ventricle as the origin of CSF pulsation is questionable. Neurol Med Chir (Tokyo). 2018;58(1):23–31.
37. Haughton V, Mardal KA. Spinal fluid biomechanics and imaging: an update for Neuroradiologists. Am J Neuroradiol. 2014;35(10):1864–9.
38. Daouk J, Bouzerar R, Balcdent O. Heart rate and respiration influence on macroscopic blood and CSF flows. Acta Radiol Stockh Swed 1987. 2017;58(8):977–82.
39. Yamada S, Miyazaki M, Yamashita Y, Ouyang C, Yui M, Nakahashi M, et al. Influence of respiration on cerebrospinal fluid movement using magnetic resonance spin labeling. Fluids Barriers CNS. 2013;10(1):36.
40. Matsumae M, Hirayama A, Atsumi H, Yatsushiro S, Kuroda K. Velocity and pressure gradients of cerebrospinal fluid assessed with magnetic resonance imaging. J Neurosurg. 2014;120(1):218–27.
41. Sandrone S, Moreno-Zambrano D, Kipnis J, van Gijn J. A (delayed) history of the brain lymphatic system. Nat Med. 2019;25(4):538–40.
42. Oliver G, Kipnis J, Randolph GJ, Harvey NL. The lymphatic vasculature in the 21st century: novel functional roles in homeostasis and disease. Cell. 2020;182(2):270–96.
43. Lundberg N. The Saga of the Monro-Kellie doctrine. In: Ishii S, Nagai H, Brock M, editors. Intracranial Pressure V. Berlin, Heidelberg: Springer; 1983. p. 68–76.
44. Dunn LT. Raised intracranial pressure. J Neurol Neurosurg Psychiatry. 2002;73 Suppl 1(Suppl 1):i23–7.
45. Brumback RA. Anatomic and physiologic aspects of the cerebrospinal fluid space. In: Herndon RM, Brumback RA, editors. The cerebrospinal fluid. Boston, MA: Springer US; 1989. p. 15–43. https://doi.org/10.1007/978-1-4613-1591-9_2.
46. Leinonen V, Vanninen R, Rauramaa T. Cerebrospinal fluid circulation and hydrocephalus. Handb Clin Neurol. 2017;145:39–50.
47. Goudie C, Burr J, Blaikie A. Incidence of idiopathic intracranial hypertension in fife. Scott Med J. 2019;64(2):62–6.
48. Ding JY, Kreipke CW, Speirs SL, Schafer P, Schafer S, Rafols JA. Hypoxia-inducible factor-1alpha signaling in aquaporin upregulation after traumatic brain injury. Neurosci Lett. 2009;453(1):68–72.
49. Nehring SM, Tadi P, Tenny S. Cerebral edema. In: StatPearls. Treasure Island, FL: StatPearls Publishing; 2022. http://www.ncbi.nlm.nih.gov/books/NBK537272/.
50. Williamson MR, Wilkinson CM, Dietrich K, Colbourne F. Acetazolamide mitigates intracranial pressure spikes without affecting functional outcome after experimental hemorrhagic stroke. Transl Stroke Res. 2019;10(4):428–39.
51. Feigin VL, Lawes CMM, Bennett DA, Barker-Collo SL, Parag V. Worldwide stroke incidence and early case fatality reported in 56 population-based studies: a systematic review. Lancet Neurol. 2009;8(4):355–69.
52. Zoerle T, Lombardo A, Colombo A, Longhi L, Zanier ER, Rampini P, et al. Intracranial pressure after subarachnoid hemorrhage. Crit Care Med. 2015;43(1):168–76.
53. Siler DA, Gonzalez JA, Wang RK, Cetas JS, Alkayed NJ. Intracisternal administration of tissue plasminogen activator improves cerebrospinal fluid flow and cortical perfusion after subarachnoid hemorrhage in mice. Transl Stroke Res. 2014;5(2):227–37.
54. Li Y, Chen J, Chopp M. Cell proliferation and differentiation from ependymal, subependymal and choroid plexus cells in response to stroke in rats. J Neurol Sci. 2002;193(2):137–46.

55. Preston D, Simpson S, Halm D, Hochstetler A, Schwerk C, Schroten H, et al. Activation of TRPV4 stimulates transepithelial ion flux in a porcine choroid plexus cell line. Am J Physiol Cell Physiol. 2018;315(3):C357–66.
56. Jie P, Lu Z, Hong Z, Li L, Zhou L, Li Y, et al. Activation of transient receptor potential Vanilloid 4 is involved in neuronal injury in middle cerebral artery occlusion in mice. Mol Neurobiol. 2016;53(1):8–17.
57. Dong Q, Li J, Wu QF, Zhao N, Qian C, Ding D, et al. Blockage of transient receptor potential vanilloid 4 alleviates myocardial ischemia/reperfusion injury in mice. Sci Rep. 2017;7:42678.
58. Trillo-Contreras JL, Ramírez-Lorca R, Hiraldo-González L, Sánchez-Gomar I, Galán-Cobo A, Suárez-Luna N, et al. Combined effects of aquaporin-4 and hypoxia produce age-related hydrocephalus. Biochim Biophys Acta Mol basis Dis. 2018;1864(10):3515–26.
59. Verkman AS, Anderson MO, Papadopoulos MC. Aquaporins: important but elusive drug targets. Nat Rev Drug Discov. 2014;13(4):259–77.
60. Frydenlund DS, Bhardwaj A, Otsuka T, Mylonakou MN, Yasumura T, Davidson KGV, et al. Temporary loss of perivascular aquaporin-4 in neocortex after transient middle cerebral artery occlusion in mice. Proc Natl Acad Sci USA. 2006;103(36):13532–6.

Cerebral Hemodynamics

4

Priyadarshini Mishra

4.1 Introduction

Cerebral hemodynamics refer to the examination of cerebral blood flow (CBF) both at rest and in response to a variety of intrinsic and extrinsic factors. It is crucial for maintaining brain function and involves the regulation of blood flow, blood pressure, and oxygen and nutrient delivery to the brain. Any alterations in cerebral hemodynamics can have significant effects on the brain and can contribute to neurological disorders.

4.1.1 Special Needs of the Brain

- The brain has a high metabolic rate and requires a constant supply of oxygen and glucose to function properly. It accounts for approximately 20% of the oxygen consumption at rest. Moreover, the brain is exquisitely sensitive to hypoxia, with irreversible damage occurring within minutes of cerebral ischemia [1, 2].
- Different areas of the brain are activated at different times, and, therefore, there is a requirement to adjust local blood supply with local demand.
- The brain needs a secure internal environment to perform its functions.

P. Mishra (✉)
AIIMS Bhubaneswar, Bhubaneswar, Odisha, India

4.1.2 Unique Features of Cerebral Circulation

- Despite its small size, accounting for only 2% of body weight, the brain receives a significant proportion of the cardiac output, approximately 15–20%. This translates to a cerebral blood flow rate of 55 ml/min/100 gm of brain tissue [3, 4].
- Blood vessels: The brain is supplied with blood by two major pairs of arteries: the internal carotid arteries and the vertebral arteries (Fig. 4.1). These arteries branch and form a circle at the base of the brain called the circle of Willis. The blood supply to the brain is divided into two main systems: the anterior circulation, which is supplied by the internal carotid arteries, and the posterior circulation, which is supplied by the vertebral arteries. The anterior circulation supplies blood to the frontal, parietal, and temporal lobes of the brain, whereas the posterior circulation supplies blood to the brainstem, cerebellum, and occipital lobe [5]. The circle of Willis provides a safety net of anastomoses, which can maintain perfusion in case one of the extracranial arteries is blocked [6, 7].

Arteries from the circle of Willis divide and branch to traverse the surface of the brain as pial arteries. These give rise to penetrating arteries,

H. Prabhakar et al. (eds.), *Principles and Practice of Neurocritical Care*,
https://doi.org/10.1007/978-981-99-8059-8_4

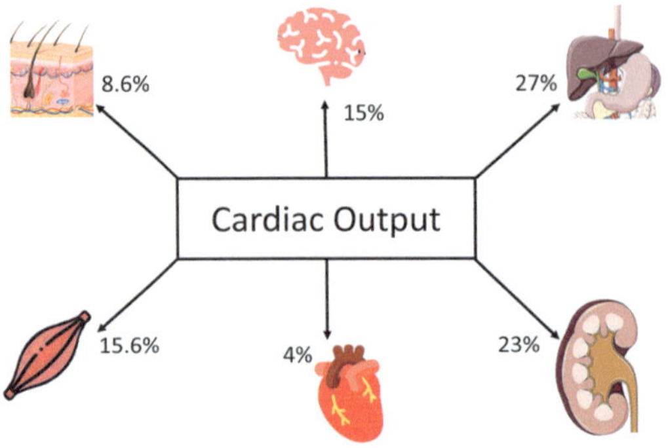

Fig. 4.1 Distribution of cardiac output

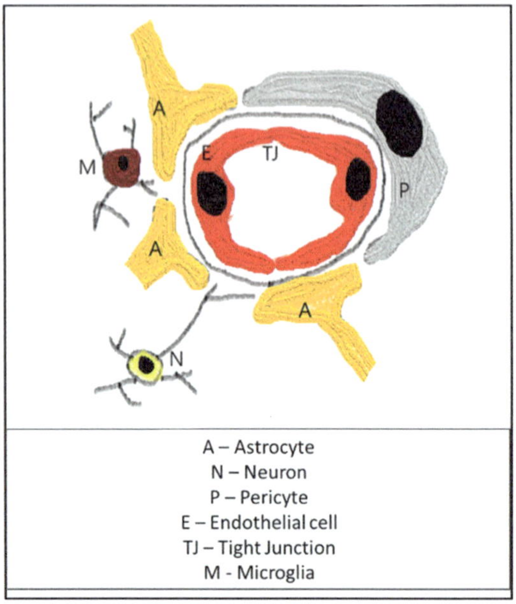

Fig. 4.2 The blood–brain barrier showing continuous capillaries with tight junctions, pericytes, end feet of astrocytes, neurons, and microglia

which ultimately form the parenchymal arteries in the substance of the brain [8, 9].

The cerebral venous system is composed of dural sinuses and cerebral veins that allow for drainage of venous outflow from the brain. There are two groups of valveless veins: the superficial cortical veins and the deep or central veins. The former is situated on the surface of the cortex and drains the cerebral cortex and subcortical white matter, whereas the latter includes subependymal veins, internal cerebral veins, basal vein, and the great vein of Galen, draining the brain's interior. The cortical veins and deep veins anastomose and empty into the superior sagittal sinus (SSS), which then flows to the sigmoid sinuses and jugular veins [10].

- The blood–brain barrier: The blood vessels in the brain are surrounded by a specialized barrier that regulates the exchange of molecules between the blood and the brain, protecting the brain from harmful substances [11, 12]. An illustration of the blood–brain barrier is provided in Fig. 4.2, but the details of its functions are beyond the scope of this chapter. The proximity of the endothelium, astrocytes, pericytes, and neurons (neurovascular unit) allows for regulation of blood flow according to the local needs of the brain.
- Innervation: Extra-parenchymal pial vessels are supplied with sympathetic and parasympathetic nerve fibers from the superior cervical ganglion, otic and sphenopalatine ganglion, and sensory fibers from the trigeminal ganglion [13]. Parenchymal vessels have intrinsic supply from intracerebral neurons from the locus ceruleus, raphae nucleus, basal forebrain, etc. [9, 14, 15]. This difference in innervation pattern from the peripheral nervous system allows autonomic regulation of only larger arteries but not the parenchymal arteries, which respond to local neuronal activity (Fig. 4.3).

4.1.3 Determinants of Cerebral Blood Flow

Assuming brain blood flow to be laminar and uniform through non-distensible tubes:

$$\text{Cerebral perfusion pressure} = \text{mean arterial pressure}(\text{MAP}) - \text{central venous pressure}(\text{CVP})$$

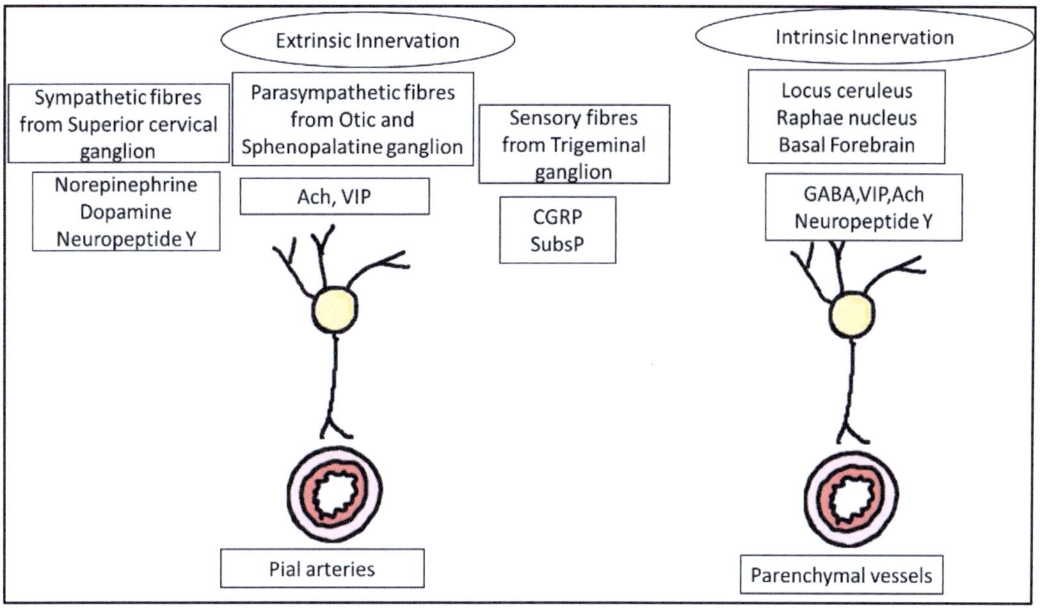

Fig. 4.3 Extrinsic and intrinsic innervation of the cerebral vasculature (Ach: Acetylcholine, VIP: Vasoactive Intestinal Peptide, CGRP: Calcitonin Gene-Related Peptide, GABA: Gamma-aminobutyric acid)

Venous pressure is directly influenced by intracranial pressure (ICP) [16], therefore

$$\text{Cerebral perfusion pressure}(\text{CPP}) = \text{MAP} - \text{ICP}$$

ICP is normally extremely low (<15 mmHg); therefore, CPP more closely follows changes in MAP, except in situations where the ICP is raised.

$$\text{Cerebral blood flow } (\text{CBF}) = \text{CPP} / \text{resistance}$$

According to Poiseuille's law,

$$\text{Resistance} = 8\eta L / \pi r^4,$$

where η is the viscosity, $L$is the length, and r is the radius.

From Poiseuille's equation, we can conclude that two factors will affect resistance, i.e., viscosity and radius. However, the changes in radius will cause a fourfold change in resistance, thus making it an extremely important factor for controlling blood flow.

4.2 Regulation of Cerebral Blood Flow

Early experiments by Monro indicated that there is no active regulation of blood flow through the brain [17, 18]. Rather, blood flow in the rest of the body is regulated to maintain cerebral blood flow. This idea was supported by leading scientists like Bayliss [19]. In their 1890 paper, "On the Regulation of the Blood-supply of the Brain," Roy and Sherrington used a variety of experimental techniques to investigate the mechanisms by which the brain maintains a constant blood flow in the face of changes in systemic blood pressure [20]. One of their key findings was that cerebral blood vessels are able to constrict or dilate in response to changes in transmural pressure, an effect they attributed to the "myogenic tone" in the vessel walls. They also proposed that there may be additional mechanisms, such as metabolic factors or neural signals, that contribute to the regulation of cerebral blood flow. Roy and Sherrington's work on cerebral autoregulation helped establish the importance of this phenomenon for normal brain function and paved the way for further research in this area. Their findings continue to influence the current understanding of the complex mechanisms that regulate CBF in health and disease.

4.2.1 Regulation of Cerebral Blood Flow Can Be Divided into Four Categories (Fig. 4.4)

1. **Autoregulation**

   Lassen compiled the results of 11 studies to produce the graph of autoregulation that we are familiar with. He determined the autoregulatory range of CBF to be 50–150 mmHg [22]. Although the Lassen autoregulation curve is a widely used tool for understanding cerebral autoregulation, there is some controversy regarding its interpretation and clinical application. One issue is that the autoregulatory plateau may not be a true plateau but rather a range of MAP over which CBF is relatively constant, with some degree of variability. However, this range is an average of 11 different studies and variations in individual subjects were not recorded.

   Numerous animal studies have confirmed the concept of an autoregulation curve, demonstrating that within a certain range of mean arterial pressure (MAP), cerebral blood flow (CBF) remains relatively constant [23–31]. However, the studies differed in methods of creating variations in blood pressure. Moreover, in humans, traditionally, it took almost 10 min to measure changes in CBF and the values determined were for net average changes of blood pressure and CBF [21]. Therefore, the classic curve of Lassen may now be referred to as the static autoregulation (Fig. 4.5a) of CBF as it reflects a steady-state relationship between blood pressure and CBF [32–36]. Recent studies have shown a much smaller autoregulatory range of blood pressure within subject analysis [37, 38], with a hysteresis existing between increased and decreased blood pressure where CBF with hypertension is better regulated as compared to that with hypotension [37, 39].

   Exploring the role of temporality, it was reported that with rapid changes in blood pressure, there is greater variability in CBF. Rapid changes in blood pressure lead to reduced buffering capacity and, gradually, a state is reached where changes in blood pressure lead to similar changes in CBF. This dynamic autoregulation (Fig. 4.5b) can be measured by correlating changes in blood flow velocity measured with transcranial Doppler (TCD) with blood pressure changes [32–36, 40]. Recently, transfer function analysis has been used, which computes the coherence between blood pressure changes and CBF changes [41].

   Clinically, caution must be exercised when relating CBF with mean arterial pressure, and

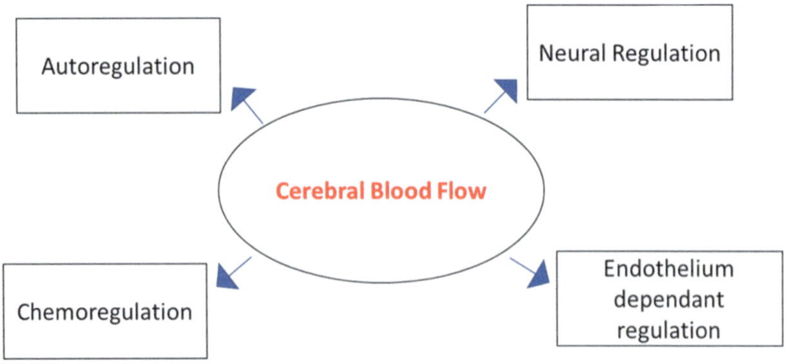

Fig. 4.4 Mechanisms of regulation of cerebral blood flow [21]

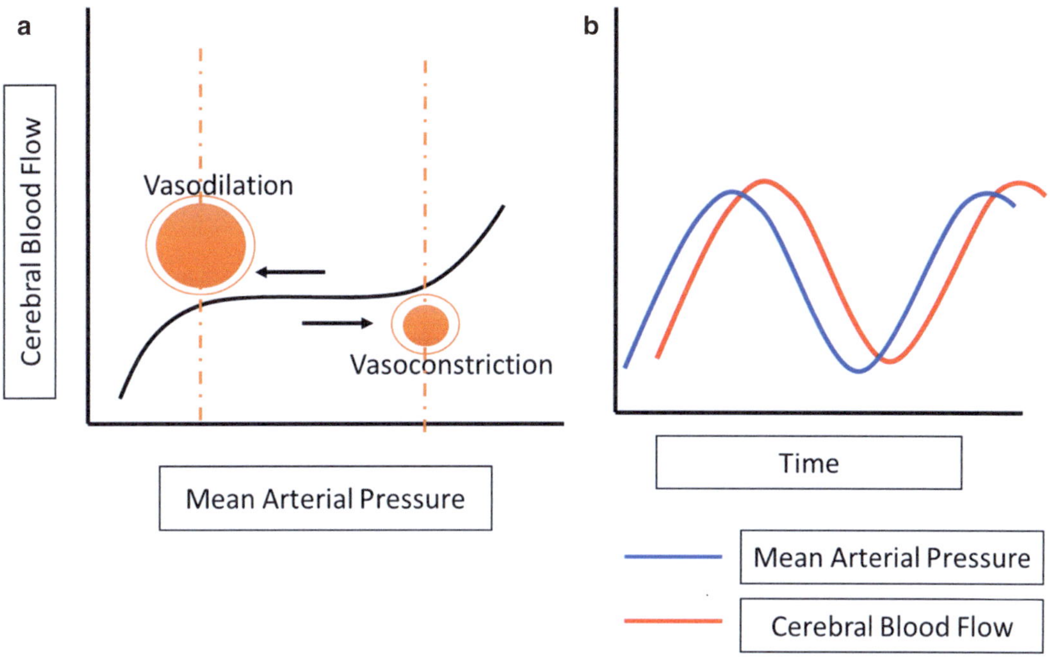

Fig. 4.5 (**a**) Static autoregulation commonly seen in situations where changes in blood pressure are more gradual. (**b**) Dynamic autoregulation in case of rapid changes in blood pressure. (Modified from Sainbhi et al. [42]; copyright © 2022 Sainbhi, Gomez, Froese, Slack, Batson, Stein, Cordingley, Alizadeh, and Zeiler)

the rate of change in MAP should also be considered when monitoring CBF.

Mechanisms of Autoregulation

Myogenic Tone

The primary mechanism of autoregulation is the generation of vascular tone and reactivity with changes in blood pressure [43–46]. It was reported that such changes occurred in the absence of any innervation and change in metabolism. The pial arteries and the parenchymal arterioles have smooth muscles, which respond to stretch. An increase in blood pressure causes increased vascular tone and reactivity. This is achieved through activation of calcium channels on the vascular smooth muscles, which leads to phosphorylation of myosin light-chain kinase, which then leads to contraction of smooth muscles. The probable mechanisms by which these calcium channels are activated are integrins, mechanosensitive G protein-coupled receptors (GPCRs), and stretch-activated ion channels (Fig. 4.6). This increase in myogenic tone and reactivity with an increase in blood pressure is modulated by the opening up of calcium-activated potassium channels, which resist the change in tone [47, 48].

Metabolic Changes

Along with the myogenic response, cerebral metabolism is also tightly coupled with CBF [49, 50]. When there is decreased blood pressure, change in oxygen, carbon dioxide, and pH levels and release of vasoactive peptides like H^+, K^+, and adenosine can lead to vasodilation and increase in CBF [51].

CBF autoregulation testing has multiple clinical uses, such as identifying patients with impaired autoregulation due to stroke, subarachnoid hemorrhage, or traumatic brain injury. It can guide clinical management and predict outcomes. Additionally, it can be used to monitor CBF during surgery for patients at a high risk of cerebral ischemia, evaluate interventions for cerebrovascular disease or traumatic brain injury, and assess the risk of poor neurological outcomes. This aids in prognostication and clinical decision-making.

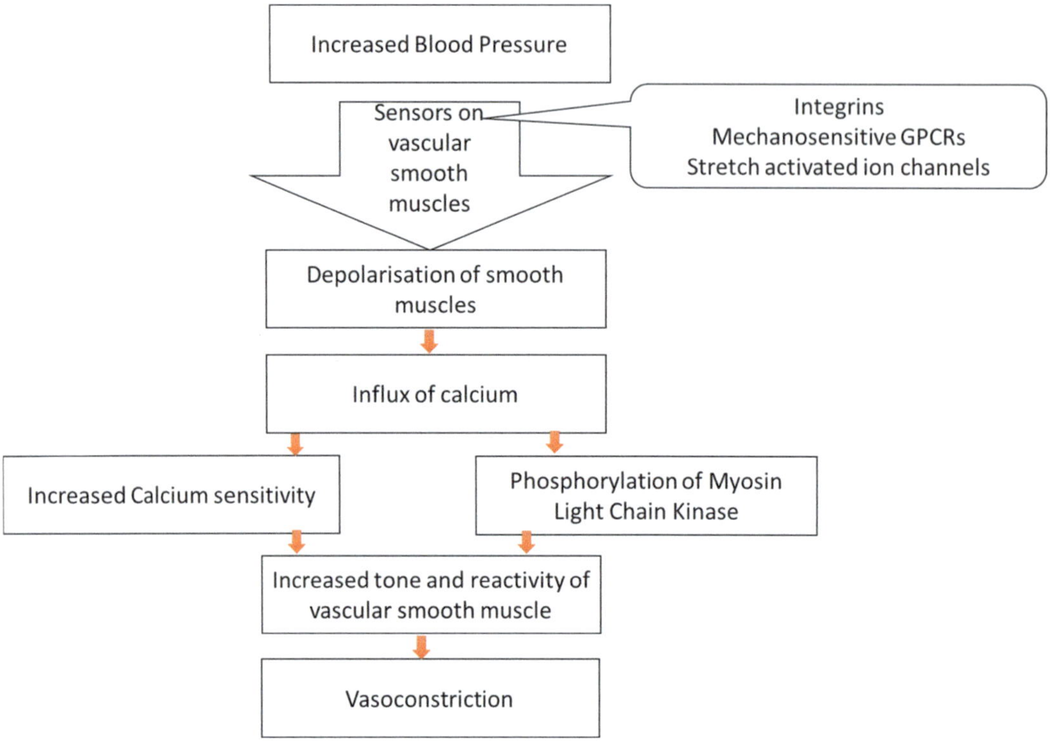

Fig. 4.6 Mechanism of myogenic autoregulation

Early methods of testing autoregulation included inducing pressure changes by the Valsalva maneuver, postural changes and deflation of pressurized thigh cuff, or, alternatively, by pharmacological agents like halothane [52–55].

Several techniques can be used to assess cerebral autoregulation. Transcranial Doppler (TCD) ultrasonography is a noninvasive method that measures blood flow velocity in intracranial arteries to indirectly estimate cerebral blood flow. This technique can assess the dynamic range of autoregulation by measuring changes in blood flow velocity in response to changes in blood pressure induced by a vasoactive drug or head-up tilt. Another noninvasive method is the cerebral blood flow autoregulation index (ARI), which uses beat-to-beat arterial blood pressure and transcranial Doppler blood flow velocity data to calculate the ARI. This index is an indicator of the strength and speed of autoregulation and can monitor changes over time. Near-infrared spectroscopy (NIRS) can measure changes in cerebral oxygenation to indirectly estimate cerebral blood flow and assess the static and dynamic range of autoregulation. More invasive and expensive techniques, such as positron emission tomography (PET) and functional magnetic resonance imaging (fMRI), directly measure cerebral blood flow and metabolism and can also be used to assess the dynamic range of autoregulation.

2. **Chemoregulation**

Carbon dioxide (CO_2) is a potent vasodilator and can cause changes in CBF when its levels in the blood change. Inhalation of 7% carbon dioxide leads to 100% increase in cerebral blood flow [56]. Harper and Glass (1965) defined relative CO_2 reactivity as the percentage change in CBF at a definite $PaCO_2$ of 40 mmHg divided by the $PaCO_2$ difference from 40 mmHg [57]. They observed a 100% increase in CBF in normotensive dogs when they raised the $PaCO_2$ from 40 to 80 mmHg, resulting in a relative CO_2 reactivity of 2.5%/

mmHg, which is consistent with other studies [58, 59]. Conversely, when CO_2 levels decrease, such as during hypocapnia, the CBF decreases to maintain a proper balance of oxygen and carbon dioxide in the brain [60]. Smaller arterioles are more sensitive to changes in carbon dioxide levels [61, 62].

Experiments have shown that severe hypotension significantly reduces CO_2 reactivity and that hypercapnia impairs the autoregulation response to hypotension [63]. The cerebrovascular bed has limited dilation capacity, and both arterial carbon dioxide tension ($PaCO_2$) and cerebral perfusion pressure (CPP) can deplete cerebral autoregulatory reserve in combination [57, 64]. Therefore, the response to one physiological variable no longer occurs when maximal vasodilation/vasoconstriction happens in response to changes in the other physiological variable.

The mechanisms underlying the effects of CO_2 on CBF are not fully understood, but acidosis resulting from increased $PaCO_2$ is mainly responsible for the vasodilation. Activation of acid-sensing ion channel 1 has been implicated as a sensor for the decreased pH [65, 66]. In addition, CO_2 can also activate signaling pathways involving nitric oxide (NO), prostaglandins, and other molecules to further increase CBF [67, 68].

Clinically, measurement of CO_2 reactivity can be used to assess the integrity of cerebrovascular regulation in patients with cerebrovascular disease or traumatic brain injury. This can provide important information about the risk of ischemia or other neurological complications and guide clinical management.

Effects of Hypoxia

A reduction in saturation below 80% and PaO_2 below 50 mmHg can cause vasodilation [33]. In response to hypoxia, there may be a redistribution of blood flow within the brain, with increased flow to areas that are more metabolically active and require more oxygen. In order to maintain adequate oxygen supply to the brain, hypoxia can stimulate an increase in the cerebral metabolic rate of oxygen consumption ($CMRO_2$), which can help extract more oxygen from the blood. Anaerobic metabolism, leading to extracellular acidosis and accumulation of metabolites, is responsible for vasodilation in hypoxia [69].

Hypoxia can impair cerebral autoregulation and lead to a loss of the normal compensatory response to changes in systemic blood pressure, which can increase the risk of cerebral ischemia or hemorrhage.

3. **Neuronal Regulation**

The extrinsic innervation of the cerebral vasculature includes sympathetic, parasympathetic, and sensory neurons that innervate the larger pial arteries. Sympathetic innervation plays a crucial role in preventing an increase in blood flow following an increase in peripheral blood pressure, thereby protecting against disruption of the blood–brain barrier and cerebral edema [27, 70, 71]. It is particularly effective during acute increases in blood pressure, protecting cerebral blood flow and the blood–brain barrier [27, 70, 72]. The role of extrinsic parasympathetic innervation is still a subject of debate, but it may play a role in dynamic autoregulation [73]. Trigeminal innervation has been implicated in the pathogenesis of migraine and has been shown to increase blood flow during vasospasm while also being protective toward neurons [74, 75]. Additionally, it can increase cerebral blood flow in the absence of pressure changes [76].

The intrinsic innervation of the cerebral vasculature is primarily by neurons originating from the brainstem and other nuclei. At the level of parenchymal vessels, a functional unit known as the neurovascular unit is formed by the neurons, astrocytes, and vascular cells. The neurons release several neurotransmitters, including acetylcholine, norepinephrine, and serotonin, which act on the receptors located on the astrocytes, endothelium, and smooth muscle cells to regulate their tone [13]. Furthermore, neuronal activity increases the calcium concentration in astrocytes, leading to the release of vasoactive substances such as potassium,

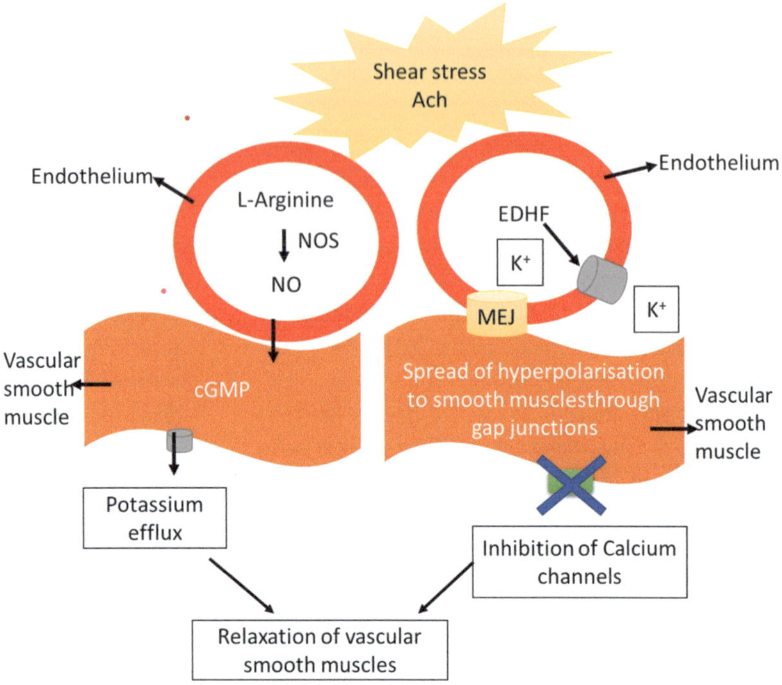

Fig. 4.7 The mechanism of action of nitric oxide and endothelium-derived hyperpolarizing factor (EDHF). *MEJ* myoendothelial junction; *NOS* nitric oxide synthase

20-hydroxyeicosatetraenoic acid (20-HETE), and prostacyclin, resulting in vasodilation [77].

4. **Endothelium-Dependent Regulation**

   The endothelium can regulate vascular smooth muscle contraction through release of signaling molecules and myoendothelial gap junctions. The endothelium produces vasoactive factors like nitric oxide (NO), prostacyclin, and endothelium-derived hyperpolarizing factor (EDHF), which can significantly affect vascular tone and therefore cerebral blood flow [78]. The mechanism of action of nitric oxide and EDHF is illustrated in Fig. 4.7.

4.3 Alterations of Cerebral Blood Flow Regulation in Health and Disease

4.3.1 Effect of Aging

Cerebral blood flow (CBF) tends to decrease with age, although the extent and pattern of this decline can vary depending on a number of factors. Some of the key changes in CBF with age include a reduction in CBF velocity as reported in studies which have shown that mean blood flow velocity in the major cerebral arteries decreases by around 0.5% per year after early adulthood [79–81]. This has been attributed to changes in cerebrovascular reactivity wherein there is decline in the ability of vessels to dilate in response to carbon dioxide. Other causes may be decreased baroreflex sensitivity and cerebral atrophy with aging. However, autoregulation seems to be largely unimpaired with aging.

4.3.2 Effect of Posture

Standing from a supine posture can cause a fall in blood pressure due to pooling of blood in the extremities. There are currently two differing opinions regarding the effect of gravity on CBF. One opinion suggests that the pressure difference on the arterial side is balanced by that on the venous side, resulting in no net effect on CBF. This theory is based on the concept of a closed-loop system, in which the pressure at either end of a length of rigid tubing is determined by the vertical position of these ends [82, 83]. However, arguments against this theory are that the comparison is flawed as the cerebral circulation has nonrigid tubing and also a wide range of vessel diameters [84–86]. Measuring the effect of posture on CBF is complex and challenging. For example, changing from a supine to an upright position affects multiple factors that also influence CBF, such as blood pressure, central blood volume, $PaCO_2$, and intracranial pressure (ICP) [87, 88]. Despite these challenges, studies have shown that CBF decreases in human subjects between supine and standing positions, suggesting that the hydrostatic gradient may indeed affect CBF. However, dynamic autoregulation can modify the effect of a change in perfusion pressure on CBF.

4.3.3 Effect of Exercise

Sedentary behavior and prolonged sitting can reduce cerebral blood flow, which may be attributed to reduced reactivity to $PaCO_2$ [89–92]. Exercise can cause changes in blood pressure, cardiac output, and oxygen consumption, all of which may cause changes in cerebral blood flow. There is a biphasic change in cerebral blood flow with exercise. It has been seen that cerebral blood flow increases by up to 60% of maximal exercise and then plateaus off and falls to resting levels with more severe exercise [80]. This may be accounted for by changes in metabolism and $PaCO_2$ [93]. Exercise does not seem to have any effect on cerebral autoregulation. Regular exercising helps improve local cerebral blood flow [94].

4.3.4 Effect of Hypertension

There is a common belief that hypertension can alter the autoregulatory range for cerebral blood flow. However, scientific evidence suggests otherwise. Several studies have demonstrated that both static and dynamic autoregulation remain intact in hypertension, even when treated with antihypertensive medications. The autoregulatory curve does not shift to a higher autoregulatory range, and a reduction in blood pressure with treatment may not result in reduced cerebral blood flow due to hypertension [95–100]. Therefore, reducing antihypertensive medication to prevent a decrease in cerebral blood flow may not be beneficial. However, it is important to note that malignant hypertension can result in autoregulation failure [101].

4.3.5 Effect of Stroke

A stroke due to any cause, ischemic or hemorrhagic, can impair autoregulation [102]. Monitoring changes in the autoregulation with time after a stroke can guide treatment protocols. The degree of autoregulation dysfunction and its changes over time after a stroke may be influenced by the size of the core and penumbra regions as well as the manner in which reperfusion occurs [103–105]. The severity and location of stroke can influence the extent to which autoregulation is affected, with autoregulation being the most affected in brain stem and subcortical strokes compared to cortical strokes [106]. The effects also vary with the subject group and the method of measurement of autoregulation. Some studies report deterioration of autoregulation within the first 5 days after stroke, whereas some report a period of 28 days of declining autoregulation [107, 108]. Other studies report impaired dynamic regulation for a period up to 6 months [109]. A reduced Transfer Function Analysis (TFA) phase and ARI indicate poor prognosis [110, 111]. Individualization of optimal blood pressure can improve outcomes in stroke.

4.3.6 Effect of Anesthesia

Anesthetic agents can have significant effects on cerebral blood flow (CBF). The effects of anesthetics on CBF depend on various factors, including the anesthetic agent used, the depth of anesthesia, and the patient's underlying health conditions. For example, inhalational anesthetics such as desflurane, isoflurane, and sevoflurane have been shown to cause an increase in CBF, which can lead to an increase in intracranial pressure (ICP) and cerebral blood volume (CBV) [112, 113]. This effect is believed to be due to the vasodilatory properties of these anesthetics. On the other hand, intravenous anesthetics such as propofol and barbiturates have been shown to cause a decrease in CBF, which may help reduce ICP and CBV. Ketamine has a direct vasodilation effect, leading to increased cerebral blood flow. Etomidate and dexmedetomidine cause reduction in cerebral blood flow by promoting vasoconstriction [112, 114].

In conclusion, cerebral hemodynamics is a complex field that plays a critical role in maintaining adequate cerebral blood flow and oxygen delivery to the brain. Despite significant advances in our knowledge of cerebral hemodynamics, there still remain lacunae in certain areas. Some of the specific goals for future research in this field can include developing novel noninvasive imaging techniques for measuring CBF, which can provide more accurate and precise measurements, identifying novel biomarkers for early detection of cerebrovascular diseases such as genetic markers, circulating microRNAs, etc., and investigating the role of lifestyle interventions, such as exercise and dietary modifications, in improving CBF and cerebrovascular function and reducing the risk of cerebrovascular diseases.

References

1. Jain V, Langham MC, Wehrli FW. MRI estimation of global brain oxygen consumption rate. J Cereb Blood Flow Metab. 2010;30(9):1598–607. http://www.ncbi.nlm.nih.gov/pubmed/20407465.
2. Vavilala MS, Lee LA, Lam AM. Cerebral blood flow and vascular physiology. Anesthesiol Clin North Am. 2002;20(2):247–64, v. http://www.ncbi.nlm.nih.gov/pubmed/12165993.
3. Ito H, Kanno I, Kato C, Sasaki T, Ishii K, Ouchi Y, et al. Database of normal human cerebral blood flow, cerebral blood volume, cerebral oxygen extraction fraction and cerebral metabolic rate of oxygen measured by positron emission tomography with 15O-labelled carbon dioxide or water, carbon monoxide and oxygen. Eur J Nucl Med Mol Imaging. 2004;31(5):635–43. http://www.ncbi.nlm.nih.gov/pubmed/14730405.
4. del Zoppo GJ, Sharp FR, Heiss W-D, Albers GW. Heterogeneity in the penumbra. J Cereb Blood Flow Metab. 2011;31(9):1836–51. http://www.ncbi.nlm.nih.gov/pubmed/21731034.
5. Purves D, Augustine GJ, Fitzpatrick D, Hall WC, LaManita A-S, White LE, editors. Neuroscience. 6th ed. New York: Sinauer Associates; 2018.
6. Liebeskind DS. Collateral circulation. Stroke. 2003;34(9):2279–84. https://doi.org/10.1161/01.STR.0000086465.41263.06.
7. Hossmann K-A. Pathophysiology and therapy of experimental stroke. Cell Mol Neurobiol. 2006;26(7–8):1055–81. https://doi.org/10.1007/s10571-006-9008-1.
8. Rennels ML, Nelson E. Capillary innervation in the mammalian central nervous system: an electron microscopic demonstration. Am J Anat. 1975;144(2):233–41. http://www.ncbi.nlm.nih.gov/pubmed/1180237.
9. Cohen Z, Molinatti G, Hamel E. Astroglial and vascular interactions of noradrenaline terminals in the rat cerebral cortex. J Cereb Blood Flow Metab. 1997;17(8):894–904. https://doi.org/10.1097/00004647-199708000-00008.
10. Cipolla MJ. The cerebral circulation. Colloq Ser Integr Syst Physiol From Mol to Funct. 2009;1(1):1–59. https://access.portico.org/stable?au=pgg3gvb7b84.
11. Roggendorf W, Cervós-Navarro J. Ultrastructure of arterioles in the cat brain. Cell Tissue Res. 1977;178(4):495. https://doi.org/10.1007/BF00219571.
12. Abbott NJ. Inflammatory mediators and modulation of blood-brain barrier permeability. Cell Mol Neurobiol. 2000;20(2):131–47. http://www.ncbi.nlm.nih.gov/pubmed/10696506.
13. Hamel E. Perivascular nerves and the regulation of cerebrovascular tone. J Appl Physiol. 2006;100(3):1059–64. http://www.ncbi.nlm.nih.gov/pubmed/16467392.
14. Estrada C, Mengual E, González C. Local NADPH-diaphorase neurons innervate pial arteries and lie close or project to intracerebral blood vessels: a possible role for nitric oxide in the regulation of cerebral blood flow. J Cereb Blood Flow Metab. 1993;13(6):978–84. http://www.ncbi.nlm.nih.gov/pubmed/8408322.
15. Bleys RL, Cowen T. Innervation of cerebral blood vessels: morphology, plasticity, age-related, and Alzheimer's disease-related neurodegeneration. Microsc Res Tech. 2001;53(2):106–18. http://www.ncbi.nlm.nih.gov/pubmed/11301486.
16. Aaslid R, Lindegaard K-F. Cerebral hemodynamics. In: Transcranial Doppler sonography. Vienna: Springer Vienna; 1986. p. 60–85. https://doi.org/10.1007/978-3-7091-8864-4_5.

17. Monro A. Observations on the structure and functions of the nervous system, illustrated with tables. L Med J. 1783;4(2):113–35.
18. Friedland RP, Iadecola C. Roy and Sherrington (1890): a centennial reexamination of "on the regulation of the blood-supply of the brain". Neurology. 1991;41(1):10–4. http://www.ncbi.nlm.nih.gov/pubmed/1985272.
19. Bayliss WM, Hill L, Gulland GL. On intracranial pressure and the cerebral circulation: part I. Physiological; Part II Histological J Physiol. 1895;18(4):334–62. http://www.ncbi.nlm.nih.gov/pubmed/16992260.
20. Roy CS, Sherrington CS. On the regulation of the blood-supply of the brain. J Physiol. 1890;11(1–2):85–158. http://www.ncbi.nlm.nih.gov/pubmed/16991945.
21. Claassen JAHR, Thijssen DHJ, Panerai RB, Faraci FM. Regulation of cerebral blood flow in humans: physiology and clinical implications of autoregulation. Physiol Rev. 2021;101(4):1487–559. http://www.ncbi.nlm.nih.gov/pubmed/33769101.
22. LASSEN NA. Cerebral blood flow and oxygen consumption in man. Physiol Rev. 1959;39(2):183–238. http://www.ncbi.nlm.nih.gov/pubmed/13645234.
23. Faraci FM, Heistad DD, Mayhan WG. Role of large arteries in regulation of blood flow to brain stem in cats. J Physiol. 1987;387:115–23. http://www.ncbi.nlm.nih.gov/pubmed/3116212.
24. Harper SL, Bohlen HG, Rubin MJ. Arterial and microvascular contributions to cerebral cortical autoregulation in rats. Am J Phys. 1984;246(1 Pt 2):H17–24. http://www.ncbi.nlm.nih.gov/pubmed/6696087.
25. Heistad DD, Marcus ML, Abboud FM. Role of large arteries in regulation of cerebral blood flow in dogs. J Clin Invest. 1978;62(4):761–8. http://www.ncbi.nlm.nih.gov/pubmed/701475.
26. Hoffman WE, Edelman G, Kochs E, Werner C, Segil L, Albrecht RF. Cerebral autoregulation in awake versus isoflurane-anesthetized rats. Anesth Analg. 1991;73(6):753–7. http://www.ncbi.nlm.nih.gov/pubmed/1952176.
27. Marcus ML, Heistad DD. Effects of sympathetic nerves on cerebral blood flow in awake dogs. Am J Phys. 1979;236(4):H549–53. http://www.ncbi.nlm.nih.gov/pubmed/434219.
28. Strandgaard S, MacKenzie ET, Sengupta D, Rowan JO, Lassen NA, Harper AM. Upper limit of autoregulation of cerebral blood flow in the baboon. Circ Res. 1974;34(4):435–40. http://www.ncbi.nlm.nih.gov/pubmed/4363762.
29. Dalkara T, Irikura K, Huang Z, Panahian N, Moskowitz MA. Cerebrovascular responses under controlled and monitored physiological conditions in the anesthetized mouse. J Cereb Blood Flow Metab. 1995;15(4):631–8. http://www.ncbi.nlm.nih.gov/pubmed/7790412.
30. Jones JV, Fitch W, MacKenzie ET, Strandgaard S, Harper AM. Lower limit of cerebral blood flow autoregulation in experimental renovascular hypertension in the baboon. Circ Res. 1976;39(4):555–7. http://www.ncbi.nlm.nih.gov/pubmed/963839.
31. Tuor UI, Farrar JK. Pial vessel caliber and cerebral blood flow during hemorrhage and hypercapnia in the rabbit. Am J Phys. 1984;247(1 Pt 2):H40–51. http://www.ncbi.nlm.nih.gov/pubmed/6742212.
32. Panerai RB. Assessment of cerebral pressure autoregulation in humans—a review of measurement methods. Physiol Meas. 1998;19(3):305–38. http://www.ncbi.nlm.nih.gov/pubmed/9735883.
33. van Beek AH, Claassen JA, Rikkert MGO, Jansen RW. Cerebral autoregulation: an overview of current concepts and methodology with special focus on the elderly. J Cereb Blood Flow Metab. 2008;28(6):1071–85. http://www.ncbi.nlm.nih.gov/pubmed/18349877.
34. Tiecks FP, Lam AM, Aaslid R, Newell DW. Comparison of static and dynamic cerebral autoregulation measurements. Stroke. 1995;26(6):1014–9. http://www.ncbi.nlm.nih.gov/pubmed/7762016.
35. Panerai RB. Cerebral autoregulation: from models to clinical applications. Cardiovasc Eng. 2008;8(1):42–59. http://www.ncbi.nlm.nih.gov/pubmed/18041584.
36. Panerai RB, Dawson SL, Eames PJ, Potter JF. Cerebral blood flow velocity response to induced and spontaneous sudden changes in arterial blood pressure. Am J Physiol Heart Circ Physiol. 2001;280(5):H2162–74. http://www.ncbi.nlm.nih.gov/pubmed/11299218.
37. Numan T, Bain AR, Hoiland RL, Smirl JD, Lewis NC, Ainslie PN. Static autoregulation in humans: a review and reanalysis. Med Eng Phys. 2014;36(11):1487–95. http://www.ncbi.nlm.nih.gov/pubmed/25205587.
38. Tan CO. Defining the characteristic relationship between arterial pressure and cerebral flow. J Appl Physiol. 2012;113(8):1194–200. http://www.ncbi.nlm.nih.gov/pubmed/22961266.
39. Willie CK, Tzeng Y-C, Fisher JA, Ainslie PN. Integrative regulation of human brain blood flow. J Physiol. 2014;592(5):841–59. http://www.ncbi.nlm.nih.gov/pubmed/24396059.
40. Panerai RB, Eames PJ, Potter JF. Variability of time-domain indices of dynamic cerebral autoregulation. Physiol Meas. 2003;24(2):367–81. http://www.ncbi.nlm.nih.gov/pubmed/12812422.
41. Giller CA. The frequency-dependent behavior of cerebral autoregulation. Neurosurgery. 1990;27(3):362–8. http://www.ncbi.nlm.nih.gov/pubmed/2234328.
42. Sainbhi AS, Gomez A, Froese L, Slack T, Batson C, Stein KY, et al. Non-invasive and minimally-invasive cerebral autoregulation assessment: a narrative review of techniques and implications for clinical research. Front Neurol. 2022;13:872731. http://www.ncbi.nlm.nih.gov/pubmed/35557627.
43. De Silva TM, Faraci FM. Microvascular dysfunction and cognitive impairment. Cell Mol Neurobiol.

2016;36(2):241–58. http://www.ncbi.nlm.nih.gov/pubmed/26988697.
44. Peixoto AJ. Acute severe hypertension. N Engl J Med. 2019;381(19):1843–52. http://www.ncbi.nlm.nih.gov/pubmed/31693807.
45. De Silva TM, Modrick ML, Dabertrand F, Faraci FM. Changes in cerebral arteries and parenchymal arterioles with aging: role of rho kinase 2 and impact of genetic background. Hypertens (Dallas, Tex 1979). 2018;71(5):921–7. http://www.ncbi.nlm.nih.gov/pubmed/29531174.
46. Elhusseiny A, Hamel E. Muscarinic—but not nicotinic—acetylcholine receptors mediate a nitric oxide-dependent dilation in brain cortical arterioles: a possible role for the M5 receptor subtype. J Cereb Blood Flow Metab. 2000;20(2):298–305. http://www.ncbi.nlm.nih.gov/pubmed/10698067.
47. Harraz OF, Hill-Eubanks D, Nelson MT. PIP2: a critical regulator of vascular ion channels hiding in plain sight. Proc Natl Acad Sci USA. 2020;117(34):20378–89. http://www.ncbi.nlm.nih.gov/pubmed/32764146.
48. Knot HJ, Nelson MT. Regulation of arterial diameter and wall [Ca2+] in cerebral arteries of rat by membrane potential and intravascular pressure. J Physiol. 1998;508(Pt 1):199–209. http://www.ncbi.nlm.nih.gov/pubmed/9490839.
49. Buxton RB, Uludağ K, Dubowitz DJ, Liu TT. Modeling the hemodynamic response to brain activation. NeuroImage. 2004;23(Suppl 1):S220–33. http://www.ncbi.nlm.nih.gov/pubmed/15501093.
50. Sokoloff L. Energetics of functional activation in neural tissues. Neurochem Res. 1999;24(2):321–9. http://www.ncbi.nlm.nih.gov/pubmed/9972882.
51. Iadecola C. The neurovascular unit coming of age: a journey through neurovascular coupling in health and disease. Neuron. 2017;96(1):17–42. http://www.ncbi.nlm.nih.gov/pubmed/28957666.
52. Pickard JD, Matheson M, Patterson J, Wyper D. Prediction of late ischemic complications after cerebral aneurysm surgery by the intraoperative measurement of cerebral blood flow. J Neurosurg. 1980;53(3):305–8. http://www.ncbi.nlm.nih.gov/pubmed/7420145.
53. Tiecks FP, Haberl RL, Newell DW. Temporal patterns of evoked cerebral blood flow during reading. J Cereb Blood Flow Metab. 1998;18(7):735–41. http://www.ncbi.nlm.nih.gov/pubmed/9663503.
54. Claassen JAHR, Levine BD, Zhang R. Dynamic cerebral autoregulation during repeated squat-stand maneuvers. J Appl Physiol. 2009;106(1):153–60. http://www.ncbi.nlm.nih.gov/pubmed/18974368.
55. Aaslid R, Lindegaard KF, Sorteberg W, Nornes H. Cerebral autoregulation dynamics in humans. Stroke. 1989;20(1):45–52. https://doi.org/10.1161/01.STR.20.1.454.
56. Kety SS, Schmidt CF. THE EFFECTS OF ALTERED ARTERIAL TENSIONS OF CARBON DIOXIDE AND OXYGEN ON CEREBRAL BLOOD FLOW AND CEREBRAL OXYGEN CONSUMPTION OF NORMAL YOUNG MEN. J Clin Invest. 1948;27(4):484–92. http://www.ncbi.nlm.nih.gov/pubmed/16695569.
57. Harper AM, Glass HI. Effect of alterations in the arterial carbon dioxide tension on the blood flow through the cerebral cortex at normal and low arterial blood pressures. J Neurol Neurosurg Psychiatry. 1965;28(5):449–52. http://www.ncbi.nlm.nih.gov/pubmed/5838479.
58. Flohr H-W, Brock M, Christ R, Heipertz R, Pöll W. Arterial pCO2 and blood flow in different parts of the central nervous system of the anesthetized cat. In: Cerebral blood flow. Berlin, Heidelberg: Springer Berlin Heidelberg; 1969. p. 86–8. https://doi.org/10.1007/978-3-642-85860-4_28.
59. von Kummer R. Local vascular response to change in carbon dioxide tension. Long term observation in the cat's brain by means of the hydrogen clearance technique. Stroke. 1984;15(1):108–14. http://www.ncbi.nlm.nih.gov/pubmed/6420942.
60. Reivich M. ARTERIAL PCO2 AND CEREBRAL HEMODYNAMICS. Am J Phys. 1964;206:25–35. http://www.ncbi.nlm.nih.gov/pubmed/14117646.
61. Faraci FM, Brian JE. Nitric oxide and the cerebral circulation. Stroke. 1994;25(3):692–703. http://www.ncbi.nlm.nih.gov/pubmed/7510430.
62. Golding EM, Steenberg ML, Contant CF, Krishnappa I, Robertson CS, Bryan RM. Cerebrovascular reactivity to CO(2) and hypotension after mild cortical impact injury. Am J Phys. 1999;277(4):H1457–66. http://www.ncbi.nlm.nih.gov/pubmed/10516183.
63. Czosnyka M, Harris NG, Pickard JD, Piechnik S. CO2 cerebrovascular reactivity as a function of perfusion pressure—a modelling study. Acta Neurochir. 1993;121(3–4):159–65. http://www.ncbi.nlm.nih.gov/pubmed/8512014.
64. Harper AM. Autoregulation of cerebral blood flow: influence of the arterial blood pressure on the blood flow through the cerebral cortex. J Neurol Neurosurg Psychiatry. 1966;29(5):398–403. http://www.ncbi.nlm.nih.gov/pubmed/5926462.
65. Kontos HA, Raper AJ, Patterson JL. Analysis of vasoactivity of local pH, PCO2 and bicarbonate on pial vessels. Stroke. 1977;8(3):358–60. http://www.ncbi.nlm.nih.gov/pubmed/16363.
66. Faraci FM, Taugher RJ, Lynch C, Fan R, Gupta S, Wemmie JA. Acid-sensing ion channels: novel mediators of cerebral vascular responses. Circ Res. 2019;125(10):907–20. http://www.ncbi.nlm.nih.gov/pubmed/31451088.
67. Iadecola C. Does nitric oxide mediate the increases in cerebral blood flow elicited by hypercapnia? Proc Natl Acad Sci. 1992;89(9):3913–6. https://doi.org/10.1073/pnas.89.9.3913.
68. Pickard JD, Mackenzie ET. Inhibition of prostaglandin synthesis and the response of baboon cerebral circulation to carbon dioxide. Nat New Biol. 1973;245(145):187–8. http://www.ncbi.nlm.nih.gov/pubmed/4200498.
69. Phillis JW. Adenosine and adenine nucleotides as regulators of cerebral blood flow: roles of acidosis, cell swelling, and KATP channels. Crit Rev

Neurobiol. 2004;16(4):237–70. http://www.ncbi.nlm.nih.gov/pubmed/15862108.
70. Faraci FM, Mayhan WG, Werber AH, Heistad DD. Cerebral circulation: effects of sympathetic nerves and protective mechanisms during hypertension. Circ Res. 1987;61(5 Pt 2):II102–6. http://www.ncbi.nlm.nih.gov/pubmed/3664981.
71. Heistad DD. Protection of cerebral vessels by sympathetic nerves. Physiologist. 1980;23(5):44–9. http://www.ncbi.nlm.nih.gov/pubmed/6777790.
72. Zhang R, Zuckerman JH, Iwasaki K, Wilson TE, Crandall CG, Levine BD. Autonomic neural control of dynamic cerebral autoregulation in humans. Circulation. 2002;106(14):1814–20. http://www.ncbi.nlm.nih.gov/pubmed/12356635.
73. Hamner JW, Tan CO, Tzeng Y-C, Taylor JA. Cholinergic control of the cerebral vasculature in humans. J Physiol. 2012;590(24):6343–52. http://www.ncbi.nlm.nih.gov/pubmed/23070700.
74. Waeber C, Moskowitz MA. Migraine as an inflammatory disorder. Neurology. 2005;64(10 Suppl 2):S9–15. http://www.ncbi.nlm.nih.gov/pubmed/15911785.
75. Bolay H, Reuter U, Dunn AK, Huang Z, Boas DA, Moskowitz MA. Intrinsic brain activity triggers trigeminal meningeal afferents in a migraine model. Nat Med. 2002;8(2):136–42. http://www.nature.com/articles/nm0202-136.
76. Edvinsson L, Uddman R, Juul R. Peptidergic innervation of the cerebral circulation. Role in subarachnoid hemorrhage in man. Neurosurg Rev. 1990;13(4):265–72. https://doi.org/10.1007/BF00346363.
77. Filosa JA, Bonev AD, Nelson MT. Calcium dynamics in cortical astrocytes and arterioles during neurovascular coupling. Circ Res. 2004;95(10):e73–81. http://www.ncbi.nlm.nih.gov/pubmed/15499024.
78. Sercombe R, Hardebo JE, Kåhrström J, Seylaz J. Amine-induced responses of pial and penetrating cerebral arteries: evidence for heterogeneous responses. J Cereb Blood Flow Metab. 1990;10(6):808–18. http://www.ncbi.nlm.nih.gov/pubmed/1976641.
79. Leenders KL, Perani D, Lammertsma AA, Heather JD, Buckingham P, Healy MJ, et al. Cerebral blood flow, blood volume and oxygen utilization. Normal values and effect of age. Brain. 1990;113:27–47. http://www.ncbi.nlm.nih.gov/pubmed/2302536.
80. Braz ID, Flück D, Lip GYH, Lundby C, Fisher JP. Impact of aerobic fitness on cerebral blood flow and cerebral vascular responsiveness to CO2 in young and older men. Scand J Med Sci Sports. 2017;27(6):634–42. http://www.ncbi.nlm.nih.gov/pubmed/26993209.
81. Ainslie PN, Cotter JD, George KP, Lucas S, Murrell C, Shave R, et al. Elevation in cerebral blood flow velocity with aerobic fitness throughout healthy human ageing. J Physiol. 2008;586(16):4005–10. http://www.ncbi.nlm.nih.gov/pubmed/18635643.
82. Munis JR, Lozada LJ. Giraffes, siphons, and starling resistors. Cerebral perfusion pressure revisited. J Neurosurg Anesthesiol. 2000;12(3):290–6. http://www.ncbi.nlm.nih.gov/pubmed/10905578.
83. Hicks JW, Badeer HS. Siphon mechanism in collapsible tubes: application to circulation of the giraffe head. Am J Phys. 1989;256(2 Pt 2):R567–71. http://www.ncbi.nlm.nih.gov/pubmed/2916707.
84. Sakas DE, Moskowitz MA, Wei EP, Kontos HA, Kano M, Ogilvy CS. Trigeminovascular fibers increase blood flow in cortical gray matter by axon reflex-like mechanisms during acute severe hypertension or seizures. Proc Natl Acad Sci USA. 1989;86(4):1401–5. http://www.ncbi.nlm.nih.gov/pubmed/2919186.
85. Dawson EA, Secher NH, Dalsgaard MK, Ogoh S, Yoshiga CC, González-Alonso J, et al. Standing up to the challenge of standing: a siphon does not support cerebral blood flow in humans. Am J Physiol Regul Integr Comp Physiol. 2004;287(4):R911–4. http://www.ncbi.nlm.nih.gov/pubmed/15191903.
86. Gisolf J, Gisolf A, van Lieshout JJ, Karemaker JM. The siphon controversy: an integration of concepts and the brain as baffle. Am J Physiol Regul Integr Comp Physiol. 2005;289(2):R627–9. http://www.ncbi.nlm.nih.gov/pubmed/16014453.
87. Gisolf J, van Lieshout JJ, van Heusden K, Pott F, Stok WJ, Karemaker JM. Human cerebral venous outflow pathway depends on posture and central venous pressure. J Physiol. 2004;560(Pt 1):317–27. http://www.ncbi.nlm.nih.gov/pubmed/15284348.
88. Wieling W, Van Lieshout JJ, Ten Harkel AD. Dynamics of circulatory adjustments to head-up tilt and tilt-back in healthy and sympathetically denervated subjects. Clin Sci (Lond). 1998;94(4):347–52. http://www.ncbi.nlm.nih.gov/pubmed/9640339.
89. Carter SE, Draijer R, Holder SM, Brown L, Thijssen DHJ, Hopkins ND. Regular walking breaks prevent the decline in cerebral blood flow associated with prolonged sitting. J Appl Physiol. 2018;125(3):790–8. http://www.ncbi.nlm.nih.gov/pubmed/29878870.
90. Claassen JAHR, Levine BD, Zhang R. Cerebral vasomotor reactivity before and after blood pressure reduction in hypertensive patients. Am J Hypertens. 2009;22(4):384–91. http://www.ncbi.nlm.nih.gov/pubmed/19229191.
91. Wheeler MJ, Dunstan DW, Smith B, Smith KJ, Scheer A, Lewis J, et al. Morning exercise mitigates the impact of prolonged sitting on cerebral blood flow in older adults. J Appl Physiol. 2019;126(4):1049–55. http://www.ncbi.nlm.nih.gov/pubmed/30730813.
92. Zlatar ZZ, Hays CC, Mestre Z, Campbell LM, Meloy MJ, Bangen KJ, et al. Dose-dependent association of accelerometer-measured physical activity and sedentary time with brain perfusion in aging. Exp Gerontol. 2019;125:110679. http://www.ncbi.nlm.nih.gov/pubmed/31382010.
93. Siebenmann C, Sørensen H, Jacobs RA, Haider T, Rasmussen P, Lundby C. Hypocapnia during hypoxic exercise and its impact on cerebral oxygenation, ventilation and maximal whole body O_2

uptake. Respir Physiol Neurobiol. 2013;185(2):461–7. http://www.ncbi.nlm.nih.gov/pubmed/22922610.
94. Lehmann N, Villringer A, Taubert M. Colocalized white matter plasticity and increased cerebral blood flow mediate the beneficial effect of cardiovascular exercise on long-term motor learning. J Neurosci. 2020;40(12):2416–29. http://www.ncbi.nlm.nih.gov/pubmed/32041897.
95. Lipsitz LA, Mukai S, Hamner J, Gagnon M, Babikian V. Dynamic regulation of middle cerebral artery blood flow velocity in aging and hypertension. Stroke. 2000;31(8):1897–903. http://www.ncbi.nlm.nih.gov/pubmed/10926954.
96. Strandgaard S. Autoregulation of cerebral blood flow in hypertensive patients. The modifying influence of prolonged antihypertensive treatment on the tolerance to acute, drug-induced hypotension. Circulation. 1976;53(4):720–7. http://www.ncbi.nlm.nih.gov/pubmed/815061.
97. Strandgaard S, Paulson OB. Cerebral autoregulation. Stroke. 1984;15(3):413–6. http://www.ncbi.nlm.nih.gov/pubmed/6374982.
98. Strandgaard S, Paulson OB. Regulation of cerebral blood flow in health and disease. J Cardiovasc Pharmacol. 1992;19(Suppl 6):S89–93. http://www.ncbi.nlm.nih.gov/pubmed/1382171.
99. Croall ID, Tozer DJ, Moynihan B, Khan U, O'Brien JT, Morris RG, et al. Effect of standard vs intensive blood pressure control on cerebral blood flow in small vessel disease: the PRESERVE randomized clinical trial. JAMA Neurol. 2018;75(6):720–7. http://www.ncbi.nlm.nih.gov/pubmed/29507944.
100. Foster-Dingley JC, Moonen JEF, de Craen AJM, de Ruijter W, van der Mast RC, van der Grond J. Blood pressure is not associated with cerebral blood flow in older persons. Hypertens (Dallas, Tex 1979). 2015;66(5):954–60. http://www.ncbi.nlm.nih.gov/pubmed/26351027.
101. Immink RV, van den Born B-JH, van Montfrans GA, Koopmans RP, Karemaker JM, van Lieshout JJ. Impaired cerebral autoregulation in patients with malignant hypertension. Circulation. 2004;110(15):2241–5. http://www.ncbi.nlm.nih.gov/pubmed/15466625.
102. Aries MJH, Elting JW, De Keyser J, Kremer BPH, Vroomen PCAJ. Cerebral autoregulation in stroke: a review of transcranial Doppler studies. Stroke. 2010;41(11):2697–704. http://www.ncbi.nlm.nih.gov/pubmed/20930158.
103. Jordan JD, Powers WJ. Cerebral autoregulation and acute ischemic stroke. Am J Hypertens. 2012;25(9):946–50. http://www.ncbi.nlm.nih.gov/pubmed/22573015.
104. Ma H, Guo Z-N, Sun X, Liu J, Lv S, Zhao L, et al. Hematoma volume is a predictive factor of disturbed autoregulation after spontaneous intracerebral hemorrhage. J Neurol Sci. 2017;382:96–100. http://www.ncbi.nlm.nih.gov/pubmed/29111029.
105. Reinhard M, Rutsch S, Lambeck J, Wihler C, Czosnyka M, Weiller C, et al. Dynamic cerebral autoregulation associates with infarct size and outcome after ischemic stroke. Acta Neurol Scand. 2012;125(3):156–62. http://www.ncbi.nlm.nih.gov/pubmed/21470192.
106. Meyer JS, Shimazu K, Fukuuchi Y, Ouchi T, Okamoto S, Koto A. Impaired neurogenic cerebrovascular control and dysautoregulation after stroke. Stroke. 1973;4(2):169–86. http://www.ncbi.nlm.nih.gov/pubmed/4702305.
107. Reinhard M, Roth M, Guschlbauer B, Harloff A, Timmer J, Czosnyka M, et al. Dynamic cerebral autoregulation in acute ischemic stroke assessed from spontaneous blood pressure fluctuations. Stroke. 2005;36(8):1684–9. http://www.ncbi.nlm.nih.gov/pubmed/16020768.
108. Eames PJ, Robinson TG, Panerai RB, Potter JF. The systemic haemodynamic and cerebral autoregulatory effects of bendrofluazide in the subacute post-stroke period. J Hypertens. 2004;22(10):2017–24. http://www.ncbi.nlm.nih.gov/pubmed/15361775.
109. Novak V, Yang ACC, Lepicovsky L, Goldberger AL, Lipsitz LA, Peng C-K. Multimodal pressure-flow method to assess dynamics of cerebral autoregulation in stroke and hypertension. Biomed Eng Online. 2004;3(1):39. http://www.ncbi.nlm.nih.gov/pubmed/15504235.
110. Gong X, Liu J, Dong P, Zhang P, Li N, Zhao X, et al. Assessment of dynamic cerebral autoregulation in patients with basilar artery stenosis. PLoS One. 2013;8(10):e77802. http://www.ncbi.nlm.nih.gov/pubmed/24124620.
111. Salinet AS, Silva NC, Caldas J, de Azevedo DS, De-Lima-Oliveira M, Nogueira RC, et al. Impaired cerebral autoregulation and neurovascular coupling in middle cerebral artery stroke: influence of severity? J Cereb Blood Flow Metab. 2019;39(11):2277–85. http://www.ncbi.nlm.nih.gov/pubmed/30117360.
112. Slupe AM, Kirsch JR. Effects of anesthesia on cerebral blood flow, metabolism, and neuroprotection. J Cereb Blood Flow Metab. 2018;38(12):2192–208. http://www.ncbi.nlm.nih.gov/pubmed/30009645.
113. Gao Y-R, Ma Y, Zhang Q, Winder AT, Liang Z, Antinori L, et al. Time to wake up: studying neurovascular coupling and brain-wide circuit function in the un-anesthetized animal. NeuroImage. 2017;153:382–98. http://www.ncbi.nlm.nih.gov/pubmed/27908788.
114. Minhas JS, Rook W, Panerai RB, Hoiland RL, Ainslie PN, Thompson JP, et al. Pathophysiological and clinical considerations in the perioperative care of patients with a previous ischaemic stroke: a multidisciplinary narrative review. Br J Anaesth. 2020;124(2):183–96. http://www.ncbi.nlm.nih.gov/pubmed/31813569.

Part III

Monitoring in Neurocritical Care

Intracranial Pressure Monitoring

5

Gunchan Paul, Birinder Singh Paul, and Guneet Singh

5.1 Introduction

Intracranial pressure (ICP) is the staple of neurocritical care as it is an indicator of dysfunctional intracranial compliance. Management of elevated ICP is critical for improved clinical outcome. Intracranial disease or pathology involves complex pathophysiological cascades of events that alter cerebral blood flow, cerebral oxygenation, and metabolism beyond intracranial pressure. ICP thus constitutes an essential part of this multimodal monitoring and is by far the most applied monitoring parameter. ICP is measured in diverse neurological conditions, not only for monitoring of therapy but also for risk stratification and prognostication [1].

The pathophysiological rationale for measuring ICP is based on the historical concept of the Scottish anatomist Alexander Monro and the compatriot surgeon George Kellie in the eighteenth century [2]. The doctrine stated that the volume of intracranial contents is constant as it is surrounded by a rigid skull. An increase in volume of any of three compartments within the skull (brain parenchyma, cerebrospinal fluid (CSF), blood) or the presence of a fourth component (mass, intracranial bleed) must be compensated by decreasing the volume of the other compartment (Fig. 5.1). As the brain parenchyma is incompressible, ICP is initially maintained by balancing the in-and-out flow of the fluid compartment, namely, the arterial and venous blood flow, as well as production and drainage of cerebrospinal fluid (CSF). However, this is a temporary compensation with a finite reserve that depends on the compliance of the system. Once the intracranial reserve mechanisms are exhausted, a rapid rise in ICP occurs [3]. Hence, ICP measurement reflects the changes in the intracranial volume based on the intracranial condition.

G. Paul (✉)
Critical Care Medicine, Dayanand Medical College & Hospital, Ludhiana, Punjab, India

B. S. Paul
Department of Neurology, Dayanand Medical College & Hospital, Ludhiana, Punjab, India

G. Singh
Manipal Hospitals, Patiala, Punjab, India

H. Prabhakar et al. (eds.), *Principles and Practice of Neurocritical Care*,
https://doi.org/10.1007/978-981-99-8059-8_5

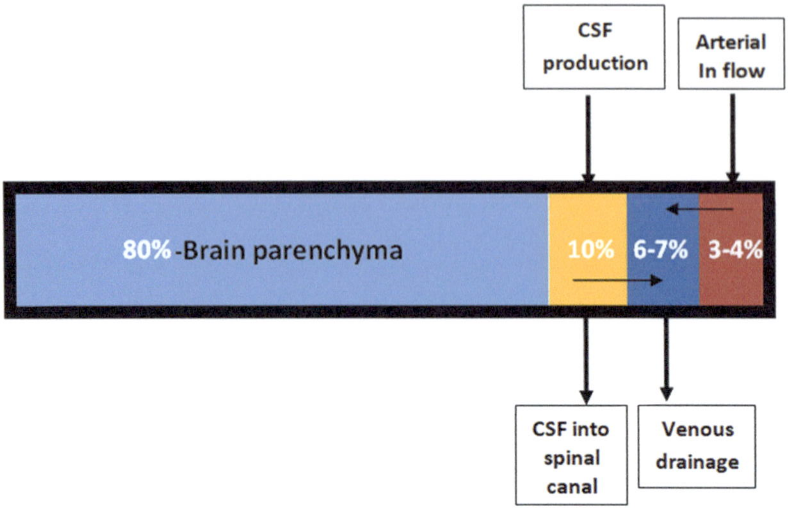

Fig. 5.1 The Monro–Kellie model for the contents of the intracranial compartment. A rigid skull (black rectangle) encloses the brain (80%), CSF (10%), venous blood (6–7%), and arterial blood (3–4%). The upper arrow depicts arterial blood flowing into the venous system through the capillaries. The lower arrow depicts that CSF is absorbed into the venous system

5.2 ICP Waveform: Physiological and Pathological Trends

The ICP waveform is pulsatile in nature, and time-averaged ICP measurement over 30 min during natural sleep is the "gold standard" for conscious patients [4]. Mean ICP varies from 5 to 15 mmHg in healthy adults in supine position and negative of 10 mmHg in vertical position (never exceeding 15 mmHg). It is normally 3–7 mmHg in children and 1.5–6 mmHg in infants, though, in a pediatric population, it may vary depending upon age. Mean ICP varies under normal physiological conditions such as change in posture and cardiovascular and respiratory variations [5].

The ICP waveform is important because its morphology provides clues to the pressure–volume relationship within the cranium. There are different waves in the normal vascular ICP waveform (Fig. 5.2a). The P1 wave (percussion wave) reflects the arterial pulsations into the CSF. P2 (tidal wave) is the reflection of arterial pulsations by the brain tissue and surrogate of the true ICP, whereas P3 (dicrotic wave) is due to the closure of the aortic valve [6].

As described by Hammer [7] the systolic uprise of the ICP waveform represents the arterial activity, whereas the descending part of the curve is the representation of venous pressure (Fig. 5.2b) [7]. An increase in the amplitude of P1 can be seen in hypertensive patients (Fig. 5.2c).

Under normal conditions, the peak of P1 is more than that of P2, indicating a compliant brain. The reversal of the P1:P2 ratio is a sensitive marker of decreases in the compliance of the brain (Fig. 5.2d), which is followed by rounding off of the waveform with a further rise in ICP (Fig. 5.2e) [8]. The other changes visible in dysfunctional intracranial compliance include an increase in the amplitude of vascular (cardiac) pulsations along with a decrease in the amplitude of respiratory variations (described below). These changes are clinically important as they alert the neurophysician to initiate urgent steps to control ICP.

The ICP trace has three types of variations: (1) the respiratory variations in the ICP waveform, which mirror changes in the intrathoracic pressure and have an amplitude in the range of 2–10 mmHg (Fig. 5.2f-W2), (2) cardiac variations, which correlate with pressure dynamics and have a frequency in the range of 1–4 mmHg [9] (Fig. 5.2f-W1), and, (3) lastly, slow vasogenic waves from the blood vessels, which are characteristically produced due to a rise in ICP and were described by Lundberg as A, B, and C waves [10] (Fig. 5.2g). A Lundberg A wave denotes the highest rise in ICP (mmHg) and persists for 5–10 min, thus representing a severe

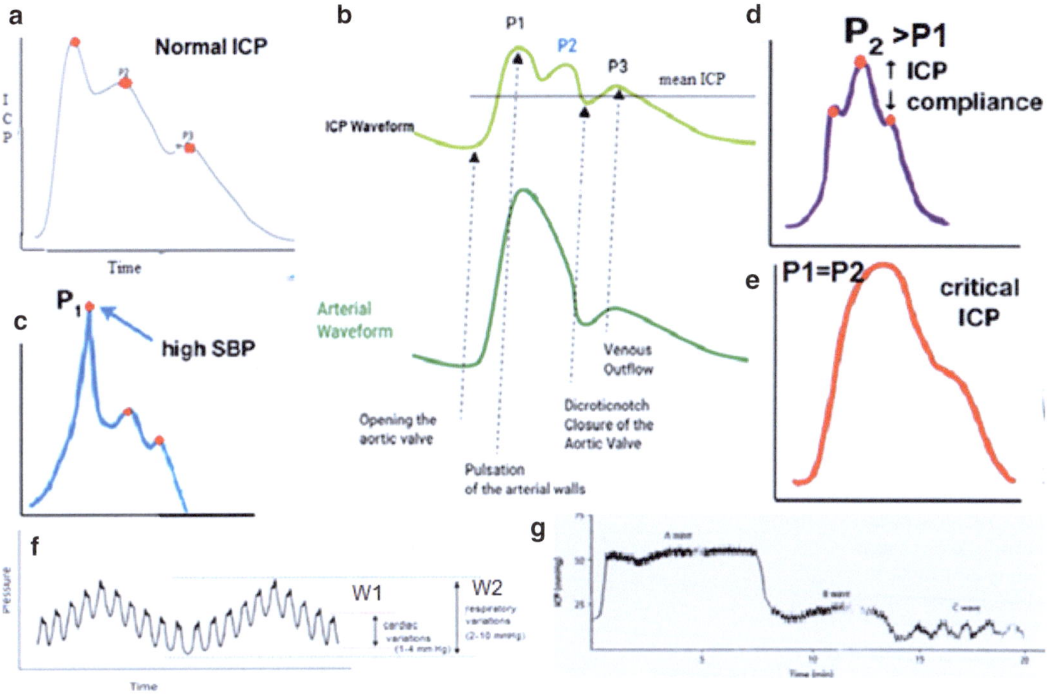

Fig. 5.2 (**a**) A normal ICP waveform with the P1 percussion wave, the P2 tidal wave, and the P3 dicrotic wave. (**b**) The relationship between the ICP waveform and the arterial pulse waveform (**c**) A raised P1 can be normally seen in hypertensive patients. (**d**) A raised P2 is an indicator of raised ICP and decreased intracranial compliance. (**e**) With critical elevation in ICP, the curve becomes rounded off with no clear distinction between the P1, P2, and P3 peaks. (**f**) The W1 waveform is generated by the cardiac cycle and the W2 waveform by the respiratory cycle. (**g**) Lundberg A (plateau), B, and C waves

degree of cerebral ischemia and impending brain herniation [11]. A Lundberg B wave persists for a shorter duration (1–2 min), is rhythmic in nature, and occurs with an ICP rise of not more than 20–30 mmHg [12, 13]. A Lundberg C wave occurs with blood pressure fluctuations produced by baro- and chemoreceptors and is not of any clinical significance.

5.3 Intracranial Pressure–Volume Relationship: Intracranial Compliance

When any pathological condition causes an increase in intracranial volume, CSF egresses from the ventricle or cerebral convexities into the dural venous sinuses. According to the Monro–Kellie doctrine, the brain has a volume of reserve of about 60–80 mL in young persons and 100–140 mL in the elderly population due to the ongoing cerebral atrophy [14]. Further addition of intracranial volume may exhaust the reserve mechanism and result in compression of the brain parenchyma and vascular structures. There is a nonlinear relationship between changes in intracranial pressure and intracranial volume (Fig. 5.3a). This mathematical relationship of change in ICP due to change in intracranial volume is termed "intra-compliance" ($ICC = \Delta P/\Delta V$) in the literature, but "elastance" is the correct term for this relationship [15]. However, compliance and elastance are the reciprocal of each other ($E = 1/C$), and both terms are often used.

At the flat portion of the curve, the buffering capacity is good, with the intracranial compartment adjusting a large change in intracranial volume without a corresponding significant increase in intracranial pressure, i.e., it has low elastance

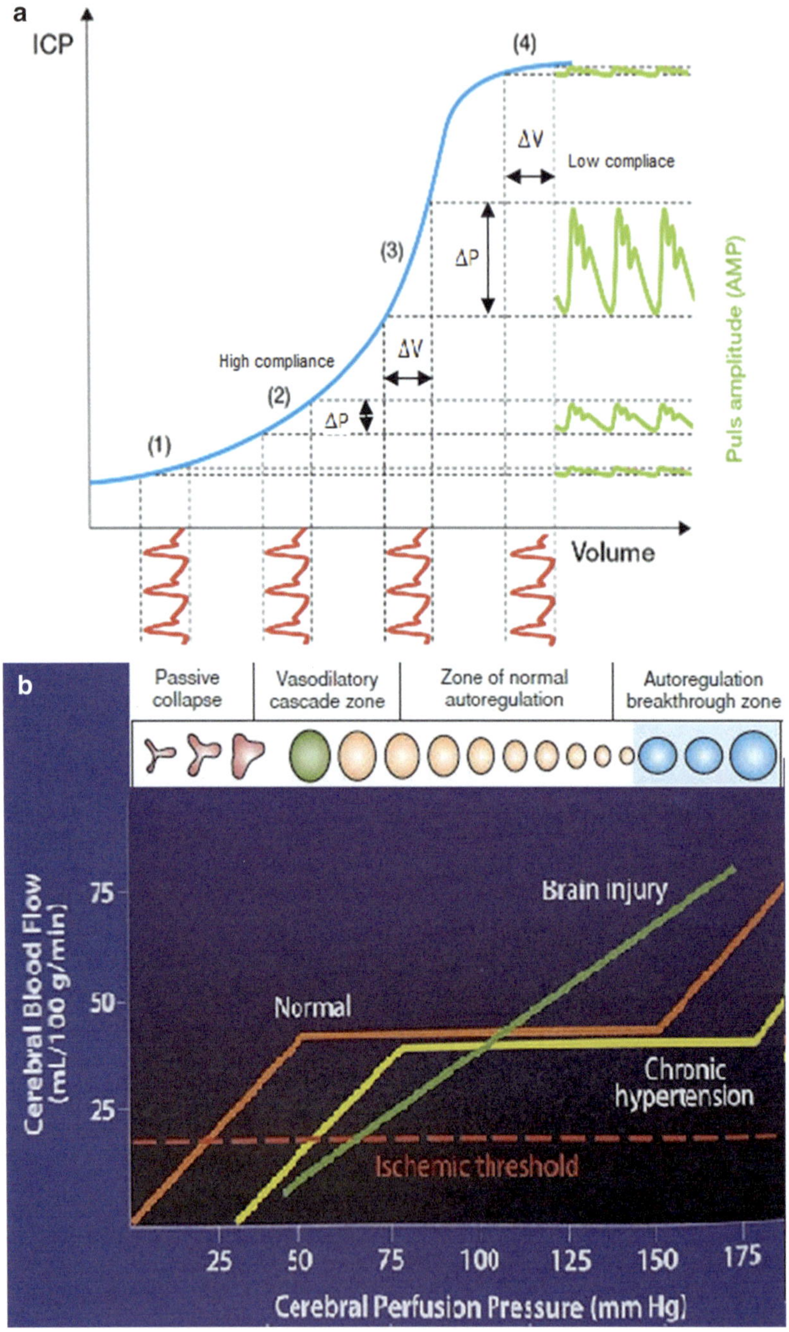

Fig. 5.3 (**a**) The intracranial pressure–volume curve depicts the nonlinear relationship between intracranial volume and pressure. At the flat portion of the curve, pressure–volume has good buffering capacity or high compliance, i.e., a small increase in intracranial blood volume during the cardiac beat (1 mL) causes a small single wave amplitude ((2) portion of the graph). However, at the vertical portion of the curve, the same net intracranial blood volume change during the cardiac beat (1 mL) causes a much larger ICP wave amplitude ((3) portion of the graph), depicting low compliance. (**b**) Cerebral autoregulation capacity

and high compliance. However, as the volume keeps increasing, the curve takes a steep uprise, and, in the vertical portion of the curve, a small change in the intracranial volume is accompanied by a marked rise in ICP, i.e., the pressure–volume reserve capacity is low (high elastance and low compliance) [16, 17]. A small increase in intracranial blood volume during the cardiac beat (about 1 mL) causes a small wave amplitude of <3–4 mmHg the flat portion of the curve, but the same volume results in a larger ICP amplitude at the vertical portion of the curve, as shown in Fig. 5.3a.

This pressure–volume curve is also affected by the nature of the expanding component. When an increase in volume is due to brain parenchyma lesions (tumors, space occupying lesion (SOL)), the pressure rise is more gradual than when the expansion is due to excess of blood or CSF (hemorrhage or hydrocephalous) in the brain.

5.4 ICP Interplay with Cerebral Perfusion Pressure (CPP)

Cerebral perfusion pressure is equivalent to the difference between the mean arterial blood pressure and mean ICP (CPP = MAP-ICP). Additionally, cerebral blood flow (CBF) is closely linked to CPP. CBF is equal to CPP divided by cerebrovascular resistance (CVR), i.e., CBF=CPP/CVR. Under normal conditions, CBF remains constant across a range of CPP (50–150 mmHg) by the mechanism of autoregulation [18]. In other words, within this range, as CPP increases, CRV also increases to keep CBF constant, but when limits are crossed above and below this range, cerebral edema and hypoperfusion may ensue, respectively (Fig. 5.3b). Interestingly, autoregulation is an energy-dependent process that occurs at the arteriolar level.

The risk of cerebra ischemia in cases of brain injury (stroke, hemorrhage, trauma) may be multifold. First, the ability to autoregulate may be lost and CBF becomes linearly related to CPP. This linear relationship may be detrimental to patients with brain injury since a decrease in CPP may drop below the critical CBF threshold of 20 mL/100 g/min, the ischemic threshold. Second, elevated ICP may hamper cerebral blood flow and compromise the adequate supply of energy required for brain metabolism, thus threatening CNS function. Additionally, elevations in ICP may cause pressure gradients on the central nervous system structures, resulting in herniation of the brain tissue relative to the meninges.

The basic idea of monitoring ICP is to predict CPP, as a CPP-oriented approach is used in many neuro-ICUs for management of critically ill patients. However, overzealous use of CPP-based management may led to cerebral hyperemia, vasogenic edema, and cardiopulmonary consequences. In light of these complications, there has been in shift in the initial attempts to maintain CPP of 70 mmHg to 60 mmHg [19]. It was an initial belief that as long as CPP is maintained, ICP was of no value. However, newer studies show that increased ICP has toxic effects on the brain independent of perfusion and a cutoff of 20 mmHg was established for intracranial hypertension. The most recent Brain Trauma Foundation guidelines have raised the cutoff to 22 mmHg for intervention [20].

5.5 ICP Measurement

5.5.1 Historical Perspective

Heinrich Quincke, in 1891, measured lumbar cerebrospinal fluid pressure via lumbar pressure [21]. This was the first indirect measurement of ICP. About half a century later, in 1950, Pierre Janny from France published his thesis on ICP monitoring, and, 10 years later, Nils Lundberg from Sweden measured ICP via ventricular puncture and described the classical Lundberg waves of the ICP [22, 23]. Since then, ICP measurement via ventricularly placed catheters based on a fluid-filled system is regarded as the gold standard.

5.5.2 Current Practice

The invasive nature, dependence on surgical expertise for insertion, and associated complications have all limited the application of ICP monitoring in clinical practice. With advancements in technology, dedicated ICP microtransducers, based on different technologies were introduced, but they are still considered as research tools and are routinely used in only few institutes. The indications of ICP monitoring are listed in Table 5.1. The current clinical practice utilizes only the mean ICP value (static pressure). A new concept of pulsatile ICP analysis, which refers to the pressure changes in ICP with each cardiac cycle, is emerging [24]. A single ICP wave is characterized by an increase in pressure from diastolic minimum pressure to systolic maximum pressure (Fig. 5.4). The attributes established from this single ICP wave are single wave amplitude (difference between diastolic and systolic pressure), rise time (time from diastolic to systolic peak), and rise time coefficient (amplitude divided by rise time, measure of steepness of the ICP waveform). The most widely applied attributes are the relative peaks of P1, P2, and P3. The American National Standards Institute/Association for the Advancement of Medical Instruments state that ICP monitoring devices should provide an accuracy of ±2 mmHg in the range of 0–20 mmHg. Moreover, the maximum error should not exceed 10% in the range of 20–100 mmHg [25].

Table 5.1 Indications of intracranial pressure monitoring

Indications of intracranial pressure monitoring
• Traumatic brain injury
• Hemorrhage – Intracranial hemorrhage – Subarachnoid hemorrhage
• Cerebral edema
• Cerebral abscess
• Hydrocephalus
• Hepatic encephalopathy
• Cerebral ischemia

5.5.3 Invasive ICP Monitoring

ICP monitoring can be performed by invasive and noninvasive approaches. Invasive methods include fluid-filled systems and implantable microtransducers.

(a) **Fluid-Filled Ventricular Catheters**

The placement of a catheter directly into the ventricles, known as the External ventricular drain (EVD) technique, is the gold standard and is also used to standardize other methods of ICP measurement [26]. Moreover, it provides an opportunity for therapeutic CSF drainage, and, hence, this method of ICP monitoring is used in patients who also need CSF drainage (Fig. 5.5a). Additionally, EVD can be used for intraventricular insertion of drugs (antibiotics) or drainage of hemorrhage.

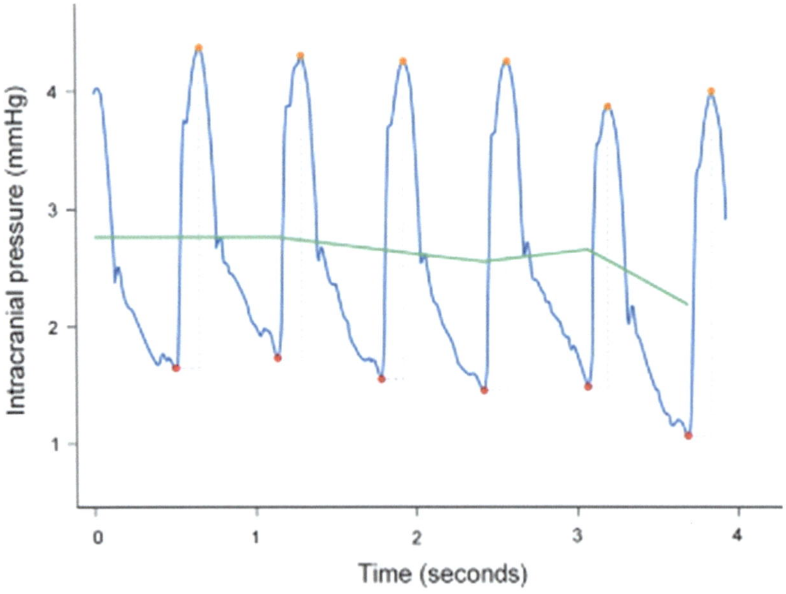

Fig. 5.4 The static ICP or mean ICP is an absolute pressure value measured against the reference point, depicted here by the horizontal line. The pulsatile ICP includes the pressure changes occurring during the cardiac cycle, with a single ICP wave characterized by an increase from diastolic minimum to peak systolic pressure, depicted here as dots

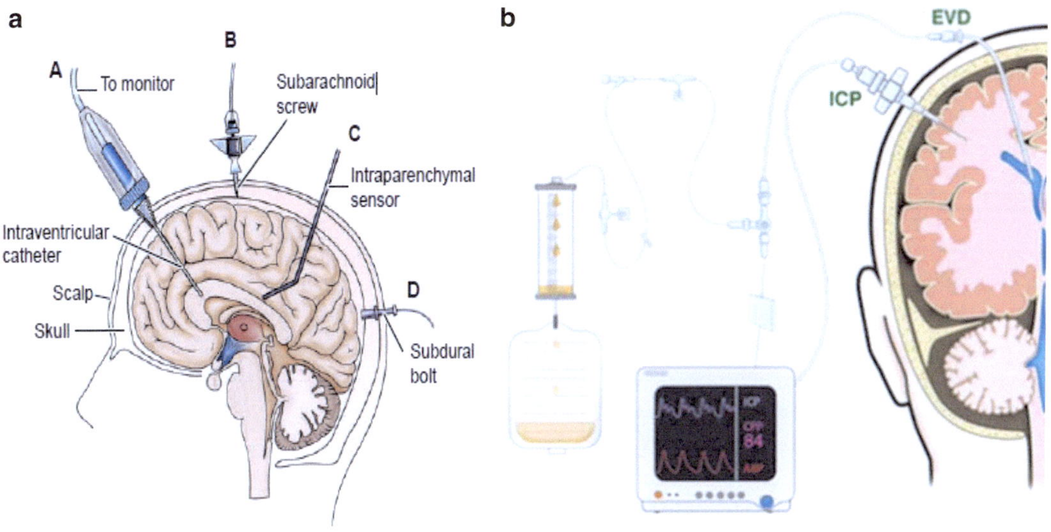

Fig. 5.5 (**a**) Sites for intracranial pressure monitoring. (**b**) The EVD is the most commonly accessed site in clinical practice that can be simultaneously used for CSF drainage also

The drain inserted into either of the lateral ventricles is connected to the strain gauge transducer through saline-filled tubing. The transducer converts the transmitted pressure wave into an electric signal, which is then displayed on the monitor screen. Although this fluid-coupled device is considered to be the most accurate form of ICP measurement, it has several limitations [27]. First, those related to the invasive nature of the procedure are misplacement of the catheter in ventricles, hemorrhage, and infections. The risk of hemorrhage during and after insertion is only 5–7%, whereas the risk of infection increases tremendously after 5 days. Various modalities applied to reduce the risk of infection include antibiotic and silver-impregnated catheters, subcutaneous placement of catheters, shortening the use of EVD to less than 5 days, and use of a sterile technique for EVD insertion. However, use of elective antibiotics and routine change of catheters is not prudent to prevent EVD-related infections [28]. Second, fluid-filled catheters have complications related to the zero level. Ideally, the foramen of Monro should be taken as the zero level, but, in routine clinical practice, zeroing of the transducer is performed at the external auditory meatus. However, the external presence of this assembly for ICP monitoring offers the advantage of recalibration. Third, inaccuracies are related to the fluid-filled system itself, i.e., the presence of air bubbles, kinks, clots, debris, etc. limit the quality of the signal obtained on the monitor screen.

(b) **Dedicated Implantable ICP Sensors**

In this era of advancing technology, the other invasive form of ICP monitoring includes a wide variety of devices based on microtransducer technology [29]. The catheter tip loaded with either a fiberoptic sensor or a balloon (pneumatic sensors) or a strain gauge device can be placed at numerous anatomical locations such as in the brain parenchyma and the epidural, subdural, or subarachnoid spaces (Fig. 5.5b).

The most commonly used IP sensor, a Camino transducer, is a fiberoptic transducer that has a displaceable mirror at its tip. With changes in ICP, the intensity of light reflected by the mirror varies and is reflected along the fiberoptic cable [30]. The Codman microsensor, the Raumedic Neurovent-P and S-type sensors, and the Pressio sensor are based on the piezoelectric strain gauze technology. With changes in ICP, the electric resistance of the diaphragm alters, which is used to calculate the ICP [31]. Pneumatic sensors, such as Spiegelberg ICP monitors, have a ballooned tip and changes in ICP are detected by changes in the pressure exerted on the balloon by the surrounding tissue [32].

The most common location of these microtransducers is the right frontal cortex parenchyma, although other sites can also be opted for depending upon the pathology of the brain. These devices have good correlation with intraventricular devices for measuring ICP, along with the advantage of a markedly reduced risk of hemorrhage and infections. Additionally, they are free from artifacts in measurement associated with the fluid coupling system. Their accuracy and reliability have been validated in the literature, making these ICP sensors good alternatives to intraventricular drainage catheters.

However, their use is limited by the fact that they are expensive, single-use, require neurosurgical expertise for placement, and lack recalibration after placement, resulting in drift or baseline jumps. This drift only applies to the mean ICP and not to the ICP waveforms. Moreover, there is an inability to simultaneously drain the CSF as with intraventricular devices. However, the newer versions of the catheters allowing for therapeutic CSF drainage, automatic drift correction, and low cost have made these monitors more popular in neurocritical care centers [33]. Still, one of the criticisms for all these implantable ICP sensors is that they reflect local pressure, which may be misleading as pressure in the skull may not be uniform, especially in pathological conditions such as trauma or intracranial hemorrhage

5.5.4 Noninvasive Techniques

1. **Ocular**

   I. **Pupillometry**

   Historically, an oval pupil was suggestive of high ICP, indicating brain herniation; however, no numerical value of ICP has been associated with pupillary size. Moreover, pupil size was measured using a ruler, which cannot measure pupillary contractions. However, advancements in technology have led to the development of a novel automatic pupillometer, based on infrared technology [34]. This device is accurate and more reliable than the manual method for measuring pupil size and can even detect subtle changes in reactivity of the pupil. It has been reported that a decrease of pupillary constriction velocity is associated with intracranial hypertension (ICP > 20 mmHg). Normally, there is 34% decrease in the size of the pupil to light reaction as against a 20% decrease in size in TBI, which is suggestive of raised ICP [35]. An increase in ICP causes mechanical compression in the pathway of the third nerve, and inhibiting pupillary reactivity as pupillary fibers lie outermost and are sensitive to pressure changes.

   The neurological pupillary index (NPi) is derived by algorithmically transforming the seven parameters involved in the pupillary light reflex and quantifies pupillary reactivity. Although there is evidence of an inverse relationship between ICP with abnormal pupillary reactivity, it is weak and not statistically significant, with one study showing that elevated ICP resulted in lower NPi values and contraction velocity, with no effect on pupil size [36]. Hence, the role of pupillometry in quantifying ICP is controversial but may be used as a screen for detecting patients with dysfunctional intracranial compliance.

II. **Visual Evoked Potential (VEP)**

VEPs are an accurate representation of the visual pathway. Mechanical compression of the brainstem or blood vessels, caused by increased ICP, can cause cerebral ischemia. This results in impaired brain tissue metabolism and subsequently affects the electric conduction reflected in the VEP. York et al., in 1981, demonstrated a clear relation between increasing ICP and shift in latency of the N2 wave [37]. This is followed by a decrease in wave amplitude and increasing wave width with increasing ICP and brain herniation. Devices based on VEP have been developed to measure ICP and is a sensitive, noninvasive method to detect cerebral cortical insults [38]. Single measurement is complete in less than a minute, and the average of three readings taken over 15 min is used as the final measurement of ICP. Its use has been studied in patients with subarachnoid hemorrhage, hypertensive intracerebral hemorrhage (ICH)-induced ICP elevation, and craniocerebral trauma [39]. However, VEP cannot be used for ICP assessment in patients with frontal lobe hematoma, retinal damage, and optic neuropathy.

III. **Visual Ophthalmodynamometry (ODM)**

The retinal artery and vein are directly observable vessels in the human body. It is observed that spontaneous pulsations of the central retinal vein (CRV) are common and can also be induced by increasing the intraocular pressure (IOP) by compressing the eyeball [40]. Ophthalmodynamometry (ODM) was first used by Baurmann to record the threshold force to induce these pulsations in the CRV, and it was found that in patients with elevated ICP, more pressure was required to trigger these pulsations [41]. Later, Firsching et al., in their study, reported that this force/IOP was equal to CRV pressure and had a linear correlation with ICP [42]. The idea of predicting ICP with cenrtral retinal vein pressure (CRVP) was thus feasible, and Quefurth defined an algorithm based on a multivariate model to improve the accuracy of ICP evaluation while using ODM [43]. This required the simultaneous use of ODM, an ophthalmoscope, and a tonometer by two operators together; hence, it was rarely used in clinical practice.

Ophthalmodynamometry for ICP measurement is safe, reliable, cheap, and feasible but is a static method that cannot be used for continuous monitoring. It can predict raised ICP with high probability. The accuracy of this method needs validation in further studies but has great clinical potential.

IV. **Optic Nerve Sheath Diameter (ONSD)**

The optic nerve sheath is an extension of the dura mater, and the subarachnoid space surrounding the optic nerve is contiguous with the intracranial subarachnoid space. Harvey, in 1968, first suggested that CSF pressure in the intracranial space was consistent with CSF pressure in the optic nerve sheath [44]. When ICP increases, intracranial CSF flows

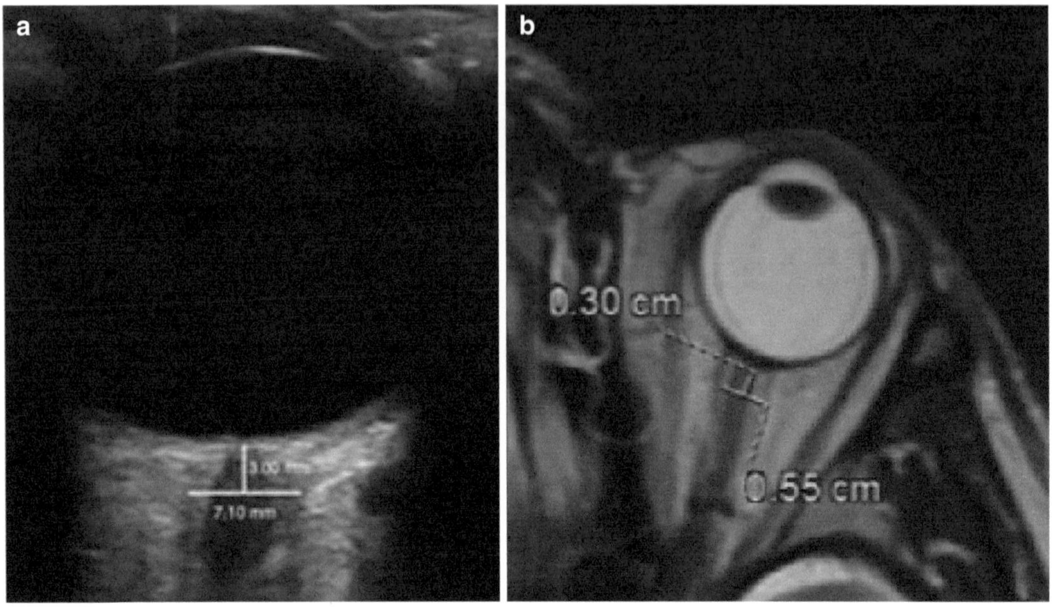

Fig. 5.6 (**a**) Ultrasound images in B-mode showing the cross-sectional cut of the optic nerve from the anterior transbulbar approach. ONSD is determined by measuring the diameter from the inner edge to the inner edge of the optic nerve sheath at 3 mm behind the globe, using the optic disc as a reference point. (**b**) Measuring of ONSD with MR imaging

through the optic canal into the subarachnoid space around the optic nerve dilating the space. This can be imaged using ultrasonography or computed tomography (CT) or magnetic resonance imaging (MRI) and is the rational for optic nerve sheath diameter (ONSD) to be used as a surrogate for invasive ICP monitoring.

ONSD measurement using ultrasound is performed by placing a high-frequency, high-resolution (13–7.5 MHz) linear probe on the closed eye with the patient lying in a supine relaxed position. A clear film adhesive strip can be placed over the eye for added protection. The probe has to be adjusted in order to ideally display the point of entrance of the optic nerve into the ocular globe, seen on the screen as "dark meets dark" (the nerve meets vitreous without interposition of the thick echogenic posterior sclera) [45]. The ONSD is determined by measuring the diameter from the inner edge to the inner edge of the optic nerve sheath at 3 mm behind the globe, using the optic disc as a reference point (Fig. 5.6a). The anterior section of the nerve sheath is most reflective of changes in ICP as it is loosely bound, and the posterior regions show markedly less dilatation [46]. The average of three or more measurements using horizontal and vertical approaches are used to calculate the final value of ONSD. Many studies have demonstrated a linear relationship between ONSD and ICP, indicating a value of >5 mm as a threshold for determining elevated ICP [47]. There is also significant and immediate reduction in ONSD following therapy, indicating a rapid response to changes in ICP. Among other methods of noninvasive ICP monitoring, ONSD is a safe, reliable, reproducible, dynamic, real-time reflection of ICP with low inter-observer variability. It is a skill easy to acquire, with experienced sonologists requiring about ten scans, whereas nonphysicians or novice ultrasound users may need 25 scans.

However, it may be false positive (increased ONSD without an increase in ICP) in cases of optic neuritis, arachnoid cyst of the optic nerve, optic nerve trauma, or nerve sheath glioma. It is contraindicated in Graves' disease, sarcoidosis, inflammation, and tumors of the eye. Despite limitations, ONSD has been established as a sensitive, bedside screening tool for detecting raised ICP, where access to invasive monitoring is not available [48].

V. **IOP Measurement**

Increased venous pressure in cavernous sinus can be transmitted through the superior ophthalmic vein to the episcleral ophthalmic vein. Hence, IOP increases linearly with ICP, and various studies have attempted to correlate them. However, the majority of the studies have unequivocally proven a poor association and do not support tonometry as a form of noninvasive modality of ICP monitoring [49]. A comparison of noninvasive methods of ICP monitoring by ocular methods is provided in Table 5.2.

2. **Auditory**

(a) **Distortion Product Otoacoustic Emissions (DPOAESs)**

Noninvasive monitoring of ICP is plausible through the auditory system as it is with the ophthalmic system. This is because of the connections between the cochlear fluids in the perilymphatic space and CSF that changes in ICP are also transmitted to the inner ear [50]. Distortion product otoacoustic emissions (DPOAEs) are a form of otoacoustic signal, transmitted from the cochlear aqueduct in the inner ear to the external ear

Table 5.2 Comparison of noninvasive methods of ICP monitoring by ocular methods

Method	Equipment	Continuous monitoring	Quantitative	Limitations
1. Pupillometry	Automatic pupillometer	No	No	Pupillary reactivity is affected by numerous factors
2. Flash visual evoked potentials (FVEPd)	Electroencephalogram	No	No	Not suitable for patients with frontal lobe hematoma, retinal damage, or optic neuropathy
3. Ophthalmodynamometry		No	No	Central retinal venous pulsations may be normally absent in some patients
4. Optic nerve sheath diameter (ONSD)	Ultrasonography/ computed tomography magnetic resonance imaging	No	No	Baseline differences in ONSD between individuals based on gender, age, and ethnicity
5. IOP	Tonometer	No	No	Not a reliable parameter for ICP assessment. It may be falsely raised in cavernous sinus pathology

canal. The signal is measured in the external auditory canal using the auditory-based measurement and is especially large at low frequencies. This new clinical tool has a good correlation with invasive methods and may be used in future to predict ICP noninvasively [51].

(b) **Tympanic Membrane Displacement**

Similar to the aforementioned concept, changes in ICP are transmitted to the cochlear fluid that affect the stapes excursions because of the proximity of the stapes to the oval window. Consequently, these changes in ICP cause tympanic membrane displacement (TMD) that can be measured in response to auditory stimulation. These tympanic membrane infrasonic emissions and TMD provide an insight into intracranial pressure dynamics [52]. Although this does not provide specific ICP values, it may be a good screening tool for follow-up of patients with elevated ICP. However, it can only be performed in patients with an intact stapedial reflex, normal middle ear pressure, and a patent cochlear aqueduct.

3. **Imaging**

Imaging techniques (CT, MRI) that are used for diagnostic purposes can also provide qualitative information about ICP, although information is limited to only that particular time frame [53]. Changes in CT suggestive of raised ICP include loss of gray–white mater differentiation, basal cistern and ventricular effacement, and midline shift.

Imaging of the optic nerve sheath on CT and MRI can also be used to evaluate patients with elevated ICP (Fig. 5.6b). Studies have shown that ONSD measured on MRI has a superior predictive value for increased ICP as compared to the classical findings of elevated ICP [54]. Advances in MRI technology have also led to the assessment of pulsatile differences in net transcranial blood and CSF flow to estimate mean ICP. Similarly, the CT-determined ratio of CSF volume to total intracranial volume has been used to determine elevated ICP in a small series of TBI patients [55]. However, CT may also be normal in the presence of raised ICP, suggesting that it is not a sensitive and reliable tool. Other disadvantages of imaging for ICP assessment include radiation exposure and problems of transportation of critically ill patients.

4. **Transcranial Doppler (TCD)**

The use of TCD has been extensively explored in neurological fields, and TCD-derived indices have been correlated with ICP [56]. TCD is a bedside, low-cost, noninvasive technique to evaluate cerebral hemodynamics. A 2-MHz probe is used for insonating the middle cerebral artery (MCA) through the temporal window, although other windows, including the transorbital, occipital, and submandibular windows, may also be used. The flow velocity in the MCA determined by TCD, along with arterial blood pressure and pulsatility index, have been computed to develop a formula to predict ICP (PI–ICP = 10.93 × PI–1.28) [57]. Although computational modeling-based ICP estimates correlate reasonably well with invasive measurements, they are limited by inter- and intra-observer variability, point of care, and noncontinuous assessment. Moreover, a poor window of the skull in about 15% patients precludes assessment by TCD. Hence, it may be used as an adjunct to neuromonitoring in critically ill patients, but its use as a surrogate marker for noninvasive ICP monitoring is ambiguous.

5. **Tissue Resonance Analysis (TRA)**

A tissue resonance analysis (TRA) device is a computerized, portable device for the noninvasive monitoring and measurement of ICP [58]. According to this, the ultrasound signal reflected from the third ventricle is digitally processed to obtain a high-resolution echopulsogram, which is visually equivalent to ICP waves obtained invasively. ICP measured by the ultrasound TRA technique, initially developed by Michaeli et al., showed good correlation with invasive ICP; however, there have been very few studies following the initial promise [59].

6. **Electroencephalogram**

   Based on the concept proposed by Amantini et al. that neurophysiological changes precede ICP change, electroencephalogram (EEG) was extensively explored as a noninvasive method for ICP monitoring [60]. Later, Chen et al. performed analysis of specific parameters from the EEG power spectrum and calculated the pressure index (PI) using self-designed software [61]. The PI obtained from EEG analysis correlated with ICP measured by lumbar puncture (LP). However, further studies are needed to support this correlation.

7. **Near-Infrared Spectroscopy**

   Near-infrared spectroscopy (NIRS), is an optical, noninvasive method to quantify the concentration of oxygenated hemoglobin (HbO) and deoxygenated hemoglobin (Hb) based on the principle of differential absorption of light in the vicinity of the infrared spectrum [62]. NIRS was used by Kampfl et al. to assess changes in regional cerebral oxygen saturation (rSO_2) in patients with TBI, reporting significantly lower NIRS values in patients with elevated ICP [63]. Hence, NIRS-based alterations in cerebral microcirculation, CBF, CBV, tissue oxygenation, and, consequently, intracranial pressure suggest that it may be an additional diagnostic tool for ICP monitoring.

5.6 Future Avenues for ICP Monitoring

Although ICP monitoring has been used as a tool for surveillance and diagnosis, its clinical utility is a matter of debate despite the robust scientific literature. The main reason for this is the constraints and weaknesses of the current ICP measurement approaches, which mainly lack signal quality control [64].

Since changes in intracranial pressure is just one of the several parameters in the pathological brain, its monitoring should be incorporated with other parameters like CBF, cerebral oxygenation, and metabolism. Although ICP monitoring will provide global assessment, other devices will provide more information of the pathological site.

Currently, there are no noninvasive devices that generates a continuous source signal for ICP monitoring. At best, a single value of ICP is obtained, indicating whether ICP is raised or not. Hence, continuous, noninvasive, new, yet unknown, source signals need to be developed. Research should focus on developing implantable, miniature, biodegradable sensors with wireless technology so that long-term ICP monitoring is feasible. Moreover, with advancements in machine learning and artificial intelligence, digitally stored ICP patterns based on source signals could be used to generate algorithms to foresee clinical adverse events. They would be ideal for monitoring patients with brain injury or disease as well as diagnosing individuals with neurological complaints.

References

1. Mokri B. The Monro-Kellie hypothesis: applications in CSF volume depletion. Neurology. 2001;56:1746–8.
2. Monro A. Observations on the structure and functions of the nervous system. Edinbourgh, UK: Creech and Johnson; 1783.
3. Kellie G. Appearances observed in the dissection of two individuals; death from cold and congestion of the brain. Trans Med Chir Soc Edinbrugh. 1824;1:84.
4. Cushing H. The third circulation in studies in intracranial physiology and surgery. London, UK: Oxford University Press; 1926.
5. Kjällquist A, Lundberg N, Pontén U. Respiratory and cardiovascular changes during rapid spontaneous variations of ventricular fluid pressure in patients with intracranial hypertension. Acta Neurol Scand. 1964;40:291–317.
6. Czosnyka M, Pickard JD. Monitoring and interpretation of intracranial pressure. J Neurol Neurosurg Psychiatry. 2004;75(6):813–21.
7. Hamer J, Alberti E, Hoyer S, Wiedemann K. Influence of systemic and cerebral vascular factors on the cerebrospinal fluid pulse waves. J Neurosurg. 1977;46:36 45. https://doi.org/10.3171/jns.1977.46.1.0036.
8. Telano LN, Baker S. Physiology, cerebral spinal fluid. In: StatPearls. Stat Pearls Publishing; Treasure Island, FL. 2022.
9. Chapman PH, Cosman ER, Arnold MA. The relationship between ventricular fluid pressure and body

position in normal subjects and subjects with shunts: a telemetric study. Neurosurgery. 1990;26:181–9.
10. Lundberg N, Troupp H, Lorin H. Continuous recording of the ventricular-fluid pressure in patients with severe acute traumatic brain injury. A preliminary report. J Neurosurg. 1965;22:581–90. https://doi.org/10.3171/jns.1965.22.6.0581.
11. Hall A, O'Kane R. The best marker for guiding the clinical management of patients with raised intracranial pressure—the rap index or the mean pulse amplitude? Acta Neurochir. 2016, 158, 1997–2009. Spiegelberg, A.; Preuß, M.; Kurtcuoglu, V. B-waves revisited. Interdiscip. Neurosurg. 2016;6:13–7.
12. Lemaire JJ, Khalil T, Cervenansky F, Gindre G, Boire JY, Bazin JE, Irthum B, Chazal J. Slow pressure waves in the cranial enclosure. Acta Neurochir. 2002;144:243–54.
13. Gjerris F, Brennum J, Paulson OB, Gjerris F, Sørensen PS. The cerebrospinal fluid, intracranial pressure and herniation of the brain. In: Paulson OB, Gjerris F, Sørensen PS, editors. Clinical neurology and neurosurgery. Copenhagen: FADL's Forlag Aktieselskab; 2004. p. 179–96.
14. Czosnyka M, Citerio G. Brain compliance: the old story with a new 'et cetera'. Intensive Care Med. 2012;38:925–7. https://doi.org/10.1007/s00134-012-2572-6.
15. Jin SC, Choi BS, Kim JS. The RAP index during intracranial pressure monitoring as a clinical guiding for surgically treated aneurysmal subarachnoid hemorrhage: consecutive series of single surgeon. Acute Crit Care. 2019;34(1):71–8. https://doi.org/10.4266/acc.2019.00437.
16. Czosnyka M, Smielewski P, Timofeev I, et al. Intracranial pressure: more than a number. Neurosurg Focus. 2007;22(5):E10. https://doi.org/10.3171/foc.2007.22.5.11.
17. Donnelly J, Budohoski KP, Smielewski P, Czosnyka M. Regulation of the cerebral circulation: bedside assessment and clinical implications. Crit Care. 2016;20:129.
18. Steiner LA, Czosnyka M, Piechnik SK, et al. Continuous monitoring of cerebrovascular pressure reactivity allows determination of optimal cerebral perfusion pressure in patients with traumatic brain injury. Crit Care Med. 2002;30:733–8.
19. Rosner MJ, Rosner SD, Johnson AH. Cerebral perfusion pressure: management protocol and clinical results. J Neurosurg. 1995;83:949–62. https://doi.org/10.3171/jns.1995.83.6.0949.
20. Carney N, Totten AM, O'Reilly C, Ullman JS, Hawryluk GW, Bell MJ, Bratton SL, Chesnut R, Harris OA, Kissoon N, Rubiano AM, Shutter L, Tasker RC, Vavilala MS, Wilberger J, Wright DW, Ghajar J. Guidelines for the management of severe traumatic brain injury, fourth edition. Neurosurgery. 2017;80:6–15. https://doi.org/10.1227/NEU.0000000000001432.
21. Quincke H. Die Lumbar punction des hydrocephalus. Berl Clin Wschr. 1891;28:929–33.
22. Janny P: La pression intra-cranienne chez l'homme. Methode d'enregistrement–Etude de ses variations et de ses rapports avec les signes cliniques et ophtalmologiques. Thesis; 1950.
23. Lundberg N. Continuous recording and control of ventricular fluid pressure in neurosurgical practice. Acta Psychiatr Scand Suppl. 1960;36:1–193.
24. Wagshul ME, Eide PK, Madsen JR. The pulsating brain: a review of experimental and clinical studies of intracranial pulsatility. Fluids Barrier CNS. 2011;8:5.
25. Kawoos U, McCarron RM, Auker CR, Chavko M. Advances in intracranial pressure monitoring and its significance in managing traumatic brain injury. Int J Mol Sci. 2015;16(12):28979–97. https://doi.org/10.3390/ijms161226146.
26. Abdoh MG, Bekaert O, Hodel J, Diarra SM, Le Guerinel C, Nseir R, Bastuji-Garin S, Decq P. Accuracy of external ventricular drainage catheter placement. Acta Neurochir. 2012;154:153–9.
27. Tavakoli S, Peitz G, Ares W, Hafeez S, Grandhi R. Complications of invasive intracranial pressure monitoring devices in neurocritical care. Neurosurg Focus. 2017;43:E6.
28. Brain Trauma Foundation; American Association of Neurological Surgeons; Congress of Neurological Surgeons; Joint Section on Neurotrauma and Critical Care, AANS/CNS, Bratton SL, Chestnut RM, Ghajar J, McConnell Hammond FF, Harris OA, Hartl R, Manley GT, Nemecek A, Newell DW, Rosenthal G, Schouten J, Shutter L, Timmons SD, Ullman JS, Videtta W, Wilberger JE, Wright DW. Guidelines for the management of severe traumatic brain injury. IV. Infection prophylaxis. J Neurotrauma. 2007;24(Suppl 1):S26–31. https://doi.org/10.1089/neu.2007.9992.
29. Zhong J, Dujovny M, Park HK, Perez E, Perlin AR, Diaz FG. Advances in ICP monitoring techniques. Neurol Res. 2003;25:339–50.
30. Gelabert-Gonzalez M, Ginesta-Galan V, Sernamito-Garcia R, Allut AG, Bandin-Dieguez J, Rumbo RM. The Camino intracranial pressure device in clinical practice. Assessment in a 1000 cases. Acta Neurochir. 2006;148:435–41.
31. Koskinen LO, Olivecrona M. Clinical experience with the intraparenchymal intracranial pressure monitoring Codman MicroSensor system. Neurosurgery. 2005;56:693–8.
32. Chambers IR, Siddique MS, Banister K, Mendelow AD. Clinical comparison of the Spiegelberg parenchymal transducer and ventricular fluid pressure. J Neurol Neurosurg Psychiatry. 2001;71:383–5.
33. Abraham M, Singhal V. Intracranial pressure monitoring. J Neuroanaesthesiol Crit Care. 2015;2:193–203. https://doi.org/10.4103/2348-0548.165039.
34. Ong C, Hutch M, Barra M, Kim A, Zafar S, Smirnakis S. Effects of osmotic therapy on pupil reactivity: quantification using Pupillometry in critically ill neurologic patients. Neurocrit Care. 2019;30:307–15.

35. Taylor WR, Chen JW, Meltzer H, Gennarelli TA, Kelbch C, Knowlton S, Richardson J, Lutch MJ, Farin A, Hults KN, et al. Quantitative pupillometry, a new technology: normative data and preliminary observations in patients with acute head injury. Technical note. J Neurosurg. 2003;98:205–13.
36. Stevens AR, Su Z, Toman E, Belli A, Davies D. Optical pupillometry in traumatic brain injury: neurological pupil index and its relationship with intracranial pressure through significant event analysis. Brain Inj. 2019;33:1032–8.
37. York DH, Pulliam MW, Rosenfeld JG, Watts C. Relationship between visual evoked potentials and intracranial pressure. J Neurosurg. 1981;55:909–16.
38. Zhong JI, Li Y, Minhui X, Yihua Z. Realization of a comprehensive non-invasive detection of intracranial pressure analyzer based upon FVEP and TCD. Acta Neurochir Suppl. 2012;114:127–9.
39. Yu F, Zhao Y, Zhang Y, Luan X, Wu Y. Clinical application of intracranial pressure monitoring based on flash visual evoked potential in treatment of patients with hypertensive intracerebral hemorrhage. Sq: Res; 2020.
40. Coccius EA. Ueber die Anwendung des Augen-Spiegels Nebst Angabe Eines Neuen Instrumentes. Immanuel Müller: Leipzig, Germany; 1853.
41. Khan MN, Shallwani H, Khan MU, Shamim MS. Noninvasive monitoring intracranial pressure—a review of available modalities. Surg Neurol Int. 2017;8:51.
42. Firsching R, Schutze M, Motschmann M, Behrens-Baumann W. Venous opthalmodynamometry: a noninvasive method for assessment of intracranial pressure. J Neurosurg. 2000;93:33–6.
43. Querfurth HW, Arms SW, Lichy CM, Irwin WT, Steiner T. Prediction of intracranial pressure from noninvasive transocular venous and arterial hemodynamic measurements: a pilot study. Neurocrit Care. 2004;1:183–94.
44. Hayreh SS. Pathogenesis of oedema of the optic disc. Doc Ophthalmol. 1968;24:289–411.
45. del Saz-Saucedo P, Redondo-Gonzalez O, Mateu-Mateu A, Huertas-Arroyo R, Garcia-Ruiz R, Botia-Paniagua E. Sonographic assessment of the optic nerve sheath diameter in the diagnosis of idiopathic intracranial hypertension. J Neurol Sci. 2016;361:122–7.
46. Kim SE, Hong EP, Kim HC, Lee SU, Jeon JP. Ultrasonographic optic nerve sheath diameter to detect increased intracranial pressure in adults: a meta-analysis. Acta Radiol. 2019;60:221–9.
47. Kishk NA, Ebraheim AM, Ashour AS, Badr NM, Eshra MA. Optic nerve sonographic examination to predict raised intracranial pressure in idiopathic intracranial hypertension: the cut-off points. Neuroradiol J. 2018;31:490–5.
48. Koziarz A, Sne N, Kegel F, Nath S, Badhiwala JH, Nassiri F, Mansouri A, Yang K, Zhou Q, Rice T, et al. Bedside optic nerve ultrasonography for diagnosing increased intracranial pressure: a systematic review and meta-analysis. Ann Intern Med. 2019;171:896–905.
49. Rosenberg JB, Shiloh AL, Savel RH, Eisen LA. Non-invasive methods of estimating intracranial pressure. Neurocrit Care. 2011;15:599–608. https://doi.org/10.1007/s12028-011-9545-4.
50. Bershad EM, Urfy MZ, Pechacek A, McGrath M, Calvillo E, Horton NJ, Voss SE. Intracranial pressure modulates distortion product otoacoustic emissions: a proof-of-principle study. Neurosurgery. 2014;75:445–54; discussion 454–5. https://doi.org/10.1227/NEU.0000000000000449.
51. Sakka L, Thalamy A, Giraudet F, Hassoun T, Avan P, Chazal J. Electrophysiological monitoring of cochlear function as a non-invasive method to assess intracranial pressure variations. Acta Neurochir Suppl. 2012;114:131–4. https://doi.org/10.1007/978-3-7091-0956-4_24.
52. Stettin E, Paulat K, Schulz C, Kunz U, Mauer UM. Noninvasive intracranial pressure measurement using infrasonic emissions from the tympanic membrane. J Clin Monit Comput. 2011;25:203–10. https://doi.org/10.1007/s10877-011-9297-x.
53. Sekhon MS, Griesdale DE, Robba C, McGlashan N, Needham E, Walland K, Shook AC, Smielewski P, Czosnyka M, Gupta AK, et al. Optic nerve sheath diameter on computed tomography is correlated with simultaneously measured intracranial pressure in patients with severe traumatic brain injury. Intensive Care Med. 2014;40:1267–74.
54. Geeraerts T, Newcombe VF, Coles JP, Abate MG, Perkes IE, Hutchinson PJ, Outtrim JG, Chatfield DA, Menon DK. Use of T2-weighted magnetic resonance imaging of the optic nerve sheath to detect raised intracranial pressure. Crit Care. 2008;12:R114.
55. Soliman I, Johnson G, Gillman LM, Zeiler FA, Faqihi F, Aletreby WT, Balhamar A, Mahmood NN, Ahmad Mumtaz S, Alharthy A, et al. New optic nerve sonography quality criteria in the diagnostic evaluation of traumatic brain injury. Crit Care Res Pract. 2018;2018:3589762.
56. Bouzat P, Francony G, Declety P, Genty C, Kaddour A, Bessou P, Brun J, Jacquot C, Chabardes S, Bosson JL, Payen JF. Transcranial Doppler to screen on admission patients with mild to moderate traumatic brain injury. Neurosurgery. 2011;68:1603–9; discussion 1609–10. https://doi.org/10.1227/NEU.0b013e31820cd43e.
57. Wakerley BR, Kusuma Y, Yeo LL, Liang S, Kumar K, Sharma AK, Sharma VK. Usefulness of transcranial Doppler-derived cerebral hemodynamic parameters in the noninvasive assessment of intracranial pressure. J Neuroimaging. 2015;25:111–6. https://doi.org/10.1111/jon.12100.
58. Goto T, Furihata K, Hongo K. Natural resonance frequency of the brain depends on only intracranial pressure: clinical research. Sci Rep. 2020;10(1):2526. https://doi.org/10.1038/s41598-020-59376-7.
59. Michaeli D, Rappaport ZH. Tissue resonance analysis; a novel method for noninvasive monitoring of intracranial pressure. Technical note. J

Neurosurg. 2002;96:1132–7. https://doi.org/10.3171/jns.2002.96.6.1132.
60. Amantini A, Fossi S, Grippo A, Innocenti P, Amadori A, Bucciardini L, Cossu C, Nardini C, Scarpelli S, Roma V, Pinto F. Continuous EEG-SEP monitoring in severe brain injury. Neurophysiol Clin. 2009;39:85–93. https://doi.org/10.1016/j.neucli.2009.01.006.
61. Chen H, Wang J, Mao S, Dong W, Yang H. A new method of intracranial pressure monitoring by EEG power spectrum analysis. Can J Neurol Sci. 2012;39:483–7.
62. Ghosh A, Elwell C, Smith M. Review article: cerebral near-infrared spectroscopy in adults: a work in progress. Anesth Analg. 2012;115:1373–83. https://doi.org/10.1213/ANE.0b013e31826dd6a6.
63. Kampfl A, et al. Near infrared spectroscopy (NIRS) in patients with severe brain injury and elevated intracranial pressure. A pilot study. Acta Neurochir. 1997;Suppl. 70:112–4. https://doi.org/10.1007/978-3-7091-6837-0_35.
64. Evensen KB, Eide PK. Measuring intracranial pressure by invasive, less invasive or non-invasive means: limitations and avenues for improvement. Fluids Barriers CNS. 2020;17(1):34. https://doi.org/10.1186/s12987-020-00195-3.

6 Cerebral Blood Flow Monitoring

J. S. Rahul and Gaurav Kakkar

6.1 Introduction

For an organ measuring roughly 2% of the total body weight, the brain needs an average of 50 mL blood for every 100 g of brain tissue per minute, accounting for 15% of the total cardiac output. The need for a constant blood supply to maintain the normal function and structure of the brain owing to its high metabolic rate renders cerebral perfusion an extremely crucial cog in brain homeostasis. The brain's inability to store oxygen or glucose makes the role of constant cerebral blood flow (CBF) all the more vital.

Of late, cerebral blood flow (CBF) monitoring has become an integral part of the neurosciences and is an important aspect of cerebral homeostasis, as mentioned, since the description of the Monro–Kellie doctrine (originally, the Monro–Kellie article). The earliest documented attempts at measuring CBF were made in the nineteenth century [1]. The mathematical principles of measuring cardiac output using a pressure difference in the oxygen content of arterial and venous blood were laid out by Adolf Fick in 1870, which eventually proved vital when Kety used these principles for CBF measurement, thus paving the way for a newer avenue in the neurosciences [2].

6.2 Arterial Supply of the Brain

The brain's arterial supply may be divided into anterior and posterior circulation, primarily constituting a pair of internal carotid arteries (ICAs) and vertebral arteries (VAs), respectively (Fig. 6.1). The right common carotid artery branches out of the brachiocephalic trunk, whereas the left common carotid artery is a direct branch of the arch of the aorta, which, in turn, divides into the internal carotid artery (ICA) and the external carotid artery (ECA) in the neck. The ICA on both sides enters the cranial cavity at the skull base through the carotid canal and is a major contributor to the anterior cerebral blood flow by further dividing at various locations in the brain.

Vertebral arteries, owing to their lesser pressure, arise from the subclavian arteries on both sides, eventually joining the vertebral artery from the opposite side to primarily form the basilar artery, and are the primary components of the vertebrobasilar system [3].

J. S. Rahul · G. Kakkar (✉)
Department of Neuroanaesthesiology and Neurocritical Care, Amrita School of Medicine, Faridabad, Haryana, India
e-mail: rahul@fbd.amrita.edu; gauravkakkar@fbd.amrita.edu

H. Prabhakar et al. (eds.), *Principles and Practice of Neurocritical Care*,
https://doi.org/10.1007/978-981-99-8059-8_6

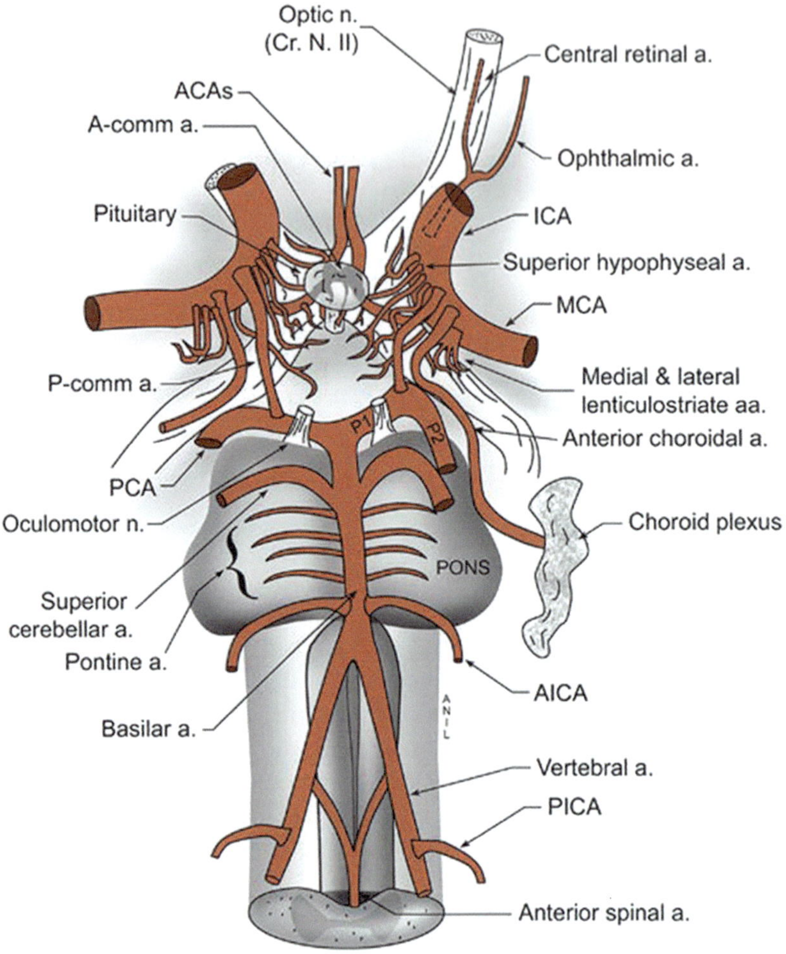

Fig. 6.1 Arterial supply of the brain

6.3 The Physiological Aspects of Cerebral Blood Flow

6.3.1 Cerebral Physiology and CBF

Owing to its nonexistent storage capacity, the brain predominantly relies on the incoming CBF for both its function and maintenance. Cerebral perfusion is essential for the delivery of oxygen, which is needed for neuronal activity, maintenance, and metabolism of energy substrates, thus rendering CBF a critical variable in brain function and viability. CBF enables the delivery of oxygen and energy substrates while aiding in the removal of products of brain metabolism. A constant CBF is warranted as both hypoperfusion (lower CBF) and hyperperfusion (higher CBF) can have undesirable effects on the brain [4].

CBF, by definition, is the amount of blood volume that flows per unit mass per unit of time in the brain tissue, which is typically expressed in units of milliliters of blood per 100 g of the brain tissue. The normal average CBF in adults in resting state is about 50 mL/100 g/min, [5] with an average blood flow (BF) of 80 mL/100 g/min in the gray matter owing to higher metabolic and functional needs and about 20 mL/100 g/min in the white matter [6].

As mentioned, CBF is coupled to brain metabolism and oxygen extraction. The cerebral metabolic rate of oxygen ($CMRO_2$) is usually in the range of 3–3.5 mL of O_2 per 100 mL of blood. Hence, with an increasing $CMRO_2$, CBF increases directly to facilitate a continuous blood supply to keep up with the growing needs.

In relation to the $CMRO_2$, CBF can be expressed as

$$\text{CBF} = \text{CMRO2} \div \text{AVDO2},$$

where $AVDO_2$ is the arteriovenous difference of oxygen, which can act as an index for oxygen extraction. Normal $AVDO_2$ is 6.5 mL of O_2/100 mL of blood [7].

Other important physiological determinants of CBF are the opposing forces laid out by the brain vasculature in the form of cerebrovascular resistance (CVR), which also has an impact on the amount of blood that eventually reaches the brain. The relationship between CBF and CVR can be represented with the equation:

$$\text{CBF} \equiv \frac{\text{CPP}}{\text{CVR}}.$$

where

- CPP is cerebral perfusion pressure, which is the difference between the mean arterial pressure (MAP) and intracranial pressure.
- CVR is the opposing force governed by the diameter and length of the blood vessels and blood viscosity.

To simplify, within the autoregulatory limits, increasing diameters of vessels tend to augment CBF, and vice versa; longer vascular segments tend to alleviate CBF, and lower viscosity within physiological limits tends to help maintain CBF [8].

6.3.2 Factors Affecting CBF [9]

The cerebral vasculature is extensively innervated neurally with a complex interplay between endothelial and neurotransmitter activity. The number of extrinsic and intrinsic factors has a bearing on the cerebral blood flow at a given point in time, of which neurogenic, humoral, and myogenic processes are some of the most important physiological mechanisms that govern CBF [10]. The extrinsic and intrinsic factors governing CBF are explained in brief as follows:

Intrinsic Factors

1. **Myogenic Regulation**

   This is the intrinsic response of smooth muscle cells in cerebral and pial arterioles to changes in mean arterial pressure (MAP). It is often considered a protective mechanism against excessive pressure fluctuations at the capillary level to maintain a constant flow. The myogenic mechanism can be simply explained by the mathematical formula pressure = flow x resistance. Going by this formula, to maintain a constant blood flow to the brain despite pressure fluctuations, cerebral vessels tend to offer an intrinsic resistance to limit the effect of pressure fluctuations on cerebral blood flow. In other words, within the autoregulatory limits, increasing diameters of vessels tend to augment CBF, and vice versa. This is brought about by the opening of calcium channels in the vessels secondary to the stretching of the blood vessels due to transmural pressure, which leads to vasoconstriction [11–13].

   Myogenic regulation and its complex interplay with other factors play a particularly important role in cerebral autoregulation (CA). With respect to blood pressure, owing to myogenic regulation, the mean arterial pressure of 60–160 mmHg guarantees a constant CBF, beyond which the CBF becomes pressure-passive.

2. **Metabolic Regulation or Flow Metabolism Coupling**

   Local cerebral metabolism and its effect on local brain perfusion have been well-known for more than a century [14]. Mediated by various vasoactive substances, metabolic regulation is driven by the balance between cerebral metabolism (demand) and oxygen delivery through cerebral blood flow (supply). In principle, this is a negative feedback control system that seeks to balance cerebral blood flow with demand. When tissue demands exceed blood flow, it leads to the release of tissue metabolites such as nitric oxide (NO), K^+ ions, endothelin, H^+ ions, prostaglandins, lactate, etc., which facilitate vasodilatation and increase blood flow to facilitate increased uptake of oxygen and glucose. This coupling is a product of the anatomical and metabolic relationship between neurons, glial cells, and cortical penetrating arterioles. This is explained by the neuron–glia metabolic coupling, which is essentially an excited brain needing blood for homeostasis and functioning [15–17].

3. **Neurogenic Regulation**

   According to neurogenic theory, perivascular neurons contribute to the autoregulatory effects on cerebral arterioles [18]. This theory suggests that two distinct mechanisms exist in the neural control of CBF, which is mediated by the superior cervical ganglion (sympathetic), the sphenopalatine ganglion (vagus parasympathetic), and the trigeminal ganglion that innervate the major cerebral blood vessels. Sympathetic stimulations are known to have a cerebral vasoconstrictive effect, whereas parasympathetic stimulations are known to be associated with the vasodilatory effect.

Extrinsic Factors Affecting CBF

1. **The partial pressure of arterial CO_2**: $PaCO_2$ is known to have powerful vasodilatory effects on the cerebral vessels. With a 1-mmHg increase in $PaCO_2$, there is an approximately 3–6% increase in CBF, and a 1-mm decrease in $PaCO_2$ causes a 1–3% decrease in CBF [19]. The major vessels of the neck, intracranial vessels, and pial arterioles are sensitive to changes in $PaCO_2$. The exact mechanism by which $PaCO_2$ acts is not known; however, it is believed to exert action by directly acting on the smooth muscle of the blood vessels. This relation is known to exist in a physiological $PaCO_2$ range of 20–80 mmHg [20].
2. **Effects of partial pressure of arterial oxygen**: Under physiological conditions, unlike $PaCO_2$, PaO_2 does not majorly affect CBF. A predominant effect on CBF is known to occur when PaO_2 falls below 50 mmHg. The effects of PaO_2 changes also depend on $PaCO_2$ levels. Under hypercapnic conditions, there is increased sensitivity, and under hypocapnia conditions, there is reduced sensitivity to hypoxia [21]. The postulated mechanisms for this association are believed to be (1) products of metabolism in the extracellular fluid (ECF), (2) stimulus from local neurovascular coupling, or (3) adenosine.
3. **Effect of hematocrit (Hct)**: Studies have shown that an Hct >44 increases blood viscosity and reduces CBF, whereas an Hct <28 increases CBF. However, overtly bringing down hematocrit for the sake of CBF might not be tolerated by the brain owing to the decreased oxygen content in the blood due to reduced hemoglobin caused by the hemodilution [22, 23].
4. **Effect of temperature**: Hyperthermia affects CBF by increasing it by 6–7% for every increase of 1 °C, whereas hypothermia has the opposite effect [24, 25]. This was the rationale behind using a strategy of neuroprotection with the aim to reduce brain metabolism and, in turn, CBF. However, sufficient evidence now exists against the routine use of hypothermia in most brain pathologies and clear evidence of the detrimental effects of hyperthermia has also been well-established [26–28].

6.3.3 Cerebral Autoregulation (CA)

Within the context of the physiological concepts of cerebral blood flow, CA is an essential homeostatic process of CBF regulation for changing CPP trends. Both intrinsic and extrinsic factors may have an influence on CBF at a given point; however, the brain's ability to ensure a fixed amount of CBF by altering its CVR as mentioned in previous sections, in a nutshell, is what cerebral autoregulation really is.

In the previous century, Bayliss, Hill, and Gulland concluded in *The Journal of Physiology* that "In all physiological conditions a rise in arterial pressure accelerates the flow of blood through the brain, and a fall slackens it." [29] However, in a 1959 landmark publication by Lansen, it was shown that at wide ranges of blood pressure (~ 60–150 mmHg), CBF remained stable, thus debunking a 60-year-old myth [30]. However, this magic figure, as we widely study, has been questioned in the past owing to concerns related to its methodology [31]. Drummond suggested that instead of a window bracket, the only safe approach for an individual patient is that no less than 75% of his or her resting MAP should be assumed to be the lower limit of autoregulation [31]. This eventually led to the concept of individualized CPP-based targeting as opposed to the standard blanket MAP range, especially in pathological brains. An individualized assessment to determine each patient's "optimal" CPP is considered more vital than mere ranges [32–35]. This led to the concept of multimodal neuromonitoring, which is an essential aspect of ensuring an optimal CPP, which goes beyond the concept of this chapter [36].

Testing for cerebral autoregulation is an important cog in a neurocritical setting to look for normalcy in the brain's ability to keep its flow intact. Testing for CA is an area of great interest and can be divided into static and dynamic CA testing. In static CA methods, measurements of MAP and CBF were taken only at baseline (i.e., before the MAP was changed) and after the effect of the challenging mechanism was complete (usually after minutes to hours). Hence, static CA methods failed to study the temporal evolution of the transition in MAP and CBF as they reached their steady-state values. Moreover, these methods suggested CA as a concept to be an all-or-none phenomenon (i.e., either it was present (if CBF recovered to the initial value) or absent (if CBF passively followed the MAP change). This led to the need for dynamic autoregulation testing, which could assess the CBF changes in response to MAP in a matter of seconds.

6.4 Cerebral Blood Flow Monitoring

6.4.1 General Concepts

Some important physical concepts that might help the readers understand the nuances of CBF monitoring are discussed here [37] (Fig. 6.2).

Fick's Principle

Fick's principle, developed in 1870, states that "the total uptake of (or release of) a substance by the peripheral tissues is equal to the product of the blood flow to the peripheral tissues and the arterial-venous concentration difference (gradient) of the substance." This principle, which was originally developed to calculate cardiac output, formed the basis for researchers over the years to use diffusible and physiologically inert materials or tracers to calculate individual organ perfusion, including the brain [38].

Hence, we measure the following as

$$\text{QBt} = \text{Qat} - \text{QVt}$$

where

- QBt is the quantity of tracer taken up by the brain.
- QAt is the quantity of tracer delivered to the brain by the arterial blood.
- QVt is the quantity of tracer inside the venous blood.

Based on Fick's principle,

$$\text{QBt} = \text{CBF} \times f\left(A - V\right)\text{dt}$$

where *A* and *V* are arterial and venous concentrations of the tracer material introduced, respectively.

CBF is cerebral blood flow over time (dt).

This formula can be rearranged to calculate CBF as

$$\text{CBF} = \text{QBt} / f\left(A - V\right)\text{dt}$$

It is important to consider that the molecule or substance used needs to be inert and should not have any reaction.

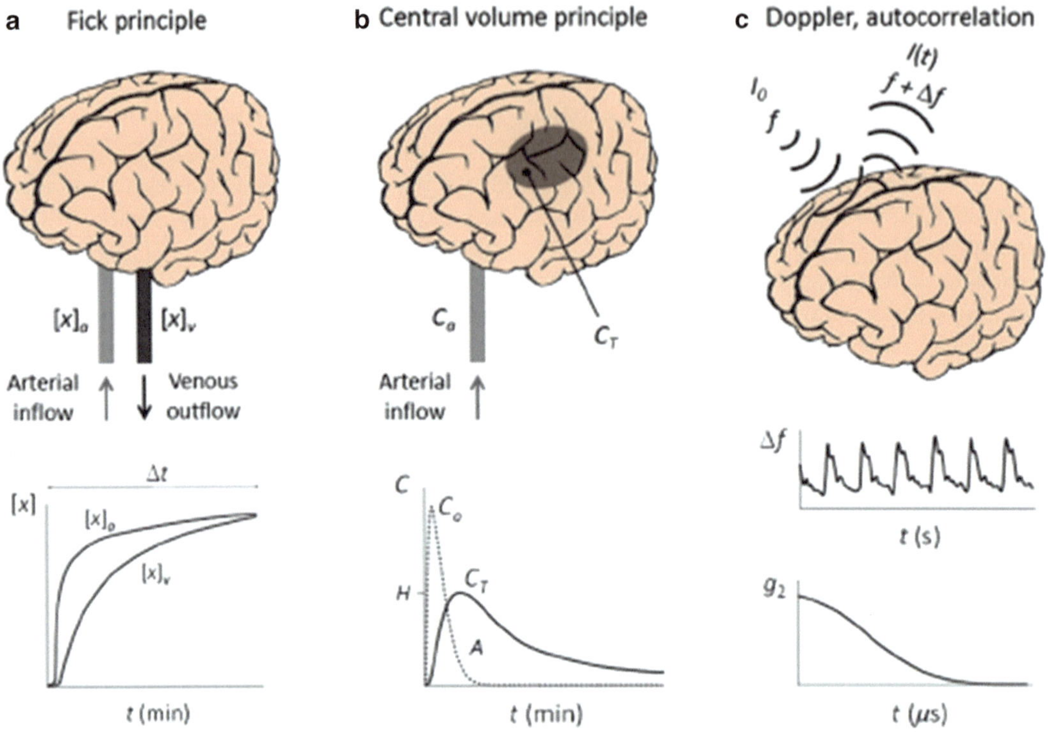

Fig. 6.2 Cerebral blood flow and autoregulation: current measurement techniques and prospects for noninvasive optical methods. (Image source: Fantini et al.)

The Central Volume Principle [37]

The central volume principle, unlike the aforementioned Fick's principle, does not depend on the tracer concentration in venous blood. It purely depends on the tracer concentration that could be directly measured in the brain volume of interest (VOI). A tracer substance that often mixes thoroughly with blood is used, whose concentration in the brain tissue at a given time is derived using both a concentration in the arterial blood and the tracer transit time to reach the VOI in the brain. Impulse residual function, which represents the tracer fraction that remains in the VOI after a given time, is calculated. The infused tracer concentration, the rate of reaching the VOI, and the residual concentration over a given period are all used to calculate the tracer's mean transit time (MTT), which plays an important role in organ perfusion estimates—in this case, CBF. How the method of estimation varies while using a diffusible or a nondiffusible tracer is beyond the scope of this chapter.

The central volume principle is the basis for most of the nuclear medicine, X-ray-, and magnetic resonance imaging (MRI)-based techniques [37].

Doppler Effect and Intensity Fluctuations [37]

Doppler application, using ultrasound (US) or optical waves that interact with the brain tissue at a certain frequency, leads to a frequency shift and a decay rate of the detected wave. The frequency shift is a manifestation of the Doppler effect, whereas intensity fluctuations can be characterized by their decay rate. Blood flow velocity (BFV) and, therefore, CBF are directly related to the Doppler shift (Δf) and to the rate of decay. Hence, it is important to note that Doppler and autocorrelation methods do not measure CBF directly but essentially yield blood flow velocity (Doppler ultrasound in large vessels and laser Doppler flowmetry (LDF) and diffuse correlation spectroscopy (DCS) in microcirculation), which can be eventually used to extrapolate to CBF measurements.

Clinicians need to note that this method purely represents blood flow velocity in the vessels and capillaries alone and not necessarily in the brain tissue per se. This information is vital to keep in mind when interpreting the results. As mentioned, this method is employed by Doppler ultrasound, laser Doppler flowmetry, and diffuse correlation spectroscopy techniques.

6.4.2 Cerebral Blood Flow Monitoring Techniques

Several measurement technologies have evolved over the years to evaluate CBF. Some of the important and most clinically relevant techniques are discussed in this section.

Direct Techniques

A. **The Kety–Schmidt Arteriovenous Difference Method** [39]

Kety and Schmidt, in their landmark work published in 1945, used inhaled nitrous oxide (N_2O) as a freely diffusible intravascular tracer. Inhaled N_2O was measured both from the femoral artery, which was used as the uptake concentrations to the brain, and from the right internal jugular vein, which was used as the uptake end venous concentration to the brain. Readings were obtained in 10 min from the beginning of the inhalation till a steady state was achieved, which was represented by equalization of concentration in both samples. The time taken to reach this steady state was indirectly used to extrapolate CBF by plotting N_2O concentrations in both arterial and venous samples (Fig. 6.3), using the previously mentioned Fick's principle method. CBF is calculated as the quantity of tracer (N_2O) removed by the brain by variations in concentrations over a given time.

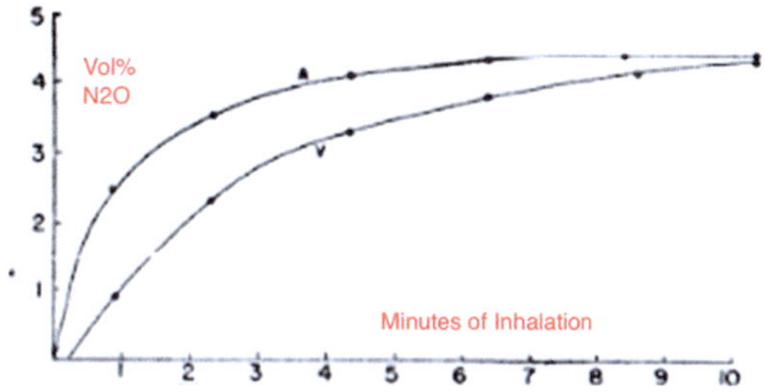

Fig. 6.3 Kety and Schmidt found a value of 62 ± 12 mL/100 g/min in 11 human subjects [39]

Despite being considered a gold standard, some of the drawbacks of the Kety–Schmidt technique are as follows:

- It is invasive.
- It requires repeated blood sampling.
- It is needed for N_2O inhalation and its associated complications.
- It overestimates CBF due to recirculation and diffusion of N_2O.
- It estimates only global CBF and does not take regional CBF (rCBF) measurement, which is important in pathological states.

B. **Radioactive Tracing for CBF Using Fick's Principle**

Radioactive tracers (^{133}Xe and ^{85}Kr) are used to overcome these limitations with N_2O. Xenon has been widely studied in the context of inhalation, intravenous injection, or intra-arterial injection to measure global and regional CBF [40–43]. ^{133}Xe is known to be a good choice for a tracer because of its low solubility in blood, ease of diffusion through cell membranes and the blood–brain barrier (BBB), lack of metabolism, and ease of elimination.

Using these isotopes, radioactivity is measured with an extracranial detector positioned on the patient's scalp to detect radioactive decay values, which are then plotted on a graph over time. Calculating the area under the curve of such variables can yield the CBF.

Furthermore, the utility has been expanded to measure regional CBF using a semilogarithmic scale and a technique called "logarithmic stripping," which can identify a two-compartmental model defined by different curves. The first curve describes the slow component corresponding to white matter blood flow, whereas the second much steeper curve describes a fast component corresponding to gray matter blood flow.

C. **The Jugular Thermodilution Technique** [44]

In the jugular thermodilution technique, as an alternative to intravascular tracers, cold saline, whose temperature is known and constant, is injected at a fixed rate through a thermodilution catheter placed retrograde into the internal jugular vein with the tip positioned at the jugular bulb. The heat lost by the blood equals the heat gained by the cold fluid, which is distally measured by the thermistor system. A graph is then formulated based on the change in the temperature between the saline indicator and the blood mixed with the indicator for jugular blood flow (JBF) (not cerebral blood flow) computation using the formula:

$$\mathrm{JBF} = \mathrm{Fi} \times 1.1 \times [\mathrm{Tm} - \mathrm{Ti}] / [\mathrm{Tb} - \mathrm{Tm}]$$

where Fi = flow rate of the indicator, 1.1 = constant for saline, Tm = temperature of the mixture, Tb = temperature of blood, and Ti = temperature of the indicator in Celsius. Thereafter, CBF is calculated in mL/min/100 g using the formula:

$$\mathrm{JBF} \times 2 \times \frac{100}{\text{Brain weight in grams}}$$

The jugular thermodilution technique is an able bedside technique that can be used in critical care patients for continuous or intermittent monitoring with reasonable amounts of accuracy compared to the gold-standard techniques [45]. It is safe and does not need radioactive or toxic trace elements, both of which are its biggest advantages. However, there are a few minor drawbacks such as:

- The need for jugular vein catheterization and associated complications.
- The need for injection of a fluid indicator, which can be a limiting factor in patients who cannot handle much fluid load.
- CBF is an extrapolated value based on JBF.

6.4.3 Imaging-Based CBF Techniques

With technological advancements in today's day and age, imaging technologies provide one of the largest sources of noninvasive or semi-invasive imaging modalities. Despite the perceived advantage of being minimally invasive, image-based CBF calculations generally provide a snapshot of the CBF alone.

X-Ray-Based Techniques

A. **Xenon-Enhanced Computed Tomography (CT)** [46]

In this method, patients are advised to inhale 30% xenon, an inert, radiopaque, nonradioactive gas, which can diffuse freely across the BBB. Considering its radiopaque nature, xenon's radiodensity is appreciable on CT imaging, and, with subsequent scanning, changes in radiodensity are studied to quantify CBF. The presence and clearance of xenon from various brain regions (gray and white matter) can be used to plot brain washout curves. These curves have varied washout compartments, which help in identifying different washout rates in each part of the brain. Since the tracer concentration in the brain can be assessed based on radiodensity, the need for venous sampling as seen with Fick's principle is not warranted.

Xenon-enhanced CT offers other advantages like simultaneously evaluating for BBB's integrity, as a gross indicator of cerebral perfusion apart from CBF quantification. Despite being an imaging-based study (which is often considered to provide a mere snapshot), xenon-enhanced CT can also be used in dynamic studies to evaluate therapy or in cerebrovascular reserve assessment. With the advent of portable CT machine-enabled systems, it is now possible to conduct these studies in the operating room (OR) as well as in neurocritical care settings [47].

However, a major limitation of Xe-enhanced CT is its difficulty in assessing CBF in the posterior fossa and infratentorial regions and highly sensitive motion artifacts [48].

B. **CT Perfusion (CTP)**

Over time, CTP, which was originally developed for evaluating an ischemic stroke, was extended for its usefulness in patients with traumatic brain injury (TBI) to identify hypoperfusion. It works on the central volume principle in which a nondiffusible iodinated contrast agent is introduced into the bloodstream and its concentration changes with sequential CT imaging (often performed at 1-s apart). Time–concentration curves of the contrast bolus are constructed, which are used to generate relevant data such as cerebral blood volume (CBV), mean transit time (MTT), cerebral blood flow (CBF), and time to peak (TTP) [49, 50].

The central volume principle using CTP can be used to express CBF using CBV and MTT as CBF = CBV ÷ MTT. Despite the existing methodology of quantitative CBF assessment using said variables, CTP is still largely considered a qualitative monitor for CBF. Questions remain regarding the accuracy and reproducibility of CBF assessment using CTP because of which it is seldom used alone to monitor CBF assessment and is more of a suggestive aid for CBF than an absolute indicator.

MRI-Based Techniques

A. **Perfusion-Weighted MRI**

MRI measurements of CBF can be brought about by gadolinium boluses to estimate CBF. Gadolinium contrast remains intravascular in an intact BBB; hence, after a bolus dosing, the presence of a contrast in the vascular spaces brings about a magnetic field gradient between the capillaries with the contrast and the surrounding tissues. This drop in intensity grows with subsequent imaging, leading to gradual signal intensity loss, especially in T2-weighted imaging [51]. This drop in signal is majorly dependent on the intravascular concentration, which is used to calculate CBV (proportional to the A-V concentration gradient of the contrast) and mean transit time, which is used to quantitate CBF using the central volume principle, CBF = CBV/MTT [52].

Perfusion-weighted imaging has been safely used as a quantitative indicator of CBF in the past where an average global CBF of 55 ± 5 mL/100 g/min has been elucidated in healthy human subjects [53]. Compared to CT, perfusion-weighted MRI studies produce superior functional images and also have a lesser incidence of contrast adverse effects. However, in patients with impaired kidney injury, it is known to cause nephrogenic systemic fibrosis [54]. Several gadolinium-free contrast materials have been investigated like organic radical contrast agents (ORCAs), which are said to have lower cytotoxicity and higher biodegradability, thus rendering a lower side effect profile [55]. However, their applications in CBF assessment are currently lacking. On the other hand, a few drawbacks such as longer duration, patient shifting concerns, and claustrophobia do pose a concern. Hence, currently, MR perfusion lacks widespread agreement as an investigative tool and as a sole CBF monitor owing to its practical and technical limitations; however, it can be used as a suggestive tool wherever feasible.

B. **Arterial Spin Labeling (ASL)**

In comparison to perfusion MRI, ASL does not use any extrinsic contrast, thus rendering it a noninvasive technique. By applying MR-based radio-frequency inversion pulses, arterial blood water is magnetically labeled and used as an intrinsic contrast. Because water is diffusible across the BBB, these labeled water molecules enter the brain tissues and alter the total tissue magnetization in the region of interest (ROI), leading to a reduction in MR signal and image intensity, which is captured by an MR image called the "tag" image. After some time, another T1 image, called the control image, is acquired in the same slice but without magnetization; this image has a higher signal intensity than the tag image due to the lack of the negative effect caused by labeled water molecules. Using a subtraction process, this difference in signal intensity and magnetization is used to plot a perfusion map to deduce CBF [56]. Hence, to simplify, ASL measures local CBF by quantifying the decrease in tissue magnetization caused by the inflow of magnetically labeled blood that carries negative magnetization due to inversion.

ASL provides reliable and reproducible CBF data without any risk of contrast administration or ionizing radiation, which means that it can be safely used for CBF assessment across all age groups. ASL is used to assess various perfusion defects like hemispheric perfusion deficits, postischemic hyperperfusion, or perfusion–diffusion mismatches [57]. It remains one of the forerunners of CBF evaluation and monitoring in the near future as a standard of practice owing to its noninvasive nature, low signal-to-noise ratio per unit time, and reduced ionizing risks [58]. However, the biggest drawback of ASL is its underestimation of CBF, especially if the flow to the tissue has associated unspecified collateral pathways, which may need addressing in the future.

Ultrasonography (USG)-Based Techniques

A. **Transcranial Doppler (TCD)**

TCD uses a 2-MHz probe to determine the blood flow velocity (not CBF directly) of the basal cerebral arteries based on the principles of Doppler shift. It is a real-time, noninvasive, bedside analyzer of blood flow velocity, which could serve as an important surrogate for CBF (qualitatively). In TCD, the sound waves emitted by the probe are reflected off the moving red blood cells (RBCs), which are captured back by the transducer to analyze the RBC velocity, which, in turn, is a function of blood flow velocity [59].

The major advantages of TCD use include being bedside and noninvasive, having a smaller learning curve, use of portable machines, low cost, and lack of radiation exposure. However, considering that only the major vessels are being studied and represented, its estimation of CBF may be widely inaccurate. The correlation between CBF and blood flow velocity is highly variable and may often get confounded in various disease processes, vessel caliber, and operator dependence [60]. Vessel characteristics play a huge role in their correlation, for example, a decrease in vessel caliber can increase BFV (suggesting hyperemia) in the face of decreasing CBF. Therefore, it is important to note that not all increments in Cerebral Blood Flow Velocity (CBFV) necessitate an increase in CBF, or vice versa [61].

TCD is not a quantitative flow monitor in mL/100 g/min; instead, it provides suggestive information, which, based on clinical correlation, can elucidate meaningful interpretations. Few situations in which TCD changes may reflect changes in CBF may be seen in conditions with abrupt changes in arterial flows [62]. TCD has been used to monitor CBF in patients with cardiopulmonary bypass, carotid endarterectomy, head injury, vasospasm, and brain death and in post-resuscitation survivors [63, 64].

B. **Transit Time Ultrasonic Flowmetry**

This is an intraoperative ultrasound technique to measure flow in an isolated blood vessel using a perivascular flow probe in a surgical setting. This probe is placed longitudinally along the vessel length while an acoustic reflector is placed on the opposite side. The probe measures the transit times of the ultrasonic waves in both directions (upstream and downstream) concerning the blood flow. The difference in transit times recorded is proportional to the blood volumes in the vessel and is used to estimate the vessel blood flow. CBF calculations can be derived by estimating the brain tissue mass supplied by the artery in contention. However, VBF is only a relative measure of CBF. This technique has been used in the quantification of blood flow through individual vessels during aneurysm surgeries but is not a monitor for CBF assessment per se [65].

C. **Thermal Diffusion Flowmetry (TDF)**

TDF uses heat or a temperature gradient to measure blood flow through tissues, referred to as the heat or thermal clearance method. It works on the assumption that thermal conductivity without flow is constant; hence, the degree of heat dissipation would be proportional to blood flow through the organ of interest [66]. TDF uses an invasive cortical probe comprising two metallic thermistors placed on the cortical tissue, which uses the aforementioned technique to measure the regional blood flow in the brain parenchyma over a spherical volume of 20–30 mm^3 [67]. Among the two thermistors, the neural plate is the passive one, which measures brain temperature, and the heated plate is an active plate placed at a higher temperature, whose measure of temperature changes helps in regional CBF calculation.

Despite its invasiveness, TDF is a simple and effective technique providing real-time, continuous CBF assessment. Although it covers an extremely small area of interest, it provides valuable information about the areas of concern in specific disease pathologies. CBF values obtained using TDF are often relative; however, when calibrated with ^{133}Xe or Xe-enhanced CT, absolute CBF can be measured.

In neurocritical care settings, TDF has been used to check for CA in TBI patients and also to assess regional blood flow in aneurysmal surgery patients [68, 69]. Despite its advantages, TDF is associated with local tissue damage, bleeding, infections and sensitivity to movements, and temperature, which cause significant artifacts.

6.4.4 Optical Techniques

A. **Laser Doppler Flowmetry (LDF)** [70, 71]

LDF is a continuous monitoring technique based on the Doppler principle to measure relative changes in CBF [72, 73]. It is an invasive technique in which a flexible fiberoptic probe is inserted through a burr hole or craniotomy, emitting monochromatic light in a wavelength range of 670–810 nm, which gets scattered by various tissues in the path. The nonmoving brain tissues will reflect this light with the same wavelengths, whereas the moving RBCs will cause a Doppler shift, which gets picked by the photodetector. This Doppler shift of light is proportional to the velocity and the number of RBCs involved in the interaction, which is translated into a time-varying voltage that is used to compute CBF. Hence, at an acceptable hemoglobin range, the shift change is purely considered due to the speed or flow.

Clinically, LDF has been used to assess CA, CO_2 reactivity, and responses to therapeutic interventions [67, 74].

The advantages of LDF, such as being continuous, bedside, dynamic, and non-radioactive, are often overshadowed by its disadvantages, such as its ability to analyze only a small sample volume of the brain, (assessed to be about 1 mm^3), under-representation of CBF when measuring ischemic zones, higher movement artifacts, and, most importantly, its invasive nature and associated complications [75]. Hence, caution should be exercised when making assumptions about global CBF purely based on LDF values. Another major drawback that could be a reason for its lower popularity could be that CBF is not expressed as absolute flow values (milliliters/grams/minute) but in LD units relative to the initial values.

B. **Diffuse Correlation Spectroscopy (DCS)**

DCS has a similar functional principle to LDF but uses near-infrared (NIR) light, is a noninvasive device, which is placed on the subject's head, and also covers a greater tissue volume than does LDF [76]. Like LDF,

NIR light is scattered by the background brain tissue and moving RBCs, which is measured by the optical detector system. The intensity of the reflected light detected is run through an autocorrelator system that computes the intensity based on the photon's (NIR light) arrival time, which is used to derive the blood flow index (BFI) using the correlation diffusion equation and the Brownian diffusion coefficient. This blood flow index, in comparison with baseline BFIs, is used to assess CBF changes. It is important to remember that relative changes in blood flow have been considered to be more accurate using DCS than absolute quantification [77].

DCS is a relatively newer method for CBF monitoring, which has been reasonably studied in neurocritical patients and neonates [78–80]. Currently, DCS shows immense promise to be a portable, low-cost monitor in near future with diverse clinical and bedside indications [81, 82].

DCS has been used with NIR spectroscopy (NIRS) monitors as well [83].

C. **Near-Infrared Spectroscopy (NIRS)** [84]

NIRS is an optical, noninvasive, bedside monitor used to indirectly estimate brain oxygenation and perfusion. It works on the principle similar to that mentioned in the previous section. Near Infrared Light (NIR) light is emitted onto the brain tissue through a scalp probe, which is eventually detected by a photodetector, usually at a distance of 4–7 cm from the emitter. Using Beer–Lambert's law, cerebral hemodynamics can be quantified based on the relative concentrations of chromophores inside the area of interest [85]. It is a diffuse optical method, which is sensitive to differential absorption rates of NIR light by oxyhemoglobin, [HbO_2], and deoxyhemoglobin [Hb]. This is used to compute rSo^2, which is an essential indicator of brain oxygenation. Normal rSo^2 is 60–80%, and a decrease to below 47% has been associated with ischemia, which could act as an indirect, qualitative CBF monitor.

NIRS technologies are used as quantitative CBF monitors using tracer tracking techniques in which endogenous oxyhemoglobin (HbO) or exogenous indocyanine green (ICG) is used. With oxyhemoglobin, a brief lowering of the inspired oxygen fraction followed by a steep rise leads to a sudden rise in oxyhemoglobin concentration in the blood, which acts as a bolus that can be used to extrapolate CBF using Fick's principle [86]. Similar quantification can be performed after ICG administration and using Fick's principle [87]. In a few instances, DCS was used to quantitate relative CBF changes in combination with ICG and time-resolved NIRS measurements [88].

D. **Optical Microangiography (OMAG)** [89]

OMAG is an emerging noninvasive technique for measuring tissue blood flow by producing three-dimensional (3D) images of blood perfusion based on endogenous light scattering due to moving blood tissues. Hence, the biggest advantage is the nonutility of exogenous contrast material. However, clinical studies are lacking in their routine utility.

6.4.5 Nuclear Medicine-Based Techniques

1. **Positron Emission Tomography (PET)**

PET is an imaging technique that provides in vivo quantitative measurements of CBF and various other metabolic parameters using positron emitter radiotracers. After the administration of radiotracers, PET detects the concentration inside the tissues based on the gamma rays emitted by the colliding positrons. These data are processed using algorithms to reconstruct a map of each reaction, which is graphically reconstructed into a PET image [90]. As opposed to the CT perfusion mentioned above, PET uses diffusible tracers like ^{15}O-labeled water for CBF quantification and (^{18}F)-2-fluoro-2-deoxy-D-glucose for the quantitative determination of the cerebral metabolic rate of glucose utilization [91, 92]. Following the injection of the desired amount of tracers, emission scans are repeated for radioactivity usually for 10 min and images are acquired.

The main advantage of PET is its high-resolution images expressing quantitative measurements of CBF and metabolism because of which it is currently considered the gold standard for studying cerebral hemodynamics. However, high cost, logistic unavailability, and patient transport concerns have made it a cumbersome task to measure CBF, especially in intensive care patients.

2. **Single-Photon Emission Computed Tomography (SPECT)**

SPECT is a functional nuclear imaging modality like PET in which instead of a positron emitter, a gamma emitter radiotracer is used, examples of which are hexamethylpropyleneamine oxime (HMPAO) or ethyl cysteine dimer (ECD), labeled with the radioisotope technetium-99 m [93]. These radiotracers pass through the BBB and are metabolized and retained intracellularly. This retention is proportional to CBF that can be formulated based on gamma emissions, which the SPECT scanner picks up to generate a three-dimensional image [94]. By comparing the photo emissions of different brain regions, relative CBF can be assessed. Hence, SPECT provides a semi-quantitative CBF measurement. Other advantages of SPECT are that it is noninvasive and produces accurate values of both global CBF and rCBF. However, the disadvantages of PET such as being expensive along with its logistical issues, bear true for SPECT as well.

SPECT/CT is a newer imaging modality that upholds a dual functionality, providing both functional and anatomical information for a single examination.

6.4.6 Monitoring Cerebral Autoregulation

CA testing remains the single most essential feature in the neurocritical management of pathological brains. Various techniques of CA testing have been proposed, which can be grouped as follows:

A. **TCD-Based Analysis for CA**

TCD provides a dynamic, continuous assessment of CA in patients while analyzing cerebral blood velocity changes in response to changes in MAP. This is based on determining the correlation coefficient between blood flow velocity (BFV) and arterial blood pressure (ABP) in real time. As mentioned in the previous sections, when CA is intact, despite fluctuations in blood pressure, BFV will remain constant. In other words, the lack of correlation between BFV and ABP denotes an intact autoregulation.

Similarly, when CA is disrupted, there would be a positive correlation between BFV and ABP, that is, an increase in ABP would increase BFV, and vice versa. TCD guidance to assess CA has been widely used in the past in TBI and stroke patients [32, 95].

B. **ICP-Based Autoregulation Testing for CA**

Under normal circumstances, ICP stays in the normal range despite blood pressure changes due to the presence of intact cerebral autoregulation. In patients with cerebral dysregulation, as seen in brain injuries, there is an increase in ICP secondary to an increase in ABP. This principle led to the development of the cerebrovascular Pressure Reactivity Index (PRx), which studies the dynamic correlation between ICP and ABP to assess the presence or absence of cerebral autoregulation [34]. This principle has been used to determine an "optimal CPP" to enable perfusion without inadvertently increasing ICP in head injury patients [33]. PRx-guided management in such patients has been associated with better outcomes.

These indices prove crucial in choosing the right amount of CPP targets since effective head injury management involves a delicate balance between avoiding hypotension-associated hypoperfusion and hypertension-associated edema/ICP, which was historically deemed difficult [34].

6.4.7 Newer Advances

Microwave-Based CBF Analysis

After being introduced to detect strokes, tumor bleeds, etc., microwave technologies have shown potential as a monitoring device for cerebral circulation [96–98].

1. **Microwave Detection of Temperature and Conductivity**

   Microwave radiometry is used to sense thermal radiation emitted by the brain secondary to changes in blood flow. This is a multi-antenna setup placed on the head for sensing radiation and uses these received signals for detecting blood flow variations. Fluid movements within the organ such as the brain would produce thermal changes, which are used to compute flow across the organ [99].
2. **Microwave Detection of Blood Volume**

   In this approach, blood volume change is detected to extrapolate blood flow. Similar to the previous technique, scalp antennas detect changes in blood volume between the antennae located around the head by detecting electromagnetic (EM) propagation. The time of flight (ToF) calculated between the antennae reflects the local changes in blood volume, which, in turn, helps calculate the blood flow.

This technique was originally used to detect brain hemorrhage, which has further shown promise in CBF detection [97].

Ultrasound-Tagged (UT)-NIRS

Newer techniques such as ultrasound-tagged NIRS to compute blood flow using a phenomenon called the acousto-optic effect have been developed, in which a low-power US transducer is used to modulate NIR photons. This modulation exerts a Doppler effect on the blood flow. [100, 101] Simply put, when tagged NIR photons collide with blood, it leads to a frequency shift that is used as an indicator of BF. This UT-NIRS system is said to be an able real-time technique, with additional features such as adjusting depth, which can change the focus point of the US transducer with a modifiable area of interest. UT-NIRS provides a cerebral flow index (CFI), a unitless number from 0 to 100, which reflects CBF [102]. Despite the seeming advantages, UT-NIRS has not been validated. Few isolated validation studies, which were conducted with other non-invasive devices like TCD, have shown that the cerebral flow velocity index with UT-NIRS detected changes in CBF only during hypercarbia, but not hypocarbia, in healthy subjects. Thus, more studies are needed for its validation [100].

6.5 Conclusion

Currently, various technologies with varied working principles are available for cerebral blood flow monitoring in the perioperative period and in the intensive care unit (ICU). There is a range of options for CBF measurements in terms of quantification, noninvasiveness, portability, and rapidity. However, the one perfect monitor that has all the above attributes while making data readily available at the bedside, is still oblivious.

With the rapidly emerging technologies, multimodality in monitoring, and widespread data integration systems, the role of CBF monitoring has become more essential than ever. Growing technological advancements show significant potential for research and development to develop ideal, portable, low-cost, real-time CBF and CA monitoring devices in future. These monitors will not only help us understand the clinical course but may also aid in understanding various neurological conditions and their overall outcomes at a much larger scale.

References

1. Jensen P. Uber die blutversorgung des gehirns pfluegers. Arch Ges Physiol. 1904;103:171–95.
2. Kety SS. Blood-tissue exchange methods. Theory of blood tissue exchange and its applications in measurement of blood flow. Methods Med Res. 1960;8:223–7.
3. Purves D, Augustine GJ, Fitzpatrick D, et al., editors. Neuroscience. 2nd ed. Sunderland, MA: Sinauer Associates; 2001. The blood supply of the brain and spinal cord.

4. Tzeng YC, Ainslie PN. Blood pressure regulation IX: cerebral autoregulation under blood pressure challenges. Eur J Appl Physiol. 2014;114:545–59.
5. Lassen NA. Normal average value of cerebral blood flow in younger adults is 50 ml/100 g/min. J Cereb Blood Flow Metab. 1985;5:347–9.
6. Vavilala MS, Lee LA, Lam AM. Cerebral blood flow and vascular physiology. Anesthesiol Clin N Am. 2002;20:247–64.
7. Kety SS, Schmidt CF. The effects of altered arterial tensions of carbon dioxide and oxygen on cerebral blood flow and cerebral oxygen consumption of normal young men. J Clin Invest. 1948;27(4):484–92.
8. Ursino M, Lodi CA. A simple mathematical model of the interaction between intracranial pressure and cerebral hemodynamics. J Appl Physiol (1985) 1997;82(4):1256–1269.
9. Peterson EC, Wang Z, Britz G. Regulation of cerebral blood flow. Int J Vasc Med. 2011;2011:823525.
10. Kuschinsky M. Coupling of blood flow and metabolism in the brain. J Basic Clin Physiol Pharmacol. 1990;1:191–201.
11. Heistad DD, Marcus ML, Abboud FM. Role of large arteries in regulation of cerebral blood flow in dogs. J Clin Invest. 1978;62:761–8.
12. Gokina NI, Park KM, McElroy-Yaggy K, Osol G. Effects of rho kinase inhibition on cerebral artery myogenic tone and reactivity. J Appl Physiol. 2005;98:1940–8.
13. Knot HJ, Nelson MT. Regulation of arterial diameter and wall [Ca2+] in cerebral arteries of rat by membrane potential and intravascularpressure. J Physiol. 1998;508:199–209.
14. Roy CS, Sherrington CS. On the regulation of the blood-supply of the brain. J Physiol. 1890;11:85–158.
15. Magistretti PJ. Neuron–glia metabolic coupling and plasticity. J Exp Biol. 2006;209:2304–11.
16. Girouard H, Iadecola C. Neurovascular coupling in the normal brain and in hypertension, stroke, and Alzheimer disease. J Appl Physiol. 2006;100:328–35.
17. Bor-Seng-Shu E, et al. Cerebral hemodynamics: concepts of clinical importance. Arq Neuropsiquiatr. 2012;70:357–65.
18. Iadecola. Neurovascular regulation in the normal brain and in Alzheimer's disease. Nat Rev Neurosci. 2004;5:347–60.
19. Battisti-Charbonney A, Fisher J, Duffin J. The cerebrovascular response to carbon dioxide in humans. J Physiol. 2011;589:3039–48.
20. Hggendal E, Johansson B. Effects of arterial carbon dioxide tension and oxygen saturation on cerebral blood flow autoregulation in dogs. Acta Physiol Scand Suppl. 1965;258:27–53.
21. Ogoh S, Sato K, Nakahara H, Okazaki K, Subudhi AW, Miyamoto T. Effect of acute hypoxia on blood flow in vertebral and internal carotid arteries. Exp Physiol. 2013;98:692–8.
22. Massik J, Tang YL, Hudak ML, Koehler RC, Traystman RJ, Jones MD Jr. Effect of hematocrit on cerebral blood flow with induced polycythemia. J Appl Physiol. 1987;62(1090–6):38.
23. Crystal GJ, Salem MR. Myocardial and systemic hemodynamics during isovolemic hemodilution alone and combined with nitroprusside-induced controlled hypotension. Anesth Analg. 1991;72:227–37.
24. Ehrlich MP, McCullough JN, Zhang N, Weisz DJ, Juvonen T, Bodian CA, Griepp RB. Effect of hypothermia on cerebral blood flow and metabolism in the pig. Ann Thorac Surg. 2002;73:191–7.
25. Nybo L, Mller K, Volianitis S, Nielsen B, Secher NH. Effects of hyperthermia on cerebral blood flow and metabolism during prolonged exercise in humans. J Appl Physiol. 1985;93:58–64.
26. Clifton GL, Valadka A, Zygun D, et al. Very early hypothermia induction in patients with severe brain injury (the National Acute Brain Injury Study: hypothermia II): a randomised trial. Lancet Neurol. 2011;10(2):131–9. https://doi.org/10.1016/S1474-4422(10)70300-8.
27. Andrews PJ, Sinclair HL, Rodriguez A, et al. Hypothermia for intracranial hypertension after traumatic brain injury. N Engl J Med. 2015;373(25):2403–12. https://doi.org/10.1056/NEJMoa1507581.
28. Truettner JS, Bramlett HM, Dalton Dietrich W. Hyperthermia and mild traumatic brain injury: effects on inflammation and the cerebral vasculature. J Neurotrauma. 2018;35:940–52.
29. Bayliss WM, Hill L, Gulland GL. On intracranial pressure and the cerebral circulation: part I. Physiological; Part II. Histological J Physiol. 1895;18:334–62.
30. Lassen NA. Cerebral blood flow and oxygen consumption in man. Physiol Rev. 1959;39:183–238.
31. Drummond JC. The lower limit of autoregulation: time to revise our thinking? Anesthesiology. 1997;86(6):1431–3.
32. Czosnyka M, Smielewski P, Piechnik S, Steiner LA, Pickard JD. Cerebral autoregulation following head injury. J Neurosurg 2001;95(5):756–63. 35.
33. Steiner LA, Czosnyka M, Piechnik SK, et al. Continuous monitoring of cerebrovascular pressure reactivity allows determination of optimal cerebral perfusion pressure in patients with traumatic brain injury. Crit Care Med 2002;30(4):733–8.36.
34. Zweifel C, Lavinio A, Steiner LA, et al. Continuous monitoring of cerebrovascular pressure reactivity in patients with head injury. Neurosurg Focus. 2008;25(4):E2. 37.
35. Czosnyka M, Brady K, Reinhard M, Smielewski P, Steiner LA. Monitoring of cerebrovascular autoregulation: facts, myths, and missing links. Neurocrit Care. 2009;10(3):373–86. https://doi.org/10.1007/s12028-008-9175-7.
36. De Georgia MA, Deogaonkar A. Multimodal monitoring in the neurological intensive care unit. Neurologist. 2005;11(1):45–54.
37. Fantini S, Sassaroli A, Tgavalekos KT, Kornbluth J. Cerebral blood flow and autoregulation: cur-

rent measurement techniques and prospects for noninvasive optical methods. Neurophoton. 2016;3(3):031411. https://doi.org/10.1117/1.NPh.3.3.031411.
38. Torbey MT, Bhardwaj A. Cerebral blood flow physiology and monitoring. In: Suarez JI, editor. Critical care neurology and neurosurgery. Humana Press Inc.; 2004.
39. Kety SS, Schmidt CF. The determination of cerebral blood flow in man by the use of nitrous oxide in low concentrations. Am J Phys. 1945;143:53–66.
40. Obrist WD, Thompson HK Jr, King CH, et al. Determination of regional cerebral blood flow by inhalation of 133-xenon. Circ Res. 1967;20(1):124–35.
41. Obrist W, Thompson H, Wang H. A subtraction method for determining CBF by xenon-133 inhalation. Neurology. 1970;20(4):411.
42. Obrist W, Thompson HJ, Wang H, Wilkinson W. Regional CBF estimated by 133-xenon inhalation. Stroke. 1975;6(3):245–56.
43. Obrist WD, Wilkinson WE. Regional cerebral blood flow measurement in humans by xenon-133 clearance. Cerebrovasc Brain Metab Rev. 1990;2(4):283–327.
44. Wilson EM, Halsey JH. Bilateral jugular venous blood flow by thermal dilution. Stroke. 1970;1:348–55.
45. Mélot C, Berré J, Moraine JJ, Kahn RJ. Estimation of cerebral blood flow at the bedside by continuous jugular thermodilution. J Cereb Blood Flow Metab. 1996;16:1263–70.
46. Johnson DW, et al. Stable xenon CT cerebral blood flow imaging: rationale for and role in clinical decision making. AJNR. 1991;12:201–13.
47. Sturnegk P, Mellergard P, Yonas H, Theodorsson A, Hillman J. Potential use of quantitative bedside CBF monitoring Xe-CT for decision making in neurosurgical intensive care. Br J Neurosurg. 2007;21(4):332–9.
48. Carlson AP, Brown AM, Zager E, Uchino K, Marks MP, Robertson C, et al. Xenon-enhanced cerebral blood flow at 28% xenon provides uniquely safe access to quantitative, clinically useful cerebral blood flow information: a multicenter study. AJNR Am J Neuroradiol. 2011;32(7):1315–20.
49. Leiva-Salinas C, Provenzale JM, Wintermark M. Responses to the 10 most frequently asked questions about perfusion CT. AJR Am J Roentgenol 2011;196(1):53–60. 143.
50. Hoeffner EG, et al. Cerebral perfusion CT: technique and clinical applications. Radiology. 2004;231:632–44.
51. Xiao YD, Paudel R, Liu J, Ma C, Zhang ZS, Zhou SK. MRI contrast agents: classification and application (review). Int J Mol Med. 2016;38(5):1319–26.
52. Østergaard L, et al. High-resolution measurement of cerebral blood flow using intravascular tracer bolus passages. Part I: mathematical approach and statistical analysis. Magn Res Med. 1996;36:715–25.
53. Li T-Q, et al. Quantification of cerebral blood flow by bolus tracking and artery spin tagging methods. Magn Res Imag. 2000;18:503–12.
54. Marckmann P, Skov L, Rossen K, Dupont A, Damholt MB, Heaf JG, et al. Nephrogenic systemic fibrosis: suspected causative role of gadodiamide used for contrast-enhanced magnetic resonance imaging. J Am Soc Nephrol. 2006;17(9):2359–62.
55. Lee H, Shahrivarkevishahi A, Lumata JL, Luzuriaga MA, Hagge LM, Benjamin CE, et al. Supramolecular and bio macromolecular enhancement of metal-free magnetic resonance imaging contrast agents. Chem Sci. 2020;11(8):2045–50.
56. Van Laar PJ, van der Grond J, Hendrikse J. Brain perfusion territory imaging: methods and clinical applications of selective arterial spin-labelling MR imaging. Radiology. 2008;246:354–64.
57. Chen J, Licht DJ, Smith SE, Agner SC, Mason S, Wang S, et al. Arterial spin labelling perfusion MRI in pediatric arterial ischemic stroke: initial experiences. J Magn Reson Imaging. 2009;29(2):282–90.
58. Telischak NA, Detre JA, Zaharchuk G. Arterial spin labelling MRI: clinical applications in the brain. J Magn Reson Imaging. 2015;41(5):1165–80.
59. Brauer P, Kochs E, Werner C, et al. Correlation of transcranial Doppler sonography mean flow velocity with cerebral blood flow in patients with intracranial pathology. J Neurosurg Anesthesiol. 1998;10(2):80–5.
60. Bishop CC, Powell S, Rutt D, Browse NL. Transcranial Doppler measurement of middle cerebral artery blood flow velocity: a validation study. Stroke. 1986;17:913–5.
61. Otis S. Chapter 4: Pitfalls in transcranial Doppler diagnosis. In: Babikian V, Wechsler L, editors. Transcranial Doppler ultrasonography. St. Louis: Mosby; 1993. p. 39–50.
62. Kofke W, Brauer P, Policare R, Penthany S, Barker D, Horton J. Middle cerebral artery blood flow velocity and stable xenon-enhanced computed tomographic blood flow during balloon test occlusion of the internal carotid artery. Stroke. 1995;26:1603–6.
63. Salvadori A, Pasquier P, Jarrassier A, Schaal JV, Mérat S. Transcranial Doppler to measure cerebral blood flow in management of traumatic brain injury. Injury. 2014;45:1801–2.
64. Jimenez CF, Padro PP, Garcia AS, Venegas JC. Cerebral blood flow is measured by transcranial doppler ultrasound during manual chest wall or automated LUCAS-2 compressions during cardiopulmonary resuscitations. Emergencias. 2012;24:47–9.
65. Charbel FT, et al. Quantitative assessment of vessel flow integrity for aneurysm surgery. J Neurosurg. 1999;91:1050–4.
66. Carter LP. Thermal diffusion flowmetry. Neurosurg Clin N Am. 1996;7(4):749–54.
67. Bhatia A, Gupta AK. Neuromonitoring in the intensive care unit. I. Intracranial pressure and cerebral blood flow monitoring. Intensive Care Med.

2007;33(7):1263–71. https://doi.org/10.1007/s00134-007-0678-z.
68. Rosenthal G, et al. Incorporating a parenchymal thermal diffusion cerebral blood flow probe in bedside assessment of cerebral autoregulation and vasoreactivity in patients with severe traumatic brain injury. J Neurosurg. 2011;114(1):62–70.
69. Verdú-López F, González-Darder JM, González-López P, Botella Macia L. Using thermal diffusion flowmetry in the assessment of regional cerebral blood flow in cerebral aneurysm microsurgery. Neurocirugia (Astur). 2010;21(5):373–80.
70. Rajan V, Varghese B, van Leeuwen TG, et al. Review of methodological developments in laser Doppler flowmetry. Lasers Med Sci. 2009;24(2):269–83.
71. Haberl RL, Villringer A, Dirnagl U. Applicability of laser-Doppler flowmetry for cerebral blood flow monitoring in neurological intensive care. Acta Neurochir Suppl (Wien). 1993;59:64–8.
72. Dirnagl U, et al. Continuous measurement of cerebral cortical blood flow by laser-Doppler flowmetry in a rat stroke model. J Cereb Blood Flow Metab. 1989;9:589–56.
73. Stern MD. In vivo evaluation of microcirculation by coherent light scattering. Nature. 1975;254:56–8.
74. Kirkpatrick PJ, et al. Continuous monitoring of cortical perfusion by laser Doppler flowmetry in ventilated patients with a head injury. J Neurol Neurosurg Psychiatry. 1994;57(11):1382–8.
75. Le Roux P. Invasive neurological and multimodality monitoring in the neuro ICU. In: Layon AJ, Gabrielli A, Friedman WA, editors. Textbook of Neurointensive care. London: Springer; 2013. p. 127–45.
76. Durduran T, Yodh AG. Diffuse correlation spectroscopy for non-invasive, micro-vascular cerebral blood flow measurement. NeuroImage. 2014;85:51–63.
77. Buckley EM, et al. Diffuse correlation spectroscopy for measurement of cerebral blood flow: future prospects. Neurophotonics. 2014;1(1):011009.
78. Selb J, Wu K-C, Sutin J, Lin P-YI, Farzam P, Bechek S, et al. Prolonged monitoring of cerebral blood flow and autoregulation with diffuse correlation spectroscopy in neurocritical care patients. Neurophotonics. 2018;5(4):045005.
79. Ferradal SL, Yuki K, Vyas R, Ha CG, Yi F, Stopp C, et al. Non-invasive assessment of cerebral blood flow and oxygen metabolism in neonates during hypothermic cardiopulmonary bypass: feasibility and clinical implications. Sci Rep. 2017;7(1):44117.
80. Ferrari M, Quaresima V. The future of noninvasive neonatal brain assessment: the measure of cerebral blood flow by diffuse correlation spectroscopy in combination with near-infrared spectroscopy oximetry. J Perinatol. 2021;41(11):2690–1.
81. Khalid M, Khalid M, Milej D, Milej D, Rajaram A, Rajaram A, et al. Development of a stand-alone DCS system for monitoring absolute cerebral blood flow. Biomed Opt Express. 2019;10(9):4607–20.
82. Tamborini D, Stephens KA, Wu MM, Farzam P, Siegel AM, Shatrovoy O, et al. Portable system for time-domain diffuse correlation spectroscopy. IEEE Trans Biomed Eng. 2019;66(11):3014–25.
83. Kim MN, Durduran T, Frangos S, et al. Noninvasive measurement of cerebral blood flow and blood oxygenation using near-infrared and diffuse correlation spectroscopies in critically brain-injured adults. Neurocrit Care. 2009;12(2):173–80.
84. Mahajan C, Rath GP, Bithal PK. Advances in neuromonitoring. Anesth Essays Res. 2013;7(3):312–8.
85. Korhonen V, Myllylä T, Kirillin MY, Popov AP, Bykov AV, Gorshkov AV, et al. Light propagation in NIR spectroscopy of the human brain. IEEE J Sel Top Quantum Electron. 2014;20(2):1–10.
86. Elwell CE, et al. Quantification of adult cerebral hemodynamics by near-infrared spectroscopy. J Appl Physiol. 1994;77(6):2753–60.
87. Roberts I, et al. Estimation of cerebral blood flow with near-infrared spectroscopy and indocyanine green. Lancet. 1993;342:1425.
88. Verdecchia K, et al. Quantifying the cerebral metabolic rate of oxygen by combining diffuse correlation spectroscopy and time-resolved near-infrared spectroscopy. J Biomed Opt. 2013;18(2):027007.
89. Jia Y, Alkayed N, Wang RK. Potential of optical microangiography to monitor cerebral blood perfusion and vascular plasticity following traumatic brain injury in mice in vivo. J Biomed Opt. 2009;14:040505.
90. Townsend D. Physical principles and technology of clinical PET imaging. Ann Acad Med Singap. 2004;33(2):133–45.
91. Derdeyn CP. Positron emission tomography imaging of cerebral ischemia. Neuroimaging Clin N Am. 2005;15(2):341–50.
92. Kudomi N, Hirano Y, Koshino K, Hayashi T, Watabe H, Fukushima K, et al. Rapid quantitative CBF and CMRO2 measurements from a single PET scan with sequential administration of dual-15 O-labeled tracers. J Cereb Blood Flow Metab. 2013;33(3):440–8.
93. Rasulo F, Matta B, Varanini N. Cerebral blood flow monitoring. In: Prabhakar H, editor. Neuromonitoring techniques. London, UK: Academic Press; 2018. p. 31–56.
94. Nemoto H, Nakai Y, Hatakeyama R, Shikano N, Jesmin S, Yamaguchi N. Measurement of cerebral blood flow with 99mTc-ECD SPECT and its potential clinical implications—analyzing the relationships between CBF and lifestyle disease. Kaku Igaku. 2012;49(4):329–40.
95. Joshi B, Brady K, Lee J, et al. Impaired autoregulation of cerebral blood flow during rewarming from hypothermic cardiopulmonary bypass and its potential association with stroke. Anesth Analg. 2010;110(2):321–8.
96. Tournier P, Bonazzoli M, Dolean V, Rapetti F, Hecht F, Nataf F, et al. Numerical modelling and high-speed parallel computing: new perspectives on tomographic microwave imaging for brain stroke

detection and monitoring. IEEE Antennas Propag Mag. 2017;59(5):98–110.
97. Mesri HY. Localization of haemorrhage site in stroke patients using multichannel microwave measurements. In: 2012 Annual international conference of the IEEE engineering in medicine and biology society; 28 Aug–1 Sept 2012; San Diego, CA, USA: IEEE; 2012. pp. 5927–5930.
98. Saleeb DA, Helmy RM, Areed NFF, Marey M, Abdulkawi WM, Elkorany AS. A technique for the early detection of brain cancer using a circularly polarized reconfigurable antenna array. IEEE Access. 2021;9:133786–94.
99. Groumpas E, Koutsoupidou M, Karanasiou IS, Papageorgiou C, Uzunoglu N. Real-time passive brain monitoring system using nearfield microwave radiometry. IEEE Trans Biomed Eng. 2020;67(1):158–65.
100. Lipnick MS, Cahill EA, Feiner JR, Bickler PE. Comparison of transcranial Doppler and ultrasound-tagged near-infrared spectroscopy for measuring relative changes in cerebral blood flow in human subjects. Anesth Analg. 2018;126(2):579–87.
101. Racheli N, Ron A, Metzger Y, Breskin I, Enden G, Balberg M, et al. Non-invasive blood flow measurements using ultrasound-modulated diffused light. In: Proc SPIE 8223 Photons Plus Ultrasound: Imaging and Sensing; 21–26 January 2012; San Francisco, CA: SPIE Press; 2012. p. 822332A.
102. Tsalach A, Schiffer Z, Ratner E, Breskin I, Zeitak R, Shechter R, et al. Depth selective acousto-optic flow measurement. Biomedical. Opt Express. 2015;6:4871.

Jugular Venous Oximetry

7

Nidhi Singh, Sabina Regmi, and Ankur Luthra

7.1 Introduction

Prompt detection and avoidance of secondary brain injury is the basis of the management of neurocritical patients. Multimodal monitoring of the brain encompasses various modalities for real-time functional analysis of cerebral physiology. Jugular venous oximetry, i.e., monitoring of jugular bulb venous oxygen saturation, is one such bedside neuromonitor that detects the adequacy of cerebral perfusion [1]. Jugular venous oxygen saturation ($SjVO_2$) provides a global overview of oxygen supply versus demand for the brain by analyzing cerebral venous outflow.

Jugular venous oximetry is to cerebral circulation what mixed venous oximetry is to systemic circulation. $SjVO_2$ measured in the jugular bulb provides information about the balance between cerebral oxygen supply and demand analogous to mixed venous oxygen saturation measured in the pulmonary artery, which reflects the balance between systemic oxygen supply and consumption.

7.2 History

In 1927, Myerson et al. sampled the jugular bulb by direct percutaneous puncture and analyzed the human cerebral venous blood for the first time [2]. Gibbs et al., in 1945, demonstrated $SjVO_2$ to be similar when both right and left jugular bulbs were simultaneously sampled [3]. In 1953, Seldinger described a practical, wire-guided approach to catheter insertion into an artery [4]. This paved the way for indirect sampling of the jugular bulb via catheters inserted into the proximal internal jugular vein (IJV) and then passed distally upward into the jugular bulb. Gejrot and Lindbom performed retrograde jugularography to demonstrate any pathology of the vessels using a polyethylene catheter inserted into the IJV with the Seldinger technique [5].

7.3 Relevant Anatomy

The veins that drain blood from the brain join to form valveless venous channels called cranial sinuses. The deoxygenated blood from the brain passes through the right and left sigmoid sinuses, which run forward as respective IJVs in the pos-

N. Singh
Department of Anesthesiology, Sanjay Gandhi Postgraduate Institute of Medical Sciences, Lucknow, India

S. Regmi
Consultant Neuroanesthesia, Neo Multispeciality Hospital, Noida, India

A. Luthra (✉)
Department of Anesthesia and Intensive Care, Postgraduate Institute of Medical Education and Research, Chandigarh, India

H. Prabhakar et al. (eds.), *Principles and Practice of Neurocritical Care*,
https://doi.org/10.1007/978-981-99-8059-8_7

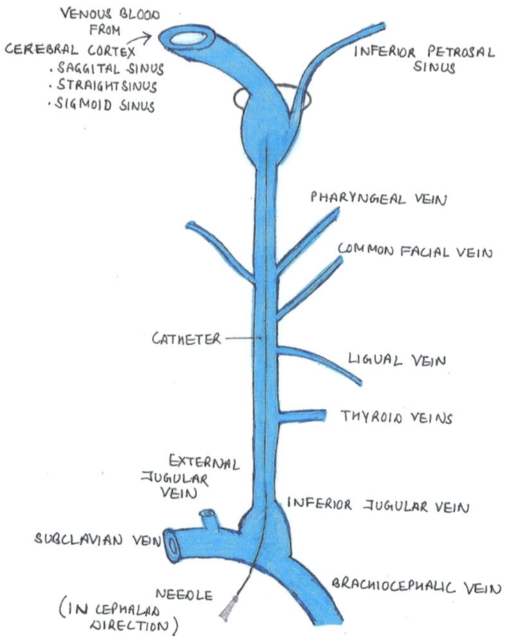

Fig. 7.1 A simplified anatomy of the jugular bulb with a jugular venous catheter in situ

terior part of the jugular foramen on each side. Each IJV has two expanded parts: the superior and the inferior jugular bulbs (Fig. 7.1). The superior jugular bulb lies at the upper end of the IJV just below the skull base. As the superior jugular bulb is less contaminated by extracerebral venous return, it is an ideal site for $SjVO_2$ sampling. The venous outflow from both cerebral hemispheres intermixes at the jugular bulb with around 70% of blood from the ipsilateral side and 30% from the contralateral side [6]. Blood from the extracranial circulation joins the IJV a few centimeters below the jugular bulb. Drainage is asymmetric and mostly right-dominant [7]. The IJV runs down the neck within the carotid sheath just lateral to the vagus nerve and carotid artery, where it is cannulated.

7.4 Site of Monitoring

The side of the dural venous sinus with predominant venous drainage has to be determined before inserting the jugular venous catheter. For a precise inference of global and hemispheric cerebral oxygenation, Lam et al. stressed the importance of monitoring the dominant jugular bulb as early as 1996 [8]. When both the cerebral hemispheres are affected by injury or the injury is diffuse, the catheter is typically positioned on the dominant side, i.e., usually the right side. For focal/unilateral injuries, the preferred side of catheterization remains contentious. Due to the propensity for cerebral venous blood to drain through the ipsilateral IJV, it is rational to catheterize the IJV on the side of the focal brain lesion, even when it is not dominant. Table 7.1 shows various methods to determine the dominant side of venous drainage.

Table 7.1 Methods to determine the dominant side of venous drainage

	Method	What to assess	Interpretation
1.	Ultrasonography	Size (diameter) of the IJV	Larger size is the dominant side
2.	Computed tomography	Size of the jugular foramen	Larger size is the dominant side
3.	Cerebral angiography	Caliber of the IJV	Larger caliber is the dominant side
4.	Transient sequential manual compression of either IJV (neck compression test [8])	Look for the side with a greater ICP rise with compression (needs ICP monitor in situ)	A greater rise in ICP on the dominant side

IJV internal jugular vein; *ICP* intracranial pressure

7.5 Insertion of a Jugular Bulb Catheter

Monitoring of $SjVO_2$ is an invasive technique. Before catheter insertion, coagulation abnormalities, cervical spine injury, and systemic or local site infection have to be ruled out. Written informed consent should be obtained beforehand. The patient is positioned supine, with the neck neutral or turned slightly to the contralateral side. A 15° head down position or slight head rotation to the opposite side may improve the visualiza-

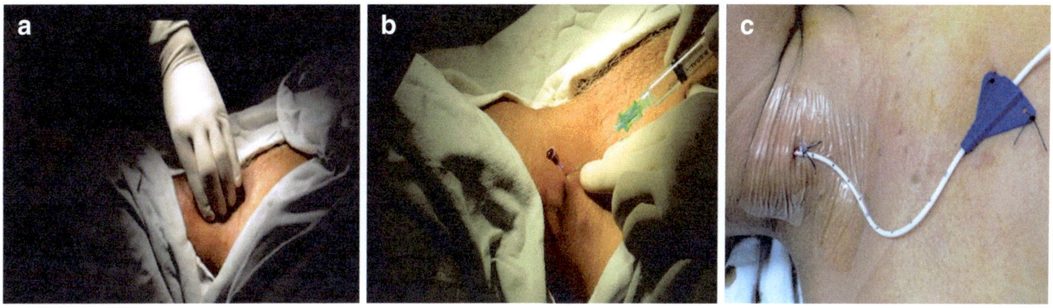

Fig. 7.2 Landmark-guided insertion of a jugular venous catheter. (**a**) Identifying the IJV lateral to the carotid artery at the apex of the triangle formed by the two heads of the sternocleidomastoid muscle. (**b**) Pilot puncture and needle insertion in the cephalad direction. (**c**) The final position of the jugular venous catheter after fixation

tion of the IJV but should be used judiciously in patients with poor intracranial compliance. Using all aseptic precautions, the junction between the sternal and clavicular heads of the sternocleidomastoid muscle is identified and the local anesthetic is infiltrated if the patient is awake.

The technique of insertion is almost similar to that of central venous catheterization (Fig. 7.2). However, unlike central venous catheterization, the operator stands in the axillary space facing the head end to advance the needle, guide wire, and catheter in a cephalad direction. The skin is punctured under ultrasound guidance with an introducer needle, through which a J-shaped guide wire is passed into the jugular bulb and advanced no further than 2–3 cm past the site of needle introduction. The catheter is passed over the guide wire in a cephalad direction till resistance is appreciated at the jugular bulb. An alert patient may report a sensation in the ipsilateral jaw or ear as the catheter lies against the base of the skull, indicating that the catheter tip is in the jugular bulb. Preferably, the catheter tip is inserted at a distance measured (beforehand) from the needle introduction point to the level of the mastoid process (approximately the level of the jugular bulb) until resistance is met. The catheter is accordingly pulled back for about 0.5–1 cm. A pressurized heparinized flush system maintains the patency of the catheter and reduces the degree of wall artifacts. If required, a central venous line can also be inserted on the same side; however, the antegrade central venous catheterization should precede retrograde cannulation.

7.6 Avoidance of Extracranial Contamination

Several veins carrying extracerebral blood, like the facial and retromandibular veins, open into the IJV a few centimeters below the jugular bulb. Hence, rapid aspiration may lead to contamination of jugular bulb blood, with extracerebral blood resulting in up to 25% high $SjVO_2$ values. Therefore, jugular venous blood sampling is recommended to be performed at rates less than 2 mL/min, especially in patients with compromised cerebral blood flow (CBF) [9]. To minimize contamination from extracerebral blood, it is also important to have the catheter in close proximity to the roof of the jugular bulb. Even a difference of 2 cm can result in contamination as high as 10% [10].

After catheter insertion, a radiographic assessment confirms the correct catheter placement. On a lateral radiograph of the neck, the tip of the catheter should lie just above the disc of C1/C2, at the level of and just medial to the mastoid process (Fig. 7.3). In 1995, Bankier et al. suggested confirmatory bony landmarks on anteroposterior skull radiographs after studying computed tomography (CT) scans of cadavers in whom $SjVO_2$ catheters were inserted [11]. An accurately placed tip should be cephalad to the line extending from the atlantooccipital joint space and caudal to the lower margin of the orbit. The tip of the catheter should lie above an imaginary line connecting the tips of the mastoid processes. Hayman et al. proposed using over-penetrated

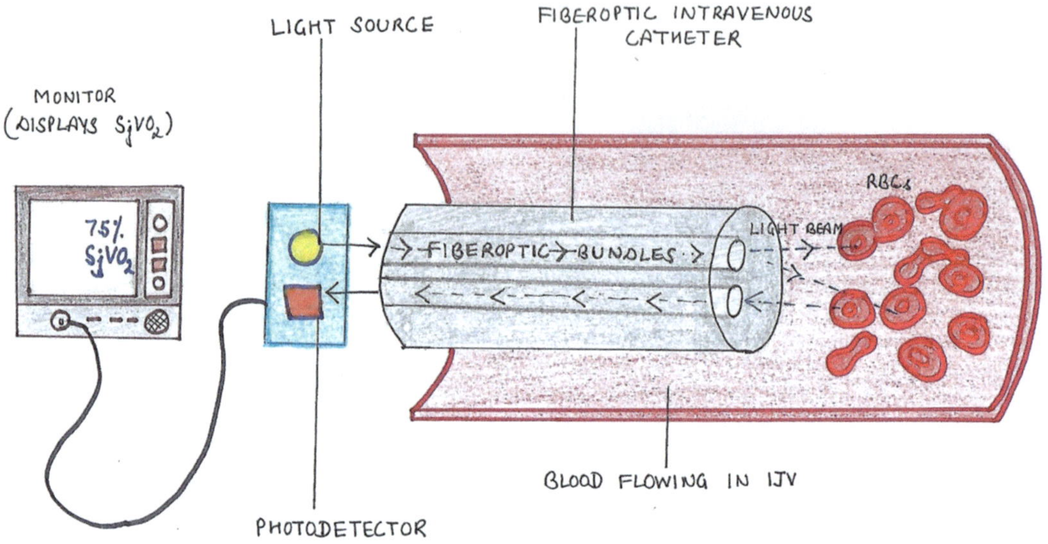

Fig. 7.3 The principle of reflection spectrophotometry

lateral radiographs for the assessment of jugular bulb catheters [12]. Intraoperatively, fluoroscopy is used to quickly confirm the position of the catheter tip.

7.7 Intermittent and Continuous Monitoring

The various methods of sampling venous blood are (Table 7.2) as follows:

1. *Direct*: The jugular bulb is punctured directly using a needle inserted 1 cm below and 1 cm anterior to the mastoid process. This technique is obsolete now.
2. *Intermittent/indirect/alternate monitoring*: Serial blood sampling is performed using an intravenous catheter.
3. *Continuous monitoring*: Continuous measurement is performed using spectrophotometric catheters.

The underlying principle of continuous monitoring is reflection spectrophotometry using a fiberoptic catheter (Fig. 7.4). The oximetry catheters meant for $SjVO_2$ measurement contain fiberoptic bundles that transmit two wavelengths of light, i.e., red and infrared, from an external light source toward the blood flowing across the catheter tip. The light is then reflected off the erythrocytes within the blood via another fiberoptic bundle onto a photodetector. Based on the differential absorption properties of the two wavelengths of light on the deoxyhemoglobin/oxyhemoglobin state of the erythrocytes, $SjVO_2$ can be ascertained by analyzing the reflected

Table 7.2 Monitoring methods

Intermittent monitoring	Continuous monitoring
Serial blood sampling	Continuous blood sampling
Uses conventional intravascular catheters	Uses fiberoptic oximetry catheters
Allows repetitive sampling of $SjVO_2$ without repeated needle puncture	Allows uninterrupted monitoring
Jugular venous blood gas analysis	Spectrophotometric determination
Cheaper	Expensive
Keeps the rate of blood aspiration <2 ml/min to avoid extracranial contamination	Since continuous, avoids errors due to rapid sampling
Comparison with an arterial sample allows determination of arteriovenous content difference in oxygen, glucose, and lactate	Detects isolated hypoperfusion events

$SjVO_2$ jugular venous oxygen saturation

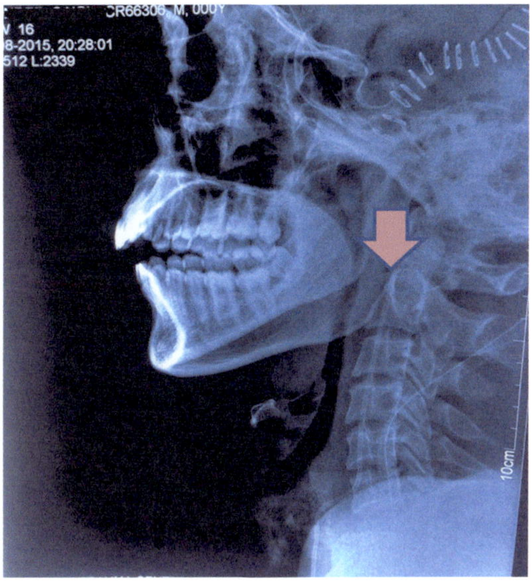

Fig. 7.4 A lateral radiograph of the cervical spine showing a jugular bulb catheter positioned with its tip cephalad to the inferior border of the first cervical vertebra

Table 7.3 Spectrophotometric catheters

Baxter–Edwards system (Edslab Sat II, Baxter–Edwards Critical Care Division, Irvine, California, USA)	Abbott system (Opticath Oximetrix, Abbott Critical Care System, Abbott Park, Illinois, USA)
Has two light-emitting diodes and employs two wavelengths of light	Uses three wavelengths of light
Calibrated against the patient's blood sample (in vivo)	May be calibrated in vivo (against the patient's blood) or in vitro (built-in calibration)
The hemoglobin value must be manually entered for each $SjVO_2$ value	The hemoglobin value is automatically obtained from the absorption spectrum
Minimal drift	Minimal drift, minimal artifact interference
Inaccurate when the hemoglobin values are unstable like with massive hemorrhage	Used in patients with a rapidly varying hemoglobin concentration, e.g., during cardiopulmonary bypass

$SjVO_2$ jugular venous oxygen saturation

non-absorbed light. Table 7.3 shows the commonly available spectrophotometric catheters. These 4F double-lumen catheters should be continuously flushed with saline at 2–4 mL/h to maintain patency.

7.8 Complications

Jugular bulb catheter placement is not without risks. The immediate complications are related to the procedure and depend on the experience of the operator. Ultrasound-guided IJV identification decreases the incidence of vascular complications, i.e., carotid artery puncture and hematoma formation. Pulmonary complications include pneumothorax, venous thrombosis, and air embolism. Delayed complications include device malfunction, vein thrombosis, central venous stenosis, and infection [13]. To avoid infections, a relevant "bundle approach" should be followed just like central venous catheterization, i.e., hand hygiene, use of complete barrier precaution, chlorhexidine skin antisepsis, an aseptic technique for blood sampling, and daily review of catheter necessity [15]. Goetting et al. found jugular bulb catheterization to be safe in head-injured patients with elevated intracranial pressure [14].

7.9 The Fundamental Concepts of Jugular Venous Oximetry

Jugular venous oximetry is a quantitative monitor that assesses cerebral perfusion. It represents the percentage of oxygenated hemoglobin at the level of the jugular bulb. $SjVO_2$ reflects the global balance between cerebral oxygen supply and demand as per the Fick principle.

When CBF = cerebral blood flow,

CaO_2 = arterial oxygen content, $CjVO_2$ = jugular venous oxygen content.

SaO_2 = arterial oxygen saturation, $SjVO_2$ = jugular venous oxygen saturation.

PaO_2 = arterial partial pressure of oxygen, $PjVO_2$ = jugular venous partial pressure of oxygen, Hb = hemoglobin.

Cerebral oxygen supply (DO_2) and consumption ($CMRO_2$) can be calculated from the following equations:

$$DO_2 = CBF \times CaO_2$$

$$CMRO_2 = CBF \times (CaO_2 - CjVO_2)$$

The difference between arterial oxygen content and venous oxygen content is represented as $CaO_2 - CjVO_2$ or $AVDO_2$ (arteriovenous oxygen difference).

$$AVDO_2 = CaO_2 - CjVO_2 = CMRO_2 / CBF$$

Now,

$$CaO_2 = (Hb \times 1.34 \times SaO_2) + 0.003 \times PaO_2$$

$$CjVO_2 = (Hb \times 1.34 \times SjVO_2) + 0.003 \times PjVO_2$$

$$AVDO_2 = Hb \times 1.34 (SaO_2 - SjVO_2)$$

As the dissolved oxygen is minimal and Hb concentration is constant in arterial and venous blood, the oxygen content is directly proportional to oxygen saturation. Hence, $AVDO_2$ is largely determined by the gradient between SaO_2 and $SjVO_2$. Under these conditions, the $SjVO_2$ is an accurate reflection of $AVDO_2$. The normal value of $AVDO_2$ is 4–8 mL O_2/100 mL blood. If $CMRO_2$ remains constant, then changes in $AVDO_2$ reflect the changes in CBF.

If $AVDO_2$ ↓es (i.e., <4 mL O_2/100 mL), brain O_2 supply > demand (hyperaemic or luxuriant state)
If $AVDO_2$ ↑es (i.e., >8 mL O_2/100 mL), brain O_2 demand > supply (hypoperfusion or ischemic state)

If cerebral metabolic demand increases without a concomitant increase in CBF, then a greater amount of oxygen will be extracted from the blood. There will be a proportional decrease in jugular venous oxygen content, leading to the widening of $AVDO_2$. Hence, $SjVO_2$ provides an indirect estimate of the use of oxygen by the brain. It is important to note that $AVDO_2$ and $SjVO_2$ move in opposite directions.

↑ oxygen demand → ↑ O_2 extraction from brain → ↓ $SjVO_2$ → ↑ $AVDO_2$ (global cerebral ischemia).
↑ oxygen supply → ↓ O_2 extraction from brain → ↑ $SjVO_2$ → ↓ $AVDO_2$ (hyperaemia).

Clinically, a decrement in $SjVO_2$ indicates an imbalance between cerebral oxygen demand and supply, which is attributed to a relative rise in $CMRO_2$ or a decline in CBF. The normal value of $SjVO_2$ is approximately 55–75%. These values are lower than those of systemic mixed venous oxygen saturation and suggest higher oxygen requirements of the normal brain. Notably, $SjVO_2$ is affected by respiratory variables, circulatory dynamics, metabolic factors, hemoglobin concentration, and arterial partial pressure of oxygen and carbon dioxide [15]. Hence, any fluctuations in $SjVO_2$ levels must be interpreted in light of these factors. When faced with a low $SjVO_2$, it is paramount to establish the cause and intervene accordingly. Table 7.4 shows the clinical factors affecting $SjVO_2$, and Fig. 7.5 shows the algorithm for the management of jugular venous desaturation.

Table 7.4 Clinical factors affecting jugular venous oxygen saturation

Decrease in $SjVO_2$		Increase in $SjVO_2$	
Decreased O_2 delivery	Increased O_2 consumption	Increased O_2 delivery	Decreased O_2 consumption
↑ ICP, ↓CPP ↓ $EtCO_2$ Vasospasm ↓ BP ↓ SaO_2 Anemia Hemorrhage	Fever Pain Light plane of anesthesia Seizures Shivering	↓ ICP, ↑ CPP ↑ $EtCO_2$ Vasodilation ↑ BP ↑ PaO_2	Coma Hypothermia Sedation Cerebral infarction Brain death

$SjVO_2$ jugular venous oxygen saturation; *ICP* intracranial pressure; *CPP* cerebral perfusion pressure; *$EtCO_2$* end-tidal carbon dioxide concentration; *BP* blood pressure; *SaO_2* arterial oxygen saturation; *PaO_2* arterial partial pressure of oxygen

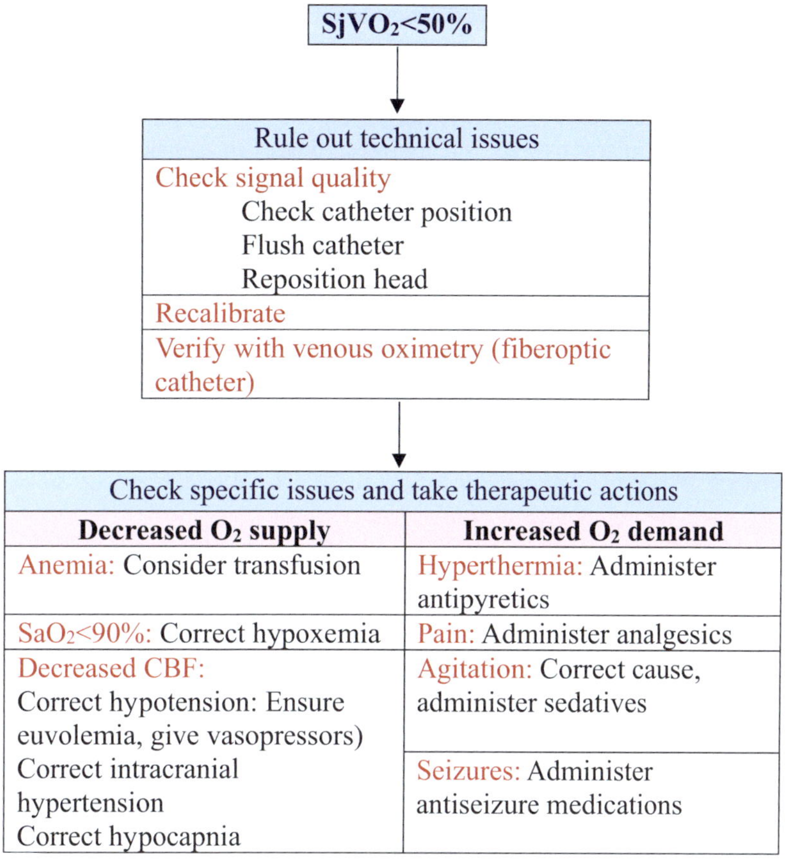

Fig. 7.5 The algorithm for management of jugular venous desaturation

7.10 Clinical Applications of $SjVO_2$

The bulk of data available on the use of $SjVO_2$ in neurocritical care are in traumatic brain injury (TBI) patients. $SjVO_2$ monitoring has also been explored in the management of subarachnoid hemorrhage, neurosurgery, cardiac surgery, and neuroprognostication after cardiac arrest.

7.10.1 Traumatic Brain Injury

Intracranial and systemic causes like raised intracranial pressure, hypocarbia, arterial hypoxemia, and reduced mean arterial pressure that trigger ischemia have been linked to a fall in $SjVO_2$ [16]. $SjVO_2$ monitoring helps diagnose early ischemia due to the insults mentioned hitherto [17–20]. An early study performed on 150 patients showed abnormal $SjVO_2$ in 38% of TBI patients within the first 12 h with a predominance of systemic insults [21]. Hence, timely insertion of $SjVO_2$ is recommended as cerebral perfusion pressure is critically reduced in the first 12 h of head injury. $SjVO_2$ monitoring correlates well with cerebral perfusion pressure and hence can be used as a surrogate to identify patients at risk of ischemia to take appropriate actions to maintain cerebral homeostasis [22].

In addition to this, $SjVO_2$ monitoring can guide hyperventilation therapy and fluid management in TBI patients [18, 23–25]. The Brain Trauma Foundation guidelines (fourth edition) recommend avoiding hyperventilation in the first 24 h of TBI [26]. If need be, hyperventilation can be used in cases of impending herniation as a temporary measure guided by $SjVO_2$ or brain tissue oxygen ($PbtO_2$) monitoring to prevent debilitating ischemia due to hypocapnia.

$SjVO_2$ monitoring also aids in predicting the outcome of head-injured patients. Multiple prospective observational studies in TBI patients reported improvement of the Glasgow Outcome Scale at 3 or 6 months with $SjVO_2$ and $AVDO_2$ monitoring [27, 28]. In addition, episodes of desaturation during $SjVO_2$ or $AVDO_2$ monitoring were associated with unfavorable outcomes in the form of cerebral infarction, mortality, and morbidity [29, 30].

Lactate oxygen index (LOI) is another important parameter that can be measured with jugular venous oximetry. An increased LOI to >0.08 indicates failing neuronal aerobic metabolism and increased anaerobic metabolism with the production of lactate. It is calculated by the formula LOI = −AVDL (arteriovenous difference of lactate) (mmol/lit) × 2.24/$AVDO_2$ (ml/dl). LOI along with AVDL and $AVDO_2$ is a reliable predictor of cerebral blood flow for a favorable neurological outcome [29].

7.10.2 Subarachnoid Hemorrhage

Cerebral vasospasms and delayed cerebral ischemia are important complications of subarachnoid aneurysmal hemorrhage that affect the outcome. Jugular venous monitoring helps predict vasospasms in aneurysmal subarachnoid hemorrhage patients. In a small cohort of 14 patients, Heran et al. demonstrated that an increase in $AVDO_2$ was predictive of a clinically evident vasospasm in aneurysmal subarachnoid hemorrhage patients occurring after hours to days [31]. This provided a therapeutic window for prophylactic management of vasospasms to improve patient outcomes. $SjVO_2$ monitoring helps determine the minimal blood pressure that should be maintained to avoid hypoperfusion during intracranial aneurysm surgery [32].

7.10.3 Cardiac Surgeries

Patients undergoing cardiac surgeries on cardiopulmonary bypass are particularly vulnerable to cognitive dysfunction during the rewarming phase of cardiopulmonary bypass. The oxygen delivery during cardiopulmonary bypass (CPB) is relatively fixed. During the initiation of CPB, the temperature starts dropping. The cerebral oxygen demand decreases as a result of decreased cerebral metabolism due to hypothermia. This is known as luxuriant perfusion, and the $SjVO_2$ values remain high. However, during the rewarming phase, cerebral metabolism and oxygen demand also increase. The $SjVO_2$ values are decreased in the background of constant oxygen supply. $SjVO_2$ monitoring may have a role in predicting cerebral hypoxia and in the prevention of postoperative cognitive dysfunction during the rewarming phase; however, the evidence is weak [33].

7.10.4 Neuroprognostication after Cardiac Arrest

In a retrospective analysis of 40 out-of-hospital cardiac arrest patients, [34] found an association between unfavorable outcomes and high mean $SjVO_2$ (75%) values. This is likely due to the underutilization of oxygen by irreversibly damaged neurons. An unfavorable outcome was associated with $SjVO_2$ values above mixed venous oxygen saturation in acutely comatose patients admitted to the intensive care unit post cardiac arrest [35]. A study by van der Hoeven et al., however, failed to show any significant difference in $SjVO_2$ values between patients with good and poor neurological outcomes a few hours after cardiac arrest in resuscitated comatose patients [36].

A mismatch between demand and supply has also been reported in pediatric patients aged between 1 and 4 years undergoing elective cardiac surgeries as evidenced by $SjVO_2$ monitoring [37]. A significant drop in $SjVO_2$ values was observed during onset, 20 min post cardiopulmonary bypass, coronary reperfusion, and during the separation and rewarming phases of cardiopulmonary bypass.

7.10.5 Effect of Anesthetics on $SjVO_2$

A prospective randomized trial was conducted in severe TBI patients who received either propofol or sevoflurane as maintenance anesthesia [38]. The $SjVO_2$ values were found to be comparable between both the groups. However, the mean arterial pressure was significantly reduced in patients who received propofol. On the contrary, in another randomized controlled trial, including 20 brain tumor patients, 50% of patients who received propofol anesthesia showed signs of hypoperfusion as assessed by $SjVO_2$ monitoring [39]. The same was not demonstrated in patients who received isoflurane or nitrous oxide anesthesia. Bhardwaj et al. compared $SjVO_2$ recordings of 13 patients receiving propofol with 14 patients receiving desflurane in aneurysmal subarachnoid hemorrhage patients [40]. Desflurane use was associated with hyperemia (>74%) as compared to the propofol group in which the values were within the normal range (55–75%) at all times. However, these differences in $SjVO_2$ values between groups had no influence on the intraoperative brain condition.

Intravenous agents like propofol are cerebral vasoconstrictors that maintain cerebral flow during metabolism coupling. Inhalational agents cause direct cerebral vasodilation, especially at a higher minimal alveolar concentration, and result in luxury perfusion. This is reflected as an increase in $SjVO_2$ values. Even though the data pertaining to $SjVO_2$ values with the use of propofol is ambiguous, the goal is to maintain normal mean arterial pressure to prevent cerebral desaturation.

7.11 Limitations

Monitoring $SjVO_2$ is an invasive procedure with multiple complications. $SjVO_2$, being a global measure, has high specificity but low sensitivity for ischemia, i.e., a normal saturation may not denote focal areas of ischemia; however, a low saturation points toward low flow. Sampling for $SjVO_2$ determination is also prone to extracerebral contamination of blood and monitoring errors because of catheter position. Besides, monitoring with jugular oximetry is unsuitable for patients with infratentorial (brainstem, cerebellum) involvement [15, 41].

7.12 Conclusions

Jugular venous oximetry is an invasive yet practical and convenient bedside neuromonitor to assess cerebral oxygenation and brain perfusion. Detecting periods of cerebral desaturation enables clinicians to take appropriate actions, thereby ameliorating secondary brain injury. Before modifying management following $SjVO_2$ alterations, one needs to be wary of technical and equipment issues. Amalgamating information obtained by jugular oximetry with other neuromonitors like brain tissue oxygen tension, near-infrared spectroscopy, and microdialysis complements standard management protocols to improve patient outcomes. Finally, but importantly, all these modalities are there to assist us in clinical decision-making to improve neurological outcomes. However, one must not forget that the clinician is the best monitor.

References

1. Yang MT. Multimodal neurocritical monitoring. Biom J. 2020;43(3):226–30. https://doi.org/10.1016/j.bj.2020.05.005.
2. Myerson A, Halloran, Hirsch HL. Techniques for obtaining blood from the internal jugular vein and internal carotid artery. Arch Neurol Psychiatr. 1927;17(6):807–8. https://doi.org/10.1001/archneurpsyc.1927.02200360087006.
3. Gibbs EL, Lennox WG, Gibbs FA. Bilateral internal jugular blood. Am J Psychiatry. 1945;102(2):184–90. https://doi.org/10.1176/ajp.102.2.184.
4. Seldinger SI. Catheter replacement of the needle in percutaneous arteriography; a new technique. Acta Radiol. 1953;39(5):368–76. https://doi.org/10.3109/00016925309136722.
5. Gejrot T, Lindbom Å. Venography of the internal jugular vein and the transverse sinuses (retrograde jugularography). Acta Otolaryngol (Stockh). 1960;52(sup158):180–6. https://doi.org/10.3109/00016486009122416.
6. Shenkin HA. Dynamic anatomy of the cerebral circulation. Arch Neurol Psychiatr. 1948;60(3):240. https://doi.org/10.1001/archneurpsyc.1948.02310030021002.
7. Chaikittisilpa N, Vavilala MS, Lele AV. Jugular venous oximetry. In: Prabhakar H, editor. Neuromonitoring techniques. 1st ed. San Diego: Elsevier Inc; 2018. p. 57–75.
8. Lam JM, Chan MS, Poon WS. Cerebral venous oxygen saturation monitoring: is dominant jugular bulb cannu-

lation good enough? Br J Neurosurg. 1996;10(4):357–64. https://doi.org/10.1080/02688699647276.
9. Matta BF, Lam AM. The rate of blood withdrawal affects the accuracy of jugular venous bulb. Oxygen saturation measurements. Anesthesiology. 1997;86(4):806–8. https://doi.org/10.1097/00000542-199704000-00010.
10. White H, Baker A. Continuous jugular venous oximetry in the neurointensive care unit—a brief review. Can J Anaesth J Can Anesth. 2002;49(6):623–9. https://doi.org/10.1007/BF03017393.
11. Bankier AA, Fleischmann D, Windisch A, et al. Position of jugular oxygen saturation catheter in patients with head trauma: assessment by use of plain films. AJR Am J Roentgenol. 1995;164(2):437–41. https://doi.org/10.2214/ajr.164.2.7839985.
12. Hayman LA, Fahr LM, Taber KH, Hughes CL, Ritter AM, Robertson C. Radiographic assessment of jugular bulb catheters. Emerg Radiol. 1995;2(6):331–8. https://doi.org/10.1007/BF02615896.
13. Coplin WM, O'Keefe GE, Grady MS, et al. Thrombotic, infectious, and procedural complications of the jugular bulb catheter in the intensive care unit. Neurosurgery. 1997;41(1):101–7; discussion 107–109. https://doi.org/10.1097/00006123-199707000-00022.
14. Goetting MG, Preston G. Jugular bulb catheterization does not increase intracranial pressure. Intensive Care Med. 1991;17(4):195–8. https://doi.org/10.1007/BF01709876.
15. Bhardwaj A, Bhagat H, Grover V. Jugular venous oximetry. J Neuroanaesth Crit Care. 2015;02(03):225–31. https://doi.org/10.4103/2348-0548.165046.
16. Gopinath SP, Robertson CS, Contant CF, et al. Jugular venous desaturation and outcome after head injury. J Neurol Neurosurg Psychiatry. 1994;57(6):717–23. https://doi.org/10.1136/jnnp.57.6.717.
17. Gupta AK, Hutchinson PJ, Al-Rawi P, et al. Measuring brain tissue oxygenation compared with jugular venous oxygen saturation for monitoring cerebral oxygenation after traumatic brain injury. Anesth Analg. 1999;88(3):549. https://doi.org/10.1213/00000539-199903000-00016.
18. Thiagarajan A, Goverdhan PD, Chari P, Somasunderam K. The effect of hyperventilation and hyperoxia on cerebral venous oxygen saturation in patients with traumatic brain injury. Anesth Analg. 1998;87(4):850–3. https://doi.org/10.1097/00000539-199810000-00019.
19. Sb L, Ja M, El T, Pl R. Cerebral oxygenation monitoring by near-infrared spectroscopy is not clinically useful in patients with severe closed-head injury: a comparison with jugular venous bulb oximetry. Crit Care Med. 1996;24(8):1334. https://doi.org/10.1097/00003246-199608000-00011.
20. Murr R, Schürer L. Correlation of jugular venous oxygen saturation to spontaneous fluctuations of cerebral perfusion pressure in patients with severe head injury. Neurol Res. 1995;17(5):329. https://pubmed.ncbi.nlm.nih.gov/8584122/.
21. De Deyne C, Decruyenaere J, Calle P, et al. Analysis of very early jugular bulb oximetry data after severe head injury: implications for the emergency management? Eur J Emerg Med Off J Eur Soc Emerg Med. 1996;3(2):69–72. https://doi.org/10.1097/00063110-199606000-00002.
22. Vigué B, Ract C, Benayed M, et al. Early SjvO2 monitoring in patients with severe brain trauma. Intensive Care Med. 1999;25(5):445–51. https://doi.org/10.1007/s001340050878.
23. Fortune JB, Feustel PJ, Weigle CGM, Popp AJ. Continuous measurement of jugular venous oxygen saturation in response to transient elevations of blood pressure in head-injured patients. J Neurosurg. 1994;80(3):461–8. https://doi.org/10.3171/jns.1994.80.3.0461.
24. Matta BF, Lam AM, Mayberg TS. The influence of arterial oxygenation on cerebral venous oxygen saturation during hyperventilation. Can J Anaesth J Can Anesth. 1994;41(11):1041–6. https://doi.org/10.1007/BF03015651.
25. Chan KH, Miller JD, Dearden NM, Andrews PJ, Midgley S. The effect of changes in cerebral perfusion pressure upon middle cerebral artery blood flow velocity and jugular bulb venous oxygen saturation after severe brain injury. J Neurosurg. 1992;77(1):55–61. https://doi.org/10.3171/jns.1992.77.1.0055.
26. Brain Trauma Foundation. http://braintrauma.org/guidelines/guidelines-for-the-management-of-severe-tbi-4th-ed#/. Accessed 12 July 2022.
27. Cruz J. The first decade of continuous monitoring of jugular bulb oxyhemoglobinsaturation: management strategies and clinical outcome. Crit Care Med. 1998;26(2):344–51. https://doi.org/10.1097/00003246-199802000-00039.
28. Le Roux PD, Newell DW, Lam AM, Grady MS, Winn HR. Cerebral arteriovenous oxygen difference: a predictor of cerebral infarction and outcome in patients with severe head injury. J Neurosurg. 1997;87(1):1–8. https://doi.org/10.3171/jns.1997.87.1.0001.
29. Robertson CS, Narayan RK, Gokaslan ZL, et al. Cerebral arteriovenous oxygen difference as an estimate of cerebral blood flow in comatose patients. J Neurosurg. 1989;70(2):222–30. https://doi.org/10.3171/jns.1989.70.2.0222.
30. Robertson C. Desaturation episodes after severe head injury: influence on outcome. Acta Neurochir Suppl (Wien). 1993;59:98–101. https://doi.org/10.1007/978-3-7091-9302-0_17.
31. Heran NS, Hentschel SJ, Toyota BD. Jugular bulb oximetry for prediction of vasospasm following subarachnoid hemorrhage. Can J Neurol Sci J Can Sci Neurol. 2004;31(1):80–6. https://doi.org/10.1017/s0317167100002870.
32. Moss E, Dearden NM, Berridge JC. Effects of changes in mean arterial pressure on SjO2 during cerebral aneurysm surgery. Br J Anaesth. 1995;75(5):527–30. https://doi.org/10.1093/bja/75.5.527.

33. Schell RM, Kern FH, Reves JG. The role of continuous jugular venous saturation monitoring during cardiac surgery with cardiopulmonary bypass. Anesth Analg. 1992;74(5):627–9. https://doi.org/10.1213/00000539-199205000-00001.
34. Richter J, Sklienka P, Chatterjee N, Maca J, Zahorec R, Burda M. Elevated jugular venous oxygen saturation after cardiac arrest. Resuscitation. 2021;169:214–9. https://doi.org/10.1016/j.resuscitation.2021.10.011
35. Zarzuelo R, Castañeda J. Differences in oxygen content between mixed venous blood and cerebral venous blood for outcome prediction after cardiac arrest. Intensive Care Med. 1995;21(1):71–5. https://doi.org/10.1007/BF02425158.
36. van der Hoeven JG, de Koning J, Compier EA, Meinders AE. Early jugular bulb oxygenation monitoring in comatose patients after an out-of-hospital cardiac arrest. Intensive Care Med. 1995;21(7):567–72. https://doi.org/10.1007/BF01700161.
37. Hu Z, Xu L, Zhu Z, Seal R, McQuillan PM. Effects of hypothermic cardiopulmonary bypass on internal jugular bulb venous oxygen saturation, cerebral oxygen saturation, and Bispectral index in pediatric patients undergoing cardiac surgery: a prospective study. Medicine (Baltimore). 2016;95(2):e2483. https://doi.org/10.1097/MD.0000000000002483.
38. Chauhan R, Panda N, Bhagat H, et al. Comparison of propofol and sevoflurane on cerebral oxygenation using jugular venous oximetry (SjVo2) in patients undergoing surgery for traumatic brain injury. Asian J Neurosurg. 2020;15(03):614–9. https://doi.org/10.4103/ajns.AJNS_348_19.
39. Jansen GF, van Praagh BH, Kedaria MB, Odoom JA. Jugular bulb oxygen saturation during propofol and isoflurane/nitrous oxide anesthesia in patients undergoing brain tumor surgery. Anesth Analg. 1999;89(2):358–63. https://doi.org/10.1097/00000539-199908000-00021.
40. Bhardwaj A, Bhagat H, Grover VK, et al. Comparison of propofol and desflurane for postanaesthetic morbidity in patients undergoing surgery for aneurysmal SAH: a randomized clinical trial. J Anesth. 2018;32(2):250–8. https://doi.org/10.1007/s00540-018-2474-z.
41. Schell RM, Cole DJ. Cerebral monitoring: jugular venous oximetry. Anesth Analg. 2000;90(3):559–66. https://doi.org/10.1097/00000539-200003000-00012.

EEG for the Intensivist: Basics

8

Atampreet Singh

8.1 Introduction

EEG is a cheap, noninvasive, bedside investigation which gives electrical activity monitoring for diagnosis of seizures and epilepsy. The main indications for EEG in ICU are: encephalopathy, seizure disorders, hypoxic and traumatic brain injuries, cerebral structural abnormalities, coma, and last but not the least neuroprognostication in brain death and severe brain damage patients [1]. It also has therapeutic indications, such as determining the depth of anesthesia in induced coma and the cessation of nonconvulsive status epilepticus by anticonvulsant or anesthetic agents [1].

Seizures are a very common complication in patients in the intensive care unit (ICU) but usually are under-recognized and mostly electrographic without any clinical correlates. Nonconvulsive seizures occur in almost one-third of patients in the ICU, with high mortality [2–4]. There has been huge increase in the use of EEG in ICU in the last 20 years or so, but it is still underutilized investigation in ICU settings [5].

Patterns that are frequently encountered in critical care include slow (wave) activity, frontal intermittent rhythmic delta activity (FIRDA), triphasic waves, epileptiform patterns and periodic discharges (PDs), suppression, and burst suppression [6].

A. Singh (✉)
Department of Neurology and Epilepsy, Fortis Hospital, Greater Noida, Uttar Pradesh, India

8.2 Basics of EEG

The EEG records electrical activity generated by cerebral neurones, in the form of potential differences between electrodes positioned over the scalp. The EEG is digitized, amplified (as in a healthy adult, it is typically 20–100 mV), filtered to remove or reduce noise (usually from 0.3 to 70 Hz), and displayed as waveforms of varying frequencies (Table 8.1). Interpretation of these waveforms is usually by visual inspection but can be performed by quantitative analysis of the frequency, amplitude, topographical distribution, cross-correlation, and reactivity; these analyses enable an objective assessment of cerebral activity.

Standard recording typically uses 21 electrodes, applied according to the international 10–20 classification system, over the frontal (F), temporal (T), central (C), parietal (P), and occipital (O) regions. Even-numbered electrodes relate to the right hemisphere and odd ones to the left,

Table 8.1 EEG waveforms in the healthy adult population (usually lower frequency activity is higher in amplitude and vice versa)

Waveform	Frequency (Hz)	Location
Gamma	>30	Somatosensory cortex
Beta	13–30	Frontal
Alpha	8–12	Occipital
Theta	4–7	Diffuse
Delta	<4	Diffuse

H. Prabhakar et al. (eds.), *Principles and Practice of Neurocritical Care*,
https://doi.org/10.1007/978-981-99-8059-8_8

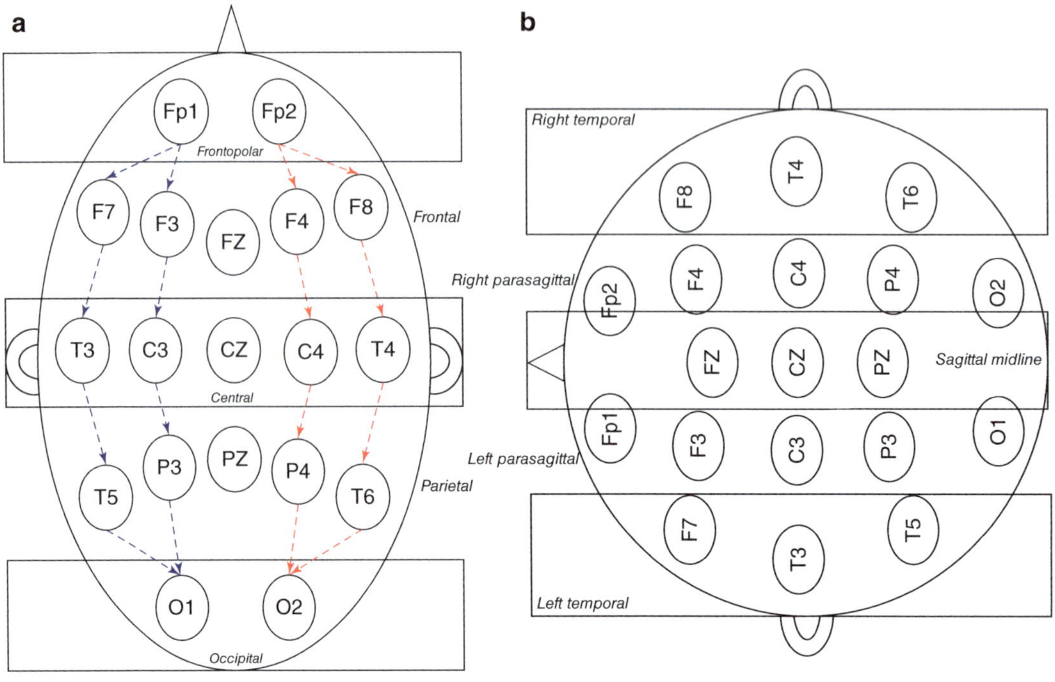

Fig. 8.1 The International 10–20 system. Panel (**a**) demonstrates the five primary transverse planes, while panel (**b**) shows the five primary sagittal planes. In panel (**a**), the bipolar or "double banana" montage is demonstrated with blue (left) and red (right) dashed arrows. *C* central; *F* frontal; *Fp* frontopolar; *O* occipital; *P* parietal; *T* temporal

whilst a post-fixed z refers to the midline (Fig. 8.1). A standard recording is usually 40–45 min in duration. With the 10–20 system, epileptologists have developed myriad electrode configurations (also called "montages") to compare different voltages on the scalp. This is done to aid localization and is why interpreters often switch between montages in a single EEG.

Surface EEG remains the most common method to detect seizures in the ICU using page-by-page visual inspection of the recording. This is usually done on-site or remotely by a neurophysiologist with EEG reading expertise [7]. The EEG signal reflects the recording of electrophysiological activity which are generated primarily by cortical layers 3 and 5. The EEG potentials are displayed in channels. In a bipolar montage, each displayed waveform represents the difference in potential between two electrodes. An upward deflection represents a negative difference, which indicates a spike and wave discharge and is considered to be epileptogenic and a downward deflection represents a positive difference [8].

8.3 Important Terminology

The term "epileptiform" can confuse clinicians. It simply means "pertaining to epilepsy" or "resembling epilepsy." Importantly, it does not mean the patient has had or is having a clinical (visible) or sub-clinical (nonvisible) seizure. "Spikes" and "sharp waves" are also commonly mentioned on EEG reports. The difference between the two is their duration: if a waveform is less than 70 ms in duration, it is a spike, whereas if it is between 70 and 200 ms, it is a sharp wave. If spikes or sharp waves occur frequently and in a specific area, it indicates an area of potential seizure activity. Use of the term "generalized" refers to activity in both hemispheres but does not mean that it is clear where the activity started. In addition to frequency, amplitude, and shape, EEG waveforms are classified by the area on the scalp in which they are recorded.

8.4 Various Patterns Seen in EEG

8.4.1 Normal Adult EEG

1. The Awake

   EEG (or normal EEG) is characterized by an alpha rhythm: a symmetrical 8–12 Hz pattern best seen in the leads from the posterior scalp (Figs. 8.2 and 8.3). It is therefore also referred to as the "posterior dominant rhythm." Alpha activity is increased in amplitude during relaxed wakefulness and is reactive if the patient is mentally alert or with eye opening, it attenuates. Normal alpha activity is rarely seen in ICU settings, but it might be seen over the anterior head regions like alpha coma or spindle coma which have prognostic significance in patients with anoxia coma or diffuse CNS disease.

   Points to Remember

   (a) A normal EEG with a reactive alpha activity in ICU virtually rules out a diffuse brain dysfunction.
   (b) The aim should be to classify the abnormality in EEG if abnormal.

2. Slowing

   Slow waves usually are of theta (4-7 Hz) and delta frequency (<4 Hz) activity and should be there for a significant period (i.e.,

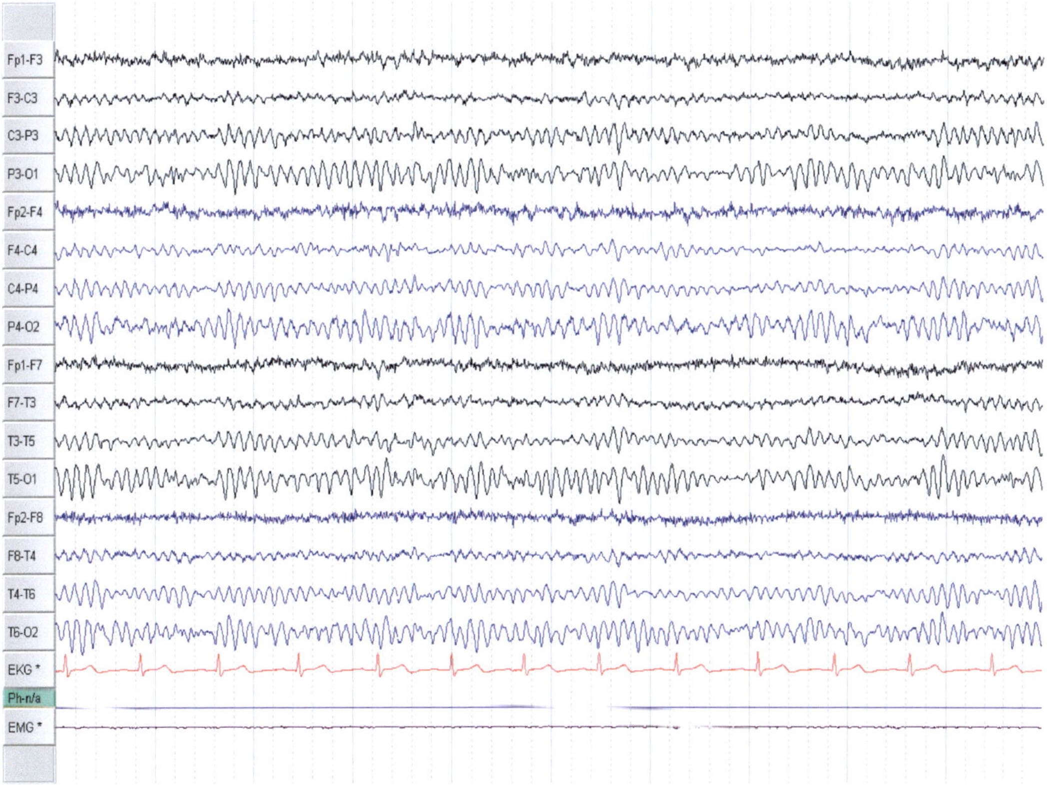

Fig. 8.2 Normal alpha rhythm. EEG demonstrating a normal alpha rhythm at 9.5–10 Hz with waxing, and waning alpha activity indicates spindling a normal phenomenon. LFF at 1 Hz, HFF at 70 Hz, Sensitivity at 10 μV

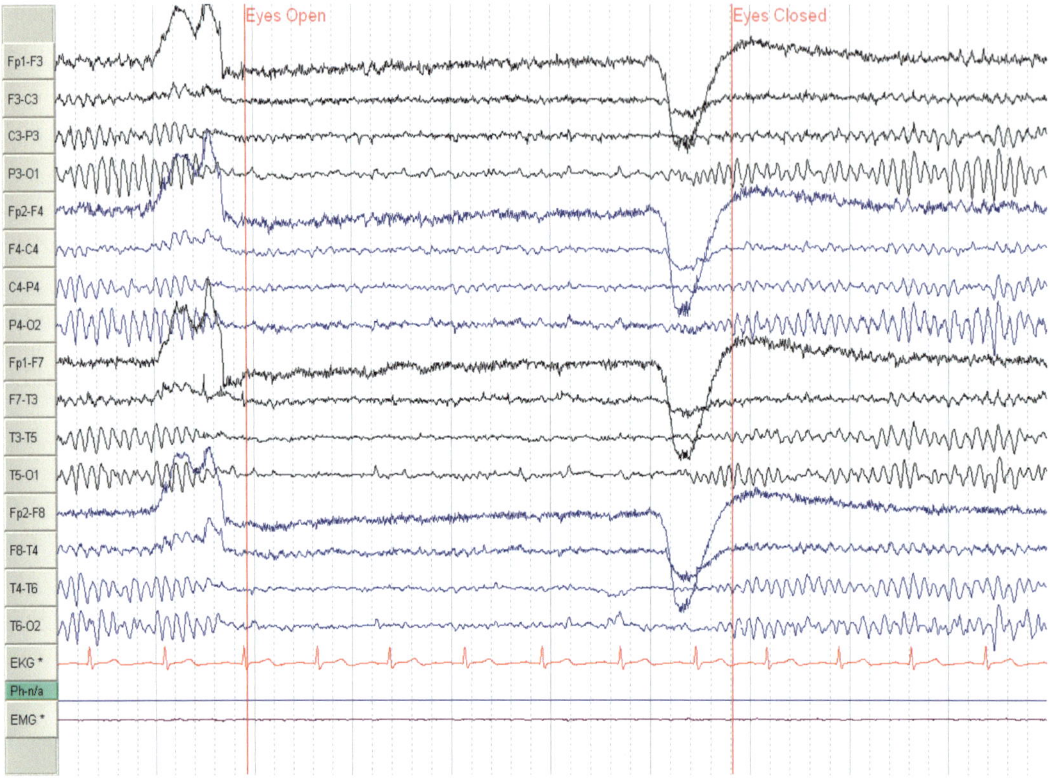

Fig. 8.3 Normal alpha rhythm. EEG demonstrating a normal reactive alpha rhythm at 10–10.5 Hz with eye closure and eye opening. LFF = 1 Hz, HFF = 70 Hz, Sensitivity = 10 μV

approximately >50%) of a recording in an awake patient is considered to be pathological. Slowing whether focal or diffuse usually suggests encephalopathy. More slow the frequency, more severe is the encephalopathy. In cases of mild to moderate encephalopathy, there will be mild theta slowing at 5–7 Hz, as shown in Fig. 8.4.

When the EEG is having persistent, diffuse delta activity, it is termed as polymorphic delta activity (PDA) in Fig. 8.5, implying that it is asymmetric in frequency, distribution, and amplitude. The presence of diffuse EEG slowing, severe slowing, or PDA rarely pinpoints the diagnosis. It is a nonspecific EEG pattern and occurs in various clinical situations, the most common of which are hepatic failure, renal failure, sepsis, drug intoxications, hypoxia, and head trauma. It is usually nonprognostic, which however, reflects the underlying pathology more than the EEG tracing.

It is the focal slowing as shown in Fig. 8.6, which is more relevant and specific indicating a lesion in the underlying brain parenchyma like abscesses, hematomas, tumors, cerebral ischemia, and recovery from a focal seizure [9, 10]. A pure cortical lesion causes a decrease in EEG waveform amplitude rather than slowing which points to a transmitted rhythm in a subcortical lesion.

Frontal intermittent rhythmic delta activity (FIRDA) is fairly regular, approximately sinusoidal or sawtooth waves, occurring in intermittent bursts at 1.5–2.5 Hz synchronously over the frontal regions (occasionally unilaterally), as shown in Fig. 8.7. FIRDA is most commonly associated with mild to moderate

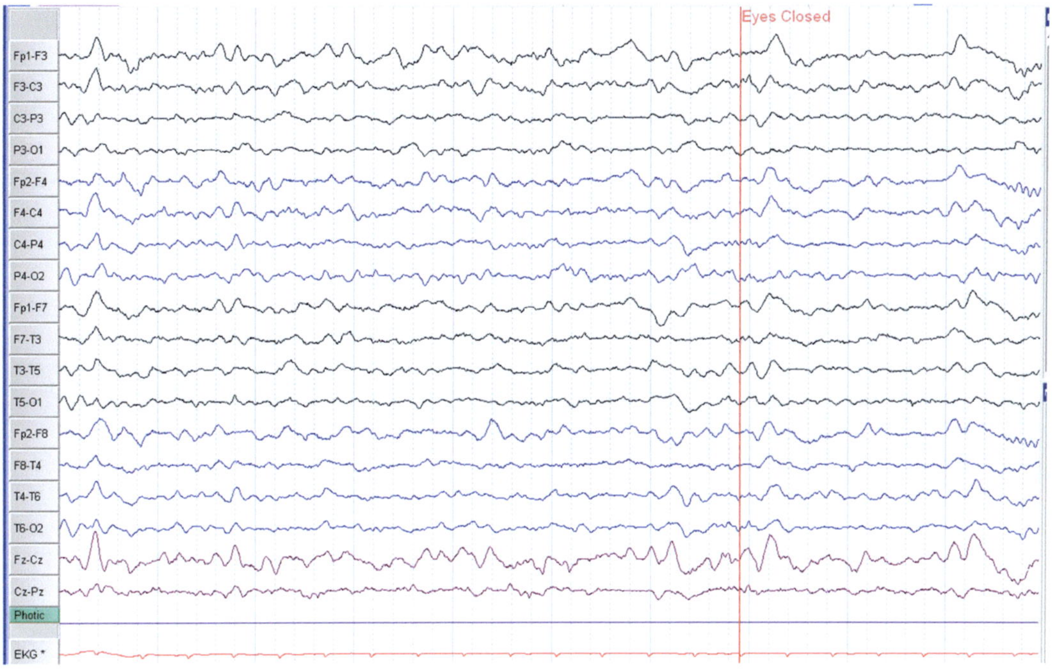

Fig. 8.4 Diffuse slowing. EEG demonstrating diffuse slowing in the theta range of frequencies at 5–6 Hz

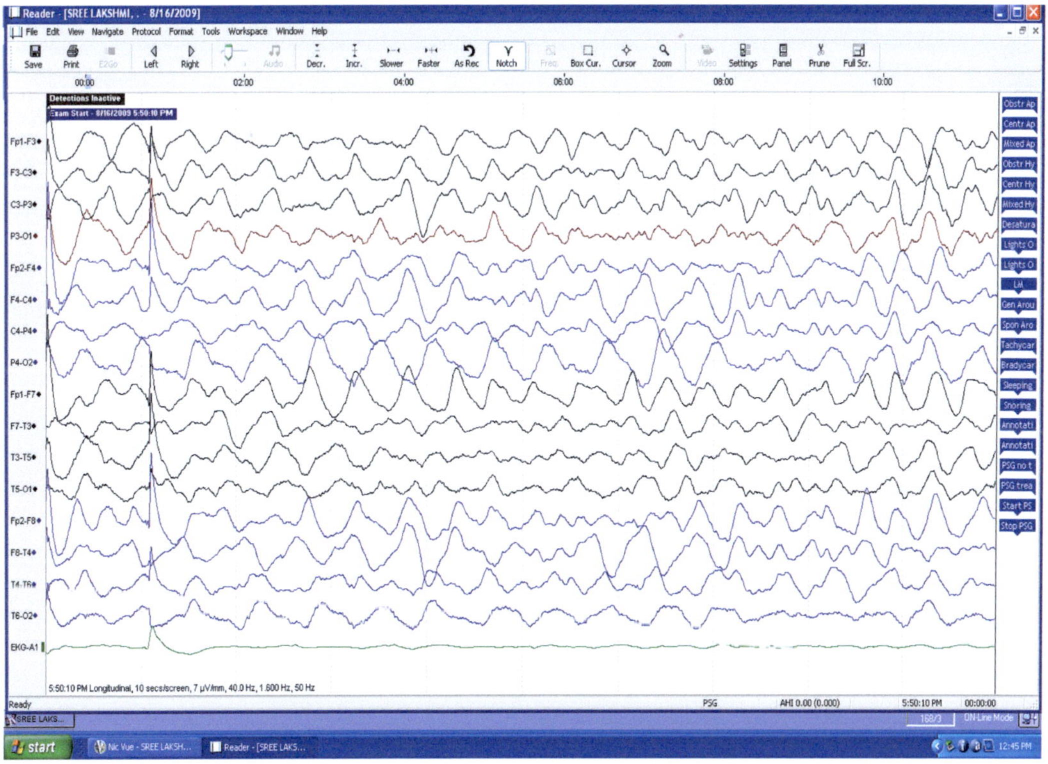

Fig. 8.5 Diffuse slowing. EEG demonstrating diffuse slowing in the delta range of frequencies (2–3 Hz in this example) which at times is polymorphic delta activity or PDA

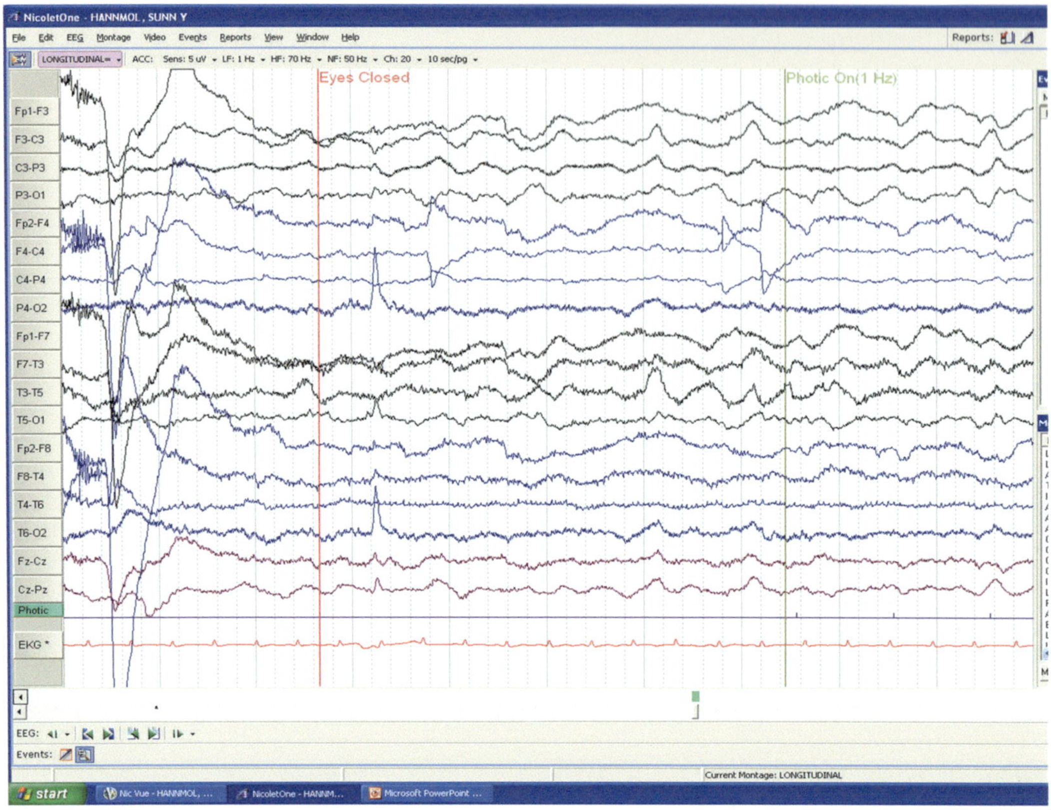

Fig. 8.6 Left Hemispheric slowing. Bipolar montage EEG demonstrating left hemispheric polymorphic delta slowing at 3-4 Hz more so over the left frontotemporal region

unspecified encephalopathy in responsive patients, often with metabolic derangement and cerebrovascular disease.

Points to Remember

(a) Polymorphic delta activity (PDA) is a non-specific EEG finding and points to a diffuse encephalopathy with no much prognostic value.
(b) Severe encephalopathy leads to more slow EEG.
(c) Focal slowing indicates a focal parenchymal lesion with more subcortical involvement.
(d) FIRDA is focal delta activity with more of diffuse encephalopathy involvement and rarely has localizing value.

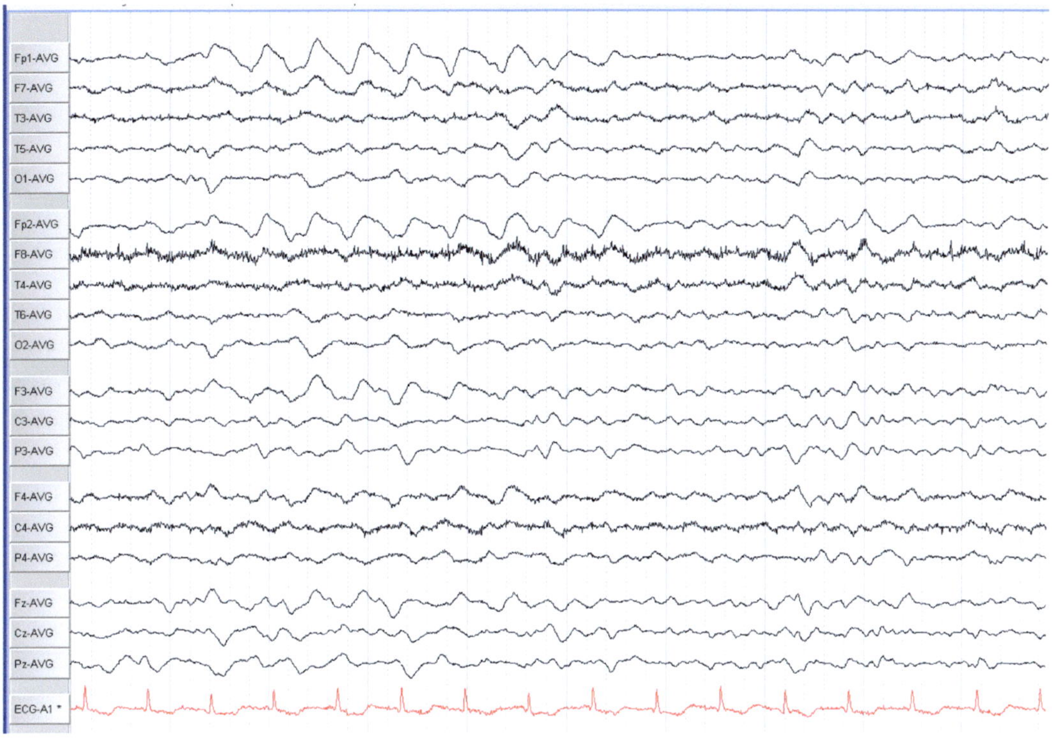

Fig. 8.7 Frontal intermittent rhythmic delta activity (FIRDA) appears as intermittent symmetrical rhythmic delta activity over frontal regions more over the left side at frequency of 2.5–3 Hz. Average referential montage with sensitivity 7 μV, LFF 1 Hz, HFF 70 Hz

8.5 Pattern 3: Periodic Epileptiform Discharges (PEDs)

PEDs are repeating waveforms of relatively uniform morphology, duration, and quantifiable interdischarge interval, occupying the majority of the recording. PEDs are described by their topography and interdischarge interval, usually 0.3 s to several seconds, which can provide clues to their etiology [11, 12]. Topographic descriptions include lateralized periodic discharges (LPDs), bilateral independent periodic discharges (BIPDs), and generalized periodic discharges (GPDs) [6]. In response to an alerting event, stimulus-induced rhythmic ictal or periodic discharges (SIRPIDs) have been described in comatose patients.

8.5.1 Periodic Lateralized Epileptiform Discharges or Lateralized Periodic Discharges

When a PED is lateralized, it is termed as a PLED. PLEDs are epileptiform complexes that recur every 1–2 s (Fig. 8.8). A recent term for them is lateralized periodic discharges (LPDs) instead of PLEDS. Though LPDs are epileptiform in appearance, they are not necessarily indicative of an ongoing active seizures. They are usually transient and cease within next few days to weeks. It indicates an acute, destructive lesion of the underlying brain parenchyma, with acute stroke being the most common followed by herpes encephalitis, autoimmune encephalitis, and rapidly expanding tumors [13]. The literature

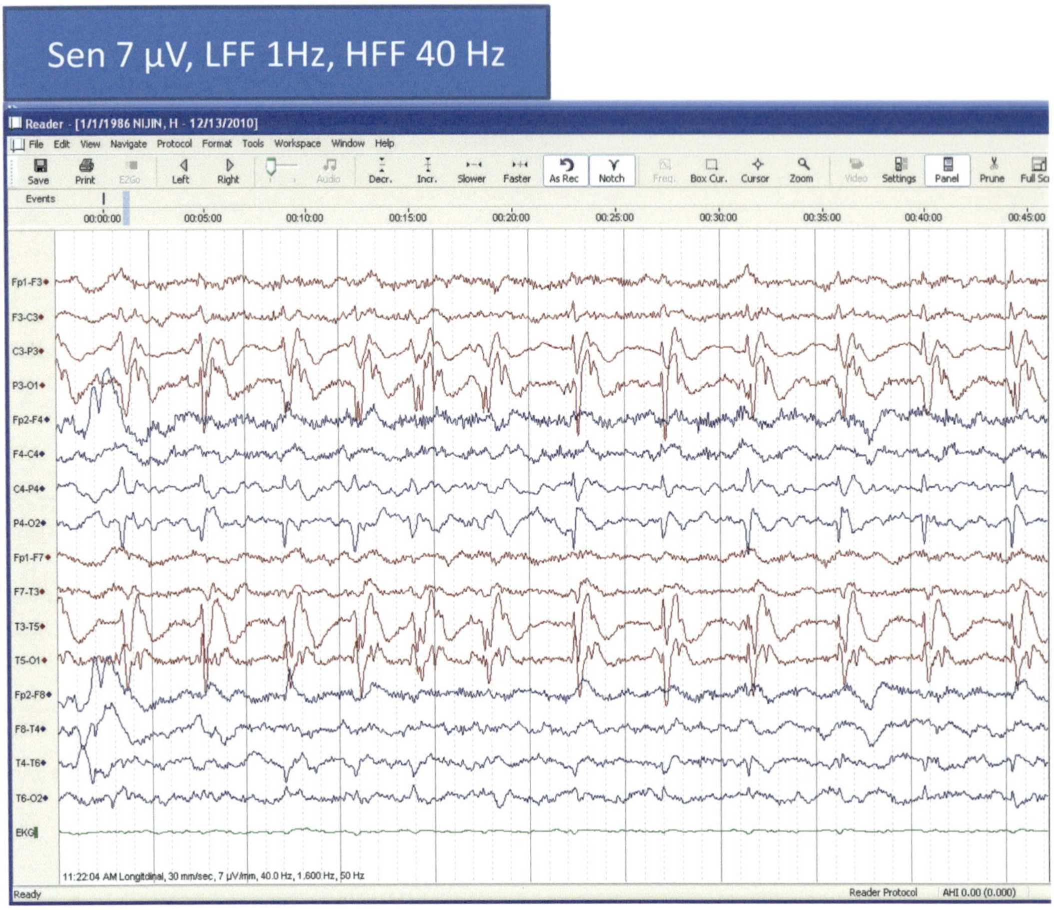

Fig. 8.8 Left-sided LPDs. EEG showing LPDs over the left hemisphere maximum over the posterior head region on the left side

suggests that up to 90% of patients with LPDs will experience seizures during the course of their illness [13]. When a patient with LPDs has an electrographic seizure (ES), the EEG typically becomes faster and more rhythmic [11].

Points to Remember

1. LPDs are indicative of an acute, destructive lesion of the brain parenchyma.
2. LPDs do not mean that the patient is seizing but do indicate a high risk of developing a seizure.
3. A repeat EEG is recommended, and sometimes patients might require brief treatment with AEDs.

8.5.2 Bilateral Independent Periodic Lateralized Epileptiform Discharges

BIPDs refers to the presence of two independent, asynchronous, lateralized discharges in both hemispheres, as shown in Fig. 8.9 [11]. BIPDs are associated with a more diffuse or multifocal process at high risk of developing clinical seizures [14, 15]. Common pathologies include hypoxic ischemic encephalopathy (HIE), severe hypoglycemia, central nervous system (CNS) infections, and HSE [13]. BIPDs are also frequently associated with seizures and often a poor neurological prognosis.

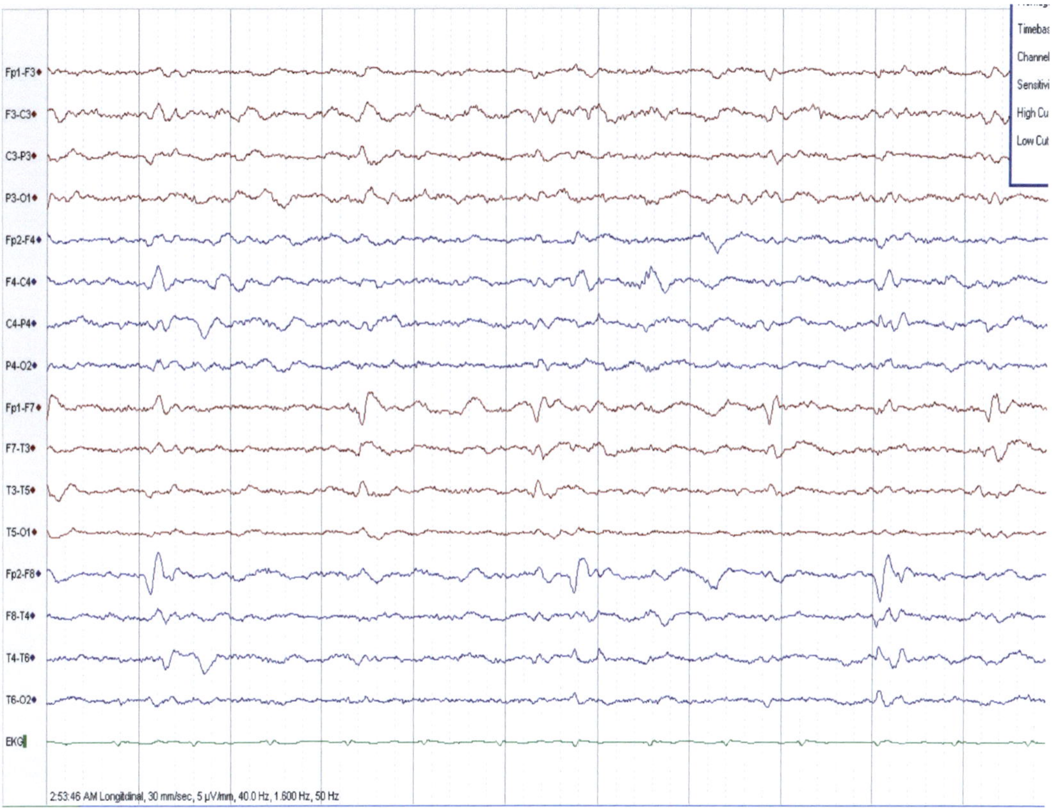

Fig. 8.9 BIPDs. The patient shown here had right basal ganglia bleed with midbrain extension and hypoxic brain damage

Points to Remember

1. Like PLEDs, BIPDs indicate an acute, destructive lesion; however, the process is often more diffuse.
2. Patients with BIPDs are at high risk of developing clinical seizures.
3. BIPDs indicate a worse prognosis, when compared to LPDs.

8.5.3 Generalized Periodic Discharges

When PEDs occur across both hemispheres, and when those discharges are synchronous and symmetrical, they are called GPEDs (Fig. 8.10). They usually indicate diffuse dysfunction of underlying cerebrum. Common causes are anoxic brain damage, Creutzfeldt–Jacob disease, Hashimoto's encephalopathy, drug intoxication, and end-stage Alzheimer's disease, [16] highly associated with seizures, with almost 50% going on to have seizures during their acute illness.

Points to Remember

1. GPEDs result from various illnesses and indicate diffuse cerebral dysfunction that is usually severe.
2. They are highly associated with progression to clinical seizures.

8.5.4 Stimulus-Induced Periodic, Rhythmic, or Ictal Discharges (SIRPIDs)

In some critically ill patients, the EEG is altered by stimuli such as suctioning, background noise,

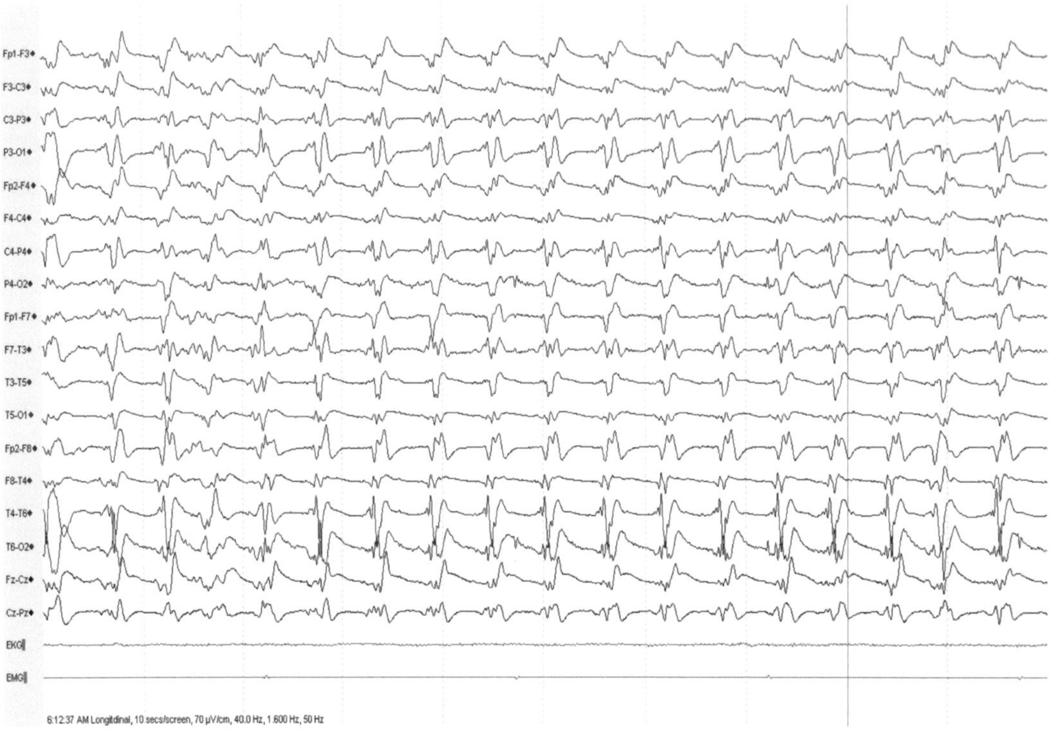

Fig. 8.10 GPEDs. EEG demonstrating GPEDs (2 per second) in a patient with generalized seizure disorder with status epilepticus

and pain. These are known as "alerting stimuli." These can create periodic discharges or frank electrographic seizures (ESs), which can either be focal or generalized (Fig. 8.11). The duration and amplitude of the SIRPIDs pattern often correlate with the duration and intensity of the stimulus [17]. Hence, a prolonged video-EEG recordings will be more helpful in ICUs if available. Discrimination between ictal and non-ictal activity can prove difficult. Clinical significance is uncertain, but overall outcome is poor.

Points to Remember

1. In comatose patients, rhythmic periodic or ictal discharges can arise in the context of alerting stimuli.
2. SIRPIDs may not correlate with any obvious clinical change, but on occasions clinical seizures do occur and often associated with poor prognosis.

8.5.5 Triphasic Waves

Triphasic waves are seen many toxic/metabolic encephalopathies, the classical disease being hepatic encephalopathy [18]. They are generalized, periodic, symmetric, and bisynchronous (across both hemispheres) (Fig. 8.12). The waves often appear blunt, which gave rise to the alternate term "blunt spike and wave." Triphasic waves tend to recur at a rate of about 1 or 2 per

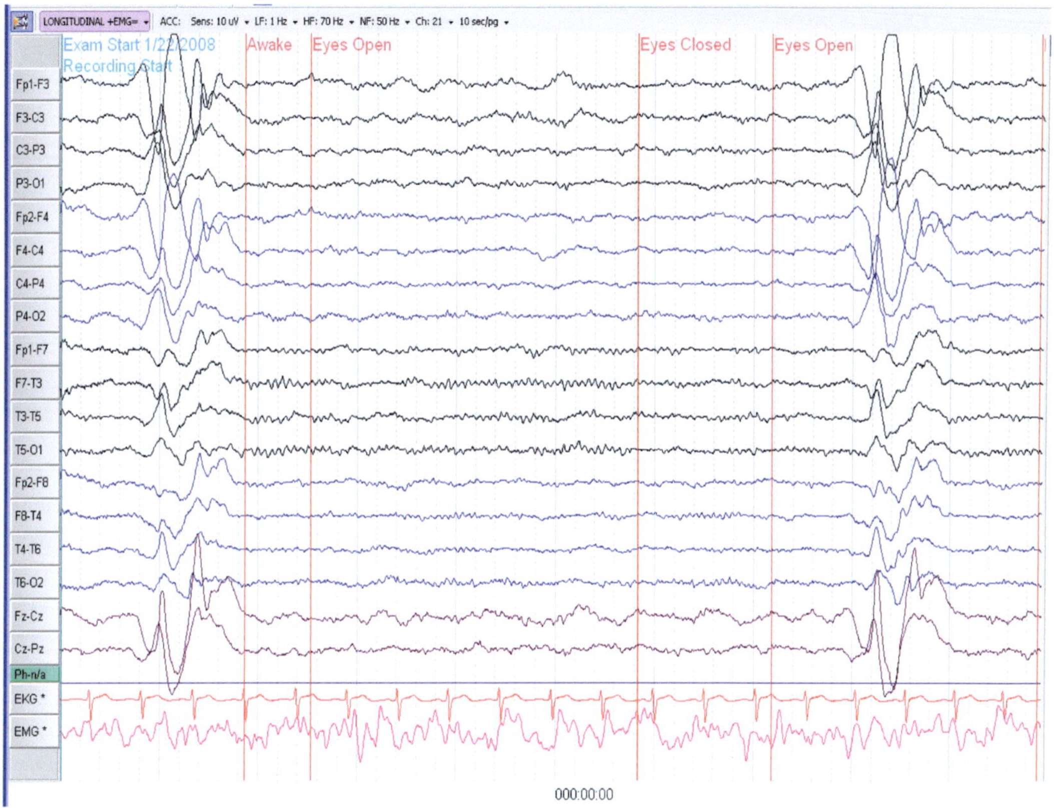

Fig. 8.11 SIRPIDs. In this example, generalized discharges developed on altering stimuli to open and close eyes consistent with SIRPIDs. The patient was comatose on ventilator following hypoxic brain damage

second and often wax and wane during the recording. Classically, triphasic waves of metabolic encephalopathy often appear similar to nonconvulsive status epilepticus on EEG [18]. Benzodiazepines will obliterate both patterns. As such, these two patterns can only be accurately distinguished post hoc, namely, depending on whether the patient clinically improves [19].

Points to Remember

1. Triphasic waves are seen in various toxic/metabolic encephalopathies, not just hepatic encephalopathy.
2. Triphasic waves appear similar to the EEG pattern seen with nonconvulsive status epilepticus.

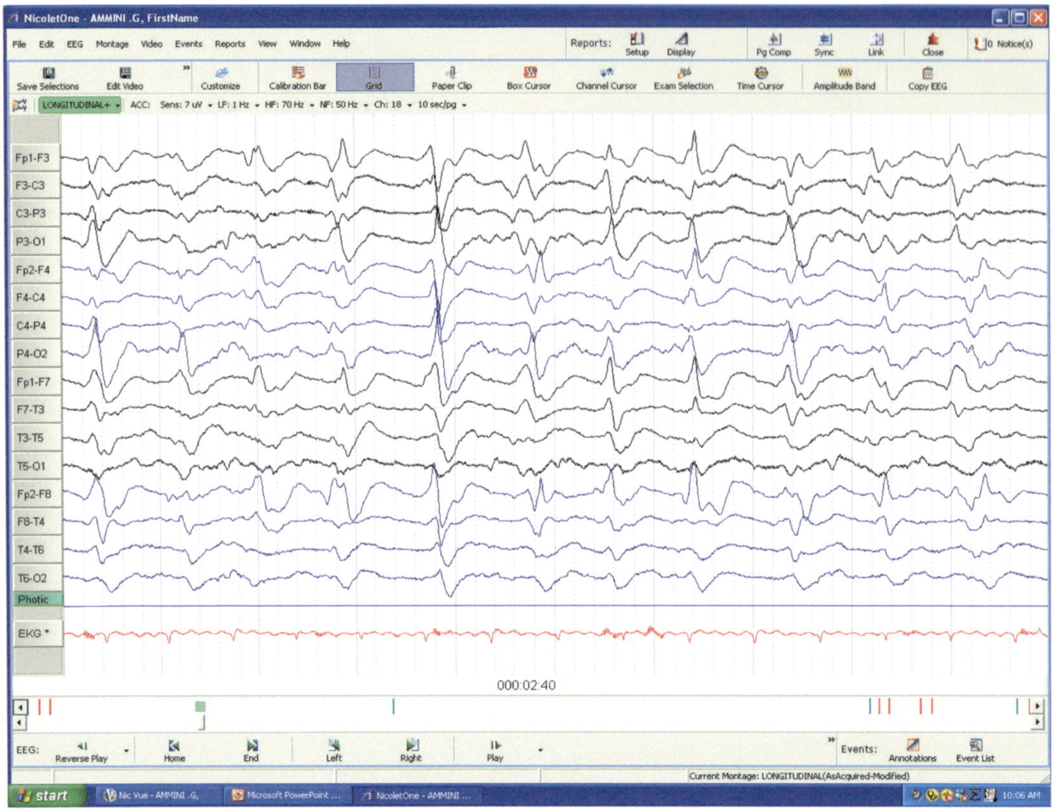

Fig. 8.12 Triphasic waves occurring with a periodicity of 1–2 Hz are symmetrical positive sharp transients (downward deflection) preceded and followed by relatively low amplitude negative waves (upward deflection), dominant over frontal cortex with an anterio-posterior lag

8.6 Pattern 4: Burst-Suppression Pattern (BSP)

Burst-suppression is characterized by periods of high-voltage EEG activity, alternating with periods of suppressed electrical activity usually below 10 uV (Fig. 8.13). When more than 50% of the record consists of attenuation or suppression, this pattern has recently been defined as burst suppression [12]. It indicates diffuse cerebral dysfunction indicating poor outcomes as it is exclusively seen in deeply comatose patients [20]. It can be seen following cerebral anoxia post cardiac arrest or head trauma, drug intoxications, [21, 22] severe hypothermia and can also be seen in patients on very high sedation [23].

Intensivists may titrate sedatives to achieve BSP in patients with resistant status epilepticus or intractable intracranial hypertension. It usually indicates maximal sedation, and further dosing will only increase drug-related side effects without added clinical benefit.

Points to Remember

1. Burst suppression typically indicates a poor prognosis and never points to an etiology.
2. Pharmacologic sedation can also produce this EEG pattern.

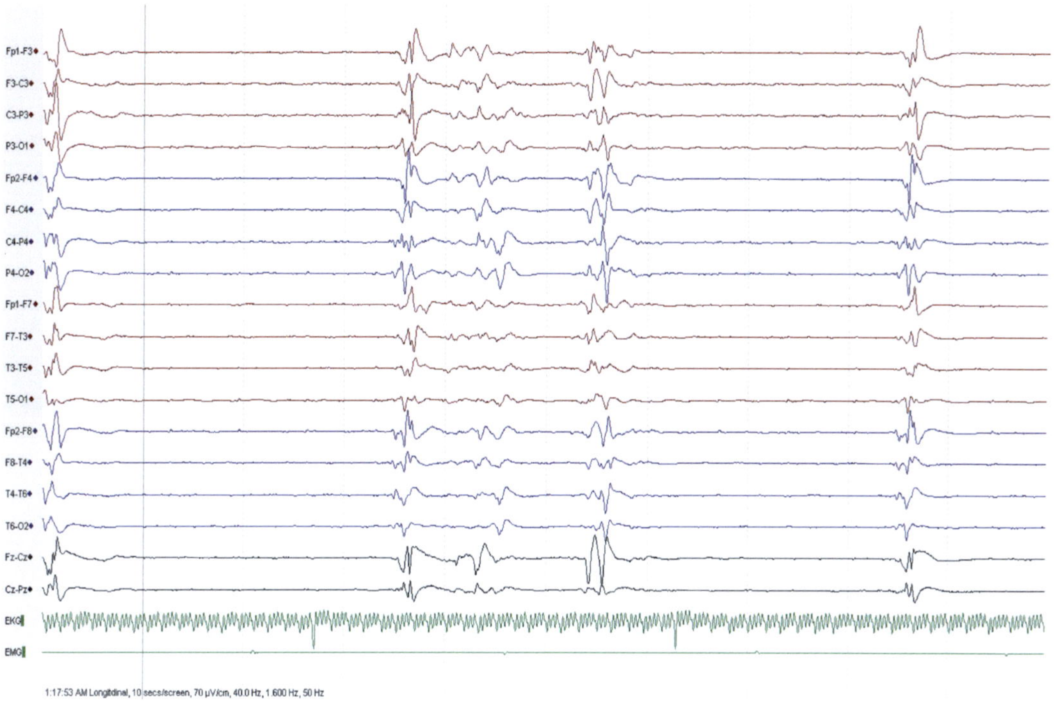

Fig. 8.13 Burst suppression. EEG showing burst suppression in a patient with status epilepticus and achieved with propofol

8.7 Pattern 5: Electrographic Seizures

ESs are commonly seen in patients with altered mental status and coma. ESs can be associated with motor movements (e.g., subtle ocular movements, facial twitches), but most are not. A short EEG of 30–60 mins does not add much to our cause of altered sensorium; hence, a continuous EEG is increasingly requested by clinicians, in order to detect those with nonconvulsive (i.e., nonvisible or subclinical) status epilepticus [21, 24]. The risk of NCSE is higher in patients with underlying epilepsy, those presenting with a generalized tonic-clonic seizures, or following intracranial hemorrhage [21, 24].

EEG patterns are classified into two main types, first one is classified according to their localization into generalized, lateralized, bilateral independent, and multifocal patterns. Second pattern is classified according to their waveform morphology into periodic discharges (PDs), rhythmic delta activity (RDA), and spike-and-wave or sharp-and-wave (SW) (Fig. 8.14). The PD pattern is defined as the repeated occurrence of the same paroxysmal discharge at a relatively constant interval. The RDA pattern is defined as the persistence of a high-amplitude waveform of ≤4 Hz, without interval between discharges. The SW pattern is defined as the persistence of spike/sharp waves followed by slow waves [12].

Salzburg EEG criteria were developed a shown in Fig. 8.15 (and have been validated) for diagnosing nonconvulsive ES activity in the critically ill [25]. Each of the following three EEG patterns supports the diagnosis of nonconvulsive ES: [1] sharp waves or spikes occurring at >2.5 Hz for any 10 s period (Fig. 8.16); [2] epileptiform activity occurring at <2.5 Hz but with spatiotemporal evolution (change in frequency, voltage, and/or locational spread); or [3] improvement in the electroclinical status following an intravenous AED trial (e.g., benzodiazepine).

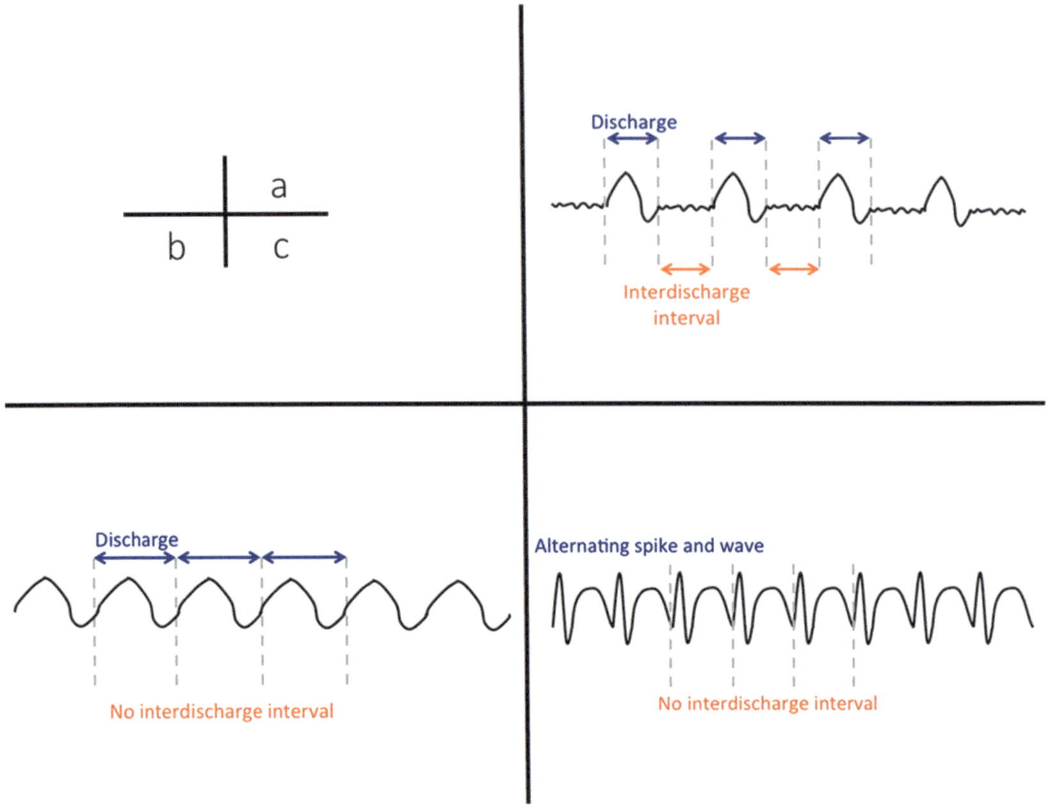

Fig. 8.14 EEG pattern associated with NCSE. a: periodic discharges. b: rhythmic delta activity. c: spike-and-wave

There is considerable debate as to the best treatment of subclinical (or electrographic only) NCSE, as there is a risk benefit assessment which must be considered on an individual basis.

8.7.1 Focal Electrographic Seizures

Many non-diffuse cortical pathologies can be associated with electrocerebral irritation and can result in focal ESs. These include stroke, encephalitis, brain abscesses, brain tumors, and post-traumatic gliosis [11]. Focal ESs usually occur hemispherically (Fig. 8.17) and are often restricted to a particular region. They can evolve from PLEDs or arise de novo.

8.7.2 Generalized Electrographic Seizures

Generalized ESs can occur in focal brain disease and patients with idiopathic/cryptogenic epilepsy [21, 24]. Sometimes, it is the focal ES leading to the spread and presenting as generalized ES (Fig. 8.18).

Points to Remember

1. Focal ES occurs hemispherically and is commonly seen in localized pathologies and may arise from LPDs.
2. Generalized ESs usually occur in patients with underlying generalized epilepsy, and focal pathologies can also cause.

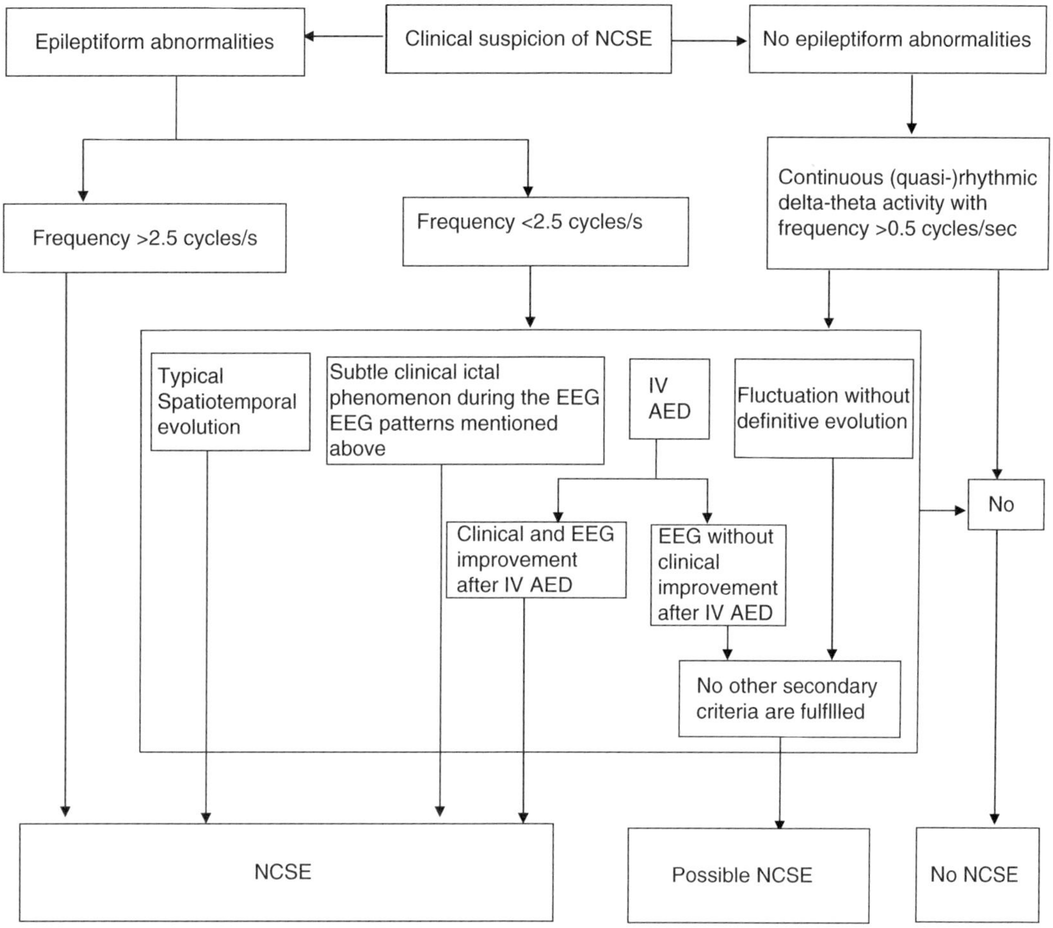

Fig. 8.15 Modified Salzburg consensus for NCSE. (From Leitinger et al., Lancet Neurol 2016;15:1054–62)

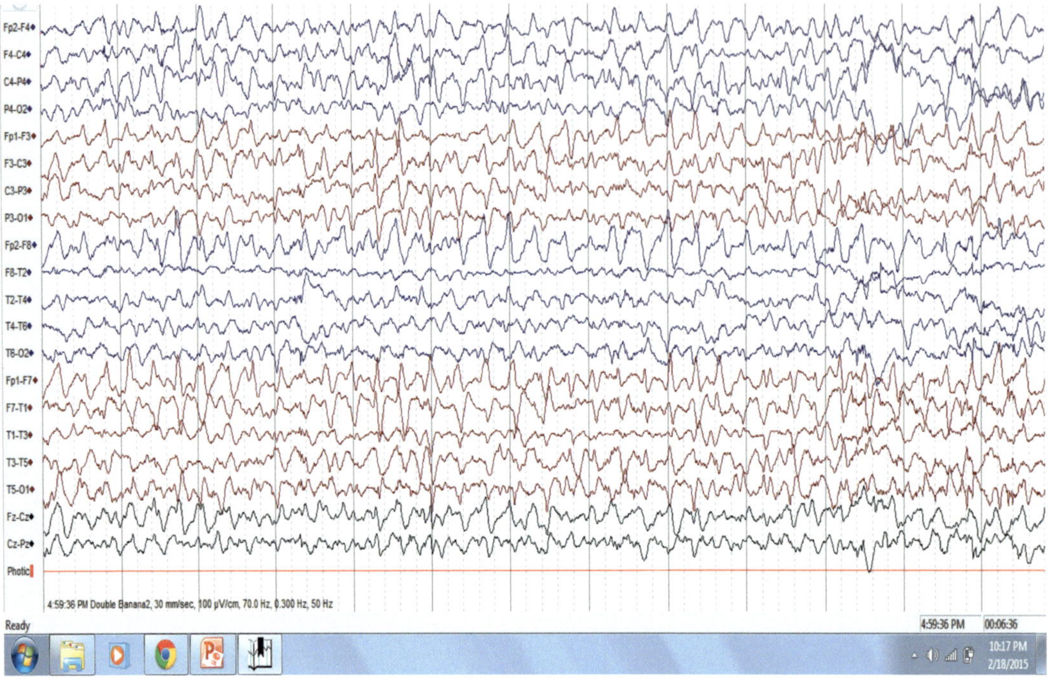

Fig. 8.16 NCSE. EEG demonstrating GPEDs at >2.5 Hz with an evolving rhythm in a patient with status epilepticus

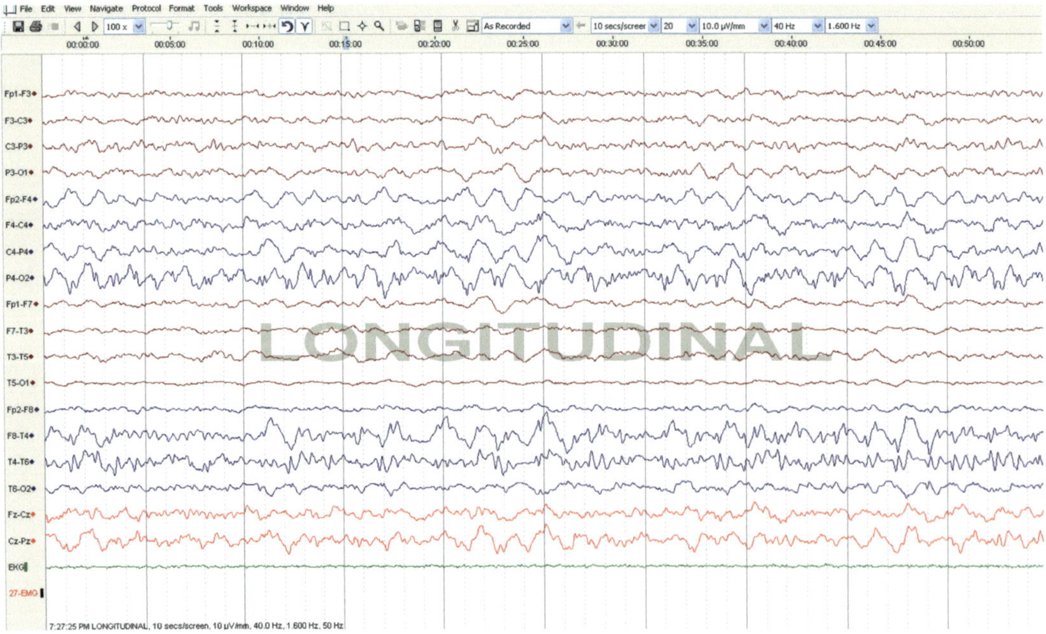

Fig. 8.17 Focal electrographic seizure. EEG demonstrating a focal electrographic seizure over the right temporoparietal region

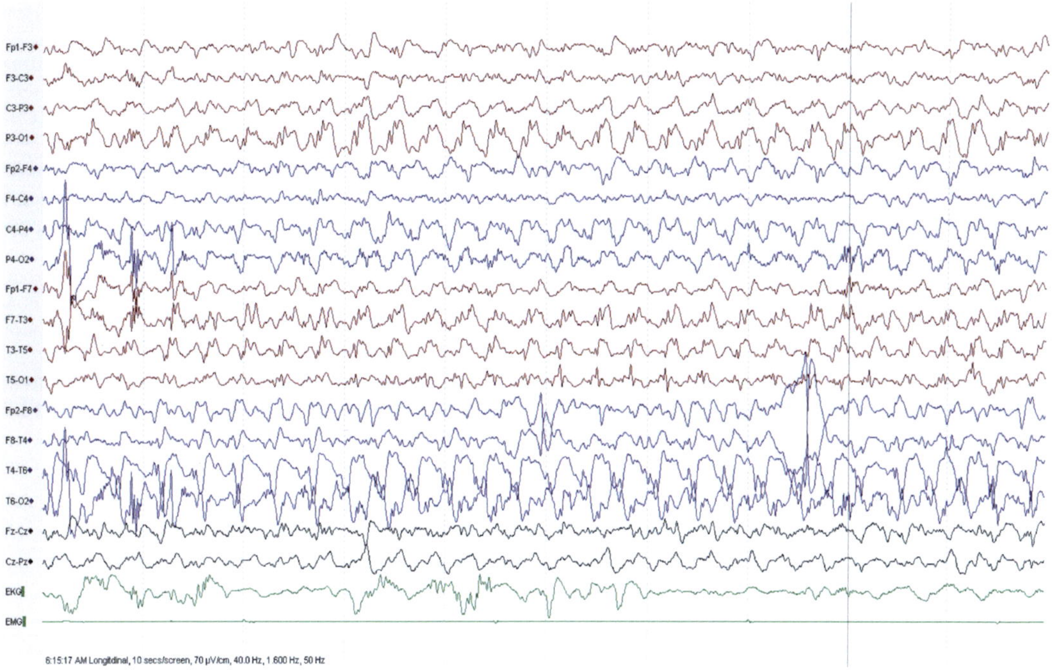

Fig. 8.18 Generalized electrographic seizure. Generalized electrographic seizure in a comatose patient with an underlying primary generalized epilepsy

8.8 Continuous EEG

Continuous EEG (cEEG), with or without video, is a relatively new entrant in the ICU, whereby cerebral EEG alongside clinical behavior is recorded over a period ranging from hours to weeks. It can be used to identify NCS and NCSE and hence is increasing in clinical applications. In cases of refractory status epilepticus, it is also used to guide depth of anesthesia, with evidence of burst suppression acting as a surrogate marker for adequate depth of anesthesia. It is also used to distinguish non-epileptic events that may closely mimic epileptic seizures.

However, cEEG is still a field of active clinical research, and more evidence is required to establish its cost-effectiveness. cEEG is also resource-intensive and often requires an epilepsy expert for its interpretation.

References

1. Limotai C, Ingsathit A, Thadanipon K, McEvoy M, Attia J, Thakkinstian A. How and whom to monitor for seizures in an ICU: a systematic review and meta-analysis. Crit Care Med. 2019;47(4):e366–73.
2. Pandian JD, Cascino GD, So EL, Manno E, Fulgham JR. Digital video-electroencephalographic monitoring in the neurological-neurosurgical intensive care unit: clinical features and outcome. Arch Neurol. 2004;61(7):1090–4.
3. Claassen J, Taccone FS, Horn P, et al. Recommendations on the use of EEG monitoring in critically ill patients: consensus statement from the neurointensive care section of the ESICM. Intensive Care Med. 2013;39(8):1337–51.
4. Herman ST, Abend NS, Thomas P. Bleck et al consensus statement on continuous EEG in critically ill adults and children, part I: indications. J Clin Neurophysiol. 2015;32:87–95.
5. Hill CE, Blank LJ, Thibault D, et al. Continuous EEG is associated with favorable hospitaliza-

tion outcomes for critically ill patients. Neurology. 2019;92(1):e9–e18.
6. Kane N, Acharya J, Benickzy S, et al. Glossary of terms most commonly used by clinical electroencephalographers and updated proposal for the report format of the EEG findings. Revision 2017. Clin Neurophysiol Pract. 2017;2:170–85.
7. Caricato A, Melchionda I, Antonelli M. Continuous electroencephalography monitoring in adults in the intensive care unit. Crit Care. 2018;22(1):75.
8. Society ACN. Guideline 1: minimum technical requirements for performing clinical electroencephalography. Am J Electroneurodiagnostic Technol. 2006;46(3):198–204.
9. Schaul N. Pathogenesis and significance of abnormal nonepileptiform rhythms in the EEG. J Clin Neurophysiol. 1990;7:229–48.
10. Huppertz HJ, Hof E, Klisch J, et al. Localization of interictal delta and epileptiform EEG activity associated with focal epileptogenic brain lesions. NeuroImage. 2001;13:15–28.
11. Brenner RP, Schaul N. Periodic EEG patterns: classification, clinical correlation, and pathophysiology. J Clin Neurophysiol. 1990;7:249–67.
12. Hirsch LJ, LaRoche SM, Gaspard N, et al. American clinical neurophysiology Society's standardized critical care EEG terminology: 2012 version. J Clin Neurophysiol. 2013;30:1–27.
13. Pohlmann-Eden B, Hoch DB, Cochius JI, et al. Periodic lateralized epileptiform discharges–a critical review. J Clin Neurophysiol. 1996;13:519–30.
14. Orta DS, Chiappa KH, Quiroz AZ, et al. Prognostic implications of periodic epileptiform discharges. Arch Neurol. 2009;66:985–91.
15. Lawn ND, Westmoreland BF, Sharbrough FW. Multifocal periodic lateralized epileptiform discharges (PLEDs): EEG features and clinical correlations. Clin Neurophysiol. 2000;111:2125–9.
16. Husain AM, Mebust KA, Radtke RA. Generalized periodic epileptiform discharges: etiologies, relationship to status epilepticus, and prognosis. J Clin Neurophysiol. 1999;16:51–8.
17. Hirsch LJ, Claassen J, Mayer SA, et al. Stimulus induced rhythmic, periodic, or ictal discharges (SIRPIDs): a common EEG phenomenon in the critically ill. Epilepsia. 2004;45:109–23.
18. Fountain NB, Waldman WA. Effects of benzodiazepines on triphasic waves: implications for nonconvulsive status epilepticus. J Clin Neurophysiol. 2001;18:345–52.
19. Boulanger JM, Deacon C, Lecuyer D, et al. Triphasic waves versus nonconvulsive status epilepticus: EEG distinction. Can J Neurol Sci. 2006;33:175–80.
20. Amzica F. What does burst suppression really mean? Epilepsy Behav. 2015;49:234–7.
21. Young GB. The EEG in coma. J Clin Neurophysiol. 2000;17:473–85.
22. De Rubeis DA, Young GB. Continuous EEG monitoring in a patient with massive carbamazepine overdose. J Clin Neurophysiol. 2001;18:166–8.
23. Akrawi WP, Drummond JC, Kalkman CJ, et al. A comparison of the electrophysiologic characteristics of EEG burst-suppression as produced by isoflurane, thiopental, etomidate, and propofol. J Neurosurg Anesthesiol. 1996;8:40–6.
24. Brenner RP. The interpretation of the EEG in stupor and coma. Neurologist. 2005;11:271–84.
25. Leitinger M, Trinka E, Gardella E, et al. Diagnostic accuracy of the Salzburg EEG criteria for nonconvulsive status epilepticus: a retrospective study. Lancet Neurol. 2016;15:1054–62.

9 Transcranial Doppler

Amit Goyal and Vasudha Singhal

9.1 Introduction

Transcranial doppler (TCD) is a valuable tool for the bedside evaluation of major intracranial vessels, including arteries of the circle of Willis. Introduced in clinical practice by Rune Aaslid and colleagues [1], TCD is a reliable, noninvasive, real-time technique, allowing dynamic monitoring of the cerebral blood flow (CBF) velocity. TCD relies on the pulsed-wave Doppler technique to insonate cerebral vessels and evaluate red blood cell (RBC) velocity inside the vessel. In current clinical practice, it is commonly used in conditions like stroke, traumatic brain injury (TBI), and aneurysmal subarachnoid hemorrhage (aSAH) [2–4]. This chapter discusses the principle, technique, clinical applications, and the limitations of TCD in detail.

9.2 Physical Principle

TCD measures blood flow velocities (FVs) in cerebral vessels by using the *Doppler principle*. Observed by the physicist Christian Andreas Doppler, the Doppler principle states that a change in the frequency of a reflected wave (Doppler shift, f_d) is directly proportional to the velocity of the reflector. In simple words, when ultrasound wave strikes the RBC in a vessel, the reflected wave undergoes a change in frequency, called the Doppler shift (f_d), that is directly proportional to the RBC velocity. If RBC is flowing in the direction of the observer (probe), the reflected wave will have a higher frequency than the incident pulse frequency, whereas if the RBC is moving away from the observer, the reflected wave will have a frequency lower than the incident frequency. The following equation derived from this principle is the basis of calculating CBF velocity (CBF-V) by TCD:

$$v = \frac{(c \times fd)}{2 \times f0 \times \cos\theta}$$

where c is the speed of the incident wave, f_d is the Doppler shift, $f0$ is the incident pulse frequency, and θ is the angle of the reflector relative to the ultrasound probe [5].

Doppler shift (f_d) is dependent on the angle of insonation (between the emitted wave and the reflector, i.e., RBC). The maximum Doppler shift is detected at an angle of 0 and 180° (Cos 0° = 1, Cos 180° = −1), while it is zero at an angle of 90°. Since getting an insonation angle of 0 or 180° is nearly impossible, the detected FV is a close approximation of the true CBF-V (lower the angle of insonation, more accurate is the CBF-V). Thus, during consecutive measurements, any change in the measured FV reflects a similar change in the true CBF-V, provided that

A. Goyal · V. Singhal (✉)
Department of Neuroanesthesiology and Critical Care, Medanta, Gurgaon, Haryana, India

H. Prabhakar et al. (eds.), *Principles and Practice of Neurocritical Care*,
https://doi.org/10.1007/978-981-99-8059-8_9

the angle of insonation and diameter of the vessels are unchanged.

The common factors known to affect the diameter of the cerebral vessels include acute blood gas changes, blood pressure variation, and anesthetic agents, amongst others. Studies using TCD have, however, shown that a change in the arterial carbon dioxide tension ($PaCO_2$), blood pressure, and intravenous anesthetic agents have a limited effect on the diameter of the basal cerebral arteries [6–9]. Inhalational anesthetic agents and vasoactive drugs, at the same time, may have a variable effect on the basal artery diameter [10–13].

9.3 Transcranial Doppler (TCD) Versus Transcranial Color-Coded Duplex Sonography (TCCD)

TCD uses *pulsed wave Doppler* to insonate vessels at different depths, and the reflected wave is processed to provide a spectral waveform with peak systolic and end diastolic flow velocities (FV_s and FV_d) (Fig. 9.1). The newer machines include the power-motion mode Doppler (PMD) (introduced by Mark Moehring) [14], allowing simultaneous display of the flow intensity and direction over 6 cm of intracranial space (Fig. 9.1). This system uses multiple gates and insonates the entire length of a vessel, as compared to the single gate TCD which provides information of a small intracranial sample volume. PMD is combined with a single-channel spectral analysis, making it easier for the operator to select a desired depth on the PMD screen and obtain a spectral waveform (Fig. 9.1).

TCCD, on the other hand, uses the *phased array ultrasound* probe. It combines color-coded Doppler with bi-dimensional pulsed wave doppler to provide brain imaging, along with a cerebral vascular map (Fig. 9.2a) and flow velocities (duplex ultrasonography) (Fig. 9.2b). Compared to TCD, it has the advantage of better visualization and easy identification of cerebral vessels, better spatial resolution, and imaging of other parenchymal structures and pathologies (hematoma, tumors, etc.). However, it provides only basic hemodynamic parameters including FV_s,

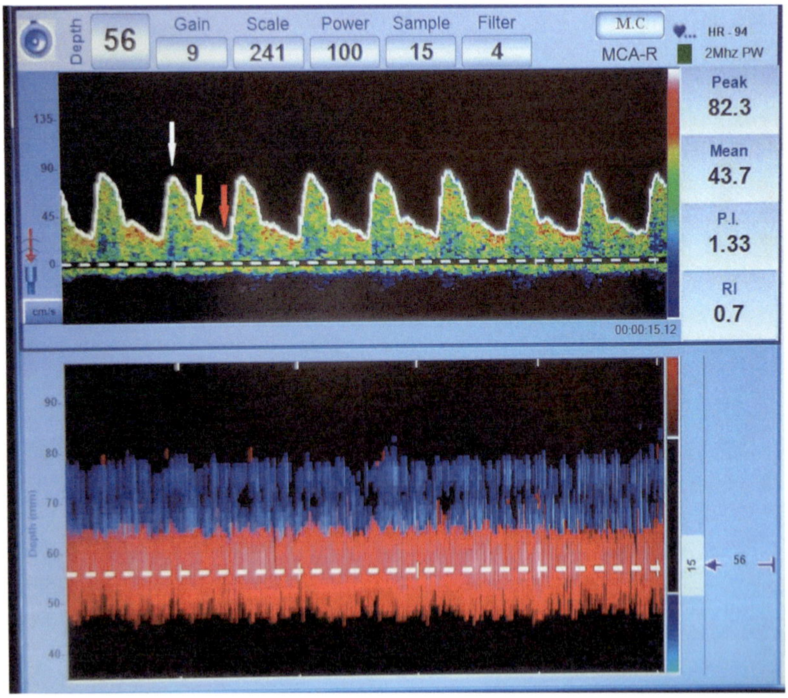

Fig. 9.1 Upper panel: Transcranial doppler spectral waveform showing peak systolic (white arrow), dicrotic notch (yellow arrow), and end-diastolic (red arrow) flow velocities of middle cerebral artery (upward trace). Lower panel: Power motion mode doppler (PMD) displaying color coded flow signals and directions (blue, flow away from the probe; red, flow toward the probe) at different depths

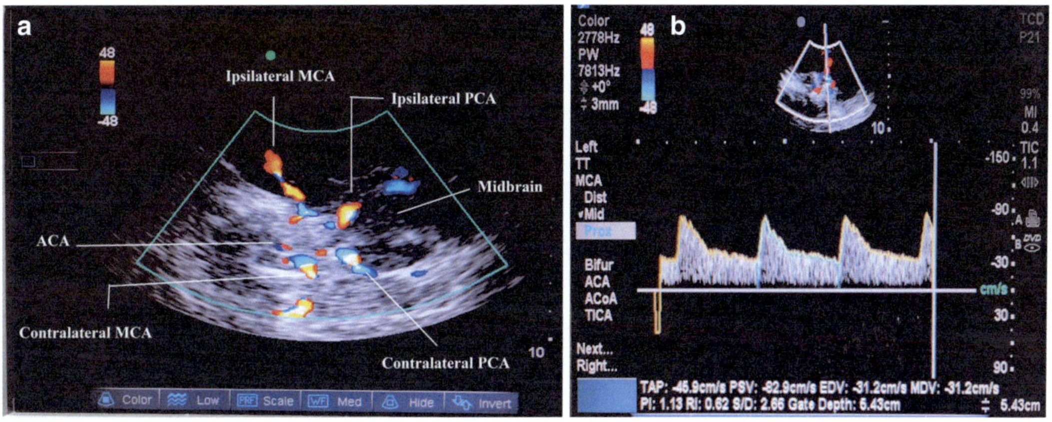

Fig. 9.2 Transcranial color-coded duplex (TCCD) showing the circle of Willis through the temporal window (**a**) and pulsed wave doppler waveform of MCA (**b**). *ACA* anterior cerebral artery; *MCA* middle cerebral artery; *PCA* posterior cerebral artery

FV_d, mean flow velocity (FV_m), and indices including pulsatility index (PI) and resistivity index (RI). Advanced parameters such as cerebral autoregulation indices and critical closing pressure cannot be derived from a TCCD.

9.4 Technique of TCD

An ultrasound probe with a frequency of ≤2 MHz is used to penetrate the skull acoustic windows (thin bony parts of the skull or foramina). There are four such acoustic windows:

1. **Transtemporal window** (Fig. 9.3a): Located above the zygomatic arch between tragus and the lateral eye canthus. This is the most commonly used window to insonate the Middle Cerebral Artery (MCA) (Fig. 9.1), the Anterior Cerebral Artery (ACA) (Fig. 9.4), the terminal Internal Carotid Artery (ICA) (Fig. 9.5), and the Posterior Cerebral Artery (PCA). It can be further divided into anterior, middle, and posterior part, allowing for an easier insonation of different vessels, although the middle window allows for the maximum reduction in the insonation angle. However, this window may be inadequate in 10–20% of population, especially older women with hyperostosis or osteoporosis [15, 16].
2. **Suboccipital (transforaminal) window** (Fig. 9.3b): Insonated through the gap between the occipital bone and the atlas vertebra. It is used to insonate the Vertebral Artery (VA) and the Basilar Artery (BA) (Fig. 9.6).
3. **Submandibular window** (Fig. 9.3c): Insonation done through the submandibular area adjacent to the angle of mandible. It is used to insonate the extracranial ICA (EICA).
4. **Transorbital window** (Fig. 9.3d): Obtained through the thin orbital plate and the bony defect of the optic foramina and superior orbital fissure. It is used to insonate the Ophthalmic Artery (OA) and the ICA siphon. Care should be exercised while using the transorbital window—the eyelid should be closed and covered with a clear dressing in order to avoid exposure to the gel; and the power output should be reduced to 10% (<17 mW/cm^2), so as to minimize damage to the orbital contents. Repeated use of this window also has a theoretical risk of inducing cataract.

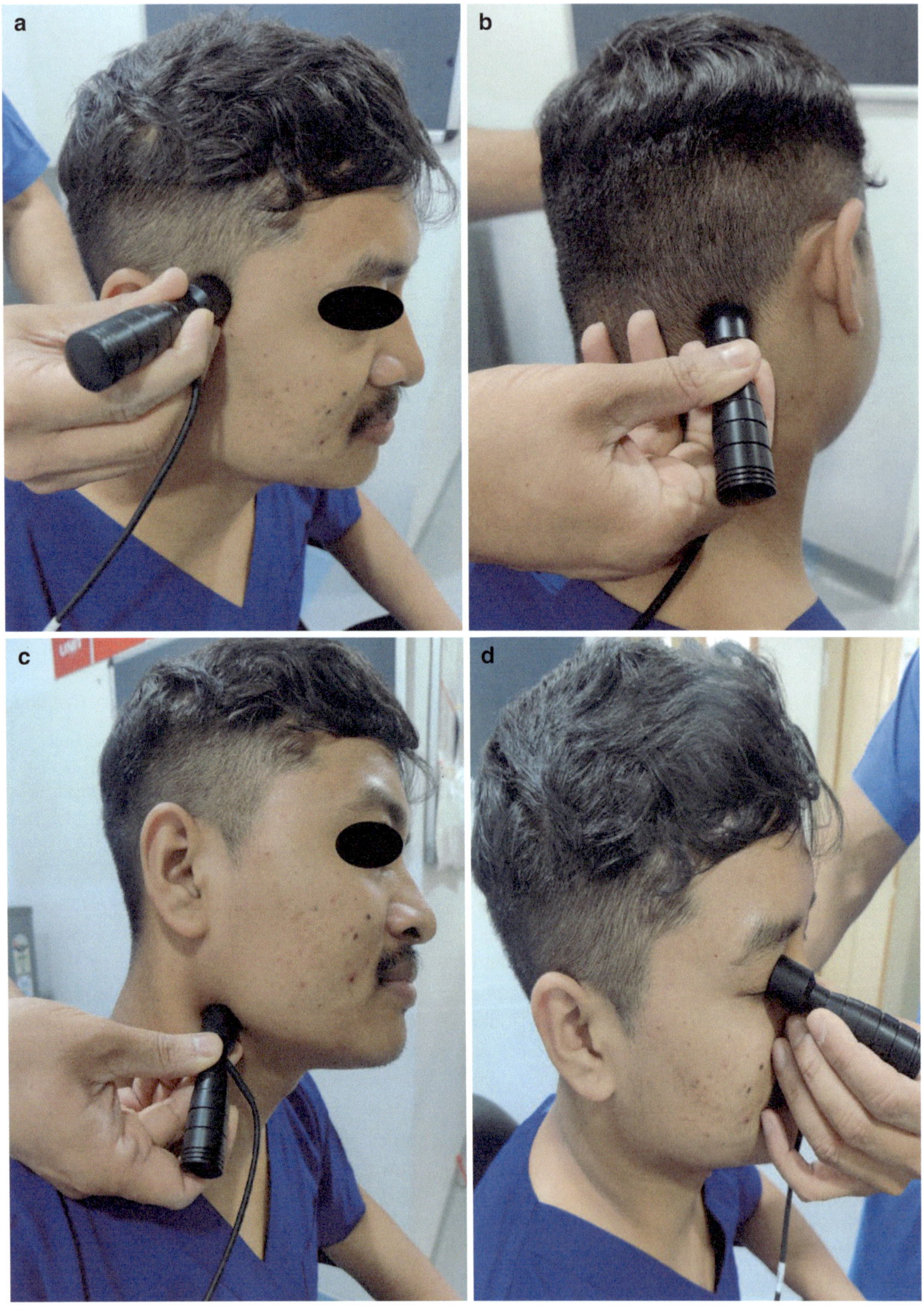

Fig. 9.3 Acoustic windows used for transcranial doppler examination. (**a**) Transtemporal window; (**b**) Suboccipital window; (**c**) Submandibular window; (**d**) Transorbital window

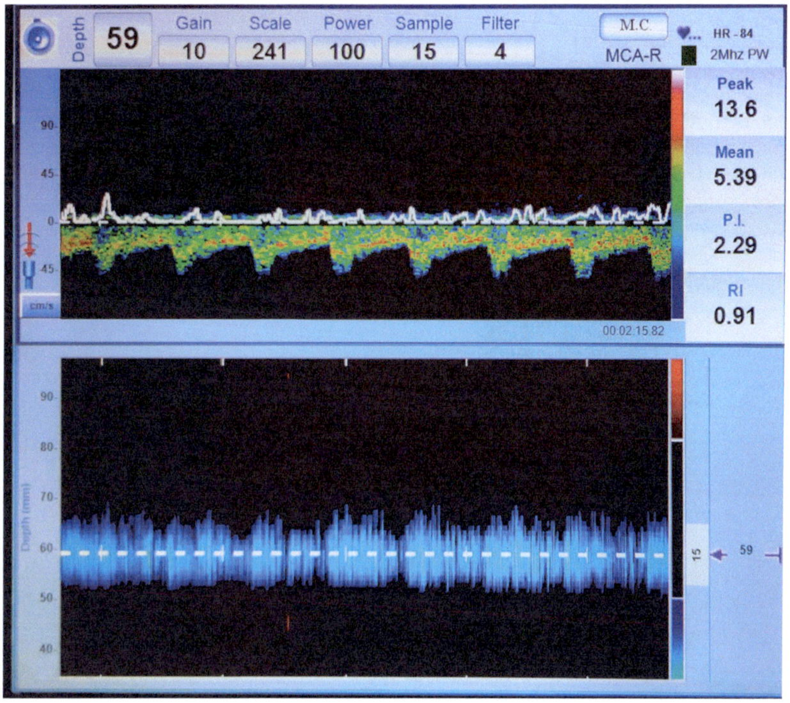

Fig. 9.4 Transcranial doppler spectral waveform showing flow velocities of anterior cerebral artery (downward trace) with power motion mode doppler (PMD) showing flow against the probe at a depth of 60 mm

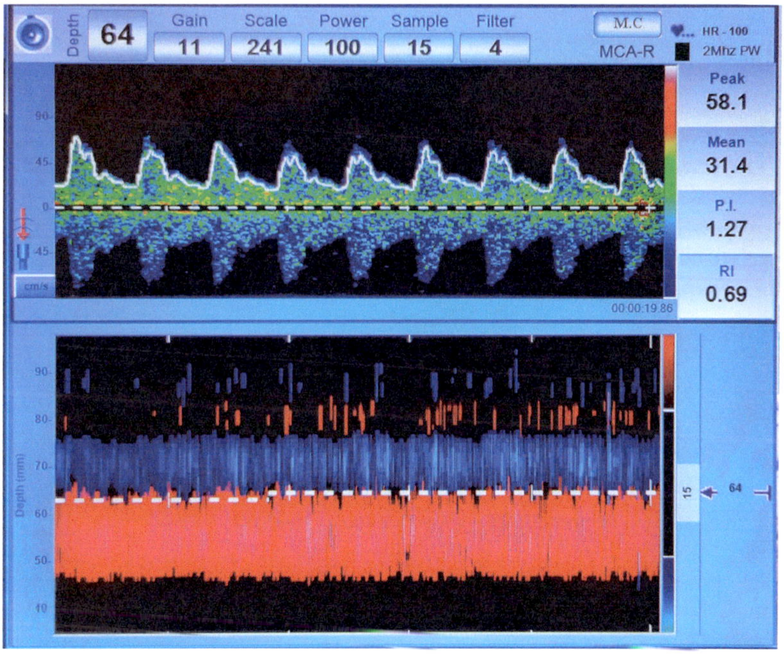

Fig. 9.5 Transcranial doppler spectral waveform showing bifurcation of terminal internal carotid artery (both upward and downward trace) with power motion mode doppler (PMD) showing flow toward and away from the probe at depth of around 65 mm

Identification of the cerebral arteries depends on the acoustic window, probe angle, insonation depth, and the blood flow direction (toward or away from the probe). Additionally, dynamic maneuvers, such as compression of the proximal ICA and tapping over the bony landmarks, can be used to induce waveform changes and identification of the vessels [17]. Common identification characteristics of the cerebral arteries on TCD are summarized in Table 9.1.

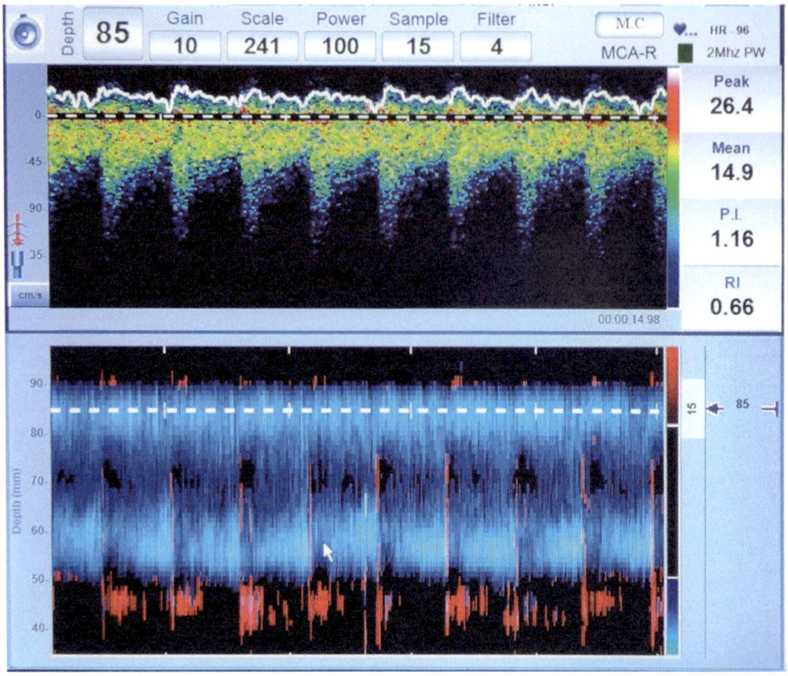

Fig. 9.6 Transcranial doppler spectral waveform showing flow velocity of basilar artery (downward trace) with power motion mode doppler (PMD) showing flow against probe at depth of 80–90 mm through the transforaminal window

Table 9.1 Common identification characteristics of cerebral arteries on TCD examination

Artery	Acoustic window	Probe angle	Depth (mm)	Flow direction	Effect of carotid compression	Adult FV_m (cm/s)
ICA (terminal)	Transtemporal	Straight/ superior	55–65	Bi-directional	Decrease	41 ± 11
MCA	Transtemporal	Straight	40–60	Towards	Decrease	55 ± 12
ACA	Transtemporal	Anterio-superior	60–70	Away	Decrease	50 ± 11
PCA-P1[a]	Transtemporal	Posterior	65–70	Towards	No change	39 ± 10
PCA-P2	Transtemporal	Posterior	65–70	Away	No change	40 ± 10
ICA (siphon)	Ophthalmic	Medial and upward	60–80	Towards/away	Decrease	41 ± 11
OA	Ophthalmic	Medial and upward	45–60	Towards	Decrease	21 ± 5
VA[b]	Suboccipital	Superior and laterally	50–70	Away	No change	38 ± 10
BA	Suboccipital	Superior and medially	80–100	Away	No change	41 ± 10
Extracranial ICA	Submandibular	Superior and medially	40–60	Away	Decrease	30 ± 9

ICA internal carotid artery; *MCA* middle cerebral artery; *ACA* anterior cerebral artery; *PCA-P1* first segment of posterior cerebral artery; *PCA-P2* second segment of posterior cerebral artery; *OA* ophthalmic artery; *VA* vertebral artery; *BA* basilar artery

[a] P1 may be hypoplastic and difficult to insonate in fetal PCA origin

[b] While insonating VA, flow toward probe may be detected, suggesting the extradural portion of VA. More superior angulation of probe can help insonating intradural VA [18]

9.5 Spectral Waveform Analysis

Similar to the arterial pressure waveform, a normal TCD waveform consists of a sharp systolic upstroke with a peak systole, and a gradual downstroke with dicrotic notch and a positive end diastolic flow (Fig. 9.1). FV_s and FV_d are recorded from the highest and lowest velocities in a cycle, respectively, whereas FV_m is calculated as the area under the velocity–time curve during that cycle. The systolic component of the TCD waveform depends upon the upstream factors, including cardiac output, arterial blood pressure, and carotid diameter, whereas the diastolic component is determined by the downstream resistance. The spectral waveform analysis provides a deeper understanding of the physiological and pathological hemodynamic changes. Therefore, prior to making any judgement from the TCD, it is important to obtain a spectral waveform with a good signal strength. Spectral envelop shows power distribution of each frequency shift (determined by the number of RBCs with that velocity), with color code similar to the color scale on graph (red depicting highest power/number of RBCs, and blue depicting lowest power/number of RBCs). Therefore, the spectral envelope of a normal caliber vessel with a good signal strength shows a higher power distribution over most of the waveform.

In proximal steno-occlusive diseases (pathology between the insonated segment and the heart), the loss of pressure head due to occlusion leads to a shallow systolic upstroke followed by a slow diastolic downstroke (blunted appearance), along with an increased FV_d (due to dilatation distal to the occlusion). This morphology may also be seen in low cardiac output conditions (differentiated by its presence in all the vessels, and not just one). In distal steno-occlusive diseases, the velocities increase to maintain the flow through the narrowed segment creating turbulence. The spectral waveform shows a sharp upstroke with a high peak systolic (FV_s) and mean flow velocities (FV_m), and a brisk downstroke with a low FV_d (external pressure opposes forward flow during diastole), with or without symmetrical artifact on either side of the baseline (due to turbulence) (Fig. 9.8a) [19]. With worsening stenosis, FV_s begins to decrease after crossing a critical limit of the reduced vessel diameter [20]. Due to turbulence (scattering of RBCs), spectral envelop of the stenosed vessel shows a disproportionately high power distribution along the lower velocities and lower power along the systolic phase.

9.6 TCD Indices

1. **Mean flow velocity** (FV_m): FV_m is the main parameter of TCD as it correlates best with the CBF [21]. It is calculated using FV_s and FV_d.

$$FV_m = [FV_s + (FV_d \times 2)]/3$$

   Normal ranges of FV_m in different cerebral arteries are mentioned in Table 9.1. Since there is a significant variability within the same individual, it is important to perform serial measurements rather than obtaining a single value [22]. Physiologic factors determining FV_m include the patient's age, sex, hematocrit, mean arterial pressure (MAP), fever, metabolic factors like $PaCO_2$, pregnancy, exercise, and the state of brain activity [23]. Differential diagnosis of the changes in cerebral blood flow velocity is mentioned in Table 9.2 [23].
2. **Lindegaard Ratio (LR)**: LR allows for the differentiation between vasospasm and hyperdynamic circulation, by comparing the FV_m in MCA with the ipsilateral EICA (LR = MCA FV_m/EICA FV_m) [24]. LR > 3 indicates vasospasm (it increases further with the increased severity of vasospasm) [25], whereas LR <3 indicates hyperdynamic circulation. A modified LR ratio for the ACA (Sloan's hemi-

Table 9.2 Conditions affecting cerebral blood flow velocity

Increased flow velocity	Decreased flow velocity
Vasospasm Hyperemia Hyperdynamic circulation Loss of cerebral autoregulation Hypercarbia Vessel stenosis Volatile anesthetic agents Sickle cell anemia Arterio-venous malformation Bacterial meningitis Pre-eclampsia	Hypotension Low cardiac output state Reduced CBF Raised ICP Brain death Hypocapnia Intravenous anesthetic agents (except ketamine) Hypothermia Fulminant hepatic failure

CBF cerebral blood flow; *ICP* intracranial pressure

Table 9.3 TCD grading of vasospasm

Vasospasm in MCA	FV_m (cm/s)	LR
Mild	120–149	3–6
Moderate	150–199	3–6
Severe	>200	>6
Vasospasm in BA	**FV_m (cm/s)**	**SR**
Mild	70–85	2–2.49
Moderate	>85	2.5–2.99
Severe	>85	>3

MCA middle cerebral artery; *BA* basilar artery; *FV_m* mean flow velocity; *LR* lindegaard ratio; *SR* Sviri ratio

spheric ratio) and the posterior circulation (Sviri's ratio) has also been defined (Table 9.3) [26, 27].

3. **Pulsatility index (PI)**: Gosling's pulsatility index describes the pulsatility of the TCD waveform. It is a numerical representation of the change in the pulsatile character of the cerebral blood vessel, with a change in the upstream or downstream resistance. With increase in the downstream resistance (e.g., in raised ICP), the FV_s increases and the FV_d reduces (indicated by a sharp rise in the systolic upstroke and a rapid decline in the diastolic downstroke), thereby increasing the pulsatility and PI (Fig. 9.8a). In cases of proximal stenosis, the distal resistance reduces, with a reduction in FV_s and an increase in the FV_d, thereby reducing the pulsatility or PI. Pulsatility index is calculated as:

$$PI = (FVs - FV_d) / FV_m$$

Since, this ratio removes the effect of Cos θ, PI is independent of the angle of insonation. The normal range of PI is 0.5–1.19 [28]. It is <0.5 in proximal steno-occlusive conditions and vasospasm and > 1.19 in conditions with an increased downstream resistance, like raised ICP and brain stem death [29]. PI <0.5 is also seen in an arterio-venous malformation, due to a decreased distal resistance.

PI and cerebrovascular resistance (CVR) do not change proportionally in all scenarios. PI decreases with a reduction in CVR due to hypercapnia. However, it increases with a reduction in CVR due to low cerebral perfusion pressure (CPP), more disproportionately when autoregulatory reserve is compromised [30, 31]. Therefore, PI-guided assessment of CVR should be interpreted carefully.

Along with the assessment of CVR, PI can also be used for the noninvasive assessment of ICP and CPP [32]. It increases linearly with ICP. PI changes approximately 2.4% with each 1 mm Hg change in ICP [33]. However, its accuracy as an estimator of ICP has been challenged [34, 35].

4. **Resistivity index (RI)**: Also known as Pourcelot index, it is calculated as:

$$RI = (FVs - FV_d) / FV_s$$

An increased RI reflects similar hemodynamic disturbances as mentioned for an abnormal PI, and a RI >0.8 indicates high downstream resistance.

5. **Microembolic signals (MES)**: MES are high intensity transient signals produced when a microemboli passes through the insonated vessel. They are defined by the following criteria:
   (a) transient character (typically <300 ms),
   (b) high intensity (amplitude >3 dB above background—appears bright),
   (c) typically unidirectional and random appearance in the cardiac cycle,
   (d) audible as "snaps or chirps".

9.7 Assessment of Cerebral Hemodynamics by TCD

1. **Assessment of cerebrovascular reactivity to CO_2**: Cerebral vessels change their diameter in response to changes in $PaCO_2$, with hypercarbia causing vasodilation and hypocapnia causing vasoconstriction. Therefore, TCD can be used to assess changes in CBF and FV with respect to changes in $PaCO_2$.
   (a) **Breath holding index (BHI)**: This index is used to detect impaired cerebral vasomotor reserve (VMR) to predict cerebral ischemia in patients with steno-occlusive disease of the internal carotid artery. It is evaluated by using the breath holding-induced hypercapnia as a vasodilatory stimulus [36–38]. It is calculated as:

$$\text{BHI} = \left[\left(\max \text{FV}_{\text{m}} - \min \text{FV}_{\text{m}}\right) \times 100 / \min \text{FV}_{\text{m}}\right] / \text{breath hold time in seconds.}$$

   A BHI >0.6 is normal, >0.2 to 0.6 is impaired and <0.2 is severely impaired.
   (b) **CO_2 index VMR challenge**: Similar to BHI, it is also based on hypercapnia-induced cerebral vasodilation. Cerebral blood flow velocity (CBFV) is estimated at baseline, after hypercapnia, and after hypocapnia. It is calculated as ((hypercapnia CBFV − hypocapnia CBFV)/baseline CBFV) × 100. A value >70% is considered normal, 40–70% is mild impairment, 15–40% is moderate impairment, and <15% is severe impairment [38, 39].
2. **Assessment of cerebral autoregulation**: Cerebral autoregulation is a protective mechanism of the brain to maintain a relatively constant CBF with respect to changes in CPP between 50 and 150 mmHg. It may be impaired in various pathologies or with the use of anesthetic agents.
   (a) **Static autoregulatory index**: It is defined as a percentage change in CVR with respect to a percent change in CPP (achieved pharmacologically using phenylephrine infusion). It ranges from 0 to 1; 0 implies complete loss of autoregulation, and 1 implies intact autoregulation. If it is tested using MAP rather than CPP, results may be erroneous due to "false autoregulation." This means that in the absence of autoregulation, increase in MAP will increase the ICP keeping the CPP relatively constant, thereby giving a false sense of an intact autoregulation.
   (b) **Dynamic autoregulation (leg-cuff deflation) test**: This test monitors the recovery of CBFV after drop in MAP with the deflation of a thigh cuff (inflated 50 mmHg above SBP for 3 min). Normal recovery rate should be approximately 20% per second [40].
   (c) **Transient hyperemic response ratio (THRR)**: This is measured by observing a change in the CBFV with respect to compression of the common carotid artery for 5–8 s. THRR is calculated as a ratio of the hyperemic CBFV (after compression release) to the baseline CBFV (pre-compression) [41]. A normal response will consist of a reduced CVR after compression, with a resulting increase in the CBFV compared to the baseline FV (Fig. 9.7). A THRR of 1.1 is considered as the threshold of a normal response. The results may be affected by the compression technique, and there is an associated risk of thromboembolism in patients with a carotid disease.
   (d) **Mx and Sx index**: Mean flow index (Mx) and systolic flow index (Sx) are correlation coefficient indices between FV_m/FV_s and CPP. Time averaged samples of FV and CPP are analyzed for the continuous

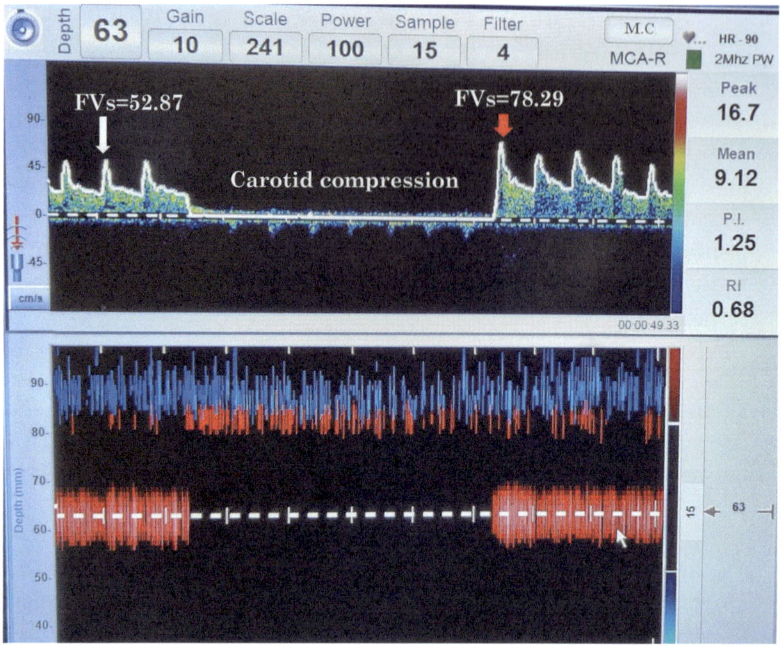

Fig. 9.7 Transcranial doppler spectral waveform showing a transient hyperemic response (THR) consisting of an increase in the flow velocity after release of the carotid compression (white arrow: baseline; red arrow: hyperemic response)

monitoring of CVR. A positive value indicates intact autoregulation, whereas a negative or 0 value implies disrupted autoregulation [42].

3. **Noninvasive estimation of CPP/ICP**: Since invasive ICP monitoring is not always feasible due to its invasiveness, cost and associated risks (hemorrhage, infection, etc.), TCD can be used for the noninvasive estimation of CPP and ICP based on the understanding of the relationship between the CBF and ICP (CPP = MAP − ICP). Aaslid et al. were the first to conduct a noninvasive CPP estimation, based on Fourier's analysis of the arterial blood pressure (ABP) and the MCA velocity waveform [43]. Later, Czosnyka et al. used the time-averaged mean, systolic and diastolic velocities from the MCA for CPP estimation, and compared the TCD-based estimation of CPP with the invasively measured CPP [21]. They concluded that the noninvasive estimation of CPP by TCD may be of value in situations where monitoring relative changes in CPP may benefit, without the need for an invasive ICP monitoring.

TCD-based measurement of CBFV can help in the indirect, noninvasive estimation of CPP, based on the relationship between MAP, CBF, and autoregulatory status. This is critical in conditions like traumatic brain injury (TBI), cerebral infarction, and carotid steno-occlusive conditions, where inadequate or an extremely high perfusion can be harmful.

Hypoperfusion: TCD-based low CBFV can help in the early diagnosis of hypoperfusion and identifying the ABP threshold to avoid cerebral ischemia. Reduced CBFV can be found in proximal steno-occlusive diseases, systemic circulatory failure, and severe TBI. **Critical closing pressure** (CrCP) indicates the level of ABP below which the CBF ceases. It is determined by the opening forces (ABP) and the closing forces (vascular tone and ICP) [44, 45]. By comparing the CBFV waveform with the ABP waveform, CrCP can be estimated as an intercept point of a regression line between ABP and CBFV. This intercept is the value of ABP at which the CBF reaches zero [46, 47].

Hyperperfusion: Increased CBFV may not necessarily indicate a downstream resistance. Hyperemia secondary to hypercapnia or a raised MAP (combined with impaired autoregulation) should be suspected. Global hyperperfusion can be ruled out with monitoring of MAP, $PaCO_2$ levels, status of autoregulation, increased CBFV in more than one vessel territory, and a Lindegaard ratio <3. In post carotid revascularization patients, TCD can be used for the early diagnosis and management of the "hyperperfusion syndrome." [48]

Raised ICP leads to characteristic changes in the cerebral blood flow pattern and TCD waveform morphology in the following sequence [49, 50]:

(a) **Increased pulsatility**: As discussed earlier, increased downstream resistance leads to a sharp systolic upstroke with an increased systolic FV and a sharp downstroke with blunting of the diastolic FV. This leads to an increase in the PI and RI (Fig. 9.8a) [32].

(b) **Oscillating waveform** (Fig. 9.8b): With further increase in ICP above the diastolic pressure, flow reversal during diastole is seen, leading to zero cerebral perfusion (equal systolic forward flow and diastolic retrograde flow) and a catastrophic ischemia ensues.

(c) **Short systolic spikes** (Fig. 9.8c): In extreme cases, ICP approaches systolic pressure with reduction in systolic forward flow and absent diastolic flow. TCD waveform shows systolic spikes with peak FV <50 cm/s and duration <200 ms.

(d) **Intracranial circulatory arrest**: Further increases in ICP lead to a circulatory arrest, with TCD showing no flow. Since inadequate acoustic window can also lead to the absence of a doppler signal, this state should only be considered if the presence of flow from the same window by the same operator was confirmed previously.

PI also shows a significant correlation with the CPP and ICP (within a range of 5–40 mmHg) and is elevated with an elevation in the ICP [32].

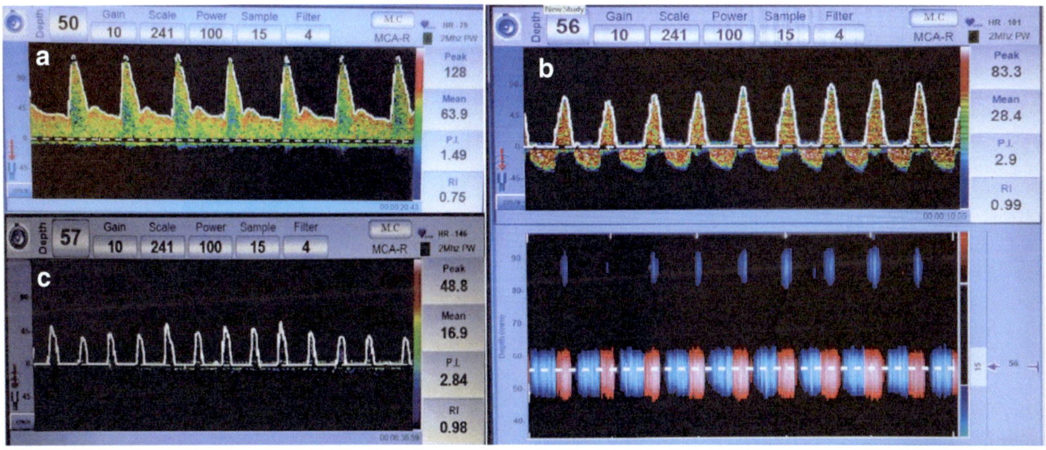

Fig. 9.8 (**a**) Transcranial doppler spectral waveform of a patient with middle cerebral artery (MCA) occlusion, showing a sharp systolic upstroke with increased systolic FV, and a sharp downstroke with reduced diastolic FV. The pulsatility is increased, indicating an increased downstream resistance (raised ICP); (**b**) Spectral waveform showing oscillating flow pattern (flow reversal during diastolic phase) in a brain dead patient. It can be noted that the power motion mode doppler (PMD) is displaying bi-colored flow signals due to different flow directions during systole and diastole; (**c**) Spectral waveform showing short systolic spikes with an absent diastolic flow in the same patient after 2 h

9.8 Clinical Uses

TCD has various clinical applications (listed in Table 9.4).

1. **Traumatic brain injury (TBI)**: Closed head injury with an intracranial hematoma and mass effect is associated with a raised ICP and a reduced CPP, leading to a poor neurological outcome if not addressed timely. TCD can be used to monitor CBF changes, noninvasive ICP estimation, management of CPP, and prognostication in TBI.

   CBF has different phases in TBI—cerebral hypoperfusion (day 0), hyperemia (day 1–3), and vasospasm (day 4–15) [51]. TCD-guided cerebral autoregulation assessment and CBF targets can help to restore normal perfusion and prevent secondary brain injury. A raised ICP causes sequential changes in the FV and distinct waveform patterns (described above). Various formulae for noninvasive estimation of CPP and ICP have been suggested, though they lack validation [23, 52]. It is therefore recommended to use TCD for the assessment of trends in cerebral hemodynamics, rather than the absolute values [52]. TCD-derived ICP values have shown to accurately exclude intracranial hypertension with a high negative predictive value [53, 54].

   A low FV <35 cm/s, accompanied by a high PI, indicates cerebral ischemia in the early stages of TBI and is associated with a poor outcome [55]. Similarly, impaired cerebral autoregulation in the early stages is also associated with a poor neurological outcome in TBI [56].
2. **Subarachnoid hemorrhage (SAH)**: Subarachnoid hemorrhage is known to cause cerebral vasospasm between days 4 and 15 of the ictus. By definition, vasopasm refers to the abnormal and reversible narrowing of the proximal cerebral arteries, associated with a delayed cerebral ischemia (DCI) and development of neurological deficits. Although digital subtraction angiography (DSA) is considered the gold standard for the diagnosis of vasospasm, TCD is very frequently used in the neurocritical care setting for this purpose. Since vasospasm is an evolving process, compared to angiography, bedside TCD monitoring can help in the dynamic surveillance of cerebral hemodynamics as well as the effect of various interventions.

   When compared to angiography, TCD is shown to be reliable in the detection of MCA and BA vasospasm. However, the sensitivity for ACA and PCA vasospasm is inferior [57–59]. TCD can detect vasospasm by showing a focal or diffuse increase in the CBFV and a high Lindegaard ratio (Table 9.3). MCA FVm <120 cm/s and > 120 cm/s can reliably predict the absence or presence of vasospasm, with higher velocities indicating a higher degree of vasospasm. Other than absolute values, the rate of increase in the FVm (rise of >20% or >65 cm/s/day) may also predict DCI and a poor outcome [60]. Another criteria to predict patients with symptomatic large vessel vasospasm (who are at risk of distal hypoperfusion and thus DCI) are a high FVm with a reduced PI (due to compensatory distal vasodilatation following hypoperfusion) (Fig. 9.9). At the same time, high FVm alone is a better predic-

Table 9.4 Clinical applications of TCD

Neurocritical care:
1. TBI
2. SAH with vasospasm
3. Raised ICP
4. Brain stem death
Ischemic cerebrovascular disease
1. Extra- or intra-cranial carotid occlusion
2. Arteriovenous malformation
3. Sickle cell disease
Peri-procedural
1. Carotid endarterectomy or stenting
2. Carotid revascularization (thrombolysis and thrombectomy)
3. Coronary artery bypass grafting
Miscellaneous
1. Sepsis
2. Liver failure
3. Cardiac arrest
4. Detection of right to left shunts
5. Research purposes

TBI traumatic brain injury; *SAH* subarachnoid hemorrhage; *ICP* intracranial pressure

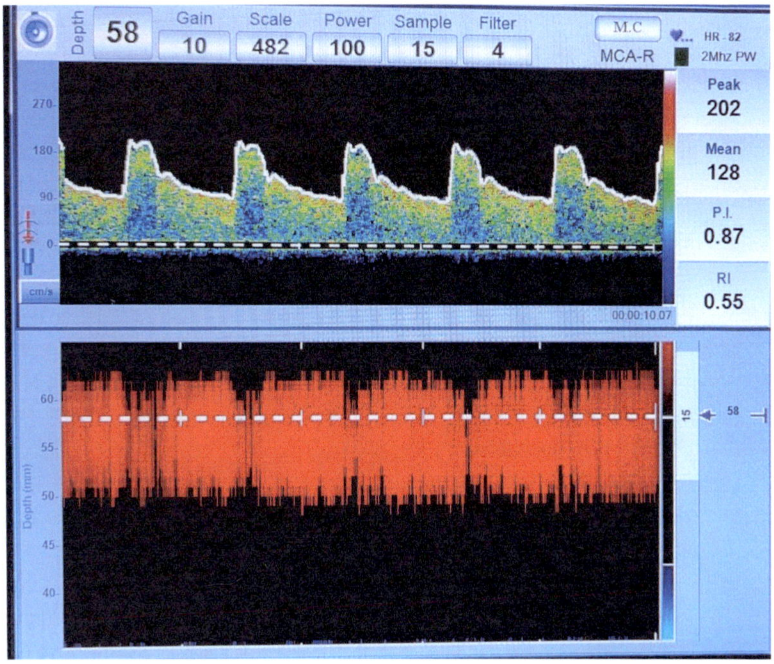

Fig. 9.9 Transcranial doppler spectral waveform of a patient with subarachnoid hemorrhage, showing high middle cerebral artery (MCA) mean flow velocity with reduced pulsatility index, indicating vasospasm

tor of angiographic vasospasm regardless of clinical symptoms [61].

3. **Acute ischemic stroke (AIS)**: TCD can be used for the diagnosis of steno-occlusive diseases, response to treatment, and prognostication in AIS. It has a higher sensitivity and specificity for the diagnosis of ICA and MCA occlusion as compared to posterior circulation arteries [62]. Serial TCD measurements can be used to monitor the status of flow through the occlusion, before and after thrombolysis [63].

   TCD TIBI (Thrombolysis in Brain Ischemia) grading [TIBI waveforms graded as: 0, absent; 1, minimal; 2, blunted; 3, dampened; 4, stenotic; and 5, normal] correlates with the stroke severity, clinical improvement, and mortality in patients treated with intravenous thrombolysis [64]. Since arterial recanalization precedes the clinical improvement, TCD TIBI grading can be used to predict outcome after thrombolysis. A meta-analysis has shown that full recanalization observed with TCD within 6 h of symptom onset in AIS was associated with clinical improvement within 48 h and a good functional outcome at 3 months [65]. In addition, rapid recanalization (improvement in TIBI grade) within 30 min is associated with better short-term outcome, as compared to a slow (>30 min) improvement in the TIBI grade [66]. TCD can also be used to detect early re-occlusion (decreased flow signal ≥1 TIBI grade) after intravenous thrombolysis. This was seen to occur more commonly in patients with partial recanalization earlier and was associated with neurological worsening and higher in-hospital mortality [67].

   Apart from the TCD TIBI grading, site and extent of occlusion can also predict the recanalization and outcome. Clinical response (recanalization and good long-term outcome) to thrombolysis is seen most in distal MCA > proximal MCA > BA > terminal ICA [68, 69].

4. **Sickle cell disease**: Patients with sickle cell disease are at an increased risk of cerebrovascular accidents, including acute ischemic stroke, especially in the border zones [70]. Therefore, regular TCD screening is recommended in children with sickle cell disease by the measurement of time-averaged mean maximum CBFV in bilateral basal cerebral arteries. CBFV <170 cm/s is considered

acceptable, whereas a CBFV >200 cm/s is recommended as the threshold for blood transfusion to reduce the risk of ischemic stroke in asymptomatic patients [71, 72].

5. **Carotid endarterectomy (CEA)**: Patients undergoing CEA are at a risk of perioperative stroke, due to cerebral hypoperfusion during carotid cross-clamping and embolization during dissection phase. Intraoperative TCD monitoring of MCA can help in the detection of both hemodynamic and embolic complications, by monitoring the MCA-FV and the presence of microembolic signals (MESs) [73, 74]. Drop in the MCA-FV (>50%) during carotid cross-clamping indicates the need of an immediate shunt placement. Changes in the MCA-FV has a higher specificity than MES for the prediction of perioperative stroke [74]. TCD monitoring should also be continued in the postoperative period for the detection of shunt occlusion, embolic episodes, and hyperperfusion syndrome [75].
6. **Brain stem death**: TCD is used to confirm the diagnosis of brain stem death by showing the state of cerebral circulatory arrest, producing various spectral waveform morphologies (described above) [76]:
   (a) Oscillating waveform (Fig. 9.8b).
   (b) Short systolic spikes (Fig. 9.8c).
   (c) Intracranial circulatory arrest.
7. **Miscellaneous uses**:

   Sepsis: Majority of patients with sepsis develop septic encephalopathy, which usually manifests as delirium or altered sensorium. TCD can play a significant role in identifying septic patients who are at a risk of cerebral dysfunction and cerebral hemodynamic derangement. The pathophysiology may involve severely depressed cerebral autoregulation and increased microvascular resistance, putting these patients at risk of cerebral hypo/hyper-perfusion [77]. TCD can be used to measure the CBFV and relate it to changes in the ABP (positive correlation with a depressed autoregulation and negative correlation with an intact autoregulation). Impaired cerebral autoregulation and a high PI in the early stage (within 24 h) of sepsis may indicate impending cerebral dysfunction [78]. TCD-guided management of cerebral hemodynamics can also mitigate functional cerebral hypoxia.

   Liver failure: Similar to sepsis, severe liver dysfunction also results in an impaired microvascular dysfunction and cerebral autoregulation. In addition, ammonia may cause neuroinflammation and cerebral edema, increasing the ICP [79]. TCD can be used to detect a raised ICP and guide management to prevent further neurological injury. TCD can demonstrate evolving changes in spectral waveform and FV with the progression of the disease. MCA-FV is reduced with an increased PI and correlates well with the ICP [80].

   Cardiac arrest: Neurological dysfunction is the main cause of significant disability (ranging from mild cognitive dysfunction to vegetative state) in survivors. Hypoxic ischemic injury along with vasogenic and cytotoxic edema, and microvascular dysfunction are the pathophysiological processes involved in the secondary brain injury [81]. Post resuscitation care focuses on preventing and limiting these processes.

   Within the first 30 min of the return of spontaneous circulation (ROSC), local perfusion deficits (no or low flow areas) coexist with areas of vasoparalysis and subsquent hyperemia [82]. Hypotension, especially if cerebral autoregulation is deranged in the early ROSC period, decreases global CBF, leading to cerebral ischemia. On the other hand, hyperemia can lead to reperfusion injury and a raised ICP. Serial assessment of CBF with TCD, during and after cardio-pulmonary resuscitation (CPR), can help in the optimization of CPP as well as in the prognostication of cardiac arrest patients.

   During CPR, maximum systolic FV during chest compression reflects cerebral perfusion and may guide in improving the quality of chest compressions [83]. Progressive deterioration of the CBFV to the point of absence of forward flow may help in deciding about the termination of CPR. However, insonation of MCA during CPR may be difficult or affected by artifact signals.

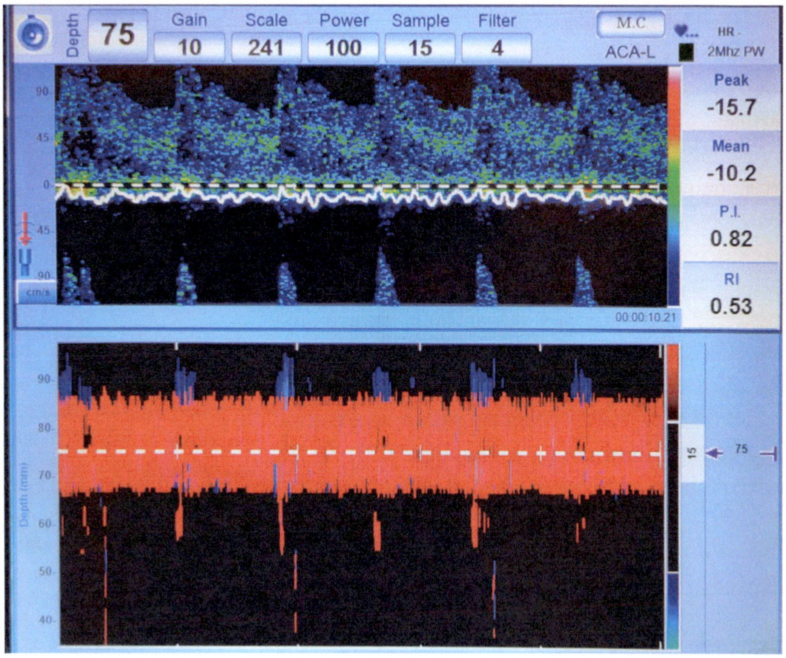

Fig. 9.10 Transcranial doppler spectral waveform showing aliasing artifact (wrapping of wave peak around scale and appearing at the bottom of the screen)

After ROSC is achieved, ABP targets can be chosen, based on the status of cerebral autoregulation and CBFV. Persistent high CrCP, together with a hypodynamic pattern (high PI and low CBFV) or a hyperdynamic pattern (high CBFV and low PI) in the first 24 h of ROSC, indicates a poor neurological recovery [84, 85].

9.9 Limitations of TCD

- TCD or TCCD requires ultrasound waves to penetrate the skull, but 10–20% patients may have an inadequate trans-temporal window (especially older women) [16, 86].
- Operator must be aware of the fact that only 18–20% of the population represents a complete circle of Willis, and up to 50% show anomalies like vessel hypoplasia, fetal PCA origin, dissection, and vascular malformaitons [87].
- The learning curve for TCD or TCCD is steep. TCD involves the identification of cerebral arteries blindly on the basis of spectral display, insonation depth, and flow direction.
- Continuous monitoring is difficult to perform, as it depends on constant probe position and angle of insonation. However, if given a choice between TCD and TCCD, continuous imaging is still possible with TCD due to a smaller probe size which can be mounted on a headframe. On the other hand, TCCD probe is larger and heavier, which requires a manual holding.
- TCD tends to overestimate ICP with the available formulae, and their applicability in focal intracranial pathologies (AIS, vasospasm) is still unclear [88, 89].
- TCD assessment can be affected by various artifacts such as motion artifacts, aliasing (Fig. 9.10), mirror image artifact, or bruits. Aliasing can be corrected by increasing the scale.
- TCD may be associated with a risk of injury to the ocular contents while insonating the transorbital window, due to thermal effect and mechanical strain produced by ultrasound waves.

9.10 Summary

TCD is an essential tool in a neuro-physician's armamentarium, allowing bedside, noninvasive, real-time, and reproducible assessment of cerebral hemodynamics, not only in neurocritical care but also in other clinical conditions as well. It also has a promising role in clinical research. Along with various indices, spectral waveform analysis also provides remarkable information regarding the cerebrovascular state. Instead of an absolute single value, it is recommended to assess trends in the CBFV. Operator should be aware of the several limitations associated with TCD, mainly the possibility of an inadequate window.

References

1. Aaslid R, Markwalder TM, Nornes H. Non-invasive transcranial Doppler ultrasound recording of flow velocity in basal cerebral arteries. J Neurosurg. 1982;57:769.
2. Sarkar S, Ghosh S, Ghosh SK, Collier A. Role of transcranial Doppler ultrasonography in stroke. Postgrad Med J. 2007;83(985):683–9. https://doi.org/10.1136/pgmj.2007.058602.
3. Fatima N, Shuaib A, Chughtai TS, Ayyad A, Saqqur M. The role of transcranial Doppler in traumatic brain injury: a systemic review and meta-analysis. Asian J Neurosurg. 2019;14(3):626–33. https://doi.org/10.4103/ajns.AJNS_42_19.
4. Kumar G, Shahripour RB, Harrigan MR. Vasospasm on transcranial Doppler is predictive of delayed cerebral ischemia in aneurysmal subarachnoid hemorrhage: a systematic review and meta-analysis. J Neurosurg. 2016;124(5):1257–64. https://doi.org/10.3171/2015.4.JNS15428.
5. Aaslid R. The Doppler principle applied to measurement of blood flow velocity in cerebral arteries. In: Vienna RA, editor. Transcranial Doppler sonography. New York: Springer; 1986. p. 22–38.
6. Huber P, Handa J. Effect of contrast material, hypercapnia, hyperventilation, hypertonic glucose and papaverine on the diameter of the cerebral arteries: angiographic determination in man. Investig Radiol. 1967;2:17.
7. Markwalder TM, Grolimund P, Seiler RW, et al. Dependency of blood flow velocity in the middle cerebral artery on end-tidal carbon dioxide partial pressure: a transcranial ultrasound Doppler study. J Cereb Blood Flow Metab. 1984;4:368.
8. Newell WD, Aaslid R, Lam AM, et al. Comparison of flow and velocity during dynamic autoregulation testing in humans. Stroke. 1994;25:793.
9. Schregel W, Schafermeyer H, Muller C, et al. The effect of halothane, alfentanil and propofol on blood flow velocity, blood vessel cross section and blood volume flow in the middle cerebral artery. Anaesthesist. 1992;41:21.
10. Matta BF, Lam AM. Isoflurane and desflurane do not dilate the middle cerebral artery appreciably. Br J Anaesth. 1995;74:486P.
11. Krishnakumar M, Ramesh V, Goyal A, et al. Clinical visualization of cerebral vasodilatation by desflurane. Can J Anesth/J Can Anesth. 2020;67:605–6. https://doi.org/10.1007/s12630-020-01596-6.
12. Matta BF, Lam AM, Mayberg TS, et al. The cerebrovascular response to carbon dioxide during sodium nitroprusside- and isoflurane-induced hypotension. Br J Anaesth. 1995;74:296.
13. Dahl A, Russell D, Nyberg-Hansen R, et al. Effect of nitroglycerin on cerebral circulation measured by transcranial Doppler and SPECT. Stroke. 1989;20:1733.
14. Moehring MA, Spencer MP. Power M-mode transcranial Doppler ultrasound and simultaneous single gate spectrogram. Ultrasound Med Biol. 2002;28:49–57.
15. Marinoni M, Ginanneschi A, Forleo P, Amaducci L. Technical limits in transcranial Doppler recording: inadequate acoustic windows. Ultrasound Med Biol. 1997;23(8):1275–7. https://doi.org/10.1016/s0301-5629(97)00077-x.
16. Babikian VL, Feldmann E, Wechsler LR, et al. Transcranial Doppler ultrasonography: year 2000 update. J Neuroimaging. 2000;10(2):101–15. https://doi.org/10.1111/jon2000102101.
17. Nicoletto HA, Burkman MH. Transcranial Doppler series part II: performing a transcranial Doppler. Am J Electroneurodiagnostic Technol. 2009;49(1):14–27.
18. Hennerici M, Rautenberg W, Sitzer G, Schwartz A. Transcranial Doppler ultrasound for the assessment of intracranial arterial flow velocity—part 1. Examination technique and normal values. Surg Neurol. 1987;27(5):439–48. https://doi.org/10.1016/0090-3019(87)90251-5.
19. Bathala L, Mehndiratta MM, Sharma VK. Transcranial doppler: technique and common findings (part 1). Ann Indian Acad Neurol. 2013;16(2):174–9. https://doi.org/10.4103/0972-2327.112460.
20. Alexandrov AV, Brodie DS, McLean A, Hamilton P, Murphy J, Burns PN. Correlation of peak systolic velocity and angiographic measurement of carotid stenosis revisited. Stroke. 1997;28(2):339–42. https://doi.org/10.1161/01.str.28.2.339.
21. Czosnyka M, Matta BF, Smielewski P, Kirkpatrick PJ, Pickard JD. Cerebral perfusion pressure in head-injured patients: a noninvasive assessment using transcranial Doppler ultrasonography. J Neurosurg. 1998;88(5):802–8. https://doi.org/10.3171/jns.1998.88.5.0802.
22. Venkatesh B, Shen Q, Lipman J. Continuous measurement of cerebral blood flow velocity using transcranial Doppler reveals significant moment-to-moment variability of data in healthy volunteers and in patients with subarachnoid hemorrhage.

Crit Care Med. 2002;30(3):563–9. https://doi.org/10.1097/00003246-200203000-00011.
23. White H, Venkatesh B. Applications of transcranial Doppler in the ICU: a review. Intensive Care Med. 2006;32(7):981–94. https://doi.org/10.1007/s00134-006-0173-y.
24. Lindegaard KF, Nornes H, Bakke SJ, Sorteberg W, Nakstad P. Cerebral vasospasm after subarachnoid haemorrhage investigated by means of transcranial Doppler ultrasound. Acta Neurochir Suppl (Wien). 1988;42:81–4. https://doi.org/10.1007/978-3-7091-8975-7_16.
25. Aaslid R, Huber P, Nornes H. Evaluation of cerebrovascular spasm with transcranial Doppler ultrasound. J Neurosurg. 1984;60:37–41.
26. Sviri GE, Ghodke B, Britz GW, Douville CM, Haynor DR, Mesiwala AH, et al. Transcranial Doppler grading criteria for basilar artery vasospasm. Neurosurgery. 2006;59:360–6.
27. Topcuoglu MA. Transcranial Doppler ultrasound in neurovascular diseases: diagnostic and therapeutic aspects. J Neurochem. 2012;123(Suppl 2):39–51. https://doi.org/10.1111/j.1471-4159.2012.07942.x.
28. Gosling RG, King DH. Arterial assessment by Doppler-shift ultrasound. Proc R Soc Med. 1974;67(6 Pt 1):447–9.
29. Czosnyka M, Richards HK, Whitehouse HE, Pickard JD. Relationship between transcranial Doppler-determined pulsatility index and cerebrovascular resistance: an experimental study. J Neurosurg. 1996;84(1):79–84. https://doi.org/10.3171/jns.1996.84.1.0079.
30. Nicoletto HA, Burkman MH. Transcranial Doppler series part III: Interpretation. Am J Electroneurodiagnostic Technol. 2009;49:244–59.
31. Ursino M, Giulioni M, Lodi CA. Relationships among cerebral perfusion pressure, autoregulation, and transcranial Doppler waveform: a modeling study. J Neurosurg. 1998;89:255–66.
32. Bellner J, Romner B, Reinstrup P, Kristiansson KA, Ryding E, Brandt L. Transcranial Doppler sonography pulsatility index (PI) reflects intracranial pressure (ICP). Surg Neurol. 2004;62(1):45–51. https://doi.org/10.1016/j.surneu.2003.12.007.
33. Homburg AM, Jakobsen M, Enevoldsen E. Transcranial Doppler recordings in raised intracranial pressure. Acta Neurol Scand. 1993;87:488–93.
34. Behrens A, Lenfeldt N, Ambarki K, Malm J, Eklund A, Koskinen LO. Transcranial Doppler pulsatility index: not an accurate method to assess intracranial pressure. Neurosurgery. 2010;66(6):1050–7. https://doi.org/10.1227/01.NEU.0000369519.35932.F2.
35. Figaji AA, Zwane E, Fieggen AG, Siesjo P, Peter JC. Transcranial Doppler pulsatility index is not a reliable indicator of intracranial pressure in children with severe traumatic brain injury. Surg Neurol. 2009;72(4):389–94. https://doi.org/10.1016/j.surneu.2009.02.012.
36. Markus HS, Harrison MJ. Estimation of cerebrovascular reactivity using transcranial Doppler, including the use of breath-holding as the vasodilatory stimulus. Stroke. 1992;23(5):668–73. https://doi.org/10.1161/01.str.23.5.668.
37. Müller M, Voges M, Piepgras U, Schimrigk K. Assessment of cerebral vasomotor reactivity by transcranial Doppler ultrasound and breath-holding. A comparison with acetazolamide as vasodilatory stimulus. Stroke. 1995;26(1):96–100. https://doi.org/10.1161/01.str.26.1.96.
38. Naqvi J, Yap KH, Ahmad G, Ghosh J. Transcranial Doppler ultrasound: a review of the physical principles and major applications in critical care. Int J Vasc Med. 2013;2013:629378. https://doi.org/10.1155/2013/629378.
39. Nicoletto HA, Boland LS. Transcranial Doppler series part v: specialty applications. Am J Electroneurodiagnostic Technol. 2011;51(1):31–41.
40. Tiecks FP, Lam AM, Aaslid R, Newell DW. Comparison of static and dynamic cerebral autoregulation measurements. Stroke. 1995;26:1014–9.
41. Smielewski P, Czosnyka M, Kirkpatrick P, Pickard JD. Evaluation of the transient hyperemic response test in head-injured patients. J Neurosurg. 1997;86(5):773–8. https://doi.org/10.3171/jns.1997.86.5.0773.
42. Czosnyka M, Smielewski P, Kirkpatrick P, Menon DK, Pickard JD. Monitoring of cerebral autoregulation in head-injured patients. Stroke. 1996;27(10):1829–34. https://doi.org/10.1161/01.str.27.10.1829.
43. Aaslid R, Lundar T, Lindegaard K-F, et al. Estimation of cerebral perfusion pressure from arterial blood pressure and transcranial Doppler recordings. In: Miller JD, Teasdale GM, Rowan JO, et al., editors. Intracranial Pressure VI. Berlin: Springer; 1986. p. 226–9.
44. Nichol J, Girling F, Jerrard W, Claxton EB, Burton AC. Fundamental instability of the small blood vessels and critical closing pressures in vascular beds. Am J Phys. 1951;164(2):330–44. https://doi.org/10.1152/ajplegacy.1951.164.2.330.
45. Dewey RC, Pieper HP, Hunt WE. Experimental cerebral hemodynamics. Vasomotor tone, critical closing pressure, and vascular bed resistance. J Neurosurg. 1974;41(5):597–606. https://doi.org/10.3171/jns.1974.41.5.0597.
46. Donnelly J, Czosnyka M, Harland S, et al. Cerebral haemodynamics during experimental intracranial hypertension. J Cereb Blood Flow Metab. 2017;37(2):694–705. https://doi.org/10.1177/0271678X16639060.
47. Varsos GV, Kasprowicz M, Smielewski P, Czosnyka M. Model-based indices describing cerebrovascular dynamics. Neurocrit Care. 2014;20(1):142–57. https://doi.org/10.1007/s12028-013-9868-4.
48. Moniche F, Escudero-Martínez I, Mancha F, et al. The value of transcranial Doppler sonography in Hyperperfusion syndrome after carotid artery stenting: a Nationwide prospective study. J Stroke. 2020;22(2):254–7. https://doi.org/10.5853/jos.2020.00682.

49. Hassler W, Steinmetz H, Gawlowski J. Transcranial Doppler ultrasonography in raised intracranial pressure and in intracranial circulatory arrest. J Neurosurg. 1988;68(5):745–51.
50. Klingelhöfer J, Conrad B, Benecke R, Sander D. Intracranial flow patterns at increasing intracranial pressure. Klin Wochenschr. 1987;65(12):542–5.
51. Martin NA, Patwardhan RV, Alexander MJ, et al. Characterization of cerebral hemodynamic phases following severe head trauma: hypoperfusion, hyperemia, and vasospasm. J Neurosurg. 1997;87(1):9–19. https://doi.org/10.3171/jns.1997.87.1.0009.
52. Saqqur M, Zygun D, Demchuk A. Role of transcranial Doppler in neurocritical care. Crit Care Med. 2007;35(5 Suppl):S216–23.
53. Rasulo FA, Bertuetti R, Robba C, et al. The accuracy of transcranial Doppler in excluding intracranial hypertension following acute brain injury: a multicenter prospective pilot study. Crit Care. 2017;21(1):44. https://doi.org/10.1186/s13054-017-1632-2.
54. Rasulo FA, Calza S, Robba C, et al. Transcranial Doppler as a screening test to exclude intracranial hypertension in brain-injured patients: the IMPRESSIT-2 prospective multicenter international study. Crit Care. 2022;26(1):110. https://doi.org/10.1186/s13054-022-03978-2.
55. Van Santbrink H, Schouten JW, Steyerberg EW, Avezaat CJ, Maas AI. Serial transcranial Doppler measurements in traumatic brain injury with special focus on the early posttraumatic period. Acta Neurochir. 2002;144(11):1141–9. https://doi.org/10.1007/s00701-002-1012-8.
56. Le Roux P, Menon DK, Citerio G, et al. Consensus summary statement of the international multidisciplinary consensus conference on multimodality monitoring in Neurocritical care: a statement for healthcare professionals from the Neurocritical care society and the European Society of Intensive Care Medicine. Intensive Care Med. 2014;40(9):1189–209. https://doi.org/10.1007/s00134-014-3369-6.
57. Lysakowski C, Walder B, Costanza MC, Tramèr MR. Transcranial Doppler versus angiography in patients with vasospasm due to a ruptured cerebral aneurysm: a systematic review. Stroke. 2001;32(10):2292–8. https://doi.org/10.1161/hs1001.097108.
58. Sloan MA, Burch CM, Wozniak MA, et al. Transcranial Doppler detection of vertebrobasilar vasospasm following subarachnoid hemorrhage. Stroke. 1994;25(11):2187–97. https://doi.org/10.1161/01.str.25.11.2187.
59. Wozniak MA, Sloan MA, Rothman MI, et al. Detection of vasospasm by transcranial Doppler sonography. The challenges of the anterior and posterior cerebral arteries. J Neuroimaging. 1996;6(2):87–93. https://doi.org/10.1111/jon19966287.
60. Tsivgoulis G, Alexandrov AV, Sloan MA. Advances in transcranial Doppler ultrasonography. Curr Neurol Neurosci Rep. 2009;9(1):46–54. https://doi.org/10.1007/s11910-009-0008-7.
61. Rajajee V, Fletcher JJ, Pandey AS, et al. Low pulsatility index on transcranial Doppler predicts symptomatic large-vessel vasospasm after aneurysmal subarachnoid hemorrhage. Neurosurgery. 2012;70(5):1195–206. https://doi.org/10.1227/NEU.0b013e3182417dca.
62. Demchuk AM, Christou I, Wein TH, et al. Accuracy and criteria for localizing arterial occlusion with transcranial Doppler. J Neuroimaging. 2000;10(1):1–12.
63. Rasulo FA, De Peri E, Lavinio A. Transcranial Doppler ultrasonography in intensive care. Eur J Anaesthesiol Suppl. 2008;42(42):167–73.
64. Demchuk AM, Burgin WS, Christou I, et al. Thrombolysis in brain ischemia (TIBI) transcranial Doppler flow grades predict clinical severity, early recovery, and mortality in patients treated with intravenous tissue plasminogen activator. Stroke. 2001;32(1):89–93. https://doi.org/10.1161/01.str.32.1.89.
65. Stolz E, Cioli F, Allendoerfer J, Gerriets T, Del Sette M, Kaps M. Can early neurosonology predict outcome in acute stroke?: a metaanalysis of prognostic clinical effect sizes related to the vascular status. Stroke. 2008;39(12):3255–61. https://doi.org/10.1161/STROKEAHA.108.522714.
66. Alexandrov AV, Burgin WS, Demchuk AM, El-Mitwalli A, Grotta JC. Speed of intracranial clot lysis with intravenous tissue plasminogen activator therapy: sonographic classification and short-term improvement. Circulation. 2001;103(24):2897–902. https://doi.org/10.1161/01.cir.103.24.2897.
67. Alexandrov AV, Grotta JC. Arterial reocclusion in stroke patients treated with intravenous tissue plasminogen activator. Neurology. 2002;59(6):862–7. https://doi.org/10.1212/wnl.59.6.862.
68. Saqqur M, Uchino K, Demchuk AM, et al. Site of arterial occlusion identified by transcranial Doppler predicts the response to intravenous thrombolysis for stroke. Stroke. 2007;38(3):948–54. https://doi.org/10.1161/01.STR.0000257304.21967.ba.
69. Allendoerfer J, Goertler M, von Reutern GM. Neurosonology in acute ischemic stroke study group. Prognostic relevance of ultra-early doppler sonography in acute ischaemic stroke: a prospective multicentre study. Lancet Neurol. 2006;5(10):835–40. https://doi.org/10.1016/S1474-4422(06)70551-8.
70. Adams RJ, McKie VC, Carl EM, Nichols FT, Perry R, Brock K, et al. Long-term stroke risk in children with sickle cell disease screened with transcranial Doppler. Ann Neurol. 1997;42:699–704.
71. Adams RJ, McKie VC, Hsu L, Files B, Vichinsky E, Pegelow C, et al. Prevention of a first stroke by transfusions in children with sickle cell anemia and abnormal results on transcranial Doppler ultrasonography. N Engl J Med. 1998;339:5–11.
72. Adams RJ. TCD in sickle cell disease: an important and useful test. Pediatr Radiol. 2005;35:229–34.
73. Ackerstaff RG, Moons KG, van de Vlasakker CJ, et al. Association of intraoperative transcranial dop-

pler monitoring variables with stroke from carotid endarterectomy. Stroke. 2000;31(8):1817–23. https://doi.org/10.1161/01.str.31.8.1817.
74. Udesh R, Natarajan P, Thiagarajan K, et al. Transcranial Doppler monitoring in carotid endarterectomy: a systematic review and meta-analysis. J Ultrasound Med. 2017;36(3):621–30. https://doi.org/10.7863/ultra.16.02077.
75. Yun WS. Cerebral monitoring during carotid endarterectomy by transcranial Doppler ultrasonography. Ann Surg Treat Res. 2017;92(2):105–9. https://doi.org/10.4174/astr.2017.92.2.105.
76. Ducrocq X, Braun M, Debouverie M, Junges C, Hummer M, Vespignani H. Brain death and transcranial Doppler: experience in 130 cases of brain dead patients. J Neurol Sci. 1998;160(1):41–6. https://doi.org/10.1016/s0022-510x(98)00188-9.
77. Crippa IA, Subirà C, Vincent JL, et al. Impaired cerebral autoregulation is associated with brain dysfunction in patients with sepsis. Crit Care. 2018;22(1):327. https://doi.org/10.1186/s13054-018-2258-8.
78. Pierrakos C, Attou R, Decorte L, et al. Transcranial Doppler to assess sepsis-associated encephalopathy in critically ill patients. BMC Anesthesiol. 2014;14:45. https://doi.org/10.1186/1471-2253-14-45.
79. Reynolds AS, Brush B, Schiano TD, Reilly KJ, Dangayach NS. Neurological monitoring in acute liver failure. Hepatology. 2019;70(5):1830–5. https://doi.org/10.1002/hep.30760.
80. Kawakami M, Koda M, Murawaki Y. Cerebral pulsatility index by transcranial Doppler sonography predicts the prognosis of patients with fulminant hepatic failure. Clin Imaging. 2010;34(5):327–31. https://doi.org/10.1016/j.clinimag.2009.09.006.
81. Nolan JP, Neumar RW, Adrie C, et al. Post-cardiac arrest syndrome: epidemiology, pathophysiology, treatment, and prognostication. A Scientific Statement from the International Liaison Committee on Resuscitation; the American Heart Association Emergency Cardiovascular Care Committee; the Council on Cardiovascular Surgery and Anesthesia; the Council on Cardiopulmonary, Perioperative, and Critical Care; the Council on Clinical Cardiology; the Council on Stroke. Resuscitation. 2008;79(3):350–79. https://doi.org/10.1016/j.resuscitation.2008.09.017.
82. Hossmann KA. Reperfusion of the brain after global ischemia: hemodynamic disturbances. Shock. 1997;8(2):95–103. https://doi.org/10.1097/00024382-199708000-00004.
83. Lewis LM, Stothert JC Jr, Gomez CR, et al. A noninvasive method for monitoring cerebral perfusion during cardiopulmonary resuscitation. J Crit Care. 1994;9(3):169–74. https://doi.org/10.1016/0883-9441(94)90013-2.
84. Álvarez-Fernández JA. Doppler transcraneal en el coma tras parada cardíaca [Transcranial Doppler ultrasound use in post-cardiac arrest coma]. Rev Neurol. 2011;53(9):545–54.
85. Van den Brule JM, Vinke E, van Loon LM, van der Hoeven JG, Hoedemaekers CW. Middle cerebral artery flow, the critical closing pressure, and the optimal mean arterial pressure in comatose cardiac arrest survivors-an observational study. Resuscitation. 2017;110:85–9. https://doi.org/10.1016/j.resuscitation.2016.10.022.
86. Moppett IK, Mahajan RP. Transcranial Doppler ultrasonography in anaesthesia and intensive care. Br J Anaesth. 2004;93:710–24.
87. Iqbal S. A comprehensive study of the anatomical variations of the circle of Willis in adult human brains. J Clin Diagn Res. 2013;7(11):2423–7. https://doi.org/10.7860/JCDR/2013/6580.3563.
88. Robba C, Goffi A, Geeraerts T, et al. Brain ultrasonography: methodology, basic and advanced principles and clinical applications. A narrative review. Intensive Care Med. 2019;45(7):913–27. https://doi.org/10.1007/s00134-019-05610-4.
89. Modrzejewska M. Guidelines for ultrasound examination in ophthalmology. Part III: Color Doppler ultrasonography. J Ultrason. 2019;19(77):128–36. https://doi.org/10.15557/JoU.2019.0019.

Evoked Response Monitoring

10

Vignesh Rajasekaran, Praveen Chander, and Devachandran Jayakumar

10.1 Introduction

Evoked response monitoring is an electrophysiological technique to interrogate the integrity of neural pathways. Although any neural pathway can be tested using this technique, sensory pathway interrogation is more commonly performed than motor. Administering a sensory stimulus and tracing the signal to the cortex reveal the intactness of the pathway. Visual, auditory, and somatosensory are the commonly monitored sensory pathways in clinical practice. In critical care, somatosensory evoked potential (SSEP) testing is regularly employed in neuroprognostication [1]; therefore, somatosensory evoked potential monitoring will be discussed in detail in this chapter.

10.2 Applied Anatomy

When a mixed motor and sensory nerve like the median nerve (or posterior tibial in the lower limb) is stimulated by an electrical impulse, the impulse travels up (normal sensory conduction called orthodromic) and down (conduction in the opposite direction called antidromic) the nerve from the point of stimulation through large diameter, fast conducting sensory fibers. The antidromic impulse travels via group 1a muscle afferents; their stimulation leads to a motor response (e.g., abduction of the thumb with median nerve stimulation; plantar flexion of the toes with posterior tibial stimulation). This confirms the delivery of the electrical impulse. The orthodromic impulse travels through group 2 cutaneous afferents. With their nuclei in the dorsal root ganglia, these first-order neurons travel up the ipsilateral dorsal column to reach the gracile and cuneate nuclei in the distal brain stem. The post synaptic second-order neurons from these nuclei decussate in the medulla travel through the contralateral medial lemniscus to reach the ventral posterior lateral (VPL) nucleus of the thalamus. The third-order neurons from VPL, through the thalamocortical projection, reach the sensory cortex situated in the postcentral gyrus [2].

10.3 Basics of Recording

10.3.1 Montages

Systematically arranged recording channels involving multiple electrodes to receive and display neuroactivity are called montages. During

V. Rajasekaran · D. Jayakumar (✉)
Department of Critical Care, Dr. Kamakshi Memorial Hospital, Chennai, Tamil Nadu, India

P. Chander
Department of Neurology, Dr. Kamakshi Memorial Hospital, Chennai, Tamil Nadu, India

H. Prabhakar et al. (eds.), *Principles and Practice of Neurocritical Care*,
https://doi.org/10.1007/978-981-99-8059-8_10

SSEP recording, bipolar and referential are the two montages commonly used [3, 4].

In bipolar montage, the electrodes are placed close to each other; both are active and receive impulses. Therefore, the signals received by them are similar. When these signals pass through a differential amplification system, only the signals that are different between the two electrodes are amplified. This "common mode rejection" is useful while recording cortical potentials.

In the referential montage, an inactive reference electrode is placed well away from the active recording electrode. Situated away from the head, the reference electrode remains silent but contributes to unwanted noise in the recording by picking up muscle activity. As the distance between the two electrodes increases, the addition of noise to the recording increases [3–5].

10.3.2 Nearfield and Far-Field Potentials [3, 5]

If the active electrode is placed directly over the signal generator (e.g., electrode placed over the upper limb area of somatosensory cortex), a large amplitude, predominantly negative signal is recorded. This recording is location-sensitive (i.e., change in the location of the recording electrode changes the signal). The potentials recorded by these electrodes are called near-field potentials, and they are recorded using bipolar montages.

In contrast, when the active electrode records signals from multiple distant generators covering many sites, the signals will be of low amplitude and non-location-sensitive. These far-field signals are generally positive, monophasic, and observed well in referential montages. A combination of near-field and far-field recordings is required to record and interpret SSEP.

10.3.3 Nomenclature, Amplitude, and Latency

SSEP record is a plot of voltage against time. After the initial stimulation artifact, a series of upward and downward waves are recorded. The waves are denoted by an alphabet and a numeric. The alphabet is generally N or P depending on the polarity of the recorded signal (Negative is up and Positive is down). The numeric that follows N and P denotes the post stimulus latency of the signal in milliseconds (e.g., N20—Negative wave recorded as an upstroke after 20 msecs after stimulation). Amplitude of a signal is measured from the peak of a wave to the trough of the wave that follows, and latency is denoted by the time from stimulation to the peak or the time between two peaks (interpeak latency) [5, 6]. Commonly monitored SSEPs are short latency evoked potentials; therefore, the total analysis time is set at 50 ms for upper limb and 100 ms for lower limb. The long latency evoked responses are not regularly used but have some value in specific conditions in critical care [1].

10.4 Recording Technique

10.4.1 Upper Limb

Median nerve (and occasionally ulnar) is stimulated in the upper limb. The stimulating electrodes are placed 2 cm apart and 2 cm proximal to the wrist crease (Fig. 10.1), between the palmaris longus and flexor carpi radialis tendons (EEG electrodes are used in critical care and needle electrodes in the operating room). Cathode is positioned proximal with a distal anode to prevent anodal block. Monophasic square-wave electrical pulses of 15–20 mA at a frequency of approximately 5 Hz are delivered from a constant current stimulator [5]. The location and current intensity are adjusted to get a visible motor twitch distally (e.g., abduction of the thumb). The American Clinical Neurophysiology Society (ACNS) recommends a four-channel montage for SSEP recording [7].

The recording electrodes for upper limb SSEP are placed as follows (Table 10.1) [3, 4]:

1. Erb's point (2 cm above the midpoint of the clavicle) on both sides. The stimulating side is denoted Epi (Erb's point ipsilateral) and the opposite side EPc (Erb's point contralateral/

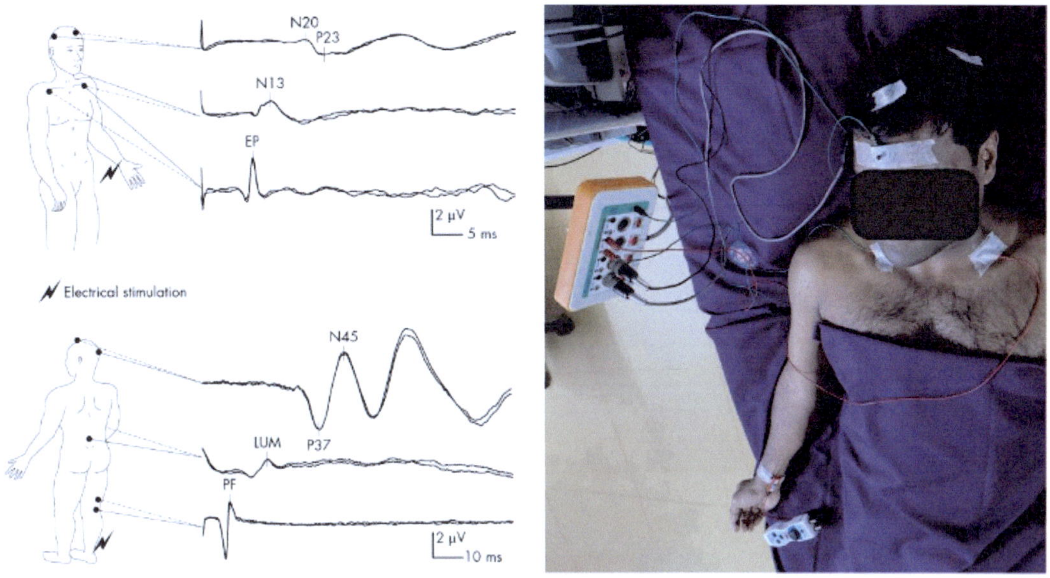

Fig. 10.1 Illustration on the left gives the location of the electrodes and their respective potentials. (Reproduced with permission from Walsh et al. 2005.) The picture on the right shows the arrangement of electrodes, stimulator, and the four-channel setup for recording

Table 10.1 Upper limb SSEP: Electrode placement and recorded waves (Modified with permission from Markand, Springer Inc. 2020)

Channel	Recommended montage	Type of potential	Recorded wave
Four	CPi–CPc	Near-field	N20
Three	CPi–EPc	Far-field	N18
Two	C5–EPc	Near-field	N13
One	EPi–EPc	Near-field	N9

referential). EPi electrode records the potentials traveling through the brachial plexus called N9 (peak recorded 9 ms after stimulation) [8].

2. An active electrode on the C5 spinous process (counted upward from the prominent C7 spinous process) with a reference electrode on the contralateral Erb's point to record the signals from the cervical cord called N13.
3. Active electrode at CPi (Centroparietal ipsilateral) with a reference at EPc to record the subcortical far-field potentials called N18.
4. The cortical electrodes placed between C3 and P3 (left) and C4 and P4 (right) of a 10–20 electrode placement system are represented CPi or CPc based on the side of stimulation. They record the near-field signals from the upper limb area of the sensory cortex with a peak at 20 ms called N20 (Fig. 10.2).

10.4.2 Lower Limb

Posterior tibial nerve (occasionally common peroneal) is used to record the lower limb SSEP. Two stimulating electrodes with the cathode placed midway between the posterior border of medial malleolus and medial edge of Achilles tendon and the anode placed 2–3 cm distally on the side of the ankle are used to stimulate the tibial nerve (Fig. 10.3). The technique of stimulation is the same as upper limb, except that the stimulation frequency is lower in lower limb SSEP (2 Hz instead of 5) [4]. Higher stimulating current may be required if the foot is edematous.

The recording electrodes for lower limb SSEP are placed as follows (Table 10.2):

1. Two electrodes 2–3 cm apart (Pfd for distal popliteal and Pfp for proximal popliteal) in

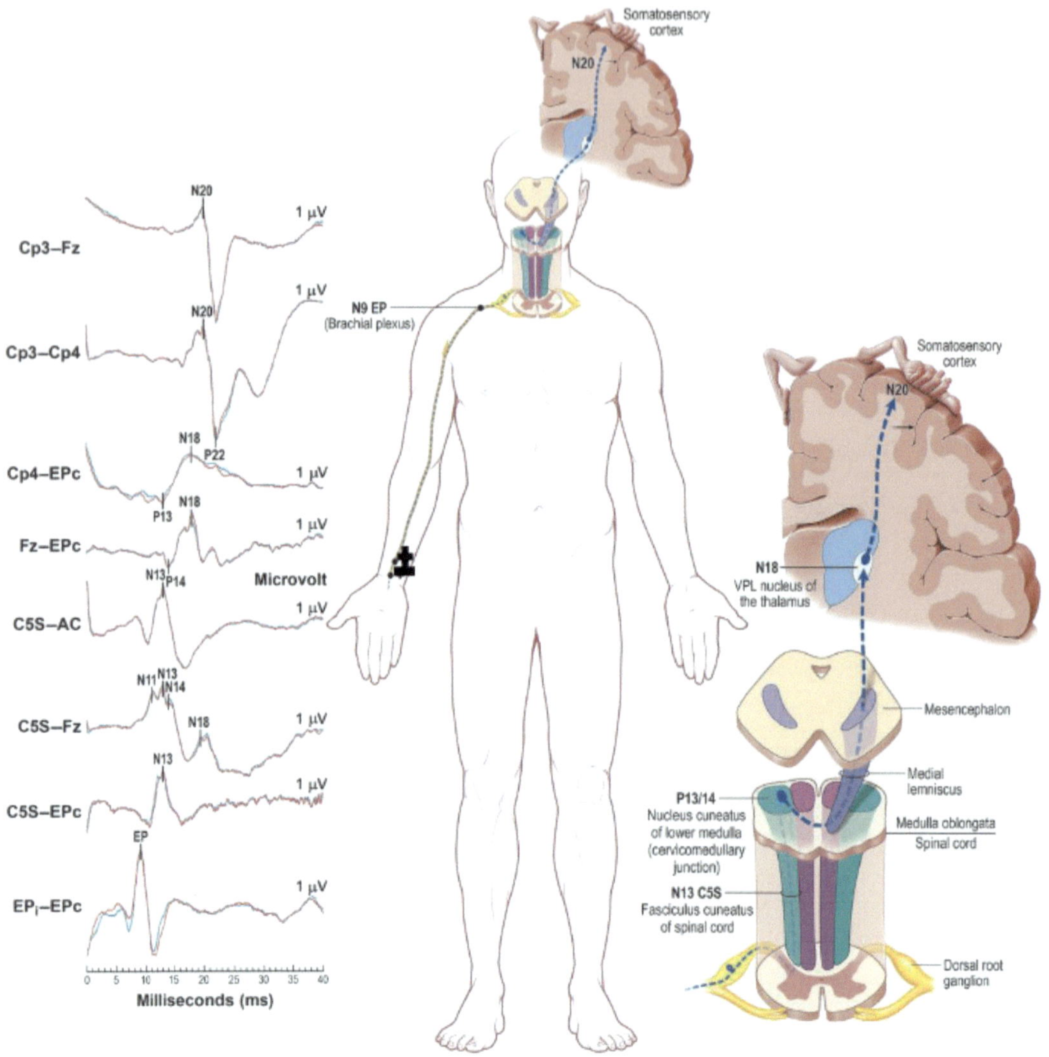

Fig. 10.2 Median nerve SSEP with relevant neuroanatomy. (Reproduced with permission from Muzyka et al., Elsevier Inc.)

the ipsilateral popliteal region midway between the hamstring tendons to record the traveling N7. The impulse recorded by these electrodes confirms the adequacy of stimulation [3].

2. An active electrode on the T12 spine with a reference electrode on the contralateral iliac crest (ICc) is to record the far-field N22 from the lumbar spinal cord.
3. C5 electrode as reference with the active electrode placed in the frontopolar (FPz) area to record the far-field low-amplitude subcortical potentials (N34).
4. An electrode placed between Cz and Pz called CPz of a 10–20 electrode placement system with a reference at FPz to record the near-field signal P37 reaching the lower limb area of the sensory cortex.

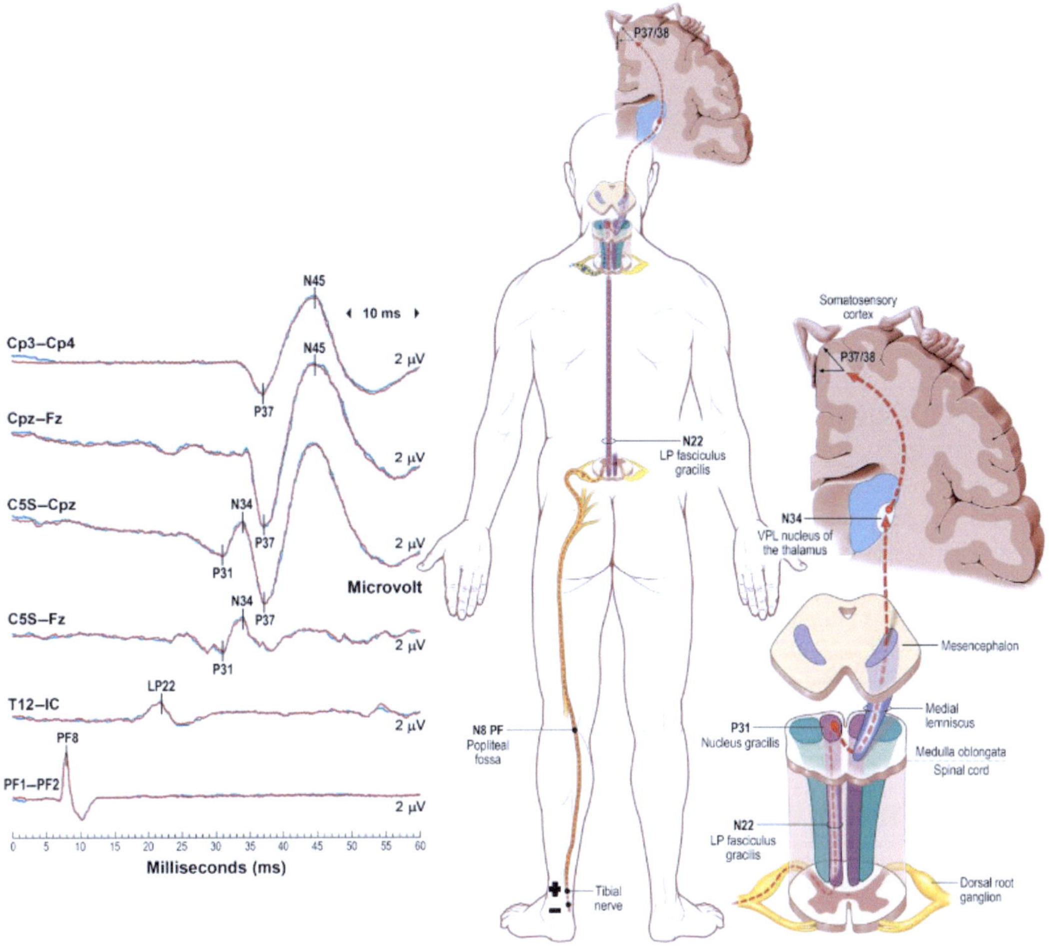

Fig. 10.3 Posterior tibial nerve SSEP with relevant neuroanatomy. (Reproduced with permission from Muzyka et al., Elsevier Inc.)

Table 10.2 Lower limb SSEP: Electrode placement and recorded waves (Modified with permission from Markand, Springer Inc. 2020)

Channel	Recommended montage	Type of potential	Recorded wave
Four	CPz–FPz	Near-field	P37
Three	C5–FPz	Far-field	N34
Two	T12–ICc	Near-field	N22
One	Pfd–Pfp	Near-field	N7

10.5 Interpretation

Since the sensory evoked response is very small (1–2 µV) compared to EEG (10–1000 µV), several hundred to thousand stimuli (typically 500–2000 pulses) are administered to obtain a record [6]. Using signal averaging and amplification techniques, the strength of the signal is improved relative to the noise to obtain a good record.

After the initial spike from the stimulation, depending on the location of interception, N9, 13, 18, and 20 are recorded for the median nerve SSEP test and N7, 22, 34, and P37 are recorded for the posterior tibial SSEP. During pathological states, these waves can be absent, their amplitude might decrease, or latency increases. Interpretation of these three findings is given below.

10.6 Prolongation of Latency

When there is a pathology affecting conduction, the latency gets prolonged. While interpreting SSEP waveforms, both the absolute latency from stimulation and the inter peak latency (IPL) between waves are useful in localizing the site of the pathology. As a general rule, if the latency is three standard deviations more than normal, it is considered clinically significant [3, 4].

10.7 Changes in Amplitude

Amplitude of the waves is affected by multiple factors. There are no clear guidelines on interpretating changes in the amplitude of the waves in critical care. The intraoperative practice of using 50% reduction in amplitude as abnormal cannot be extrapolated to the critical care setting because of the technical-, patient-, and pathology-related differences between these two settings [5].

10.8 Absence of Waves

10.8.1 Upper Limb (Table 10.3)

- If all the four waves are absent in either limb, it is usually due to a technical issue in the stimulator. SSEPs are usually recorded by technologists, and critical care is a non-neurophysiological environment; therefore, care must be taken while setting up, stimulating, and recording impulses.
- If the peripheral and subcortical impulses are present and cortical N20 alone is absent, it indicates a block at the level of somatosensory cortex or thalamocortical projection, provided that technical issues like improperly placed electrode etc. are ruled out [9].
- If the peripheral impulses (N9 and 13) are present and central impulses are absent (N18 and 20), it indicates a conduction block in the intracranial sensory fibers above the foramen magnum [9].
- If N9 is present and all other impulses are either delayed or absent, it reflects a conduction block proximal to the brachial plexus. The interpeak latencies might help decipher the location of the block.
- If the peripheral impulse is absent (absent N9) but the cervical and central impulses are present, it is a normal SSEP [9]. Sometimes, the presence of neuropathy might prolong the N20 latency when N9 is absent. This is an abnormal SSEP.

Table 10.3 Upper limb SSEP interpretation (Modified with permission from Muzyka et al., Elsevier Inc. 2019)

Median nerve SSEP	Location of the block	Interpretation
Bilateral N20 absent, but all other potentials present	Sensory cortex or thalamocortical projection	Abnormal
N18 and N20 absent; N9 and N13 present	Central sensory fibers (above foramen magnum)	Abnormal
N9 absent; all other potentials present	No pathology	Normal
N9 present; others absent	Proximal to brachial plexus	Abnormal
All potentials absent	Likely technical fault	None

10.8.2 Lower Limb (Table 10.4)

- As with median nerve, if the peripheral, cord, and subcortical impulses are present and cortical p37 alone is absent, it indicates a block at the level of somatosensory cortex or thalamocortical projection.
- If the cortical and subcortical potentials (P37 and N34) are absent, but N7 and N22 are present, it indicates a pathology in the spinal cord above lumbar level. Corroborating with cervical cord potentials from median nerve stimulation will help localization [9].
- When only N7 is recordable with absent or delayed proximal potentials, the lesion can be anywhere proximal to the peripheral nervous system. Again, checking the median nerve potentials is warranted.

Table 10.4 Lower limb SSEP interpretation (Modified with permission from Muzyka et al., Elsevier Inc. 2019)

Posterior tibial SSEP	Location of the block	Interpretation
Bilateral P37 absent, but all other potentials including N34 present	Sensory cortex, thalamocortical projection	Abnormal
P37 and N34 absent; N7 and N22 present	Sensory fibers proximal to lumbar cord (correlate with median nerve SSEP to locate the site)	Abnormal
N7 absent; all other potentials present with normal IPL	No pathology	Normal
All potentials absent	Likely technical fault	None

10.9 Factors Affecting SSEPs

Length of the limb and age affect the recording with taller individuals and elderly having slightly prolonged latencies. In tall individuals, the absolute latency is prolonged but the interpeak latency remains normal. Hypothermia has been shown to slow the rate of conduction; therefore, it is prudent to wait till normothermia before doing SSEPs after cardiac arrest [10]. Unlike anesthesia, critical care sedation has very little effect on N20 potentials [11]; in patients where the noise level is high from muscle potentials, sedation and paralysis can be employed to obtain better N20 recordings.

10.10 Indications and Common Applications in Critical Care

10.10.1 Prognostication After Cardiac Arrest [12–18]

Bilateral absent N20 responses strongly predict poor neurological outcome or death in comatose patients following cardiac arrest (Fig. 10.4). With very low false positive rate in the majority of published studies (FPR 0%, CI95% (0.001–0.047), SSEPs are quite useful in predicting poor outcome after return of spontaneous circulation (ROSC). Conversely, the presence of N20 waveform is not predictive of a good outcome. Although sensory tracts have no influence over the level of consciousness, it is the damage to the surrounding neuronal structures from hypoxia or anoxia that affects consciousness. This is probably the reason why only 50% of the patients regain consciousness even when the N20 waveforms are present after ROSC. If hypothermia is employed in post cardiac arrest care, it is better to record SSEPs after 72 h after rewarming. Since the current evidence favors fever prevention and not active cooling after cardiac arrest, SSEPs can be recorded as early as 24 h after ROSC.

To improve the prognostic value of SSEP, recent studies assessed the peak-to-peak amplitude of N20/P25 complex among patients with bilateral presence of N20. For poor outcome prediction, a low-voltage amplitude (between 0.40 and 1 μV) improved sensitivity from 30% to 50% compared to bilateral N20 absence, with a high specificity (93–100%). Conversely, a high N20–P25 amplitude (>2.30 to 4 μV) predicts a favorable outcome with a high specificity (85–96%), but a moderate sensitivity (30–61%). A recent study highlighted that N20–P25 presented a higher prognostic value (AUC = 0.85) compared to N20-baseline (AUC = 0.70). Standardization of the method (i.e., SSEP N20-baseline or N20–P25 peak-to-peak measure) might be a useful prognostic marker.

10.10.2 Prognostication After Traumatic Brain Injury [1, 19–21]

SSEP can be used to determine the prognosis after traumatic brain injury (TBI). Performed at day 3 and using a 6-point ordinal scale to grade the SSEP outcome, it was found that patients with bilateral absent cortical response had poor neurological outcome, whereas patients with normal cortical response had good neurological outcome. It must be remembered that cerebral oedema might affect the SSEP recordings in the

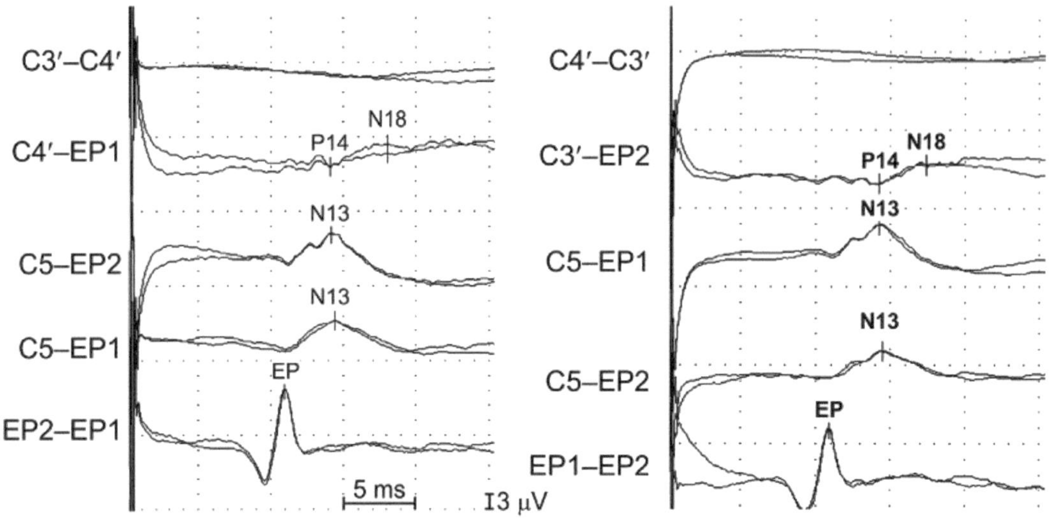

Fig. 10.4 Bilateral absent N20 waveforms with preserved N18, N13, and N9. (Reproduced with permission from Muzyka et al., Elsevier Inc. 2019)

initial days after trauma; bilateral absence of N20 in the initial test has been associated with recovery in about 15% of cases; therefore, follow up SSEP might be required to accurately prognosticate outcomes after TBI.

10.11 Other Uses

Bilateral absent SSEPs might be associated with poor neurological recovery after ischemic or hemorrhagic stroke, but the available evidence is not sufficient enough to recommend SSEPs to prognosticate outcomes in this population [1].

In patients with spinal cord injury, early presence or appearance of lower limb SSEPs after the injury is associated with functional recovery but the absence does not indicate a lack of recovery. Similarly, the absence of cortical responses in patients with cervical cord injury might indicate poor neurologic outcome [22].

10.12 Multimodal Monitoring [23, 24]

Instead of using SSEP as a single prognostic indicator, it is advisable to include SSEP as part of a multimodal strategy to prognosticate. The recent ILCOR guidelines recommend combining clinical, imaging, laboratory, and evoked responses to prognosticate neurologic outcomes after ROSC.

10.13 Other Evoked Responses in Critical Care [25]

Brian stem auditory evoked responses are rarely used in critical care. As an add on ancillary test to SSEP, it may be used diagnose brain stem death. Visual evoked potentials (VEPs) require a cooperative patient and a checkerboard to record responses. Although flashing lights can be used in comatose patients, the utility of VEP in critical care is quite limited.

References

1. Xiong W, Eccher M, Geocadin R. Evoked potentials in neurocritical care. In: Neurocritical care monitoring. Demos Medical Publishing, LLC; 2015.
2. Walsh P, Kane N, Butler S. The clinical role of evoked potentials. J Neurol Neurosurg Psychiatry. 2005;76(ii):16–22.
3. Muzyka I, Estephan B. Somatosensory evoked potentials. In: Clinical neurophysiology: basis and technical aspects, Handbook of clinical neurology series, vol. 160. 1st ed. Elsevier; 2019. p. 523–40.

4. Markand O. Somatosensory evoked potentials. In: Clinical evoked potentials. Springer Nature Switzerland; 2020. p. 325–480.
5. Carter J, Stevens C. Somatosensory evoked potentials. In: Clinical neurophysiology. 3rd ed. Oxford; 2009. p. 257–69.
6. Sloan T, Jameson L, Janik D, Koht A. Evoked potentials. In: Cottrell and Patel's neuroanesthesia. 6th ed. Elsevier; 2017. p. 114–26.
7. Guideline 9C: guidelines on short-latency auditory evoked potentials. J Clin Neurophysiol. 2006;23(2):157–67.
8. MacDonald D, Dong C, Quatrale R, Sala F, Skinner S, Soto F, et al. Recommendations of the International Society of Intraoperative Neurophysiology for intraoperative somatosensory evoked potentials. Clin Neurophysiol. 2019:161–79.
9. Berger J, Blum A. Somatosensory evoked potentials. In: The clinical neurophysiology primer. 1st ed. Humana Totowa, NJ; 2007. p. 485–97.
10. Rothstein T. SSEP retains its value as predictor of poor outcome following cardiac arrest in the era of therapeutic hypothermia. Crit Care. 2019;23(327):1–7.
11. Cloostermans M, Horn J, van Putten M. The SSEP on the ICU: current applications and pitfalls. Neth J Crit Care. 2013;17(1):5–9.
12. Kane N, Oware A. Somatosensory evoked potentials aid prediction after hypoxic–ischaemic brain injury. Pract Neurol. 2015:1–9.
13. Koenig M, Kaplan P. Clinical applications for EPs in the ICU. J Clin Neurophysiol. 2015;32(6):472–80.
14. Sandroni C, Cronberg T, Sekhon M. Brain injury after cardiac arrest: pathophysiology, treatment, and prognosis. Intensive Care Med. 2021;47:1393–414.
15. Sandroni C, D'Arrigo S, Cacciola S, Hoedemaekers C. Prediction of poor neurological outcome in comatose survivors of cardiac arrest: a systematic review. Intensive Care Med. 2020;46(10):1803–51.
16. Sandroni C, D'Arrigo S, Nolan J. Prognostication after cardiac arrest. Crit Care. 2018;22(150):1–9.
17. Sandroni C, D'Arrigo S, Cacciola S. Prediction of good neurological outcome in comatose survivors of cardiac arrest: a systematic review. Intensive Care Med. 2022;48:389–413.
18. Lachance B, Wang Z, Badjatia N. Somatosensory evoked potentials and neuroprognostication after cardiac arrest. Neurocrit Care. 2020;32:847–57.
19. Sun Y, Yu J, Wu J, Wu X, Yuan Q. Predictive value of SSEP for patients with severe traumatic brain injury. Clin Neurosurg. 2014;61(1):171–4.
20. Houlden DA, Taylor A, Feinstein A, Midha R, Bethune A, Stewart C, Schwartz ML. Early SSEP grades in comatose traumatic brain injury patients predict cognitive and functional outcome. Crit Care Med. 2010;38(1):167–74.
21. Sleigh J, Havill J, Frith R, Kersel D, Marsh N, Ulyatt D. Somatosensory evoked potentials in severe traumatic brain injury: a blinded study. J Neurosurg. 1999;91(4):577–80.
22. Spiess M, Schubert M, Kliesch U, group E-SS, et al. Evolution of tibial SSEP after traumatic spinal cord injury. Clin Neurophysiol. 2008;119(5):1051–61.
23. Youn CS, Park KN, Kim SH, Lee BK, Kronberg T. External validation of the 2020 ERC/ESICM prognostication strategy algorithm after cardiac arrest. Crit Care. 2022;26(95):1–9.
24. Nolan JP, Sandroni C, Bottiger BW, Cariou A. Post resuscitation care. Resuscitation. 2021;161:220–69.
25. Rosenthal E. The utility of EEG, SSEP and other neurophysiologic tools to guide neurocritical care. Neurotherapeutics. 2012;9:24–36.

Near Infrared Spectroscopy

11

Indu Kapoor

11.1 Introduction

Various bedside methods for cerebral monitoring are introduced in neurointensive care unit (NICU) for neurological or neurosurgical critically ill patients. Early diagnosis and treatment of abnormalities in cerebral perfusion, cerebral metabolism, or cerebral oxygenation are the main objective of the treating clinician in NICU to prevent further brain injury, termed as "secondary brain insult." These cerebral monitors can be further divided into either invasive or noninvasive monitors (Table 11.1). Near-infrared spectroscopy (NIRS)-based cerebral oximetry is an important part of multimodel monitoring in neurocritically ill patients to measure cerebral oxygenation. NIRS uses the near-infrared spectrum of light to penetrate skin, subcutaneous tissue, bone, and finally brain tissue, to estimate oxy-/deoxyhemoglobin concentration changes and oxidation status of cytochrome c oxidase, and, finally, to measure the cortical regional oxygen saturation (rSO_2) [1]. The bifrontal light-emitting diodes placed on the forehead at 4 cm apart provide information about oxygen saturation within the frontal lobe (Fig. 11.1) [2]. These probes contain a fiber optic light source and light detectors. Light sources release light in the infrared range through a process of either stimulated emission of radiation or through light-emitting diodes (Fig. 11.2) [2]. The threshold for cerebral ischemia is set at <50% or 20% drop from the base-

Table 11.1 Bedside cerebral monitors used in neurointensive care unit

Monitoring	Invasive	Noninvasive
Intracranial pressure	Intraventricular catheter Intraparenchymal catheter Extraventricular drain (EVD)	Optic nerve sheath diameter (ONSD)
Electrical activity	Electroencephalography [EEG]	–
Oxygenation	Brain tissue oxygen tension ($PbtO_2$) Juglar venous oximetry ($SjvO_2$)	Near-infrared spectroscopy (NIRS)
Blood flow	–	Transcranial Doppler (TCD)
Metabolism	Microdialysis	–

I. Kapoor (✉)
Department of Neuroanesthesiology and Critical Care, AIIMS, New Delhi, India

H. Prabhakar et al. (eds.), *Principles and Practice of Neurocritical Care*,
https://doi.org/10.1007/978-981-99-8059-8_11

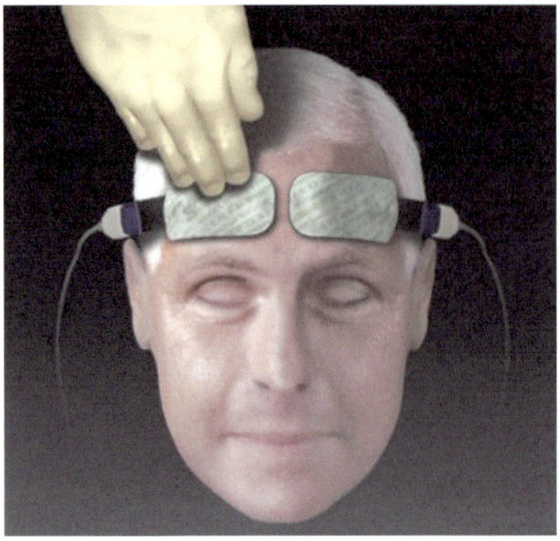

Fig. 11.1 INVOS (In Vivo Optical Spectroscopy) sensor placement on the patients' forehead. (Picture taken from the INVOS Cerebral/Somatic Oximeter Operations Manual, Covidien 2010) [2]. [*With permission from: Murniece S, Soehle M, Vanags I, Mamaja, B. Near Infrared Spectroscopy Based Clinical Algorithm Applicability During Spinal Neurosurgery and Postoperative Cognitive Disturbances. Medicina. 2019, 55, 179*]

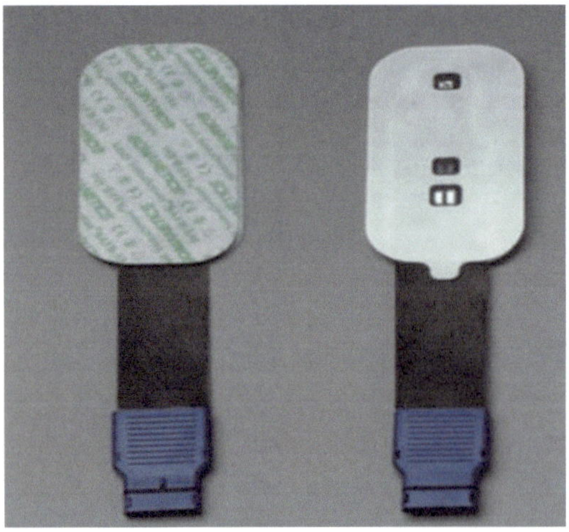

Fig. 11.2 INVOS sensor. (Picture taken from The INVOS Cerebral/Somatic Oximeter Operations Manual, Covidien 2010) [2]. [*With permission from: Murniece S, Soehle M, Vanags I, Mamaja, B. Near Infrared Spectroscopy Based Clinical Algorithm Applicability During Spinal Neurosurgery and Postoperative Cognitive Disturbances.* Medicina. *2019,* 55, *179*]

line value [3]. Rather than the absolute value, it would be useful to have a continuous data on trends of relative change from baseline. Brain tissue hypoxia has been associated with worse outcome. That makes the cerebral oxygenation monitoring an important pillar of cerebral care in neurocritically ill patients in NICU. Various cerebral oxygenation monitors are available in the market (Table 11.1) NIRS-based cerebral oximetry is a noninvasive cerebral oxygenation monitor and is easy to use or interpret.

11.2 Factors Affecting NIRS-Based Cerebral Oximetry Readings

The values of NIRS-based cerebral oximetry are affected by a number of factors which include cerebral blood flow, extra-cerebral blood flow, cerebral metabolic rate of oxygen consumption, arterial blood oxygen content, thickness of skull bone, and contamination from extracranial tissues [4]. Among other factors which might affect the NIRS values are indocyanine green, methylene blue, and different vasopressors [4–7]. The vasopressors are the most commonly used drug in NICU. Studies have shown that these drugs can affect the frontal lobe cerebral oxygenation. The short-acting vasopressors like phenylephrine or ephedrine are administered in relatively large quantities. Despite the fact that both vasopressor agents effectively elevate mean blood pressure, there is increasing evidence that frontal lobe rSO_2, measured by NIRS, decreases during the administration of phenylephrine, while it remains unaffected during ephedrine use [6, 7]. If there is a possibility to choose between phenylephrine and ephedrine to correct hypotension induced by anesthesia, ephedrine is the drug that preserves rSO_2 [6]. Despite these findings, the above studies had been performed in anesthetized patients where these short-acting vasopressors are used to treat anesthesia-induced hypotension. To date, the effect of vasopressors on rSO_2 has not been studied in neurocritically ill patients. It would be interesting to observe the effect of vasopressors on frontal lobe rSO_2 in critically ill patients in NICU.

11.3 Clinical Application of NIRS-Based Cerebral Oximetry in NICU

Cerebral Autoregulation Monitoring: NIRS-based cerebral oximetry measures rSO_2 which can be used as a surrogate of cerebral blood flow (CBF) to measure cerebral autoregulation [8, 9]. Unlike transcranial doppler (TCD), NIRS provides continuous output with minimal operator intervention while monitoring autoregulation. A significant correlation and agreement has been found between TCD-based mean velocity index (Mx) and cerebral oximetry index (COx) in adult patients undergoing cardiopulmonary bypass [8], where COx is calculated by the moving correlation between the slow waves of rSO_2 and mean arterial pressure (MAP). *Rivera and colleagues* reported a good correlation and agreement of NIRS-derived COx with previously validated TCD-based method for monitoring cerebral autoregulation [10]. In their study, functional autoregulation was indicated when COx approached zero (i.e., no correlation between $rScO_2$ and arterial blood pressure), while COx approaching 1 indicated impaired autoregulation [10]. They suggested that COx may be an acceptable substitute for Mx monitoring in patients with acute intracranial injury. *Steiner* et al compared tissue oxygenation index (TOI) recorded with NIRS as an index of cerebral autoregulation with traditional TCD-based FV to monitor autoregulation [11]. Both the indices showed significant correlation with each other while monitoring for autoregulation. The authors concluded that NIRS-based index can be used for continuous assessment of cerebral autoregulation in adult patients.

Subarachnoid Hemorrhage [SAH]: Poor-grade SAH patients have higher mortality rates ranging from 34 to 77%, although the mortality rate in patients with good-grade SAH is <10 to 20% [12]. Delayed cerebral ischemia (DCI) is one of the major contributors toward poor neurological outcome after SAH [13]. Hence, early diagnosis and treatment of DCI are critical to achieving good clinical outcome. TCD is routinely used to detect vasospasm in SAH patients. TCD monitoring is highly expert-dependent, and also the acoustic window is absent in around 10% of the individuals. NIRS can be used as a continuous bedside tool to detect ischemia in SAH patients who are at risk of DIC. Taussky and colleagues observed a good correlation between NIRS oxygenation and regional cerebral blood flow in a perfusion computed tomography imaging study of eight stroke patients (SAH, $n = 6$; ischemic stroke, $n = 1$; intracerebral hemorrhage, $n = 1$) in the critical care unit [14]. Park et al. examined the diagnostic value of NIRS in DCI involving patients with poor-grade SAH [15]. They found that the patients with DCI experienced a greater decrease in rSO_2 levels than patients without DCI beyond 3 days after the ictus. Authors concluded that NIRS might be a promising tool for real-time detection of DCI in patients with poor-grade SAH at the bedside. As per a retrospective and monocentric study in a neurointensive care unit over an 18-month period where authors included patients who were admitted to the neurointensive care unit with severe brain injury after nontraumatic SaH and were equipped with a brain tissue oxygen tension $PbtO_2$ probe, they observed that there is lack of significant correlation between $PbtO_2$ and NIRS measurements [16]. NIRS was unable to detect $PbtO_2$ values <20 mmHg, and percentage changes in NIRS were unable to detect a decrease in $PbtO_2 \geq 10\%$. There is no evidence that NIRS could be a substitute for $PbtO_2$ monitoring in patients with nontraumatic subarachnoid hemorrhage.

Traumatic Brain Injury: In traumatic brain injury (TBI) patients, the secondary injury is closely linked to insufficient oxygen delivery to the brain. Red blood cell (RBC) transfusion in

TBI patients is routinely done to treat anemia. However, the exact neurophysiological effect of RBC transfusion on frontal lobe oxygen saturation using NIRS-based cerebral oximetry has not been studied adequately. Previous studies have invasively monitored $PbtO_2$ in severe TBI patients undergoing a transfusion of RBCs, with their concomitant potential adverse effects and variable changes in $PbtO_2$ [17, 18]. $PbtO_2$ monitoring is an invasive procedure and is associated with many complications like bleeding, injury to brain, infection etc. NIRS-based cerebral oximetry being a noninvasive technique of monitoring brain oxygenation is devoid of all these complications. Maccredie et al. monitored the change in rSO_2 values in TBI patients using NIRS-based cerebral oximetry [19]. They found a significantly different mean pre- and post-transfusion hemoglobin concentration; however, the NIRS-based cerebral oximetry did not detect a measurable impact on rSO_2 in patients receiving RBC transfusion. Further, a large prospective trial with a large sample size could help evaluate the effect of RBC transfusion on NIRS values.

Stroke: Various imaging modalities like CT scan, magnetic imaging resonance (MRI), positron emission tomography (PET), ultrasound, microdialysis have been used to estimate the cerebral blood flow in malignant middle cerebral artery (MCA) infarction [20–25]. One exception is NIRS, a technology that has been evolved over the past years and repeatedly considered to obtain continuous data of cerebral oxygenation. However, there are some concerns with NIRS which include penetration depth, contamination from extracranial tissues, and poor topographic resolution. Another important concern is that rSO_2 may estimate cerebral blood volume but cannot be equated to cerebral blood flow [26] because of various contributions of other vascular compartments as well extracranial tissues. Terborg et al. however were able to measure cerebral perfusion at the bedside using Indocyanin Green tracer in 13 patients with acute ischemic infarction utilizing bilateral NIRS measurements and reported increased time to peak values with good sensitivity and specificity [27]. Damian and Schlosser use simultaneous bilateral NIRS monitoring in 24 patients with space-occupying or malignant MCA infarction and rSO_2. They found that the differences in oxygen saturation (rSO2-diff) values between the infarcted and non-infarcted sides were predictive of outcomes with narrowing of rSO2-diff predictive of clinical deterioration [28]. They hypothesize that the narrowing is either due to "steal" with collateral flow to the infarcted side attempting to compensate for low ipsilateral blood volume or due to decreased oxygen consumption on the non-infarcted side from progressive edema.

Neurological Outcome: NIRS monitoring as a noninvasive toll along with serum neuromarkers like neuron-specific enolase (NSE), S100beta, glial fibrillary acidic protein (GFAP), brain-derived neurotropic factor (BDNF) can also be used to assess the adverse neurological outcome in patients undergoing non-neurosurgical procedures [29–31]. *Subbaswami* et al found a significant correlation between mean rSO_2 and S100beta, a recognized marker of neurological injury in critically ill children with at least one organ failure [32]. Authors believed that future large trials can be done to determine if this technology is predictive of long-term neurological outcome.

References

1. Ghosh A, Elwell C, Smith M. Cerebral near-infrared spectroscopy in adults: a work in progress. Anesth Analg. 2012;115:1373–83.
2. Murniece S, Soehle M, Vanags I, Mamaja B. Near infrared spectroscopy based clinical algorithm applicability during spinal neurosurgery and postoperative cognitive disturbances. Medicina. 2019;55:179.
3. Obrig H. NIRS in clinical neurology—a "promising" tool? NeuroImage. 2014;85:535–46.
4. Barud M, Dabrowski W, Siwicka-Gieroba D, Robba C, Bielacz M, Badenes R. Usefulness of cerebral oximetry in TBI by NIRS. J Clin Med. 2021;10:2938.
5. Yoo KY, Baek HY, Jeong S, Hallacoglu B, Lee J. Intravenously administered indocyanine green may cause falsely high near-infrared cerebral oximetry readings. J Neurosurg Anesthesiol. 2015;27:57–60.
6. Nissen P, Brassard P, Jørgensen TB, Secher NH. Phenylephrine but not ephedrine reduces frontal lobe oxygenation following anesthesia induced hypotension. Neurocrit Care. 2010;12:17–23.

7. Meng L, Cannesson M, Alexander BS, Yu Z, Kain ZN, Cerussi AE, et al. Effect of phenylephrine and ephedrine bolus treatment on cerebral oxygenation in anaesthetized patients. Br J Anaesth. 2011;107:209–17.
8. Brady K, Joshi B, Zweifel C, Smielewski P, Czosnyka M, Easley RB, et al. Real-time continuous monitoring of cerebral blood flow autoregulation using near-infrared spectroscopy in patients undergoing cardiopulmonary bypass. Stroke. 2010;41:1951–6.
9. Brady KM, Lee JK, Kibler KK, Smielewski P, Czosnyka M, Easley RB, et al. Continuous time-domain analysis of cerebrovascular autoregulation using near-infrared spectroscopy. Stroke. 2007;38:2818–25.
10. Rivera-Lara L, Geocadin R, Zorrilla-Vaca A, Healy R, Radzik BR, Palmisano C, et al. Validation of near-infrared spectroscopy for monitoring cerebral autoregulation in comatose patients. Neurocrit Care. 2017;27:362–9.
11. Steiner LA, Pfister D, Strebel SP, Radolovich D, Smielewski P, Czosnyka M. Near-infrared spectroscopy can monitor dynamic cerebral autoregulation in adults. Neurocrit Care. 2009;10:122–8.
12. Komotar RJ, Schmidt JM, Starke RM, Claassen J, Wartenberg KE, Lee K, et al. Resuscitation and critical care of poor-grade subarachnoid hemorrhage. Neurosurgery. 2009;64:397–410.
13. Jeon JS, Sheen SH, Hwang G, Kang SH, Heo DH, Cho YJ. Intravenous magnesium infusion for the prevention of symptomatic cerebral vasospasm after aneurysmal subarachnoid hemorrhage. J Korean Neurosurg Soc. 2012;52:75–9.
14. Taussky P, O'Neal B, Daugherty WP, Luke S, Thorpe D, Pooley RA, et al. Validation of frontal near-infrared spectroscopy as noninvasive bedside monitoring for regional cerebral blood flow in brain-injured patients. Neurosurg Focus. 2012;32:E2.
15. Park JJ, Kim Y, Chai CL, Jeon JP. Application of near-infrared spectroscopy for the detection of delayed cerebral ischemia in poor-grade subarachnoid hemorrhage. Neurocrit Care. 2021;35:767–74.
16. de Courson H, Proust-Lima C, Tuaz E, Georges D, Verchère E, Biais M. Relationship between brain tissue oxygen and near-infrared spectroscopy in patients with nontraumatic subarachnoid hemorrhage. Neurocrit Care. 2022;37:620–8.
17. Zygun DA, Nortje J, Hutchinson PJ, Timofeev I, Menon DK, Gupta AK. The effect of red blood cell transfusion on cerebral oxygenation and metabolism after severe traumatic brain injury. Crit Care Med. 2009;37:1074–8.
18. Smith MJ, Stiefel MF, Magge S, Frangos S, Bloom S, Gracias V, et al. Packed red blood cell transfusion increases local cerebral oxygenation. Crit Care Med. 2005;33:1104–8.
19. McCredie VA, Piva S, Santos M, Xiong W, de Oliveira Manoel AL, Rigamonti A, et al. The impact of red blood cell transfusion on cerebral tissue oxygen saturation in severe traumatic brain injury. Neurocrit Care. 2017;26:247–55.
20. Krieger DW, Demchuk AM, Kasner SE, Jauss M, Hantson L. Early clinical and radiological predictors of fatal brain swelling in ischemic stroke. Stroke. 1999;30:287–92.
21. Kasner SE, Demchuk AM, Berrouschot J, Schmutzhard E, Harms L, Verro P, et al. Predictors of fatal brain edema in massive hemispheric ischemic stroke. Stroke. 2001;32:2117–23.
22. Thomalla G, Kucinski T, Shcoder V, Fiehler J, Knab R, Zeumer H, et al. Prediction of malignant middle cerebral artery infarction by early perfusion and diffusion weighted magnetic resonance imaging. Stroke. 2003;34:1892–900.
23. Bartels E, Bitterman H. Transcranial contrast imaging of cerebral perfusion in patients with space-occupying intracranial lesions. J Ultrasound Med. 2006;25:499–507.
24. Gerriets T, Stolz E, Konig S, Babacan S, Fiss I, Jauss M, et al. Sonographic monitoring of midline shift in space-occupying stroke. An early outcome predictor. Stroke. 2001;32:442–7.
25. Dohmen C, Bosche B, Graf R, Staub F, Kracht L, Sobesky J, et al. Prediction of malignant course in MCA infarction by PET and microdialysis. Stroke. 2003;34:2152–8.
26. Hargroves D, Tallis R, Pomeroy V, Bhalla A. Near-infrared spectroscopy in stroke: from research to clinical practice. (correspondence). Stroke. 2004;35:2430.
27. Terborg C, Bramer S, Harscher S, Simon M, Witte O. Bedside assessment of cerebral perfusion reductions in patients with acute ischaemic stroke by near-infrared spectroscopy and indocyanine green. J Neurol Neurosurg Psychiatry. 2004;75:38–42.
28. Damian MS, Schlosser R. Bilateral near infrared spectroscopy in space-occupying middle cerebral artery stroke. Neurocrit Care. 2007;6:165–73.
29. Sanchez-de-Toledo J, Chrysostomou C, Munoz R, Lichtenstein S, Sao-Avilés CA, Wearden PD, et al. Cerebral regional oxygen saturation and serum neuromarkers for the prediction of adverse neurological outcome in pediatric cardiac surgery. Neurocrit Care. 2014;21:133–9.
30. Abdul-Khaliq H, Schubert S, Stoltenburg-Didinger G, Huebler M, Troitzsch D, Wehsack A, et al. Release patterns of astrocytic and neuronal biochemical markers in serum during and after experimental settings of cardiac surgery. Restor Neurol Neurosci. 2003;21:141–50.
31. Herrmann M, Ebert AD, Galazky I, Wunderlich MT, Kunz WS, Huth C. Neurobehavioral outcome prediction after cardiac surgery: role of neurobiochemical markers of damage to neuronal and glial brain tissue. Stroke. 2000;31:645–50.
32. Subbaswamy A, Hsu AA, Weinstein S, Bell MJ. Correlation of cerebral near infrared spectroscopy and neurological markers in critically ill children. Neurocrit Care. 2009;10:129–35.

12 Brain Tissue Oxygenation

Toby Jeffcote and Andrew Udy

12.1 Introduction: The Physiology of Brain Oxygen

The brain has remarkably high metabolic activity. It also lacks capacity to store energy. As such it is fundamentally reliant on the continuous provision of energy substrates and oxygen from the blood. It is for this reason that an organ representing only 2% of body weight receives 18% of the cardiac output and uses up to 20% of systemic oxygen supply.

The importance of adequate perfusion to the survival of cerebral tissue is illustrated by the devastating effects of pathophysiological states that interrupt the brains blood supply. The prototypical example of this pathology is ischemic stroke in which the interruption of blood supply to a tissue region results in ischemia, hypoxia, metabolic distress, and tissue necrosis unless blood supply is re-established.

Brain tissue ischemia and hypoxia are also key features of traumatic brain injury (TBI) and sub-arachnoid hemorrhage (SAH). However, these diseases differ from ischemic stroke in two key respects:

1. They are complex multi-faceted pathologies in which ischemia is one of several overlapping factors that contribute to tissue stress and damage.
2. The management of these diseases may require extended periods of care in the neurocritical care unit with sedative medications limiting the availability of clinical examination to indicate tissue hypoxia and guide treatment.

The need for insights into tissue blood flow and brain tissue oxygenation has led to the development of invasive techniques for brain tissue oxygen monitoring. A technique that is gaining recognition for its ability to guide effective treatment in such circumstances.

12.1.1 Systemic Determinants of Brain Oxygen

Adequate brain tissue oxygenation can only be achieved if there is sufficient oxygen delivery. The two pillars of oxygen delivery to the CNS are arterial oxygen content (hemoglobin concentration, blood oxygen saturation, and the arterial partial pressure of oxygen) and cerebral blood flow (CBF). It is important to note that the

T. Jeffcote · A. Udy (✉)
Department of Intensive Care and Hyperbaric Medicine, Alfred Health, Melbourne, VIC, Australia

Australia New Zealand Intensive Care Research Centre, Monash University, Melbourne, VIC, Australia
e-mail: andrew.udy@monash.edu

H. Prabhakar et al. (eds.), *Principles and Practice of Neurocritical Care*,
https://doi.org/10.1007/978-981-99-8059-8_12

maintenance of each of these pillars relies upon the function of multiple organ systems.

12.1.2 Arterial Oxygen Content

The oxygenation of arterial blood is achieved through the combined function of the neuromuscular, respiratory, cardiovascular, and hematological systems. Dysfunction of any single organ system may lead to deficiencies in brain oxygenation.

The neuromuscular system underlies the ability to maintain extrathoracic airway patency and respiratory muscle function, both of which drive lung ventilation. The lung parenchyma provides the structural apparatus necessary for gas exchange. This consists of the branching airways of the lung and the many alveoli responsible for oxygen absorption. The hematological system serves to maintain red blood cell structure and function and a hemoglobin level sufficient to transport oxygen throughout the body. The cardiovascular system plays a vital role in the transport of de-oxygenated blood through the lung to enable its oxygenation.

12.1.3 Cerebral Blood Flow

The arterial network of the cardiovascular system and the vasculature of the brain work in a coordinated fashion to transport oxygenated blood to the brain. Given the unique metabolic and vascular demands of the brain, this network must meet three key requirements [1]:

1. Provision of at least 100 mL/min of oxygenated blood per 100 g of tissue
2. Responsiveness to dynamic changes in metabolic demand from different brain regions
3. Protection of the brain parenchyma from potentially harmful variations in systemic blood pressure

The maintenance of cardiac output, flow metabolism coupling, and cerebral autoregulation work in concert to achieve these goals. While a detailed discussion of these topics is beyond the scope of this chapter, it is important to note that significant dysfunction of one or more of the inter-reliant organ systems, providing arterial oxygenation and cerebral blood flow can significantly impact brain tissue oxygenation.

12.1.4 Capillary Oxygen Delivery

The delivery of oxygenated blood to the penetrating arterioles of the brain provides the blood flow to perfuse the rich capillary networks of cerebral tissue. The relationship between capillary perfusion and tissue oxygenation was originally described by Krogh in terms of a simplified cylindrical capillary within a homogenously respiring tissue cylinder [2]. He proposed that oxygen would diffuse away from the capillary in a uniform fashion resulting in a linear decrease in capillary oxygen tension along the length of the capillary. Krogh's model was a significant first step toward understanding oxygen delivery, and its basic principles have been confirmed in cerebral tissue with advanced neuroimaging techniques [3].

The model is, however, an over-simplification of cerebral oxygen supply in that it assumes uniform oxygen delivery and consumption. The Krogh model also proposes capillary recruitment as a means of increasing tissue oxygen delivery, whereas experimental evidence points toward an increase in vessel diameter as the main means of increased brain tissue oxygen. This introduces a convective element of oxygen delivery, i.e., increased flow will steepen Krogh's diffusion gradient and increase tissue oxygen delivery [4]. Recent evidence also identifies capillary transit time heterogeneity as a significant factor governing the effective delivery of oxygen to meet tissue needs [5].

12.1.5 Oxygen Diffusion

The final stage in the pathway of delivery of oxygen to the intracellular mitochondria is that of diffusion through the capillary wall and cell membranes. Oxygen is highly lipid soluble and unpolarized and under normal physiological conditions is assumed to diffuse rapidly down a concentration gradient through capillary walls and cell membranes enabling its ready utilization by intracellular mitochondria [6]. It is important to note, however, that oxygen is poorly soluble in both cytosolic and interstitial fluid [6] and its transport to mitochondria may be significantly impeded by the altered tissue conditions of acute neurological pathologies which may include interstitial oedema, increased intercapillary distance, capillary transit time heterogeneity [7], and microvascular occlusion [8].

12.2 Brain Tissue Oxygen Monitoring

Several methods exist for the measurement of brain oxygenation including Jugular Venous Oximetry (SJVO2) and Near-Infrared Spectroscopy—both of which are discussed in other chapters of this book. Brain tissue oxygen ($PbtO_2$) monitoring has emerged as the most commonly used modern technique due to its accuracy, ease of use, and ability to demonstrate dynamic changes to brain oxygen levels.

Brain tissue oxygen monitoring involves placement of monitoring probes in the brain parenchyma to obtain a direct measure of the partial pressure of oxygen in the extracellular space surrounding the probe. Measurement techniques based on the Clark principle and on oxygen-sensitive optical dyes are both used in clinical practice.

The Clark electrode-based technique consists of two electrodes in electrolyte solution housed in a protective cover with a diffusible membrane window to the brain parenchyma. Oxygen diffuses across the membrane to contact the gold polarographic cathode inducing a flow of electrons directly proportional to the oxygen concentration. The optical technique utilizes wavelength analysis of oxygen-induced photochemical reactions to estimate local oxygen concentration. One of the more commonly used systems is a combined temperature and brain tissue oxygen catheter, attached to a Licox® monitor (Integra lifesciences ltd). This probe combines a Clarks electrode (reading surface area = 18 mm^2, oxygen sensing length 7 mm [9]) and a thermocouple for internal calibration of readings to brain temperature (see Fig. 12.1).

12.2.1 Normal Values for Brain Oxygen Levels

$PbtO_2$ values are a measure of tissue oxygenation in the region surrounding the probe. Readings primarily reflect the relative proliferation of arterial and

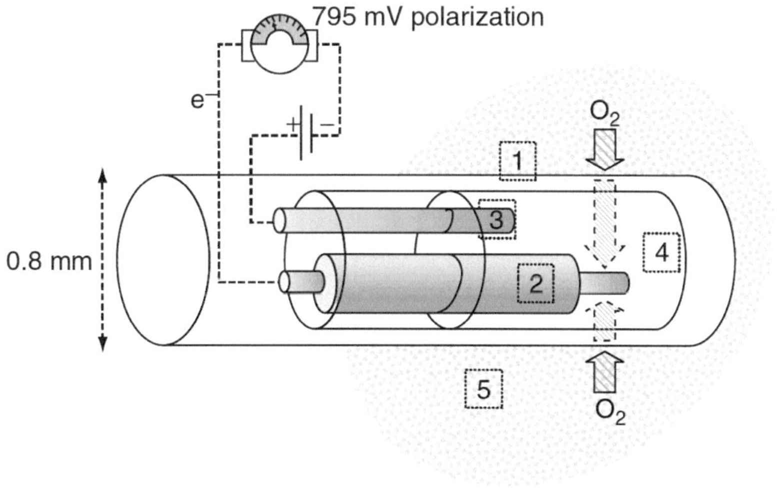

Fig. 12.1 Licox Clark electrode for brain tissue oxygen monitoring [10]. (1) Protective covering. (2) Gold working electrode. (3) Ag/AgCl reference/counter electrode. (4) Ionic solution. (5) Brain parenchyma

venous vessels in the immediate vicinity of the probe. Under normal conditions, arterial PO_2 is approximately 90 mmHg and venous PO_2 is approximately 30 mmHg. The normal value of $PbtO_2$ is in the region of 40 mmHg [10], reflecting the fact that 70% of the cortical vasculature is venous.

There is no universally accepted PbtO2 value indicative of ischemia [10], and indeed these values may vary according to tissue physiology and methods of defining ischemia. The most commonly quoted ischemic tissue oxygen values derived from Positron Emission Tomography (PET) scanning data are equivalent to between 10 and 15 mmHg [11], and a value of 8.5 mmHg translates to 50% $sjVO_2$ [12]. Despite the variability of values denoting ischemia, $PbtO_2$ values <5 mmHg are associated with cell death [13].

The close relationship between PbtO2 values and cerebral blood flow (CBF) has led some authors to investigate the technology as a means of monitoring cerebral perfusion. Xenon CT studies and studies using $PbtO_2$ probes paired with CBF probes have confirmed that with a stable inspired oxygen concentration (fiO_2), $PbtO_2$ correlates well with CBF [14–16]. However, while Jaeger et al. found significant correlations between $PbtO_2$ and CBF in all patients studied, the strength of this correlation was highly variable between patients. This variability may represent differences in local anatomy, tissue pathology, probe placement, and/or the electrophysiological status of the monitored tissue (see below). These considerations mean that estimations of dynamic changes to CBF based on PbtO2 can only be inferred from relative changes to baseline values as opposed to absolute values of PbtO2 indicating levels of cerebral perfusion.

12.3 Methodological Issues with Clinical Monitoring of pbtO2

12.3.1 Systemic Determinants of PbtO2

As previously discussed, brain tissue oxygenation levels are a function of multiple systemic factors with the function and dysfunction of upstream organ systems likely to have profound effects on PbtO2 levels [17]. In addition to this, patients managed in the intensive care unit are often reliant on multiple methods of organ support (such as mechanical ventilation). The need to manipulate these organ supports in the course of clinical care, e.g., increase in fraction of inspired oxygen, represents a significant source of factors that may confound our interpretation of PbtO2 readings.

12.3.2 The Balance of Supply and Demand

Levels of oxygen in the brain will be determined by the balance of oxygen supply (see above) and oxygen demand. Cerebral tissue is extremely metabolically active at baseline, and this activity will further increase in certain physiological (e.g., activation of specific brain regions associated with cognition) and pathophysiological states (e.g., epileptic seizure [18] or cortical spreading depolarization [19]).

12.3.3 Local Tissue Factors Influencing PbtO2 Readings

PbtO2 readings therefore are a dynamic reflection of systemic oxygenation, global and local cerebral blood flow, and the balance of oxygen supply and demand in local tissue. A related issue that must be considered when interpreting PbtO2 values in clinical scenarios involving TBI or SAH is that local pathophysiology may have a profound influence on cerebral blood flow and oxygen diffusion characteristics in the sampling region (see Fig. 12.2). Placement of PbtO2 probes within or near brain contusions or in tissue previously compressed by hematoma result in low PbtO2 readings that do not reflect more global tissue oxygenation [20]. Similarly, placement of PbtO2 probes in SAH will provide tissue oxygenation data for a limited arterial perfusion territory and may not detect ischemia in other territories.

Recommendations for probe placement in TBI include placement within the sub-cortical

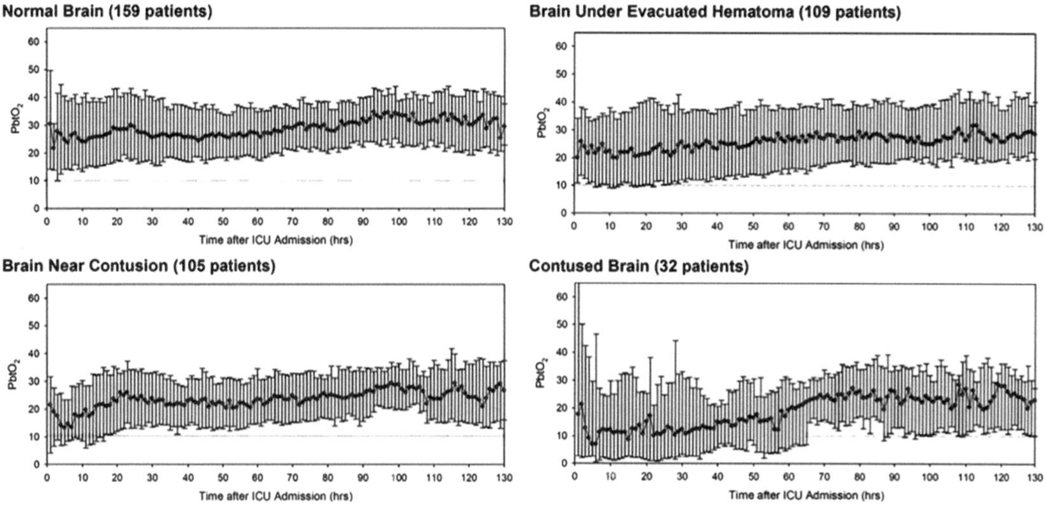

Fig. 12.2 Variations in PbtO2 values associated with different tissue conditions in moderate to severe TBI [20]

white matter in the hemisphere with the highest burden of disease [21]. It is also crucial to perform CT imaging of probe placement in order to correctly interpret PbtO2 readings in the context of local tissue conditions [22].

12.4 Brain Tissue Oxygen Monitoring in TBI

12.4.1 Ischemia as a Component of Secondary Brain Injury in TBI

One of the guiding principles of neurointensive care is that ischemia is a major cause of secondary brain injury after TBI. This practice is based on over 30 years of pathologic observations documenting that brain infarction is almost universally noted in fatal TBI and persistent vegetative state [23]. These observations have been confirmed in histopathological studies of TBI in the modern era of protocolized goal-directed TBI care [24]. Functional imaging studies of cerebral blood flow and oxygenation following TBI are complicated by multiple confounding factors that are not present in ischemic stroke. This has led to debate as to the extent of ischemia in TBI and the role that it plays in secondary brain injury. Indeed, some authors argue that while brain tissue hypoxia and low cerebral blood flow (CBF) are common after TBI, they are a consequence rather than a cause of tissue injury [23]. Countering this view is the clear demonstration of increased oxygen extraction fraction early after TBI [25] and diffusion hypoxia, which continues several days post-injury [26, 27]. Further, the robust association between low $PbtO_2$ and increased lactate/pyruvate ratios (measured by microdialysis) indicates that hypoxic episodes lead to impaired tissue metabolism [28]. In these studies, low $PbtO_2$ precedes increased lactate/pyruvate ratio, and the use of normobaric hyperoxia, and/or CPP augmentation, results in normalization of $PbtO_2$ and lactate/pyruvate ratios. These studies indicate that correction of tissue hypoxia in the early stages can affect brain metabolism, thereby potentially salvaging tissue at risk [28]. The strong association (see below) between duration of hypoxia and functional outcome also supports the hypothesis that unrecognized brain tissue hypoxia leads to further brain injury, and correction of this may improve outcomes.

12.4.2 Mechanisms of Brain Hypoxia and Dysoxia

It is well established that tissue within brain contusions is hypoxic [29] and that brain tissue oxygen levels are reduced in brain regions that have been compressed with mass lesions associated with brain trauma, e.g., sub-dural hematoma [20]. The nature of this tissue hypoxia is multifactorial with capillary transit time heterogeneity, swelling of astrocytic end-feet, capillary compression, pericyte dysfunction, vasoactive effects of blood breakdown products, blood viscosity, and intracranial hypertension all contributing to reductions in local blood flow and oxygen availability [7].

It is important, however, to recognize that ischemia or reduced blood flow does not account for all of the changes to metabolism and oxygen utilization in cerebral tissue following traumatic injury. Recent evidence demonstrating hypoxic brain regions distal from radiographically identified traumatic lesions [27] has highlighted the need for a more wide-reaching conceptualization of brain hypoxia and dysoxia. One such framework describes a more generalized failure of cerebral oxidative metabolism or "Brain shock." The concept offers a framework for understanding widespread changes to oxygen utilization following TBI by highlighting the additional factors of diffusion limitation, mitochondrial uncoupling, microvascular shunting, extraction, and hypermetabolism [8].

12.4.3 Identification of Brain Hypoxia with PbtO2

Low PbtO2 is common after TBI, with investigators demonstrating that 70–86% of monitored patients have $PbtO_2$ measurements below 20 mmHg within the first few days after traumatic injury [30, 31]. In one series, 57% of patients had $PbtO_2$ values lower than 15 mmHg, 42% had values lower than 10 mmHg, and values lower than 5 mmHg were noted in 22% [30]. In 17 TBI patients with $PbtO_2$ monitors placed in normal appearing brain, Longhi et al. noted moderate hypoxia ($PbtO_2$ 10–19 mmHg) 23% of the time and severe hypoxia ($PbtO_2$ < 10 mmHg) another 11% of the time [21]. The median episode of moderate hypoxia lasted 50 min, and the median episode of severe hypoxia lasted 39 min [21]. In a 30 patient TBI study at a tertiary trauma center in Victoria, Australia [32], it was demonstrated that the mean duration of brain hypoxic episodes ($PbtO_2$ < 15 mmHg) with standard care (Group 1, $n = 10$) was 106 min and overall brain tissue hypoxia was present for 10% of the monitoring time.

It has also been reported that most episodes of regional cerebral hypoxia would not have been detected and would have gone untreated using standard monitoring (only 3% of these episodes were associated with an elevated ICP and only 33% were associated with a CPP <65 mmHg, in one series) [31].

12.4.4 Outcomes Associated with Low $PbtO_2$

Available data indicate that $PbtO_2$ values below a critical threshold are associated with unfavorable neurologic outcomes. Bardt et al. found that the odds ratio (OR) of severe disability or death was 10.8 (95% CI 2.09–55.7, $P = 0.004$) for patients with $PbtO_2$ under 10 mmHg for >30 min [33]. Van den Brink reached similar conclusions, reporting an OR of 3.8 (95% CI 1.6–8.4, $P = 0.002$) for death in patients with >30 min of hypoxia ($PbtO_2$ < 10 mmHg) [30]. Valadka et al. concluded that mortality increased linearly with the duration of time that $PbtO_2$ was below 15 mmHg [34]. Further, physiological studies suggest that mitochondria need an intracellular oxygen tension of 1.5 mmHg to support ATP synthesis, a level corresponding to tissue O_2 tensions between 15 and 20 mmHg [35]. Brain tissue hypoxia is also associated with variables known to be related to poor outcome, such as poor GCS and poor CT score [36]. In a historical cohort-matched study, 52 patients were treated with normobaric hyperoxia (100% oxygen for 24 h), which resulted in higher $PbtO_2$ tensions, lower ICP, improvement in biochemical parameters such as glutamate, lactate, lactate/pyruvate ratio, and a trend toward improved outcomes at 3 and 6 months, when compared to 112 historical controls [37]. Finally, Stiefel and colleagues published the results of a non-randomized trial (using historical controls), which concluded that $PbtO_2$-directed management lowered mortality from 44% to 25% ($P < 0.05$) [38].

12.4.5 Protocolized Approach to Brain Hypoxia

Observational evidence indicates that interventions such as ventilator adjustments that raise the partial arterial pressure of oxygen (PaO_2) and carbon dioxide ($PaCO_2$), increasing CPP, or red blood cell (RBC) transfusion to raise the hemoglobin (Hb) concentration [39] are associated with the reversal of detected brain tissue hypoxia [40]. Bohman et al. reported that medical management successfully reversed 72% of cerebral hypoxia episodes, usually through ventilator adjustments, CPP augmentation, and sedation [41].

Formalization of these interventions into a $PbtO_2$ optimization algorithm have also been demonstrated to reduce the duration of brain tissue hypoxia [32]. In 30 TBI patients managed at a tertiary trauma center in Victoria, Australia, it was demonstrated that periods of cerebral hypoxia were significantly reduced ($P = 0.01$) in patients (Group 2, $n = 20$) where a brain tissue oxygen-guided algorithm was employed (see Fig. 12.3).

Additionally, several forms of PbtO2 optimization algorithms are currently being utilized as part of three large randomized controlled trials of PbtO2 management in TBI (see below). The results of these studies will be able to definitively assess the impact of such algorithms on patient outcome in TBI.

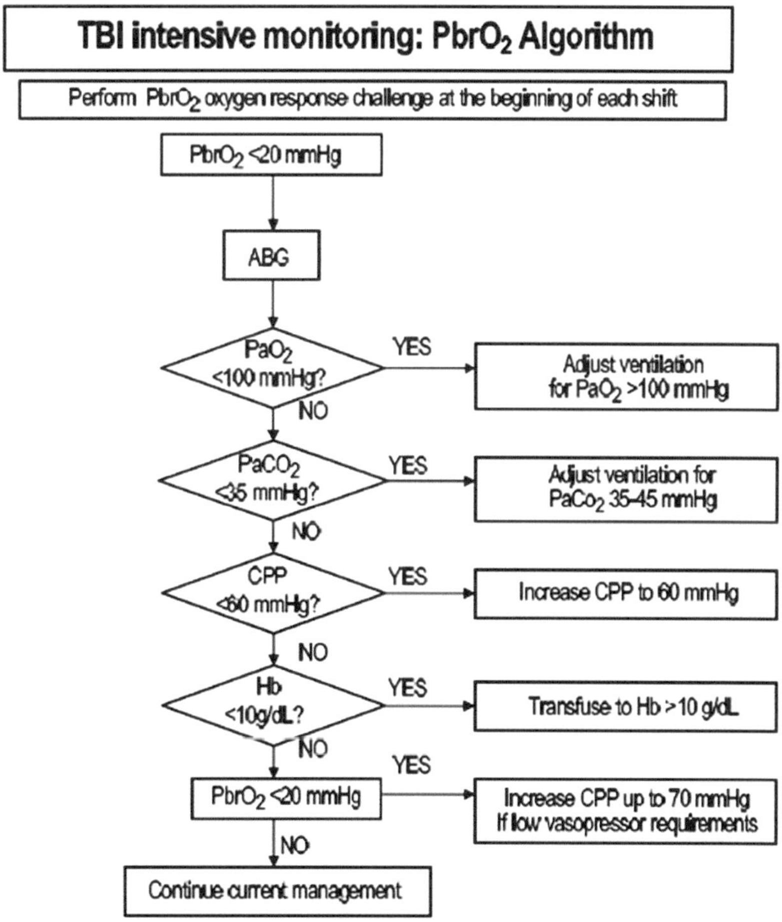

Fig. 12.3 PbtO2 optimization algorithm from Adamides et al. [32]

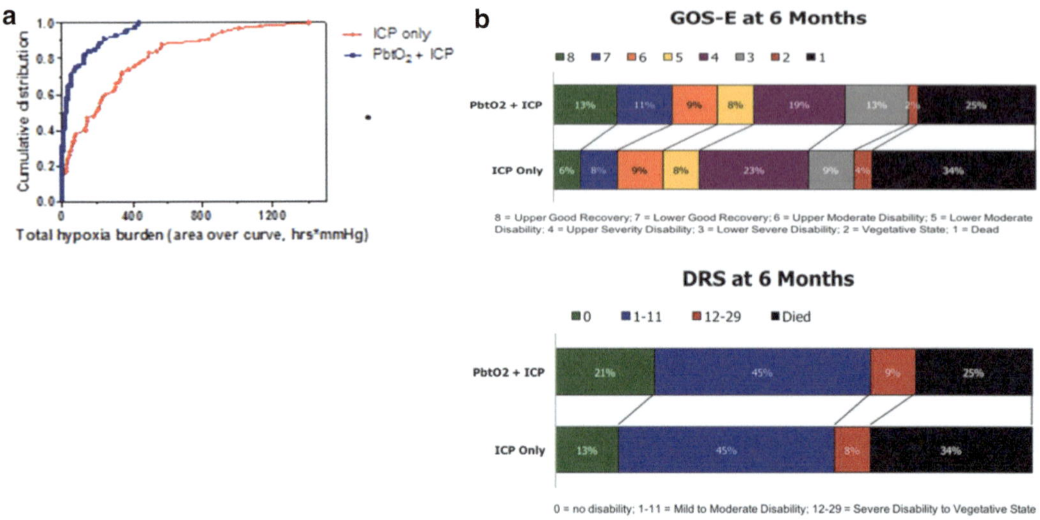

Fig. 12.4 (**a**) Comparison of total hypoxia burden in PbtO2 and ICP group versus ICP only group. (**b**) 6 month Extended Glasgow Outcome score for PbtO2 and ICP group versus ICP only group

12.4.6 Randomized Trials of PbtO2-Based Management in TBI

The Brain Oxygen Optimization in Severe TBI Phase II (BOOST-2) study has recently been completed [42]. This two-arm, single-blind prospective randomized controlled trial was conducted in ten ICUs in the USA. Patients with severe TBI who required ICP monitoring were enrolled and randomized to either ICP or ICP plus $PbtO_2$ monitoring and optimization. The primary hypothesis was that a neurointensive care management strategy informed by $PbtO_2$ as well as ICP values would reduce the total burden of cerebral hypoxia. Secondary hypotheses related to safety, feasibility, and non-futility. The target sample size of the study was 182 participants, and the trial was stopped early by the DSMB for efficacy in the primary outcome after the enrolment of 122 subjects (see Fig. 12.4).

This encouraging result led to the development of three large phase 3 trails of PbtO2 monitoring in TBI (BOOST 3, BONANZA, and OXY TC) and fits into an emerging picture of benefit from PbtO2 management that has also been confirmed in two systematic reviews and meta-analyses of the available literature [43, 44].

12.5 Brain Tissue Oxygen Monitoring in SAH

Sub-arachnoid hemorrhage (SAH) is a devastating disease with a hospitalization rate of 14.5 per 100,000 per year in the USA and an overall case fatality rate of 25–50% [45]. The pathology of SAH differs markedly from TBI, but the two pathologies share two characteristics:

1. The risk of delayed secondary neurological injury from ischemia and hypoperfusion following the initial insult.
2. The reduced availability of neurological examination to guide treatment in the setting of reduced conscious state or sedative infusions.

These two factors have driven investigations into the use of pbtO2 monitoring in SAH.

12.5.1 Mechanisms of Brain Injury in SAH

Eighty percentage of SAH results from the rupture of intra-cranial aneurysms; this initial release of arterial blood at systemic blood pressure results in a sudden increase in intra-cranial pressure which may cause a transient decrease in cerebral perfusion pressure resulting in a transient episode of cerebral ischemia. This initial ictus may also result in intra-parenchymal hemorrhage, brain shift, and cerebral herniation syndromes [46].

Between approximately day 3 and day 21 following aneurysm rupture, patients are at risk of delayed cerebral ischemia (DCI). This complication of SAH occurs in approximately 30% of SAH cases [47]. DCI and the cerebral infarctions that result from DCI are one of the most important indicators of adverse outcomes following SAH [48].

The pathophysiology of DCI is characterized by a complex interplay of factors including, angiographic vasospasm, microvascular constriction, blood–brain barrier disruption, formation of microthrombi, inflammation, and cortical spreading ischemia [46].

12.6 PbtO2 Monitoring in SAH

Patients with mild to moderate severity SAH can be monitored for DCI with serial neurological examination which will reveal focal neurological deficits in affected individuals. With increased SAH severity, the incidence of reduced levels of consciousness increases alongside the need for artificial airway support, mechanical ventilation, and sedation. These factors increase the difficulty of performing neurological examinations and accurately interpreting their results. This has led to the introduction of intra-cranial monitoring that aims to identify DCI in this patient group.

12.6.1 Evidence for PbtO2 Use in SAH

Multiple factors that exacerbate tissue hypoxia and metabolic distress in SAH have been identified. These include anemia [49], hypocapnia [50], reduced PaO2 [51], and compromised cardiovascular function [52]. PbtO2 monitoring has been successfully leveraged to demonstrate the effectiveness of various clinical interventions such as red blood cell transfusion [53, 54], controlled hypercarbia [55], and augmentation of the cardiac index [52] in achieving the goal of increasing brain tissue oxygenation.

This evidence leads inevitably to the question of whether augmentation of PbtO2 leads to improved patient outcomes. Much of the available evidence for the use of PbtO2 monitoring to guide clinical decision-making in SAH comes from small-scale observational studies, and large randomized controlled trials of the technique are notably absent from the literature. Veldeman et al. demonstrated improved outcomes associated with PbtO2-guided SAH management in both poor grade [56] and good grade [57] SAH. Bogossian et al. showed improved outcomes with PbtO2-guided SAH management but importantly, only in comparison with those patients managed with the aim of controlling raised intracranial pressure [58]. The use of a protocolized approach to PbtO2 optimization similar to that seen in TBI has also been demonstrated to be feasible and effective but did not demonstrate a relationship between low PbtO2 readings and poor outcome. The study was not designed to demonstrate differences in outcome as it did not include a control group [59].

In summary, the evidence for the use of PbtO2-guided therapy in SAH is mixed and PbtO2 monitoring in SAH may only be useful in selected patients with the most severe pathologies [56, 60]. One major question regarding the use of PbtO2 in SAH is methodological. Angiographic vasospasm and many of the other factors underpinning ischemia in SAH are localized to discrete arterial territories. This means that DCI may occur in brain regions remote from the local sampling region of the PbtO2 probe and therefore remain undetected. Given the localized nature of many forms of DCI, it is unclear whether a local measure of PbtO2 is sufficient to identify DCI.

12.7 The Future of Brain Oxygen Monitoring in Acute Brain Injury

12.7.1 Indices of Auto-regulation

PbtO2 monitoring is emerging as a valuable adjunct to other neuromonitoring techniques. PbtO2 reflects tissue oxygenation and can be used as a surrogate marker of cerebral blood flow [61]. The ability to detect dynamic changes to tissue perfusion has led to attempts to utilize PbtO2 values to assess cerebral

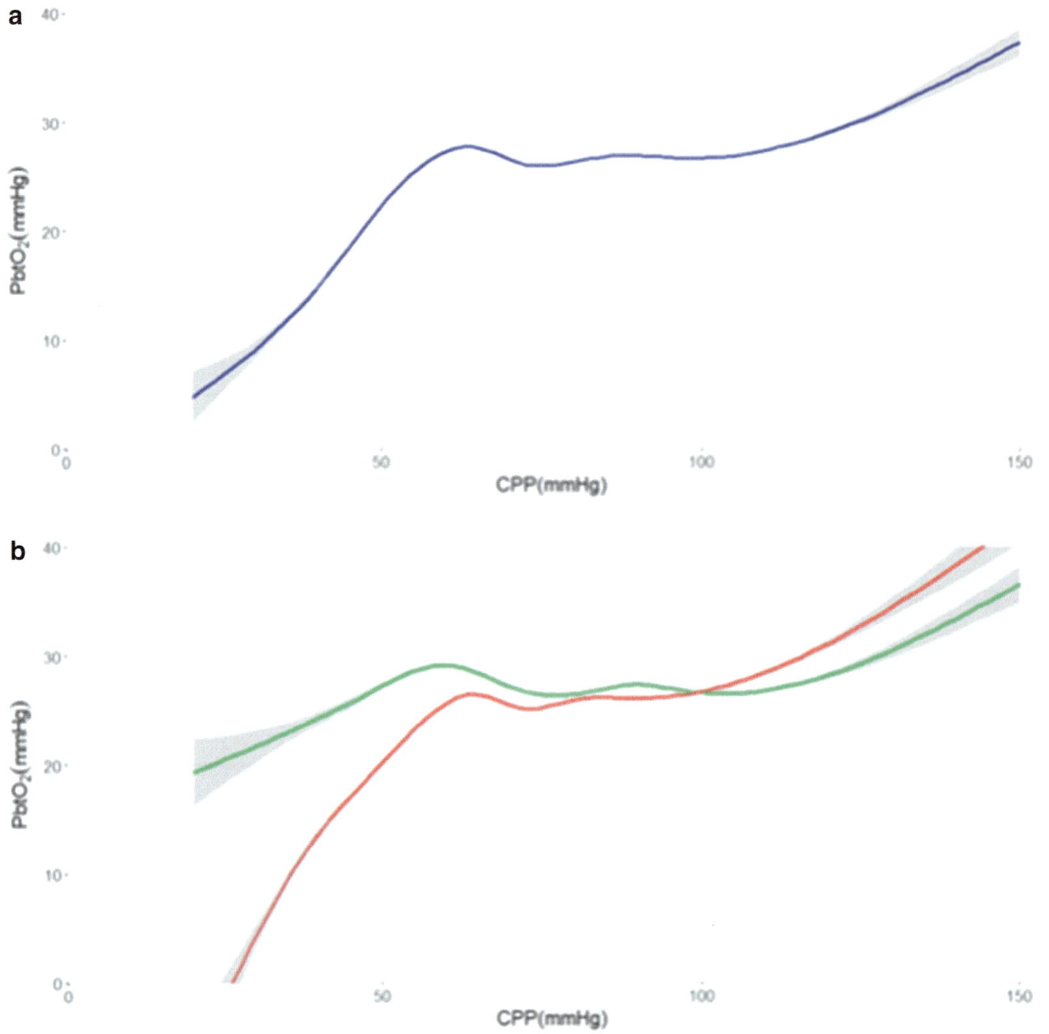

Fig. 12.5 (**a**) The relationship of PbtO2 to cerebral perfusion pressure in a cohort of patients with severe TBI ($n = 77$). (**b**) The relationship of PbtO2 to cerebral perfusion pressure according in the setting of intact (green curve) and disrupted (red curve) cerebral auto-regulation [62]

auto-regulation and the adequacy of cerebral perfusion pressure in acute brain injury. Gomez and colleagues [62] were able to define cerebral autoregulation curves (see Fig. 12.5) with the use of cumulative PbtO2 and CPP values derived from a TBI cohort. They were also able to demonstrate variability of the auto-regulatory plateau depending on autoregulatory function (as assessed by the pressure reactivity index). They were unable, however, to define autoregulatory function with PbtO2 and CPP values from individual patients.

Jaeger et al. have utilized a technique similar to the pressure reactivity index to successfully derive a measure of cerebral auto-regulatory function—the oxygen reactivity index (ORx) in both TBI [63, 64] and SAH [65] cohorts. These findings are important as they offer the possibility of measuring autoregulatory function based on a measure of cerebral blood flow. Unfortunately, these findings have not been replicated by other others, indicating that significant methodological issues remain to be resolved for these techniques [66]. Despite these issues, PbtO2-derived indices have the potential to significantly improve personalization of cerebral perfusion pressure targets in acutely brain injured patients [62].

12.7.2 Use of PbtO2 Monitoring in CSD

Another emerging application of PbtO2 monitoring is in combination with electrophysiological monitoring modalities such as Electrocorticography (ECoG). Of particular note is the ability of PbtO2 readings to identify changes in the cortical microvascular responses to cortical spreading depolarization (CSD). First discovered by Aristides Leao in 1944 [67], CSD waves are mass depolarizations of cortical neurons and glia triggered by noxious stimuli that result in an episodic silencing of the electrical activity in the cortex [68]. These waves are associated with secondary brain injury in multiple acute neurological pathologies including ischemic and hemorrhagic stroke, TBI, and SAH [19].

Spreading depolarization occurs as a result of the near complete breakdown of the ionic gradients across the cell membranes of cortical neurons. Given that approximately 50% of the brains usage of energy results from the maintenance of trans-membrane sodium concentration gradients [68], it follows that the re-establishment of these gradients to enable tissue recovery is an extremely energy intensive process requiring increased tissue blood flow.

Under normal conditions, CSD triggers an increase in tissue blood flow of greater than 100% of baseline—termed spreading hyperemia. However, under certain pathological conditions, this normal hemodynamic response can be inverted resulting in reduced tissue blood flow at the height of tissue stress and demand for metabolites—termed spreading ischemia [69]. This process is thought to contribute significantly to secondary brain injury in both SAH and TBI [70]. PbtO2 readings have been utilized to identify and characterize the hemodynamic responses to CSD and could in theory be used to guide tar geted treatments of spreading ischemia including systemic hypertension [71], hyperoxia [72], or pharmaceutical NMDA receptor blockade, e.g., by Ketamine [73].

12.8 Conclusions

Acute brain injuries such as TBI and SAH are complex multi-faceted pathologies that evolve over time. This evolution may involve extension of tissue damage beyond the areas damaged by the initial insult. Serious injuries managed in the neurocritical care unit will also typically render patients unconscious and clinically un-assessable. This lack of clinical accessibility means that clinicians are reliant on invasive methods to assess tissue health and function and identify secondary insults in order to provide the optimal environment for tissue recovery.

Brain tissue oxygen monitoring is an imperfect tool, it requires invasive placement in brain parenchyma, readings are influenced by multiple systemic and local factors, and to date there is no level 1 evidence supporting its use. Despite these limitations, PbtO2 is emerging as an important method for increasing both our understanding of brain pathologies and our ability to respond effectively to episodes of cerebral hypoxia. Whether this approach significantly improves functional outcomes following acute brain injury remains uncertain, although this question will be greatly informed by ongoing clinical trials nearing completion.

References

1. Hirsch S, Reichold J, Schneider M, Szekely G, Weber B. Topology and hemodynamics of the cortical cerebrovascular system. J Cereb Blood Flow Metab. 2012;32(6):952–67.
2. Krogh A. The number and distribution of capillaries in muscles with calculations of the oxygen pressure head necessary for supplying the tissue. J Physiol. 1919;52(6):409–15.
3. Kasischke KA, Lambert EM, Panepento B, Sun A, Gelbard HA, Burgess RW, et al. Two-photon NADH imaging exposes boundaries of oxygen diffusion in cortical vascular supply regions. J Cereb Blood Flow Metab. 2011;31(1):68–81.
4. Ellsworth ML, Ellis CG, Goldman D, Stephenson AH, Dietrich HH, Sprague RS. Erythrocytes: oxygen sensors and modulators of vascular tone. Physiology (Bethesda). 2009;24:107–16.

5. Jespersen SN, Ostergaard L. The roles of cerebral blood flow, capillary transit time heterogeneity, and oxygen tension in brain oxygenation and metabolism. J Cereb Blood Flow Metab. 2012;32(2):264–77.
6. Pias SC. How does oxygen diffuse from capillaries to tissue mitochondria? Barriers and pathways. J Physiol. 2021;599(6):1769–82.
7. Ostergaard L, Engedal TS, Aamand R, Mikkelsen R, Iversen NK, Anzabi M, et al. Capillary transit time heterogeneity and flow-metabolism coupling after traumatic brain injury. J Cereb Blood Flow Metab. 2014;34(10):1585–98.
8. Lazaridis C. Brain shock-toward pathophysiologic phenotyping in traumatic brain injury. Crit Care Explor. 2022;4(7):e0724.
9. Beynon C, Kiening KL, Orakcioglu B, Unterberg AW, Sakowitz OW. Brain tissue oxygen monitoring and hyperoxic treatment in patients with traumatic brain injury. J Neurotrauma. 2012;29(12):2109–23.
10. Nortje J, Gupta AK. The role of tissue oxygen monitoring in patients with acute brain injury. Br J Anaesth. 2006;97(1):95–106.
11. Johnston AJ, Steiner LA, Coles JP, Chatfield DA, Fryer TD, Smielewski P, et al. Effect of cerebral perfusion pressure augmentation on regional oxygenation and metabolism after head injury. Crit Care Med. 2005;33(1):189–95; discussion 255–7.
12. Kiening KL, Unterberg AW, Bardt TF, Schneider GH, Lanksch WR. Monitoring of cerebral oxygenation in patients with severe head injuries: brain tissue PO2 versus jugular vein oxygen saturation. J Neurosurg. 1996;85(5):751–7.
13. De Georgia MA. Brain tissue oxygen monitoring in Neurocritical care. J Intensive Care Med. 2015;30(8):473–83.
14. Menzel M, Doppenberg EM, Zauner A, Soukup J, Reinert MM, Clausen T, et al. Cerebral oxygenation in patients after severe head injury: monitoring and effects of arterial hyperoxia on cerebral blood flow, metabolism and intracranial pressure. J Neurosurg Anesthesiol. 1999;11(4):240–51.
15. Valadka AB, Hlatky R, Furuya Y, Robertson CS. Brain tissue PO2: correlation with cerebral blood flow. Acta Neurochir Suppl. 2002;81:299–301.
16. Jaeger M, Soehle M, Schuhmann MU, Winkler D, Meixensberger J. Correlation of continuously monitored regional cerebral blood flow and brain tissue oxygen. Acta Neurochir. 2005;147(1):51–6; discussion 6.
17. Rosenthal G, Hemphill JC, Sorani M, Martin C, Morabito D, Meeker M, et al. The role of lung function in brain tissue oxygenation following traumatic brain injury. J Neurosurg. 2008;108(1):59–65.
18. Suh M, Ma H, Zhao M, Sharif S, Schwartz TH. Neurovascular coupling and oximetry during epileptic events. Mol Neurobiol. 2006;33(3):181–97.
19. Winkler MK, Chassidim Y, Lublinsky S, Revankar GS, Major S, Kang EJ, et al. Impaired neurovascular coupling to ictal epileptic activity and spreading depolarization in a patient with subarachnoid hemorrhage: possible link to blood-brain barrier dysfunction. Epilepsia. 2012;53 Suppl 6(06):22–30.
20. Ponce LL, Pillai S, Cruz J, Li X, Julia H, Gopinath S, et al. Position of probe determines prognostic information of brain tissue PO2 in severe traumatic brain injury. Neurosurgery. 2012;70(6):1492–502; discussion 502–3.
21. Longhi L, Pagan F, Valeriani V, Magnoni S, Zanier ER, Conte V, et al. Monitoring brain tissue oxygen tension in brain-injured patients reveals hypoxic episodes in normal-appearing and in peri-focal tissue. Intensive Care Med. 2007;33(12):2136–42.
22. Le Roux P, Menon DK, Citerio G, Vespa P, Bader MK, Brophy G, et al. The International Multidisciplinary Consensus Conference on Multimodality Monitoring in Neurocritical Care: evidentiary tables: a statement for healthcare professionals from the Neurocritical Care Society and the European Society of Intensive Care Medicine. Neurocrit Care. 2014;21(Suppl 2):S297–361.
23. Adams JH, Jennett B, McLellan DR, Murray LS, Graham DI. The neuropathology of the vegetative state after head injury. J Clin Pathol. 1999;52(11):804–6.
24. Adams JH, Jennett B, Murray LS, Teasdale GM, Gennarelli TA, Graham DI. Neuropathological findings in disabled survivors of a head injury. J Neurotrauma. 2011;28(5):701–9.
25. Coles JP, Fryer TD, Smielewski P, Chatfield DA, Steiner LA, Johnston AJ, et al. Incidence and mechanisms of cerebral ischemia in early clinical head injury. J Cereb Blood Flow Metab. 2004;24(2):202–11.
26. Menon DK, Coles JP, Gupta AK, Fryer TD, Smielewski P, Chatfield DA, et al. Diffusion limited oxygen delivery following head injury. Crit Care Med. 2004;32(6):1384–90.
27. Veenith TV, Carter EL, Geeraerts T, Grossac J, Newcombe VF, Outtrim J, et al. Pathophysiologic mechanisms of cerebral ischemia and diffusion hypoxia in traumatic brain injury. JAMA Neurol. 2016;73(5):542–50.
28. Nortje J, Coles JP, Timofeev I, Fryer TD, Aigbirhio FI, Smielewski P, et al. Effect of hyperoxia on regional oxygenation and metabolism after severe traumatic brain injury: preliminary findings. Crit Care Med. 2008;36(1):273–81.
29. Sarrafzadeh AS, Kiening KL, Bardt TF, Schneider GH, Unterberg AW, Lanksch WR. Cerebral oxygenation in contusioned vs. nonlesioned brain tissue: monitoring of PtiO2 with Licox and Paratrend. Acta Neurochir Suppl. 1998;71:186–9.
30. van den Brink WA, van Santbrink H, Steyerberg EW, Avezaat CJ, Suazo JA, Hogesteeger C, et al. Brain oxygen tension in severe head injury. Neurosurgery. 2000;46(4):868–76; discussion 76–8.
31. Gracias VH, Guillamondegui OD, Stiefel MF, Wilensky EM, Bloom S, Gupta R, et al. Cerebral cortical oxygenation: a pilot study. J Trauma. 2004;56(3):469–72; discussion 72–4.
32. Adamides AA, Cooper DJ, Rosenfeldt FL, Bailey MJ, Pratt N, Tippett N, et al. Focal cerebral oxygenation

and neurological outcome with or without brain tissue oxygen-guided therapy in patients with traumatic brain injury. Acta Neurochir. 2009;151(11):1399–409.
33. Bardt TF, Unterberg AW, Hartl R, Kiening KL, Schneider GH, Lanksch WR. Monitoring of brain tissue PO2 in traumatic brain injury: effect of cerebral hypoxia on outcome. Acta Neurochir Suppl. 1998;71:153–6.
34. Valadka AB, Gopinath SP, Contant CF, Uzura M, Robertson CS. Relationship of brain tissue PO2 to outcome after severe head injury. Crit Care Med. 1998;26(9):1576–81.
35. Zauner A, Daugherty WP, Bullock MR, Warner DS. Brain oxygenation and energy metabolism: part I-biological function and pathophysiology. Neurosurgery. 2002;51(2):289–301; discussion 2.
36. Dunham CM, Ransom KJ, Flowers LL, Siegal JD, Kohli CM. Cerebral hypoxia in severely brain-injured patients is associated with admission Glasgow coma scale score, computed tomographic severity, cerebral perfusion pressure, and survival. J Trauma. 2004;56(3):482–9; discussion 9–91.
37. Tolias CM, Reinert M, Seiler R, Gilman C, Scharf A, Bullock MR. Normobaric hyperoxia—induced improvement in cerebral metabolism and reduction in intracranial pressure in patients with severe head injury: a prospective historical cohort-matched study. J Neurosurg. 2004;101(3):435–44.
38. Stiefel MF, Spiotta A, Gracias VH, Garuffe AM, Guillamondegui O, Maloney-Wilensky E, et al. Reduced mortality rate in patients with severe traumatic brain injury treated with brain tissue oxygen monitoring. J Neurosurg. 2005;103(5):805–11.
39. Zygun DA, Nortje J, Hutchinson PJ, Timofeev I, Menon DK, Gupta AK. The effect of red blood cell transfusion on cerebral oxygenation and metabolism after severe traumatic brain injury. Crit Care Med. 2009;37(3):1074–8.
40. Kiening KL, Hartl R, Unterberg AW, Schneider GH, Bardt T, Lanksch WR. Brain tissue pO2-monitoring in comatose patients: implications for therapy. Neurol Res. 1997;19(3):233–40.
41. Bohman LE, Heuer GG, Macyszyn L, Maloney-Wilensky E, Frangos S, Le Roux PD, et al. Medical management of compromised brain oxygen in patients with severe traumatic brain injury. Neurocrit Care. 2011;14(3):361–9.
42. Okonkwo DO, Shutter LA, Moore C, Temkin NR, Puccio AM, Madden CJ, et al. Brain oxygen optimization in severe traumatic brain injury phase-II: a phase II randomized trial. Crit Care Med. 2017;45(11):1907–14.
43. Gouvea Bogossian E, Diosdado A, Barrit S, Al Barajraji M, Annoni F, Schuind S, et al. The impact of invasive brain oxygen pressure guided therapy on the outcome of patients with traumatic brain injury: a systematic review and meta-analysis. Neurocrit Care. 2022;37(3):779–89.
44. Hays LMC, Udy A, Adamides AA, Anstey JR, Bailey M, Bellapart J, et al. Effects of brain tissue oxygen (PbtO(2)) guided management on patient outcomes following severe traumatic brain injury: a systematic review and meta-analysis. J Clin Neurosci. 2022;99:349–58.
45. Lawton MT, Vates GE. Subarachnoid hemorrhage. N Engl J Med. 2017;377(3):257–66.
46. Macdonald RL. Delayed neurological deterioration after subarachnoid haemorrhage. Nat Rev Neurol. 2014;10(1):44–58.
47. Dorsch N. A clinical review of cerebral vasospasm and delayed ischaemia following aneurysm rupture. Acta Neurochir Suppl. 2011;110(Pt 1):5–6.
48. Rosengart AJ, Schultheiss KE, Tolentino J, Macdonald RL. Prognostic factors for outcome in patients with aneurysmal subarachnoid hemorrhage. Stroke. 2007;38(8):2315–21.
49. Kurtz P, Schmidt JM, Claassen J, Carrera E, Fernandez L, Helbok R, et al. Anemia is associated with metabolic distress and brain tissue hypoxia after subarachnoid hemorrhage. Neurocrit Care. 2010;13(1):10–6.
50. Williamson CA, Sheehan KM, Tipirneni R, Roark CD, Pandey AS, Thompson BG, et al. The association between spontaneous hyperventilation, delayed cerebral ischemia, and poor neurological outcome in patients with subarachnoid hemorrhage. Neurocrit Care. 2015;23(3):330–8.
51. Grensemann J, Mader MM, Westphal M, Kluge S, Czorlich P. Hyperoxia is dose-dependently associated with an increase of unfavorable outcomes in ventilated patients with aneurysmal subarachnoid hemorrhage: a retrospective cohort study. Neurocrit Care. 2022;37(2):523–30.
52. Rass V, Bogossian EG, Ianosi BA, Peluso L, Kofler M, Lindner A, et al. The effect of the volemic and cardiac status on brain oxygenation in patients with subarachnoid hemorrhage: a bi-center cohort study. Ann Intensive Care. 2021;11(1):176.
53. Dhar R, Zazulia AR, Derdeyn CP, Diringer MN. RBC transfusion improves cerebral oxygen delivery in subarachnoid hemorrhage. Crit Care Med. 2017;45(4):653–9.
54. Kurtz P, Helbok R, Claassen J, Schmidt JM, Fernandez L, Stuart RM, et al. The effect of packed red blood cell transfusion on cerebral oxygenation and metabolism after subarachnoid hemorrhage. Neurocrit Care. 2016;24(1):118–21.
55. Westermaier T, Stetter C, Kunze E, Willner N, Holzmeier J, Weiland J, et al. Controlled hypercapnia enhances cerebral blood flow and brain tissue oxygenation after aneurysmal subarachnoid hemorrhage: results of a phase 1 study. Neurocrit Care. 2016;25(2):205–14.
56. Veldeman M, Albanna W, Weiss M, Park S, Hoellig A, Clusmann H, et al. Invasive multimodal Neuromonitoring in aneurysmal subarachnoid hemorrhage: a systematic review. Stroke. 2021;52(11):3624–32.
57. Veldeman M, Albanna W, Weiss M, Conzen C, Schmidt TP, Clusmann H, et al. Treatment of delayed cerebral ischemia in good-grade subarachnoid hem-

orrhage: any role for invasive Neuromonitoring? Neurocrit Care. 2021;35(1):172–83.
58. Gouvea Bogossian E, Diaferia D, Ndieugnou Djangang N, Menozzi M, Vincent JL, Talamonti M, et al. Brain tissue oxygenation guided therapy and outcome in non-traumatic subarachnoid hemorrhage. Sci Rep. 2021;11(1):16235.
59. Rass V, Solari D, Ianosi B, Gaasch M, Kofler M, Schiefecker AJ, et al. Protocolized brain oxygen optimization in subarachnoid hemorrhage. Neurocrit Care. 2019;31(2):263–72.
60. Gouvea Bogossian E, Battaglini D, Fratino S, Minini A, Gianni G, Fiore M, et al. The role of brain tissue oxygenation monitoring in the Management of Subarachnoid Hemorrhage: a scoping review. Neurocrit Care. 2023;39:229.
61. Radolovich DK, Czosnyka M, Timofeev I, Lavinio A, Kim DJ, Jaeger M, et al. Transient changes in brain tissue oxygen in response to modifications of cerebral perfusion pressure: an observational study. Anesth Analg. 2010;110(1):165–73.
62. Gomez A, Sekhon M, Griesdale D, Froese L, Yang E, Thelin EP, et al. Cerebrovascular pressure reactivity and brain tissue oxygen monitoring provide complementary information regarding the lower and upper limits of cerebral blood flow control in traumatic brain injury: a CAnadian high resolution-TBI (CAHR-TBI) cohort study. Intensive Care Med Exp. 2022;10(1):54.
63. Jaeger M, Dengl M, Meixensberger J, Schuhmann MU. Effects of cerebrovascular pressure reactivity-guided optimization of cerebral perfusion pressure on brain tissue oxygenation after traumatic brain injury. Crit Care Med. 2010;38(5):1343–7.
64. Jaeger M, Schuhmann MU, Soehle M, Meixensberger J. Continuous assessment of cerebrovascular autoregulation after traumatic brain injury using brain tissue oxygen pressure reactivity. Crit Care Med. 2006;34(6):1783–8.
65. Barth M, Woitzik J, Weiss C, Muench E, Diepers M, Schmiedek P, et al. Correlation of clinical outcome with pressure-, oxygen-, and flow-related indices of cerebrovascular reactivity in patients following aneurysmal SAH. Neurocrit Care. 2010;12(2):234–43.
66. Dengler J, Frenzel C, Vajkoczy P, Horn P, Wolf S. The oxygen reactivity index and its relation to sensor technology in patients with severe brain lesions. Neurocrit Care. 2013;19(1):74–8.
67. Leao AA. Further observations on the spreading depression of activity in the cerebral cortex. J Neurophysiol. 1947;10(6):409–14.
68. Dreier JP. The role of spreading depression, spreading depolarization and spreading ischemia in neurological disease. Nat Med. 2011;17(4):439–47.
69. Dreier JP, Major S, Manning A, Woitzik J, Drenckhahn C, Steinbrink J, et al. Cortical spreading ischaemia is a novel process involved in ischaemic damage in patients with aneurysmal subarachnoid haemorrhage. Brain. 2009;132(Pt 7):1866–81.
70. Ayata C, Lauritzen M. Spreading depression, spreading depolarizations, and the cerebral vasculature. Physiol Rev. 2015;95(3):953–93.
71. Dreier JP, Victorov IV, Petzold GC, Major S, Windmuller O, Fernandez-Klett F, et al. Electrochemical failure of the brain cortex is more deleterious when it is accompanied by low perfusion. Stroke. 2013;44(2):490–6.
72. Sonn J, Mayevsky A. Responses to cortical spreading depression under oxygen deficiency. Open Neurol J. 2012;6:6–17.
73. Hertle DN, Dreier JP, Woitzik J, Hartings JA, Bullock R, Okonkwo DO, et al. Effect of analgesics and sedatives on the occurrence of spreading depolarizations accompanying acute brain injury. Brain. 2012;135(Pt 8):2390–8.

13 Brain Microdialysis

Mayank Tyagi, Charu Mahajan, Indu Kapoor, and Hemanshu Prabhakar

13.1 Introduction

Cerebral microdialysis (CMD) is a minimally invasive means of providing bedside continuous monitoring of cerebral extracellular fluid, which can potentially detect secondary injuries occurring at the subcellular and molecular levels. During the early period, these changes can otherwise go undetected by the neurological exam and conventional hemodynamic monitoring [1]. CMD is a promising clinical research tool that has contributed significantly to identify and better understand post-injury brain metabolic distress mechanisms. These can be posttraumatic glycolysis, energy dysfunction, post-aneurysmal early brain injury, cerebral edema, neuroinflammation, cortical spreading depression, and subclinical seizures, before the systemic manifestations of an intracranial catastrophe appear [2, 3]. CMD metabolites (namely lactate/pyruvate ratio, glucose, and glycerol) can be used to monitor the brain response to specific interventions, assess the extent of injury, identify potential novel biomarkers of injury and prognosis, and help to refine novel therapeutic approaches and drug effects on downstream targets [2]. Over the last decade, CMD, in combination with multimodal monitoring [intracranial pressure (ICP) and brain tissue oxygenation ($PbtO_2$)], has been used for the management of "secondary systemic and cerebral insults" in brain-injured patients. These include patients with severe traumatic brain injury (sTBI), aneurysmal subarachnoid hemorrhage (aSAH), intracerebral hemorrhage (ICH), intracranial tumors, acute ischemic stroke, epilepsy, and other neurological diseases [4–7]. Consensus statement on microdialysis monitoring in neurocritical care helps guide individualized intensive care therapy of comatose brain-injured patients [8]. This review focuses on specific technical aspects related to CMD monitoring in neurocritical care patients, aiming to discuss the role of CMD to optimize intensive care and improve our understanding of the complex disease mechanisms occurring after severe brain injury.

13.2 The Principle of Microdialysis

The MD catheter consists of a shaft, semipermeable end, and double-lumen tube (with an inlet and outlet tubing) that allows the fluid to pass through it (Fig. 13.1). The semipermeable membrane at its tip allows the exchange of substances, which is the key to providing information about

M. Tyagi
Department of Neuroanaesthesiology, Fortis, Noida, India

C. Mahajan (✉) · I. Kapoor · H. Prabhakar
Department of Neuroanaesthesiology and Critical Care, AIIMS, New Delhi, India

H. Prabhakar et al. (eds.), *Principles and Practice of Neurocritical Care*,
https://doi.org/10.1007/978-981-99-8059-8_13

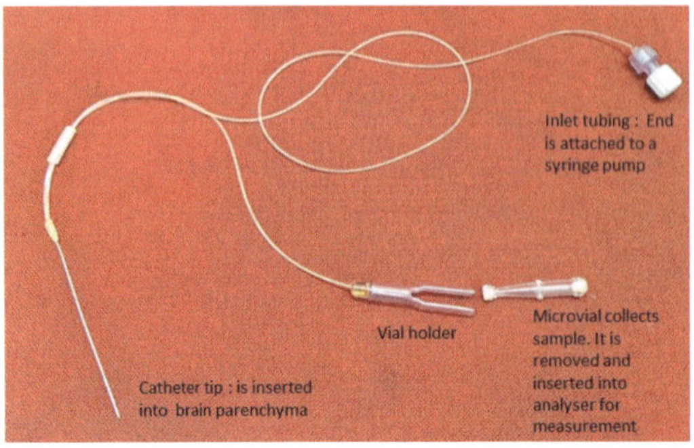

Fig. 13.1 A standard cerebral microdialysis catheter

the extracellular environment in the brain. This membrane performs sampling dialysis of the surrounding interstitial fluid yielding neurochemical information about the extracellular tissue surrounding the catheter [6, 9]. The catheter (except the distal end) is made of polyurethane and has a maximum outer diameter of 0.9–1 mm. The distal end of the catheter has a 1–3 cm long semipermeable membrane having a diameter of 0.6 mm. Through the inlet tubing, a solution is perfused continuously with a physiological solution at ultra-low flow rates (0.1–2.0 μL/min) using a perfusion pump [7]. The artificial CSF is isotonic, similar in composition and pH to brain interstitial fluid. Artificial CSF lacks proteins and neurotransmitters, which enable these substances to be retrieved from brain tissue via microdialysate (fluid collected after exchange of substances). However, an adequate amount of cations (Na+, K+, Ca2+, and Mg2+) are present in artificial CSF, preventing their depletion from the surrounding tissue [6]. The semipermeable membrane permits the exchange of substances with molecular weight <20 kDa. Newer types of MD catheters (CMA 71) enable the collection of larger molecules having a molecular weight of up to 100 kDa [10]. The perfusate flow rate varies from 0.1 to 3.0 μL/min. The perfusate reaches the distal end of the probe, which is placed in the brain tissue (Fig. 13.2), where molecules below the cut-off size of the semipermeable membrane (20 kDa) diffuse along the concentration gradient from the extracellular space into the catheter. This collected fluid, known as "microdialysate," moves along the outlet tubing and gets collected in chambers called "microvial" (Fig. 13.1). These microvials are then placed on the bedside monitor and analyzed for point-of-care parameters (Fig. 13.3) [11]. These microvials are changed every 60 min, allowing up to 70% equilibration across the semipermeable membrane [12].

Intracranial catheter insertion may cause small hemorrhages locally around the tip, causing macrophage infiltration and mild astrogliosis [13]. Catheters should be placed in the penumbra region to help determine the metabolic state of the "at-risk area" in SAH patients (most likely the parent vessel territory affected by vasospasm) and in the right frontal region (non-dominant hemisphere) in patients with diffuse axonal injury after TBI. In patients with focal mass lesions, one catheter should be placed in the penumbra (peri-contusional tissue), and a second may be placed in uninjured or "normal" tissue for comparison [8]. The area of brain tissue covered by the catheter is only 1.5 cm^2 which necessitates proper placement. Hence, timely optimization of cerebral perfusion pressure, oxygenation, and glucose may help in salvaging the penumbra region. The catheter can be inserted into the cerebral tissue either via craniotomy (during open surgery), twist drill hole, or via cranial access device (bolt) (Fig. 13.4). Catheter position can be verified using computed tomography (located by its radiopaque gold tip) or magnetic resonance imaging (Fig. 13.5).

The measurable key substances can be categorized as [14]:

1. *Energy-related metabolites:* e.g., glucose, lactate, pyruvate, lactate/pyruvate ratio, adenosine, and xanthine.
2. *Neurotransmitters:* e.g., glutamate, aspartate, and γ-aminobutyric acid (GABA).
3. *Markers of tissue damage and neuroinflammation*: e.g., glycerol, potassium, and cytokines (IL-6).
4. *Exogenous substances*: e.g., administered drugs. Table 13.1 summarizes the key cerebral microdialysis analytes, their normal ranges, and potential causes of derangements (obtained with a 10-mM semipermeable membrane with a perfusion rate of 0.3 μL/min) [1, 11].

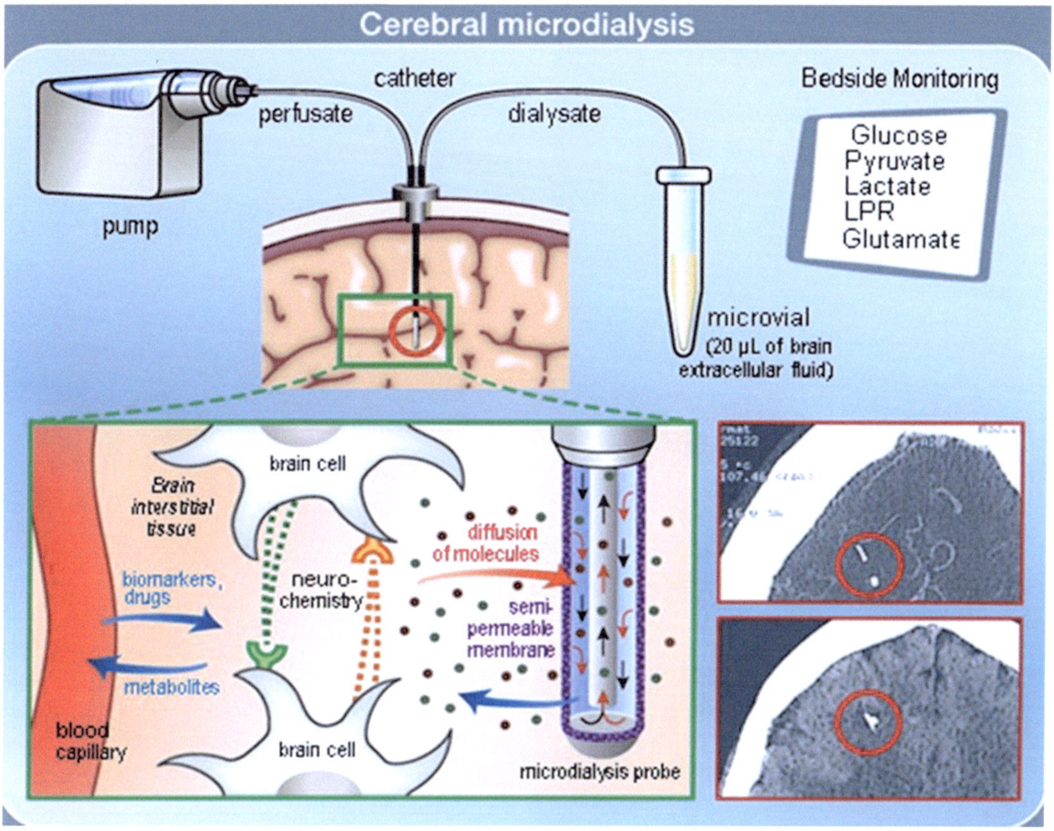

Fig. 13.2 Process of cerebral microdialysis: The syringe pump delivers perfusion fluid through the outer tube down to the tip (red circle), where the dialysis membrane allows bidirectional diffusion (driven by the concentration-dependent diffusion system) between the perfusate and the extracellular fluid of the brain parenchyma (subcortical white matter). The lower right side image shows head CT scan with microdialysis catheter in-situ

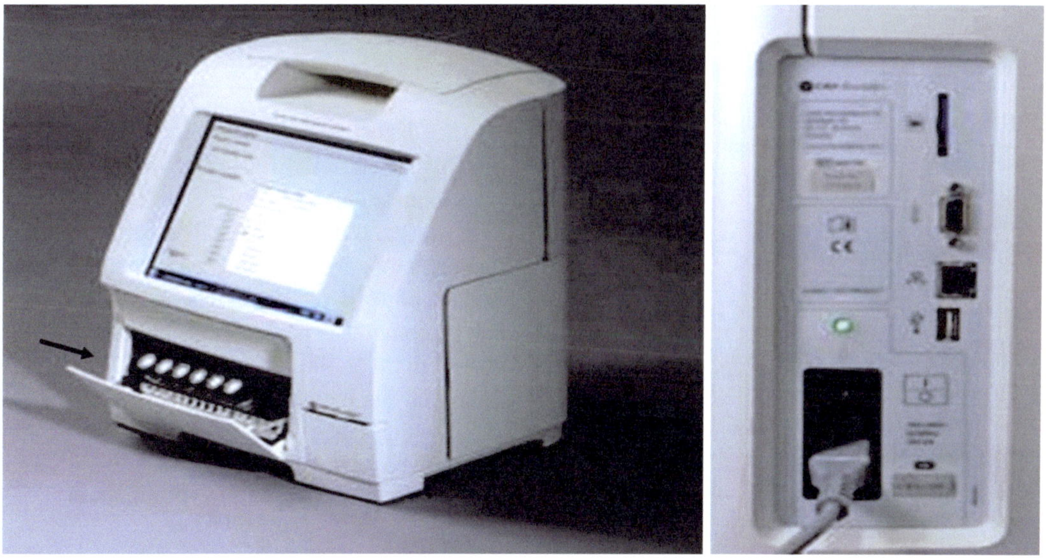

Fig. 13.3 Cerebral microdialysis analyzer. Black arrow shows site of insertion of microvials for analysis

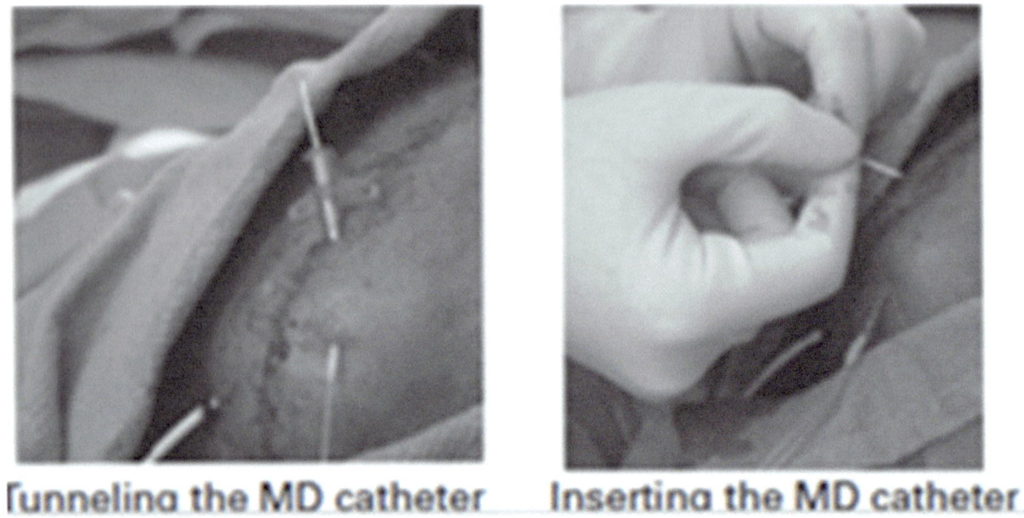

Fig. 13.4 Showing microdialysis catheter insertion and tunnelling technique

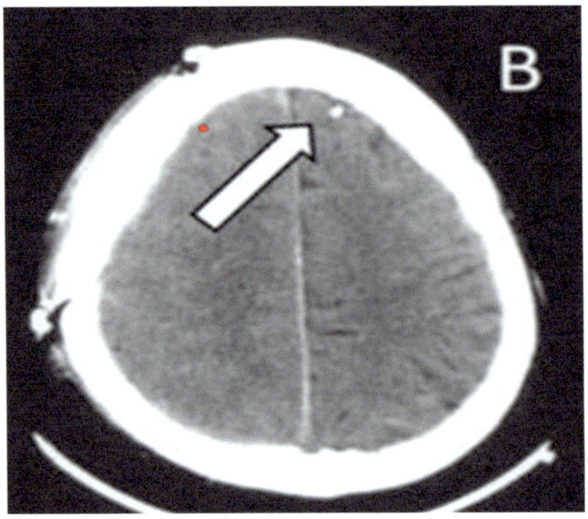

Fig. 13.5 Axial computed tomography showing an arrow pointing at the gold tip of the catheter

13.3 Factors Affecting Solute Recovery

Extraction fraction is the ratio between the analyte concentrations in the microdialysate and the ECF [15]. Several mechanical and tissue-related factors impact extraction fraction or solute recovery. The extraction fraction increases with the flow of the analyte across the CMD membrane. The flow, in turn, depends on several components of the CMD setup, as expressed by the following equation:

$$I = A \times P \times (\Delta c / \Delta z)$$

where I is the flow of the analyte (mol/s)

A is the area of diffusion
P denotes the membrane permeability (cm^2/s)
Δc is the concentration gradient across the membrane, and
Δz is the distance across which diffusion occurs (i.e., membrane thickness).

The diffusion area depends on the probe's dimensions; faster diffusion rates are observed with longer lengths and wider lumens catheters than shorter, thinner probes. The permeability of the membrane is determined by membrane material and porosity. Commercially available clinical CMD membranes have a molecular weight filter cut-off of 20 or 100 kDa. FDA-approved 20-kDa microdialysis membrane is the most commonly used, which can collect glucose, pyruvate, lactate, glycerol, glutamate, and other small hydrophilic molecules. The 100-kDa membranes are

Table 13.1 Summary of cerebral microdialysis analytes, their normal ranges, and potential causes of derangements (obtained with a 10-mM semipermeable membrane with a perfusion rate of 0.3 μL/min)

CMD analytes	Normal range	Possible causes of decreased analyte level	Possible causes of increased analyte level
Lactate	2.9 + 0.9 mmol/L	Not clinically applicable	Poor outcome, Acute FND, DCI Global cerebral edema Cerebral hypermetabolism Mitochondrial dysfunction
Pyruvate	166 + 47 μmol/L	DCI Cerebral hypoglycemia	Cerebral hypermetabolism Mitochondrial dysfunction
Lactate pyruvate ratio	23 + 4	Not clinically applicable	Acute FND Poor outcome 12–16 h before DCI Systemic hypoglycemia Mitochondrial dysfunction
Glucose	1.7 + 0.9 mmol/L	Acute FND Poor outcome 12–16 h before DCI Systemic hypoglycemia	Hyperemia Systemic hyperglycemia Cerebral hypometabolism
Glutamate	16 + 16 mmol/L	Not clinically applicable	DCI Excitotoxicity Poor outcome
Glycerol	82 + 44 μmol/L	Not clinically applicable	DCI Poor outcome Cerebral hypoglycemia Mitochondrial dysfunction Mainly on days 1–2 after SAH

DCI delayed cerebral ischemia; *FND* focal neurological deficits; *SAH* subarachnoid hemorrhage

not yet FDA-approved but have the advantage of recovering larger molecules such as inflammatory cytokines [1]. Relative recovery of large molecules can be significantly improved by using colloid in the perfusate (e.g., albumin or dextran) [16, 17]. Dextrans with molecular weight 40–250 kDa may leak through the catheter, potentially disturbing the interstitial microenvironment and resulting in regional swelling; this can be avoided with high molecular weight dextrans. Also, colloid perfusate having higher oncotic pressure can cause a higher fluid influx into the catheter, potentially dehydrating the extracellular space [8, 16, 18]. This can be resolved using human serum albumin (an alternative colloid to dextran), which has been shown to recover larger cytokines without significantly dehydrating the extracellular environment [17]. The third driving force for solute flow is the concentration gradient across the dialysate and the ECF, which can be changed by varying the solute concentration in the perfusate.

13.3.1 Flow Rate of Perfusate

The flow rate of the perfusate also impacts the recovery of molecules. The extraction fraction is inversely related to the perfusate flow rate. The lower the perfusate flow rate, the more time is available for the substance to move across the semipermeable membrane to increase the extraction fraction [19]. For most clinical applications, the flow rate of 0.3 μL/min is recommended to achieve detectable concentrations of analytes in microdialysate (about 70% for the most commonly assessed molecules) [20]. Almost 100% recovery may be achieved through a 3 cm long semipermeable membrane with a 0.1 μL/min perfusion speed. For intraoperative CMD, a higher flow rate of 1–2 μL/min is usually employed to quicken the recovery of microdialysate and shorten the event detection time. It is recommended not to analyze the first 6 h of microdialysate since it is confounded by the micro-trauma induced during the catheter insertion and the initial perfusate flushing [21].

13.3.2 Characteristics of Semipermeable Membrane

The materials commonly used for the semipermeable membrane are regenerated cellulose, polyacrylonitrile, polycarbonate ether, or polyarylethersulfone. The higher the surface area of the semipermeable membrane, more is the recovery rate. The length of the membrane is usually 10 mm, but theoretically, by using a longer membrane of 30 mm, 100% recovery may be achieved. Besides probe shape and length, membrane porosity, and perfusate flow rate, properties of the brain tissue and analytes also influence the recovery of substances.

13.3.3 Characteristics of Analyte

The molecular weight of the analyte and hydrophilicity also impact diffusion. The diffusion of substances increases proportionally with lower molecular weight substances, and hence a higher recovery rate is obtained [22].

13.3.4 Temperature

The temperature of the environment affects the diffusion coefficient. A 1–2% increase in the diffusion coefficient is seen for every 1 °C increase in temperature and so is the velocity of molecular movement and diffusion of the solutes.

13.3.5 Tissue Factors

Generally, an aqueous medium offers less resistance to diffusion than solid tissues [1, 22]. Diffusion in tissues may be slowed by increased diffusion path and binding of the analyte to cell proteins. This may be responsible for the difference between in vitro and in vivo recovery rates. The hydrophilicity and weight of the analyte impact diffusion; where lower weight and hydrophilic molecules are recovered in higher quantities.

13.4 Clinical Applications of Microdialysis in Brain Injury

13.4.1 Aneurysmal Subarachnoid Hemorrhage

While CMD is not currently an essential component of standard post-SAH care, it can still provide useful information regarding bioenergetic metabolism inside the post-SAH brain. The average metabolite concentrations and treatment recommendations based on CMD monitoring for various acute brain injuries, including SAH, have been given by the international microdialysis forum [8, 23]. Table 13.2 summarizes the main advances of CMD since the 2004 consensus statement. Hutchinson et al. stated that CMD could be used as a primary monitoring device in patients with poor-grade SAH, allowing clinicians to detect secondary neurological deterioration [8].

Delayed cerebral ischemia (DCI) occurs in approximately 30% of patients with SAH, commonly occurring between days 3 and 14 after the aneurysm rupture [24]. The deficits of DCI are reversible but can lead to brain infarctions and significant morbidity and mortality when left untreated [25]. Besides vasospasm, several factors have been proposed to contribute to the development of DCI, such as microthrombi formation, inflammatory responses, and cortical spreading depolarization (CSD) [26]. Early brain injury (EBI) applies to neuronal damage incurred within 72 h from the initial hemorrhage; its manifestations include ICP surge, activation of inflammatory cascades, triggering of death receptor pathways, blood–brain barrier breakdown leading to early global cerebral edema and early vasospasm [27, 28]. EBI is now believed to be an important cause

Table 13.2 Summary of advances since the consensus 2004 [21]

	2004 consensus statement [21]	2014 consensus statement [8]
Microdialysis methodology	Monitoring small molecules using a 10-mm 20-kDa catheter Focus on microdialysis metabolites as a marker of ischemia and cell damage	Advances in monitoring large molecules, with experience in using 100-kDa membrane and colloid for perfusate [16, 84, 85]. Novel applications of microdialysis for monitoring and understanding brain pathology following SAH and TBI
Reference values	Not defined	Pathological thresholds defined for glucose, lactate, and the LPR [64, 86, 87]
Tiered approach to microdialysis metabolites for clinical application	Not defined	Glucose and LP ratio more clinically useful than glutamate and glycerol in TBI and SAH patients
Guidance for microdialysis-directed management	Not given	Suggested therapeutic interventions for when glucose is low (<0.2 mM) and for when the LP ratio indicates ischemia ± tissue hypoxia
Monitoring in SAH	Guidance on catheter placement in the tissue at risk	Two principal indications for microdialysis monitoring are defined: 1. As a primary monitoring device in mechanically ventilated patients 2. As a monitor of patients with a secondary neurological deterioration
Monitoring in TBI	Guidance on catheter placement in focal or diffuse injury	Guidance on single or multiple catheter placement based on whether the injury is focal or diffuse and based on the aims of microdialysis monitoring

TBI traumatic brain injury; *SAH* subarachnoid hemorrhage

of mortality and disability in patients with aSAH [1].

Based on published data, several biochemical patterns of ischemia have also been identified to predict DCI. Sharp cerebral glucose reduction and elevated ECF lactate correlate poorly with DCI and functional outcome; compared to ECF lactate, LPR is a much more sensitive marker for impending tissue ischemia [29, 30]. A rise in LPR, followed by an increase in glutamate level, is observed when the CMD probe is placed in close proximity to impending infarction. The rise in glutamate is almost always seen when LPR >25 [30]. Increase in LPR and lactate to glycerol ratio (L/G) greater than 20% and a subsequent 20% increase in glycerol within one day are observed when the CMD probe is located near the parent vessel of the ruptured aneurysm, with 94% sensitivity and 88% specificity for predicting DCI [29]. During the late phase of aSAH, metabolic profiling using CMD has shown a similar pattern as the early phase after SAH [11]. Interestingly, in addition to the reduction in glucose and elevation of lactate, glutamate, and glycerol, an aggravation of energy crisis is reflected by a further increase in LPR, which can be detected during this delayed phase after SAH and may be partially due to the decreased level of pyruvate, suggesting the occurrence of delayed cerebral ischemia [11, 23, 31]. Sarrafzadeh et al. conducted a prospective, controlled study in 97 SAH patients, suggesting CMD to be a safe technique for monitoring regional cerebral ischemia. They found that the changes in metabolites (low cerebral glucose level with significant elevations in LPR, lactate, glutamate, and glycerol) indicative of cerebral ischemia preceded the onset of symptomatic vasospasm in 83% of the patients having delayed ischemic neurologic deficit [32]. Later, the author found similar result in another prospective study in 44 SAH patients, with extreme pathological CMD concentrations indicative of irreversible tissue damage, development of cerebral infarction and permanent neurological deficits [33].

Another aspect of post-SAH pathophysiology is the proinflammatory cytokines that play a central role in neuroinflammation after brain injury. Using CMD in 14 comatose patients, Hanafy et al. established the relationship between the increased extracellular TNF-α levels, higher brain interstitial fluid glucose levels, incidence of larger aneurysm size >6 mm, and intraventricular hemorrhage after SAH [34]. The TNF-α level (aSAH days 4–6) in extracellular space also correlates with the severity of radiographic vasospasm after aSAH [35]. Interleukin (IL)-6 is another predominant proinflammatory cytokine in the context of SAH. An increased level of IL-6 in extracellular fluid reflects a pronounced proinflammatory trigger response after SAH. Interestingly, the elevation of IL-6 is also accompanied by a higher LPR ratio and indicates the subsequent occurrence of DCI in symptomatic patients [36]. Graetz et al. studied 24 aSAH patients and noted the presence of strong activation of proinflammatory trigger (elevated IL-6 and C-reactive protein) in patients with intracranial hypertension (ICP ˃20 mmHg) [37]. In addition, a higher level of CMD matrix metalloproteinase-9 in extracellular space is observed in poor-grade SAH and vasospasm, and in patients with sTBI [20, 38–40]. Preliminary data by Helbok and authors also established a potential link between high CMD p-tau181 level and poor functional outcome (modified Rankin Scale ≥4), cognitive impairment, brain metabolic distress, and delayed cerebral infarction in 22 consecutive aSAH patients using multimodal neuromonitoring [41].

CMD biomarkers can facilitate risk prediction and optimization of management, which is essential for the future of precision medicine in SAH. Biomarkers may enable a proactive approach and preventive actions, which is extremely important in neurocritical care, as secondary brain injuries may lead to severe disability or death. To date, no molecular biomarker has been validated in SAH patients due to the high variability of individual values from different anatomical compartments of biospecimen origin, irregular schedules for biospecimen acquisition, and lack of standardization in biospecimen storage and processing. These factors pose significant barriers to biomarker validation and translation into clinical practice. In addition to the article proposing the standard CMD reporting recommendations [42], a more comprehensive meta-analysis might be required for further standardizing the reporting of CMD results from both clinical and experimental studies to synergize the large body of research efforts into larger datasets to facilitate biomarker validation and translation. Indeed, more research is essential to allow us to build a more robust consensus for the use of CMD in management of patients with SAH or other types of brain injury, rather than limiting it only for research purpose. Two recent scoping systematic reviews have addressed the potential value of microdialysis cytokines in sTBI and poor-grade SAH. Although preliminary studies support the feasibility of measurements and associations of CMD cytokines and neurophysiologic outcomes, evidence is limited and further larger prospective multicenter studies need to be conducted [43, 44].

13.4.2 Traumatic Brain Injury

Secondary injuries following sTBI include activation of proinflammatory cascades, generation of free radical species and excitatory amino acids leading to a regional reduction in brain oxidative metabolism, altered glucose metabolism, worsening neurochemistry, and widespread metabolic perturbations [45, 46]. During this acute period, secondary events such as seizures or elevated ICP can place additional energy demand, compromising the metabolic reserve of the tissue [47]. Here, we will focus on key biochemical processes that impact outcomes after TBI and are attractive targets for directed therapies. Placement of a CMD catheter in a recoverable area helps understand the pathophysiology of injury and guides the therapeutic interventions. Incorporating multimodal monitoring such as brain tissue oxygenation, jugular venous oximetry, and CPP in intensive care unit along with CMD can be helpful in optimizing therapy for salvaging the vulnerable

Table 13.3 Summary of clinical cerebral microdialysis studies [2]

Studies	Summary of main results	Clinical utility	Reference
Observational studies			
Glycemic control	Moderate (6.1–8 mM) vs tight (4–6 mM) glycemic control is associated with more episodes of low CMD glucose. (Kurtz et al. [52] analyzed 46 comatose patients with brain injury; randomized controlled study by Vespa et al. [88] in 13 TBI patients; Helbok et al. [89] analyzed 28 poor-grade SAH patients, respectively)	Guiding insulin management	[52, 88, 89]
Cerebral perfusion	Cerebral hypoperfusion is associated with increased brain metabolic distress (low CMD glucose/high LPR), as analyzed by Ronquest et al. in 3 patients with inoperable malignant glioma	Early cerebral ischemia detection	[90]
Hemoglobin level	Hb < 9 g/dL is associated with increased brain metabolic distress (analyzed by Kurtz et al. in 34 SAH patients)	Management of red blood cell transfusion	[91]
Interventional studies			
Succinate	Intracerebral succinate is associated with reduced brain metabolic distress (studied by Jalloh et al. in 9 sTBI patients using 2,3-13C2 succinate)	Potential for cerebral microdialysis biomarkers to be used as surrogate endpoints in clinical trials (phase II)	[69]
Mechanistic studies			
CSD	CSD is associated with low CMD glucose (analyzed by Roger et al. in 6 brain injured patients)	Monitoring and testing the efficacy of new therapeutic interventions targeted at reducing seizure episodes and CSD	[92, 93]
Seizures	Electrographic seizures are associated with increased brain metabolic distress (analyzed by Vespa et al. in 34 TBI patients)		[94]
Neuroinflammation	Identification of inflammatory cytokines (IL-6, IL-8, and TNF-α) following acute brain injury (two systematic scoping reviews conducted by Zeiler et al. in TBI and SAH patients)	Establishment of new therapeutic intervention targeted at attenuating the proinflammatory cascade	[43, 44]
Neurodegeneration	Relationship of tau proteins with MRI axonal degeneration and patient outcome (studied by Magnoni et al. in 19 severe closed-head TBI patients)	Selecting patient for interventional studies targeted at decreasing neurodegeneration	[95]

CMD cerebral microdialysis; *CPP* cerebral perfusion pressure; *CSD* cortical spreading depression; *FiO2* fraction of inspired oxygen; *Hb* hemoglobin; *IL* interleukin; *L/P* lactate/pyruvate ratio; *MRI* magnetic resonance imaging; *TBI* traumatic brain injury; *TNF* tumor necrosis factor; *SAH* subarachnoid hemorrhage

tissue. Table 13.3 summarizes the main results of clinical CMD studies and their clinical utility and potential implications.

The brain, under normal conditions, derives most of its energy from the oxidative metabolism of glucose. However, within 24 h after the initial insult, a transient period of increased cerebral glucose uptake is seen due to two potential mechanisms: hyperglycolysis (to meet the high energy demands of restoring ionic balance and cell membrane potential in the injured neurons) and the pentose phosphate pathway (PPP) (to mitigate oxidative stress) [1]. This hypermetabolism phenomenon usually follows a prolonged period of global glucose metabolic depression, which may last 2–4 weeks [48–51]. Some evidence suggests that severe glucose hypometabolism is associated with low levels of consciousness and poor functional outcome [50, 51]. Glucose hypometabolism could be related to reduced cerebral extracellular glucose, another abnormal metabolic phenomenon seen after TBI and a marker for poor outcomes [52]. Vespa et al. studied 2708 CMD samples from 30 moderate and sTBI patients and analyzed them for glucose, lactate, pyruvate, LPR, and lactate/glucose ratio. Very low extracellular glucose levels (less than 0.2 mmol/L, frequently ranging 18–30% daily for up to 7 days post-injury) and increased lactate/glucose ratio, despite lack of increased lactate, are associated with poor 6-month outcomes [53]. Similarly, in another study, authors assessed 1260 CMD samples from 12 TBI patients demonstrating high extracellular lactate and low glucose. They suggested these as good biomarkers for monitoring brain tissue metabolism and integrity indicative of severe neurological damage and poor outcome [54]. Vespa et al. found that tight intensive insulin therapy was associated with increased incidence of elevated glutamate, lactate/pyruvate ratio, and global oxygen extraction fraction, causing more episodes of low cerebral extracellular glucose level in TBI patients than liberal glycemic control. Taken together, aggressive glucose control should be avoided in TBI patients to prevent depleting cerebral glucose availability and exacerbating metabolic stress [55]. Lactate concentration in CMD should always be interpreted, considering the LPR to distinguish between anaerobic metabolism and hyper-metabolism [56, 57]. Bullock et al. analyzed CMD samples from 80 sTBI patients and found the outcome worse in patients with high dialysate excitatory amino acid levels (approximately 10–20 times higher in contused cortex in comparison with the non-contused cortex). Sustained high ICP and poor outcomes were significantly correlated with glutamate levels of more than 20 μmol/L. [58]

High extracellular glutamate level is often seen in TBI, leading to the hypothesis that glutamate-mediated excitotoxicity is a major contributor to neuronal damage following traumatic injury [59, 60]. Whether extracellular glutamate concentrations in TBI correlate with prognosis and functional outcome is debatable [61]. Chamoun et al. prospectively evaluated CMD glutamate levels (over 120 h) from 165 sTBI patients with GCS ≤ 8 and found that patients with a glutamate level > 20 μmol/L had a mortality rate of 30.3%, whereas glutamate <20 μmol/L was associated with a mortality rate of 18% [61]. Hejčl et al. studied 20 patients with an sTBI utilizing intracranial pressure (ICP), cerebral perfusion pressure (CPP), brain tissue oxygenation, and CMD monitoring and documented a significant association between high ICP/low CPP, increased LPR, and increased mortality/poor GOS at 3–6 months [62]. They also demonstrated a significant association between raised LPR and low $PbtO_2$ [62]. Timofeev et al. prospectively analyzed 97 TBI patients and observed that the relationship between neurochemistry parameters and CPP depends on the state of cerebrovascular reactivity (pressure reactivity index). In patients with impaired autoregulation, a decrease in cerebral perfusion and oxygenation was associated with deranged neurochemistry variables [63]. Extracellular metabolic markers measured by CMD were independently associated with the neurologic outcome following TBI [64]. Specific interventions in neuroglycopenic TBI patients, such as glucose administration, can prevent secondary insults in at-risk brain tissue [65]. Direct succinate supplementation via CMD improved brain chemistry/energy metabolism and better redox status in TBI patients by decreasing LPR and improving glucose utilisation [66–69].

13.4.3 Acute Ischemic Stroke

Patients with acute ischemic stroke require careful monitoring to detect any deterioration due to the development of edema of the infarcted tissue. Berger et al., in one of the earliest reports, demonstrated the use of CMD in a patient with a large hemispheric stroke, revealing neurochemical alterations to precede clinical signs of intracranial catastrophe [70]. In a prospective observational study of 24 patients with large MCA infarction (˃2/3 of MCA territory), authors found that average concentrations of glutamate, glycerol, and LPR were lower in the patients receiving hypothermia (33°C) or undergoing hemicraniectomy than in those managed conservatively [71]. Same authors also demonstrate that moderate hypothermia (33 °C) applied as rescue therapy in 12 large hemispheric strokes (>2/3 of MCA territory) patients decreases glutamate and other extracellular metabolic substances (glycerol, lactate, and pyruvate) in the "tissue at risk" area of the infarct but not within the infarct core [72].

13.4.4 Brain Tumor

CMD helps study the neurochemical analysis of brain tumors and associated changes in response to treatment. The concentration of extracellular neurotransmitters, metabolites, amino acids, proteases, and adenosine has been seen to vary between a normal brain and tumor tissue. Roslin et al. conducted a study in 15 high-grade astrocytoma patients using CMD and observed low glucose and high lactate values with necrotic tissue showing higher levels of glutamate and glycerol [73]. Xu et al. studied CMD in 8 non-secreting pituitary adenoma patients, providing valuable information regarding tissue damage during brain retraction and developing optimal retraction neurosurgical techniques. It presents a picture of pronounced incomplete cerebral ischemia evident in CMD as raised LPR, lactate, glutamate, and glycerol [74]. Blood–CSF, blood–brain, and blood tumor barrier determine the effective delivery of systemically administered drugs. The delivered drug reaches the target tissue in varied concentrations depending on its lipid solubility, molecular weight, protein binding, and state of these barriers. CMD has been used to measure the drug concentration in tumor tissue and interstitial space surrounding brain tumors to understand interpatient variability. Thus, CMD has been used to analyze drug neuro-pharmacokinetics, real-time measurement of unbound drugs near the site of action in the brain, and monitor the therapeutic effect [75]. Delivery of chemotherapy drugs directly into intracranial tumoral tissue through CMD (retro-dialysis) has been carried out in certain brain tumor patients [76–78].

13.4.5 Epilepsy

An underlying imbalance between excitatory and inhibitory neurotransmitters may lead to epileptic discharges. CMD has also been used to study the neurochemical milieu of epileptic foci. An increase in extracellular aspartate, glutamate, glycine, and serine associated with spontaneous and electrically induced seizures has been observed [79]. Ronne-Engstrom et al. demonstrated direct evidence of elevations of extracellular aspartate, glutamate, glycine, and serine in association with both spontaneous and electrically induced seizures in 7 patients undergoing epilepsy surgery for medically intractable epilepsy [80].

13.5 Other Applications of Cerebral Microdialysis

Several neuropsychiatric disorders and neurodegenerative diseases, such as Alzheimer's and Parkinson, involve an imbalance of acetylcholine, dopamine, norepinephrine, and serotonin. CMD makes it possible to study both their level and the effect of therapeutic drugs on these neurotransmitters [81, 82]. Interestingly, CMD use also demonstrates increased endogenous brain lactate production with hyperglycolysis found in patients with fulminant hepatic failure who later developed high ICP [83].

13.6 Future Applications

Direct measurement of brain metabolic function, various metabolites, neurotransmitters, biomarkers, and drugs via CMD has shed light on various unexplored mechanisms underlying dysfunction and recovery in SAH and TBI. There is growing interest in the utilization of CMD for targeted drug delivery in TBI patients, such as to guide nutrition; for the development of hypertonic lactate as a therapeutic agent, and the possibility of a ketogenic diet for TBI patients. However, these fields are still in their infancy and require further research to establish their impact on survival. Based on data obtained from CMD, specific interventions like blood glucose increment, ICP-directed therapy, brain oxygen optimization, and/or seizure control can be instituted to minimize or prevent secondary insults. Thus, microdialysis measurements of brain metabolic function provide clinically valuable information that other monitoring adjuncts cannot provide in the standard ICU setting.

References

1. Zhou T, Kalanuria A. Cerebral microdialysis in neurocritical care. Curr Neurol Neurosci Rep. 2018;18:1–1.
2. Carteron L, Bouzat P, Oddo M. Cerebral microdialysis monitoring to improve individualised neurointensive care therapy: an update of recent clinical data. Front Neurol. 2017;8:601.
3. Carpenter KL, Young AM, Hutchinson PJ. Advanced monitoring in traumatic brain injury: microdialysis. Curr Opin Crit Care. 2017;23(2):103–9.
4. Le Roux P, Menon DK, Citerio G, Vespa P, Bader MK, Brophy GM, Diringer MN, Stocchetti N, Videtta W, Armonda R, Badjatia N. Consensus summary statement of the international multidisciplinary consensus conference on multimodality monitoring in neurocritical care: a statement for healthcare professionals from the Neurocritical Care Society and the European Society of Intensive Care Medicine. Neurocrit Care. 2014;21:1–26.
5. Le Roux P, Menon DK, Citerio G, Vespa P, Bader MK, Brophy GM, Diringer MN, Stocchetti N, Videtta W, Armonda R, Badjatia N. Consensus summary statement of the international multidisciplinary consensus conference on multimodality monitoring in neurocritical care: a statement for healthcare professionals from the Neurocritical Care Society and the European Society of Intensive Care Medicine. Intensive Care Med. 2014;40(9):1189–209. https://doi.org/10.1007/s00134-014-3369-6.
6. Mahajan C, Rath GP. Cerebral microdialysis. J Neuroanaesthesiol Crit Care. 2015;2(03):232–9.
7. Prabhakar H, editor. Neuromonitoring techniques: quick guide for clinicians and residents. Elsevier Science; 2017.
8. Hutchinson PJ, Jalloh I, Helmy A, Carpenter KL, Rostami E, Bellander BM, Boutelle MG, Chen JW, Claassen J, Dahyot-Fizelier C, Enblad P. Consensus statement from the 2014 international microdialysis forum. Intensive Care Med. 2015;41:1517–28.
9. Peerdemsan SM, Girbes AR, Vandertop WP. Cerebral microdialysis as a new tool for neurometabolic monitoring. Intensive Care Med. 2000;26(6):662.
10. Zeiler FA, Thelin EP, Helmy A, Czosnyka M, Hutchinson PJ, Menon DK. A systematic review of cerebral microdialysis and outcomes in TBI: relationships to patient functional outcome, neurophysiologic measures, and tissue outcome. Acta Neurochir. 2017;159:2245–73.
11. Helbok R, Kofler M, Schiefecker AJ, Gaasch M, Rass V, Pfausler B, Beer R, Schmutzhard E. Clinical use of cerebral microdialysis in patients with aneurysmal subarachnoid hemorrhage—state of the art. Front Neurol. 2017;8:565.
12. Hutchinson PJ, O'Connell MT, Al-Rawi PG, Maskell LB, Kett-White R, Gupta AK, Richards HK, Hutchinson DB, Kirkpatrick PJ, Pickard JD. Clinical cerebral microdialysis: a methodological study. J Neurosurg. 2000;93(1):37–43.
13. Bhatia A, Gupta AK. Neuromonitoring in the intensive care unit. II. Cerebral oxygenation monitoring and microdialysis. Intensive Care Med. 2007;33:1322–8.
14. Johnston AJ, Gupta AK. Advanced monitoring in the neurology intensive care unit: microdialysis. Curr Opin Crit Care. 2002;8(2):121–7.
15. Chefer VI, Thompson AC, Zapata A, Shippenberg TS. Overview of brain microdialysis. Curr Protoc Neurosci. 2009;47(1):7–1.
16. Hillman J, Åneman O, Anderson C, Sjögren F, Säberg C, Mellergård P. A microdialysis technique for routine measurement of macromolecules in the injured human brain. Neurosurgery. 2005;56(6):1264–70.
17. Helmy A, Carpenter KL, Menon DK, Pickard JD, Hutchinson PJ. The cytokine response to human traumatic brain injury: temporal profiles and evidence for cerebral parenchymal production. J Cereb Blood Flow Metab. 2011;31(2):658–70.
18. Chu J, Koudriavtsev V, Hjort K, Dahlin AP. Fluorescence imaging of macromolecule transport in high molecular weight cut-off microdialysis. Anal Bioanal Chem. 2014;406:7601–9.
19. Wages SA, Church WH, Justice JB. Sampling considerations for on-line microbore liquid chromatography of brain dialysate. Anal Chem. 1986;58(8):1649–56.
20. Helbok R, Schiefecker AJ, Beer R, Dietmann A, Antunes AP, Sohm F, Fischer M, Hackl WO, Rhomberg P, Lackner P, Pfausler B. Early brain injury after aneurysmal subarachnoid hemorrhage: a multimodal neuromonitoring study. Crit Care. 2015;19:1–9.
21. Bellander BM, Cantais E, Enblad P, Hutchinson P, Nordström CH, Robertson C, Sahuquillo J, Smith M, Stocchetti N, Ungerstedt U, Unterberg A. Consensus

meeting on microdialysis in neurointensive care. Intensive Care Med. 2004;30:2166–9.
22. Kendrick KM, De La Riva C, Hinton M, Baldwin BA. Microdialysis measurement of monoamine and amino acid release from the medial preoptic region of the sheep in response to heat exposure. Brain Res Bull. 1989;22(3):541–4.
23. Spencer P, Jiang Y, Liu N, Han J, Li Y, Vodovoz S, Dumont AS, Wang X. Update: microdialysis for monitoring cerebral metabolic dysfunction after subarachnoid hemorrhage. J Clin Med. 2020;10(1):100.
24. Roos YB, De Haan RJ, Beenen LF, Groen RJ, Albrecht KW, Vermeulen M. Complications and outcome in patients with aneurysmal subarachnoid haemorrhage: a prospective hospital based cohort study in The Netherlands. J Neurol Neurosurg Psychiatry. 2000;68(3):337–41.
25. Schmidt JM, Rincon F, Fernandez A, Resor C, Kowalski RG, Claassen J, Connolly ES, Fitzsimmons BF, Mayer SA. Cerebral infarction associated with acute subarachnoid hemorrhage. Neurocrit Care. 2007;7:10–7.
26. Rowland MJ, Hadjipavlou G, Kelly M, Westbrook J, Pattinson KT. Delayed cerebral ischaemia after subarachnoid haemorrhage: looking beyond vasospasm. Br J Anaesth. 2012;109(3):315–29.
27. Sabri M, Lass E, Macdonald RL. Early brain injury: a common mechanism in subarachnoid hemorrhage and global cerebral ischemia. Stroke Res Treat. 2013;2013:394036.
28. Claassen J, Carhuapoma JR, Kreiter KT, Du EY, Connolly ES, Mayer SA. Global cerebral edema after subarachnoid hemorrhage: frequency, predictors, and impact on outcome. Stroke. 2002;33(5):1225–32.
29. Skjøth-Rasmussen J, Schulz M, Kristensen SR, Bjerre P. Delayed neurological deficits detected by an ischemic pattern in the extracellular cerebral metabolites in patients with aneurysmal subarachnoid hemorrhage. J Neurosurg. 2004;100(1):8–15.
30. Persson L, Valtysson J, Enblad P, Wärme PE, Cesarini K, Lewén A, Hillered L. Neurochemical monitoring using intracerebral microdialysis in patients with subarachnoid hemorrhage. J Neurosurg. 1996;84(4):606–16.
31. Peerdeman SM, van Tulder MW, Vandertop WP. Cerebral microdialysis as a monitoring method in subarachnoid hemorrhage patients, and correlation with clinical events: a systematic review. J Neurol. 2003;250:797–805.
32. Sarrafzadeh AS, Sakowitz OW, Kiening KL, Benndorf G, Lanksch WR, Unterberg AW. Bedside microdialysis: a tool to monitor cerebral metabolism in subarachnoid hemorrhage patients? Crit Care Med. 2002;30(5):1062–70.
33. Sarrafzadeh A, Haux D, Sakowitz O, Benndorf G, Herzog H, Kuechler I, Unterberg A. Acute focal neurological deficits in aneurysmal subarachnoid hemorrhage: relation of clinical course, CT findings, and metabolite abnormalities monitored with bedside microdialysis. Stroke. 2003;34(6):1382–8.
34. Hanafy KA, Grobelny B, Fernandez L, Kurtz P, Connolly ES, Mayer SA, Schindler C, Badjatia N. Brain interstitial fluid TNF-α after subarachnoid hemorrhage. J Neurol Sci. 2010;291(1–2):69–73.
35. Hanafy KA, Stuart RM, Khandji AG, Connolly ES, Badjatia N, Mayer SA, Schindler C. Relationship between brain interstitial fluid tumor necrosis factor-α and cerebral vasospasm after aneurysmal subarachnoid hemorrhage. J Clin Neurosci. 2010;17(7):853–6.
36. Sarrafzadeh A, Schlenk F, Gericke C, Vajkoczy P. Relevance of cerebral interleukin-6 after aneurysmal subarachnoid hemorrhage. Neurocrit Care. 2010;13:339–46.
37. Graetz D, Nagel A, Schlenk F, Sakowitz O, Vajkoczy P, Sarrafzadeh A. High ICP as trigger of proinflammatory IL-6 cytokine activation in aneurysmal subarachnoid hemorrhage. Neurol Res. 2010;32(7):728–35.
38. Roberts DJ, Jenne CN, Léger C, Kramer AH, Gallagher CN, Todd S, Parney IF, Doig CJ, Yong VW, Kubes P, Zygun DA. Association between the cerebral inflammatory and matrix metalloproteinase responses after severe traumatic brain injury in humans. J Neurotrauma. 2013;30(20):1727–36.
39. Sarrafzadeh A, Copin JC, Bengualid DJ, Turck N, Vajkoczy P, Bijlenga P, Schaller K, Gasche Y. Matrix metalloproteinase-9 concentration in the cerebral extracellular fluid of patients during the acute phase of aneurysmal subarachnoid hemorrhage. Neurol Res. 2012;34(5):455–61.
40. Guilfoyle MR, Carpenter KL, Helmy A, Pickard JD, Menon DK, Hutchinson PJ. Matrix metalloproteinase expression in contusional traumatic brain injury: a paired microdialysis study. J Neurotrauma. 2015;32(20):1553–9.
41. Helbok R, Schiefecker A, Delazer M, Beer R, Bodner T, Pfausler B, Benke T, Lackner P, Fischer M, Sohm F, Hackl W. Cerebral tau is elevated after aneurysmal subarachnoid haemorrhage and associated with brain metabolic distress and poor functional and cognitive long-term outcome. J Neurol Neurosurg Psychiatry. 2015;86(1):79–86.
42. Chou SH, Macdonald RL, Keller E. Biospecimens and molecular and cellular biomarkers in aneurysmal subarachnoid hemorrhage studies: common data elements and standard reporting recommendations. Neurocrit Care. 2019;30:46–59.
43. Zeiler FA, Thelin EP, Czosnyka M, Hutchinson PJ, Menon DK, Helmy A. Cerebrospinal fluid and microdialysis cytokines in severe traumatic brain injury: a scoping systematic review. Front Neurol. 2017;8:331.
44. Zeiler FA, Thelin EP, Czosnyka M, Hutchinson PJ, Menon DK, Helmy A. Cerebrospinal fluid and microdialysis cytokines in aneurysmal subarachnoid hemorrhage: a scoping systematic review. Front Neurol. 2017;8:379.
45. Werner C, Engelhard K. Pathophysiology of traumatic brain injury. Br J Anaesth. 2007;99(1):4–9.
46. Prins M, Greco T, Alexander D, Giza CC. The pathophysiology of traumatic brain injury at a glance. Dis Model Mech. 2013;6(6):1307–15.

47. Vespa P, Bergsneider M, Hattori N, Wu HM, Huang SC, Martin NA, Glenn TC, McArthur DL, Hovda DA. Metabolic crisis without brain ischemia is common after traumatic brain injury: a combined microdialysis and positron emission tomography study. J Cereb Blood Flow Metab. 2005;25(6):763–74.
48. Carpenter KL, Jalloh I, Gallagher CN, Grice P, Howe DJ, Mason A, Timofeev I, Helmy A, Murphy MP, Menon DK, Kirkpatrick PJ. 13C-labelled microdialysis studies of cerebral metabolism in TBI patients. Eur J Pharm Sci. 2014;57:87–97.
49. Jalloh I, Carpenter KL, Grice P, Howe DJ, Mason A, Gallagher CN, Helmy A, Murphy MP, Menon DK, Carpenter TA, Pickard JD. Glycolysis and the pentose phosphate pathway after human traumatic brain injury: microdialysis studies using 1, 2-13C2 glucose. J Cereb Blood Flow Metab. 2015;35(1):111–20.
50. Kato T, Nakayama N, Yasokawa Y, Okumura A, Shinoda J, Iwama T. Statistical image analysis of cerebral glucose metabolism in patients with cognitive impairment following diffuse traumatic brain injury. J Neurotrauma. 2007;24(6):919–26.
51. Wu HM, Huang SC, Hattori N, Glenn TC, Vespa PM, Yu CL, Hovda DA, Phelps ME, Bergsneider M. Selective metabolic reduction in gray matter acutely following human traumatic brain injury. J Neurotrauma. 2004;21(2):149–61.
52. Kurtz P, Claassen J, Schmidt JM, Helbok R, Hanafy KA, Presciutti M, Lantigua H, Connolly ES, Lee K, Badjatia N, Mayer SA. Reduced brain/serum glucose ratios predict cerebral metabolic distress and mortality after severe brain injury. Neurocrit Care. 2013;19:311–9.
53. Vespa PM, McArthur D, O'Phelan K, Glenn T, Etchepare M, Kelly D, Bergsneider M, Martin NA, Hovda DA. Persistently low extracellular glucose correlates with poor outcome 6 months after human traumatic brain injury despite a lack of increased lactate: a microdialysis study. J Cereb Blood Flow Metab. 2003;23(7):865–77.
54. Sanchez JJ, Bidot CJ, O'Phelan K, Gajavelli S, Yokobori S, Olvey S, Jagid J, Garcia JA, Nemeth Z, Bullock R. Neuromonitoring with microdialysis in severe traumatic brain injury patients. In: Brain edema XV 2013. Springer Vienna. p. 223–7.
55. Vespa P, Boonyaputthikul R, McArthur DL, Miller C, Etchepare M, Bergsneider M, Glenn T, Martin N, Hovda D. Intensive insulin therapy reduces microdialysis glucose values without altering glucose utilisation or improving the lactate/pyruvate ratio after traumatic brain injury. Crit Care Med. 2006;34(3):850–6.
56. Sahuquillo J, Merino MA, Sánchez-Guerrero A, Arikan F, Vidal-Jorge M, Martínez-Valverde T, Rey A, Riveiro M, Poca MA. Lactate and the lactate-to-pyruvate molar ratio cannot be used as independent biomarkers for monitoring brain energetic metabolism: a microdialysis study in patients with traumatic brain injuries. PLoS One. 2014;9(7):e102540.
57. Sala N, Suys T, Zerlauth JB, Bouzat P, Messerer M, Bloch J, Levivier M, Magistretti PJ, Meuli R, Oddo M. Cerebral extracellular lactate increase is predominantly nonischemic in patients with severe traumatic brain injury. J Cereb Blood Flow Metab. 2013;33(11):1815–22.
58. Bullock R, Zauner A, Woodward JJ, Myseros J, Choi SC, Ward JD, Marmarou A, Young HF. Factors affecting excitatory amino acid release following severe human head injury. J Neurosurg. 1998;89(4):507–18.
59. Globus MY, Alonso O, Dietrich WD, Busto R, Ginsberg MD. Glutamate release and free radical production following brain injury: effects of posttraumatic hypothermia. J Neurochem. 1995;65(4):1704–11.
60. Zauner A, Bullock R. The role of excitatory amino acids in severe brain trauma: opportunities for therapy: a review. J Neurotrauma. 1995;12(4):547–54.
61. Chamoun R, Suki D, Gopinath SP, Goodman JC, Robertson C. Role of extracellular glutamate measured by cerebral microdialysis in severe traumatic brain injury. J Neurosurg. 2010;113(3):564–70.
62. Hejčl A, Bolcha M, Procházka J, Hušková E, Sameš M. Elevated intracranial pressure, low cerebral perfusion pressure, and impaired brain metabolism correlate with fatal outcome after severe brain injury. J Neurol Surg Part A Centr Eur Neurosurg. 2012;73(01):10–7.
63. Timofeev I, Czosnyka M, Carpenter KL, Nortje J, Kirkpatrick PJ, Al-Rawi PG, Menon DK, Pickard JD, Gupta AK, Hutchinson PJ. Interaction between brain chemistry and physiology after traumatic brain injury: impact of autoregulation and microdialysis catheter location. J Neurotrauma. 2011;28(6):849–60.
64. Timofeev I, Carpenter KL, Nortje J, Al-Rawi PG, O'Connell MT, Czosnyka M, Smielewski P, Pickard JD, Menon DK, Kirkpatrick PJ, Gupta AK. Cerebral extracellular chemistry and outcome following traumatic brain injury: a microdialysis study of 223 patients. Brain. 2011;134(2):484–94.
65. Sharma H, McGinnis JP, Kabotyanski KE, Gopinath SP, Goodman JC, Robertson C, Navarro JC. Cerebral microdialysis and glucopenia in traumatic brain injury: a review. Front Neurol. 2023;14:1017290.
66. Rajagopalan S, Baker W, Mahanna-Gabrielli E, Kofke AW, Balu R. Hierarchical cluster analysis identifies distinct physiological states after acute brain injury. Neurocrit Care. 2022;2:630–9.
67. Stovell MG, Mada MO, Helmy A, Carpenter TA, Thelin EP, Yan JL, Guilfoyle MR, Jalloh I, Howe DJ, Grice P, Mason A. The effect of succinate on brain NADH/NAD+ redox state and high energy phosphate metabolism in acute traumatic brain injury. Sci Rep. 2018;8(1):11140.
68. Khellaf A, Garcia NM, Tajsic T, Alam A, Stovell MG, Killen MJ, Howe DJ, Guilfoyle MR, Jalloh I, Timofeev I, Murphy MP. Focally administered succinate improves cerebral metabolism in traumatic brain injury patients with mitochondrial dysfunction. J Cereb Blood Flow Metab. 2022;42(1):39–55.
69. Jalloh I, Helmy A, Howe DJ, Shannon RJ, Grice P, Mason A, Gallagher CN, Stovell MG, van der Heide S, Murphy MP, Pickard JD. Focally perfused succinate potentiates brain metabolism in head injury patients. J Cereb Blood Flow Metab. 2017;37(7):2626–38.

70. Berger C, Annecke A, Aschoff A, Spranger M, Schwab S. Neurochemical monitoring of fatal middle cerebral artery infarction. Stroke. 1999;30(2):460–3.
71. Berger C, Kiening K, Schwab S. Neurochemical monitoring of therapeutic effects in large human MCA infarction. Neurocrit Care. 2008;9:352–6.
72. Berger C, Schäbitz WR, Georgiadis D, Steiner T, Aschoff A, Schwab S. Effects of hypothermia on excitatory amino acids and metabolism in stroke patients: a microdialysis study. Stroke. 2002;33(2):519–24.
73. Roslin M, Henriksson R, Bergström P, Ungerstedt U, Tommy BA. Baseline levels of glucose metabolites, glutamate and glycerol in malignant glioma assessed by stereotactic microdialysis. J Neuro-Oncol. 2003;61:151–60.
74. Xu W, Mellergård P, Ungerstedt U, Nordström CH. Local changes in cerebral energy metabolism due to brain retraction during routine neurosurgical procedures. Acta Neurochir. 2002;144:679–83.
75. Blakeley J, Portnow J. Microdialysis for assessing intratumoral drug disposition in brain cancers: a tool for rational drug development. Expert Opin Drug Metab Toxicol. 2010;6(12):1477–91.
76. Liu L, Zhang X, Lou Y, Rao Y, Zhang X. Cerebral microdialysis in glioma studies, from theory to application. J Pharm Biomed Anal. 2014;96:77–89.
77. Ronquist G, Hugosson R, Sjölander U, Ungerstedt U. Treatment of malignant glioma by a new therapeutic principle. Acta Neurochir. 1992;114:8–11.
78. Pierce CF, Kwasnicki A, Lakka SS, Engelhard HH. Cerebral microdialysis as a tool for assessing the delivery of chemotherapy in brain tumor patients. World Neurosurg. 2021;145:187–96.
79. During MJ, Spencer DD. Extracellular hippocampal glutamate and spontaneous seizure in the conscious human brain. Lancet. 1993;341(8861):1607–10.
80. Ronne-Engström E, Hillered L, Flink R, Spännare BO, Ungerstedt U, Carlson H. Intracerebral microdialysis of extracellular amino acids in the human epileptic focus. J Cereb Blood Flow Metab. 1992;12(5):873–6.
81. Panin F, Cathala A, Piazza PV, Spampinato U. Coupled intracerebral microdialysis and electrophysiology for the assessment of dopamine neuron function in vivo. J Pharmacol Toxicol Methods. 2012;65(2):83–92.
82. McAdoo DJ, Wu P. Microdialysis in central nervous system disorders and their treatment. Pharmacol Biochem Behav. 2008;90(2):282–96.
83. Tofteng F, Jorgensen L, Hansen BA, Ott P, Kondrup J, Larsen FS. Cerebral microdialysis in patients with fulminant hepatic failure. Hepatology. 2002;36(6):1333–40.
84. Helmy A, Carpenter KL, Skepper JN, Kirkpatrick PJ, Pickard JD, Hutchinson PJ. Microdialysis of cytokines: methodological considerations, scanning electron microscopy, and determination of relative recovery. J Neurotrauma. 2009;26(4):549–61.
85. Hillered L, Dahlin AP, Clausen F, Chu J, Bergquist J, Hjort K, Enblad P, Lewén A. Cerebral microdialysis for protein biomarker monitoring in the neurointensive care setting–a technical approach. Front Neurol. 2014;5:245.
86. Stein NR, McArthur DL, Etchepare M, Vespa PM. Early cerebral metabolic crisis after TBI influences outcome despite adequate hemodynamic resuscitation. Neurocrit Care. 2012;17:49–57.
87. Nikaina I, Paterakis K, Paraforos G, Dardiotis E, Chovas A, Papadopoulos D, Brotis A, Komnos A. Cerebral perfusion pressure, microdialysis biochemistry, and clinical outcome in patients with spontaneous intracerebral hematomas. J Crit Care. 2012;27(1):83–8.
88. Vespa P, McArthur DL, Stein N, Huang SC, Shao W, Filippou M, Etchepare M, Glenn T, Hovda DA. Tight glycemic control increases metabolic distress in traumatic brain injury: a randomised controlled within-subjects trial. Crit Care Med. 2012;40(6):1923–9.
89. Helbok R, Schmidt JM, Kurtz P, Hanafy KA, Fernandez L, Stuart RM, Presciutti M, Ostapkovich ND, Connolly ES, Lee K, Badjatia N. Systemic glucose and brain energy metabolism after subarachnoid hemorrhage. Neurocrit Care. 2010;12:317–23.
90. Schmidt JM, Ko SB, Helbok R, Kurtz P, Stuart RM, Presciutti M, Fernandez L, Lee K, Badjatia N, Connolly ES, Claassen J. Cerebral perfusion pressure thresholds for brain tissue hypoxia and metabolic crisis after poor-grade subarachnoid hemorrhage. Stroke. 2011;42(5):1351–6.
91. Kurtz P, Schmidt JM, Claassen J, Carrera E, Fernandez L, Helbok R, Presciutti M, Stuart RM, Connolly ES, Badjatia N, Mayer SA. Anemia is associated with metabolic distress and brain tissue hypoxia after subarachnoid hemorrhage. Neurocrit Care. 2010;13:10–6.
92. Rogers ML, Leong CL, Gowers SA, Samper IC, Jewell SL, Khan A, McCarthy L, Pahl C, Tolias CM, Walsh DC, Strong AJ. Simultaneous monitoring of potassium, glucose and lactate during spreading depolarisation in the injured human brain–proof of principle of a novel real-time neurochemical analysis system, continuous online microdialysis. J Cereb Blood Flow Metab. 2017;37(5):1883–95.
93. Hinzman JM, Wilson JA, Mazzeo AT, Bullock MR, Hartings JA. Excitotoxicity and metabolic crisis are associated with spreading depolarisations in severe traumatic brain injury patients. J Neurotrauma. 2016;33(19):1775–83.
94. Vespa P, Tubi M, Claassen J, Buitrago-Blanco M, McArthur D, Velazquez AG, Tu B, Prins M, Nuwer M. Metabolic crisis occurs with seizures and periodic discharges after brain trauma. Ann Neurol. 2016;79(4):579–90.
95. Magnoni S, Esparza TJ, Conte V, Carbonara M, Carrabba G, Holtzman DM, Zipfel GJ, Stocchetti N, Brody DL. Tau elevations in the brain extracellular space correlate with reduced amyloid-β levels and predict adverse clinical outcomes after severe traumatic brain injury. Brain. 2012;135(4):1268–80.

14 Neuroimaging: CT Scan and MRI

Anshu Mahajan and Ashima Mahajan

14.1 Introduction

Diagnostic imaging is frequently used to evaluate patients in the intensive care unit (ICU), who present with a diverse range of pathologies and are considered to be among the most critically ill patients in the hospital.

14.2 Imaging Modalities

The selection of the appropriate imaging modality is a critical first step when imaging a sick patient, as it is essential to ensure quality, safety, and appropriateness. In this article, we briefly introduce some of the most commonly used imaging modalities [1, 2].

14.2.1 Computed Tomography

Computed tomography (CT) is widely utilized for neuroimaging due to its easy availability and quick acquisition time. Noncontrast computed tomography (NCCT) head scans are typically performed to promptly assess patients for critical intracranial conditions, such as hemorrhage, herniation, infection, inflammation, infarction, and hydrocephalus. CT is frequently used in scenarios involving severe trauma, stroke, and altered mental status. Additionally, scout radiographs, performed as part of CT examinations, can be beneficial in evaluating support apparatus, craniocervical alignment, craniotomies, and surgical hardware [2]. The use of iodinated contrast should only be considered when necessary for decisions that directly impact clinical management. It is essential to take into account any allergies and impaired renal function that may affect their use in ICU patients. The American College of Radiology Manual on Contrast Media and Appropriateness Criteria offers valuable evidence-based resources on when and how to use contrast, which is particularly crucial for ICU patients [3].

- **Computed Tomography Angiography**
  CT angiography (CTA) is a diagnostic imaging procedure that involves the use of intravenous iodinated contrast during the arterial phase to provide a comprehensive assessment of potential arterial pathology, such as aneurysms, vasospasm, infarction, and vascular malformations. In critical care patients, CTA of the neck is often performed to evaluate arterial stenosis, as well as vascular injuries, including traumatic arterial injury,

A. Mahajan (✉)
Department of Neurosciences, Medanta, The Medicity, Gurgaon, Haryana, India

A. Mahajan
Department of Radiodiagnosis, Artemis Hospital, Gurgaon, Haryana, India

H. Prabhakar et al. (eds.), *Principles and Practice of Neurocritical Care*,
https://doi.org/10.1007/978-981-99-8059-8_14

dissection, and transections. This noninvasive technique can provide detailed and accurate imaging results without requiring invasive procedures, making it a valuable diagnostic tool for critical care patients [3].

CT venography (CTV) is a noninvasive diagnostic imaging technique that uses intravenous contrast to visualize the venous phase and assess potential venous pathologies. CTV of the neck can be used to evaluate the extent of clot, stenosis, and occlusion and can also be valuable in the post-traumatic setting to assess injuries resulting from blunt or penetrating trauma. Due to its noninvasive nature, CTV provides a safe and effective method for accurate and detailed imaging results, making it a useful diagnostic tool for critically ill patients [4].

- **Computed Tomography Perfusion**

  CT perfusion (CTP) is a diagnostic imaging procedure that involves the administration of iodinated contrast during dynamic imaging to evaluate acute ischemia, acute infarction, or vasospasm. This technique enables the calculation of quantitative parameters, including cerebral blood flow, cerebral blood volume, mean transit time, time to peak, and Tmax, from contrast curves to evaluate specific pathologies. By examining these parameters, clinicians can diagnose and assess the severity of cerebrovascular conditions, providing valuable information for critical care patients. Although CTP requires the administration of iodinated contrast, it provides a noninvasive means of obtaining precise and detailed imaging results without requiring invasive procedures, making it an excellent diagnostic tool for critical care patients [5].

- **Portable Computed Tomography**

  Portable CT scanners can be incredibly helpful in critical care settings by increasing scan availability and reducing the need to transport critically ill patients. Transporting patients in the ICU can be challenging, given the need for portable ventilation, intravenous sedation, and extensive supportive tubes, lines, and drains. Portable CT scanners can be especially useful for patients who are too unstable to travel, such as those on extracorporeal membrane oxygenation or ventricular assist devices. However, interpreting portable CT scans can be challenging, as they may have decreased spatial and contrast resolution and increased motion artifacts. Despite these limitations, portable CT scanners provide a noninvasive means of obtaining valuable imaging information for critical care patients without requiring invasive procedures, making them a valuable tool in the ICU [6].

14.2.2 Magnetic Resonance Imaging

Magnetic resonance imaging (MRI) is often used to further investigate CT findings, evaluate patients with persistent neurological symptoms despite normal CT or prior imaging, and for post-treatment follow-up. However, performing MRI on patients in the ICU presents several challenges, particularly related to patient safety considerations. Patients must be cleared for MRI safety, taking into account any devices, implants, foreign bodies, or prior surgeries they may have had. Monitoring equipment must also be switched to MR-compatible equipment. Patients with implanted cardiac devices such as pacemakers and defibrillators require special consideration but may be scanned after consultation with an electrophysiologist and appropriate changes to device settings, if local protocols allow. Gadolinium contrast agents should only be used when necessary to answer a specific clinical question, taking into account the patient's renal function and potential for allergic reactions. Pregnant patients are generally not given gadolinium agents due to concerns about its potential effects on the fetus. Despite these challenges, MRI can provide valuable information in critical care settings, especially when other imaging modalities have limitations or are insufficient [7, 8].

14.2.3 Basic Sequences of MRI

The selection of MRI sequences is crucial for the detection and characterization of various emergency conditions. The choice of sequences depends on the clinical signs and symptoms of the patient and the suspected pathology [9].

- **T1-weighted images** exhibit anatomical features, and when used alongside T2-weighted images, they aid in identifying lesions and evaluating the extent of contrast enhancement.
- **T2-weighted images** are ideal for detecting pathological conditions like tumor, edema, ischemia, and demyelinating disorders as they generate a strong signal.
- **FLAIR (Fluid Attenuation Inversion Recovery)** suppresses CSF signal effects and helps in the detection of subtle white matter changes or edema. FLAIR is more sensitive for early detection of ischemic changes than T2W sequence. It is also the most sensitive MR sequence for detection of subarachnoid hemorrhage.
- **Diffusion-weighted imaging (DWI)** relies on measuring the spontaneous, erratic motion of water molecules within the brain's tissues. DWI is an essential tool for detecting both ischemic stroke and non-ischemic conditions, including infections, trauma, tumors, and metabolic encephalopathy. To identify irreversibly damaged tissue cores, DWI should be the primary sequence performed.
- **Gradient Recalled Echo (GRE) or Susceptibility Weighted Imaging (SWI) sequences** are sensitive to the paramagnetic effects of blood products, which result in a signal loss phenomenon known as "blooming." These imaging techniques are particularly useful in detecting all phases of bleeding and microhemorrhages. Physicians frequently use GRE and SWI sequences in patients who have suffered acute head trauma, hemorrhagic tumors, or vascular malformations.
- **Magnetic Resonance Angiography (MRA)** is a diagnostic imaging technique used to evaluate the arterial vasculature of the brain and/or neck. The Time-of-Flight (TOF) technique allows MRA to be performed without using intravenous gadolinium contrast agents. However, contrast-enhanced or time-resolved MRA may be necessary to evaluate specific pathologies, such as vascular malformations, pseudoaneurysms, and dissections.
- **Magnetic Resonance Venography (MRV)** is a diagnostic tool that can be used to evaluate the venous vasculature of the brain and/or neck. Similar to MRA, MRV can be performed using the time-of-flight (TOF) technique without the administration of gadolinium contrast agents or with the use of gadolinium for contrast-enhanced imaging. However, TOF MRV can produce artifacts that may affect the accuracy of the results. In contrast, MRV with gadolinium contrast is preferred to accurately evaluate for dural venous sinus thrombosis.
- Although **Magnetic Resonance Spectroscopy (MRS)** is typically not performed in emergency situations, it can offer valuable insights into the metabolites present in abnormal tissue, making it a valuable tool for assessing tumors, demyelinating diseases, and infections.
- **Magnetic Resonance Perfusion (MRP)** can aid in identifying the rescuable ischemic penumbra during an ischemic stroke, evaluating the stage of specific tumors, or differentiating between radiation-induced necrosis and tumor advancement [7].

14.2.4 Digital Subtraction Angiography

Digital subtraction angiography (DSA) is still considered the gold standard for detecting cerebrovascular pathology, especially for the diagnosis of vasospasm in patients with subarachnoid hemorrhage. DSA allows for detailed evaluation of the cerebral vasculature and can also be used for therapeutic interventions such as intra-arterial vasodilation. However, CTA and MRA can be used as noninvasive alternatives to DSA in many ICU conditions.

14.3 Different Spectrum of Pathology

1. Trauma
2. Vascular pathology

3. Brain herniation patterns
4. Hydrocephalus
5. Intracranial infections/inflammatory
6. Postsurgical complications
7. Immunocompromised patients
8. Toxic/metabolic
9. Spine imaging in ICU

1. **Trauma**

   CT is the preferred imaging technique for the initial evaluation of traumatic brain injury (TBI), and neurointensivist usually orders a head CT scan immediately after the initial screening and stabilization. CT has the capability of detecting various injuries, such as skull and facial fractures, epidural hematoma (EDH), subdural hematoma (SDH), subarachnoid hemorrhage (SAH), and cerebral contusions. Furthermore, localized and diffuse cerebral swelling is commonly observed. Severe TBI often presents multiple types and locations of intracerebral hemorrhages (ICHs), unlike spontaneous intracerebral hemorrhages [10, 11]. MRI is highly sensitive and accurate in diagnosing neuronal damage in acute traumatic brain injury, including diffuse axonal injury, cortical contusions, and brainstem injury, compared to other imaging modalities. Additionally, MRI has a superior ability to detect subacute to chronic hematomas as the composition of the blood changes over time, making it a valuable tool for monitoring the progression of brain injuries [12].

   - **Hemorrhage**

     Differentiating the types of pathology that can occur within the intracranial compartments is crucial. However, it is not always possible to assign extra-axial hemorrhage to a specific compartment. Subdural hematoma is usually crescent-shaped and can cross sutures. It is primarily caused by the tearing of bridging veins. On the other hand, epidural hematoma typically appears biconvex or lens-shaped and does not cross sutures. It may cross the midline and is commonly associated with calvarial fractures. The classic description includes injury to the middle meningeal artery or midline venous structures [10]. SAH is most commonly caused by trauma. When it is traumatic in origin, it is typically found in the peripheral cerebral sulci instead of the sylvian fissures and basal cisterns. In cases of traumatic SAH, it may also be located near cerebral contusions or fractures instead of the circle of Willis. When significant subarachnoid bleeding is detected in the basal cisterns, it is important to consider the possibility of aneurysm rupture resulting from previous head trauma. Appropriate angiographic imaging should be obtained to confirm this [13]. Cerebral contusions are a significant hallmark of TBI, resulting from damaged and leaking small blood vessels, similar to contusions in other tissues. These contusions frequently initiate as multiple, scattered microhemorrhages, leading to vasogenic edema in the surrounding area (Fig. 14.1). Following the initial injury, red blood cells and plasma may continue to leak, resulting in the characteristic delayed hematoma expansion or "blossoming" of the contusion. Due to the tendency of contusions to expand, close clinical observation and follow-up imaging are recommended for all patients with cerebral contusions. Typically, contusions are found in the frontal or anterior temporal lobes due to the free-floating nature of the brain, causing it to scrape against bony prominences in the anterior and middle cranial fossae during trauma. Underlying the site of impact, so-called coup injuries may be observed, with "contrecoup" contusions located 180° from the impact due to the free-floating nature of the brain within the skull. They are usually accompanied by subarachnoid hemorrhage [11, 14]. Compared to CT imaging, MR imaging is highly sensitive in detecting both hemorrhagic and nonhemorrhagic portions of cerebral contusions, particularly when the contusions are located near the calvarium and during the acute phase of traumatic brain injury, when edema is min-

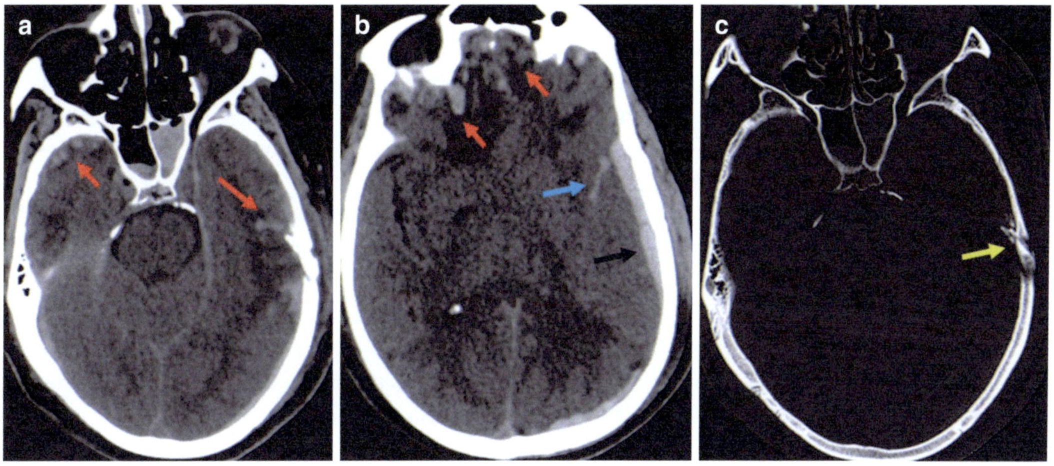

Fig. 14.1 A 37-year male with road traffic accident. Axial NCCT head (**a** and **b**) shows multiple hemorrhagic contusions with surrounding vasogenic edema in bilateral frontal and temporal region (red arrow), left temporo-parietal subdural hematoma (black arrow), and focal sub-arachnoid hemorrhage in left sylvian fissure (blue arrow). NCCT head (bone window) (**c**) shows comminuted depressed fracture of left temporal bone (yellow arrow)

Table 14.1 MR signal of intracranial blood products

	Time	Hemoglobulin degradation status	T1WI	T2WI	T2*
Hyperacute	<6 h	Oxyhemoglobin	Mild hyperintense	Very hyperintense	Peripheral hypointensity
Late acute	6–72 h	Deoxyhemoglobin	Isointense to hypointense	Hypointense	Hypointense (blooming)
Early subacute	3 days to 1 week	Intracellular methemoglobin	Very hyperintense	Hypointense	Hypointense
Late subacute	1–2 weeks to 2 months	Extracellular methemoglobin	Very hyperintense	Very hyperintense (with peripheral hypointensity)	Variable
Chronic	2 weeks to years	Hemosiderin	Hypointense	Hypointense	Hypointense

imal. Hemorrhagic components are frequently present in TBI, and the MR signal is dependent on the timing of the injury (Table 14.1). Studies have shown that MR imaging has a better ability to detect cerebral contusions than CT imaging, making it a valuable tool in the diagnostic workup of TBI [15].

- **Diffuse Axonal Injury (DAI)**

  Patients who have suffered high-energy trauma may develop diffuse axonal injury (DAI), which can present as altered mental status. DAI is caused by widespread shearing of axons due to rotational forces and is typically observed at the grey-white matter junction, corpus callosum, and brainstem. The grading of DAI has been translated to imaging by Gentry et al. [16], with stage 1 referring to lobar involvement, stage 2 indicating callosal involvement, and stage 3 indicating brainstem involvement. Some studies have proposed alternative or modified classifications to the Gentry grading system. For example, a study by Kou et al. proposed a modified grading system that included the degree of involvement of the substantia nigra in addition to the traditional brain regions assessed in the Gentry system. The study found that incorporating substantia nigra involvement into the grading system improved its ability to predict outcomes in patients with DAI. However, further research is needed to determine the optimal method for grading and predicting outcomes in DAI based on imaging findings [17–19]. While CT may show small hemorrhages, it is normal in almost half of DAI cases. On the other hand, MRI can detect both hemorrhagic and nonhemorrhagic DAI and is therefore a more sensitive test. MRI can reveal areas of abnormal T2 prolongation on T2-weighted or fluid-attenuated inversion recovery (FLAIR) images. In addition, diffusion-weighted images (DWIs) can be used to detect acute areas of nonhemorrhagic DAI that may not be visible on T2/FLAIR images alone. Imaging sequences with high sensitivity for detecting hemosiderin and other iron-containing hemoglobin breakdown products, such as gradient echo (GRE) and susceptibility-weighted (SW) sequences, can also be used to identify the presence of DAI in both the acute and chronic phases, as a small amount of bleeding is frequently present (Fig. 14.2). Therefore, in stable patients with severe and persistent impairment of consciousness, MRI should be considered for the diagnosis of DAI [18].

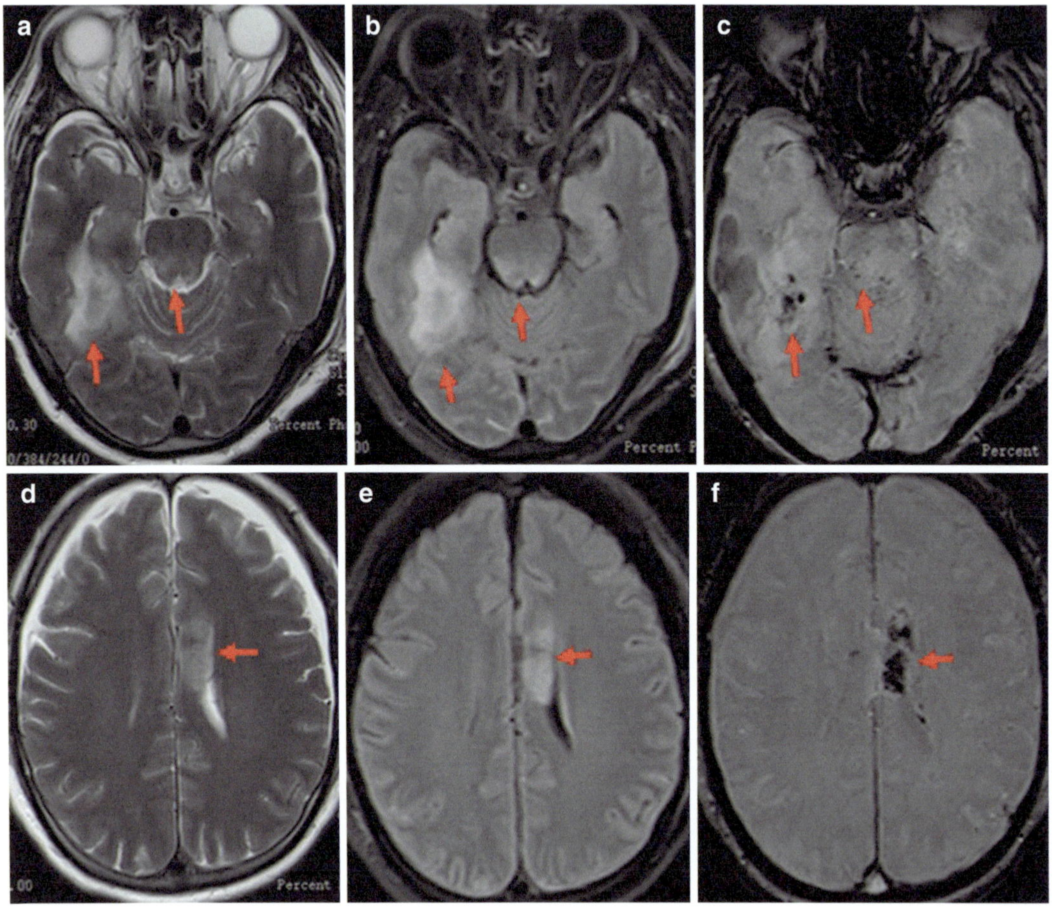

Fig. 14.2 A 45-year male with history of road traffic accident with diffuse axonal injury. T2W and FLAIR sequences (**a** and **b**) show hyperintensity in right temporal lobe at the grey-white matter junction and posterior pons (arrows). SWI sequence (**c**) shows multiple hypointense foci of hemorrhagic lesions in same locations (arrows). T2W and FLAIR sequences (**c** and **d**) show hyperintensity in body of corpus callosum on left side (arrow). SWI sequence (**f**) shows multiple hypointense foci of hemorrhagic lesions in the same location (arrow)

2. **Vascular Pathology**

ICU patients can have a range of intracranial vascular pathologies, including aneurysm, vascular malformation, ischemia, and vasospasm.

- **Aneurysmal Subarachnoid Hemorrhage**

CT is typically the first imaging technique used when SAH is suspected in patients. If acute intracranial SAH is detected through NCCT scans of the head, then the most suitable next step is to perform a CTA of the head or DSA in order to investigate any underlying vascular abnormalities. One such abnormality is a ruptured intracranial aneurysm, which can be signaled by the sudden onset of an excruciating headache, often referred to as a "thunderclap headache." This type of headache is usually accompanied by symptoms such as light sensitivity, nausea, vomiting, stiffness in the neck, and changes in mental clarity. Ruptured aneurysm results in the widespread presence of blood in the subarachnoid space, with a significant concentration in the basal cisterns and sometimes in the ventricles. Intraparenchymal bleeding may occur depending on the site of rupture and the direction of the arterial blood flow, which may indicate the location of an aneurysm. A temporal intraparenchymal hematoma of significant size with little blood in the Sylvian fissure is a common indication of a ruptured aneurysm at the bifurcation of the middle cerebral artery (MCA). Additionally, intraventricular bleeding is present in almost 20% of cases, and subdural hematoma (SDH) is also a possible outcome. The sensitivity of nonenhanced CT to the detection of subarachnoid hemorrhage is heavily impacted by both the volume of blood and the duration following the bleeding. The FLAIR imaging sequence is sensitive during the initial phase and demonstrates high signal intensity in the sulci. T2* sequences exhibit a sensitivity of 94% within 4 days but achieve full sensitivity at a later stage with excellent specificity [7, 19]. The initial imaging can predict the likelihood of vasospasm and the consequent development of delayed cerebral ischemia (DCI) based on the pattern and extent of bleeding. Patients can be classified according to the thickness of SAH and the presence of intraventricular hemorrhage, using the Fischer scale that was subsequently revised by Claassen et al. (Table 14.2). This classification can help to estimate the probability of delayed cerebral ischemia. The modified Fisher's scale ranges from 0 to 4, with higher scores corresponding to greater DCI risk [20, 21] (Fig. 14.3).

Table 14.2 The Fisher's and modified Fisher's scales for SAH

Fisher's scale		Modified Fisher's scale	
Grade	SAH appearance	Grade	Characteristics
		0	No SAH or IVH
1	No SAH visible	1	Minimal/thin SAH, no IVH in both lateral ventricles
2	Thin, diffuse SAH	2	Minimal/thin SAH, with IVH in both lateral ventricles
3	Clot or thick SAH[a]	3	Thick[b] SAH, no IVH in both lateral ventricles
4	Diffuse or none, with IPH or IVH	4	Thick[b] SAH, with IVH in both lateral ventricles

SAH subarachnoid hemorrhage; *IPH* intraparenchymal hemorrhage; *IVH* intraventricular hemorrhage

[a] Grade 3 is defined by localized clot and/or vertical layers of blood >1 mm

[b] Thick SAH is defined as blood completely filling >1 cistern or fissure

- **Spontaneous intracerebral hemorrhage**

The occurrence of sudden neurological symptoms and headache is typical in spontaneous intracerebral hemorrhage (ICH). The initial imaging modality is a noncontrast CT head, which shows a hyperdense area within the brain parenchyma. The size and location of the hemorrhage, along with the clinical history, are crucial in determining the underlying cause. Primary causes of ICH include hypertensive bleed and cerebral amyloid angiopathy (CAA). Hypertensive hemorrhages tend to more commonly occur in a deep location (gan-

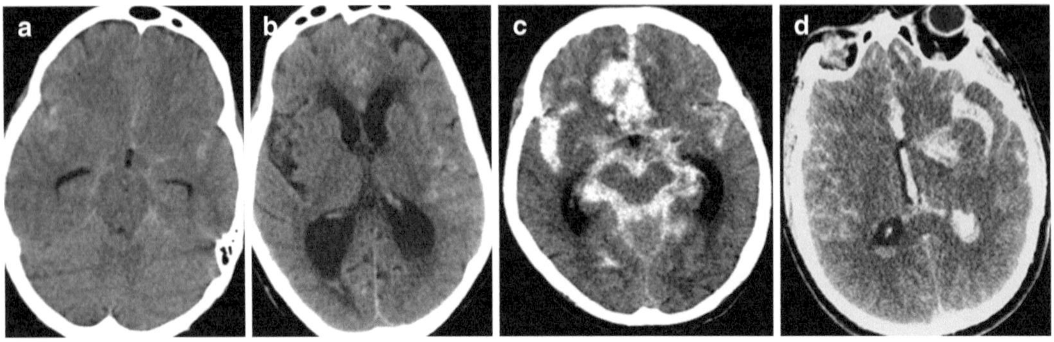

Fig. 14.3 NCCT head axial scans of different patients (**a**–**d**) shows modified Fisher grading (1–4, respectively)

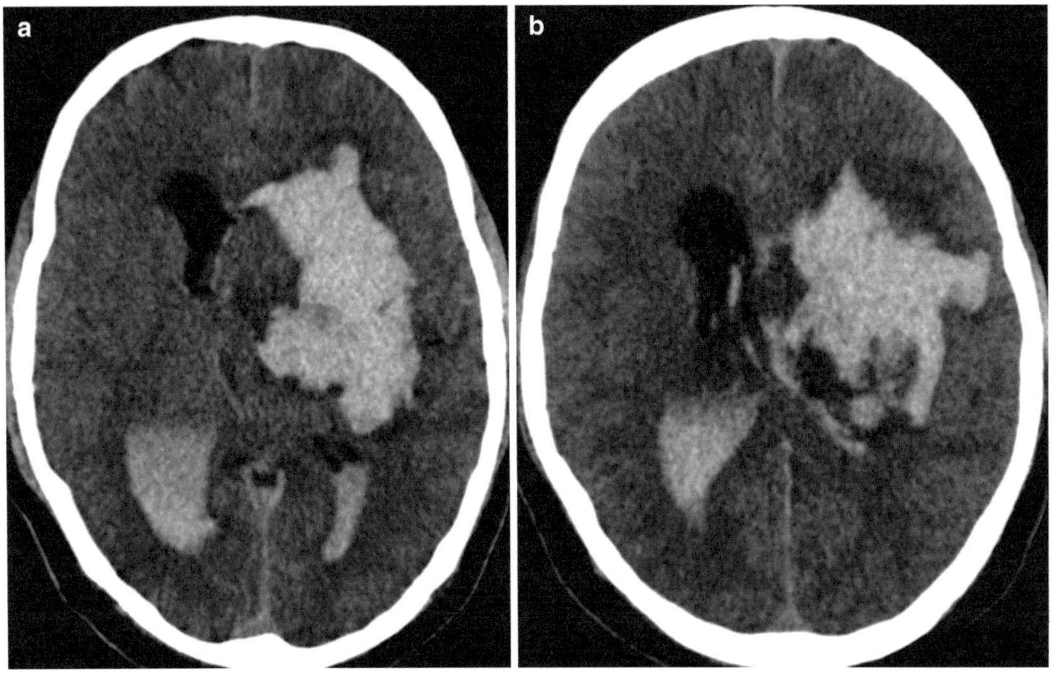

Fig. 14.4 Axial CT head (**a** and **b**) shows left-sided gangliocapsular bleed in a middle age hypertensive male patient

gliocapsular), are more common in the middle-aged group, and often have a history of hypertension. The other common sites of hypertensive bleed are thalamus, cerebellum, and pons (Fig. 14.4). On the other hand, CAA-related hemorrhages are more likely to be lobar and frequently occur in the occipital and parietal lobes in the elderly population. Secondary causes of ICH include underlying vascular malformation or structural lesion such as arteriovenous malformations (AVMs), cavernous malformations, dural AV fistulas (dAVF), and aneurysms (Fig. 14.5). Hemorrhages associated with underlying dAVF typically involve SAH in the cerebral convexity. In general, vascular imaging is necessary to rule out underlying vascular malformation in young patients presenting with spontaneous ICH in an unusual location [7, 22].

Although CT is more effective in detecting arterial vascular lesions and current bleeding, MR imaging is superior in identifying non-arterial causes and determining the age of hemorrhage (as shown in Table 14.1) (Fig. 14.6). For detecting

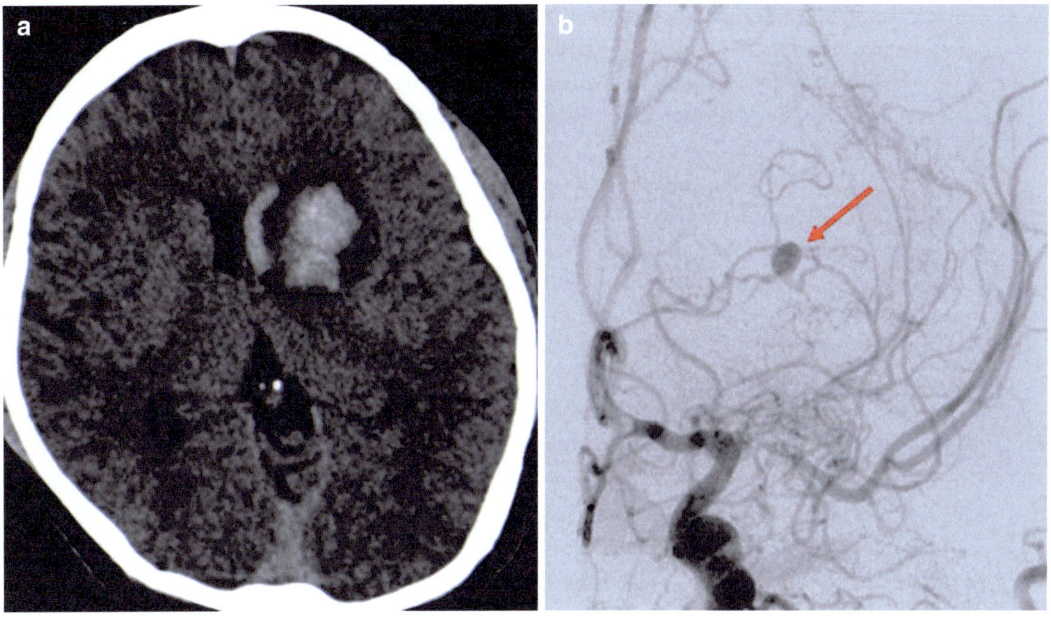

Fig. 14.5 (**a**) NCCT head axial scan shows left caudate head hematoma with intraventricular extension. (**b**) Catheter angiography (left internal carotid artery injection) shows perforator aneurysm (arrow) at the junction between the medial and lateral lenticulostriate artery

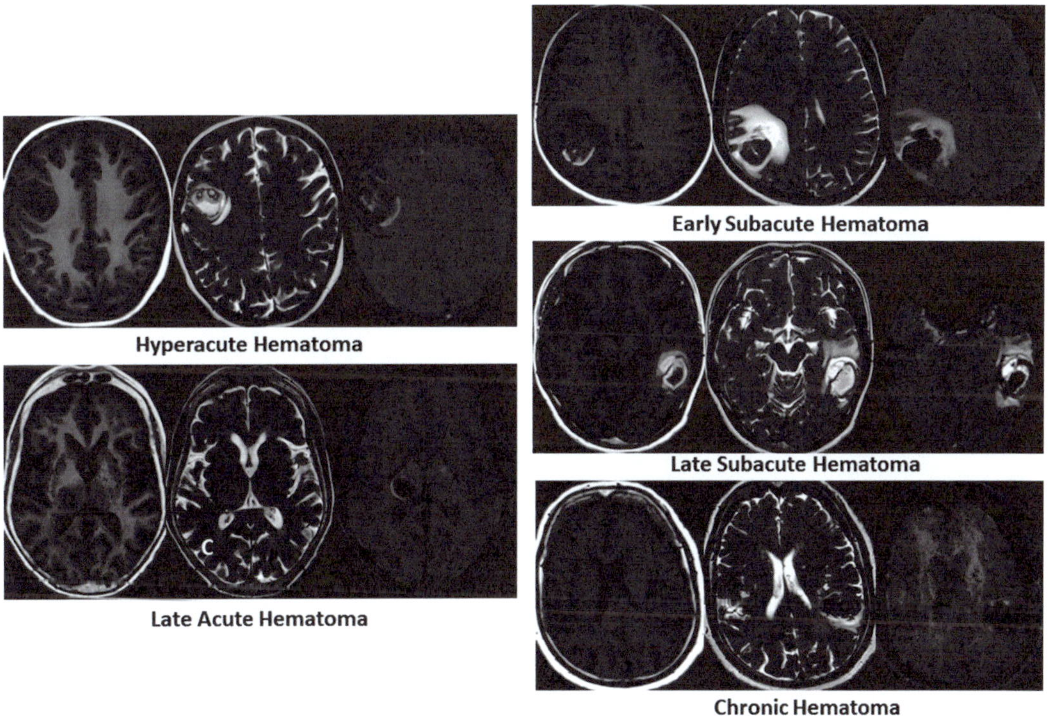

Fig. 14.6 MR signal of intracranial blood products in different stages of hematoma (T1W, T2W, and SWI sequences)

chronic blood and microhemorrhages (i.e., hemorrhages less than 10 mm in size), GRE and SWI sequences are more effective. Dynamic contrast-enhanced MR angiography is a useful tool for assessing the hemodynamics of vascular malformations, allowing for differentiation between high and low flow malformations. This technique is particularly effective in depicting the enlarged feeding arteries and draining veins, which often resemble a "bag of worms" [23, 24]. On T2-weighted images, the presence of a tangle of signal flow voids is indicative of fast and turbulent flow within the abnormal vessels and nidus. Magnetic resonance imaging (MRI) has also a greater sensitivity than other imaging modalities in identifying small cavernous malformations, which often exhibit a distinctive appearance on T2-weighted images known as "popcorn" due to the presence of blood products in different stages of degradation. These malformations can also be easily detected on gradient-echo (GRE) and susceptibility-weighted (SW) sequences [7]. Digital subtraction angiography (DSA) is recommended if an underlying small aneurysm, AVM, or dural AVF is suspected.

Tumor bleed is another potential cause of spontaneous ICH. The highest occurrence of bleeding is typically associated with primary brain tumors like glioblastoma and oligodendroglioma, as well as metastases from renal, thyroid, and choriocarcinomas. When a large ICH occurs, it can mask the presence of an underlying tumor. However, a contrast-enhanced MRI can identify the tumor separately from the hemorrhage [7, 23]. Cerebral hyperperfusion syndrome (CHS) is a serious consequence of carotid recanalization. CHS occurs in approximately 0–3% of patients undergoing this procedure. CHS typically develops within several hours to a few days after the surgery. The condition is characterized by symptoms such as intense, one-sided headaches, confusion, seizures, vision problems, neurological deficits, intracranial bleeding, and even death if left untreated (Fig. 14.7). It is essential to aggressively control blood pressure to prevent and manage the progression of CHS [25].

- **Dural Venous Thrombosis**

  Dural venous thrombosis is another pathology that can be seen in ICU patients. NCCT head may reveal hyperdense dural venous sinus or parenchymal hemorrhages in an unusual location for hemorrhagic transformation of ischemic infarction raising suspicion of hemorrhagic venous

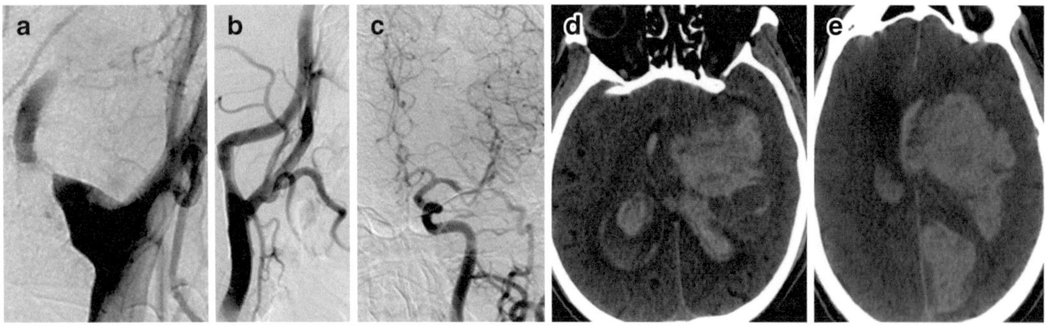

Fig. 14.7 Cerebral hyperperfusion syndrome. 75-year male hypertensive patient with symptomatic left ICA stenosis (**a**) was treated with endovascular carotid stent placement (**b**). Intracranial control angiogram demonstrates normal flow in the intracranial right ICA and middle cerebral artery (**c**). After 4 h, patient complaint of severe headache followed by sudden loss of consciousness. He was urgently intubated. His pupils were fixed and dilated. NCCT head was done which showed bleed in basal ganglia with intraventricular extension in a setting of cerebral hyperperfusion syndrome (**d** and **e**)

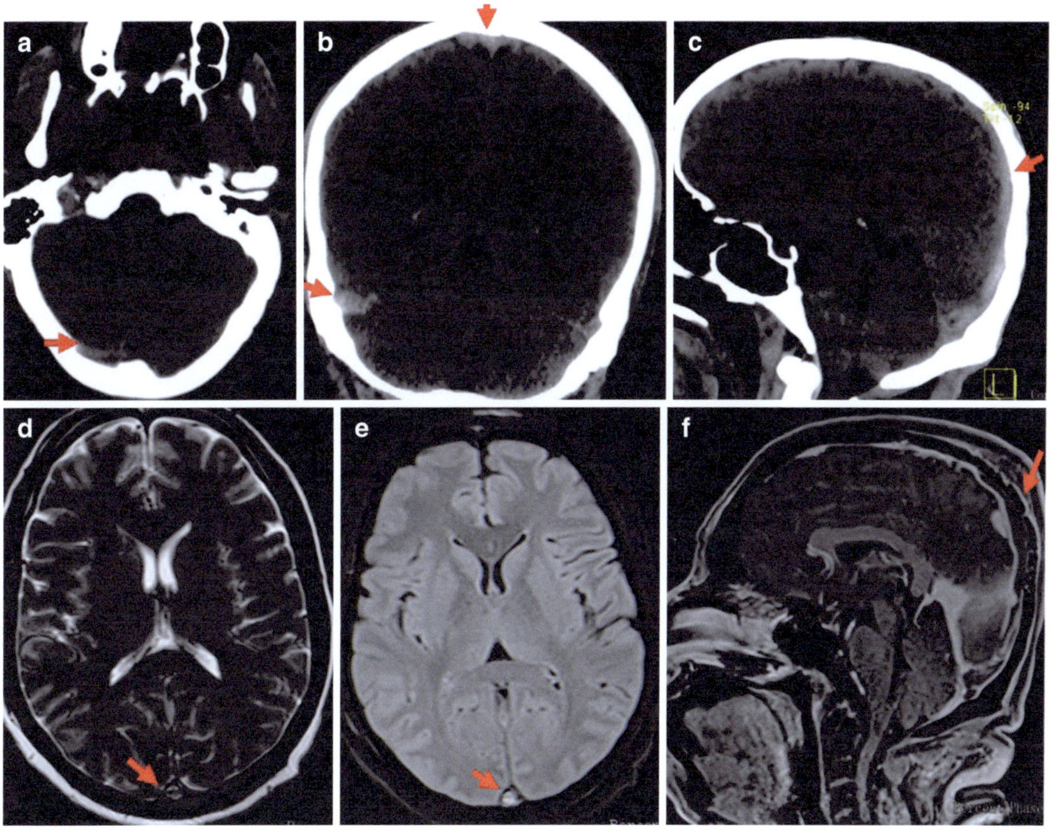

Fig. 14.8 Axial (**a**), coronal (**b**), sagittal (**c**), nonenhanced CT images show areas of abnormal hyperattenuation that are consistent with CVT (arrows) in the right transverse sinus and superior sagittal sinus. Axial T2W (**d**) and FLAIR (**e**) shows loss of signal void in superior sagittal sinus (arrow). Contrast MRI (**f**) shows filling defect in the superior sagittal sinus suggestive of sinus thrombosis (arrow)

infarction (Fig. 14.8a–c). Presence and extent of venous thrombosis can be characterized further with CTV. Compared to a CT scan, conventional MRI sequences, unenhanced time-of-flight (TOF) venography, gradient-echo (GRE), and contrast-enhanced MR venography are more sensitive in detecting venous sinus and cerebral venous thrombosis, as well as any associated brain parenchymal changes [24]. Thrombosed veins and sinuses are visible as areas of hyperintensity on conventional T1-weighted and T2-weighted sequences and as areas of hypointensity on gradient-echo (GRE) sequences due to the presence of methemoglobin. Time-of-flight (TOF) MR venography, which is highly sensitive to slow flow, is the most commonly used method for evaluating thrombosis. However, confirmation may require contrast-enhanced MRI and venography, which provides improved visualization of filling defects, recanalization changes, and dural collaterals (Fig. 14.8d–f). Parenchymal hemorrhage appears as flame-shaped areas of lobar hemorrhage that are typically located in cortical and subcortical locations. Other parenchymal changes including edema, sulcal effacement, and ventricular narrowing due to vasogenic and cytotoxic edema are also noted [7, 24].

- **Ischemic Stroke**

  Ischemic stroke is another common indication for imaging. In an in-patient setting, this need may arise due to a sudden change in a patient's mental status or new neurologic deficit. Typically, the evaluation process starts with a NCCT head scan to identify ischemic stroke patients who could receive thrombolysis treatment. The primary purpose of this scan is to detect and exclude the acute intracranial hemorrhage, but it also rules out other potential causes of a patient's symptoms, such as metastatic disease and brain tumor [26, 27]. Additionally, it provides valuable information about the size, density, and extent of the ischemic infarction. Parenchymal sign of early acute ischemia on CT is loss of gray-white differentiation (GWD) which is best viewed at a high contrast stroke window (centered at 32 HU with a width of 8 HU). Various named signs have been described in the literature: insular ribbon sign, loss of normal insular cortical hyperdensity; lentiform obscuration sign, loss of delineation of GWD of the lentiform nucleus; and disappearing basal ganglia sign, loss of GWD of the basal ganglia (Fig. 14.9a). Once the infarct is established, there is relative hypodensity of regions compared with others, cortical sulcal effacement, sylvian fissure obscuration due to localized mass effect (Fig. 14.9b). These changes are irreversible and plays an important part in prognostication [28, 29]. To quantify the degree of territorial loss, the involvement of more than one-third of the MCA territory was considered a contraindication for intravenous thrombolysis (IV-tPA). However, estimation of territorial loss by this system can be challenging with lack of interobserver reliability. Thus, The Alberta Stroke Program Early CT Score (ASPECTS) was developed to estab-

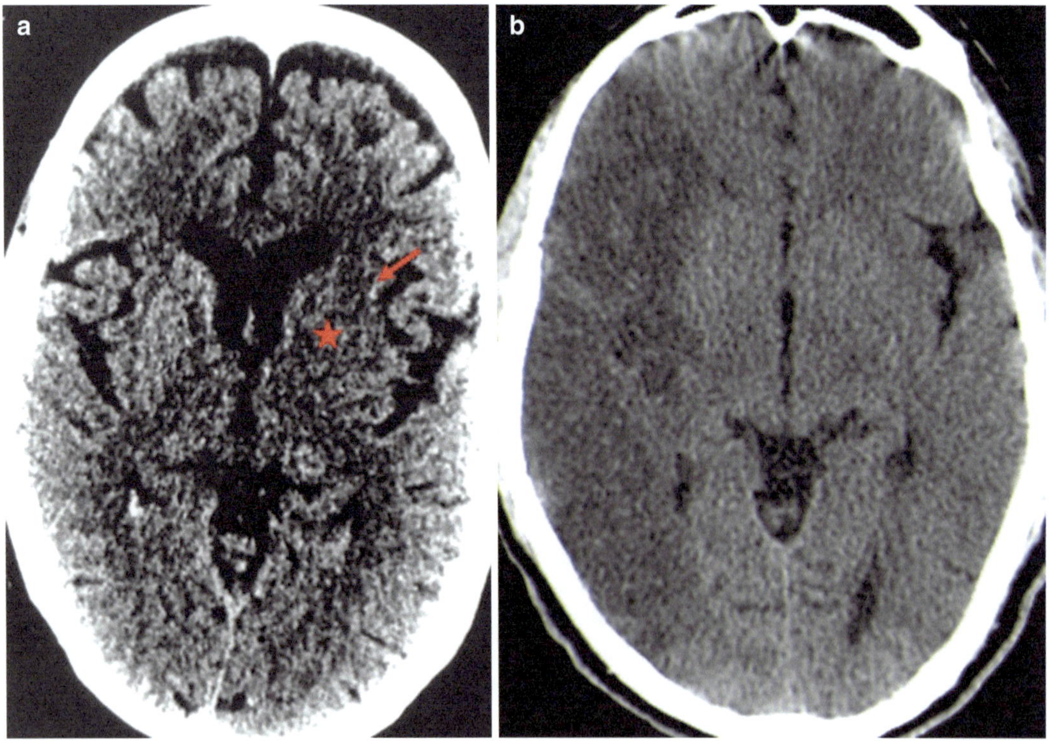

Fig. 14.9 Noncontrast CT head showing lentiform nucleus obscuration (star) and insular ribbon sign (arrow) (**a**). Noncontrast CT showed hypodensity in the right MCA territory with cortical sulcal effacement in established infarct (**b**)

lish a reproducible scoring system for early ischemic changes on nonenhanced CT due to MCA stroke. It is a ten-point quantitative topographic CT scan score used for middle cerebral artery (MCA) stroke patients. Whole MCA territory is divided into ten anatomical regions at ganglionic and supraganglionic level to be evaluated on axial images of CT scan. Three subcortical regions at the level of basal ganglia include caudate (C), lentiform nucleus (L), and internal capsule (IC). Four cortical regions at the level of basal ganglia include anterior MCA cortex (M1), lateral MCA cortex (M2), posterior MCA cortex (M3), and insular cortex (I). Three cortical regions just rostral to the basal ganglia include anterior MCA cortex (M4), lateral MCA cortex (M5), and posterior MCA cortex (M6) (Fig. 14.10). If there is a hypodensity seen in any of the above region compared to expected normal tissue density, 1 point is deducted from the initial score of 10 for every region involved [4, 7]. Lower ASPECTS scores (7 or less) are associated with a higher risk of parenchymal hemorrhage and poor functional outcomes after treatment with IV-tPA or EVT therapy. Current AHA guidelines do not recommend a score of <6 for thrombolysis or EVT based on data from randomized trials [30, 31]. MRI stroke protocol can be obtained in approximately 6 min. This include diffusion-weighted imaging (DWI), fluid-attenuated inversion recovery (FLAIR), gradient-echo (GRE), MR angiography (MRA), and perfusion imaging [32]. DWI is superior to NCCT head for detection of early ischemia as well as smaller or posterior fossa lesions. DWI is a very sensitive sequence to detect ischemia within minutes. Ischemia causes free water restricted diffusion in brain tissue, appearing as hyperintense signal. Onset of diffusion hyperintensity is usually within 30 min although reported as early as <10 min in

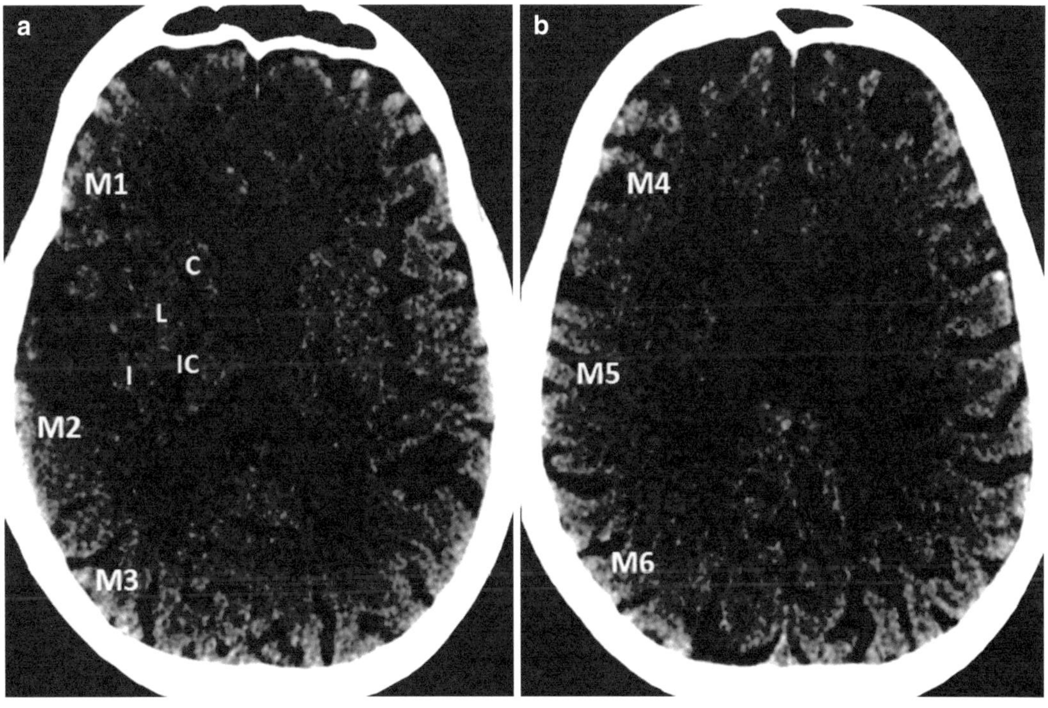

Fig. 14.10 Axial NCCT head at ganglionic and supraganglionic level (**a** and **b**) showing labeled ASPECTS regions at ganglionic and supraganglionic level

some animal studies. It provides level I evidence for assessing the ischemic core [31, 33]. Depending on institutional preference, stroke patients go on to be evaluated by a combination of CTA and CTP or MR imaging. Careful evaluation of major neck vessels for atherosclerotic changes, evaluation of bilateral internal carotid artery and bilateral vertebral artery course, branches of any filling defects, luminal attenuation may help reach a complete diagnosis as well as allow planning for a suitable intervention if indicated based on perfusion imaging. Based on CT or MR perfusion, one can quantify the ischemic penumbra. This information is then used to determine whether revascularization may provide benefits in cases of ischemic stroke [34, 35].

Vasospasm

Vasospasm is reactive narrowing of the intracranial arteries, commonly after SAH with peak at 5–14 days after initial hemorrhage. If severe enough, the vasospasm can result in alterations in cerebral perfusion, leading to ischemia/infarction (Fig. 14.11). Transcranial doppler is typically used to evaluate patients at the bedside, but CT/CTA/CTP/MRI/DSA may also be utilized for more extensive assessment, which can vary depending on institutional practices [36]. Angiographic narrowing visualized on CTA or DSA occurs in up to 70% of patients with aneurysmal SAH. Less than half of patients with radiographic vasospasm will develop clinical signs of DCI and, in up to 15% of cases, DCI can occur in the absence of radiographic vasospasm. Nonetheless, new unexplained decline in the level of consciousness or focal neurological deficit is much more likely to be due to DCI when angiographic vasospasm is present. The diagnosis is easily made on DSA and immediately treated with the direct injection of vasodilatory agents, such as nimodipine or milrinone, into constricted arteries [37].

3. **Brain Herniation Patterns**

   Understanding the different patterns of brain herniation and the complications that are commonly associated with them is essential [2].

   Subfalcine herniation is characterized by the displacement of frontal lobe, particularly

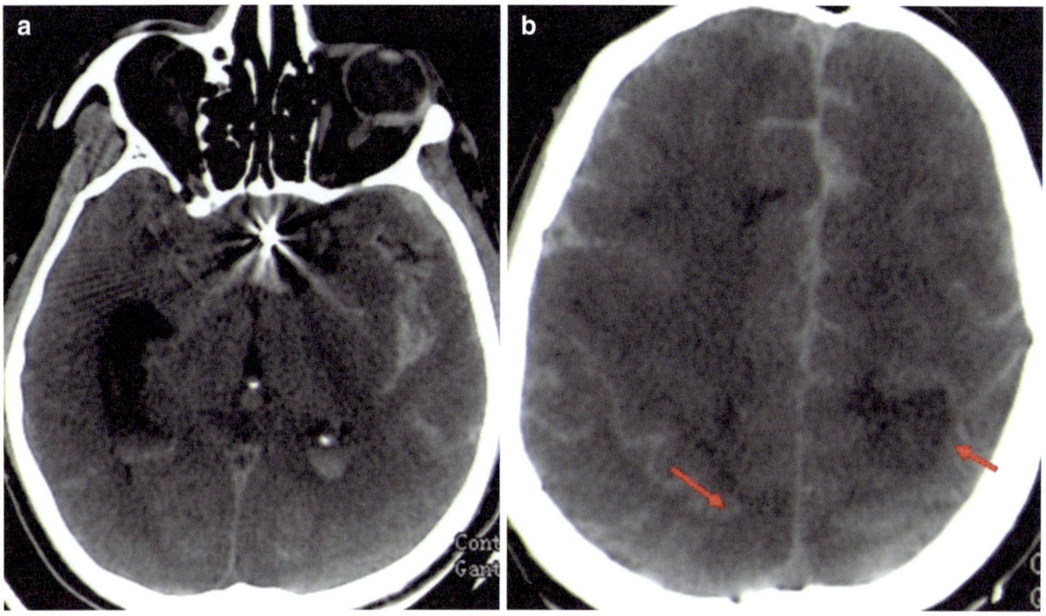

Fig. 14.11 Axial NCCT head shows Fisher grade 4 subarachnoid hemorrhage due ruptured Acom aneurysm. Coil mass with artifacts seen in situ (**a**). NCCT head was performed on sixth day from the ictus. Multiple hypodensities suggestive of infarcts noted in bilateral cerebral hemispheres due to vasospasm (**b**)

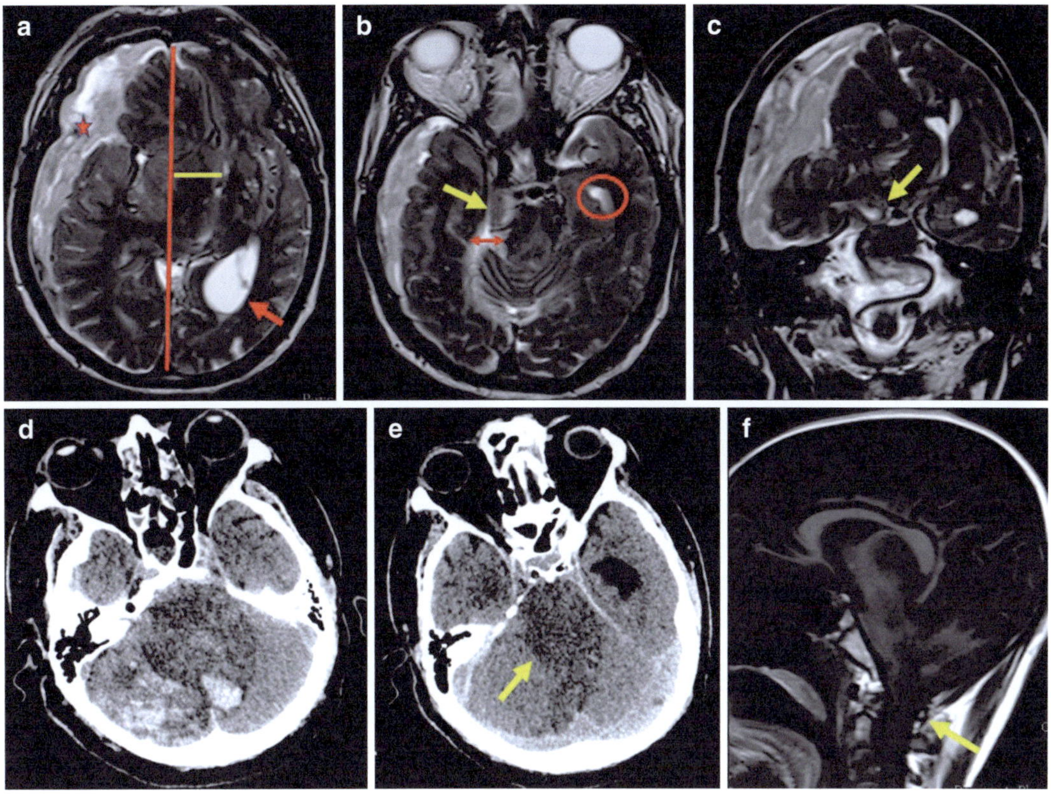

Fig. 14.12 Subfalcine herniation. Axial T2W image (**a**) shows a right subdural hematoma with mixed signal intensity that represents different blood stages (star). The hematoma results in significant midline shift toward left side. (yellow line). The right lateral ventricle is compressed, but the left lateral ventricle is dilated (arrow). T2W image axial and coronal (**b** and **c**) show the uncus displaced downward across the tentorial incisura (yellow arrow). The ipsilateral perimesencephalic cistern (double-headed arrow) is widened, and the contralateral cistern is compressed. Note the contralateral dilatation of the temporal horn of the lateral ventricle (circle). Axial CT scan (**d** and **e**) shows right cerebellar bleed with ascending transtentorial herniation. Hypoxic ischemic encephalopathy in a young patient. Sagittal T1-weighted MR image (**f**) shows tonsillar descent (arrow) with anterior brainstem displacement and effacement of the CSF in the foramen magnum

the cingulate gyrus, below the falx cerebri. This condition may lead to various complications, such as the compression of the anterior cerebral artery that can cause acute ischemia or hydrocephalus due to the compression at the foramen of Monro (Fig. 14.12a).

Transtentorial herniation presents as either unilateral or bilateral and occurs when the brain crosses the tentorium at the level of the incisura or notch. This condition has multiple subtypes:

- **Uncal herniation:** It involves the displacement of the medial portion of the anterior temporal lobe, known as the uncus, into the suprasellar cistern. This displacement leads to the effacement of the ambient cisterns and potential complications such as compression of the posterior cerebral artery or brainstem (Fig. 14.12b, c).
- **Descending transtentorial herniation**: Small hemorrhages called duret hemorrhages may be observed in the medulla or pons in this case scenario.
- **Ascending/upward transtentorial herniation:** It occurs when a cerebellar hemisphere crosses the tentorium at the level of the incisura or notch (Fig. 14.12d, e).

Extracranial/transcranial brain herniation may occur following an open calvarial fracture due to trauma or after a decompressive hemicraniectomy in cases of elevated intracranial pressure, such as after a middle cerebral artery stroke.

Cerebellar tonsillar herniation is manifested as crowding at foramen magnum due to descent of the cerebellar tonsils. However, the presence of low-lying cerebellar tonsils extending through the foramen magnum does not necessarily indicate acute brain herniation. This finding can also be caused by other conditions such as Chiari I malformation, idiopathic intracranial hypertension, or cerebrospinal fluid (CSF) hypotension and also seen in brain dead patient (Fig. 14.12f) [38].

4. **Hydrocephalus**

   Hydrocephalus is a condition characterized by the active distension of the ventricular system, resulting from the inadequate flow of cerebrospinal fluid (CSF) from its point of origin to the site of absorption. Hydrocephalus can be classified as either communicating or non-communicating/obstructive. Communicating hydrocephalus involves the enlargement of all ventricles, while non-communicating hydrocephalus affects only the ventricles located proximal to an obstruction within the ventricular system. Periventricular edema observed on CT and MR is a characteristic feature of acute or uncompensated hydrocephalus. In patients with known or suspected hydrocephalus, NCCT head is typically the initial imaging modality used. In cases where a shunt is present, the portions of the shunt hardware that are visible on CT and MR imaging should be thoroughly examined for any discontinuities. It is important to also monitor for the development of subdural hygroma on CT or MRI as a potential sequelae of overdrainage (Fig. 14.13). Hydrocephalus is a frequently occurring complication in patients with SAH. Several risk factors may predispose individuals to hydrocephalus, including a poor Hunt–Hess grade, intraventricular hemorrhage, a history of hypertension, and aneurysm rupture in the posterior circulation, which can obstruct the fourth ventricle. Hydrocephalus is also a commonly encountered condition following decompressive craniectomy for refractory intracranial hypertension in patients with traumatic brain injury (TBI) and SAH and poses significant

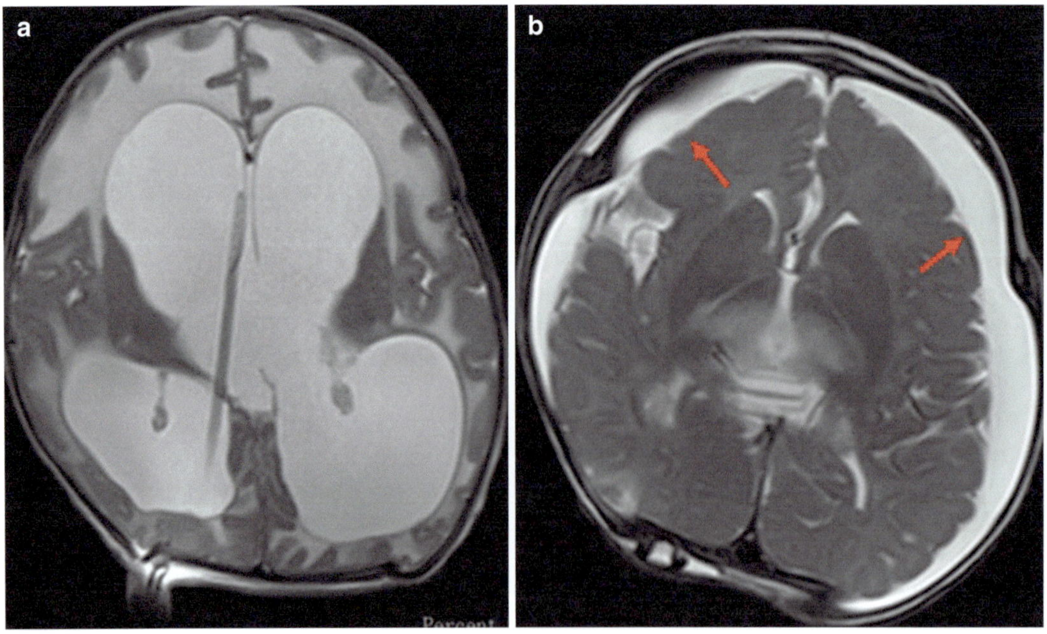

Fig. 14.13 (**a** and **b**) CSF overshunting-associated bilateral subdural hematoma (arrows)

diagnostic challenges to neurocritical care physicians [39, 40].

5. **Central Nervous System Infections/ Inflammatory Conditions**

   Diagnosing intracranial infections such as meningtis, encephalitis, and focal abscess can be difficult and is a major concern for patients in the ICU. These infections can cause alterations in mental status, which may require ICU hospitalization or can develop in patients who are already hospitalized for other reasons. In the emergency setting, most cases of infections in the central nervous system (CNS) are caused by bacteria or viruses, while fungal or parasitic etiologies are less frequently encountered [41]. Meningitis can have a spontaneous onset or be iatrogenic, such as after intracranial or spinal surgery. When there is suspicion of meningitis, initial imaging usually involves a noncontrast CT scan of the head. Although this scan has low sensitivity for detecting intracranial infections, it can help rule out masses and hemorrhage and assess for any mass effect. In some cases of infection, edema may be visible on the CT scan. Although CSF analysis is considered the "gold standard" for diagnosing bacterial meningitis, MR imaging of the brain with contrast is often the preferred method of imaging for intracranial infections, as it has high sensitivity and specificity for detecting abnormalities in the brain and meninges. Meningitis can be identified through various imaging findings, including enhancement of the leptomeninges, brain swelling, hydrocephalus, and changes in the intensity of cerebrospinal fluid (CSF) on T1 and fluid-attenuated inversion recovery (FLAIR) imaging (Fig. 14.14). In severe cases, the CSF may appear hyperintense on T1 and fail to suppress on FLAIR, often observed in the prepontine cistern and cerebral sulci. Meningitis may also advance to involve the CSF in the ventricles, leading to ventriculitis. Additional signs of a severe condition may include hyperintensity on FLAIR, restricted diffusion (suggestive of pus), and

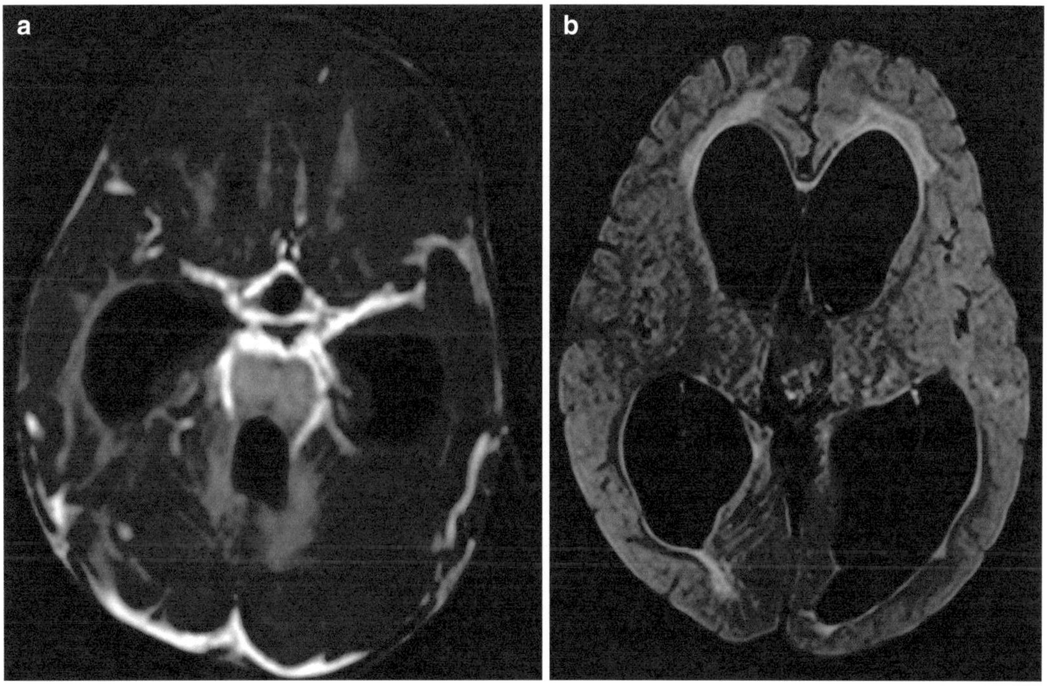

Fig. 14.14 T1W Postcontrast and FLAIR images (**a** and **b**) show thick basal meningeal enhancement with associated hydrocephalus as a sequelae of meningitis

periventricular edema or enhancement. To increase sensitivity for leptomeningeal disease, performing post-contrast fluid-attenuated inversion recovery (FLAIR) imaging can be helpful. Abnormal imaging enhancement centered on the basal cisterns, prepontine cisterns, and sylvian fissures may indicate basal meningitis, which suggests uncommon causes like tuberculosis, fungi, or sarcoidosis [42, 43]. Encephalitis refers to an intracranial infection involving the brain tissue, which can affect the cerebral hemispheres (cerebritis) or the cerebellum, presenting as abnormal T2/FLAIR hyperintensity and swelling. Cerebritis of the medial temporal lobes, whether unilateral or bilateral, requires differential diagnosis, including herpes encephalitis (Fig. 14.15). Limbic encephalitis is an immune-mediated encephalitis that sometimes accompanies systemic malignancy and has an appearance similar to herpes encephalitis, but it does not typically show enhancement. Patients suspected of having limbic encephalitis should undergo evaluation

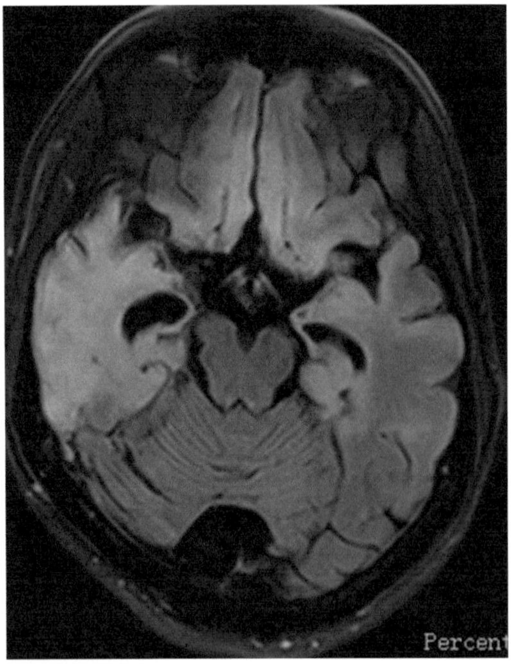

Fig. 14.15 Herpes simplex encephalitis. Bilateral fronto-temporal hyperintensities with gyral swelling on FLAIR sequence

for systemic malignancies [44, 45]. An abscess is an intracranial infection that has been contained within a single location or compartment. Pyogenic parenchymal abscess is identified by one or more fluid collections with a central region of reduced diffusion encased by a wall exhibiting T2 hypointensity and post-contrast enhancement (Fig. 14.16). Abscesses along the ventricular margin may have a thinner wall and can rupture into the ventricles, leading to ventriculitis. Multiple abscesses indicate a central source of infection, such as endocarditis or bacteremia [43]. Infections caused by nonbacterial agents, such as toxoplasmosis, may display a similar appearance, but usually lack abnormal diffusion. Abscesses located outside of the brain parenchyma, typically in the epidural space (empyema) or subdural space, are frequently associated with the local spread of infection from frontal sinusitis or mastoiditis. Their imaging characteristics are comparable, featuring a central area of reduced diffusion and a surrounding thick rim of enhancement. Epidural empyema may lead to a serious complication of dural venous sinus thrombosis [42, 43, 46]. Neurocysticercosis can lead to seizures and neurological impairments, and the imaging results are influenced by the infection's stage, the number of lesions, and the host's inflammatory reaction upon presentation. The vesicular stage demonstrates a thin-walled cyst that closely resembles cerebrospinal fluid. The scolex is most distinctly visible on MRI, appearing as a nodular "dot in a hole." In the colloidal vesicular stage, the cyst exhibits an enhancing wall and significant surrounding edema. Cerebral edema decreases during the granular nodular stage. The nodular calcified (inactive) stage is identifiable by a small calcified nodule, which is more clearly visible on CT than MRI [43].

Tuberculosis is the most widespread neurological infection in our country, and it can present with various manifestations, including acute meningitis, tuberculoma, abscess, vasculitis, infarction, and hydrocephalus. On FLAIR imaging, exudates in the sulcal spaces

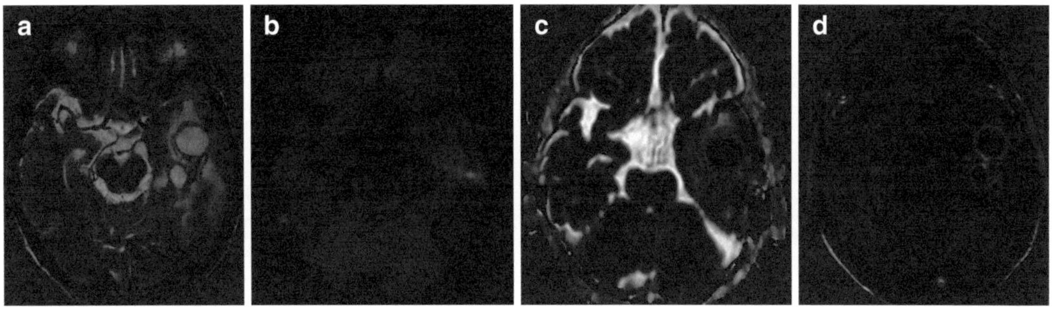

Fig. 14.16 A case of cerebral abscesses. A 55 year old man with odontogenic infections presenting with headache and two episode of seizures. T2W sequence (**a**) shows multiple cystic lesion in left temporal lobe with surrounding perilesional edema. DWI and ADC image (**b** and **c**) has central hyperintensity compatible with pus. Postcontrast T1 (**d**) shows peripheral rim enhancement compatible with abscesses

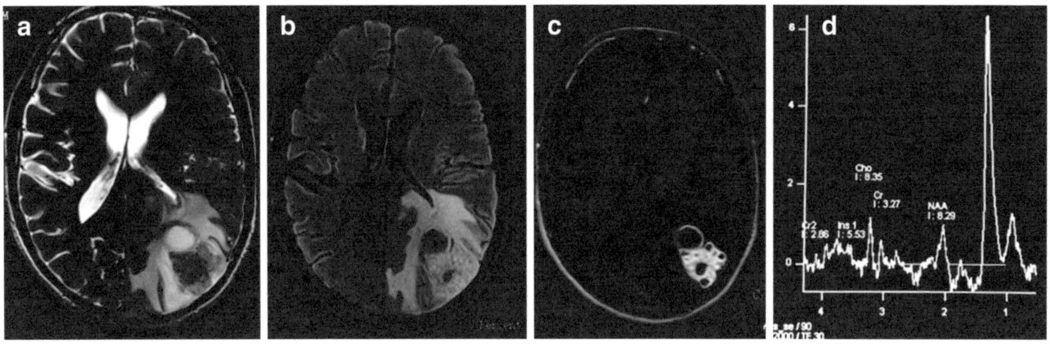

Fig. 14.17 Multiple tuberculoma in the left parietal region. Multiple conglomerate solid and cystic lesion noted in left parietal region with significant perilesional edema (T2W and FLAIR) (**a** and **b** respectively). Multiple ring enhancing lesion on T1W postcontrast (**c**). MR spectroscopy (**d**) at the site of lesion shows increased lipid peak

and basal cisterns display hyperintensity along with nodular and thick enhancement of the basal cisterns, sylvian fissure, and meninges. TB abscesses are typically hyperintense on T2-weighted/FLAIR imaging, with a T2-weighted hypointense enhancing ring that resembles pyogenic abscesses. Elevated lipid peaks on MR spectroscopy are observed due to the high lipid content of the mycolic acid within the bacteria (Fig. 14.17) [7, 43].

6. **Postsurgical Complications**

   Individuals undergoing intracranial procedures are susceptible to both early (i.e., less than 48 h) and late (lasting for days to weeks) complications. After a neurosurgery, alterations in cognitive function are typically examined using noncontrast CT scans, while magnetic resonance imaging (MRI) might be utilized subsequently if required. Direct injury during a procedure can cause early complications such as hemorrhage or infarction. Patients who undergo the removal of highly vascular masses like glioblastoma or metastases of breast, thyroid, renal, or melanoma are at higher risk of hemorrhage. Parenchymal arterial supply or draining veins can get damaged, leading to infarction that can be recognized by hypodensity and loss of gray-white differentiation on CT scans or areas of reduced diffusion on MR imaging, which can appear close to or distant from the resection area. While some devitalized tissues surrounding the resection bed are normal, larger or focal areas of restricted diffusion located near or distant from the resection bed are a cause of concern. Resection cavity may contain gelfoam, hemorrhage, or air (Fig. 14.18). Occasionally, venous occlusion

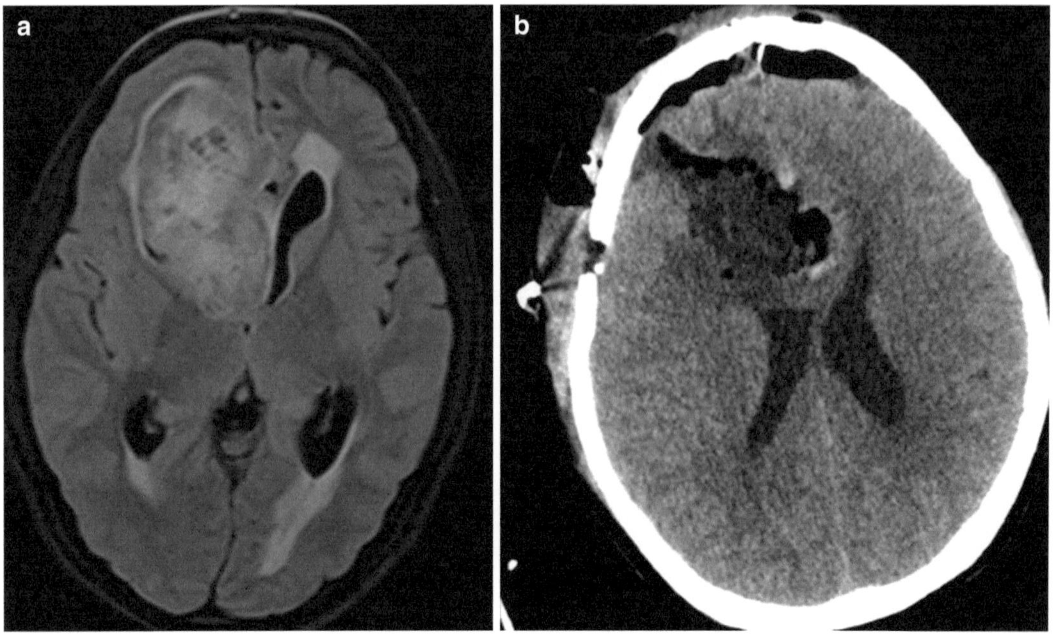

Fig. 14.18 MRI, FLAIR sequence (**a**) shows a supratentorial ependymoma. CT head (**b**) shows frontal craniotomy and excision of previously seen mass. Postoperative changes are seen in overlying scalp with air locules and subgaleal hemorrhages. Extra-axial collection mixed with hemorrhage and air foci is noted. In addition, postoperative large cavity with air foci and gel foam packing is also noted

and resulting infarction can also take place (Fig. 14.19) [47]. Another postoperative complication that is less frequent but still significant is tension pneumocephalus. This occurs when air from the sinuses or surrounding environment is drawn into the intracranial space and then trapped by a ball valve mechanism [48]. Delayed postsurgical complication such as intracranial infection can also occur. Thrombolytic treatment, which includes intravenous tissue plasminogen activator and intra-arterial interventions, can result in hemorrhagic complications that are best assessed with noncontrast CT scans. In cases where intravenous contrast leaks from abnormal vessels in the region, a phenomenon known as contrast staining occurs. This obscures the areas of infarction and mimics hemorrhage. However, contrast staining is less dense than hemorrhage and is limited to the anatomic areas of infarction. Within 24 h, it significantly decreases in density (Fig. 14.20). Stroke patients should be further evaluated using brain MR imaging, including diffusion and FLAIR, to identify infarction [49, 50]. Patients with brain tumors, including primary tumors and metastases, are prone to complications such as intracranial hemorrhage, in addition to the surgical complications discussed earlier. Another significant complication experienced by patients with tumors is the worsening of mass effect, which can lead to herniation, hydrocephalus, and ventricular entrapment. NCCT head is usually sufficient to assess tumor complications, but contrast-enhanced MR imaging (CEMRI) may be required to determine the extent of the tumor [2]. Postprocedure ischemia is a significant concern in ICU patients and can range from punctate infarcts to diffuse hypoxic injury. While CT may be useful as an initial screening tool, MR imaging with diffusion is often required to assess small infarcts and subtle indications of diffuse hypoxia. Small infarcts may not be visible on CT scans, whereas more widespread damage can manifest as brain swelling, loss of gray-white differentiation, and parenchymal hypodensities.

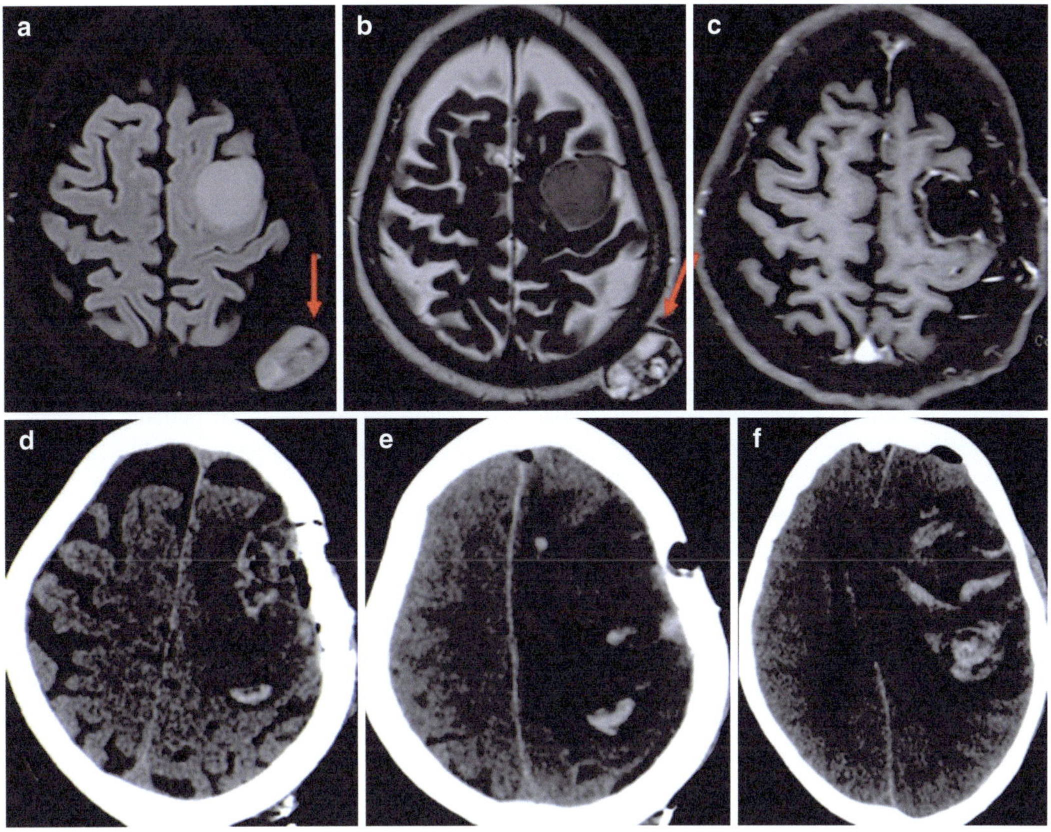

Fig. 14.19 There is a well-defined extra-axial lesion in left frontal region which shows hyperintense signal on FLAIR sequence (**a**) and hypointense signal on T2W image (**b**). Incidental trichilemmal cyst in left parietal region (arrow in **a** and **b**). Post contrast T1W image (**c**) after the resection of meningioma and trichilemmal cyst shows no residual lesion. NCCT head (**d**) reveals postoperative changes with air, mild edema, and hemorrhage on day 1. Patient became comatose on day 2. There is interval increase in the edema and hemorrhage in left cerebral hemisphere with significant midline shift toward left side (**e** and **f**). These findings are consistent with venous hemorrhagic infarct

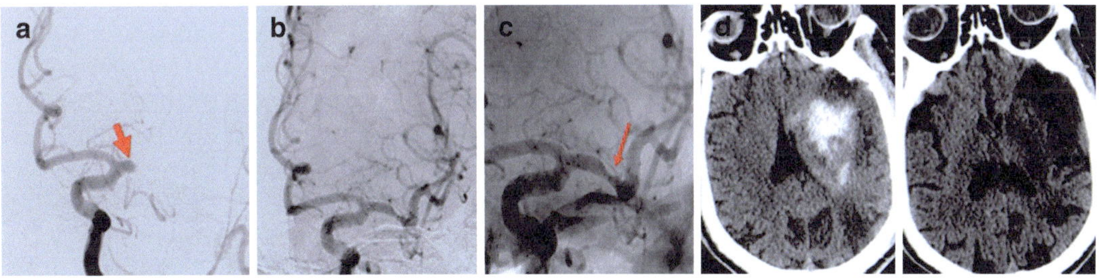

Fig. 14.20 Catheter angiography shows left middle cerebral artery occlusion (**a**). Endovascular clot removal was performed with stent retriever device (**b**). Underlying intracranial atherosclerotic disease was treated with stent deployment (**b** and **c**). Post operative 24 h CT shows hyperdensity in left ganglio-capsular region (**d**). Postoperative CT after 48 h shows resolution of contrast staining (**e**)

MR imaging findings, on the other hand, can include abnormal diffusion in areas that are sensitive to oxygen deprivation, such as the basal ganglia and cortex. Detecting diffuse hypoxic injury can be challenging because the findings are typically subtle and bilaterally symmetric [51]. Intracranial complications can result from spine procedures as well. Hemorrhages can occur in areas that are spatially distant from the surgical site due to shifts in cerebrospinal fluid (CSF) during intradural procedures. This process often leads to a remote cerebellar hemorrhage, after spinal surgery. Similar findings have been observed after surgeries within the intracranial compartment. It is recommended to search for associated dural sinus thrombosis, which can cause hemorrhagic venous infarction. Delayed postoperative complications, typically occurring from 2 days to weeks after the procedure, include a distinct set of conditions. Postoperative hemorrhage is still a possibility, but its likelihood decreases with time [52]. Postoperative infections typically weeks to months after surgery. Findings are similar to other infections of the neural axis, such as meningitis, encephalitis, and abscess, with the site of infection usually centered around the surgical site. Imaging techniques such as diffusion-weighted imaging (DWI) and post-contrast MR imaging are crucial, as focal sites of infection frequently appear hyperintense on DWI. However, postoperative blood products are also hyperintense on DWI, mimicking infection and making imaging interpretation difficult. It is possible to have a combination of both blood and infection. Postoperative infection should be suspected in cases such as increasing fluid collection, DWI hyperintensity exceeding suspected blood products on T1 and gradient-weighted imaging, increasing mass effect, and worsening edema within the parenchyma or soft tissues [53]. Another late complication that can arise after intracranial surgery is the sunken (skin) flap syndrome, which can occur after craniectomy. This condition is characterized by a paradoxical mass effect, with the midline shifting away from the side of the craniectomy [54].

7. **Immunocompromised Patients**

   Immunocompromised patients are at risk of experiencing various neurological issues, such as uncommon infections (e.g., fungal diseases, tuberculosis, and toxoplasmosis) and lymphoma. Moreover, imaging results may differ in immunocompromised and immunocompetent individuals. For instance, HIV patients with CNS lymphoma may exhibit a more diverse appearance and a lack of typical solid nodular enhancement seen in immunocompetent patients [55]. In immunocompromised patients, a rare but severe virus-mediated demyelinating syndrome known as progressive multifocal encephalopathy may occur, with characteristic imaging findings including progressively worsening bilateral white matter abnormalities that appear T1 hypointense and T2/FLAIR hyperintense and lack of post-contrast enhancement (Fig. 14.21). Furthermore, immunocompromised patients are particularly vulnerable to

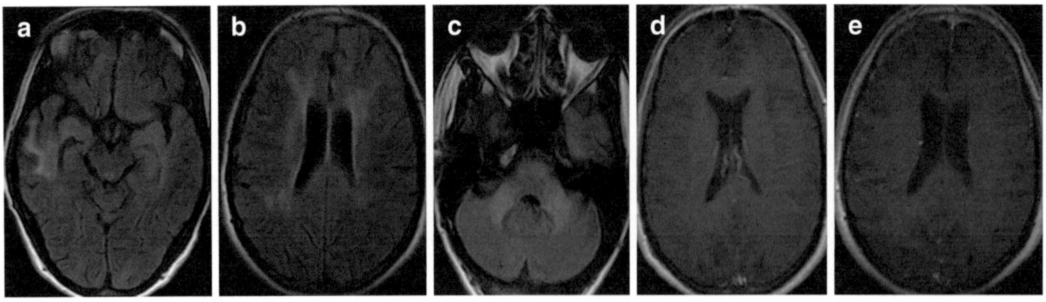

Fig. 14.21 Axial FLAIR images (**a**–**c**) shows hyperintensity of bilateral periventricular white matter, white matter of right temporal lobe and of bilateral middle cerebellar peduncles. Postcontrast T1W images (**d** and **e**) shows no enhancement of lesions

sinus diseases, notably invasive fungal sinusitis (IFS). Emergency MR imaging is often the preferred imaging modality, revealing findings such as nonenhancing nasal mucosa, enhancement/invasion outside of the sinus affecting structures such as retroantral and/or orbital fat, and likely intracranial enhancement along the leptomeninges and cavernous sinus. In immunocompromised patients, routine CT scans are advisable for identifying manifestations of IFS, particularly when fever and neutropenia are present [56].

8. **Metabolic/Toxic**

Metabolic or toxic conditions often exhibit bilaterally symmetric involvement of the basal ganglia. For example, patients with hepatic encephalopathy may display hepatocerebral degeneration, with symmetric T1 hyperintensities in the basal ganglia [57]. In Wernicke encephalopathy, caused by thiamine deficiency, imaging may reveal symmetric T2 hyperintense abnormalities in the basal ganglia, thalamus, and the tissue surrounding the cerebral aqueduct, with involvement of the mammillary bodies being a strong indication [58, 59]. Reversible Posterior Leukoencephalopathy Syndrome (PRES) refers to a neurotoxic state that can occur when the posterior circulation of the brain fails to autoregulate in response to acute changes in blood pressure. This results in hyperperfusion, which disrupts the blood–brain barrier and leads to the development of vasogenic edema, typically without infarction. The areas of the brain most commonly affected are the parietal and occipital lobes, followed by the frontal lobes and cerebellum. Additionally, the brain stem and basal ganglia may also be affected. Imaging studies reveal the presence of vasogenic edema, which is symmetric and reversible on follow-up imaging, in the affected locations. The affected areas appear hyperintense on T2W/FLAIR imaging, do not enhance with contrast, and do not show diffusion restriction (Fig. 14.22). However, atypical cases may exhibit post-contrast enhancement of adjacent cortical vessels and restricted diffusion [7].

Osmotic demyelination, which is an inflammatory condition, can occur when there are serum osmolality abnormalities, particularly rapid correction of low sodium levels. Central pontine myelinolysis, a type of osmotic demyelination, is associated with bilaterally symmetric T2 hyperintense demyelinating lesions in the pons, and extrapontine myelinolysis may be seen in the basal ganglia and subcortical white matter (Fig. 14.23) [57]. Glucose abnormalities, such as severe hypoglycemia and hyperglycemia, are frequent in ICU patients. Seizures may accompany very low blood sugar, with subtle T2 hyperintensities in the basal ganglia and cortex being the more common MRI findings. On the other hand, marked hyperglycemia, particularly nonketotic acidosis,

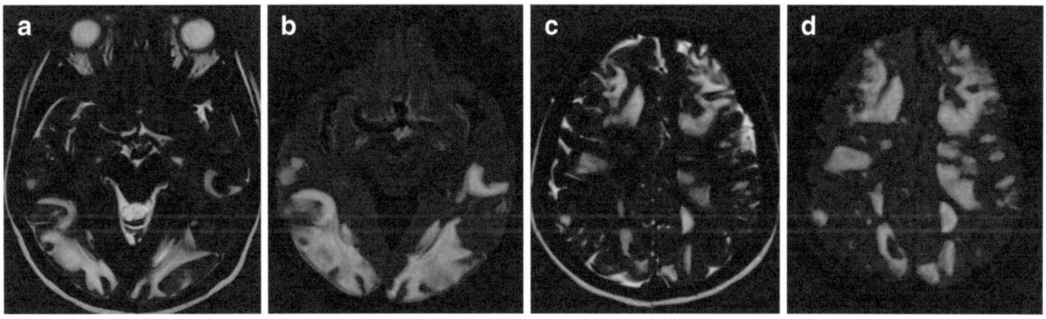

Fig. 14.22 Posterior reversible encephalopathy syndrome. T2W (**a**) and FLAIR (**b**) Symmetrical hyperintensity in parieto-occipital subcortical white matter. T2W (**c**) and FLAIR (**d**) Moderate vasogenic edema also noted in the subcortical white matter of the frontal and parietal regions

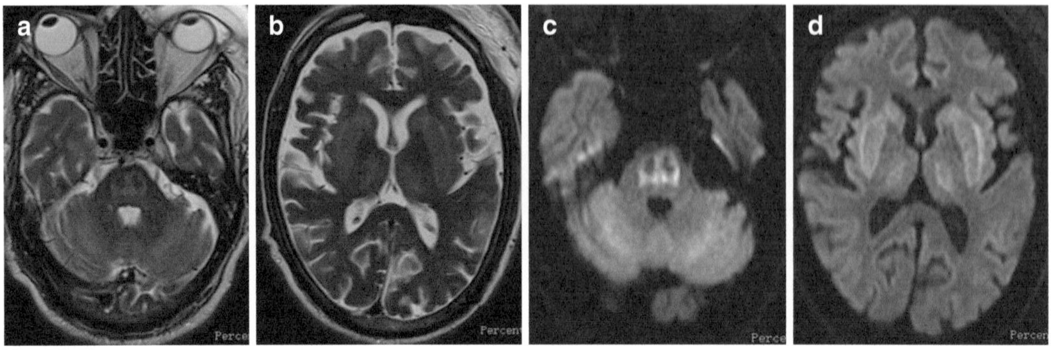

Fig. 14.23 Central pontine and extrapontine myelinolysis. (**a** and **b**) T2W hyperintense signal in central part of pons with symmetrical lesions involving basal ganglia and thalami. The peripheral fibers of pons are spared (**c** and **d**) DWI shows intense diffusion restriction

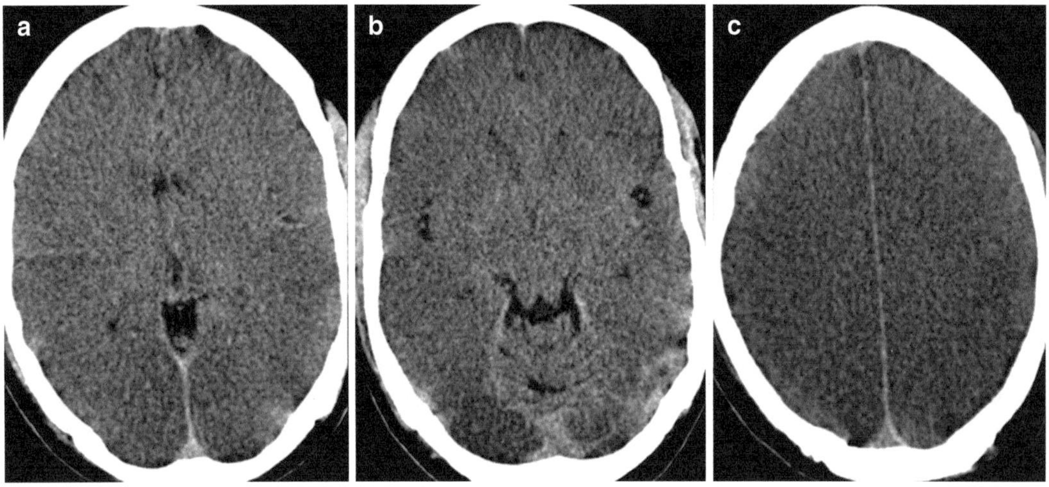

Fig. 14.24 NCCT Head (**a**–**c**). A 23-year-old man brought unconscious in emergency with history multiple drug abuse. He had poor Glasgow coma scale and was intubated urgently. CT head shows hypodensities in bilateral basal ganglia and diffuse cerebral oedema with loss of grey and white matter differentiation. Effacement of basal cistern and cortical sulci is also noted. There is high attenuation of tentorium and falx

has its own imaging findings of T1 hyperintensities in the basal ganglia. MRI findings of both hypoglycemia and hyperglycemia can be reversible. In general, toxic or metabolic abnormalities should be considered whenever symmetric brain abnormalities are detected. Sometimes, drug abuse patients who have experienced hypoxic-ischemic brain damage may exhibit diffuse cerebral edema on CT scans (Fig. 14.24) [60].

9. **Spine Imaging in ICU**

   Imaging of the spine is performed in ICU patients if there is suspicion of infection, specifically bacterial discitis osteomyelitis. CT imaging is not ideal for this purpose due to the overlap between imaging findings of degenerative changes and infection. In this context, MR imaging is typically preferred over CT. Spinal infections typically originate in the disk and spread to adjacent bone, with imaging findings including abnormal fluid signal within the disk and surrounding soft tissues, abnormal enhancement, and paraspinal or epidural abscess. Tuberculous osteomyelitis is also a possibility and should be considered in patients with relevant risk factors and spinal osteomyelitis with relative sparing of the underlying disk. Postoperative complications in the spine may include hematoma and infection [61]. Postoperative hematoma can lead to compression of the remaining spinal canal, and CT is typically the first performed in such cases, although hematoma may be difficult to visualize, especially in the presence of surgical hardware. MR imaging is often superior to CT in evaluating postoperative hematoma, although it may be degraded by metallic artifacts. In the days to weeks following surgical intervention, postoperative fluid collections in the surgical bed and epidural space may cause complications. Postoperative seroma, evolving hematoma, and abscess typically appear as T2 hyperintense fluid collections within the surgical bed. Intravenous contrast can be useful, as abscess typically has more robust surrounding enhancement and enhancement of the descending nerve roots or spinal cord which may indicate infectious arachnoiditis. DWI is an excellent sequence to detect abscess. It shows diffusion restriction and appears more hyperintense than the spinal cord on DW [2, 61]. Spinal cord infarction is a rare but serious complication of surgeries, particularly aortic repair and long-segment fusions involving the thoracic spine. Spinal cord infarction is characterized by long-segment T2 hyperintensity MRI that may involve the complete, central, and ventral portions of the cord cross section. A dorsal location of spinal cord infarction is uncommon [62].

14.4 Summary

In conclusion, performing neuroimaging on ICU patients may appear challenging, but it can be managed by being aware of the typical pathology and complications observed in these patients.

References

1. Hollingsworth TD, Duszak R Jr, Vijayasarathi A, et al. Trainee knowledge of imaging appropriateness and safety: results of a series of surveys from a large academic medical center. Curr Probl Diagn Radiol. 2019;48(1):17–21.
2. Gadde JA, Weinberg BD, Mullins ME. Neuroimaging of patients in the intensive care unit: pearls and pitfalls. Radiol Clin North Am. 2020;58(1):167–85.
3. ACR appropriateness criteria. Radiology ACo In: 2019. https://www.acr.org/Clinical-Resources/ACR-Appropriateness-Criteria.
4. Mutch CA, Talbott JF, Gean A. Imaging evaluation of acute traumatic brain injury. Neurosurg Clin N Am. 2016;27(4):409–39.
5. de Lucas EM, Sa'nchez E, Gutierrez A, et al. CT protocol for acute stroke: tips and tricks for general radiologists. Radiographics. 2008;28(6):1673–87.
6. Mangla S, Chaloopka JC, Huddle DC. Early clinical experience with a dedicated portable computer tomography scanner in a biplane neuroangiography suite: assessment of feasibility and utility in neurointerventional practice. Interv Neuroradiol. 2000;6(3):211–20.
7. Patra A, Janu A, Sahu A. MR imaging in Neurocritical care. Indian J Crit Care Med. 2019;23(Suppl 2):S104–14.
8. Webb JA, Thomsen HS, Morcos SK. The use of iodinated and gadolinium contrast media during pregnancy and lactation. Eur Radiol. 2005;15(6):1234–40.
9. Mohindra N, Neyaz Z. Magnetic resonance sequences: Practical neurological applications. Neurol India. 2015;63(2):241–9.
10. Aurangzeb A, Ahmed E, Afridi EA, et al. Frequency of extradural hematoma in patients with linear skull fracture. J Ayub Med Coll Abbottabad. 2015;27(2):314–7.
11. Currie S, Saleem N, Straiton JA, et al. Imaging assessment of traumatic brain injury. Postgrad Med J. 2016;92(1083):41–50.
12. Mittl RL, Grossman RI, Hiehle JF, et al. Prevalence of MR evidence of diffuse axonal injury in patients with mild head injury and normal head CT findings. AJNR Am J Neuroradiol. 1994;15(8):1583–9.
13. Edlow JA, Caplan LR. Avoiding pitfalls in the diagnosis of subarachnoid hemorrhage. N Engl J Med. 2000;342(01):29–36.
14. Young LA, Rule GT, Bocchieri RT, Burns JM. Biophysical mechanisms of traumatic brain injuries. Semin Neurol. 2015;35(01):5–11.
15. Diouf A, Machnowska M. Conventional MR imaging in trauma management in adults. Neuroimaging Clin N Am. 2023;33(2):235–49.
16. Gentry LR. Imaging of closed head injury. Radiology. 1994;191(1):1–17.
17. Abu Hamdeh S, Marklund N, Lannsjo M, et al. Extended anatomical grading in diffuse axonal injury using MRI: hemorrhagic lesions in the substantia Nigra and mesencephalic tegmentum indicate poor long-term outcome. J Neurotrauma. 2017;34(2):341–52.
18. Ma J, Zhang K, Wang Z, et al. Progress of research on diffuse axonal injury after traumatic brain injury. Neural Plast. 2016;2016:9746313.

19. Van Gijn J, Kerr RS, Rinkel GJ. Subarachnoid haemorrhage. Lancet. 2007;369(9558):306–18.
20. Fisher CM, Kistler JP, Davis JM. Relation of cerebral vasospasm to subarachnoid hemorrhage visualized by computerized tomographic scanning. Neurosurgery. 1980;6(01):1–9.
21. Claassen J, Bernardini GL, Kreiter K, et al. Effect of cisternal and ventricular blood on risk of delayed cerebral ischemia after subarachnoid hemorrhage: the Fisher scale revisited. Stroke. 2001;32(09):2012–20.
22. Williamson C, Morgan L, Klein JP. Imaging in neurocritical care practice. Semin Respir Crit Care Med. 2017;38(6):840–52.
23. Kidwell CS, Chalela JA, Saver JL, Starkman S, Hill MD, Demchuk AM, et al. Comparison of MRI and CT for detection of acute intracerebral hemorrhage. JAMA. 2004;292(15):1823–30.
24. Provenzale JM. CT and MR imaging of nontraumatic neurologic emergencies. Am J Roentgenol. 2000;174(2):289–99.
25. Siroos B, Harirchian MH, Kazemi Khaledi A, Ghaffarpour M, Golshani S. Cerebral hyperperfusion syndrome, an unusual but disastrous complication of carotid recanalization: a case report. J Stroke Cerebrovasc Dis. 2018;27(2):e17–9.
26. Chalela JA, Kidwell CS, Nentwich LM, Luby M, Butman JA, Demchuk AM, et al. Magnetic resonance imaging and computed tomography in emergency assessment of patients with suspected acute stroke: a prospective comparison. Lancet. 2007;369:293–8.
27. Prodi E, Danieli L, Manno C, Pagnamenta A, Pravatà E, Roccatagliata L, et al. Stroke mimics in the acute setting: role of multimodal CT protocol. AJNR Am J Neuroradiol. 2022;43(2):216–22.
28. Pressman B, Tourje E, Thompson J. An early CT sign of ischemic infarction: increased density in a cerebral artery. AJR Am J Roentgenol. 1987;149(3):583–6.
29. Mainali S, Wahba M, Elijovich L. Detection of early ischemic changes in noncontrast CT head improved with "stroke windows". ISRN Neurosci. 2014;2014:1.
30. Pexman JH, Barber PA, Hill MD, Sevick RJ, Demchuk AM, Hudon ME, et al. Use of the Alberta stroke program early CT score (ASPECTS) for assessing CT scans in patients with acute stroke. AJNR Am J Neuroradiol. 2001;22:1534–42.
31. Powers WJ, Rabinstein AA, Ackerson T, Adeoye OM, Bambakidis NC, Becker K, et al. Guidelines for the early management of patients with acute ischemic stroke: 2019 update to the 2018 guidelines for the early management of acute ischemic stroke: guideline for healthcare professionals from the American Heart Association/American Stroke Association. Stroke. 2019;50(12):e344–e41.
32. Kim HJ, Choi CG, Lee DH, Lee JH, Kim SJ, Suh DC. High-b-value diffusion-weighted MR imaging of hyperacute ischemic stroke at 1.5T. AJNR Am J Neuroradiol. 2005;26(2):208–15.
33. Srinivasan A, Goyal M, Al Azri F, Lum C. State-of-the-art imaging of acute stroke. Radiographics. 2006;26(Suppl 1):S75–95.
34. Austein F, Riedel C, Kerby T, Meyne J, Binder A, Lindner T, et al. Comparison of perfusion CT software to predict the final infarct volume after thrombectomy. Stroke. 2016;47(9):2311–7.
35. Fang H, He G, Cheng Y, Liang F, Zhu Y. Advances in cerebral perfusion imaging techniques in acute ischemic stroke. J Clin Ultrasound. 2022;50(8):1202–11.
36. Mills JN, Mehta V, Russin J, Amar AP, Rajamohan A, Mack WJ. Advanced imaging modalities in the detection of cerebral vasospasm. Neurol Res Int. 2013;2013:415960.
37. Jabbarli R, Pierscianek D, Rolz R, et al. Endovascular treatment of cerebral vasospasm after subarachnoid hemorrhage: more is more. Neurology. 2019;93:e458–66.
38. Johnson PL, Eckard DA, Chason DP, et al. Imaging of acquired cerebral herniations. Neuroimaging Clin N Am. 2002;12(2):217–28.
39. Hochstetler A, Raskin J, Blazer-Yost BL. Hydrocephalus: historical analysis and considerations for treatment. Eur J Med Res. 2022;27(1):168.
40. Papaioannou V, Czosnyka Z, Czosnyka M. Hydrocephalus and the neuro-intensivist: CSF hydrodynamics at the bedside. Intensive Care Med Exp. 2022;10(1):20.
41. Foerster BR, Thurnher MM, Malani PN, et al. Intracranial infections: clinical and imaging characteristics. Acta Radiol. 2007;48(8):875–93.
42. Jim KK, Brouwer MC, van der Ende A, et al. Cerebral abscesses in patients with bacterial meningitis. J Infect. 2012;64:236–8.
43. Duong MT, Rudie JD, Mohan S. Neuroimaging patterns of intracranial infections: meningitis, cerebritis, and their complications. Neuroimaging Clin N Am. 2023;33(1):11–41.
44. Rath TJ, Hughes M, Arabi M, et al. Imaging of cerebritis, encephalitis, and brain abscess. Neuroimaging Clin N Am. 2012;22(4):585–607.
45. Rabinstein AA. Herpes virus encephalitis in adults: current knowledge and old myths. Neurol Clin. 2017;35(4):695–705.
46. Mohan S, Jain KK, Arabi M, et al. Imaging of meningitis and ventriculitis. Neuroimaging Clin N Am. 2012;22(4):557–83.
47. Gempt J, Gerhardt J, Toth V, et al. Postoperative ischemic changes following brain metastasis resection as measured by diffusion-weighted magnetic resonance imaging. J Neurosurg. 2013;119(6):1395–400.
48. Clement AR, Palaniappan D, Panigrahi RK. Tension pneumocephalus. Anesthesiology. 2017;127(4):710.
49. Charidimou A, Turc G, Oppenheim C, et al. Microbleeds, cerebral hemorrhage, and functional outcome after stroke thrombolysis. Stroke. 2017;48(8):2084–90.
50. Amans MR, Cooke DL, Vella M, et al. Contrast staining on CT after DSA in ischemic stroke patients progresses to infarction and rarely hemorrhages. Interv Neuroradiol. 2014;20(1):106–15.

51. Muttikkal TJ, Wintermark M. MRI patterns of global hypoxic-ischemic injury in adults. J Neuroradiol. 2013;40(3):164–71.
52. Sturiale CL, Rossetto M, Ermani M, et al. Remote cerebellar hemorrhage after supratentorial procedures (part 1): a systematic review. Neurosurg Rev. 2016;39(4):565–73.
53. Dashti SR, Baharvahdat H, Spetzler RF, et al. Operative intracranial infection following craniotomy. Neurosurg Focus. 2008;24(6):E10.
54. Akins PT, Guppy KH. Sinking skin flaps, paradoxical herniation, and external brain tamponade: a review of decompressive craniectomy management. Neurocrit Care. 2008;9(2):269–76.
55. Brandsma D, Bromberg JEC. Primary CNS lymphoma in HIV infection. Handb Clin Neurol. 2018;152:177–86.
56. Horger M, Beschorner R, Beck R, et al. Common and uncommon imaging findings in progressive multifocal leukoencephalopathy (PML) with differential diagnostic considerations. Clin Neurol Neurosurg. 2012;114(8):1123–30.
57. Chokshi FH, Aygun N, Mullins ME. Imaging of acquired metabolic and toxic disorders of the basal ganglia. Semin Ultrasound CT MR. 2014;35(2):75–84.
58. Ferrara J, Jankovic J. Acquired hepatocerebral degeneration. J Neurol. 2009;256(3):320–32.
59. Manzo G, De Gennaro A, Cozzolino A, et al. MR imaging findings in alcoholic and nonalcoholic acute Wernicke's encephalopathy: a review. Biomed Res Int. 2014;2014:503596.
60. Bathla G, Hegde AN. MRI and CT appearances in metabolic encephalopathies due to systemic diseases in adults. Clin Radiol. 2013;68(6):545–54.
61. Jain NK, Dao K, Ortiz AO. Radiologic evaluation and management of postoperative spine paraspinal fluid collections. Neuroimaging Clin N Am. 2014;24(2):375–89.
62. Yadav N, Pendharkar H, Kulkarni GB. Spinal cord infarction: clinical and radiological features. J Stroke Cerebrovasc Dis. 2018;27(10):2810–21.

Brain Ultrasonography

15

Erika J. Sigman, Fahad J. Laghari, and Aarti Sarwal

15.1 Introduction

Ultrasonography is becoming increasingly accessible and widely used by practitioners to complement the physical exam and gain a better understanding of patient's physiology in critical care. The portable nature allows expeditious real-time information at point of care to improve clinical diagnostic accuracy, especially patients who are unstable and thus not safe to be transported for other advanced imaging modalities such as computed tomography (CT). It is noninvasive and without risk of radiation. While ultrasound of thorax, abdomen, and pelvis has become prevalent in critical care, brain ultrasound, also referred to as transcranial sonography or brain echography, is being increasingly used to explore intracranial pathology to aid in the diagnostics and management of critically ill patients.

Brain ultrasound has been used in pediatrics for over 50 years as a primary diagnostic imaging modality to assess the brain parenchyma and ventricular system via patent fontanels, given the critical need for avoiding radiation in this age group. Adult applications of brain ultrasound were introduced in the 1970s, with later studies exploring identification of intracranial hemorrhage as well as pathology of the ventricular system [1–3]. These applications were soon overshadowed by computed tomography (CT) and magnetic resonance imaging. With increasing survival of critically ill patients with advanced resuscitation techniques, the widespread availability of ultrasound equipment and the emergence of point-of-care ultrasound (POCUS), there has been a resurgence of interest in the evaluation of brain pathology at the bedside, otherwise known as cranial ultrasound (c-POCUS). c-POCUS is especially suitable for unstable critically ill patients unable to be transported to the CT. In this chapter, we will review the fundamentals of brain ultrasound image acquisition and various clinical applications in assessing structural brain pathology such as intracranial hemorrhage, midline shift, hydrocephalus, and postoperative evaluation. In addition, we will review orbital ultrasound for noninvasive intracranial pressure assessment via optic nerve sheath diameter measurement and papilledema detection.

E. J. Sigman
Emory University School of Medicine,
Atlanta, GA, USA
e-mail: esigman@emory.edu

F. J. Laghari
University of Rochester School of Medicine,
Rochester, NY, USA

A. Sarwal (✉)
Wake Forest University School of Medicine,
Winston-Salem, NC, USA
e-mail: asarwal@wakehealth.edu

H. Prabhakar et al. (eds.), *Principles and Practice of Neurocritical Care*,
https://doi.org/10.1007/978-981-99-8059-8_15

15.2 Principles of Brain Ultrasound

B mode ultrasound utilizing a low-frequency phase-array probe (1–3 MHz range) is used to assess brain topography using the Transcranial Doppler (TCD) preset utilizing the temporal window. An optimal preset for B mode cranial imaging is unfortunately not commercially available, and the TCD preset optimized for vascular imaging is the closest. In the absence of a TCD preset or in patients with hemicraniectomy, the abdominal preset should be used. The probe, with the index marker facing the patient's eyes, is placed on the temporal bone. The theoretical insonation line is positioned from the lateral canthus to the tragus to allow an axial section of brain to be imaged. The depth should be adjusted until the contralateral skull is seen, identified by the hyperechoic convex structure in the far field. The temporal bone is thin enough in 80–90% of adults to provide an acoustic window to the brain, albeit with some beam attenuation and distortion [4]. If a particular tissue reflects sound, it will appear hyperechoic or bright white; conversely, tissues are hypoechoic or gray, when they reflect less sound or absorb the ultrasound. Brain parenchyma is normally gray or hypoechoic. White matter has higher attenuation than gray matter, but cranial topographic studies have failed to demonstrate the ability to reliably distinguish between parenchyma structure such as gyri and sulci or white and gray matter using currently available presets. Suboccipital windows traditionally used in vertebrobasilar insonation in TCD only yield the imaging of foramen magnum and have not been explored for local pathology.

Due to artifacts from the ipsilateral skull convexity formed by petrous part of the temporal bone and lesser wing of sphenoid outlining the middle cranial fossa, there is limited interpretation of the ipsilateral brain parenchyma. Cranial details are better discernible in the contralateral brain. Skeletal landmarks of the skull base as well as many other key structures can be identified by transcranial ultrasound (Figs. 15.1, 15.2 and 15.3)

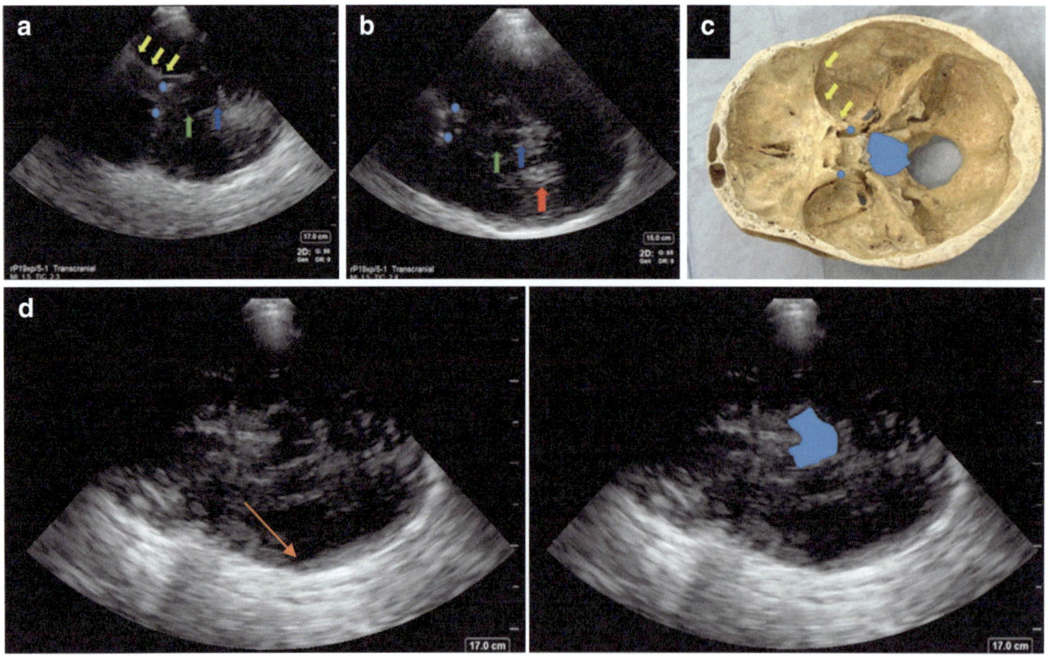

Fig. 15.1 B mode transcranial images with indicated anatomical landmarks. (**a**, **b**) B mode transcranial ultrasound images showing sphenoid wing (yellow arrows), clinoid processes (blue dots), midbrain (green arrow), basal cisterns (blue arrow), and choroid plexus situated in the temporal horn of lateral ventricle (red arrow). (**c**) is the corresponding view of the skull base from the top; the blue butterfly shape represents the location of midbrain, clinoid processes (blue dots), sphenoid wing [yellow arrows (**d**) midbrain (blue butterfly shape)] and hyperechoic curved linear structure showing the skull contralateral to insonation (orange arrow)

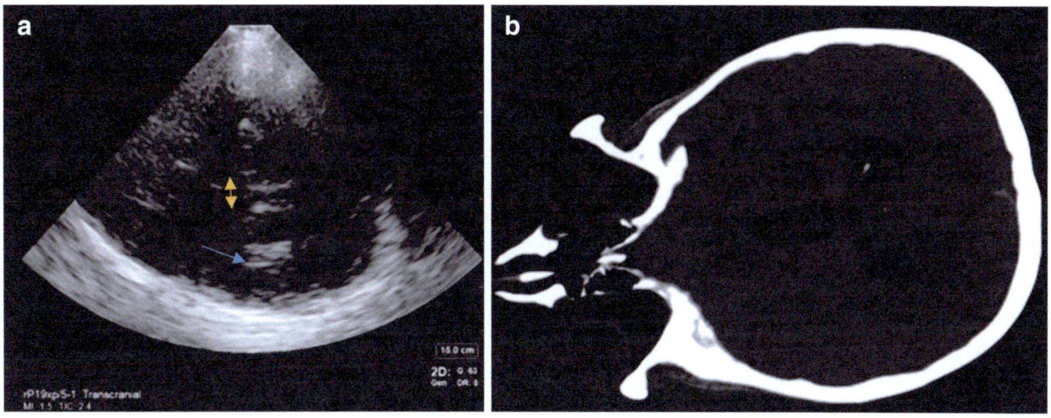

Fig. 15.2 Comparison of B mode imaging to CT in patient with hydrocephalus. (**a**) Transcranial B mode ultrasound of a patient with hydrocephalus: hypoechoic space between two hyperechoic lines representing third ventricle (yellow arrow heads), which typically cannot be seen in patients without ventriculomegaly. Choroid plexus in the lateral ventricle can also be seen (blue arrow). (**b**) Representative CT scan of the head with enlargement of third ventricle

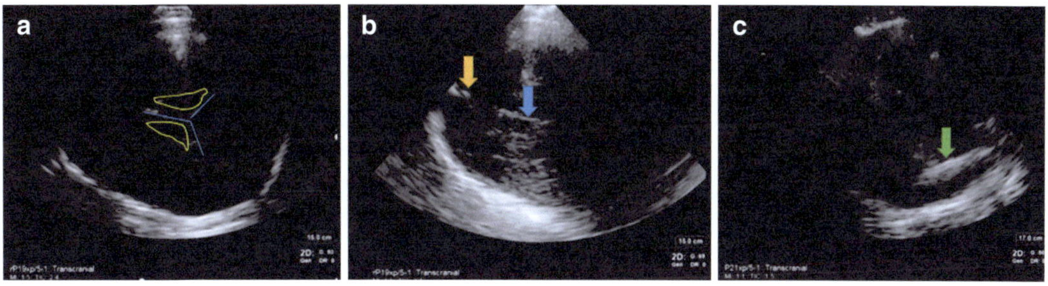

Fig. 15.3 Transcranial B mode images panel with anatomical landmarks: (**a**) yellow boundary highlights ependymal hyperechoic lining of lateral ventricles, while CSF appears hypoechoic; (**b**) crista galli (orange arrow) and hyperechoic shadow at the bottom is acoustic enhancement artifact produced by falx cerebri (blue arrow); (**c**) occipital bone with ridge (green arrow) outlining the transverse venous sinus

[3, 5]. Artifacts may limit brain ultrasound and include surgical drains, head wraps, electroencephalographic leads, and other overlying materials. Transcranial color-coded duplex sonography (TCCS) or imaging TCD also utilizes the same phased array probe as above further allowing Doppler analysis of the cerebral vasculature (discussed in Transcranial Doppler Chapter).

Using the temporal window, brain can be imaged across three different sections identified by tilting the probe from caudal to cephalad [2, 3, 5, 6]:

1. Mesencephalic: at the level of midbrain visible as a central hypoechoic structure shaped like a butterfly surrounded by hyperechoic basal cisterns (Fig. 15.1). Cerebral peduncles, colliculi, and cerebral aqueduct are discernible to allow identification of midbrain.
2. Diencephalic: at the level of third ventricle identified as central parallel hyperechoic lines with hypoechoic thalami on each side. A hyperechoic pineal gland may be visible in this plane (Fig. 15.2).
3. Ventricular plane: at the level of frontal horns of the lateral ventricle visible as hypoechoic structure lined by hyperechoic choroid plexus (Fig. 15.3).

Coronal section of the brain is feasible using the temporal window but has not been adequately described though it is being increasingly used for midline shift assessment and lateral ventricular visualization [7].

15.3 Clinical Applications

15.3.1 Midline Shift

Midline shift (MLS) is a common manifestation of mass effect wherein cerebral edema displaces the brain parenchyma. It is often a target for neuromonitoring and interventions. B mode ultrasound can be used as a point-of-care tool to assess midline shift through the identification of landmarks in patients with favorable anatomy (e.g., good temporal windows) or skull defects. Using the temporal window, the midbrain is identified by its characteristic butterfly shape. The probe is then tilted up to identify either the third ventricle or the septum pellucidum and pineal gland on ultrasound (Fig. 15.4) [3, 5, 8, 9]. The distance between the midline structure of interest and the ipsilateral skull is measured and recorded. The midline structure used for midline shift measurements depends on patient's pathology and the structure most discernible on ultrasound and may be third ventricle, septum pellucidum, posterior portion of falx cerebri or pineal gland. The maneuver is carried out again on the opposite temporal window. If there is no midline shift, these values should be essentially equal. Midline shift is calculated by subtracting the distances and dividing by two [3]. Some experts recommend using the same window to assess midline shift ipsilaterally and contralaterally since alignment of planes can be difficult by separate insonation of each window. If the same window is used for MLS, the distance from the probe position to midline structure can be measured and compared to the distance between the midline structure and contralateral skull. For either technique, radiographically significant shifts are considered to be more than 5 mm. A review and meta-analysis by Hakim et al. of over 400 patients suggests strong concordance between brain ultrasound and CT for assessment of midline shift provided a standardized protocol is used, although brain ultrasound was found to underestimate the presence of MLS compared to CT [8]. Ultrasound-based initial measurements should not replace CT for MLS measurements rather ultrasound MLS measurements can be used serially over time and used as a rapid bedside assessment for a patient too unstable for transport.

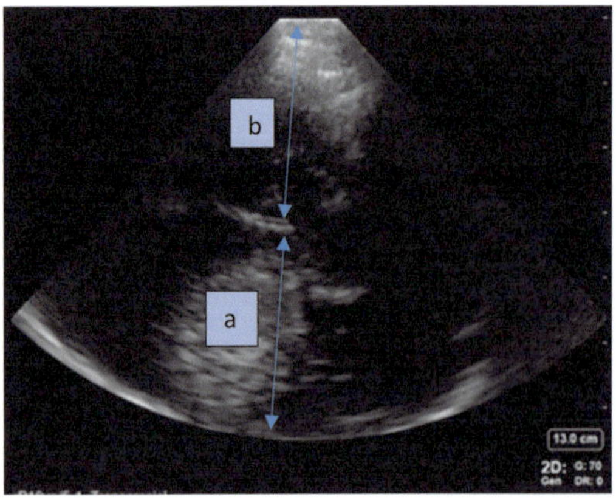

Fig. 15.4 Transcranial B mode ultrasound image for midline shift evaluation. Measurements from each skull end to the third ventricle. Unequal lengths denote midline shift and this can be measured $[a - b]/2 = \text{MLS}$

15.3.2 Intraparenchymal Hemorrhage

While computed tomography (CT) remains the gold standard for detecting intracranial hemorrhage (ICH), brain ultrasound has been explored to assess for the presence of ICH in patients who are too unstable to transport (e.g., acutely brain injured patients with refractory elevated intracranial pressure crisis or patients with hemodynamic instability). Temporal windows can reveal large acute hemorrhages in the contralateral parenchyma. The ipsilateral parenchyma is limited due to artifacts from the middle cranial fossa. By insonating both temporal windows, the provider can get an assessment of both hemispheres. Intraparenchymal hemorrhage produces a hyperechoic signal (Fig. 15.5) against the background of normal brain echogenicity [3, 5, 10–15]. Several studies have assessed the utility of ultrasound in the differentiation of ICH from ischemic

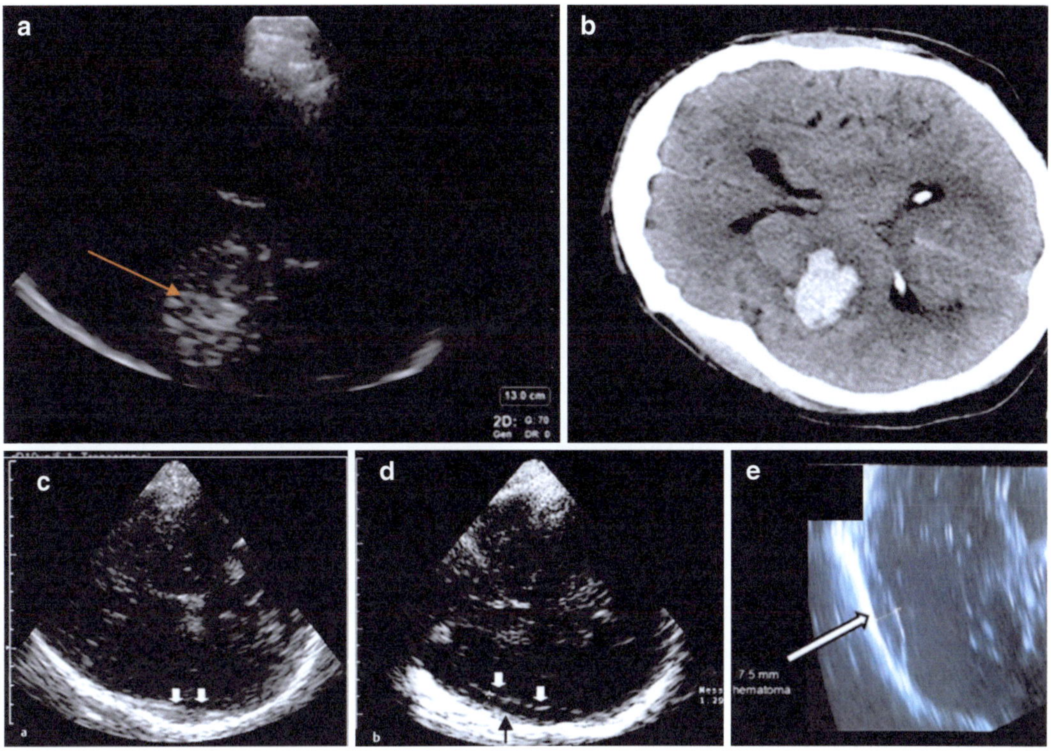

Fig. 15.5 Transcranial B mode ultrasound identifying intracranial hemorrhage. Hyperechoic intraparenchymal hemorrhage (orange arrow) (**a**), as also seen on the CT head without contrast (**b**). Transcranial B mode ultrasound of acute subdural hematoma (arrows) (**c**) and (**d**) chronic subdural hematoma (arrows). B mode ultrasound of epidural hematoma (arrow) (**e**). [Image c and d adapted with permission from Wolters Kluwer Health, Inc.: W.-D. Niesen, D. Burkhardt, J. Hoeltje, M. Rosenkranz, C. Weiller, U. Sliwka. Transcranial Grey-Scale Sonography of Subdural Haematoma in Adults. *European Journal of Ultrasound.* 27(3):251–5. https://www.thieme-connect.com/products/ejournals/abstract/10.1055/s-2006-926544. Image e is adapted under the terms of the Creative Commons Attribution License, which permits unrestricted use, distribution, and reproduction in any medium, provided the original work is properly cited. Lacerda FH, Rahhal H, Soares LJ, Ureña FDRM, Park M. Intracranial epidural hematoma follow-up using bidimensional ultrasound. Rev. Bras Ter Intensiva. 29(2):259–260. Image e—Copyright notice for publication: "This is an Open Access article distributed under the terms of the Creative Commons Attribution License, which permits unrestricted use, distribution, and reproduction in any medium, provided the original work is properly cited"]

stroke. Brain ultrasound was able to differentiate supratentorial ICH larger than 1 cm in size with specificity of 95–97% and sensitivity of 78–95% [3, 11, 14–16]. Ultrasound does not have high sensitivity for ICH smaller than 1 cm or certain locations such as high frontal lobe, high parietal lobe, and infratentorial locations. Intraventricular hemorrhage is similarly seen as hyperechoic material in the ventricles, although false positives can occur given the hyperechoic choroid plexus in the lateral ventricles. False positives can appear with other pathologies that lead to hyperechoic signals, including vasogenic edema, effacement of cisterns, tumors, and leukoencephalopathies, and these may not be discernible from hemorrhage [3, 13, 16]. Additionally, artifacts that mimic hemorrhage in cranial ultrasound have been described and include the midbrain acoustic shadow, which is the hyperechoic structure between the midbrain and contralateral skull, calcified choroid plexus and hyperechoic linear signals along the occipital bone, which is made by skull ridges in the posterior fossa [3]. Given false positives of intraparenchymal hemorrhage, the most effective application of cranial ultrasound would be to monitor the size of known intraparenchymal hemorrhage and additional parameters including midline shift (as described above) as well as changes in optic nerve sheath diameter and papilledema (described below).

15.3.3 Extra-axial Hemorrhage

In addition to the detection of intraparenchymal hemorrhage, brain ultrasound may detect extra-axial hemorrhages such as subdural hematoma (SDH) and epidural hematoma (EDH) (Note to editor: requesting permissions for SDH, EDH to be added into Fig. 15.5) [3, 17–20]. The temporal window contralateral to the affected side is used as the window to interrogate the brain. The dural border of the arachnoid space is identified as a highly echogenic structure that delineates the proximal aspect of the subdural space and is typically sharp. The space between the hyperechoic linear structure and the hyperechoic skull is the subdural space. The echogenicity of the material may help delineate whether this is acute or chronic SDH [17, 18]. The general observation is that acute SDH is hyperechoic relative to the brain and chronic SDH is hypoechoic to the brain tissue, but this correlation is not perfect and chronic SDH has been reported to look hyperechoic in some cases due to septations. Additionally, hygromas may look similar to chronic SDH on ultrasound. The size of the subdural is calculated by measuring from the inside of the contralateral skull to the inside of the most proximal area of the subdural space enlargement [13, 17, 18]. Monitoring and detection of epidural hematoma via ultrasound have been described in limited reports of patients [19, 20]. Epidural hematomas are also visualized as hyperechoic areas adjacent to the skull. EDH may be distinguished from SDH given the convex appearance of hemorrhage in EDH compared to the concave appearance of SDH. Limitations to this application of ultrasound include patients with poor temporal windows or extra-axial hemorrhages located in the posterior fossa. While ultrasound does not have enough sensitivity or specificity to rule out extra-axial hemorrhage or as a primary diagnostic study in the general population, there may be applications in the future to use it as screening tool for large acute midline shift inducing extra-axial hemorrhages. It can also be used for following the size of a hemorrhage in patients with adequate bone windows or patients who are unable to travel for a CT scan.

15.3.4 Hydrocephalus

CT is the preferred diagnostic tool for hydrocephalus, but transcranial ultrasound can be considered in an unstable patient who cannot travel. Transcranial ultrasound offers efficient serial examinations without the risk of cumulative radiation from repeated CT scans. To evaluate for hydrocephalus, the phased-array probe is placed on the temporal window to identify the midbrain, as described above. The probe is then tilted slightly cephalad to insonate the third ventricle, which appears as parallel hyperechoic lines [3]. Further tilting the probe, cephalad can reveal the frontal horns of the lateral ventricles as described above (Fig. 15.3). The ventricular system is identified by identifying hyperechoic lines generated by the ependymal lining of the ventricular system or hyperechoic signals produced by choroid plexus. Once identified, the size of the ventricles can be measured by measuring the distance between two hyperechoic lines [3, 21–24].

Obtaining normative ranges of third ventricle size is difficult because it varies between individuals depending on age and brain atrophy. However, if performed on a person and validated with the initial CT scan of the head, serial ultrasound can provide valuable information as changes in the ventricular size can indicate decreasing or increasing hydrocephalus. In 1995, Seidel et al. demonstrated a good inter-observer reliability correlation between ventricular size data obtained with brain ultrasound and that obtained with a CT scan of the head [21]. Brain ultrasound has also been used to monitor the change in the ventricular size after clamping of a ventricular drain in patients with hydrocephalus, with an increase in ventricular size of more than 5.5 cm after clamping predicting an unsuccessful EVD wean [23]. Operator skill is an important factor for measuring hydrocephalus, and other structures like the cerebral aqueduct can be mistaken for the third ventricle and provide false negatives for hydrocephalus [3, 25]. Given the skill required and strength of the available literature, we recommend against the clinical use of ultrasound for hydrocephalus until more data is available. Lateral ventricular measurements have been attempted in axial and coronal plane, but inconsistent boundaries of ventricles have impaired reliable size measurements [21].

15.3.5 Post-surgical Applications

In patients who have had craniectomy for various pathologies, ultrasound can be used to interrogate the brain parenchyma for the presence of hemorrhage, hydrocephalus, and worsening midline shift (Fig. 15.6) [3, 26–29]. In these patients, it is important to use the abdominal preset to avoid thermal injury to parenchyma as it has a lower thermal and mechanical index [26–28]. Since imaging of brain parenchyma is not limited by skull, ultrasound-derived brain parenchymal images have high resolution with good degree of details and the evaluation of parenchymal pathology and ventricular size is much more reliable. The presence of hemorrhage, hydrocephalus, and a midline shift can be evaluated as described above [26, 28, 29]. It may be most beneficial for postoperative patients to obtain a baseline B mode view of the brain tissue immediately postop and compare it to the post-operative head CT. Thereafter, serial ultrasounds can be evaluated and compared to the postoperative baseline. New findings can guide the acquisition of a CT scan of the head if a clinical suspicion arises.

Cranial ultrasound of sonolucent cranioplasty material is now being explored in postoperative craniotomy patients as a cost-effective, rapid way to monitor patients without CT scans or MRIs. Lee et al. described the placement of sonolucent covers after new ventriculoperitoneal shunt placement or endoscopic third ventriculostomy to monitor hydrocephalus in the postoperative period [30]. The ventricles were visualized by placing the probe in the coronal plane over a frontal sonolucent burr hole while directing the probe at the ipsilateral foramen of Monroe to obtain measurements of the lateral ventricle. Given the cost of sonolucent placement and additional foreign bodies in patients, only time will tell if the benefits outweigh the risks [30, 31].

15.3.6 Limitations of Brain Ultrasound

Currently available ultrasound technology does not have a preset optimized for B mode imaging of the brain parenchyma with use of TCD or abdominal preset as a surrogate. Hence, B mode imaging has several limitations. C-POCUS cannot reliably detect or discern ischemic parenchyma, encephalomalacia, subarachnoid hemorrhage, pneumocephalus, or cerebral edema, as they may appear as bright hyperechoic

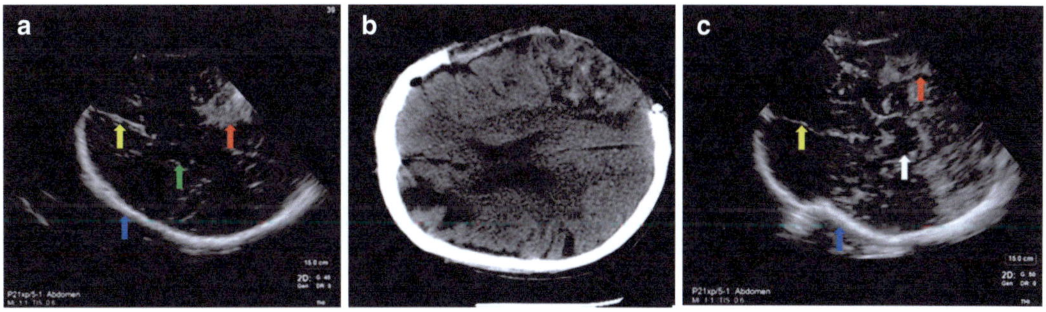

Fig. 15.6 Transcranial B mode ultrasound images in patient after hemicraniectomy. B mode images with abdominal preset (**a**, **c**): falx cerebri (yellow arrow), opposite skull (blue arrow), lateral ventricles (green arrow), midbrain (white arrow) and cerebral edema (red arrow). The corresponding CT head without contrast (**b**)

regions [3, 13, 32, 33]. Subacute intracranial hemorrhage after 5–10 days of onset, ICH less than 1 cm or in infratentorial locations may not be visible on ultrasound. Some tumors can be detected on B mode imaging, but they do not seem to be discernible from intraparenchymal hemorrhage. Recognition of expected artifacts that produce hyperechoic signals is crucial to use of brain ultrasound in screening for acute intracranial pathology [3, 25].

15.3.7 Orbital Ultrasound

There are several applications of orbital ultrasound in the neurocritical care unit, making it an extension of neuroultrasound. Orbital ultrasound can be used for noninvasive measurements of intracranial pressure using optic nerve sheath diameter and assessment of papilledema (Fig. 15.7). Ultrasound can also be used for measurements of pupillary light response and eye movements (Fig. 15.8) [3, 34–46]. Orbital ultrasound should never be performed on a patient who has a suspected glaucoma or globe injury as this could further damage the eye. Transorbital ultrasound is performed with high-frequency (5–15 MHz) linear pulses with an orbital preset. If there is no orbital present, the MI should be set to 0.2 and the TI to zero [3]. These settings are critical to ameliorating any mechanical or thermal injury to eye. The probe is placed over the

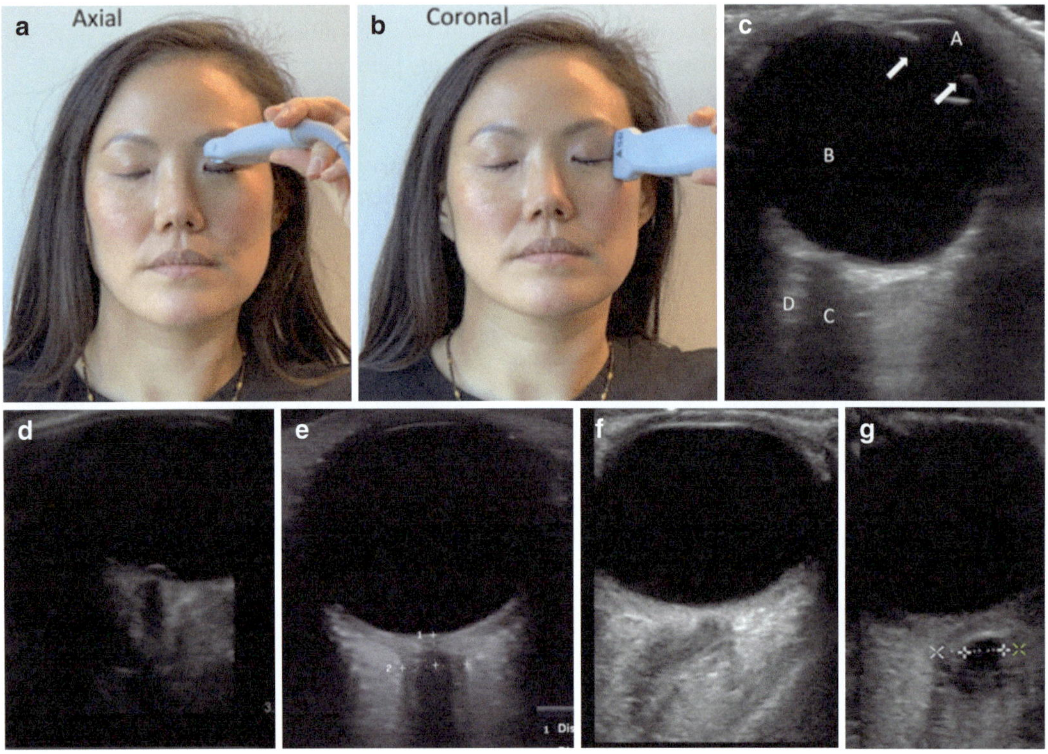

Fig. 15.7 Orbital anatomy and ONSD measurement. Two techniques of ONSD measurement: axial (**a**) and coronal (**b**). (**c**) Orbital ultrasound of axial B mode image: anterior chamber (A), borders of pupil (arrows), posterior chamber (B), optic nerve (C), and optic nerve sheath (D). (**d**) Anterior protrusion of optic disc (orange arrow) consistent with optic disease edema, (**e**) measurement of optic nerve sheath diameter taken in horizontal plane 3 mm from papilla, (**f**) anatomic variation of tortuous optic nerve (blue arrow) making it difficult to obtain ONSD measurement in some individuals. Coronal view of optic nerve sheath with "X" denoting the outer edge of sheath (**g**). [Image a, b and g adapted with permission from Wolters Kluwer Health, Inc.: Agrawal A, Cheng R, Tang J, Madhok DY. Comparison of Two Techniques to Measure Optic Nerve Sheath Diameter in Patients at Risk for Increased Intracranial Pressure. *Crit Care Med.* 47(6):e495–e501. https://journals.lww.com/ccmjournal/Abstract/2019/06000/Comparison_of_Two_Techniques_to_Measure_Optic.34.aspx]

patient's closed eye after a liberal amount of ultrasound gel is placed over the eye. Operators may choose to place a film dressing over the patient's eye to protect it from irritation. Hypoallergenic gel now commercially available though more expensive has been used in the pediatric population.

It is important for clinicians to be aware of incidental orbital pathology found on orbital ultrasound. Certain ophthalmologic findings may warrant expert evaluation and management, including retinal hemorrhage, retinal detachments, vitreous hemorrhage, and lens dislocation. These structural assessments are beyond the scope of this chapter. Point-of-care ultrasound of the orbit does not replace ophthalmology consultation but may be done as an initial evaluation while awaiting consulting services to arrive for evaluation.

15.3.8 Optic Nerve Sheath Diameter

Orbital ultrasound can be used as a noninvasive monitor of intracranial pressure when an invasive monitoring is not feasible (e.g., in the case of severe coagulopathy or limited resource settings) [3, 35, 36]. The optic nerve sheath is a continuation of the dura mater, and CSF surrounds the optic nerve contained in the optic nerve sheath. Due to this continuation and communication, gradual elevations in ICP result in an increase in the optic nerve sheath diameter (ONSD) [36]. There are different techniques for measuring the optic nerve sheath diameter (Fig. 15.8). For all techniques, the patient is supine with the head of the bed at 30° [46]. In a transverse or axial technique, the probe is placed on the eye in right to left orientation. The posterior portion of the globe

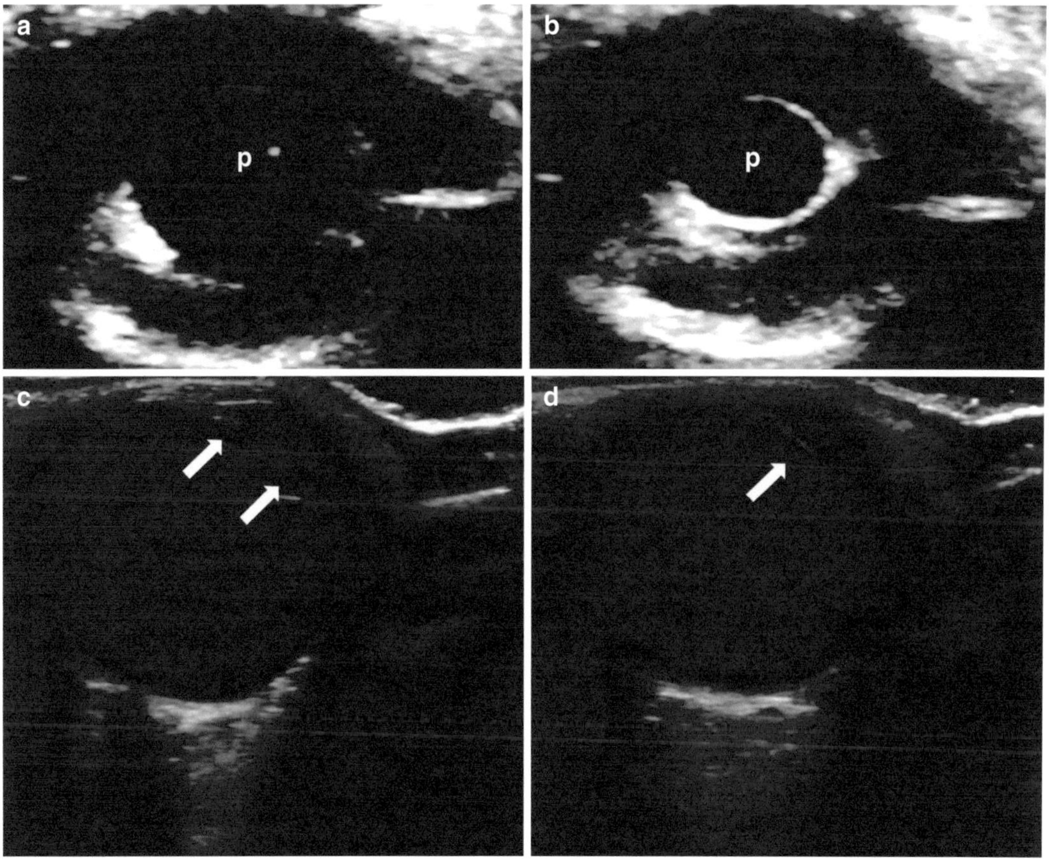

Fig. 15.8 Pupillary light reflex evaluated by ultrasound imaging. (**a**, **b**) Demonstrate coronal view of the eye with pupil (p) in the center with (**a**) prior to light stimulus and (**b**) after light stimulus. (**c**, **d**) Axial view with borders of pupil (white arrows). (**c**) Prior to light stimulus and (**d**) after light stimulus

and the retina is identified. Posterior to this area is a linear structure that corresponds to the optic nerve and its sheath. To ensure the ONSD is measured on axis, the optic nerve should be aligned with the iris [3, 47]. The ONSD is measured 3 mm behind the papilla as a horizontal line from one end of the sheath to the other. Similar measurements can be done by insonating the orbit in the sagittal plane, with probe-oriented cranial to caudad. There are variable practices regarding repeating measurements in each plane with some investigators choosing best of 3 measurements in same plane, some choosing average of 2 in axial and sagittal place with the average of these measures constituting the ONSD mean [3, 34–36, 38–43, 46, 47]. Another technique, the "coronal technique" involves placing the probe in a vertical orientation at the lateral canthus and aimed nasally and posteriorly to identify the circular optic nerve. The measurement is taken across the diameter of the optic nerve sheath [47]. Regardless of technique, the ONSD measurement is repeated for the contralateral eye.

There is significant variability of the ONSD across individuals, with observation studies reporting ONSD means from 3.5 to 5.5 mm with ranges of normal ONSD from 1.3 to 7.6 mm [35, 36, 38–43]. While there seems to be a statistical correlation between ONSD and high ICP in brain injured patients, a consistent cut-off for ONSD and elevated ICP greater than 20 mmHg that be used at bedside is not agreed upon and may range from 5.7 to 6.2 mm [3, 35, 36, 38–41]. Major differences in ONSD between the two eyes can be significant and should alert the practitioner to issues in technique, baseline anatomical differences between the two optic nerve sheaths or pathologies alternative to elevated intracranial pressure. Hyperacute changes in ICP caused by hematoma expansion may not manifest in widened ONSD compared to more gradual elevations in ICP and false negatives for ONSD are possible with elevated ICP [48]. Additionally, infiltrative optic nerve processes and individual variations can cause the ONSD to be higher than the perceived normal. Because ONSD is measured in millimeters, there can be operator variability in addition to inherent coefficient of variance induced by available resolution of ultrasound machines. Some investigators have further delineated measurements of optic nerve sheath diameters inside and outside the dura mater but ICU POCUS machines will need higher resolution imaging for using this even if this was validated on a large scale [49]. As such, ONSD has a wide range of reported sensitivity and specificity, 74–100% and 74–100% when using a cutoff of 5.5–6 mm [35, 36, 38–41], respectively. Given possible false positives and negatives, as well as operator differences, like other ultrasound techniques, ONSD should not be used in isolation to diagnose the absence or presence of elevated ICP. ONSD may become more reliable when trended over time in comparison to a person's known baseline ONSD.

15.3.9 Papilledema

Papilledema, or swelling of the disc, can be caused by increased ICP and seen on orbital ultrasound (Fig. 15.8) as elevation of the optic disc into the posterior chamber. It is caused by chronic cerebrospinal fluid buildup in the retrobulbar optic nerve sheath as a byproduct of elevated ICP. Other processes, such as inflammatory disease, calcium deposition (Drusen), infection, infiltrative diseases, extreme hypertension, and ischemic disease, can also cause an increase in optic disc height [44, 45]. The technique is the same as described for measuring the ONSD, except the operator is looking for a protuberance of the optic disc into the posterior chamber (Fig. 15.8). Optic disc height can be measured as the distance between the top of the papilla and the fundus. Optic disc height greater than 1 mm had a sensitivity of 73% and a specificity of 100% when compared to the fundoscopic evaluation of optic disc edema [44]. Several studies showed better sensitivity of detecting high ICP by ultrasonographic detection of papilledema compared to widened ONSD [38, 43]. Since hyperacute ICP elevations or very slow, gradual elevations may not cause optic disc edema, assessment of ultrasonographic papilledema should not be used in isolation to rule out increased intracranial pressure [47]. Many experts have suggested a combined approach of orbital ultrasound to assess elevations in intracranial pressure, in which the presence of both an enlarged ONSD larger than 6 mm and ultrasonographic papilledema is suggestive of an elevated ICP.

15.3.10 Eye Movements and Pupillary Light Reflex

Orbital ultrasound can also be useful to aid in physical examination of the eye in patients with periorbital swelling preventing eyelid opening or in patients after tarsorrhaphy performed for facial weakness. Using ultrasound, both extraocular movements and the pupillary light reflex can be tested. For extraocular eye movement assessment, the probe is placed over the orbit in a transverse position. The patient is then asked to look up, down, and from side to side. The pattern of eye movement can reveal restrictions in basic horizontal or vertical gaze. There are two main techniques for checking the pupillary light reflex (Fig. 15.8). One method is to place the linear probe in a transverse position over the eye. After identification of the lens, cornea, iris, and anterior chamber, the probe is tilted either cephalad or caudal until the iris and aperture of the pupil is visualized in a coronal view. The other technique is to place the probe in the traverse position over the eye with the iris and aperture of pupil visualized in an axial view. For either method, a bright light is shone into the contralateral eye and consensual pupillary constriction can be observed by ultrasound as the aperture of the pupil decreases in size [46].

15.4 Conclusions

B mode cranial ultrasound is an emerging tool that may be useful for patients too unstable to travel to CT or resource limited environments. Given the prevalence of point-of-care ultrasound equipment in critical care units and the portable nature of the machine, providers should be aware of the applications of brain ultrasound. Efforts to create better ultrasound presets to increase accuracy of B mode imaging are underway. Initiatives should also be made toward formulating a consensus after gathering data regarding the number of B mode cranial ultrasounds needed to gain proficiency or the degree of operator skill for detection of acute intracranial pathology.

References

1. Qiu W, Bouakaz A, Konofagou EE, Zheng H. Ultrasound for the brain: a review of physical and engineering principles, and clinical applications. IEEE Trans Ultrason Ferroelectr Freq Control. 2021;68(1):6–20. https://doi.org/10.1109/TUFFC.2020.3019932.
2. Blanco P, Abdo-Cuza A. Transcranial Doppler ultrasound in neurocritical care. J Ultrasound. 2018;21(1):1–16. https://doi.org/10.1007/s40477-018-0282-9.
3. Ziai WC, Cornwell CL, editors. Neurovascular sonography. Springer; 2022. https://doi.org/10.10007/978-3-030-96893-9_2.
4. Lee CH, Jeon SH, Wang SJ, et al. Factors associated with temporal window failure in transcranial Doppler sonography. Neurol Sci. 2020;41:3293–9.
5. Sarwal A, Robba C, Citerio G. Brain echography. In: Oxford textbook of neurocritical care. 2nd ed. Oxford University Press; 2016.
6. Kalanuria A, Nyquist PA, Armonda RA, Razumovsky A. Use of transcranial Doppler (TCD) ultrasound in the neurocritical care unit. Neurosurg Clin N Am. 2013;24(3):441–56. https://doi.org/10.1016/j.nec.2013.02.005. Epub 2013 Apr 17.
7. D'Andrea A, Conte M, Cavallaro M, Scarafile R, Riegler L, Cocchia R, et al. Transcranial Doppler ultrasonography: from methodology to major clinical applications. World J Cardiol. 2016;8(7):383–400. https://doi.org/10.4330/wjc.v8.i7.38.
8. Hakim SM, Abdellatif A, Ali MI, Ammar MA. Reliability of transcranial sonography for assessment of brain midline shift in adult neurocritical patients: a systematic review and meta-analysis. Minerva Anestesiol. 2021;87:467–75.
9. Stolz E, Gerriets T, Fiss I, Babacan SS, Seidel G, Kaps M. Comparison of transcranial color-coded duplex sonography and cranial CT measurements for determining third ventricle midline shift in space-occupying stroke. AJNR Am J Neuroradiol. 1999;20(8):1567–71.
10. Caballero-Lozada AF, Nanwani KL, Pavón F, Zorrilla-Vaca A, Zorrilla-Vaca C. Clinical applications of ultrasonography in neurocritically ill patients. J Intensive Care Med. 2021;36(6):627–34. https://doi.org/10.1177/0885066620905796. Epub 2020 Mar 10.

11. Seidel G, Kaps M, Dorndorf W. Transcranial color-coded duplex sonography of intracerebral hematomas in adults. Stroke. 1993;24(10):1519–27. https://doi.org/10.1161/01.str.24.10.1519.
12. Dinsmore M, Venkatraghavan L. Clinical applications of point-of-care ultrasound in brain injury: a narrative review. Anaesthesia. 2022;77(Suppl 1):69–77. https://doi.org/10.1111/anae.15604.
13. Kapoor S, Offnick A, Allen B, Brown PA, Sachs JR, Gurcan MN, Pinton G, D'Agostino R Jr, Bushnell C, Wolfe S, Duncan P, Asimos A, Sarwal A. Brain topography on adult ultrasound images: techniques, interpretation, and image library. J Neuroimaging. 2022;32(6):1013–26. https://doi.org/10.1111/jon.13031. Epub 2022 Aug 4. PMID: 35924877; PMCID: PMC9804536.
14. Sarwal A, Patel Y, Agostino R, Brown P, Wolfe SQ, Bushnell C, et al. Exploratory study to assess feasibility of intracerebral hemorrhage detection by point of care cranial ultrasound. Ultrasound J. 2022;14(1):40.
15. Seidel G, Kaps M, Dorndorf W. Transcranial color-coded duplex sonography of intracerebral hematomas in adults. Stroke. 1993;24:1519–27.
16. Bertuetti R, Gritti P, Pelosi P, Robba C. How to use cerebral ultrasound in the ICU. Minerva Anestesiol. 2020;86(3):327–40. https://doi.org/10.23736/S0375-9393.19.13852-7. Epub 2020 Jan 8.
17. Niesen WD, Burkhardt D, Hoeltje J, Rosenkranz M, Weiller C, Sliwka U. Transcranial grey-scale sonography of subdural haematoma in adults. Ultraschall Med. 2006;27(3):251–5. https://doi.org/10.1055/s--2006-926544. Epub 2006 Feb 16.
18. Niesen W-D, Rosenkranz M, Weiller C. Bedsided transcranial sonographic monitoring for expansion and progression of subdural hematoma compared to computed tomography. Front Neurol. 2018;9:374.
19. Lacerda FH, Rahhal H, Soares LJ, Ureña FDRM, Park M. Intracranial epidural hematoma follow-up using bidimensional ultrasound. Rev Bras Ter Intensiva. 2017;29(2):259–60. https://doi.org/10.5935/0103-507X.20170036. PMID: 28977267; PMCID: PMC5496762.
20. Caricato A, Mignani V, Sandroni C, Pietrini D. Bedside detection of acute epidural hematoma by transcranial sonography in a head-injured patient. Intensive Care Med. 2010;36(6):1091–2. https://doi.org/10.1007/s00134-010-1801-0. Epub 2010 Mar 6.
21. Seidel G, Gerriets T, Kaps M, Hutzelmann A. Evaluation of the ventricular system in adults by transcranial duplex sonography. J Neuroimaging. 1995;5:105. https://doi.org/10.1111/jon199552105.
22. Harrer JU, Tsivgoulis G. Transcranial sonography for monitoring hydrocephalus: an underestimated imaging modality. Neurology. 2011;76(10):852–3. https://doi.org/10.1212/WNL.0b013e31820f2e8a.
23. Kiphuth IC, Huttner HB, Struffert T, Schwab S, Köhrmann M. Sonographic monitoring of ventricle enlargement in posthemorrhagic hydrocephalus. Neurology. 2011;76(10):858–62. https://doi.org/10.1212/WNL.0b013e31820f2e0f.
24. Phillips SB, Gates M, Krishnamurthy S. Strategic placement of bedside ventriculostomies using ultrasound image guidance: report of three cases. Neurocrit Care. 2012;17:255–9.
25. Caricato A, Ioannoni E, Gelormini C. Is it really third ventricle? A pitfall in the diagnosis of hydrocephalus by brain ultrasound. Neurocrit Care. 2020;33(3):844–6. https://doi.org/10.1007/s12028-020-01060-9.
26. Bendella H, Maegele M, Hartmann A, Spreer J, Rommel N, Lefering R, et al. Cerebral ventricular dimensions after decompressive craniectomy: a comparison between bedside sonographic duplex technique and cranial computed tomography. Neurocrit Care. 2017;26(3):321.
27. Robba C, Simonassi F, Ball L, Pelosi P. Transcranial color-coded duplex sonography for bedside monitoring of central nervous system infection as a consequence of decompressive craniectomy after traumatic brain injury. Intensive Care Med. 2019;45(8):1143–4.
28. Sarwal A, Elder N. Point-of-care cranial ultrasound in a hemicraniectomy patient. Clin Pract Cases Emerg Med. 2018;2:375–7.
29. Caricato A, Mignani V, Bocci MG, Pennisi MA, Sandroni C, Tersali A, Antonaci A, de Waure C, Antonelli M. Usefulness of transcranial echography in patients with decompressive craniectomy: a comparison with computed tomography scan. Crit Care Med. 2012;40(6):1745–52. https://doi.org/10.1097/CCM.0b013e318246b6ea.
30. Lee RP, Meggyesy M, Ahn J, Ritter C, Suk I, Machnitz AJ, Huang J, Gordon C, Brem H, Luciano M. First experience with postoperative transcranial ultrasound through sonolucent burr hole covers in adult hydrocephalus patients. Neurosurgery. 2023;92(2):382–90.
31. Del Bene M, Raspagliesi L, Carone G, et al. Cranial sonolucent prosthesis: a window of opportunity for neuro-oncology (and neuro-surgery). J Neuro-Oncol. 2022;156:529–40.
32. Mäurer M, Shambal S, Berg D, et al. Differentiation between intracerebral hemorrhage and ischemic stroke by transcranial color-coded duplex-sonography. Stroke. 1998;29:2563–7.
33. Becker G, Winkler J, Hofmann E, Bogdahn U. Differentiation between ischemic and hemorrhagic stroke by transcranial color-coded real-time sonography. J Neuroimaging. 1993;3:41–7.
34. Robba C, Wong A, Poole D, Al Tayar A, Arntfield RT, Chew MS, Corradi F, Douflé G, Goffi A, Lamperti M, Mayo P, Messina A, Mongodi S, Narasimhan M, Puppo C, Sarwal A, Slama M, Taccone FS, Vignon P, Vieillard-Baron A, European Society of Intensive Care Medicine Task Force for Critical Care Ultrasonography*. Basic ultrasound head-to-toe skills for intensivists in the general and neuro intensive care unit population: consensus and expert recommendations of the European Society of Intensive Care Medicine. Intensive Care Med. 2021;47(12):1347–67. https://doi.org/10.1007/s00134-021-06486-z. Epub 2021 Oct 5. PMID: 34787687; PMCID: PMC8596353.

35. Galetta S, Byrne SF, Smith JL. Echographic correlation of optic nerve sheath size and cerebrospinal fluid pressure. J Clin Neuroophthalmol. 1989;9:79–82.
36. Robba C, Santori G, Czosnyka M, et al. Optic nerve sheath diameter measured sonographically as non-invasive estimator of intracranial pressure: a systematic review and meta-analysis. Intensive Care Med. 2018;44(8):1284–94. https://doi.org/10.1007/s00134-018-5305-7.
37. Harries A, Shah S, Teismann N, Price D, Nagdev A. Ultrasound assessment of extraocular movements and pupillary light reflex in ocular trauma. Am J Emerg Med. 2010;28(8):956–9. https://doi.org/10.1016/j.ajem.2009.06.026.
38. Lochner P, Brio F, Zedde ML, Sanguigni S, Coppo L, Nardone R, Naldi A, Sola D, Stolz E. Feasibility and usefulness of ultrasonography in idiopathic intracranial hypertension or secondary intracranial hypertension [Erratum in: BMC Neurol. 2016;16:94]. BMC Neurol. 2016;16:85. https://doi.org/10.1186/s12883-016-0594-3. PMID: 27250852; PMCID: PMC4890482.
39. Bäuerle J, Nedelmann M. Sonographic assessment of the optic nerve sheath in idiopathic intracranial hypertension. J Neurol. 2011;258(11):2014–9. https://doi.org/10.1007/s00415-011-6059-0. Epub 2011 Apr 28.
40. Irazuzta JE, Brown ME, Akhtar J. Bedside optic nerve sheath diameter assessment in the identification of increased intracranial pressure in suspected idiopathic intracranial hypertension. Pediatr Neurol. 2015;54:35.
41. Kimberly HH, Shah S, Marill K, Noble V. Correlation of optic nerve sheath diameter with direct measurement of intracranial pressure. Acad Emerg Med. 2008;15(2):201–4.
42. Potgieter DW, Kippin A, Ngu F, McKean C. Can accurate ultrasonographic measurement of the optic nerve sheath diameter (a non-invasive measure of intracranial pressure) be taught to novice operators in a single training session? Anaesth Intensive Care. 2011;39(1):95–100. https://doi.org/10.1177/0310057X1103900116.
43. Bäuerle J, Lochner P, Kaps M, Nedelmann M. Intra- and interobsever reliability of sonographic assessment of the optic nerve sheath diameter in healthy adults. J Neuroimaging. 2012;22(1):42–5. https://doi.org/10.1111/j.1552-6569.2010.00546.x. Epub 2010 Dec 1.
44. Teismann N, Lenaghan P, Nolan R, Stein J, Green A. Point-of-care ocular ultrasound to detect optic disc swelling. Acad Emerg Med. 2013;20(9):920–5. https://doi.org/10.1111/acem.12206.
45. Carter SB, Pistilli M, Livingston KG, Gold DR, Volpe NJ, Shindler KS, Liu GT, Tamhankar MA. The role of orbital ultrasonography in distinguishing papilledema from pseudopapilledema. Eye (Lond). 2014;28(12):1425–30. https://doi.org/10.1038/eye.2014.210. Epub 2014 Sep 5. PMID: 25190532; PMCID: PMC4268455.
46. Agrawal A, Cheng R, Tang J, Madhok DY. Comparison of two techniques to measure optic nerve sheath diameter in patients at risk for increased intracranial pressure. Crit Care Med. 2019;47(6):e495–501. https://doi.org/10.1097/CCM.0000000000003742. PMID: 30882482; PMCID: PMC6522267.
47. Raghunandan N, Joseph M, Nithyanandam S, Karat S. Role of ultrasonographic optic nerve sheath diameter in the diagnosis and follow-up of papilledema and its correlation with Frisén's severity grading. Indian J Ophthalmol. 2019;67(8):1310–3. https://doi.org/10.4103/ijo.IJO_1827_18.
48. Dubourg J, Javouhey E, Geeraerts T, Messerer M, Kassai B. Ultrasonography of optic nerve sheath diameter for detection of raised intracranial pressure: a systematic review and meta-analysis. Intensive Care Med. 2011;37(7):1059–68. https://doi.org/10.1007/s00134-011-2224-2.
49. Pansell J, Bell M, Rudberg P, Friman O, Cooray C. Optic nerve sheath diameter in intracranial hypertension: measurement external or internal of the dura mater? J Neuroimaging. 2023;33(1):58–66. https://doi.org/10.1111/jon.13062.

Part IV

Neuropharmacology in Neurocritical Care

16 Sedation and Analgesia

Subramanian Senthilkumaran

16.1 Introduction

Sedation and analgesia play crucial roles in the management of critically ill patients. The goals of sedation and analgesia in NCCU are to prevent pain and discomfort, reduce anxiety, facilitate mechanical ventilation, control seizures, and promote cerebral perfusion as well as to generally improve patient management. Recent developments in critical care management have placed a strong emphasis on the need to reduce ongoing deep sedation and paralysis in order to enhance outcomes and shorten intensive care unit (ICU) stays [1].

Within the context of neurocritical care, sedation serves distinct purposes in the management of acute brain injury (ABI). It works by diminishing the cerebral metabolic rate of oxygen ($CMRO_2$), cerebral blood flow (CBF), and cerebral blood volume (CBV), thus enhancing the brain's ability to withstand potential ischemic injury. Additionally, it plays a significant role in preventing intracranial hypertension and managing increased intracranial pressure (ICP) [2].

Cognitive impairment itself can cause an increase in anxiety, agitation, and restlessness. Yet, even little sedation can mask subtle neurological deterioration. Sedation regimens in NCCU should ideally be premeditated to enable repeated attainment of a high-quality neurological examination as the means of assessing patient status. Thus, it is necessary to use an interdisciplinary approach to observe and drug titration in order to reduce the impact on the neurological evaluation [3].

There are several classes of medications commonly used for sedation and analgesia in NCCU, including opioids, benzodiazepines, propofol, and dexmedetomidine. Each medication has its own unique pharmacokinetic and pharmacodynamic properties, which can influence its efficacy and side effect profile. The choice of sedative and analgesic medication depends on several factors, including the patient's underlying medical conditions, the severity of their illness, and the specific goals of treatment. In general, it is important to use the lowest effective dose of sedative and analgesic medication to minimize the risk of adverse effects [4].

16.2 Indications

It is crucial to rule out all alternate causes for agitation, disorientation, or sympathetic hyperactivity before administering any sedative in NCCU patient prior to aggressively concealing these potential symptoms and signs of a serious underlying condition [4, 5].

S. Senthilkumaran (✉)
Department of Emergency & Critical Care, Manian Medical Centre, Erode, Tamil Nadu, India

H. Prabhakar et al. (eds.), *Principles and Practice of Neurocritical Care*,
https://doi.org/10.1007/978-981-99-8059-8_16

16.2.1 General Indication

- **Agitation**: Patients with neurological conditions such as traumatic brain injury (TBI), stroke, and subarachnoid hemorrhage (SAH) may experience agitation, which can worsen their condition and lead to further brain damage. Sedation can help to calm these patients and prevent agitation.
- **Pain**: Patients in NCCU may experience pain, which can worsen their condition and lead to agitation and increased ICP.
- **Facilitate mechanical ventilation**: Patients who require mechanical ventilation may require sedation to reduce their respiratory drive and prevent agitation and patient–ventilator synchrony.
- **Diagnostic and therapeutic procedures**: Sedation may be required for diagnostic and therapeutic procedures such as computed tomography (CT) scans, magnetic resonance imaging (MRI), and lumbar punctures.

16.2.2 Brain-Specific Indications

- **Control of ICP**: The key indication for ongoing sedation in the NCCU is to avoid deleterious change in intracranial pressure and cerebral perfusion pressure (CPP). Sedatives lower ICP through multiple mechanisms. Coughing and other kinds of Valsalva are first suppressed. Second, they also reduce motoric restlessness and agitation. Thirdly, they reduce brain metabolism ($CMRO_2$). A decrease in cerebral blood flow (CBF), which is tightly regulated by $CMRO_2$, will also result in a decrease in cerebral blood volume (CBV), bringing the patient in a less steep range of the ICP/volume curve and improve the brain's tolerance to ischemia and energy dysfunction [6].
- **Status epilepticus**: Many sedatives, including benzodiazepines, propofol, and barbiturates, have intrinsic antiepileptic properties and are also used in the management of refractory status epilepticus when both first-line therapy (such as antiepileptic medications) and emergency therapy (such as benzodiazepines) are unable to control seizures [7].
- **Cerebral edema**: Patients with cerebral edema may require sedation to reduce their metabolic demand and promote cerebral perfusion.
- **Targeted temperature management**: Hypothermia is accompanied with shivering, resulting in discomfort for the patient, elevated $CMRO_2$ and elevated ICP [8].
- **Paroxysmal sympathetic hyperactivity**: It is a rare but remarkable clinical condition involving paroxysmal tachycardia, arterial hypertension, tachypnea, hyperthermia, and spasticity in response to afferent stimulation that develops after a severe acquired brain injury [9].

16.3 Selection of Sedatives and Analgesics in the NCCU [6, 10, 11]

There are several pharmacological options for sedation, and no single intravenous sedative has superior to others in improved prognosis or reduced mortality. Few studies incorporate washout intervals between the administration of several sedatives, leaving them vulnerable to confounding effects and impeding the independent assessment of each medication.

While selecting the right sedative, routes of administration, pharmacokinetics, ease of titration, and adverse effect profiles with a focus on impacts on the neurological exam, respiratory drive, and systemic or cerebral hemodynamics are all things to taken into account while treating an NCCU patient. Due to the frequent requirement for repeated neurological examinations, short-acting medicines are often recommended in the NCCU. Each has potential advantages as well as disadvantages in critically sick patients, particularly those with primary neurological disorders. Possibilities include ketamine, alpha-2 agonists, neuroleptics, barbiturates, benzodiazepines, opioids, propofol, and many others.

Eventually, a customized strategy is required, with particular drug criteria such as drug–drug interactions, drug–disease state interactions, drug reversibility, and cost-effectiveness. Selected agents and selected salient pharmacologic parameters will be described in the following sections and are summarized in Tables 16.1 and 16.2.

Table 16.1 Administration of Selected Sedatives in the Neuro-ICU

Drug	Starting dose	Titration	Half-life	Binding active metabolite	Metabolism/active metabolite
Fentanyl	25–50 mcg IV every 5–10 min	0.5 2.5 mcg/kg/h titrate every 15–30 min, up to 50 single IV 100 mcg/h infusion: 0.05–0.2 mcg/kg/min	30–60 min (single IV dose)	80–86%	Hepatic
Morphine sulfate	5–20 mg IM every 4 h	Caution: metabolites may accumulate	1.5–4.5 h IV, IM, SQ	20–30%	Hepatic/morphine-3-glucuronide morphine-6-glucuronide
Ketamine	0.1–1 mcg/kg every 10 min	Infusion: 0.05–3 mcg/kg/h	2–3 h	47%	Hepatic
Lorazepam	0.25 mg–1 mg IV every 5–30 min	Infusion: 0.01–0.1 mcg/kg/h	10–20 h	91–93%	Hepatic
Midazolam	0.5–1 mg IV every 5–30 min	Infusion; 0.25–1 mcg/kg/min	1–2.5 h	97%	Hepatic/1-hydroxymethylmidazolam
Dexmedetomidine	1 mcg/kg iv bolus over 10 min	Infusion 0.2–1 mcg/kg/h	2 h	94%	Hepatic
Phenobarbital	10 mcg IV at 100 mg/min	50 mg/min until seizures are controlled	36–117 h	20–60%	Hepatic
Propofol	1.0–2.5 mg/kg IV (anesthesia induction) 5 mcg/kg/min IV (sedation)	Increase infusion 5–10 mcg/kg/min every 5–10 min to maintenance of 25–80 mcg/kg/min, up to 100–300 mcg/kg/min	4–10 min	>90%	Hepatic and extra hepatic

Table 16.2 Key characteristics of agents commonly used for sedation in the Neuro-ICU

Drugs	Indications in the neuro-ICU	Mechanism of action	CNS effects	Advantages	Disadvantages
Propofol	• First-line sedative to treat intracranial hypertension • First-choice sedative for status epilepticus unresponsive to antiepileptic drugs • Postcardiac arrest, when rapid awakening is important	GABA-R agonist	↓ ICP	Rapid onset and short duration of action	No amnesia, especially at low doses
			↓ $CMRO_2$, ↓ CBF, preserved CO_2 reactivity and cerebral autoregulation	Clearance independent of renal or hepatic function	No analgesic effect
			↓ Cerebral electrical activity, can be used to induce EEG burst suppression (at high dose)	No significant drug interactions	Tolerance and tachyphylaxis
					↓ MAP, ↓ CPP (particularly in hypovolemic patients)
					↑ Triglycerides, ↑ caloric intake
					Propofol infusion syndrome (↓ HR, ↓ pH, ↑ lactate, ↑ CPK, myocardial failure)
Midazolam	• Second-line sedative, to be added when other sedatives are insufficient or at their maximum dose • Sedation of hemodynamically unstable patients	GABA-R agonist	↓ $CMRO_2$, ↓ CBF	Amnesia	Tolerance and tachyphylaxis

			Slight ↓ ICP	Rapid onset of effect in acutely agitated patient	Hepatic metabolism to active metabolite
			Preserved CO_2 reactivity and cerebral autoregulation	Less hemodynamic instability than propofol (may prevent CPP reductions)	May accumulate in renal dysfunction
			Antiepileptic effect		May prolong the duration of MV
					May increase ICU delirium
Barbiturates	• Rescue therapy for intracranial hypertension • Refractory or superrefractory status epilepticus	GABA-R agonist	↓↓ CBF that is proportional to the ↓↓ $CMRO_2$ (up to 60%) during burst suppression	By ↓↓ CBF and CBV, barbiturates have a strong effect on ↓↓ ICP	Hypotension, ↓↓ MAP/CPP
			↓↓ ICP	Indications for barbiturates are limited to the treatment of refractory ICP and refractory status epilepticus, titrated to the lowest effective dose; EEG may help with the titration of barbiturate therapy	Immune suppression, increased risk of infections (pneumonia)
					Adrenal dysfunction
Morphine	• Analgesia • Sedative/hypnotics in low doses	μ-Receptor agonist	↑ ICP and ↓ MAP/CPP transiently following bolus	Low cost	Low predictability to control ICP
					Histamine release
					Accumulation with hepatic/renal impairment
Fentanyl, sufentanil	• Analgesia • Tolerance of mechanical ventilation	μ-Receptor agonists	↑ ICP and ↓ MAP/CPP transiently following bolus	More potent opioid than morphine (sufentanil is 1000 × more potent than morphine)	Accumulation with hepatic impairment
			Control ICP during endotracheal suctioning		May prolong the duration of MV

(continued)

Table 16.2 (continued)

Drugs	Indications in the neuro-ICU	Mechanism of action	CNS effects	Advantages	Disadvantages
Remifentanil		μ-Receptor agonist	No changes in ICP or CBF during drug infusion	500 × more potent than morphine	Hyperalgesia at the cessation of drug infusion
				Rapid onset and short duration of action to permit neurological assessment	Limited effect to control ICP during painful procedures
				Clearance independent of renal or hepatic function	Tachyphylaxis
					Higher cost than other opiates
Dexmedetomidine	• Mild sedation, for instance in case of agitation • While weaning off other sedatives • Anxiolysis	α_2-Agonist	ICP ↓ or unchanged	Sedative, analgesic, and anxiolytic	Very limited clinical experience in patients with ABI
			CPP ↑ or unchanged	Short acting, no accumulation, patient may be frequently assessed neurologically	In non-neurointensive care population
			$SjvO_2$ unchanged	Minimal respiratory depression	• Hypotension, bradycardia
			$PbtO_2$ unchanged	May reduce incidence/ severity of delirium	• Arrhythmias including atrial fibrillation
					• Hyperglycaemia
					May require high doses; deep sedation may not be possible
					High cost

Ketamine	• Control of refractory or super refractory status epilepticus, when GABA agents are no longer effective • Neuroprotective role in acute brain injury, suppression of cortical spreading depolarizations	NMDA-R antagonist	ICP ↓ or unchanged	Short acting, fast onset	Hallucinations/emergence phenomena
			CPP ↑ or unchanged	Induces sedation, analgesia, and anesthesia	
			No change in $SjvO_2$ or cerebral blood flow velocities	Does not depress respiration	
				Hemodynamic stability, preserves MAP	
				May be used as an adjunct for refractory seizures	
				No withdrawal symptoms	
Inhaled anesthetics	Unclear	Not fully established: may act at several sites (reduction in junctional conductance; activation of Ca^{2+}-dependent ATP-ase; binding to the GABA-R, the large conductance Ca^{2+}-activated K^+ channel, and the glutamate receptor)	↓ Cerebral electrical activity, ↓ $CMRO_2$	↑ CBF in patients with cerebral ischemia (0.8% isoflurane)	↑ ICP due to ↑ CBV
			Dose-dependent effects on CBF: ↓ CBF at low concentrations, ↑ CBF at high concentrations	Rapid elimination	Myocardial depression
					Malignant hyperthermia
					Not widely available, requires specific systems and expertise
					Data very preliminary

16.4 Assessing Patients While on Sedation in the NCCU

In NCCU, neurological wake-up tests (NWTs) are frequently performed [12]. These "neurochecks" enable periodic repeated neurological examinations, which are the gold standard for neuromonitoring since they involve presenting a stimulus and assaying response. However, there is some danger associated with sedation interruption (SI). Arousing patients may exhibit disinhibited behavior in the NCCU, with exaggerated motor responsiveness, and jerky head and body movements, which do carry some risk for self-extubation if unattended.

Frequent neuroimaging studies may be necessary when a patient is over-sedated, as it can affect neuro assessment. Other issues that may arise because of over-sedation include delayed emergence, muscle disuse atrophy, respiratory depression, hypotension, venous stasis, and setup for venous thrombosis. This can negatively impact the patient's ability to stay mobile and lead to an increased time on the ventilator and in the ICU, as well as higher costs.

Alternatively, under-sedation can lead to restlessness, anxiety, pain, elevated intracranial pressure, tachycardia, and hypertension and may even cause arrhythmias and cardiac ischemia. It can also result in difficulties synchronizing with the ventilator resulting ineffective ventilation and increased oxygen consumption. Furthermore, it may cause wound disruption, increase the danger of fall, and result in the accidently removal of drains, catheters, tubes, and other devices [13].

16.5 Monitoring of Sedation and Analgesia in the NCCU

In NCCU practice, there are a variety of validated clinical sedation assessment scales. These tools, which are mostly driven by nursing staffs, are used to record the patient's status and then to monitor and modify sedation to achieve the desired outcome. The most popular tool for assessing the quality and level of sedation in adult ICU patients is the Richmond Agitation Sedation Scale and the Sedation-Agitation Scale [14]. Depending on the patient and the clinical situation, the target sedation scores on individual scales vary.

The utilization of EEG to monitor sedation in patients who are deeply sedated or have been administered neuromuscular blocking agents has been under clinical scrutiny. Studies have revealed that simplified EEG tools that provide quantitative monitoring of bispectral index (BIS) display significant correlations between BIS values and scores from the Richmond Agitation Sedation Scale and Sedation-Agitation Scale in acute brain injury patients (ABI) [15]. The use of BIS in the NCCU was hindered by the dependability issues of certain techniques (muscle artifacts and shivering) within the ICU setting. Additionally, it was originally designed to gauge the level of anesthesia in patients without any brain-related ailments. The presence of ABI could affect the BIS algorithm due to EEG changes associated with the condition rather than the sedative state [16]. The feasibility of improved monitoring of sedation in the NCCU using new EEG techniques requires further research.

Assessing the adequacy of analgesia can be particularly challenging in NCCU environment. For conscious patients, the preferred approach is to use the Numeric Rating Scale, whereas for patients who cannot respond, either the Behavioural Pain Scale [17] or the Critical Care Pain Observation Tool [18] may be used. However, there is still uncertainty about how effective these tools are for ABI patients [19]. A recently developed tool called the Nociception Coma Scale has shown promise in assessing pain levels in patients with altered sensorium [20]. In determining whether a patient's pain relief is adequate, healthcare professionals currently rely on observing indirect signs such as increased heart rate, high blood pressure, and raised intracranial pressure during painful procedures [21].

16.6 A Practical Approach for the Use of Sedation and Analgesia in the NCCU

The use of sedation and analgesia in neurocritical care requires a systematic approach that takes into consideration the patient's underlying condition, severity of the brain injury, the cerebral physiological state, mainly ICP, the level of sedation required, and the potential adverse effects of each medication. It is important to focus on promoting ventilator synchronization, controlling agitation, and managing pain effectively [22].

Below is a basic algorithm for sedation in neurocritical care:

Step 1: Assess the patient's underlying condition, including the level of consciousness, ICP, and pain level.

Step 2: Choose the appropriate sedative based on the patient's condition and level of sedation required. Some commonly used sedatives in neurocritical care include propofol, midazolam, and dexmedetomidine.

Step 3: Initiate sedation at a low dose and titrate to achieve the desired level of sedation. The goal is to achieve adequate sedation while minimizing adverse effects such as respiratory depression and hypotension.

Step 4: Monitor the patient's vital signs, including blood pressure, heart rate, and respiratory rate, and adjust the sedative dose as needed to maintain stable vital signs.

Step 5: Monitor for adverse effects of the sedative, such as respiratory depression, hypotension, and bradycardia, and adjust the dose or switch to a different sedative if necessary.

Step 6: Use analgesics as needed to control pain and minimize the need for higher doses of sedatives.

Step 7: Regularly assess the patient's level of sedation and adjust the dose as needed. Consider periodic sedation interruptions to assess the patient's neurological status and prevent oversedation.

Step 8: When discontinuing sedation, gradually wean the patient off the medication to prevent rebound agitation and withdrawal symptoms.

16.7 Withdrawal of Sedation in NCCU Patients

It is evident from various studies conducted on patients in the general ICU population that implementing sedation minimization strategies can lead to better patient outcomes [22]. Daily sedation interruption (SI) is one such strategy that has been shown to be beneficial for NICU patients [23]. This approach allows for clinical neuromonitoring and timely detection of warning neurological signs, potentially reducing mechanical ventilation duration and the need for tracheostomy. However, it is important to weigh the potential benefits against the risks of abrupt withdrawal of sedation. Daily SI trials may result in a significant increase in intracranial pressure (ICP) and reduction in cerebral perfusion pressure (CPP), particularly during the first days after injury. In addition, research has shown that abrupt SI can lead to increased levels of stress hormones like cortisol and endogenous catecholamines, as well as adrenergic activation and a slight but significant increase in ICP [24].

A practical approach would be to refraining from the use of SI for patients who are at risk of experiencing brain edema or an increase in intracranial pressure (ICP), as well as those who are receiving treatment for refractory status epilepticus or undergoing therapeutic hypothermia. For these patients, it is important to gradually withdraw sedation while closely monitoring ICP (and $PbtO_2$, if possible) levels to ensure that they remain within target ranges. In cases where ABI patients are not at risk for brain edema or elevated ICP, sedation withdrawal can proceed based on general ICU protocols, and daily use of SI is not discouraged [25]. Overall, the withdrawal of sedation in neurocritical care patients requires careful planning, monitoring, and management to ensure patient safety, comfort, and successful recovery [26].

16.8 Conclusion

In NCCU, analgesia and sedation are routinely utilized for both "general" and "neuro-specific" indications. Sedation carries several risks and, like in the general ICU, can prolong the duration of mechanical ventilation, the length of stay and impact morbidity and mortality, as well as obscure repeated neurological examination. Sedatives should be used to achieve a specific therapeutic goal, and their effectiveness and side effects should be closely monitored. Although the physiological effects of the most commonly prescribed sedatives are well established, it is usually essential to combine several agents to enhance the desired benefits and reduce the undesirable consequences.

Overall, the use of sedation in neurocritical care requires a multidisciplinary approach that involves close monitoring and frequent assessment of the patient's neurological status and vital signs. The sedation algorithm should be tailored to the severity of the ABI and therapeutic objectives (ICP, CPP, and $PbtO_2$) derived from intracranial monitoring, with the goal of maximizing analgesia and minimizing sedative dosages as necessary to achieve optimal outcomes.

References

1. Devlin JW, Skrobik Y, Gélinas C, et al. Clinical practice guidelines for the prevention and management of pain, agitation/sedation, delirium, immobility, and sleep disruption in adult patients in the ICU. Crit Care Med. 2018;46:e825–73.
2. Oddo M, Crippa IA, Mehta S, et al. Optimizing sedation in patients with acute brain injury. Crit Care. 2016;20:128.
3. Sharshar T, Citerio G, Andrews PJ, et al. Neurological examination of critically ill patients: a pragmatic approach. Report of an ESICM expert panel. Intensive Care Med. 2014;40(4):484–95.
4. Bauerschmidt A, Al-Bermani T, Ali S, Bass B, Dorilio J, Rosenberg J, Al-Mufti F. Modern sedation and analgesia strategies in Neurocritical care. Curr Neurol Neurosci Rep. 2023;23:149.
5. Seo Y, Lee HJ, Ha EJ, Ha TS. 2021 KSCCM clinical practice guidelines for pain, agitation, delirium, immobility, and sleep disturbance in the intensive care unit. Acute Crit Care. 2022;37(1):1–25.
6. Shehabi Y, Al-Bassam W, Pakavakis A, Murfin B, Howe B. Optimal sedation and pain management: a patient- and symptom-oriented paradigm. Semin Respir Crit Care Med. 2021;42(1):98–111.
7. Güiza F, Depreitere B, Piper I, et al. Visualizing the pressure and time burden of intracranial hypertension in adult and paediatric traumatic brain injury. Intensive Care Med. 2015;41(6):1067–76.
8. Glauser T, Shinnar S, Gloss D, et al. Evidence-based guideline: treatment of convulsive status epilepticus in children and adults: report of the guideline Committee of the American Epilepsy Society. Epilepsy Curr. 2016;16(1):48–61.
9. Ceric A, May TL, Lybeck A, Cronberg T, Seder DB, Riker RR, Hassager C, Kjaergaard J, Haxhija Z, Friberg H, Dankiewicz J, Nielsen N. Cardiac arrest treatment center differences in sedation and analgesia dosing during targeted temperature management. Neurocrit Care. 2023;38(1):16–25.
10. Meyfroidt G, Baguley IJ, Menon DK. Paroxysmal sympathetic hyperactivity: the storm after acute brain injury. Lancet Neurol. 2017;16(9):721–9.
11. Prabhakar H, Tripathy S, Gupta N, Singhal V, Mahajan C, Kapoor I, Wanchoo J, Kalaivani M. Consensus statement on Analgo-sedation in Neurocritical care and review of literature. Indian J Crit Care Med. 2021;25(2):126–33.
12. Mahmoud L, Zullo AR, Thompson BB, Wendell LC. Outcomes of protocolised analgesia and sedation in a neurocritical care unit. Brain Inj. 2018;32(7):941–7.
13. Musick S, Alberico A. Neurologic assessment of the Neurocritical care patient. Front Neurol. 2021;12:588989.
14. Marklund N. The neurological wake-up test-a role in Neurocritical care monitoring of traumatic brain injury patients? Front Neurol. 2017;8:540.
15. Fuller BM, Roberts BW, Mohr NM, et al. The ED-SED study: a multicenter, prospective cohort study of practice patterns and clinical outcomes associated with emergency department SEDation for mechanically ventilated patients. Crit Care Med. 2019;47(11):1539–48.
16. Heavner MS, Gorman EF, Linn DD, et al. Systematic review and meta-analysis of the correlation between bispectral index (BIS) and clinical sedation scales: toward defining the role of BIS in critically ill patients. Pharmacotherapy. 2022;42(8):67.
17. Mahmood S, El-Menyar A, Shabana A, et al. Bispectral index as a predictor of unsalvageable traumatic brain injury. Brain Inj. 2017;31:1382–6.
18. Pande RK. Behavioral pain assessment tool: yet another attempt to measure pain in sedated and ventilated patients! Indian J Crit Care Med. 2020;24(8):617–8.
19. Nazari R, Froelicher ES, Nia HS, et al. Diagnostic values of the critical care pain observation tool and the behavioral pain scale for pain assessment among unconscious patients: a comparative study. Indian. J Crit Care Med. 2022 Summer;26(4):472–6.
20. Jendoubi A, Abbes A, Ghedira S, Houissa M. Pain measurement in mechanically ventilated patients with traumatic brain injury: behavioral pain tools versus analgesia nociception index. Indian J Crit Care Med. 2017;21(9):585–8.
21. Formisano R, Contrada M, Aloisi M, et al. Nociception coma scale with personalized painful stimulation versus standard stimulus in non-communicative patients with disorders of consciousness. Neuropsychol Rehabil. 2020;30(10):1893–904.
22. Jurth C, Zimmermann V, Schaaf L, et al. Investigation of Behavioural pain scale, critical care pain observation tool, nociceptive flexion reflex and pupillary dilatation reflex as predictors of behavioural reactions to

nociceptive procedures in critically ill patients unable to self-report pain. Eur J Pain. 2022;26(10):2074–82.
23. Senthilkumaran S, Balamurugan N, Thirumalaikolundusubramanian P. A practical approach for the use of sedation and analgesia in the rural neuro intensive care. Neuro. Crit Care. 2020;21(2):67–71.
24. Sharma S, Hashmi MF, Valentino DJ III. Sedation vacation in the ICU. In: StatPearls. Treasure Island. FL: StatPearls Publishing; 2023.
25. Chen TJ, Chung YW, Chen PY, et al. Effects of daily sedation interruption in intensive care unit patients undergoing mechanical ventilation: a meta-analysis of randomized controlled trials. Int J Nurs Pract. 2022;28(2):e12948.
26. Poddar B. Withdraw sedation gently or face withdrawal syndrome! Indian J Crit Care Med. 2020;24(6):381–2.

17 Antiseizure Medications

Sulaiman Almohaish, David M. Peters Jr., and Gretchen M. Brophy

17.1 Introduction

Epilepsy and status epilepticus (SE) are both common neurologic disease states encountered in any neurocritical care unit and require aggressive treatment to halt seizure activity [1]. Epilepsy type, intensity, and etiology usually vary between one patient to another. Patients with unprovoked seizure episodes are commonly diagnosed with epilepsy, whereas when a seizure continues for at least 5 minutes, it is defined as SE and must be treated as a medical emergency [2, 3]. In many cases, the specific etiology and pathophysiology of seizures are unknown [4]. What is generally known is that seizures emerge from a sudden abnormal electrical activity in the brain which typically lead to excessive neuronal discharge and involuntary body movements [2, 3]. There are several possible causes of epilepsy and SE that include genetic mutations, infectious diseases, metabolic abnormalities, immunity-related diseases, and in some cases unknown causes [5]. Treatment strategies are generally determined based on patient-specific factors and the underlying seizure type. This chapter will discuss in detail different antiseizure medications (ASMs) that are commonly used to treat seizures and status epilepticus in neurocritical care patients.

17.2 Seizure Prophylaxis

The risk of seizures in neurocritical care patients is highly variable from one patient to another, and the risk/benefit ratio of seizure prophylaxis is not well defined in some conditions. Numerous guidelines are available describing the available literature specific to each indication for these ASMs. A summary of some of the main disease states and the recommendation for seizure prophylaxis can be found in Table 17.1.

S. Almohaish
Department of Pharmacotherapy and Outcomes Science, School of Pharmacy, Virginia Commonwealth University, Richmond, VA, USA

Department of Pharmacy Practice, Clinical Pharmacy College, King Faisal University, Al-Ahsa, Saudi Arabia

D. M. Peters Jr.
Department of Pharmacy Practice, Cedarville University School of Pharmacy, Cedarville, OH, USA

G. M. Brophy (✉)
Department of Pharmacotherapy and Outcomes Science, School of Pharmacy, Virginia Commonwealth University, Richmond, VA, USA
e-mail: gbrophy@vcu.edu

H. Prabhakar et al. (eds.), *Principles and Practice of Neurocritical Care*,
https://doi.org/10.1007/978-981-99-8059-8_17

Table 17.1 Seizure prophylaxis in neurocritical care patients [6–12]

Indication	ASM recommendation	Duration
Aneurysmal SAH	Consider levetiracetam (less cognitive effects than phenytoin)	3–7 days, though shorter durations may be preferable
Cerebral venous thrombosis	Prophylaxis not recommended	N/A
Craniotomy for tumor	Prophylaxis not recommended; patients presenting with seizures should be treated	Perioperatively, consider discontinuing ASM treatment 1–3 months after surgery for those presenting with seizures
Intracerebral hemorrhage	Prophylaxis not recommended	N/A
Ischemic stroke	Prophylaxis not recommended	N/A
Meningitis	Prophylaxis not recommended	N/A
Traumatic brain injury	Consider levetiracetam or (fos)phenytoin	7 days

17.3 Acute Treatment of Seizures

17.3.1 Benzodiazepines

Each benzodiazepine is a Gamma aminobutyric acid-A (GABA-A) agonist, but what sets each one apart from the others is their distinct pharmacokinetic profile. Benzodiazepines are crucial for managing acute seizures and SE, and their effectiveness depends on their pharmacological properties. The timing and duration of their effects can be influenced by variables such as absorption, distribution, metabolism, and excretion (Table 17.2). The fastest onset of effect and 100% bioavailability are provided by intravenous (IV) administration. For seizure management in neurocritical care, it is important to consider both the serum and central nervous system (CNS) half-lives of benzodiazepines. In the neurocritical care setting, where patients often have intravenous access, lorazepam has optimal pharmacokinetics which result in rapid and consistent therapeutic drug concentration in the CNS [13]. If lorazepam is unavailable, intravenous

Table 17.2 Benzodiazepine dose, route, and considerations in emergent therapy [14–17]

Medication	Dose (maximum)	Onset (duration of action for seizure control)	Metabolism and excretion	Half-life	CNS properties	Alternative routes of administration	Contains propylene glycol?
Lorazepam	0.1 mg/kg IV (4 mg) infused at 2 mg/min, may repeat in 5–10 min	1–10 min (approximately 12 h)	Hepatic metabolism to inactive metabolites	12 h	Slow penetration and long half-life	Not preferred	Yes
Diazepam	0.15–0.2 mg/kg IV infused at 5 mg/min (10 mg), may repeat in 5 min	1–3 min (approximately 30 min)	CYP2C19 and CYP3A4 to active metabolites and excreted renally	33–45 h	Fast penetration and short half-life	Rectal: 0.2 mg/kg Intranasal: 0.2 mg/kg (max 20 mg)	Yes
Midazolam	0.2 mg/kg IM (10 mg)	5–15 min (IM–30 min to 2 h)	CYP3A4 to active metabolite and excreted renally	3–5 h	Fast penetration and short half-life	Intravenous (very short duration of action): 0.2 mg/kg bolus Intranasal: 0.2 mg/kg (max 10 mg) Buccal: 0.5 mg/kg (max 10 mg)	No

diazepam or intramuscular midazolam should be utilized. Intravenous diazepam is extremely lipophilic and quickly redistributes out of the CNS, providing only about 30 min of seizure control. Intravenous midazolam also has a short duration of activity and would need to be given as a bolus followed by a continuous infusion [13]. Although these small time variations may appear insignificant, there are clinically relevant advantages when clinicians choose benzodiazepines with optimal pharmacokinetic profiles. When giving benzodiazepines as continuous intravenous (cIV) infusions or frequently enough for accumulation to occur, renal and hepatic function must be considered. It is important to be cautious recommending diazepam and midazolam for patients with hepatic dysfunction because the duration of their effects may be prolonged as these drugs are metabolized via CYP3A4 to active metabolites.

17.3.2 Antiseizure Medications

The goal of ASM therapy is to stop seizure activity as quickly as possible while having the least negative effects on quality of life. Neurocritical care patients are at risk of seizure due to their underlying injuries and are often prescribed ASMs for a short period of time (1–3 months) after the initial seizure. Neurocritical care patients who have experienced two or more unprovoked seizures are generally continued on ASM therapy for prolonged durations of time and followed by a neurologist in the outpatient setting [18]. A precise diagnosis and identification of seizure type is essential to choose the best ASM therapy (Table 17.3). The selection of an ASMs is also based on patient-specific factors such as age, sex, possibility of pregnancy, susceptibility to adverse effects, comorbidities, potential drug interactions, adherence, and cost of therapy. Some patients may require more than one ASM therapy and others may need only one agent to control their seizures.

Table 17.3 Common antiseizure medication treatment options for neurocritical care patients

Seizure type	ASM treatment options
Primary generalized tonic–clonic	Valproic acid, phenytoin, topiramate, levetiracetam, lacosamide, and perampanel
Secondary generalized tonic–clonic	Levetiracetam, valproic acid, phenytoin, topiramate, lacosamide, and perampanel
Focal—with or without awareness	Levetiracetam or brivaracetam, phenytoin, valproic acid, topiramate, lacosamide, and perampanel
Absence	Valproic acid and topiramate
Myoclonic, atonic/akinetic	Valproic acid, levetiracetam, and topiramate

Antiseizure medications have changed over time. First-generation ASMs have a narrow therapeutic window, requiring serum concentration monitoring to attain a desired therapeutic range and to prevent potential harm. In contrast, the newer generation ASMs do not. Most of the available ASMs' mechanisms of action can be divided into four major groups: (1) alteration of ionic conductance (sodium channel blocker or calcium channel blocker); (2) enhancement of GABAergic (inhibitory) neurotransmission; (3) suppression of glutamatergic (excitatory) neurotransmission or modulation of neurotransmitter release; and (4) unique or unknown mechanisms (Table 17.4) [19].

First-Generation Antiseizure Medications

The Food and Drug Administration (FDA) approved the following first-generation ASMs before 1978: phenobarbital, phenytoin/fosphenytoin, and valproate. Although the ASMs in this class are among the most effective at controlling seizures, they are more difficult to manage than second- or third-generation ASMs due to their complex pharmacokinetics, numerous interactions, and higher incidence of adverse effects.

Table 17.4 Antiseizure medication overview [20–34]

Medication	MOA	Dosing	Route	Dilution	Rate of administration	ADR	Monitoring/pearls
Brivaracetam	Modulates neurotransmitter release through binding to the synaptic vesicle protein SV2A	In SE: loading dose 100–200 mg Maintenance 50–100 mg BID Maximum 200 mg/day	IV push	Can administer undiluted	2 min	Sedation Fatigue Nystagmus Irritability Aggressive behavior	Dose adjustment required for patients with hepatic impairment A substrate of CYP2C19 which may be impacted by genomics May be effective in patients who fail levetiracetam
			IV piggyback	Dilute in 50–100 mL NS, D5W, or LR	15 min		
Clobazam	Increases GABA activity	Initial 5–15 mg BID then increases to the desirable effect Maximum dose: 60 mg/day	Oral	–	–	Sedation Drooling Ataxia Aggressive behavior/irritability	Can be used off-label as an adjunctive in refractory seizures Requires dose adjustment in patients with liver disease; major substrate of CYP2C19
Phenytoin (PHT)	Inhibits sodium channels	Loading dose of 15–20 mg/kg Maintenance dose of 4–5 mg/kg/day) Titrate on basis of clinical response and target serum concentration	Oral	–	–	Rash Hypotension (with loading dose) Sedation Stevens–Johnson syndrome/toxic epidermal necrolysis; higher risk in Asian patients positive for HLA-B*15021.	PHT suspension binds to enteral nutrition and feeding tube (hold enteral nutrition 1 h pre/post-dose) PHT: use IV filter, can form precipitate
			IV piggyback	Dilute in 50–100 mL of NS (incompatible with dextrose)	PHT: Administer no faster than 50 mg/min		
Fosphenytoin (FPHT)			IV piggyback	Dilute in 50–100 mL of NS or D5W	FPHT: Administer no faster than 150 mgPE/min		
			FPHT: IM injection	No dilution for IM	–		

Medication	MOA	Dosing	Route	Dilution	Rate of administration	ADR	Monitoring/pearls
Lacosamide	Inhibits sodium channels	SE: loading dose of 200–400 mg Maintenance dose: 50–200 mg BID	Oral	–	–	Dizziness Ataxia Diplopia P–R interval prolongation	Low risk of drug–drug interactions Metabolized by CYP2C19 and excreted renally Caution in patients with heart block or P–R prolongation
			IV push	Can administer undiluted	Administer at 80 mg/min		
			IV piggyback	Dilute in 50–100 mL NS, D5W, or LR	Administer over 15 min		
Levetiracetam	Modulates neurotransmitter release through binding to the synaptic vesicle protein SV2A	SE: loading dose 1000–3000 mg (or 40–60 mg/kg, maximum single loading dose 4500 mg) Maintenance 500–1500 mg BID Maximum dose 3000 mg/day	Oral	–	–	Somnolence Dizziness Behavioral symptoms (agitation, hostility, and depression)	Preferred agent in pregnancy No hepatic metabolism Requires renal adjustment Low risk for drug–drug interactions Change to alternate agent if behavioral adverse events develop
			IV push	Can administer undiluted (doses <1500 mg) or dilute in 1 mL NS per 1 mL drug	500 mg/min		
			IV piggyback	Dilute in 100 mL NS or D5W	10 min or 500 mg/min		
Perampanel	Inhibits (AMPA) glutamate receptor	Initial 2 mg daily at bedtime (not on enzyme-inducing ASMs) ***OR*** 4 mg once daily at bedtime (on enzyme-inducing ASMs) Maintenance dose is 8–12 mg/day daily at bedtime	Oral	–	–	Dizziness Somnolence Risk of falls in older adult patients Aggression/irritability	Serious or life-threatening psychiatric and behavioral adverse effects have occurred
Phenobarbital	Prolongs opening of GABA receptors	SE: Loading dose 5–15 mg/kg—May repeat loading dose once if seizures persist	Oral	–	–	Sedation Hypotension Decreased cardiac output	Loading doses for status epilepticus commonly require intubation
			IV piggyback	Dilute in 50–100 mL NS	50–100 mg/min		

(continued)

Table 17.4 (continued)

Medication	MOA	Dosing	Route	Dilution	Rate of administration	ADR	Monitoring/pearls
Medication	MOA	Dosing	Route	Dilution	Rate of administration	ADR	Monitoring/pearls
Topiramate	Inhibits sodium channels and activates GABA receptors, inhibits glutamate receptors	SE: 200–400 mg every 6 h Recommended maintenance target dosage range at 200–400 mg/day	Oral	–	–	Sedation Dizziness Difficulty concentrating Confusion Metabolic acidosis	Requires renal adjustment Phenytoin and carbamazepine may decrease concentrations
Valproate sodium (valproic acid)	Increase activity of GABA, inhibits sodium channel	SE: loading dose: 20–40 mg/kg/day Maintenance dose: 10–15 mg/kg/day Increase by 5–10 mg/kg/day to therapeutic effect or target serum concentration	Oral	–	–	Thrombocytopenia Hepatotoxicity Pancreatitis Hyperammonemia	Monitor LFTs and platelet count Severe fetal abnormalities, confirm negative pregnancy test
			IV piggyback	Dilute in 50 mL NS or D5W Undiluted administration associated with injection site pain, not recommended	6–10 mg/kg/min or over 10 min		

ADR adverse drug reaction, *AMPA* α-Amino-3-hydroxy-5-methyl-4-isoxazolepropionic acid, *D5W* 5% dextrose solution, *GABA* Gamma-aminobutyric acid, *IM* intramuscular, *LFTs* liver function tests, *LR* lactated Ringer's solution, *MOA* mechanism of action, *NS* normal saline, *SE* status epilepticus, *SV2A* synaptic vesicle glycoprotein 2A

Phenytoin (or fosphenytoin) is one of the most complicated ASMs due to its pharmacologic properties. Ninety percent of total phenytoin is protein-bound and 10% is free (unbound) in patients with normal albumin concentrations. Only the free, unbound phenytoin is pharmacologically active [22]. A total phenytoin concentration in the therapeutic range of 10–20 mg/L (mcg/mL; 40–79 mol/L) corresponds to a pharmacologically active free phenytoin concentration of 1–2 mg/L (mcg/mL; 4–8 mol/L), according to the reference ranges for total and free phenytoin concentrations [35, 36]. In order to interpret the true concentration of pharmacologically active medicine, it is crucial to know which phenytoin concentration is being utilized. Total and free phenytoin concentrations are both used in clinical practice to direct therapy. In patients with hypoalbuminemia, monitoring of free phenytoin concentrations more accurately reflects the real therapeutic concentrations. However, free phenytoin concentrations are not readily available through many laboratories and results may take days to weeks to become available. Valproate is likewise strongly bound to albumin, and the amount of valproate that is free in the serum will increase as total serum concentration increases. The total valproate concentrations might not accurately reflect the quantity of free drug that is available to make a pharmacologic impact, but free valproate concentrations are not typically ordered and total valproate concentrations are the only ones that are typically used. To help with the interpretation of total phenytoin and valproate serum concentrations, it is crucial to know the patient's serum albumin concentrations and protein status. This is very important for phenytoin since the Winter–Tozer equation

$$\left(\text{Corrected Phenytoin} = \frac{\text{Measured Total Phenytoin}}{(0.25 \times \text{Albumin}) + 0.1}\right)$$

can be used to help interpret total serum phenytoin concentrations in individuals with low protein at baseline. In clinical practice, valproate concentrations are not typically adjusted for low protein status, though it is prudent to be aware of this possibility. Phenobarbital is also highly protein bound, but this has less of a clinically meaningful impact in practice.

The cytochrome P450 (CYP450) enzymes in the liver metabolize phenytoin, which exhibits Michaelis–Menten pharmacokinetics [22]. The metabolism of phenytoin is typically linear in most persons at doses of less than 300 mg/day. A slight increase in dose might cause a disproportionally significant increase in serum concentrations which may result in toxicity [22, 35]. Some people may also experience toxicity at lower serum concentrations. Although CYP450 enzymes also catabolize phenobarbital and valproate through the liver, these drugs often exhibit linear pharmacokinetics at therapeutically useful dosages [26, 28]. As a result of their narrow therapeutic windows, phenobarbital, phenytoin, and valproate all necessitate serum concentration monitoring (Table 17.5).

ASMs from the first generation are typically considered broad-spectrum ASMs. Valproate is effective for a variety of epileptic disorders as well as seizures with both focal and generalized onset (Table 17.3) [28]. Phenytoin is very effective in controlling tonic–clonic seizures and is known to be effective in controlling focal-onset seizures, though it can exacerbate patients with generalized atypical absence seizures [22, 37–39]. Medications like valproic acid may exhibit benefit for patients with concomitant disorders, such as migraine and bipolar disorder [28]. Despite the strong efficacy of first-generation ASMs, newer generation ASMs are more commonly prescribed due to their higher tolerability, lower risk of drug interactions, and widespread availability of generic versions.

Table 17.5 Antiseizure medications pharmacokinetic characteristics

ASM	Oral absorption (%)	Half-life (h)	Time to steady state	Target serum concentration	Protein binding (%)	Volume of distribution (L/kg)
Brivaracetam	~100	9	2–3 days	N/A	<20	0.5
Clobazam	87	16–42; *N*-desmethyl (active metabolite) 71–82	3–7 days	N/A	80–90	NA
Lacosamide	100	13; increase slightly with renal impairment	2–3 days	N/A	<15	0.6
Levetiracetam	100	*Normal renal function:* 6–8; increased with renal impairment	1–1.5 days	N/A	<10	≈0.7
Perampanel	100	*Normal hepatic function*: 105	2–3 weeks	N/A	95	NA
Phenobarbital	90–100	2–4 days	8–16 days	15–40 mcg/mL	50	0.5–0.6
Phenytoin (fosphenytoin)	90–100	Varies with dose	5–30 days	Total: 10–20 mcg/mL Free: 1–2 mcg/mL	95	0.5–0.7
Topiramate	≥80	12–24	3–4 days	N/A	10–15	0.7
Valproate	100 (≈80% with divalproex ER)	10–16	2–3 days	50–150 mcg/mL	90+	0.09–0.17

Second-Generation Antiseizure Medications

The second-generation ASMs, which received FDA approval between 1993 and 2000, were created with an understanding of the drawbacks of the first-generation ASMs. Levetiracetam and topiramate are common members of this class encountered in the ICU [24, 27]. These drugs have less frequent adverse effects, relatively straightforward pharmacokinetics with fewer interactions and are thought to be equally effective at controlling seizures as first-generation ASMs.

Levetiracetam, which modulates both glutamatergic and GABA neurotransmission by modulating presynaptic neurotransmitter release via inhibition of synaptic vesicle glycoprotein 2A (SV2A), is one of the ASMs with a unique mechanism of action [24]. It is commonly regarded as a beneficial broad-spectrum ASM and is used as a first-line medication to treat focal-onset epilepsy, as well as primary generalized seizures. The most commonly cited adverse effects are behavioral, including agitation, delirium, and anxiety [24, 40]. In a recent neurocritical care study, levetiracetam-associated behavioral adverse events occurred in 46% of the patients [40]. Levetiracetam is largely removed through the kidneys, as opposed to the first-generation ASMs which are exclusively hepatically metabolized [24]. Patients with considerably impaired renal function may require dose adjustments [24, 35].

Topiramate also has multiple mechanisms of action; inhibiting sodium channels, activating GABA receptors, inhibiting glutamate receptors. Although it undergoes CYP3A4 metabolism, topiramate requires dosage adjustment in patients with renal impairment as 60% is cleared via the kidneys [27]. Topiramate can induce a metabolic acidosis due to its carbonic anhydrase inhibitor properties, especially with high doses used for refractory status epilepticus (RSE) [27]. It is often a last resort for maintenance therapy because of its impact on cognition [27]. Many patients cite difficulty concentrating, clouded thinking, or other adverse effects when taking topiramate. These adverse effects can sometimes be mitigated by increasing topiramate dosing on a very gradual titration. Topiramate can be a particularly helpful treatment option for patients with migraines, as it can help to reduce the intensity or severity of the headache. In addition, it useful for patients with comorbid obesity because it can help to reduce weight [27].

Third-Generation Antiseizure Medications

Between 2004 and 2020, the FDA authorized third-generation ASMs; these compounds can be further divided into those that are approved for general seizure indications and those that are approved for certain epilepsy conditions. In the ICU, clinicians encounter third-generation ASMs such as brivaracetam, lacosamide, perampanel, and clobazam [20, 21, 23, 25]. Even though many ASMs were only licensed for a handful of extremely specific conditions, they are frequently used off-label in refractory epilepsy after other first-line ASMs have failed.

Lacosamide has emerged as a preferred ASM among many clinicians. This is due to its simplicity of administration, the availability of intravenous doses, and minimal drug interactions [23]. It is usually well tolerated, though it can cause PR prolongation and should be utilized carefully in patients with atrial cardiovascular blocks.

Brivaracetam has a 15–30 times higher binding affinity for SV2A than levetiractam, does not bind to α-Amino-3-hydroxy-5-methyl-4-isoxazolepropionic acid (AMPA) receptors, and has fewer behavioral adverse effects [19, 20]. The CYP2C19 enzyme breaks down brivaracetam, and individuals who are poor or quick CYP2C19 metabolizers may exhibit altered brivaracetam pharmacokinetics [20]. Thus, brivaracetam dose should always be adjusted for patients with liver impairment.

Clobazam is a benzodiazepine agent that enhances GABAergic transmission. The CYP3A4 and CYP2C19 enzymes metabolize clobazam to produce an active metabolite, *N*-desmethylclobazam, which is also metabolized by CYP2C19 [21]. As a result, patients with hepatic impairment always require dose adjustment. Clobazam has the broadest use among third-generation drugs as it works on focal seizures and primary generalized epilepsies [21].

Perampanel decreases glutamatergic transmission through inhibition of the AMPA receptor. It has high protein binding (between 96 and 98%) and is predominantly removed by CYP3A4 metabolism to an inactive metabolite with a half-life of about 100 h [25]. Therefore, clinicians should try to avoid its use in patients with liver or renal impairment. While perampanel is broadly approved for focal seizures with or without generalized tonic–clonic seizures, clinicians may avoid its use due to the appearance of aggression or behavioral side effects in some patients [25].

17.4 Treatment of Medical Emergencies with Antiseizure Medications (ASMs)

In the neurocritical care unit, ASMs are most commonly used to treat convulsive or nonconvulsive SE. SE is defined as 5 min or more of seizure activity or two or more seizures without a return to baseline. Multiple guidelines have been published to outline the proper definitions, treatment strategy, and monitoring for this challenging disease state [33, 37, 41]. The most common approach to SE management distinguishes three phases of care: emergent treatment, urgent treatment, and refractory treatment. This is outlined in Fig. 17.1. This section will highlight key pharmacotherapy pearls used throughout the treatment of SE in each phase.

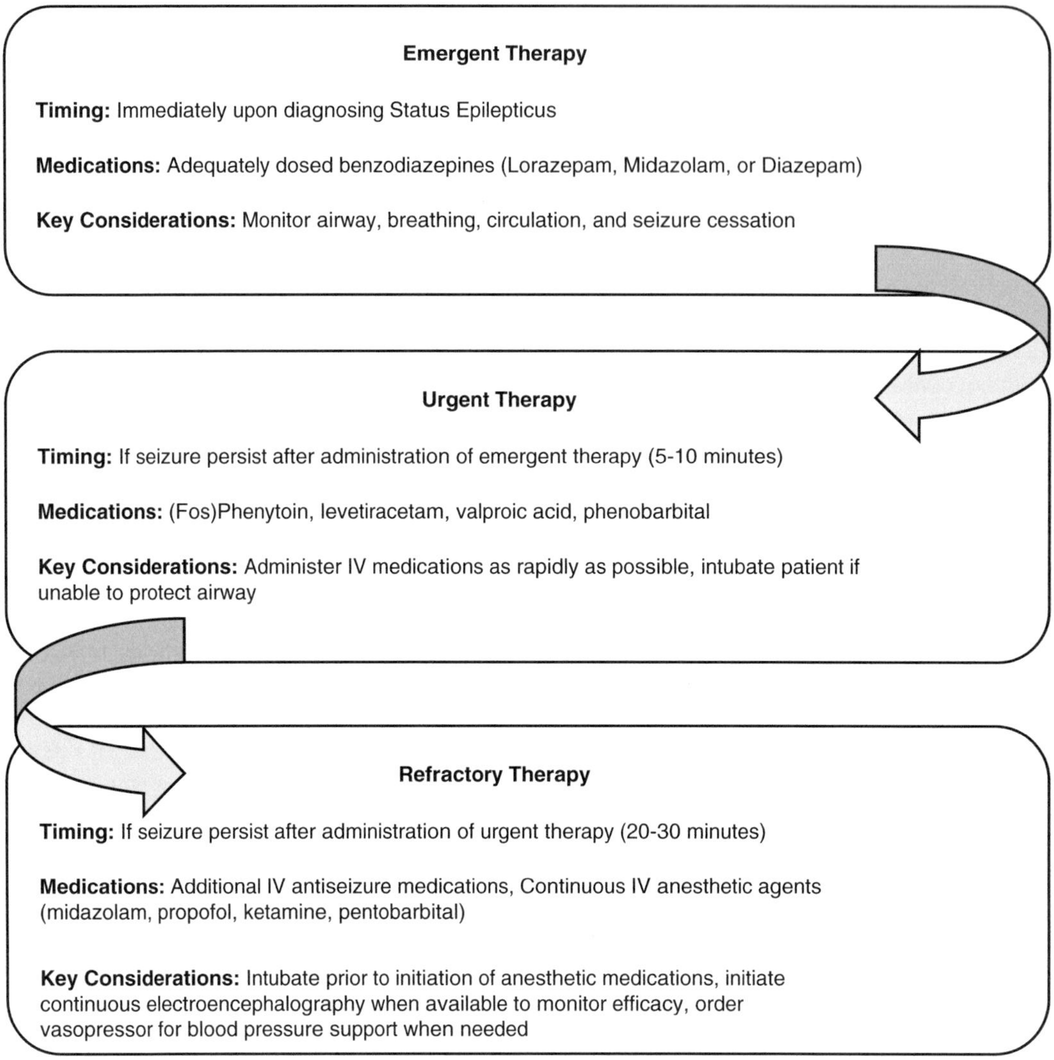

Fig. 17.1 Medication use and monitoring through phases of status epilepticus care

17.4.1 Emergent Therapy for Status Epilepticus

Benzodiazepines are the established initial treatment for seizure emergencies and SE. This was confirmed through multiple randomized controlled trials [42–44]. Two principles of therapy are to initiate benzodiazepines as rapidly as possible and to administer an adequate dose. In the prehospital and outpatient setting, utilizing benzodiazepines through routes other than intravenous is safe and effective. A randomized clinical trial displayed efficacy of intramuscular midazolam compared to intravenous lorazepam in the prehospital setting in patients without intravenous access [44]. Other benzodiazepine options exist for the lay public, such as nasal sprays, rectal suppositories, and autoinjectors [17]. Dosing is outlined in Table 17.2.

Whatever benzodiazepine is utilized, it must be given at an adequate dose. It is common for prescribers to underdose benzodiazepines, which results in higher rates of treatment failure [45–47]. The most common reason cited for underdosing benzodiazepines is the fear of respiratory depression and the need for intubation. However, patients who received inadequate doses of benzodiazepines are more likely to require respiratory support when compared to patients who received an adequate dose [48]. Therefore, an appropriate dose should always be utilized (Table 17.2).

17.4.2 Urgent Therapy for Status Epilepticus

Benzodiazepines will succeed to halt seizures in approximately 60% of patients [44, 49]. However, the 40% of patients who fail treatment will need additional pharmacologic support. Therefore, initiating an ASM is critical as the second phase of SE treatment. The clinician wants to provide an immediate therapeutic effect; therefore, these medications need to be given as an intravenous loading dose followed by maintenance therapy.

The three most used medications are phenytoin, valproic acid, and levetiracetam. When compared directly in a randomized controlled trial, all three medications exhibited similar safety and efficacy [49]. Ideally, selection will be supported by whichever medication can be procured and administered most rapidly based on practice patterns, familiarity, and availability. There are multiple strategies to improve time to medication delivery (Fig. 17.2). Levetiracetam has shown safety when administered IV Push and undiluted, improving time to administration [50, 51]. Complete administration and dilution data are included in Table 17.4.

Additional intravenous options for SE control include lacosamide and brivaracetam. Lacosamide has been trialed in status epilepticus with a common loading dose of 400 mg followed by maintenance doses of 100–200 mg twice daily in adults. Data are relatively sparse though efficacy has been shown [52, 53]. Lacosamide has been associated with arrhythmias, so electrocardiogram monitoring may be useful during loading doses. This is especially true in patients with underlying cardiac disease and/or receiving high doses. Another medication with sparse data in SE is brivaracetam. Brivaracetam has a similar mechanism of action to levetiracetam and can be administered via intravenous push over 2 min. Brivaracetam has decreased behavioral adverse effects when compared to levetiracetam but has lower levels of evidence for use in status epilepticus. Dosing is not well described, though a loading dose of 200 mg is reasonable followed by a standard maintenance dose of 50–100 mg twice daily [54, 55].

Prehospital Factors	Medication Factors
• Keep nasal, rectal or autoinjector benzodiazepine at home/school/work • Rapidly establish IV access • Maintain benzodiazpines in ambulances • Train Emergency Medical Services on diagnosis and treatment of SE	• Store ASMs in an automated dispensing unit in the Emergency Department • Order medications as STAT • Use minimal dilution medication (i.e. IV Push) • Know rate limits for administration (i.e. phenytoin, fosphenytoin, phenobarbital) • Monitor for hypotension with ASM administration (propylene glycol content) • Give fosphenytoin intramuscular if there is no IV access (slower time to onset)

Fig. 17.2 Strategies for rapid antiseizure drug administration

17.4.3 Refractory Status Epilepticus Treatment

When SE progresses despite provision of emergent and urgent therapy, it is defined as RSE. This disease state is challenging to treat and requires multiple pharmacotherapeutic interventions. Even when treated optimally mortality can exceed 20–30% [56]. The neurocritical care clinician must be familiar with the treatment philosophy of continuous intravenous (cIV) anesthesia and apply optimal pharmacotherapy to promote best outcomes for these patients.

There are three key principles for the provision of cIV anesthesia: intubation, high-dose GABA agonism, and continuous electroencephalography (cEEG) monitoring. Patients must be intubated prior to provision of an anesthetic loading dose as they will lose the ability to maintain their airway. After or during intubation, clinicians must administer a loading dose of an intravenous anesthetic, followed by a continuous IV infusion. Continuous EEG is necessary for clinicians to review the impact of cIV therapy and understand how to titrate the anesthetic medications [33].

Medications used in this treatment approach are midazolam, propofol, pentobarbital/thiopental, and ketamine. The GABA-agonizing agents (midazolam, propofol, and pentobarbital) can be used as monotherapy, whereas ketamine should be combined with one of these agents when utilized in this indication [57]. The standard dosing and monitoring parameters are outlined in Table 17.6. There is limited evidence comparing the efficacy of these agents. A key meta-analysis published in 2002 identified that efficacy was greatest for pentobarbital, but mortality was identical between agents [58]. Furthermore, pentobarbital was associated with the greatest number of adverse effects. Midazolam was associated with the least amount of hypotension but also exhibited the highest degree of breakthrough seizures.

Adverse effects are extremely prevalent when treating RSE and must be considered when selecting a cIV esthetic agent. Every agent except ketamine is associated with profound hypotension, with rates up to 80% [58–61]. As such, maintaining euvolemia and initiation of a vasopressor may be necessary to maintain adequate perfusion. Midazolam appears to be the best tolerated cIV anesthetic and is a reasonable first-line option when needed. Patients who do not respond to midazolam are candidates for propofol, pentobarbital/thiopental, or adjunctive ketamine. Pentobarbital exhibits the most adverse effects, which include ileus (10–55%), healthcare-acquired infections (32–44%), and cardiac depression [59, 61]. As such, pentobarbital is reserved for salvage therapy for most patients. Propofol is commonly used and is generally tolerated at low doses for short periods of time. However, RSE requires large doses of sedative for days or weeks and patients should be monitored for propofol-related infusion syndrome (PRIS) and increases in triglycerides. PRIS is defined as abrupt myocardial failure with possible metabolic acidosis and muscular breakdown [62]. PRIS occurs most commonly at doses greater than 80 mcg/kg/min for a prolonged duration and should be monitored with labs such as triglycerides, arterial blood gas, creatinine kinase, lactic acid, and potassium [62].

Table 17.6 Intravenous anesthetic medications for RSE [33]

Medication	Primary mechanism	Loading dose	Continuous infusion maintenance dose	Serious adverse events	Clinical considerations	Weaning recommendations
Midazolam	↑$GABA_A$	0.2 mg/kg Repeat loading doses every 3–5 min if seizures persist Maximum total loading dose 2 mg/kg	0.05–2 mg/kg/h	Hypotension, prolonged obtundation	Tachyphylaxis after prolonged infusions	50% reduction every 3 h
Propofol	↑$GABA_A$ ↓NMDA	1–2 mg/kg Repeat loading dose once in 5 min if seizures persist	20–200 μg/kg/min (use caution with doses > 80 mcg/kg/min)	Hypotension, increased triglycerides, propofol-related infusion syndrome	Monitor creatinine kinase, pH, and triglycerides if the infusion is prolonged Best option in the setting of organ dysfunction	20% reduction every 3 h
Pentobarbital	↑$GABA_A$	5–15 mg/kg Repeat loading dose if seizures persist	0.5–5 mg/kg/h	Hypotension, decreased cardiac output, ileus, increased infection risk	Contains propylene glycol, continuous infusions can result in toxicity	20% reduction every 3 h
Ketamine	↓NMDA	0.5–1 mg/kg Repeat loading dose once if seizures persist	0.5–7.5 mg/kg/h	Tachyarrhythmia, excessive salivation	Decreased hypotension risk Should be used in combination with a GABA agonist	20% reduction every 3 h

Anesthesia Weaning

Continuous IV anesthesia weaning after cEEG seizure suppression is a challenging task. The exact timing of when to wean is uncertain, but guidelines suggest 24–48 h after reaching goal burst suppression or seizure cessation is reasonable [33, 60]. Strong evidence is lacking related to how quickly a weaning attempt should occur, though expert recommendations are provided in Table 17.6 [63]. If recurrence of seizures or SE is suspected, the clinician should restart a previously effective cIV anesthetic and adjust the maintenance ASMs. It is prudent to add maintenance ASMs that match the mechanism of action of an anesthetic to which the patient has responded. For example, if seizure suppression occurs in response to midazolam, enteral clobazam may be a wise maintenance ASM choice.

17.4.4 Super-Refractory Status Epilepticus

Super-refractory status epilepticus (SRSE) is a complication of RSE defined as seizure activity that persists after 24 h of cIV therapy or seizure activity that recurs during/after weaning of cIV therapy. This disease portends a poor prognosis and requires further pharmacologic and nonpharmacologic treatment [56]. There is weak evidence for the management of this stage of SE, mostly derived from case reports/series or retrospective reviews. Typically, the clinician will adjust maintenance ASMs while attempting to wean cIV medications. There are multiple pharmacologic and nonpharmacologic approaches which are selected based on clinician preference (Table 17.7) [57]. Some therapies may be difficult to administer or require specialty physician consultation, such as inhaled anesthesia. If possible, inciting factors can be used to select a patient-specific treatment to halt seizures.

Patients with new-onset refractory status epilepticus (NORSE) are characterized by a lack of prior diagnosis of epilepsy or an acute cerebral disorder. Patients experiencing NORSE have an increased risk of SRSE and mortality [64]. These patients are more likely to suffer from autoimmune disorders, encephalitis, neoplastic disorders, or toxicologic disorders [65, 66]. Treatment pathways have been recommended, and these patients may benefit from immunologic treatments like intravenous immunoglobulin, high-dose methylprednisolone, or plasmapheresis [67].

A prominent and complicated nonpharmacologic intervention for SRSE is the ketogenic diet. The ketogenic diet limits carbohydrate intake and derives more than 90% of caloric intake from fat. It is thought that there is a direct anticonvulsant effect of ketone bodies in the CNS and that the ketogenic diet directly increases GABA concentration [68]. Pediatric patients are more likely to benefit than adults from this intervention. There are multiple considerations for medications when initiating the ketogenic diet. First, clinicians must recognize that many medications contain carbohydrates, particularly those in oral solutions or syrups. In addition, high-dose steroids can inhibit ketosis and should not

Table 17.7 Treatment options for SRSE

Pharmacologic options	Nonpharmacologic options
– Ketamine – Phenobarbital – Oral ASMs (if feeding tube present) • Topiramate • Clobazam • Perampanel – Prolonged pentobarbital infusion – Inhaled anesthesia—isoflurane – Pyridoxine (genetic epilepsy syndromes) – Magnesium (primarily eclampsia) – Autoimmune-based treatments (IVIG, steroids)	– Ketogenic diet – Electroconvulsive therapy – Vagal nerve stimulation – Therapeutic hypothermia – Magnetic stimulation

not be used concurrently. Finally, propofol should be avoided with patients on a ketogenic diet due to an increase in the risk of propofol infusion syndrome [69].

17.5 ICU Interventions Which Impact Pharmacotherapy

17.5.1 Renal Replacement Therapy

Renal replacement therapy (RRT) may need to be initiated within the neurocritical care unit for a number of reasons. RRT impacts many medications, but most prominently impacts clearance of small molecules that are not protein-bound. Levetiracetam and lacosamide are two key ASMs which are renally eliminated and must be dose-adjusted based on renal function or type of RRT. For patients on continuous renal replacement therapy, a standard dose of levetiracetam and lacosamide is recommended [70]. Patients receiving intermittent hemodialysis will receive a lower maintenance dose based on creatinine clearance. Optimally, a half dose of medication can be given after dialysis sessions for intermittent hemodialysis [71]. Another impact on medications is related to protein binding. Hemodialysis patients commonly have low serum protein, and as such, free (unbound) drug concentrations are higher than expected in these patients. Total concentrations of phenytoin and valproic acid are less reliable. This may result in the need to monitor free drug concentrations, and clinicians may need to use pharmacokinetic correction calculations [72].

17.5.2 Plasmapheresis

Plasmapheresis can be used as a treatment for NORSE or another autoimmune disease in neurocritical care patients. Plasmapheresis removes highly protein-bound medications and can make medication dosing quite challenging [73, 74]. There is evidence to support increasing the dose of topiramate when initiating plasmapheresis in a patient with RSE [64]. Additional doses might be required for clobazam or valproic acid [73]. Other medications can be dosed normally with careful monitoring of the patients' clinical response. Similar to RRT, therapeutic drug monitoring of free drug concentrations is recommended in this setting for phenytoin or valproic acid.

17.5.3 Therapeutic Hypothermia

Therapeutic hypothermia (TH) has been studied as a treatment for SE and after cardiac arrest with varying efficacy. Regardless of the reason for use, there are pharmacokinetic impacts which can be considered. The most prominent impact of TH is generalized slowing of pharmacokinetic processes that decrease medication clearance. Hepatic enzymatic metabolism diminishes significantly at hypothermic temperatures and requires conservative drug dosing or therapeutic drug monitoring [75, 76]. This is impactful on a multitude of medications, with sparse data related to ASMs. There is data to support decreased clearance of midazolam, propofol, pentobarbital, and phenobarbital which may result in prolonged sedation [75, 77, 78]. This complicates prognostication when using these agents for RSE or SRSE. Decreased clearance has been observed in maintenance of ASMs like phenytoin and topiramate, but most ASMs have no data available in this setting and require clinical judgment for dose optimization [79].

17.6 Summary

Antiseizure medications are commonly used for prophylaxis and treatment of seizures and SE in neurocritical care patients. There is increasing evidence to avoid prophylactic treatment in most acute neurologic injuries, although prophylaxis is still recommended for traumatic brain injury or aneurysmal subarachnoid hemorrhage when used for a short duration of time. Treatment of seizures is more challenging, and medications should be selected carefully. Neurocritical care providers can use knowledge of the medications pharmacokinetics and pharmacodynamics to design an optimal treatment and monitoring regimen for their patients to improve outcomes. Preferential use of newer generation medications can decrease adverse effects and drug interactions while maintaining efficacy of treatment regimens.

Status epilepticus is a common disease state encountered within the ICU and should be managed via a stepwise treatment algorithm. Benzodiazepines should be utilized first line and dosed aggressively to abort seizure activity. If benzodiazepines fail, intravenous levetiracetam, phenytoin, fosphenytoin, or valproate sodium are all acceptable treatment options. The use of continuous intravenous anesthetics is appropriate for patients who progress to RSE and require additional monitoring with cEEG when available. Clinicians treating RSE or SRSE may need to design treatment regimens that combine multiple ASMs with different mechanisms of action while attempting nonpharmacologic interventions to holistically treat the patient.

Acknowledgments No acknowledgment.

Conflict of Interest StatementDr. Brophy is a consultant for UCB, Marinus Pharmaceuticals and Ceribell and is a speaker for UCB.

References

1. Westover MB, Shafi MM, Bianchi MT, Moura LMVR, O'Rourke D, Rosenthal ES, et al. The probability of seizures during EEG monitoring in critically ill adults. Clin Neurophysiol. 2015;126(3):463–71.
2. Fisher RS, van Emde BW, Blume W, Elger C, Genton P, Lee P, et al. Epileptic seizures and epilepsy: definitions proposed by the international league against epilepsy (ILAE) and the International Bureau for Epilepsy (IBE). Epilepsia. 2005;46(4):470–2.
3. Trinka E, Cock H, Hesdorffer D, Rossetti AO, Scheffer IE, Shinnar S, et al. A definition and classification of status epilepticus—report of the ILAE task force on classification of status epilepticus. Epilepsia. 2015;56(10):1515–23.
4. Lasoń W, Chlebicka M, Rejdak K. Research advances in basic mechanisms of seizures and antiepileptic drug action. Pharmacol Rep. 2013;65(4):787–801.
5. Scheffer IE, Berkovic S, Capovilla G, Connolly MB, French J, Guilhoto L, et al. ILAE classification of the epilepsies: position paper of the ILAE Commission for Classification and Terminology. Epilepsia. 2017;58(4):512–21.
6. Hoh BL, Ko NU, Amin-Hanjani S, Chou SH-Y, Cruz-Flores S, Dangayach NS, Derdeyn CP, Du R, Hänggi D, Hetts SW, Ifejika NL, Johnson R, Keigher KM, Leslie-Mazwi TM, Lucke-Wold B, Rabinstein AA, Robicsek SA, Stapleton CJ, Suarez JI, Tjoumakaris SI, Welch BG. 2023 Guideline for the Management of Patients With Aneurysmal Subarachnoid Hemorrhage: A Guideline From the American Heart Association/American Stroke Association. Stroke. 2023 Jul;54(7):e314-e370. https://doi.org/10.1161/STR.0000000000000436. Epub 2023 May 22. Erratum in: Stroke. 2023 Dec;54(12):e516. PMID: 37212182.
7. Greenberg SM, Ziai WC, Cordonnier C, Dowlatshahi D, Francis B, Goldstein JN, Hemphill JC 3rd, Johnson R, Keigher KM, Mack WJ, Mocco J, Newton EJ, Ruff IM, Sansing LH, Schulman S, Selim MH, Sheth KN, Sprigg N, Sunnerhagen KS; American Heart Association/American Stroke Association. 2022 Guideline for the Management of Patients With Spontaneous Intracerebral Hemorrhage: A Guideline From the American Heart Association/American Stroke Association. Stroke. 2022 Jul;53(7):e282-e361. https://doi.org/10.1161/STR.0000000000000407. Epub 2022 May 17. PMID: 35579034.
8. Powers WJ, Rabinstein AA, Ackerson T, Adeoye OM, Bambakidis NC, Becker K, Biller J, Brown M, Demaerschalk BM, Hoh B, Jauch EC, Kidwell CS, Leslie-Mazwi TM, Ovbiagele B, Scott PA, Sheth KN, Southerland AM, Summers DV, Tirschwell DL. Guidelines for the Early Management of Patients With Acute Ischemic Stroke: 2019 Update to the 2018 Guidelines for the Early Management of Acute Ischemic Stroke: A Guideline for Healthcare Professionals From the American Heart Association/American Stroke Association. Stroke. 2019 Dec;50(12):e344-e418. https://doi.org/10.1161/STR.0000000000000211. Epub 2019 Oct 30. Erratum in: Stroke. 2019 Dec;50(12):e440-e441. PMID: 31662037.
9. Ferro JM, Canhão P, Bousser MG, Stam J, Barinagarrementeria F, ISCVT Investigators. Early seizures in cerebral vein and dural sinus thrombosis: risk factors and role of antiepileptics. Stroke. 2008;39(4):1152–8.
10. Wijdicks EFM, Sheth KN, Carter BS, Greer DM, Kasner SE, Kimberly WT, et al. Recommendations for the management of cerebral and cerebellar infarction with swelling. Stroke. 2014;45(4):1222–38.
11. Mikkelsen T, Paleologos NA, Robinson PD, Ammirati M, Andrews DW, Asher AL, et al. The role of prophylactic anticonvulsants in the management of brain metastases: a systematic review and evidence-based clinical practice guideline. J Neuro-Oncol. 2010;96(1):97–102.
12. Brain Trauma Foundation. https://braintrauma.org/guidelines/guidelines-for-the-management-of-

severe-tbi-4th-ed#/:guideline/11-seizure-prophylaxis. Accessed 2 Sept 2022.
13. Kienitz R, Kay L, Beuchat I, Gelhard S, von Brauchitsch S, Mann C, et al. Benzodiazepines in the management of seizures and status epilepticus: a review of routes of delivery, pharmacokinetics, efficacy, and tolerability. CNS Drugs. 2022;36(9):951–75.
14. Lorazepam Injection Insert [Internet]. https://webcache.googleusercontent.com/search?q=cache:OLkMdcRKnCMJ:https://www.accessdata.fda.gov/drugsatfda_docs/label/2006/018140s028lbl.pdf+&cd=2&hl=en&ct=clnk&gl=us. Accessed 6 Jan 2021.
15. DIAZEPAM Injection Insert [Internet]. https://webcache.googleusercontent.com/search?q=cache:GOD94rHmAFQJ:https://dailymed.nlm.nih.gov/dailymed/getFile.cfm%3Fsetid%3D7e7dd743-a87b-4ab3-b6ae-f116cd0c8b0f%26type%3Dpdf+&cd=1&hl=en&ct=clnk&gl=us. Accessed 6 Jan 2021.
16. Midazolam Injection Insert [Internet]. https://webcache.googleusercontent.com/search?q=cache:z54yylc3GggJ:https://www.accessdata.fda.gov/drugsatfda_docs/label/2017/208878Orig1s000lbl.pdf+&cd=1&hl=en&ct=clnk&gl=us. Accessed 6 Jan 2021.
17. Almohaish S, Sandler M, Brophy GM. Time is brain: acute control of repetitive seizures and status epilepticus using alternative routes of administration of benzodiazepines. J Clin Med. 2021;10(8):1754.
18. Krumholz A, Wiebe S, Gronseth GS, Gloss DS, Sanchez AM, Kabir AA, et al. Evidence-based guideline: management of an unprovoked first seizure in adults: report of the guideline development Subcommittee of the American Academy of Neurology and the American Epilepsy Society. Neurology. 2015;84(16):1705–13.
19. Rogawski MA, Löscher W, Rho JM. Mechanisms of action of antiseizure drugs and the ketogenic diet. Cold Spring Harb Perspect Med. 2016;6(5):a022780.
20. Brivaracetam Insert [Internet]. https://webcache.googleusercontent.com/search?q=cache:O5zYTbEwGWEJ:https://www.accessdata.fda.gov/drugsatfda_docs/label/2018/205836s005,205837s004,205838s003lbl.pdf&cd=1&hl=en&ct=clnk&gl=us. Accessed 6 Feb 2023.
21. Onfi® (Clobazam) Insert [Internet]. https://webcache.googleusercontent.com/search?q=cache:sDdS5BkGp1AJ:https://www.accessdata.fda.gov/drugsatfda_docs/label/2016/203993s005lbl.pdf&cd=1&hl=en&ct=clnk&gl=us. Accessed 6 Feb 2023.
22. Phenytoin Insert [Internet]. https://labeling.pfizer.com/showlabeling.aspx?id=546. Accessed 6 Feb 2023.
23. Lacosamide Insert [Internet]. https://webcache.googleusercontent.com/search?q=cache:Zi61N9IOktIJ:https://www.accessdata.fda.gov/drugsatfda_docs/label/2017/022253s039,022254s030,022255s022lbl.pdf&cd=2&hl=en&ct=clnk&gl=us. Accessed 6 Feb 2023.
24. Levetiracetam Insert [Internet]. https://webcache.googleusercontent.com/search?q=cache:jzxcGG3APCUJ:https://www.accessdata.fda.gov/drugsatfda_docs/label/2009/021035s078s080%252C021505s021s024lbl.pdf&cd=2&hl=en&ct=clnk&gl=us. Accessed 6 Feb 2023.
25. Perampanel Insert [Internet]. https://webcache.googleusercontent.com/search?q=cache:fWkw7VJWDi4J:https://www.accessdata.fda.gov/drugsatfda_docs/label/2012/202834lbl.pdf&cd=2&hl=en&ct=clnk&gl=us. Accessed 6 Feb 2023.
26. PHENOBARBITAL Insert [Internet]. https://webcache.googleusercontent.com/search?q=cache:83V4wLd2CyEJ:https://www.sandoz.ca/sites/www.sandoz.ca/files/Phenobarbital%2520Product%2520Monograph.pdf&cd=2&hl=en&ct=clnk&gl=us. Accessed 6 Feb 2023.
27. Topiramate Insert [Internet]. https://webcache.googleusercontent.com/search?q=cache:sExXpwIHq_sJ:https://www.accessdata.fda.gov/drugsatfda_docs/label/2012/020844s041lbl.pdf&cd=1&hl=en&ct=clnk&gl=us. Accessed 6 Feb 2023.
28. Depakene (Valproic Acid) Insert [Internet]. https://webcache.googleusercontent.com/search?q=cache:pZrfTmaOPNEJ:https://www.accessdata.fda.gov/drugsatfda_docs/label/2011/018081s046_18082s031lbl.pdf&cd=1&hl=en&ct=clnk&gl=us. Accessed 6 Feb 2023.
29. Davidson KE, Newell J, Alsherbini K, Krushinski J, Jones GM. Safety and efficiency of intravenous push lacosamide administration. Neurocrit Care. 2018;29(3):491–5.
30. Kellinghaus C. Lacosamide as treatment for partial epilepsy: mechanisms of action, pharmacology, effects, and safety. Ther Clin Risk Manag. 2009;5:757–66.
31. Haller JT, Bonnin S, Radosevich J. Rapid administration of undiluted intravenous levetiracetam. Epilepsia. 2021;62(8):1865–70.
32. Jense A, Douville A, Weiss A. The safety of rapid infusion levetiracetam: a systematic review. Pharmacother J Hum Pharmacol Drug Ther. 2022;42(6):495–503.
33. Brophy GM, Bell R, Claassen J, Alldredge B, Bleck TP, Glauser T, et al. Guidelines for the evaluation and management of status epilepticus. Neurocrit Care. 2012;17(1):3–23.
34. Limdi NA, Knowlton RK, Cofield SS, Ver Hoef LW, Paige AL, Dutta S, et al. Safety of rapid intravenous loading of valproate. Epilepsia. 2007;48(3):478–83.
35. Patsalos PN, Spencer EP, Berry DJ. Therapeutic drug monitoring of antiepileptic drugs in epilepsy: a 2018 update. Ther Drug Monit. 2018;40(5):526–48.
36. Hiemke C, Bergemann N, Clement HW, Conca A, Deckert J, Domschke K, et al. Consensus guidelines for therapeutic drug monitoring in neuropsychopharmacology: update 2017. Pharmacopsychiatry. 2018;51(1–02):9–62.
37. Glauser T, Shinnar S, Gloss D, Alldredge B, Arya R, Bainbridge J, et al. Evidence-based guideline: treatment of convulsive status epilepticus in children and adults: report of the guideline Committee of the American Epilepsy Society. Epilepsy Curr. 2016;16(1):48–61.

38. Kanner AM, Ashman E, Gloss D, Harden C, Bourgeois B, Bautista JF, et al. Practice guideline update summary: efficacy and tolerability of the new antiepileptic drugs II: treatment-resistant epilepsy: report of the American Epilepsy Society and the Guideline Development, Dissemination, and Implementation Subcommittee of the American Academy of Neurology. Epilepsy Curr. 2018;18(4):269–78.
39. Kanner AM, Ashman E, Gloss D, Harden C, Bourgeois B, Bautista JF, et al. Practice guideline update summary: efficacy and tolerability of the new antiepileptic drugs I: treatment of new-onset epilepsy: report of the American Epilepsy Society and the Guideline Development, Dissemination, and Implementation Subcommittee of the American Academy of Neurology. Epilepsy Curr. 2018;18(4):260–8.
40. Strein M, Holton-Burke JP, Stilianoudakis S, Moses C, Almohaish S, Brophy GM. Levetiracetam-associated behavioral adverse events in neurocritical care patients. Pharmacotherapy. 2023;43(2):122–8.
41. Meierkord H, Boon P, Engelsen B, Göcke K, Shorvon S, Tinuper P, et al. EFNS guideline on the management of status epilepticus in adults. Eur J Neurol. 2010;17(3):348–55.
42. Alldredge BK, Gelb AM, Isaacs SM, Corry MD, Allen F, Ulrich S, et al. A comparison of lorazepam, diazepam, and placebo for the treatment of out-of-hospital status epilepticus. N Engl J Med. 2001;345(9):631–7.
43. Treiman DM, Meyers PD, Walton NY, Collins JF, Colling C, Rowan AJ, et al. A comparison of four treatments for generalized convulsive status epilepticus. Veterans Affairs Status Epilepticus Cooperative Study Group. N Engl J Med. 1998;339(12):792–8.
44. Silbergleit R, Durkalski V, Lowenstein D, Conwit R, Pancioli A, Palesch Y, et al. Intramuscular versus intravenous therapy for prehospital status epilepticus. N Engl J Med. 2012;366(7):591–600.
45. Sathe AG, Underwood E, Coles LD, Elm JJ, Silbergleit R, Chamberlain JM, et al. Patterns of benzodiazepine underdosing in the established status epilepticus treatment trial. Epilepsia. 2021;62(3):795–806.
46. Rao SK, Mahulikar A, Ibrahim M, Shah A, Seraji-Bozorgzad N, Mohamed W. Inadequate benzodiazepine dosing may result in progression to refractory and non-convulsive status epilepticus. Epileptic Disord Int Epilepsy J Videotape. 2018;20(4):265–9.
47. Alvarez V, Lee JW, Drislane FW, Westover MB, Novy J, Dworetzky BA, et al. Practice variability and efficacy of clonazepam, lorazepam, and midazolam in status epilepticus: a multicenter comparison. Epilepsia. 2015;56(8):1275–85.
48. Guterman EL, Sanford JK, Betjemann JP, Zhang L, Burke JF, Lowenstein DH, et al. Prehospital midazolam use and outcomes among patients with out-of-hospital status epilepticus. Neurology. 2020;95(24):e3203–12.
49. Kapur J, Elm J, Chamberlain JM, Barsan W, Cloyd J, Lowenstein D, et al. Randomized trial of three anticonvulsant medications for status epilepticus. N Engl J Med. 2019;381(22):2103–13.
50. Morgan O, Medenwald B. Safety and tolerability of rapid administration undiluted levetiracetam. Neurocrit Care. 2020;32(1):131–4.
51. Adams T, Greathouse K. Evaluation of time to administration, benzodiazepine use, and safety of intravenous push levetiracetam in a neuro-spine intensive care unit. Neurocrit Care. 2021;35(3):789–93.
52. Husain AM, Lee JW, Kolls BJ, Hirsch LJ, Halford JJ, Gupta PK, et al. Randomized trial of lacosamide versus fosphenytoin for nonconvulsive seizures. Ann Neurol. 2018;83(6):1174–85.
53. Panda PK, Panda P, Dawman L, Sharawat IK. Efficacy of lacosamide and phenytoin in status epilepticus: a systematic review. Acta Neurol Scand. 2021;144(4):366–74.
54. Aicua-Rapun I, André P, Rossetti AO, Decosterd LA, Buclin T, Novy J. Intravenous brivaracetam in status epilepticus: correlation between loading dose, plasma levels and clinical response. Epilepsy Res. 2019;149:88–91.
55. Santamarina E, Parejo Carbonell B, Sala J, Gutiérrez-Viedma Á, Miró J, Asensio M, et al. Use of intravenous brivaracetam in status epilepticus: a multicenter registry. Epilepsia. 2019;60(8):1593–601.
56. Guterman EL, Betjemann JP, Aimetti A, Li JW, Wang Z, Yin D, et al. Association between treatment progression, disease refractoriness, and burden of illness among hospitalized patients with status epilepticus. JAMA Neurol. 2021;78(5):588–95.
57. Rai S, Drislane FW. Treatment of refractory and super-refractory status epilepticus. Neurother J Am Soc Exp Neurother. 2018;15(3):697–712.
58. Claassen J, Hirsch LJ, Emerson RG, Mayer SA. Treatment of refractory status epilepticus with pentobarbital, propofol, or midazolam: a systematic review. Epilepsia. 2002;43(2):146–53.
59. Pugin D, Foreman B, De Marchis GM, Fernandez A, Schmidt JM, Czeisler BM, et al. Is pentobarbital safe and efficacious in the treatment of super-refractory status epilepticus: a cohort study. Crit Care Lond Engl. 2014;18(3):R103.
60. Rossetti AO, Milligan TA, Vulliémoz S, Michaelides C, Bertschi M, Lee JW. A randomized trial for the treatment of refractory status epilepticus. Neurocrit Care. 2011;14(1):4–10.
61. Newey CR, Wisco D, Nattanmai P, Sarwal A. Observed medical and surgical complications of prolonged barbiturate coma for refractory status epilepticus. Ther Adv Drug Saf. 2016;7(5):195–203.
62. Corbett SM, Montoya ID, Moore FA. Propofol-related infusion syndrome in intensive care patients. Pharmacotherapy. 2008;28(2):250–8.
63. Legriel S, Oddo M, Brophy GM. What's new in refractory status epilepticus? Intensive Care Med. 2017;43(4):543–6.
64. Sculier C, Gaspard N. New onset refractory status epilepticus (NORSE). Seizure. 2019;68:72–8.

65. NORSE INSTITUTE [Internet]. NORSE INSTITUTE. https://www.norseinstitute.org. Accessed 7 Feb 2023.
66. Gaspard N, Hirsch LJ, Sculier C, Loddenkemper T, van Baalen A, Lancrenon J, et al. New-onset refractory status epilepticus (NORSE) and febrile infection-related epilepsy syndrome (FIRES): state of the art and perspectives. Epilepsia. 2018;59(4):745–52.
67. Wickstrom R, Taraschenko O, Dilena R, Payne ET, Specchio N, Nabbout R, et al. International consensus recommendations for management of new onset refractory status epilepticus (NORSE) including febrile infection-related epilepsy syndrome (FIRES): summary and clinical tools. Epilepsia. 2022;63(11):2827–39.
68. Bough KJ, Rho JM. Anticonvulsant mechanisms of the ketogenic diet. Epilepsia. 2007;48(1):43–58.
69. Thakur KT, Probasco JC, Hocker SE, Roehl K, Henry B, Kossoff EH, et al. Ketogenic diet for adults in super-refractory status epilepticus. Neurology. 2014;82(8):665–70.
70. Smetana KS, Cook AM, Bastin MLT, Oyler DR. Antiepileptic dosing for critically ill adult patients receiving renal replacement therapy. J Crit Care. 2016;36:116–24.
71. Bansal AD, Hill CE, Berns JS. Use of antiepileptic drugs in patients with chronic kidney disease and end stage renal disease. Semin Dial. 2015;28(4):404–12.
72. Kiang TKL, Ensom MHH. A comprehensive review on the predictive performance of the Sheiner–Tozer and derivative equations for the correction of phenytoin concentrations. Ann Pharmacother. 2016;50(4):311–25. https://doi.org/10.1177/1060028016628166.
73. Mahmoud SH, Buhler J, Chu E, Chen SA, Human T. Drug dosing in patients undergoing therapeutic plasma exchange. Neurocrit Care. 2021;34(1):301–11.
74. Ibrahim RB, Liu C, Cronin SM, Murphy BC, Cha R, Swerdlow P, et al. Drug removal by plasmapheresis: an evidence-based review. Pharmacotherapy. 2007;27(11):1529–49.
75. Arpino PA, Greer DM. Practical pharmacologic aspects of therapeutic hypothermia after cardiac arrest. Pharmacotherapy. 2008;28(1):102–11.
76. van den Broek MPH, Groenendaal F, Egberts ACG, Rademaker CMA. Effects of hypothermia on pharmacokinetics and pharmacodynamics: a systematic review of preclinical and clinical studies. Clin Pharmacokinet. 2010;49(5):277–94.
77. Hostler D, Zhou J, Tortorici MA, Bies RR, Rittenberger JC, Empey PE, et al. Mild hypothermia alters midazolam pharmacokinetics in normal healthy volunteers. Drug Metab Dispos Biol Fate Chem. 2010;38(5):781–8.
78. Schaible DH, Cupit GC, Swedlow DB, Rocci ML. High-dose pentobarbital pharmacokinetics in hypothermic brain-injured children. J Pediatr. 1982;100(4):655–60.
79. Empey PE, Velez de Mendizabal N, Bell MJ, Bies RR, Anderson KB, Kochanek PM, et al. Therapeutic hypothermia decreases phenytoin elimination in children with traumatic brain injury. Crit Care Med. 2013;41(10):2379–87.

18 Antibiotic Drugs

M. N. Sivakumar

18.1 Introduction

Antibiotics form the cornerstone of treating bacterial infections, and appropriate early institution of antibiotics can save lives. Neurocritical care patients are at highest risk of developing healthcare-associated infections [1] and pose a significant challenge for diagnosing and treating them. This chapter details pharmacological principles, methods, and means of antibiotic therapy used to treat community-acquired and hospital-acquired infections and their associated challenges.

18.2 Pharmacokinetics (PK) and Pharmacodynamics (PD)

The effectiveness of antimicrobial therapy depends on how the drug, the patient's body, and the infection-causing agent interact with each other [2]. The interactions are complex, making it challenging to select the appropriate antibiotic treatment. Currently, the minimum inhibitory concentration (MIC) measured in vitro is the primary factor used to choose antibiotics. However, antibiotics does not act in the bloodstream but in specific tissues where they need to be distributed. Achieving a balance between blood and tissue concentration is a difficult task. Hence, local strategies such as intrathecal and intraventricular administration are used [3].

18.2.1 PK–PD Parameters of the Major Classes of Antimicrobials

Changes in pharmacokinetic (PK) parameters due to various factors like decreased renal function, hyperdynamic state, and use of vasoactive drugs can directly impact the serum concentration of antibiotics [4]. The overall serum concentration of the drug does not always reflect its active portion. The pharmacodynamic (PD) effect of an antibiotic is determined by the unbound fraction of the drug present at the site of infection [4]. Insufficient antibiotic concentration at the target site can lead to therapeutic failures, especially for bacteria with higher in vitro MICs.

The principles of pharmacokinetics and pharmacodynamics rely on understanding the relationship between antimicrobial exposure and response. Antimicrobial drugs are classified based on PK–PD measures that predict their effectiveness (Table 18.1). It provides the most accurate representation of the effectiveness of antibiotics, depending on the specific pattern of activity of each drug. There are three main

M. N. Sivakumar (✉)
Institute of Critical Care Medicine, Royal Care Super Speciality Hospital, Coimbatore, Tamil Nadu, India

H. Prabhakar et al. (eds.), *Principles and Practice of Neurocritical Care*,
https://doi.org/10.1007/978-981-99-8059-8_18

Table 18.1 Classification of antibiotics based on pharmacodynamics [6]

Pattern of activity	Antibiotics	Goal of therapy and PK/PD parameter correlating efficacy
Concentration-dependent killing and moderate to prolonged persistent effects	Aminoglycoside Fluoroquinolones Daptomycin Ketolides Metronidazole	Maximize concentrations: C_{max}/MIC and 24 h AUC/MIC
Time-dependent killing and minimal or no persistent effects	Penicillins Cephalosporins Carbapenams Monobactam	Maximize duration of exposure: $T >$ MIC
Time-dependent killing and moderate to prolonged persistent effects	Macrolide Clindamycin Streptogramin Glycopeptide Oxazolidinone	Maximize amount of drug: 24 h AUC/MIC

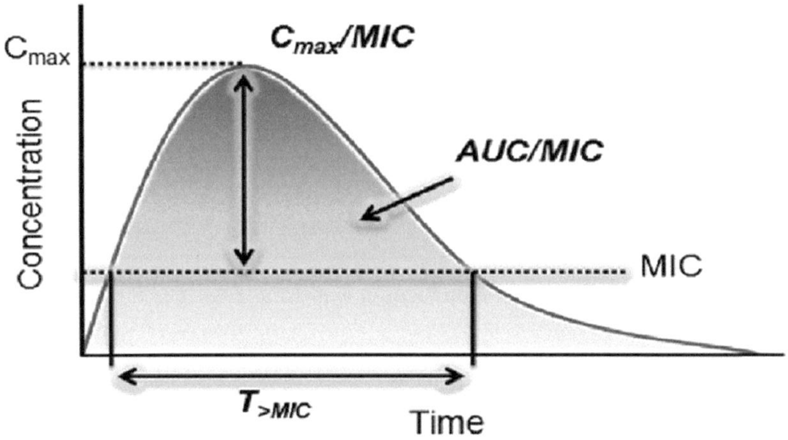

Fig. 18.1 PK/PD characteristics of antibiotics

patterns of antimicrobial activity that have been identified [5] (Fig. 18.1)

1. First pattern involves concentration-dependent killing and extended, long-lasting effects—the ratio of the highest drug concentration to the MIC (C_{max}/MIC)
2. Second pattern pertains to antimicrobials that exhibit time-dependent killing with little to no persistent effects—the time for which drug concentration remains above the MIC ($T >$ MIC)
3. Third pattern is characterized by concentration-independent killing and prolonged persistent effects—the ratio of the area under the concentration–time curve over 24 h to the MIC (24 h AUC/MIC)

18.2.2 Alterations in the PK Parameters in ICU Patients

Understanding the effects of pharmacokinetic changes in critically ill patients is crucial as these changes can affect serum and tissue antimicrobial concentrations. Clearance rate (*C*) and volume of distribution (*V*) are the primary pharmacokinetic (PK) parameters that influence drug levels and half-life (*T*1/2). Initial dosing is usually based on volume of distribution, and subsequent dosing is based on clearance rate. Physiological changes during sepsis or septic shock often alter these parameters in ICU patients [7].

In septic patients, inflammatory mediators increase capillary permeability and damages the endothelium. This, in turn, leads to fluid shift from the intravascular space and results in lower plasma and tissue concentrations of hydrophilic drugs. On the other hand, lipophilic antimicrobial concentrations are less affected due to their extensive distribution. Hypoalbuminemia is another common finding in critically ill patients that leads to an increase in the unbound fraction of a drug, which results in greater tissue distribution [8].

In sepsis, the hyperdynamic state is associated with increased renal clearance of drugs eliminated by glomerular filtration, such as beta-lactams and glycopeptides. In hepatic or renal dysfunction, the decreased clearance and metabolism of drugs result in drug/metabolite accumulation and dose reductions should be considered.

18.3 PK–PD Parameters of the Major Classes of Antimicrobials

18.3.1 Beta-lactams

Beta-lactam antibiotics like penicillin, cephalosporins, and carbapenems are widely used for treating infections in hospitals. This class of antibiotics is hydrophilic, excreted through the kidneys, has low protein binding, and has a low volume of distribution (with the exception of ceftriaxone). The effectiveness of beta-lactams depends on the time that the drug level remains above the MIC. To achieve optimal results, serum levels of beta-lactams should remain between 20 and 60% of the duration, above the MIC. This can be achieved through more frequent dosing or by extending the duration of the infusion [6].

18.3.2 Linezolid

Linezolid is an antibiotic that is part of the oxazolidinone class and works by inhibiting the initiation of bacterial protein synthesis [9]. It has moderate hydrophilicity, a moderate to low volume of distribution and a short half-life. Although it is hydrophilic, linezolid can penetrate tissues effectively and achieve satisfactory levels in the target tissues. Linezolid is a time-dependent antibiotic with a persistent post-antibiotic effect, and the best PD parameters that describe its activity are $T >$ MIC and AUC/MIC [7].

18.3.3 Vancomycin

The increase in vancomycin MICs (MIC creep) for *Staphylococcus aureus* is concerning because higher MICs can lead to lower AUC/MIC ratios and reduced vancomycin efficacy. For example, a standard dose of vancomycin (1 g every 12 h) is likely to reach target attainment with an MIC of 0.5 mg/L, but as the MIC value increases to 1.0 or 2.0 mg/L, the probability of target attainment decreases considerably. Higher vancomycin doses used to improve AUC/MIC ratios have led to increased rates of nephrotoxicity [10]. However, serum vancomycin trough level of (15–20 μg/ml) can be attained with a loading dose of 25–30 mg/kg [11].

18.4 Antibiotic Prophylaxis for Neurosurgical Patients

The primary aim of prophylaxis is to reduce postoperative surgical site infections and its related morbidity and mortality. This has to be balanced against cost, adverse effects, and emergence of antimicrobial resistance. Hence, institutions need to have local guidelines based on their flora and compliance to it has to be strictly monitored.

Table 18.2 Surgical prophylaxis recommendations [12–14]

Neurosurgery procedure	Recommendations	Antibiotic(s)	Dose/duration
"Clean" neurosurgery [craniotomy, extraventricular drains (EVD), aneurysm clipping]	Antibiotic prophylaxis is recommended	IV Cefazolin[a] 2 g or IV cefuroxime[a] 1.5 g	Single dose
Cerebrospinal fluid (CSF) shunt or drain insertion	Antibiotic prophylaxis is recommended		Single dose
Spinal surgery without implant (laminectomy, micro/discectomy, fusion, decompression, tumors, corpectomy)	Antibiotic prophylaxis is recommended		Single dose
Spinal surgery with implant	Antibiotic prophylaxis is recommended		24 h prophylaxis
Special implants Anterior cervical discectomy (ACD)/baclofen pumps)	Local recommendation is to give prophylaxis		Single dose
"**Clean, contaminated**" i.e. trans-sphenoidal (e.g. pituitary resection, repair of CSF leak, tumor debulking)	Antibiotic prophylaxis is recommended	IV Cefuroxime[a] 1.5 g then 750 mg every 8 h + IV metronidazole 500 mg every 8 h	Single dose/24 h
Penetrating intracranial injury	Antibiotic prophylaxis is recommended	IV Cefuroxime[a] 1.5 g then 750 mg every 8 h + IV metronidazole 500 mg every 8 h	To begin as soon as possible after injury and continue for 5 days postoperatively Seek advice on duration if foreign body still in situ
Base of skull fracture, CSF leak, CSF fistula	No prophylaxis recommended	–	–

[a]If anaphylaxis to cephalosporin use IV vancomycin

Table 18.3 Intravenous (IV) antibiotic dosing and redosing recommendations

Antibiotic	Dose	Administration	Redosing[a]
Cefuroxime	1.5 g	Bolus over 3–5 min	Redose 1.5 g after 3–4 h
Vancomycin	1 g	Infusion over 100–120 min in 250 mL 0.9% NS	Redose 1 g after 12 h
Metronidazole	500 mg	Infusion over 20 min	Redose 500 mg after 8 h

[a]Redosing to be considered if blood loss is more than 1500 mL and replaced with fluids

18.5 Principles of Surgical Prophylaxis

1. **Indication**

   Need for prophylaxis based on established/local guidelines (Table 18.2)

2. **Timing of Antibiotics**

   Started 60 min before skin incision (120 min for vancomycin and fluoroquinolones)

3. **Frequency of Administration**

   Single dose unless you have extensive blood loss or prolonged surgery (Table 18.3)

4. **Choice of Agent**

   (a) Use narrow spectrum whenever possible.

Table 18.4 Choices of empirical antibiotic therapy in community-acquired meningitis

Age	Bacterial pathogen	Empirical antibiotics
Age <1 month	*Streptococcus agalactiae, Escherichia coli, Listeria monocytogenes*	Amoxicillin or ampicillin plus cefotaxime or aminoglycoside
Age 2–50 years	*Streptococcus pneumoniae*[a], *Neisseria meningitidis, Hemophilus influenzae*[a], (*S. agalactiae, E. coli—age 1–23 months*)	Vancomycin plus a third-generation cephalosporin (either cefotaxime or ceftriaxone)
Age >50 years	*Streptococcus pneumoniae*[a], *Neisseria meningitidis, Listeria monocytogenes*, aerobic gram-negative bacilli	Vancomycin plus ampicillin plus a third-generation cephalosporin (either cefotaxime or ceftriaxone)
Immunocompromised patients	*S. pneumoniae*[a], *N. meningitidis, L. monocytogenes, Staphylococcus aureus, Salmonella* spp., aerobic gram-negative bacilli (including *Pseudomonas aeruginosa*)	Vancomycin plus ampicillin plus either cefepime or meropenem
Patients with recurrent meningitis	*S. pneumoniae*[a], *N. meningitidis, H. influenzae*[a]	Vancomycin plus a third-generation cephalosporin (either cefotaxime or ceftriaxone)
Patients with base of skull fracture	*S. pneumoniae*[a], *H. influenzae*[a], group A b–hemolytic streptococci	Vancomycin plus a third-generation cephalosporin (either cefotaxime or ceftriaxone)

[a]For *Streptococcus pneumoniae* and *H. influenzae* meningitis, dexamethasone 0.15 mg/kg every sixth hourly for 2–4 days is recommended ideally dexamethasone started before the first dose of antibiotic

The preferred total daily intravenous doses in patients with normal renal and hepatic function are as follows:
Neonates aged <1 week: ampicillin 150 mg/kg/day; cefotaxime 100–150 mg/kg/day; gentamicin 5 mg/kg/day. Neonates aged 1–4 weeks: ampicillin 200 mg/kg/day; gentamicin 7.5 mg/kg/day; tobramycin 7.5 mg/kg/day; amikacin 30 mg/kg/day; cefotaxime 150–200 mg/kg/day. Infants and children aged >4 weeks: vancomycin 60 mg/kg/day to achieve serum trough concentrations of 15–20 mg/mL; cefotaxime 225–300 mg/kg/day; ceftriaxone 80–100 mg/kg/day
Adults: vancomycin 30–60 mg/kg/day to achieve serum trough concentrations of 15–20 mg/mL; ceftriaxone 4 g/day; cefotaxime, 8–12 g/day; cefepime 6 g/day; ceftazidime 6 g/day; amoxicillin or ampicillin 12 g/day; penicillin 24 million units/day; meropenem 6 g/day

(b) Local resistance patterns should be considered.
(c) Alternatives for beta-lactam allergy.

18.6 Antimicrobial Therapy for Community Acquired Meningitis

Most international guidelines recommend to start treatment for bacterial meningitis as early as possible, but no later than 1 h after presentation. The choice of initial antimicrobial therapy is based on the most common bacteria that cause the disease in the region and taking into account local antimicrobial susceptibility patterns (Table 18.4). *Listeria* cover should be given for extremes of age and immunocompromised individuals. Neonates should be treated for infection with *E. coli* and *Streptococcus agalactiae*. The increase in penicillin and cephalosporin resistance in *Streptococcus pneumoniae* strains worldwide has changed the initial therapy of patients with bacterial meningitis in several regions. Meningococcal strains with reduced susceptibility to penicillin have been associated with unfavorable outcomes. The European Society of Clinical Microbiology and Infectious Diseases (ESCMID) guideline recommends vancomycin and a third-generation cephalosporin as part of the initial treatment regimen. Though in areas with very low cephalosporin resistance for *pneumococcus*, ceftriaxone alone is considered appropriate [15].

Once the causative pathogen and bacterial antimicrobial susceptibility patterns have been identified, therapy should be optimized. Individuals who have been in close contact with patients with meningococcal meningitis should receive antibiotic prophylaxis.

Table 18.5 Duration of therapy in community-acquired meningitis

Microorganisms	Duration of therapy in days
Neisseria meningitidis	7
Haemophilus influenzae	7
Streptococcus pneumoniae	10–14
Streptococcus agalactiae	14–21
Aerobic gram-negative bacilli	21
Listeria monocytogenes	21, (42 for cerebritis or brain abcess)

18.6.1 Repeat Lumbar Puncture

Repeat cerebrospinal fluid (CSF) analysis to confirm the sterilization of CSF and the improvement of CSF parameters is not necessary for patients with bacterial meningitis who have responded clinically well to antimicrobial therapy. However, for patients who have not responded well after 48 h of appropriate antimicrobial therapy, repeated CSF analysis should be performed.

18.6.2 Duration of Therapy

The duration of treatment may require customization based on causative organism and the patient's specific response to therapy. Nevertheless, the overall strategy is as follows (Table 18.5):

18.7 Healthcare-Associated Meningitis

It is usually associated with patients undergoing neurosurgery, head trauma, external ventricular drainage, and shunt surgeries. Etiology depends on local epidemiology. Commonly isolated organisms are multi-resistant or extremely resistant pathogens, including *Staphylococcus aureus, Coagulase Negative Staphylococcus, Pseudomonas aeruginosa, Acinetobacter baumannii, Klebsiella, and Propionibacterium.* Diagnostic challenges include altered clinical and CSF picture due to preexisting surgery or trauma. Infections are more with cranial than spinal surgeries [16].

Table 18.6 Dosages of drugs used in CNS infections [20]

Drug	Adult dose	Pediatric dose
Ceftriaxone	2 g 12 h	50 mg/kg 8 h
Ceftazidime	2 g q 6–8 h	50 mg/kg 8 h
Cefepime	2 g 8–12 h	50 mg/kg 12 h
Cefotaxime	2 g 6 h	50 mg/kg 6 h
Meropenem	2 g 8 h	40 mg/kg 8 h
Colistin	9 million unit loading and then 4.5 million units 12 h	150,000 units/kg loading and then 75,000 units/kg 12 h
Polymyxin B	20,000–25,000 units/kg loading and then 12,500–15,000 units/kg 12 h, single dose not to exceed 20,00,000 units	15–25,000 units/kg loading and then 5000–7500 units/kg 8 h
Fosfomycin	4 g 6 h	75–100 mg/kg/dose 6 h
Vancomycin	15 mg/kg (max 2 g) 8 h	15 mg/kg 6 h
Rifampicin	600 mg once daily	10–20 mg/kg once daily
Metronidazole	400 mg 8 h	10 mg/kg 8 h

18.8 Antimicrobial Considerations

Antibiotics penetrate into CNS, attain therapeutic concentration in CSF, and have bactericidal activity against targeted pathogen. Drugs with difficulty in attaining target concentration like vancomycin or ceftriaxone therapeutic drug monitoring in CSF are recommended [17–19]. In sicker patients, vancomycin trough level of 15–20 μg/mL is recommended. For beta-lactam anaphylaxis, aztreonam or ciprofloxacin is recommended as an alternative.

Intrathecal therapy is considered for severe ventriculitis, resistant gram-negative infections, persistently positive CSF cultures, device removal not possible, or when patient develops complications to systemic antibiotics [20]. Seizures and myoclonus are associated with antibiotics like cefepime, fluoroquinolones, and metronidazole. Aminoglycosides and Polymyxins can lead to neuromuscular blockade like effect.

Table 18.7 Treatment of healthcare-associated meningitis and ventriculitis [20]

Organism	Preferred drug	Alternative drug
Methicillin-sensitive Staphylococcus	Cloxacillin	Ceftriaxone
Methicillin-resistant Staphylococcus	Vancomycin	Linezolid/ cotrimoxazole if susceptible
Non-ESBL gram-negative	Ceftriaxone	Cefotaxime/ ceftazidime
ESBL gram-negative	Meropenem	Cotrimoxazole/ moxifloxacin
Carbapenem-resistant gram-negative	Systemic colistin/polymyxin B with (depending on susceptibility) high-dose tigecycline/ minocycline/fosfomycin/cotrimoxazole/quinolones/chloramphenicol with intraventricular/ intrathecal colistin/polymyxin/aminoglycosides	

Dosages of Drugs used in CNS infections are shown in Table 18.6.

18.9 Management of Healthcare-Associated Meningitis/ Ventriculitis

- Empirical therapy depends on local flora. Usually, antipseudomonal cephalosporin or carbapenem with vancomycin is recommended. Later, it is modified based on culture results (Table 18.7). Surgical drainage and removal of devices may be necessary.
- For carbapenem-resistant gram-negative infections, intraventricular or intrathecal therapy may be needed. Duration varies depending on the causative organism, clinical features, and CSF finding. Generally, it requires treatment for 2–3 weeks [21]. Duration is 2 weeks for gram-positive pathogens, longer if devices are retained.
- Empirical antimicrobial regimen to be adjusted if patient is colonised with (or) has an infection of another body site with resistant organism [14].

18.10 Shunt and Reservoir Infections

Treatment involves removal or externalization of the shunt and systemic antibiotics empirical therapy with fourth-generation cephalosporin or meropenem with vancomycin followed by definitive therapy. Rifampicin can be added in staphylococcal infections for synergistic action [22]. Evidence regarding intraventricular therapy is limited, can be considered in resistant-gram negatives or when CSF is not clearing. Polymyxins, vancomycin, and aminoglycosides are the drugs employed.

18.10.1 Shunt Reimplantation

Coagulase-negative Staphylococci, *Diphtheroid, or P. acnes*

No CSF abnormalities: day 3 after externalization if CSF cultures are negative at 48 h.

CSF abnormalities present: 7–10 days after the last positive CSF culture.

S. aureus or gram-negative organism: 10 days after last positive CSF culture.

18.11 Intrathecal/Intraventricular Antibiotics

Intrathecal antibiotics gain direct entry to the extracellular central nervous compartment, thereby negating all the barriers. This helps in achieving higher CSF concentration, even with small doses, unlike high intravenous dose requirements for achieving the same.

Data suggests that intraventricular administration achieves rapid distribution across the entire CSF quicker than lumbar intrathecal

Table 18.8 Dosage and adverse effects of intrathecal drugs

Antibiotic profile	Suggested adult dose	Side effect profile
Aminoglycosides	4–10 mg every 24 h	Side effects includes seizures, aseptic meningitis, painful radiculitis, and temporary hearing loss
Gentamicin		
Amikacin	30 mg every 24 h	Side effect profile similar to gentamicin
Polymyxins	10 mg every 24 h	Agitation, seizures, intraventricular hemorrhage, pain, edema, albuminuria
Colistin		
Polymyxin B	5 mg every 24 h	Similar profile as that of colistin
Glycopeptides	5–10 mg every 24 h	Red man syndrome, transient hearing loss, ataxia, CSF leukocytosis, headache, nausea
Vancomycin		

administration. Pharmacokinetic data prefers intraventricular administration of antibiotics; however, clinical studies do not show better efficacy for intraventricular administration over lumbar intrathecal administration. Intraventricular along with intravenous antibiotics use has better clinical outcome than intraventricular route alone, as per recent meta-analysis findings [23].

Aminoglycosides, colistin, and vancomycin are used more commonly via intrathecal and intraventricular route. Dosage, duration, and adverse effects of intrathecal/intraventricular antibiotics are described in Table 18.8.

Indications include:

- External and internal ventricular shunt infections.
- Infections of devices in the CNS with multidrug-resistant bacteria.
- Nosocomial meningitis and ventriculitis caused by methicillin-resistant coagulase-negative staphylococci and *Staphylococcus aureus*, vancomycin-resistant enterococci, and carbapenemase-producing gram-negative bacteria (*Acinetobacter* spp., *Klebsiella* spp., *Escherichia coli*, and *Pseudomonas aeruginosa*).

18.11.1 Factors Affecting CSF Concentration

CSF volume: CSF is present in four ventricles, aqueduct, basal cisterns, sub-arachnoid space over the cerebral convexities and in the spinal cord. Individual variations exist regarding the CSF volume present at any given time. Age-related CSF volumes changes could affect the CSF antibiotic concentration.

CSF flow: Oscillatory flow of CSF between areas determines the equilibration of the drug concentration which is variable in nature between individuals.

Drug factors: Drugs with poor intracellular penetration, with trans-capillary leakage and which undergo bulk flow elimination tend to achieve higher CSF concentration. Once daily dosage is commonly employed. Clamping the ventricular drain for 15–120 min helps to achieve better distribution of the antibiotic within the CSF compartments [24].

18.11.2 Infectious Disease Society of America (IDSA) Recommendations Includes

1. Intraventricular antimicrobial therapy should be considered for patients with healthcare-associated ventriculitis and meningiti in which the infection responds poorly to systemic antimicrobial therapy alone.
2. When antimicrobial therapy is administered via a ventricular drain, the drain should be clamped for 15–60 min to allow the agent to equilibrate throughout the CSF.
3. Dosages and intervals of intraventricular antimicrobial therapy should be adjusted based on CSF antimicrobial concentrations to 10–20 times the MIC of the causative microorganism, ventricular size, and daily output from the ventricular drain [14].

18.11.3 Adjunctive Therapy Along with Intrathecal Administration

Neuro endoscopic lavage of intraventricular cavity to remove debris and intraventricular fibrinolysis for clearing blood clots within the cavity have been tried but are not established practices. Theoretically, these practices offer superiority in terms of optimizing conditions for better antibiotic action within the ventricular cavity.

18.12 Drug to Drug Interactions (DDI)

Potential drug–drug interaction (DDI) occurs in neurocritical care patients who are on multiple medication during their stay [25]. Of these potential interactions, many could result in clinically relevant drug interactions causing adverse drug reactions (ADRs) [26]. ADRs can increase morbidity and mortality. Cardiac arrhythmias and bleeding are the commonest clinically relevant drug–drug interactions in ICU, and antibiotics per se can pose a significant problem due to their drug interactions.

18.12.1 Pharmacokinetics (PK) and Pharmacodynamics (PD) in Drug–Drug Interaction

Pharmacokinetic interactions are drug absorption, distribution, metabolism, and excretion related. Cytochrome P450 (CYP450) and enterocyte P glycoproteins are involved in these processes. Pharmacodynamic interactions are dependent on drug effect at receptors, mechanism of action, and therapeutic effects. Extent of protein binding mainly by albumin and alpha 1 acid glycoprotein and metabolism during hepatic pass play a major role in pharmacodynamic interactions.

Significant number of DDI are due to Cytochrome P450 (CYP450) enzyme induction or inhibition. CYP450 system located both in liver and extrahepatic locations could be involved in DDI. Orally administered drugs undergo both hepatic and extrahepatic changes by the CYP450 system; hence, they have major DDI chances. CYP450 functional variations occur due to age, gender, disease, and genetic polymorphism resulting in further DDI variability.

18.12.2 Carbapenems

Carbapenems does not have metabolism through CYP450 enzyme, hence exhibiting few interactions. They could cause a significant decrease in valproate concentrations and could result in breakthrough seizures. The possible mechanisms for reducing valproate concentration include reduced absorption, increased valproate glucuronidation, and reduced valproate enterohepatic recirculation. If valproate need is essential to control seizures, alternate antibiotic should replace carbapenem in those circumstances [27].

18.12.3 Erythromycin

Erythromycin strongly inhibits cytochrome P450 isoenzymes, thereby increasing the plasma levels of antiepileptics like phenytoin, phenobarbital, and carbamazepine. Erythromycin along with simvastatin if administered over prolonged period could result in rhabdomyolysis [27].

18.12.4 Linezolid

Linezolid with a weak monoamine oxidase (MAO) inhibitor action could potentially precipitate serotonergic syndrome. Buspirone, a serotonergic agent used to reduce shivering in therapeutic hypothermia, could potentiate such adverse events. Avoiding other serotonergic agents along with linezolid use should be borne in mind [27].

Drug–drug interactions in neurocritical care is a significant problem which the intensivist and clinical pharmacist should be aware of and take preventive steps to avoid clinically relevant interactions from happening.

Table 18.9 Common antibiotics and their associated encephalopathy features

Antibiotic-causing encephalopathy	Associated feature of encephalopathy
Sulphonamide	Psychosis
Quinolones	Psychosis, seizure
Macrolides	Psychosis, seizure
Procaine penicillin	Psychosis
Cephalosporins	Seizure—majority nonconvulsive, psychosis, myoclonus
Metronidazole	Psychosis, seizure
Penicillin	Seizure, myoclonus

Table 18.10 Phenotypes of AAE

Clinical phenotype	Clinical features	Investigations	Common antibiotics
Type 1 Disruption of gamma aminobutyric acid-A (GABA-A) receptor signals leading to excitotoxicity	Onset within few days of antibiotic, Common feature is myoclonus or seizure Resolution within days	Abnormal electroencephalogram (EEG) Normal magnetic resonance imaging (MRI)	Penicillin, cephalosporins
Type 2 Perturbations of dopamine (D2) and *N*-methyl-D-aspartate (NMDA) glutamate receptors	Onset within few days of antibiotic Psychosis is common Rarely seizures resolution within days	Nonspecific abnormal EEG Normal MRI	Procaine penicillin Sulfonamides Fluoroquinolones Macrolides
Type 3 Free radical formation and altered thiamine metabolism-induced damage	Onset after weeks of antibiotic Cerebellar dysfunction common Rarely seizure Resolution within months	Rarely nonspecific EEG, abnormal MRI[a]	Metronidazole (isoniazid has onset time of weeks to months, with psychosis as major presentation)

[a]Classic imaging findings include bilateral symmetric T2 hyperintense lesions in the dentate nuclei and midbrain, lesions in the corpus callosum may exhibit restricted diffusion.

18.12.5 AAE (Antibiotic-Associated Encephalopathy)

Antibiotic-Associated Encephalopathy (AAE) is relatively an underdiagnosed condition in critical care. Incidence varies from less than 1–15% [28]. Most important risk factor is renal failure, especially for cephalosporin associated encephalopathy. Hepatic dysfunction and previous history of psychiatric illness are other associated risk factors. Clinical presentations of AAE includes psychosis, seizures, and myoclonus in the order of higher to lower prevalence rate. Table 18.9 indicates the common antibiotics and their associated features of encephalopathy.

There are three clinical phenotypes of AAE based on clinical features, investigation findings, and antibiotic use (Table 18.10).

Onset of the AAE occurs within a median time of 5 days, whereas AAE induced by isoniazid and metronidazole could be delayed up to 3 weeks duration. Time to resolution after stopping the inciting antibiotic has a median time of 5 days, and metronidazole-induced AAE resolution can take up to 13 days.

18.13 Conclusion

Neurocritical care poses the challenge of diagnosing and treating both community-acquired and healthcare-associated infections. Understanding the pharmacological principles behind the antibiotic therapy, antibiotic-associated side effect profile, choosing the appropriate early therapy, and right mode of delivery play a critical role in successfully treating bacterial infection. It is vital for the entire healthcare delivery team to be aware of antimicrobial stewardship principles, especially among neurocritical care patients, as they are at highest risk of healthcare-associated infections.

References

1. Cevik MA, Yilmaz GR, Erdinc FS, Ucler S, Tulek NE. Relationship between nosocomial infection and mortality in a neurology intensive care unit in Turkey. J Hosp Infect. 2005;59(4):324–30.
2. Müller M, dela Peña A, Derendorf H. Issues in pharmacokinetics and pharmacodynamics of anti-infective agents: distribution in tissue. Antimicrob Agents Chemother. 2004;48(5):1441–53.
3. Joukhadar C, Frossard M, Mayer BX, Brunner M, Klein N, Siostrzonek P, et al. Impaired target site penetration of beta-lactams may account for therapeutic failure in patients with septic shock. Crit Care Med. 2001;29(2):385–91.
4. Scaglione F, Paraboni L. Pharmacokinetics/pharmacodynamics of antibacterials in the intensive care unit: setting appropriate dosing regimens. Int J Antimicrob Agents. 2008;32(4):294–301.
5. Asín-Prieto E, Rodríguez-Gascón A, Isla A. Applications of the pharmacokinetic/pharmacodynamic (PK/PD) analysis of antimicrobial agents. J Infect Chemother. 2015;21(5):319–29.
6. Lee DG, Shin HH. Pharmacokinetics and pharmacodynamics of antibiotics: general concepts and recent advances. Infect Chemother. 2008;40(3):140.
7. Macedo RS, Onita JH, Wille MP, Furtado GHC. Pharmacokinetics and pharmacodynamics of antimicrobial drugs in intensive care unit patients. Shock. 2013;39(Suppl 1):24–8.
8. Varghese JM, Roberts JA, Lipman J. Antimicrobial pharmacokinetic and pharmacodynamic issues in the critically ill with severe sepsis and septic shock. Crit Care Clin. 2011;27(1):19–34.
9. Pigrau C. Oxazolidinonas y glucopéptidos. Enferm Infecc Microbiol Clin. 2003;21(3):157–65.
10. Lodise TP, Lomaestro B, Graves J, Drusano GL. Larger vancomycin doses (at least 4 g/day) are associated with an increased incidence of nephrotoxicity. Antimicrob Agents Chemother. 2008;52(4):1330–6.
11. Kullar R, Davis SL, Taylor TN, Kaye KS, Rybak MJ. Effects of targeting higher vancomycin trough levels on clinical outcomes and costs in a matched patient cohort. Pharmacotherapy. 2012;32(3):195–201.
12. Scottish Intercollegiate Guidelines Network. No SG. 104. Antibiotic prophylaxis in surgery. A national clinical guideline. Edinburgh: Scottish Intercollegiate Guidelines Network; 2008.
13. Bayston R, de Louvois J, Brown EM, Johnston RA, Lees P, Pople IK. Use of antibiotics in penetrating craniocerebral injuries. "Infection in Neurosurgery" Working Party of British Society for Antimicrobial Chemotherapy. Lancet. 2000;355(9217):1813–7.
14. Tunkel AR, Hartman BJ, Kaplan SL, Kaufman BA, Roos KL, Scheld WM, et al. Practice guidelines for the management of bacterial meningitis. Clin Infect Dis. 2004;39(9):1267–84.
15. van Ettekoven CN, van de Beek D, Brouwer MC. Update on community-acquired bacterial meningitis: guidance and challenges. Clin Microbiol Infect. 2017;23(9):601–6.
16. McClelland S, Hall WA. Postoperative central nervous system infection: incidence and associated factors in 2111 neurosurgical procedures. Clin Infect Dis. 2007;45(1):55–9.
17. Beach JE, Perrott J, Turgeon RD, Ensom MHH. Penetration of vancomycin into the cerebrospinal fluid: a systematic review. Clin Pharmacokinet. 2017;56(12):1479–90.
18. Le Turnier P, Navas D, Garot D, Guimard T, Bernard L, Tattevin P, et al. Tolerability of high-dose ceftriaxone in CNS infections: a prospective multicentre cohort study. J Antimicrob Chemother. 2019;74(4):1078–85.
19. Ng K, Mabasa VH, Chow I, Ensom MHH. Systematic review of efficacy, pharmacokinetics, and administration of intraventricular vancomycin in adults. Neurocrit Care. 2014;20(1):158–71.
20. Treatment guidelines for antimicrobial use in common syndromes. 2019.
21. Dréno B, Pécastaings S, Corvec S, Veraldi S, Khammari A, Roques C. Cutibacterium acnes (*Propionibacterium acnes*) and acne vulgaris: a brief look at the latest updates. J Eur Acad Dermatol Venereol. 2018;32(Suppl 2):5–14.
22. Wilson JW, Estes LL. Mayo Clinic antimicrobial therapy. Mayo Clinic Scientific Press. 2008. http://repository.stikesbcm.ac.id/id/eprint/176/1/Mayo%20Clinic%20antimicrobial%20therap.pdf. Accessed 4 Apr 2023.
23. Ziaka M, Markantonis SL, Fousteri M, Zygoulis P, Panidis D, Karvouniaris M, et al. Combined intravenous and intraventricular administration of colistin methanesulfonate in critically ill patients with central nervous system infection. Antimicrob Agents Chemother. 2013;57(4):1938–40.
24. Nau R, Blei C, Eiffert H. Intrathecal antibacterial and antifungal therapies. Clin Microbiol Rev. 2020;33(3):10–1128.
25. Uijtendaal EV, van Harssel LLM, Hugenholtz GWK, Kuck EM, Zwart-van Rijkom JEF, Cremer OL, et al. Analysis of potential drug–drug interactions in medical intensive care unit patients. Pharmacotherapy. 2014;34(3):213–9.
26. Kane-Gill SL, Dasta JF, Buckley MS, Devabhakthuni S, Liu M, Cohen H, et al. Clinical practice guideline: safe medication use in the ICU. Crit Care Med. 2017;45(9):e877–915.
27. Spoelhof B, Farrokh S, Rivera-Lara L. Drug interactions in neurocritical care. Neurocrit Care. 2017;27(2):287–96.
28. Bhattacharyya S, Darby RR, Raibagkar P, Gonzalez Castro LN, Berkowitz AL. Antibiotic-associated encephalopathy. Neurology. 2016;86(10):963–71.

19 Antiviral Drugs

Pragyan Kumar Routray, Pragati Jena,
and Debasis Mishra

19.1 Introduction

Historically, the development of antiviral drugs has lagged behind the development of other antimicrobial agents. Since the early 1950s when the search began for antiviral agents, the demand for new antiviral strategies has increased gradually and remarkably. Multiple factors have contributed to this increasing demand and research for newer antiviral agents. The ever-increasing incidence of acute herpes infections, the prevalence of chronic viral infections such as HIV and hepatitis B and C, along with the emergence of new challenging viruses such as the SARS coronavirus causing pandemics have put an impetus to our research on antivirals. Antiviral drugs share the common property of being virustatic; they are active only against replicating viruses and do not affect latent viruses [1].

As a consequence, some infections require monotherapy for brief periods of time (e.g., acyclovir for herpes simplex virus), some need dual therapy for prolonged periods (e.g., interferon alfa/ribavirin for HCV), whereas indefinite multiple drug therapy is required in HIV. In chronic fatal illnesses such as viral hepatitis and HIV infection, potent inhibition of viral replication is very important in limiting the systemic damage. Currently, 37 chemicals, plus IFN-α in both pegylated and non-pegylated forms, have been formally approved for the treatment of viral infections and half of these agents are intended to treat HIV infections [2].

The antiviral activity can be divided into two categories:

(A) Agents directly inhibiting viruses usually at cellular level (Fig. 19.1)
(B) Agents that augment or modify host defenses to viral replication (immunomodulating agents)

(A) Direct Antiviral Mechanism:
  1. Inhibition of viral nucleic acid synthesis, e.g., acyclovir and penciclovir
  2. RNA antisense nucleotides, e.g., fomivirsen
  3. Viral entry inhibition, e.g., enfuvirtide
  4. Protease Inhibition, e.g., ritonavir and nelfinavir
  5. Integrase Inhibition, e.g., raltegravir
  6. Inhibition of uncoating of virus, e.g., amantidine
  7. Inhibition of virus release, e.g., oseltamivir

(B) Host Defense Modifier:
  1. Interferons
  2. Innate immune stimulators
  3. Sialidase inhibitors

P. K. Routray (✉) · P. Jena · D. Mishra
Critical Care, CARE Hospitals, Bhubaneswar, India

H. Prabhakar et al. (eds.), *Principles and Practice of Neurocritical Care*,
https://doi.org/10.1007/978-981-99-8059-8_19

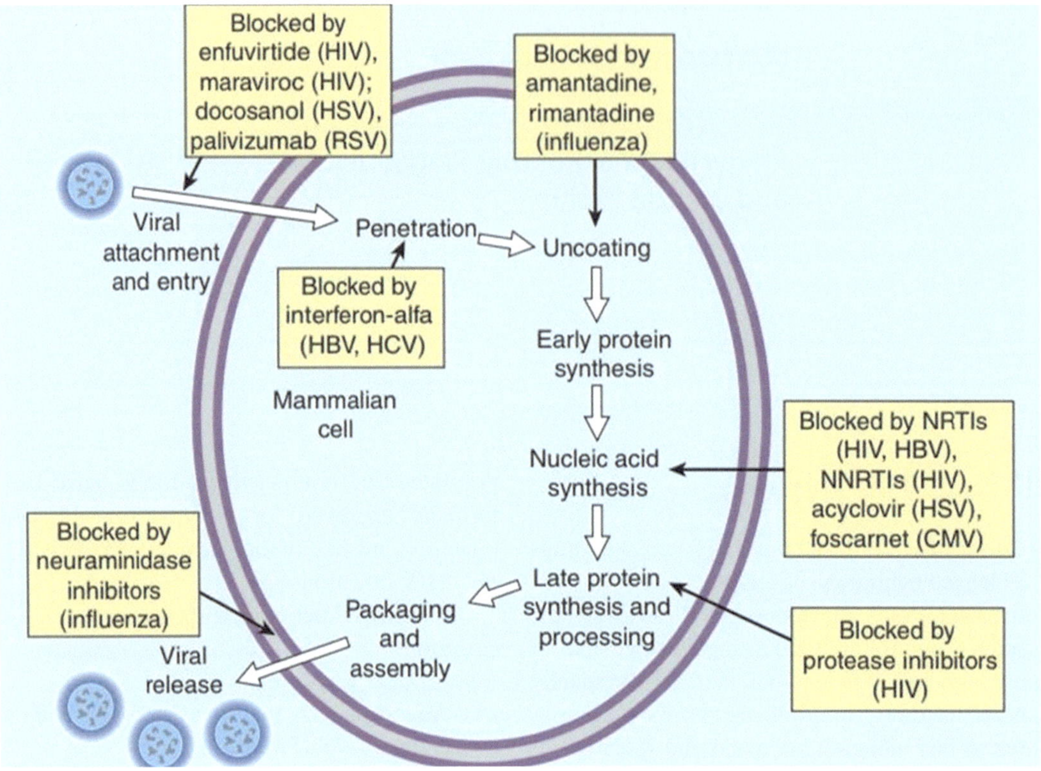

Fig. 19.1 Major sites of antiviral drug action. (Katzung BG, Trevor AJ. Pharmacology: Examination and board review. Appleton & Lange; 1993 Jan; 12thedition; 862)

This chapter mainly depicts antivirals used in neurocritical care and focuses on the interaction of antivirals and neuroscience and its application across neurocritical care ICUs.

19.2 Viruses Causing Encephalitis/Myelitis

DNA Viruses

1. *Herpes virus*
2. *Varicella zoster virus*

RNA Viruses

1. *Enterovirus*
2. *Arbovirus*
3. *West Nile Virus*
4. *Human immune deficiency (HIV) virus*

Among the DNA viruses, there are more than 100 known viruses, but only seven may produce encephalitis, namely herpes simplex virus (HSV), varicella zoster virus (VZV), Epstein-Barr virus, cytomegalovirus (CMV), HHV 6, and rarely HHV 7 and HIV 8. Herpes simplex virus (HSV) encephalitis is the most commonly diagnosed viral encephalitis in industrialized nations, with an annual incidence of 1 in 250,000–500,000. The age-specific incidence is bimodal, with peaks in the young and the elderly. Most HSV encephalitis is due to HSV-1, but about 10% is caused by HSV-2. The latter typically occurs in immunocompromised individuals and neonates, in whom it can cause a disseminated infection [3].

Varicella zoster virus (VZV) is also a relatively common cause of viral Encephalitis, especially in the immunocompromised, while cytomegalovirus (CMV) occurs almost exclusively in this group. Enteroviruses most often cause aseptic meningitis but can also be an important cause of encephalitis. Among the other causes, encephalitis associated with antibodies to the voltage-gated potassium channel complex, or *N*-methyl-D-aspartate antibody (NMDA) receptors are increasingly recognized [3]. The only commonly encountered viral meningoencephalitis with effective treatment is HSV, and empiric acyclovir should be administered until HSV infection is ruled out or a clear alternative diagnosis established.

19.3 Antivirals Practiced in Encephalitis

19.3.1 Acyclovir and Valacyclovir

HSV is the most recognized cause of infectious encephalitis worldwide. Intravenous acyclovir (10 mg/kg three times daily) should be started if the initial cerebrospinal fluid (CSF) and/or imaging findings suggest viral encephalitis, or within 6 h of admission if these results will not be available, or if the patient is very unwell or deteriorating [4]. Acyclovir is a deoxyguanosine analog which is activated by viral thymidine kinase (TK) to become inhibitor of viral DNA polymerase and DNA replication of different herpes viruses. Valacyclovir is the L-valyl ester prodrug of acyclovir. Enhanced antiherpes activity occurs when acyclovir is combined with interferon and other antivirals [5].

The prevalence of acyclovir-resistant HSV isolates is 0.7% and 14% in immunocompetent and immunocompromised patients [6].

CSF concentrations reach 20–50% of serum value. Clinical isolates of HSV, VZV resistant to acyclovir are also cross-resistant to valacyclovir, famciclovir, and ganciclovir. Foscarnet, cidofovir, and trifluridine do not require thymidine kinase activation and hence are active against acyclovir-resistant strains [7].

Intravenous infusion may be associated with reversible renal toxicity (i.e., crystalline nephropathy, or interstitial nephritis) or neurological effects (tremor, delirium, or seizures). These can be prevented with adequate hydration and slow infusion rates [7]. The neurotoxicity of acyclovir is usually described within the first 24–72 h of treatment, and there is complete recovery within 2–7 days after treatment cessation. Simultaneous use of other nephrotoxic drugs can enhance potential for nephrotoxicity. Probenecid and cimetidine decrease acyclovir clearance and increase exposure. Somnolence and lethargy are caused due to simultaneous use of acyclovir and zidovudine [8].

The CSF levels of valacyclovir is also 50% of serum value and is used for VZV encephalitis. Confusion, hallucinations, seizures, ataxia, dysarthria, hallucination, psychosis, and mania have been reported at high doses [9]. Valacyclovir toxicity occurs within 72 h of treatment and recovery after 4 days after the treatment is discontinued.

19.3.2 Ganciclovir and Valganciclovir

Ganciclovir is a potent inhibitor of viruses of the herpes family, including cytomegalovirus (CMV). The primary mechanism of ganciclovir action against CMV is inhibition of the replication of viral DNA by ganciclovir-5′-triphosphate (ganciclovir-TP). This inhibition includes a selective and potent inhibition of the viral DNA polymerase [5, 10]. Ganciclovir is metabolized to the triphosphate form by primarily three cellular enzymes: (1) a deoxyguanosine kinase induced by CMV-infected cells, (2) guanylate kinase, and (3) phosphoglycerate kinase.

Other nucleotide-metabolizing enzymes may be involved as well. The selective antiviral response associated with ganciclovir treatment is achieved because of the much weaker inhibition of cellular DNA polymerases by ganciclovir-TP.

Valganciclovir is the L-valyl ester of ganciclovir and is rapidly metabolized to ganciclovir after oral administration.

CMV infections are commonly found in patients with advanced immunosuppression due to reactivation of latent infection. It usually results in end organ complications [11]. Commonly used agents are valganciclovir and ganciclovir. CSF concentrations are approximately 50% of serum levels. Clearance of drug is linearly related to creatinine clearance. Most common adverse effects of IV formulation is myelosuppression. CNS toxicity like confusions, seizures, and psychiatry disturbances has been rarely noted.

19.3.3 Foscarnet

Foscarnet is an inorganic pyrophosphate analog that inhibits herpes viruses and HIV [5]. It directly inhibits herpesvirus DNA polymerase or HIV reverse transcriptase. Foscarnet selectivity relates to its greater inhibitory effect against herpesvirus DNA polymerase and HIV reverse transcriptase compared to cellular DNA polymerase. Foscarnet resistance is caused by point mutations in DNA polymerase of HSV and CMV or in reverse transcriptase of HIV. It can be used synergistically with acyclovir and ganciclovir to inhibit CMV and with zidovudine to inhibit HIV replication [12]. Foscarnet is available in only iv formulations, and CNS levels are 30–67% of serum value. It is effective against acyclovir-resistant HSV and VZV infections. Excretion is directly proportional to creatinine clearance [13].

Potential adverse effects include renal impairment, hypo/hypercalcemia, hypo/hyperphosphatemia, hypokalemia, and hypomagnesemia. Avoiding concurrent administration with other nephrotoxic drugs and saline preloading prevents neurotoxicity to some extent. CNS toxicity includes headache, hallucinations, and seizures.

19.3.4 Cidofovir

Cidofovir is an analog of deoxycytidine monophosphate and is phosphorylated to its active form. The diphosphate form competes with deoxycytidine triphosphate for incorporation into herpesvirus DNA [14]. The drug inhibits replication of all herpes viruses as well as poxviruses, adenovirus, papillomaviruses, and polyomaviruses. Cidofovir is approved used for CMV retinitis in patients with AIDS and CMV infection resistant to ganciclovir. It is potentially nephrotoxic requiring renal dose adjustment, and it also causes metabolic acidosis as well as glucosuria. Hence, this requires saline and probenecid administration along with the drug. Cidofovir is typically used for ganciclovir and foscarnet-resistant CMV or acyclovir and foscarnet-resistant HSV disease in immunocompromised patients [15].

19.3.5 Leteromovir

It is a dihydroquinazolin that inhibits CMV DNA terminase complex (UL51 and UL59). It is approved for adult CMV seropositive recipients of an allogenic hematopoietic stem cell transplantation and prophylaxis of CMV infection [16]. Dose modification is required with concomitant use of cyclosporine, voriconazole, sirolimus, and tacrolimus. It is neither nephrotoxic or myelosuppressive.

Table 19.1 describes major neurotropic viruses and their treatment.

Table 19.1 Neurotropic viruses and their treatment

Viruses causing encephalitis or myelitis	Antivirals
DNA viruses	
Herpes simplex virus (HSV)	IV acyclovir 10 mg/kg every 8 h for 14
Varicella zoster virus (VZV)	IV acyclovir 10 mg/kg every 8 h for 14–21 days; ganciclovir (alternative in case acyclovir is not available; preventive measures: VZV vaccination with live attenuated varicella vaccine for children: 2 doses, 12 months and 5 years; recombinant zoster vaccine for adults >50 years: 2 doses separated by 2–6 months)
Cytomegalovirus (CMV)	Ganciclovir 5 mg/kg every 12 h and foscarnet 90 mg/kg/day until symptomatic improvement in immunocompromised (B-III). Immunocompetent: same medications

Table 19.1 (continued)

Viruses causing encephalitis or myelitis	Antivirals
Epstein-Barr virus (EBV)	No specific IDSA recommendation. Supportive. Corticosteroids (C-III). Acyclovir not recommended
Human herpesvirus 6 (HHV-6)	Ganciclovir 5 mg/kg every 8 h and foscarnet 60 mg/kg every 12 h in immunocompromised persons (B-III) and immunocompetent persons
RNA viruses	
Enterovirus	Supportive; pleconaril and ribavirin under study
Influenza	Oseltamivir 75 mg twice per day for 5 days or more
Human immunodeficiency virus (acute HIV encephalitis)	ART (A-II) nucleoside reverse transcriptase inhibitors: abacavir, lamivudine, zidovudine. Integrase strand transfer inhibitors: raltegravir and dolutegravir
West Nile virus	No specific IDSA recommendation. Supportive
Eastern equine virus	No specific IDSA recommendation. Supportive
St. Louis virus	No specific IDSA recommendation. Supportive. Interferon-alpha has been previously used
Japanese encephalitis virus	No specific IDSA recommendation. Supportive. Vaccine available
La Crosse virus	No specific IDSA recommendation. Supportive
Powassan virus	No specific IDSA recommendation. Supportive. Some patients have been treated with steroids and IVIg
Jamestown canyon virus	No specific IDSA recommendation. Supportive
Tick-borne virus	No specific IDSA recommendation. Supportive. Vaccine available
Dengue	No specific IDSA recommendation. Supportive
Chikungunya	No specific IDSA recommendation. Supportive
Zika	No specific IDSA recommendation. Supportive
Rabies	No specific IDSA recommendation. Supportive. Pre-exposure vaccination schedule: 3 doses over 21 or 28 days. Post-exposure vaccination schedule: If no prior vaccination: 4 doses, first dose should be administered followed by other doses on day third, seventh and 14th. Patients should get a single dose of human rabies Ig. If previously vaccinated: Only two doses, first dose should be administered immediately and second on the third day
Lymphocytic choriomeningitis virus (LCMV)	No specific IDSA recommendation. Supportive
Mumps	No specific IDSA recommendation. Supportive. MMR vaccine: first dose at 9–15 months of age, second dose at 15 months–6 years of age and should consider one dose in young adults
Measles]	No specific IDSA recommendation. Supportive. MMR vaccine: first dose at 9–15 months of age, second dose at 15 months–6 years of age and should consider one dose in young adults. Post-measles encephalitis: corticosteroids and IVIg
Ebola	No specific IDSA recommendation. Supportive. Emerging medications: nucleoside and nucleotide analogs, nucleic acid-based drugs and immunotherapeutic drugs. Available vaccines, look promising

19.4 HIV and Antiretroviral Drugs

The neurocritical care emergencies associated with HIV are related to primarily four clinical situations:

1. HIV encephalitis
2. Opportunistic CNS infections during stages of immunosuppression
3. IRIS (immune reconstitution syndrome)
4. Antiretroviral drugs-related neuropsychiatric complications

19.4.1 HIV Encephalitis

HIV encephalitis (HIVE), also referred to as HIV-associated neurological disorder (HAND), includes a range of neurocognitive defects of varying severity following HIV infection. The clinical presentation of this condition varies from asymptomatic or minor neurocognitive impairment to severe dementia. HIV encephalopathy, also known as AIDS–dementia complex, lies at the most severe end of this spectrum. A low CD4 count and high plasma viral load are the key factors determining the development of HIV encephalitis. Patients of older age groups having an increased prevalence of cognitive deficits compared to younger populations. The classical presentation of HIV encephalitis presents in a waxing and waning pattern rather than a progressive deterioration as noted in conditions such as Alzheimer disease [17, 18]. Though HIV encephalitis is usually considered a late manifestation of HIV disease, it has also been known to occur in patients with CD4 counts of more than 350 cells/μL.

Diagnosis

Lab study: An increase in CSF protein, cell count, and the identification of HIV RNA in CSF are all noted but are often nonspecific findings related to HIV encephalopathy. In patients with HIV infection presenting with neurologic problems, CSF analysis helps rule out other opportunistic infections [19]. An extensive metabolic panel needs to be undertaken in these patients to rule out conditions related to thyroid disease, folate, B12, syphilis, and hepatic disorders, which can present with a similar neurologic presentation.

Radiology: Neuroimaging studies in patients suffering from HIV encephalopathy usually show cerebral atrophy on CT or MRI. In advanced stages of the disease, on T2-weighted sequences, multiple symmetric foci of hyperintense, nonenhancing lesions are seen predominantly in a subcortical distribution.

Management

These patients may present in neurocritical care as acute emergencies necessitating resuscitation and ventilator support. They may require pronged ICU stay and face difficult and prolonged weaning and nosocomial infections. Broad-spectrum antimicrobial coverage will be required frequently. The definitive option in managing HIV encephalitis is HART. The treatment has been shown to decrease and effectively reverse the pathologic damage caused by HIV clinically and radiographically. Drug regimens that have higher CNS penetrance have been proven to be of better effect in managing patients with HIV encephalitis. Efavirenz is usually not preferred in neurocognitive disorders owing to its many neuropsychiatric adverse effects [20].

In patients diagnosed with HIV-associated dementia in whom initiation of ART is planned, the preferred regimen is tenofovir, dolutegravir plus emtricitabine, or a combination of lamivudine, abacavir plus dolutegravir. Drugs such as lithium, memantine, and minocycline have not proven beneficial in patients with HIV encephalitis [21, 22].

HIV-Associated CD8 Encephalitis

In a UK case series and review of histopathologically confirmed cases, HIV-associated CD8-encephalitis (HIV-CD8E) is a severe inflammatory disorder dominated by infiltration of the brain by CD8+ T-lymphocytes. HIV-CD8E presents with symptoms and signs related to marked cerebral inflammation and swelling and can lead to coma and death unless treated promptly with corticosteroids. It has a more acute course than HIV encephalitis. It occurs in people with HIV, typically when the virus is apparently well controlled by antiretroviral treatment (ART). Risk events such as intercurrent infection, antiretroviral therapy interruption, immune reconstitution inflammatory syndrome (IRIS) after starting ART, and concomitant associations such as cerebrospinal fluid (CSF) HIV viral escape have been identified, but the pathogenesis of the disorder is not known [19].

Neuroimaging shows diffuse white matter changes and cerebral swelling edema. Definitive diagnosis is made on brain biopsy or at autopsy, where diffuse, predominantly white matter, infiltration by CD8+ T-cells is seen (normal brains do not have T-cells visible in the parenchyma, only within the vasculature).

HIV-CD8E is clinico-pathologically distinct from classical "HIV encephalitis (HIVE)" where pathology shows HIV-containing microglial cells on immunohistochemistry, microglial nodules, microglial giant cells, and few T-cells, which presents with a sub-acute to chronic subcortical dementia syndrome. Often this condition is clinically recognized as immune reconstitution inflammatory syndrome, but it has also been described in the context of viral escape and treatment interruption [23].

Several associations and risk events for HIV-CD8E have been previously identified including: intercurrent extra-cerebral infection or malignancy, CSF virological escape, ART treatment interruption, immune reconstitution inflammatory syndrome (IRIS), and antiretroviral drug resistance. Occasionally, HIV-CD8E occurs in patients who have never been treated with ART.

19.4.2 Opportunistic Infections

During the early stage of AIDS or stages of immunosuppression due to the marked decrease of CD4+ lymphocytes and increased HIV viral load, several opportunistic infections have the potential to affect the CNS. Most of these infections include DNA viruses such as JCV, VZV, CMV, and EBV as well as bacteria (e.g., *Mycobacterium tuberculosis*), fungi (e.g., *Cryptococcus neoformans*, *Candida albicans*, Aspergillus, Histoplasma, and Coccidioides), and parasites (e.g., *Toxoplasma gondii*).

19.4.3 IRIS

The immune reconstitution inflammatory syndrome (IRIS) leads to paradoxical worsening of an infection shortly after initiation of ART [24]. This syndrome results from improvement in the immune system and a renewed inflammatory response directed against infectious agents. Retrospective case series suggest that up to 30% of HIV patients treated with ART develop one or more inflammatory syndromes. The clinical picture follows a subacute or chronic course succeeding the initiation of ART and depend on the type of preexisting opportunistic infection. For instance, patients with a previous cryptococcal infection could develop fever, gastrointestinal symptoms, eye pain, and meningismus, while patients with *M. avium* complex may experience expansion of preexisting intracranial tuberculomas.

Although there are no well-established diagnostic criteria of IRIS, the diagnosis could be made if patients present with the following features: the presence of AIDS with a CD4 count of less than 100 cells/μL; viral or immune response to ART; absence of drug-resistant infection, bacterial infection, or drug allergy; the presence of clinical features compatible with an inflammatory disorder; and time frame consistent with IRIS [25].

19.4.4 Antiretroviral Drugs Related Neuropsychiatric Complications

One of the major complications often encountered in critical care settings for patients on ART is the syndrome of severe hepatic steatosis and lactic acidosis. It was first described in the 1990s. The syndrome is most commonly associated with nucleoside reverse transcriptase inhibitors (NRTIs), particularly didanosine and stavudine, and results from the mitochondrial toxicity of these agents [26]. The incidence of hyperlactatemia in patients taking NRTIs has been reported as high as 227 cases per 1000 person-years. Symptomatic lactic acidosis ranges from 1 to 25.2 cases per 1000 patient-years, with mortality as high as 77% [27]. Risk factors for the development of hyperlactatemia include older age, drug regimens containing stavudine or combined stavudine-didanosine, concomitant buprenorphine, creatinine clearance under 70 mL/min, and a nadir CD4 cell count less than 250 cells/μL.

Data regarding treatment outcomes are not extensive, and treatment with riboflavin, thiamine, and L-carnitine has reversed the toxicity in some case reports. One recommended regimen is to administer 50 mg of riboflavin daily with 50 mg/kg of L-carnitine and 100 mg of thiamine until the lactic acidosis resolves [27].

19.5 Antiretroviral Drugs

19.5.1 Nucleoside Reverse Transcriptase Inhibitor

These molecules are nucleoside analogs (NAs) which lack a 3-OH group, which is necessary for phosphodiester bond formation and chain elongation, and their incorporation into the newly synthesized DNA strand causes premature termination of transcription, preventing antiretroviral replication. In a similar manner, they inhibit replication of mitochondrial DNA and telomere elongation, respectively, causing peripheral neuropathy and myopathy. All drugs of this category have been associated with this side effect profile, though they have the strength of the association varies.

Didanosine and stavudine have been more strongly associated with peripheral neuropathy with increased risk when used concurrently with ribavirin, isoniazid, and vincristine. Zidovudine has more commonly been associated with myopathy and myelotoxicity.

Tenofovir disoproxil fumarate is the first-line treatment for both HIV and hepatitis B virus (HBV) infection due to its similar efficacy and significantly improved safety profile compared to other NRTIs. Peripheral neuropathy is less common with tenofovir compared to other NRTIs (especially stavudine), although it does occur. The risk is increased when it is combined with efavirenz.

Zalcitabine is associated with dose-dependent peripheral neuropathy that can be treatment limiting in 10–20% of cases and is slowly reversible after stopping the treatment. Its bioavailability reduces with antacids and metoclopramide.

19.5.2 Nonnucleoside Reverse Transcriptase Inhibitors

Efavirenz is no longer considered a first-line choice for HAART due to its psychiatric side effects, which may limit patient compliance. Since the drug was approved, it has been known to produce a variety of psychiatric issues, including sleep disturbances (insomnia, nightmares), psychotic symptomatology (visual hallucinations, derealization, and depersonalization), and mood dysregulation. Initially, the mechanism for these effects was unknown, though it was obvious that they were dose-dependent and that tolerance to the acute psychotropic effects of the drug developed a few weeks after treatment initiation.

Nevirapine is another nonnucleoside reverse transcriptase inhibitor, which, unlike efavirenz, has been infrequently associated with neuropsychiatric adverse events.

19.5.3 Protease Inhibitors

Saquinavir and ritonavir have poor blood–brain barrier (BBB) penetrance, so CNS adverse effects are unlikely. They have, however, been associated with peripheral neurotoxicity, including perioral paraesthesia, taste alteration, and hearing loss. Prolonged use may contribute to the development of dementia by promoting the pathogenesis of cerebral small vessel disease.

19.5.4 Integrase Inhibitors

Raltegravir was the first drug of this class to be approved in 2007, with elvitegravir and dolutegravir being approved in 2012 and 2013, respectively. They are among the most well-tolerated antiretroviral agents, although they have also been associated with adverse psychiatric effects, especially dolutegravir. Side effects which have been reported include insomnia, hallucinations, abnormal dreams, mood disturbances (mostly depression), fatigue, and confusion, similar to efavirenz.

19.5.5 Entry and Fusion Inhibitors

Maraviroc and enfuvirtide are the two agents belonging to this class. They are used in conjunction with other components of HAART. They are not first-line agents (mostly reserved for salvage therapy) and appear to be better tolerated compared to other antiretroviral drugs. They are well tolerated and have not been associated with treatment-limiting neuropsychiatric adverse effects. Substitution of efavirenz with one of these drugs may reduce the risk of neuropsychiatric effects, whereas substitution of an NRTI by a fusion inhibitor may partially attenuate peripheral neuropathy and myopathy without compromising treatment efficacy.

19.6 Neuropsychiatry Effects of Other Antivirals

Antiviral drugs are known to cause significant neuropsychiatric complications, ranging from irritability to severe depressive syndrome, cognitive impairment, and sleep disturbance. Neuropsychiatric side effects are defined as new neurological or psychiatric symptoms that develop during treatment or worsening of preexisting neurological or psychiatric disorders. It may be difficult to determine whether the clinical phenotype can be attributed to the viral illness itself, the immune response to it, or the drugs used to treat it.

19.6.1 Antiviral Drugs in Influenza

Oseltamivir and zanamivir are neuraminidase inhibitors, used for treating influenza by shortening the duration of the disease, relieving the symptoms and reducing the complications and transmission of influenza. Results from studies in the USA, Spain, Japan, China, and South Korea associate oseltamivir with many neuropsychiatric adverse events and abnormal behaviors such as delusions and perceptual disorders, delirium and delirium-like events, frightening episodes, abrupt anger, delirious speech, jumping or falling from a height, depressive episodes, mania, and suicidal feelings.

The mechanism involved can be attributed to inhibition of monoamine oxidase-A (MAO-A), which is related to excitatory behaviors. Another study reported that Oseltamivir sialylates a serum glycolipid that stimulates D2 dopaminergic receptor and is related to abnormal behavior reported in some children taking oseltamivir. Unchanged oseltamivir phosphate is suggested to be related to central nervous system reactions such as acute behavioral change, occurring in the early phase of treatment [28].

The US Food and Drug Administration (FDA) added a warning to the oseltamivir label in 2006 to draw attention to the risk of neuropsychiatric adverse events. In March 2007, the Japanese Ministry of Health, Labour and Welfare (MHLW) warned against the use of oseltamivir in children aged 10–19 years because of the possible cause of abnormal behavior [29].

19.6.2 Antivirals in Chronic Hepatitis B

Lamivudine and telbivudine have been associated with myopathy and peripheral neuropathy, with the incidence of these effects being similar across all age groups and both genders. The proposed mechanism underlying this reaction is the depletion of mitochondrial DNA. An interesting report of two cases of lamivudine-induced dystonia has been reported, which responded to prompt administration of anticholinergic agents and did not recur after lamivudine discontinuation [30, 31].

Moreover, patients receiving telbivudine treatment suffer from weakness in upper and lower extremities. Myopathy is characterized by creatine kinase (CK) elevation alongside muscle pain and weakness. CK elevations to more than twice the upper limit of normal are among the well-described adverse effects of nucleoside analogs (NAs), but they are not specific for myopathy and may be associated with strenuous exercise and many other illnesses.

The most frequent neuropsychiatric adverse events in clinical trials were headache (17–23%), fatigue (10–13%), and dizziness (9%), while 1–10% of patients treated with entecavir suffer from insomnia [32].

19.6.3 Antivirals in Hepatitis C

Neuropsychiatric symptoms during antiviral therapy are reported in 30–40% of chronic hepatitis C (CHC) patients treated for 6–12 months and are much more troublesome due to their insidious onset, unpredictable nature, and potentially serious consequences. The incidence of side effects is more than Hepatitis B-treated individuals.

The combination of pegylated interferon and ribavirin was the mainstay of treatment for hepatitis C infection until the approval of direct-acting antivirals (DAAs). The drugs were not well tolerated, and psychiatric disturbances were a common adverse event during treatment. Interferon is notorious for its depressogenic potential and patients treated with it commonly experienced apathy, anhedonia, loss of motivation, and depressed mood. The use of ribavirin in combination with either interferon or direct-acting antivirals may be associated with a greater incidence of psychiatric disturbances compared to monotherapy [33].

Depression is among the most common treatment-limiting side effects with the combination treatment of interferon and ribavirin. Headache, weakness, and irritability were major effects by DAAs (direct-acting antivirals) like telaprevir, ledipasvir, and sofosbuvir.

19.7 Newer/Investigational Antivirals

19.7.1 Brincidofovir

It is a phospholipid conjugate of cidofovir that is taken up by cells and converted to cidofovir. It is active against herpes viruses including ganciclovir-resistant CMV and poxvirus, adenovirus as well as polyoma virus. Although it is neither nephrotoxic or myelosuppressive, it causes potential gastrointestinal toxicity.

19.7.2 Maribavir

It is a benzimidazole that inhibits the CMV UL97 protein kinase and prevents egress of viral particles from the nucleus. In vitro it is active against most strains of ganciclovir and foscarnet-resistant CMV. It is presently being tested for CMV infection refractory to other antivirals. Dose-related taste disturbance and diarrhea occur along with rash, headache, nausea, and fever.

19.7.3 Pritelivir

It inhibits helicase–primase complex required for replication of HSV. It is being tested for acyclovir-resistant HSV infections. It has a long half-life and can be administered in once weekly doses.

19.8 Conclusion

Although the development of antivirals is at a rapid pace but apart from Herpes viruses and HIV, effective treatment of the majority of viruses is elusive. Taking into account the severity of nervous system infections by the viruses, more antivirals need to develop with newer mechanisms of action. The more important fact apart from the drug development is to curtail the potential side effects of these drugs which need to be addressed while dealing with their pharmacokinetics and pharmacodynamics.

At present, we have to focus in our present armamentarium of drugs with rapid diagnosis and treatment, if possible with multiple drugs along with immunomodulators.

References

1. Pankey GA, Sabath LD. Clinical relevance of bacteriostatic versus bactericidal mechanisms of action in the treatment of Gram-positive bacterial infections. Clin Infect Dis. 2004;38(6):864–70.
2. Clercq ED. Antivirals and antiviral strategies. Nat Rev Microbiol. 2004;2(9):704–20.
3. Solomon T, Michael BD, Smith PE, Sanderson F, Davies NW, Hart IJ, Holland M, Easton A, Buckley C, Kneen R, Beeching NJ. Management of suspected viral encephalitis in adults—Association of British Neurologists and British Infection Association National Guidelines. J Infect. 2012;64(4):347–73.
4. Michael B, Menezes BF, Cunniffe J, Miller A, Kneen R, Francis G, Beeching NJ, Solomon T. Effect

of delayed lumbar punctures on the diagnosis of acute bacterial meningitis in adults. Emerg Med J. 2010;27(6):433–8.
5. Katzung BG, Trevor AJ. Pharmacology: examination and board review. 12th ed. Appleton & Lange; 1993.
6. Stránská R, Schuurman R, Nienhuis E, Goedegebuure IW, Polman M, Weel JF, Wertheim-Van Dillen PM, Berkhout RJ, van Loon AM. Survey of acyclovir-resistant herpes simplex virus in The Netherlands: prevalence and characterization. J Clin Virol. 2005;32(1):7–18.
7. Safrin S. Antiviral agents. In: Basic and clinical pharmacology, vol. 11; 2018. p. 845–75.
8. Kimberlin DW, Whitley RJ. Antiviral therapy of HSV-1 and-2. In: Human herpesviruses: biology, therapy, and immunoprophylaxis. Cambridge: Cambridge University Press; 2007.
9. Serrano-Pozo A. Encephalopathy. In: The Wiley handbook on the aging mind and brain, vol. 18. Wiley; 2018. p. 553–90.
10. Matthews T, Boehme R. Antiviral activity and mechanism of action of ganciclovir. Rev Infect Dis. 1988;10(Supplement_3):S490–4.
11. Boeckh M, Geballe AP. Cytomegalovirus: pathogen, paradigm, and puzzle. J Clin Invest. 2011;121(5):1673–80.
12. Upadhyayula S, Michaels MG. Ganciclovir, foscarnet, and cidofovir: antiviral drugs not just for cytomegalovirus. J Pediatr Infect Dis Soc. 2013;2(3):286–90.
13. Chrisp P, Clissold SP. Foscarnet: a review of its antiviral activity, pharmacokinetic properties and therapeutic use in immunocompromised patients with cytomegalovirus retinitis. Drugs. 1991;41:104–29.
14. Magee WC, Hostetler KY, Evans DH. Mechanism of inhibition of vaccinia virus DNA polymerase by cidofovir diphosphate. Antimicrob Agents Chemother. 2005;49(8):3153–62.
15. Safrin S, Cherrington J, Jaffe HS. Clinical uses of cidofovir. Rev Med Virol. 1997;7(3):145–56.
16. Marty FM, Ljungman P, Chemaly RF, Maertens J, Dadwal SS, Duarte RF, Haider S, Ullmann AJ, Katayama Y, Brown J, Mullane KM. Letermovir prophylaxis for cytomegalovirus in hematopoietic-cell transplantation. N Engl J Med. 2017;377(25):2433–44.
17. Daliparty VM, Balasubramanya R. HIV encephalitis. In: StatPearls. StatPearls Publishing; 2021.
18. Everall IP, Hansen LA, Masliah E. The shifting patterns of HIV encephalitis neuropathology. Neurotox Res. 2005;8:51–61.
19. Lucas SB, Wong KT, Nightingale S, Miller RF. HIV-associated CD8 encephalitis: a UK case series and review of histopathologically confirmed cases. Front Neurol. 2021;12:628296.
20. Kennedy PG. Viral encephalitis: causes, differential diagnosis, and management. J Neurol Neurosurg Psychiatry. 2004;75(suppl 1):i10–5.
21. Tavazzi E, Morrison D, Sullivan P, Morgello S, Fischer T. Brain inflammation is a common feature of HIV-infected patients without HIV encephalitis or productive brain infection. Curr HIV Res. 2014;12(2):97–110.
22. Lin SP, Calcagno A, Letendre SL, Ma Q. Clinical treatment options and randomized clinical trials for neurocognitive complications of HIV infection: combination antiretroviral therapy, central nervous system penetration effectiveness, and adjuvants. In: Neurocognitive complications of HIV-infection: neuropathogenesis to implications for clinical practice. Springer; 2021. p. 517–45.
23. Morgello S. HIV neuropathology. Handb Clin Neurol. 2018;152:3–19.
24. Shelburne SA 3rd, Hamill RJ. The immune reconstitution inflammatory syndrome. AIDS Rev. 2003;5(2):67–79.
25. Sharma SK, Soneja M. HIV and immune reconstitution inflammatory syndrome (IRIS). Indian J Med Res. 2011;134(6):866.
26. Abers MS, Shandera WX, Kass JS. Neurological and psychiatric adverse effects of antiretroviral drugs. CNS Drugs. 2014;28:131–45.
27. Fink MP. Textbook of critical care. 7th ed; 2005.
28. Hama R, Bennett CL. The mechanisms of sudden-onset type adverse reactions to oseltamivir. Acta Neurol Scand. 2017;135(2):148–60.
29. Ueda N, Umetsu R, Abe J, Kato Y, Nakayama Y, Kato Z, Kinosada Y, Nakamura M. Analysis of neuropsychiatric adverse events in patients treated with oseltamivir in spontaneous adverse event reports. Biol Pharm Bull. 2015;38(10):1638–44.
30. Kayaaslan B, Guner R. Adverse effects of oral antiviral therapy in chronic hepatitis B. World J Hepatol. 2017;9(5):227.
31. Kamara DA, Smith C, Ryom L, Reiss P, Rickenbach M, Phillips A, Mocroft A, De Wit S, Law M, Monforte AD, Dabis F. Longitudinal analysis of the associations between antiretroviral therapy, viraemia and immunosuppression with lipid levels: the D: A: D study. Antivir Ther. 2016;21(6):495–506.
32. Song X, Hu Z, Zhang H. Acute dystonia induced by lamivudine. Clin Neuropharmacol. 2005;28(4):193–4.
33. Davoodi L, Masoum B, Moosazadeh M, Jafarpour H, Haghshenas MR, Mousavi T. Psychiatric side effects of pegylated interferon-α and ribavirin therapy in Iranian patients with chronic hepatitis C: a meta-analysis. Exp Ther Med. 2018;16(2):971–8.

20 Antifungal Drugs

Neeta Karmarkar, Pooja Shah,
and Kalpana Rathod

20.1 Introduction and Epidemiology

Invasive fungal infection is growing problems globally in critically ill patients which increases prolong ICU stay along with increasing morbidity and mortality.

Fungal pathogens are responsible for at least 13 million infections and 1.5 million deaths globally per years, primarily in those with some compromised immune function [1]. In these patients, infections can quickly become severe, resulting in high mortality.

Fungal infections of the central nervous system (CNS) were considered rare until the 1970s. Since few years, due to widespread use of corticosteroids, cytotoxic drugs and antibiotics and immunocompromised patients with underlying malignancy, organ transplantations, and acquired immune deficiency syndrome are all responsible factors predisposing for fungal infections either in meninges or brain. A considerable number of cases of CNS fungal infections even in immunocompetent hosts have been reported recently. CNS fungal infections comprise of a wide spectrum of clinical syndrome, including abscesses, meningitis/meningoencephalitis, focal masses (SOL), stroke/vacuities, and immune reconstitution inflammatory syndrome (IRIS). Often with delays in diagnosis due to the nonspecific symptoms of severe disease, fungal infections are chronically underdiagnosed, with a high degree of variability in the prognosis of affected patients [2].

The fungal infection can enter the CNS by following routes:

1. Hematogenous route: This is the most common way infection travel.
2. Direct implantation
   (a) Traumatic
   (b) Iatrogenic via lumbar puncture
   (c) Congenital meningomyelocele
3. Local extension: Secondary to established infection.

20.2 Classification of Fungi

1. Yeast:
   (a) Candida
   (b) Cryptococcus
   (c) Trichosporon
2. Filamentous fungi:
   (a) Rhizopus
   (b) Rhizomucor
   (c) Mucor
3. Dimorphic fungi:
   (a) Blastomyces
   (b) Histoplasma
   (c) Coccidoides
   (d) Paracoccidoides

N. Karmarkar (✉) · P. Shah · K. Rathod
Department of Neuroanaesthesiology, Nanavati Max Superspeciality Hospital,
Mumbai, Maharashtra, India

H. Prabhakar et al. (eds.), *Principles and Practice of Neurocritical Care*,
https://doi.org/10.1007/978-981-99-8059-8_20

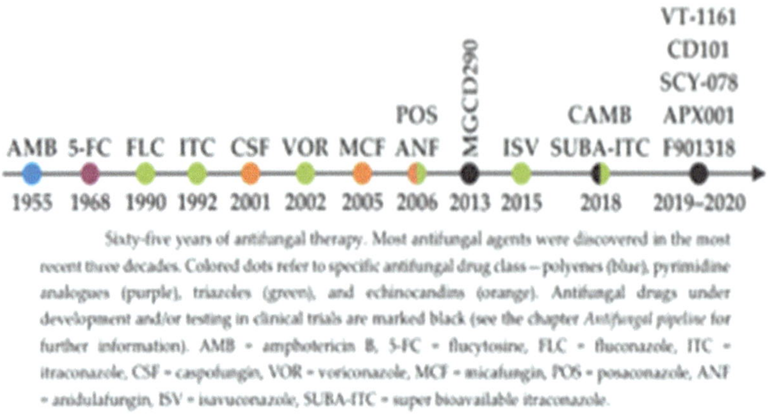

Fig. 20.1 [4]

Cryptococcus neoformans, Candida albicans, Coccidioides immitis. Histoplasma capsulatum is a common cause of fungal meningitis; Aspergillus spp., Candida spp., Zygomycetes, and some of the melanized fungi are known to cause mass lesions in brain.

Most of the fungi-causing CNS infections are saprobes with worldwide distribution; a few are geographically restricted like Coccidioides immitis. The infections reach the CNS either by the hematogenous route or by direct extension from colonized sinuses or ear canal or by direct inoculation during neurosurgical procedures.

The most common CNS fungal infection worldwide is cryptococcal meningoencephalitis. Disseminated mycosis is often associated with CNS involvement. It is estimated that between 67 and 84% of patients with invasive cryptococcosis develop CNS mycosis, 3–64% develop invasive candidiasis, 40% blastomycosis, 25% disseminated coccidioidomycosis, and 5–20% disseminated histoplasmosis, while 12% develop mucormycosis and 4–6% invasive aspergillosis [3].

20.3 Classification of Antifungal Agents

1. Polyenes
2. Triazoles
3. Echinocandins
4. Pyrimidine analog 5-flucytosine

Since the arrival of more than 200 polyenes, amphotericin B has remained the single polyene medicine of choice in the treatment of invasive fungal infections [4, 5]. 5-Flucytosine was first introduced and used as the antimetabolite in cancer treatment.

As its antineoplastic ability was low, 5-FC now serves in combinational antifungal treatment [4, 5].

Whereas fluconazole (FLC) and itraconazole (ITC) are first-generation triazoles, the second generation of triazoles, with better pharmacological biographies, include voriconazole (VOR), posaconazole (POS), and isavuconazole (ISV) [6]. Caspofungin (CSF), micafungin (MCF), and anidulafungin (ANF) represent the newest class of peptide antifungals called echinocandins. The chronology of antifungal application and development is shown in Fig. 20.1 [4]. The importance of combination therapy in the treatment of invasive fungal infections was epitomized lately [7].

20.4 Mechanism of Action

Amphotericin B is produced by the gram-positive bacterium.

Streptomyces nodosus. It has two mechanisms of action (Fig. 20.2) [4]. First, molecules of AMB merge with the ergosterol in the fungal lipid bilayer causing ergosterol sequestration. This leads to pore formation and both the ions (K^+, Mg^{2+}, Ca^{2+}, and Cl^-) and electrolyte glucose,

Fig. 20.2 [4]

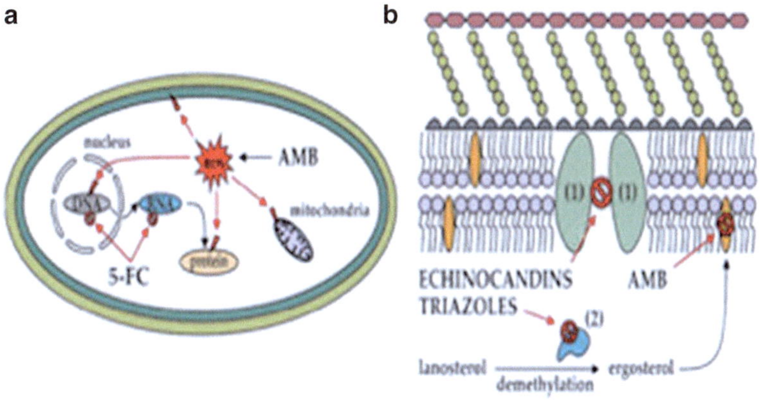

Mechanisms of actions of antifungals in the fungal cell. (**A**): In the fungal cytoplasm, AMB induces ROS formation resulting in the mitochondrial, biomembrane, DNA, and protein damage. Furthermore, 5-FC prevents DNA, RNA, and thus protein biosynthesis. (**B**): In the fungal biomembrane, 1,3-β-D-glucan synthase (1) and 14-α-demethylase (2) are inhibited by echinocandins and triazoles, respectively. Additionally, ergosterol contained in the biomembrane is sequestered by AMB, resulting in pore formation.

resulting in fungal cell death due to rapid depletion of intracellular ions. Second, AMB induces the accumulation of reactive oxygen species (ROS), resulting in DNA, protein, mitochondrial, and membrane damage [8]. The structural parts of mycosamine and hydroxyl groups at the C8, C9, and C35 positions are critical for the AMB biological activity [9].

The mechanism of action of triazoles (Fig. 20.2d–h) is based on the inhibition of the microsomal cytochrome P450 (CYP450) monooxygenase-dependent 14-α-demethylase (Fig. 20.2). The demethylation of fungal lanosterol is a two-step process involving the reduced form of nicotinamide dinucleotide phosphate (NADPH) and oxygen. As nitrogen from the triazole ring binds to the heme iron, oxidation of the methyl group is prevented. The combination of the accumulation of toxic 14-α-methylsterols and depletion of ergosterol results in the fungistatic effect.

5-Flucytosine (Fig. 20.2b) is a synthetic analog of cytosine. After administration, 5-FC is taken up by cytosine permease into the fungal cell and deaminated to 5-fluorouracil. 5-Fluorouracil is subsequently converted into 5-fluorouridine triphosphate. Unlike uridylic acid, this compound is incorporated into fungal ribonucleic acid (RNA), resulting in inhibition of protein synthesis. Besides, 5-fluorouracil can be metabolized to the 5-fluorodeoxyuridine monophosphate by uridine monophosphate pyrophosphorylase. This compound inhibits the primary source of thymidine in DNA biosynthesis, thymidylate synthetase, due to the enzyme's inability to remove the fluorine atom.

20.5 Drug Toxicities

20.5.1 Polyenes

The standard amphotericin B formulation is associated with renal toxicity, caused by the vasoconstriction of the afferent arteriole, resulting in reduced renal blood flow and glomerular filtration rate combined with tubular injury, causing loss of potassium, magnesium bicarbonates, and amino acids. To reduce renal injury, liposomal amphotericin B allows lower absorption of amphotericin B by the reticuloendothelial system, resulting in a longer stay in the bloodstream.

Amphotericin B is contraindicated in patients with renal failure. Liposomal amphotericin B and amphotericin B lipid complex are less nephrotoxic than conventional amphotericin B, allowing a higher dosage because their PK are very different [5]. Since enteral absorption is negligible for all commercially available amphotericin B formulations, they must be administered by intravenous infusion.

Infusion-related adverse events include chills, rigor, fever, hypotension or hypertension, hypoxia, nausea, vomiting, and hypokalemia and affect about half of patients treated with conventional amphotericin B.

20.5.2 Azoles

The most frequent side effects induced by triazoles include liver toxicity, prolonged QTc, and emerging resistance among fungal isolates [5]. Moreover, triazoles inhibit most of the cytochromeP450 enzymes (including the CYP34A), inducing variable drug–drug interactions. This plays a key role in metabolizing immunosuppressant drugs such as cyclosporine, tacrolimus, and sirolimus. Close therapeutic drug monitoring of both immunosuppressants and triazoles is therefore indispensable.

Fluconazole-available oral, iv. Has high bioavailability, well tolerated, active against most candida species, maintenance dose needs to reduced by 50% for patients with renal failure (creatinine clearance 11–50 ml/min).

Voriconazole-available oral, iv. Has high bioavailability, broad-spectrum antifungal, recommended as first-line treatment for invasive aspergillosis. No dosing change needed in renal failure, but accumulation of solvent sulfobutylether-b-cyclodextrin (SBECD), potentially nephrotoxic, seen after iv use. Hence, oral dosing recommended in patients with creatinine clearance below 50 ml/min. Significant interaction with sirolimus contradicates there concomitant use.

Posaconazole-wide antimycotic spectrum, iv, and oral form with high bioavailability is now available. Strong inhibitor of CYP3A4, responsible for drug–drug interactions. Mild to moderate renal or liver impairment as no relevant influence.

Isavuconazole-once a day dose, wider antifungal spectrum, excellent bioavailability and predictable PK. It can safely be used in renal failure patients without accumulation of cyclodextrin in iv. formulations. Gastrointestinal side effects (nausea, vomiting, and diarrhea) and central nervous adverse effects are possible. Most azoles cause QT interval prolongation, shortening of QT interval seen with isavuconazole. It is a moderate CYP3A4 inhibitor (Tables 20.1, 20.2, 20.3, 20.4 and 20.5).

Table 20.1 [5]

Overview on pharmacokinetics of antifungals						
Drugs	Protein binding (%)	V_d (L/kg)	C_{max} (μg/ml)	$T_{1/2}$ (h)	Elimination	Dosage
Amphotericin	95–99	0.5–2	1.7–2.8	15–27	Bile, kidney (80%)	0.3 mg/kg on day 1
					No metabolite yet identified	+ 5 mg per day until 1 mg/kg
						T_{inf} > 4 h mandatory
Liposomal amphotericin	95–99	0.05–2.2	14–29 (90)	13–24	Bile, RES long-term disposition, final elimination not yet clear, no metabolites identified	3–4 mg/kg per day
						T_{inf} > 4 h recommended
Fluconazole	12	0.7	9	30	Mainly unchanged via the kidney, tubular reabsorption	IV loading dose: 12 mg/kg once

Table 20.1 (continued)

Overview on pharmacokinetics of antifungals

Drugs	Protein binding (%)	V_d (L/kg)	C_{max} (μg/ml)	$T_{1/2}$ (h)	Elimination	Dosage
						Maintenance dose: 6 mg/kg per 24 h
Voriconazole	58	4.5	4.4	6	Hepatic metabolism involving 2C9, 2C19, and CYP3A4	IV loading dose: 6 mg/kg on day 1
					Strong inhibitor	Maintenance: 4 mg/kg per 12 h
Isavuconazole	98–99	6.5	2.6	80–120	Hepatic metabolism involving UGT, CYP3A4	IV loading dose: 200 mg day 1 and day 2
					Moderate inhibitor	Maintenance dose: 200 mg per 24 h
Caspofungin	92–97	0.3–2	10	8	Independent from cytochrome P450	IV loading dose: 70 mg
						Maintenance dose 50 mg (70 mg if body weight > 80 kg)
Anidulafungin	99	0.6	7	40–50	Spontaneous degradation in plasma	Loading dose: 200 mg (T_{inf} 180 min)
						Maintenance dose: 100 mg (T_{inf} 90 min)
Micafungin	99.9	0.3	18	13–20	CYP involved	50 mg for prophylaxis, 100 mg for candidiasis, 150 mg for esophageal candidiasis

Details and references are displayed in the text

C_{max} peak level, $T_{1/2}$ half-life, *Cl* clearance, V_d apparent volume of distribution, T_{inf} infusion time, *RES* reticuloendothelial system, *CYP* cytochrome, *UGT* urindin diphosphate glucuronsyltranferase

Table 20.2 [5]

Overview on pharmacokinetics of antifungals in patients with renal or liver failure			
Drug	Renal impairment	Liver impairment	Suggestions
Amphotericin	No indication	No dosage adjustment	
Liposomal amphotericin	Avoid (nephrotoxicity)	No dosage adjustment	ICU patients: decreased plasma levels, increased dosage?
	No dose adjustment if continuous		
Fluconazole	Dose reduction by 50% for GFR 11–50 ml/min	No dosage adjustment	Obese critically ill: actual body weight
	Enhanced dose if continuous RRT		ICU patient: enhanced doses
			Strong inhibitor of CYP3A4 and 2C9
Voriconazole	No dose adjustment	Mild to moderate hepatic impairment: 50% dose reduction,	Strong inhibitor of CYP2C0 and 2C19
	Consider SBECD accumulation during intravenous infusions		
		TDM recommended	Moderate inhibitor of CYP3A4
Isavuconazole	No dose adjustment	Enhanced levels, no dosage reduction	Moderate inhibitor of CYP3A4, P-gp, and BRCP
Posaconazole	No dose adjustment	No dose adjustment	Strong inhibitor of CYP3A4 causing drug-drug interactions
Caspofungin	No dose adjustment	Enhanced exposure in moderate hepatic impairment: dosage reduction	
		Dosage reduction in critically ill patients with liver dysfunction may cause underexposure	
&$$$;Atidulafungin	No dose adjustment	Slightly lowered concentrations but no dosage adjustment recommended	
Micafungin	No dose adjustment	Slightly lowered concentrations	Potential risk for liver tumors use only if other antifungals are not appropriate
	RRT: no dose adjustment		

Details and reference are displayed in the test

RRT renal replacement therapy, *SBECD* butylether-β-cyclodextrin, *TDM* therapeutic drug monitoring, *CYP* cytochrome, *P-gp* P-glycoprotein, *BCRP* breast cancer resistance protein, *UGT* urindin diphosphate glucronosyltranferase, *GFR* glomerular filtration rate

Table 20.3 [5]

Profile of intrinsic susceptibility and resistance of *Candida* species

Fungi	Fluconazole	Voriconazole	Amphotericin	Echinocandin
Candida albicans	S	S	S	S
Candida dubliniensis	S	S	S	S
Candida glabrata	S/R	S/R	S	S
Candida parapsilosis	S	S	S	R
Candida tropicalis	S	S	S	S
Candida krusei	R	S	S	S
Candida kefyr	S	S	S	S
Uncommon Candida species				
Candida lusitaniae	S	S	R	S
Candida auris	S	S	S	S
Candida guilliermondii	S	S	S	S/R

Green, intrinsic susceptibility of the species and first line treatment recommended; red, intrinsic resistance; yellow, susceptibility to be tested

Profile of susceptibility and resistance of *Aspergillus* species

Fungi	Fluconazole	Isavuconazole	Voriconazole	Amphotericin	Echinocandin
Aspergillus fumigatus	R	S	S	S	S/R
Aspergillus flavus	R	S	S	R	S/R
Aspergillus terreus	R	S	S	S/R	S/R
Aspergillus nidulans	R	S	S	S	S/R
Aspergillus niger	R	R	R	S	S/R
Aspergillus lentulus	R	R	R	S	S/R

Green, intrinsic susceptibility of the species and first line treatment recommended; red, intrinsic resistance; yellow, susceptibility to be tested

Table 20.4 [5]

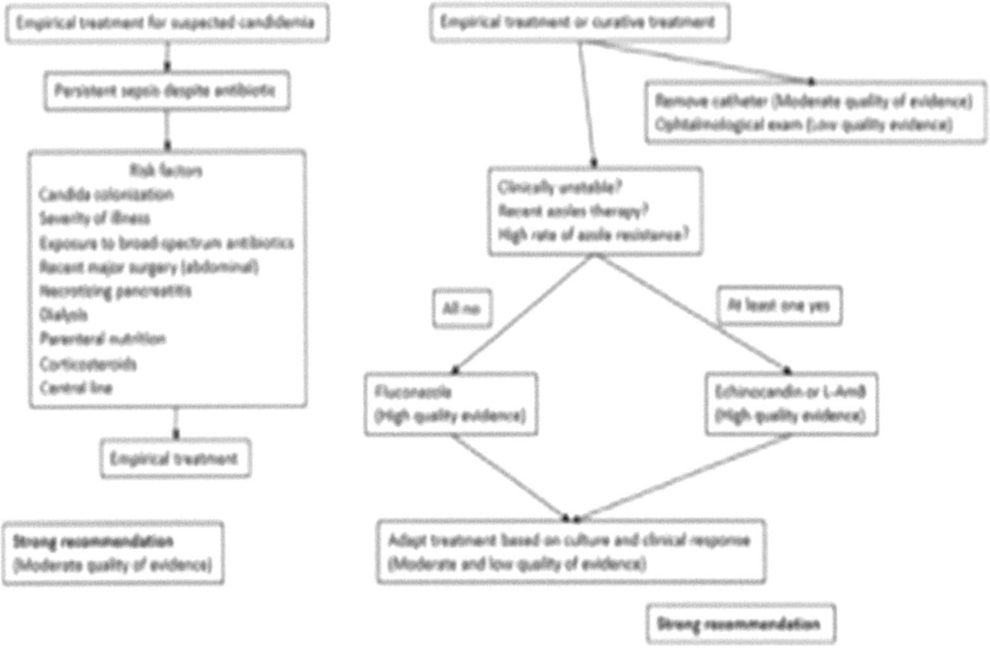

Practical guidelines for empiric and curative treatment of candidiasis adapted from the IDSA guideline

Table 20.5 [5]

Summary of practical guidelines for invasive aspergillosis	
Primary therapy	Salvage therapy
IV administration of voriconazole (6 mg/kg per 12 h at day 1 then 4 mg/kg per 12 h until improvement) followed by oral administration of voriconazole (200 mg per 12 h) or itraconazole (400–600 mg per 24 h) until resolution or stabilization of all clinical and radiological manifestations	IV administration of caspofungin (70 mg at day 1 then 50 mg) or IV administration of micafungin (100–150 mg per 24 h) until improvement followed by oral administration of voriconazole (200 mg per 12 h) or oral administration of itraconazole (400–600 mg per 24 h) until resolution or stabilization of all clinical and radiological manifestations
OR	OR
IV administration of L-amphotericin B (3–5 mg/kg per 24 h) followed by oral administration of voriconazole (200 mg per 12 h) or itraconazole (400–600 mg per 24 h) until resolution or stabilization of all clinical and radiographic manifestations	Posaconazole (200 mg per 6 h initially then 400 mg per 12 h orally after stabilization of disease)

20.6 Recommendations of Recent Guidelines

Recent guidelines for invasive candidiasis management were put forth by the Infectious Diseases Society of America (IDSA) in 2016 and by the task force of the European Society of Intensive Care medicine – European Society of Clinical Microbiology and Infectious Diseases (ESCMID) in 2019 [10].

They stated that.

20.6.1 Regarding Invasive Candidiasis

1. Antifungals cannot be used universally without clear signs or symptoms of infections (prophylaxis).
2. They supported the use of empirical antifungal treatment based on signs or symptoms of infections without certain proof of candida infection.
3. Empirical antifungal treatment with an echinocandin as the first-line agent (strong recommendation) can be used in patients with septic shock, multiple organ failure, no other causes of fever, and more than one extradigestive site of candida spp. Colonization (e.g., Mouth, throat, upper and lower respiratory tracts, skin folds, drains, operative sites, urine).
4. Fluconazole can be used in less severe patients or where there is low rate of fluconazole resistance.
5. For targeted treatment of invasive candidiasis, echinocandins should be used in patients who are likely to be infected or colonized by fluconazole resistant candida spp.
6. In clinically stable patients who have an isolate susceptible to fluconazole and have negative repeated blood cultures, transition from echinocandin to fluconazole is recommended (de-escalation). However, it is not considered in cases of difficult or impossible source control.
7. The recommended treatment duration of candidemia without metastatic complications is 14 days after the first negative blood culture.
8. For infections by azole- and echinocandin-resistant strains, lipid formulation amphotericin B (3–5 mg/kg/day) is recommended [11].

20.6.2 For Invasive Aspergillosis

The 2018 ESCMID—European Confederation of Medical Microbiology-European Respiratory Society stated that:

Early diagnosis and treatment should be based on the integration of clinical findings, risk factors, radiological data, and microbiological data.

Chest computerized tomography is the imaging of choice though classic signs are rare in ICU patients.

Common risk factors for aspergillosis are chronic obstructive pulmonary disease, steroid treatment, sepsis, and influenza-associated respiratory failure [12].

Voriconazole (2 × 6 mg/kg on day 1 and then 2 × 4 mg/kg IV) is the first-line agent. Therapeutic drug monitoring and susceptibility testing is recommended for voriconazole.

20.7 Conclusion

Fungal infections are an increasing concern in ICU patients. Hence, recent guidelines have become important. Three treatment classes are currently used for fungal infections, but data on those treatments are less in number and questions remain unanswered. Therapeutic drug monitoring is an essential option for evaluating treatment efficacy and tolerance.

Acknowledgments We would like to thank Dr. Chaleton, Dr. Cortegiani, and Dr. M Leone for permitting us to use their tables and images for the chapter.

References

1. Bongomin F, Gago S, Oladele RO, Denning DW. Global and multi-national prevalence of fungal diseases-estimate precision. J Fungi. 2017;3:57.
2. Formanek PE, Dilling DF. Advances in the diagnosis and management of invasive fungal disease. Chest. 2019;156:834–42.
3. Murthy JMK, Sundaram C. Fungal infections of the central nervous system. In: Biller J, Ferro JM, editors. Handbook of clinical neurology. New York: Elsevier; 2014. p. 1383–401.
4. Houst J, Spizek J, Havlicek V. Meta. 2020;10(3):106.
5. Chatelon J, Cortegiani A, Hammad E, Cassir N, Leone M. Choosing the right antifungal agent in ICU patients. Adv Ther. 2019;36(12):3308–20.
6. Ping B, Zhu Y, Gao Y, Yue C, Wu B. Second- versus first-generation azoles for antifungal prophylaxis in hematology patients: a systematic review and meta-analysis. Ann Hematol. 2013;92:831–9.
7. Livengood SJ, Drew RH, Perfect JR. Combination therapy for invasive fungal infections. Curr Fungal Infect Rep. 2020;14:40–9.

8. Mesa-Arango AC, Scorzoni L, Zaragoza O. It only takes one to do many jobs: Amphotericin B as antifungal and immunomodulatory drug. Front Microbiol. 2012;3:1–10.
9. Tevyashova AN, Olsufyeva E, Solovieva SE, Printsevskaya SS, Reznikova MI, Trenin AS, Galatenko OA, Treshalin ID, Pereverzeva ER, Mirchink EP, et al. Structure-antifungal activity relationships of polyene antibiotics of the amphotericin B group. Antimicrob Agents Chemother. 2013;57:3815–22.
10. Martin-Loeches I, Antonelli M, Cuenca-Estrella M, et al. ESCIM/ESCMID task force on practical management of invasive candidiasis in critically ill patients. Intensive Care Med. 2019;45:789–805.
11. Pappas PG, Kaufmann CA, Andes DR, et al. clinical practice guideline for the management of candidiasis: 2016 update by the Infectious Diseases Society of America. Clin Infect Dis. 2016;62:e1–50.
12. Ullmann AJ, Aguado JM, Arikan- Akdagli S, et al. Diagnosis and management of Aspergillus diseases: executive summary of the 2017 ESCMID-ECMM-ERS guideline. Clin Microbiol Infect. 2018;24(Suppl. 1):e1–38.

21 Antihypertensive Therapy

Paramita Basu and Suresh Ramasubban

21.1 Introduction

Antihypertensive therapy comprises medication of various classes that are used to treat hypertension. The drugs used to treat hypertension belong to different classes of compounds and are different structurally and functionally. A neurointensivist needs to be aware of antihypertensive drugs, their pharmacology, therapeutic effects, side effects, interactions with other drugs, and their role in neurocritical care. The knowledge of antihypertensive pharmacology is essential because of the common nature of hypertension which is very prevalent in the general population and hence reflects in the practice of neurointensive care. Hypertension is a very important risk factor for death and disability in India [1]. A survey by the national family health survey in 2019–2020 reported a prevalence of 24% in men and 21% among women for hypertension [2]. About, 1–2% of patients will have a hypertensive emergency in their lifetime [3]. Mortality during hospitalization for hypertensive emergencies is about 6.9% [4]. Leave aside the hypertensive emergencies, hypertension is very common among patients in the neurointensive care unit with ischemic CVA, subarachnoid hemorrhage, and elevated intracranial pressures being some of the common causes. An acute rise in blood pressure (BP) is one of the main postulated mechanisms of posterior reversible encephalopathy syndrome (PRES). Acute management of hypertension is of utmost importance in neurocritical care settings to ensure adequate cerebral perfusion and for the prevention of secondary brain injury. There is no ideal antihypertensive drug that can be used in different neurologically critical patients as a gold standard therapy.

While choosing pharmacological therapy for hypertension, a rational pathophysiological approach along with adequate analysis of the risk–benefit ratio should be adopted that includes the effect of the drug on blood volume, vascular tone, and other determinants of cardiac output (CO). Calcium channel blockers (CCB), beta-blockers (BB), and vasodilators, all agents decrease BP but through different modes of action which may be suitable or contraindicated in individual patients with different neurological crises, although some agents may be more advantageous than others with fewer adverse reaction.

In this chapter, we propose to focus on the applied pharmacology of various antihypertensives used in routine clinical practice, i.e., their therapeutic effects, side effects, and interactions with other drugs with relevance to the practice of neurocritical care.

P. Basu · S. Ramasubban (✉)
Department of Critical Care Medicine, Apollo Multispecialty Hospitals, Kolkata, India

H. Prabhakar et al. (eds.), *Principles and Practice of Neurocritical Care*,
https://doi.org/10.1007/978-981-99-8059-8_21

21.2 Definitions of Hypertension

Hypertension is defined and staged as per the suggestions of the American College of Cardiology/American Heart Association in 2017 [5]. They categorize the blood pressure (BP) measured as normal, elevated, and hypertension.

- Normal BP—systolic 130–139 mmHg or diastolic 80–89 mmHg.
- Elevated BP—systolic 120–129 mmHg and diastolic at least 90 mmHg.
- Hypertension:
  - Stage 1—systolic 130–139 mmHg or diastolic 80–89 mmHg.
  - Stage 2—systolic at least 140 mmHg or diastolic at least 90 mmHg.

A hypertensive emergency is defined as a severe elevation in blood pressure to greater than or equal to 180/120 mmHg and is associated with impending or progressive end-organ dysfunction. It is a situation wherein the immediate reduction of blood pressure is needed to prevent further organ damage, while hypertensive urgency is a situation where there is a severe elevation of blood pressure but there is no target end-organ damage. Both hypertensive emergency and hypertensive urgency are commonly encountered in the neurointensive care unit, and they need to be recognized and treated appropriately.

21.2.1 Causes of Hypertension

Most patients in neurointensive care have primary (essential) hypertension and are admitted with conditions unrelated to hypertension. However, a significant proportion of patients with essential hypertension have sustained end-organ damage due to uncontrolled hypertension and have neurological manifestations leading to admission to the ICU. Neurointensive care is unique in that a significant subset of hypertensive patients have secondary hypertension related to the presence of a space-occupying lesion and intracranial hypertension, a condition labeled as neurogenic secondary hypertension (Table 21.1). Acute hypertension in the ICU is also related to factors like pain, agitation, delirium, withdrawals, urinary retention, hypoxia, and hypercapnia. These factors need to be addressed simultaneously while considering pharmacologic therapy [6].

Table 21.1 Causes of hypertension

Type	Cause
Primary (Essential)	Idiopathic
Secondary	
Renal	Chronic kidney disease (CKD), Polycystic kidney disease, Nephritis
Vascular	Renovascular disease, Collagen vascular disease, Coarctation of aorta, Vasculitis
Hormonal	Endogenous-Hyperaldosteronism, Phaeochromocytoma, Cushing's syndrome, Hyperthyroidism, Hyperparathyroidism, Excessive growth hormone, Hypercalcemia Exogenous-Steroids, Oral contraceptive pills
Neurogenic	Raised Intracranial pressure, Space occupying lesion
Toxins	Non-steroidal medications, Alcohol, Vasopressors
Others	Obstructive sleep apnea, Pregnancy induced

21.2.2 Blood Pressure Goals in Neurocritical Care

Patients cared for in neurointensive care have diverse pathologies. Goals differ from condition to condition, but the principle is to control arterial pressure and prevent end-organ damage. The goals of BP are discussed in chapters on SAH, Ischemic CVA, ICH, and TBI.

21.2.3 Pharmacology of Antihypertensive Drugs

Blood pressure is a product of cardiac output (CO) and systemic vascular resistance (SVR) and can be reduced by drugs reducing cardiac output, SVR, or both (Fig. 21.1). CO is manipulated by

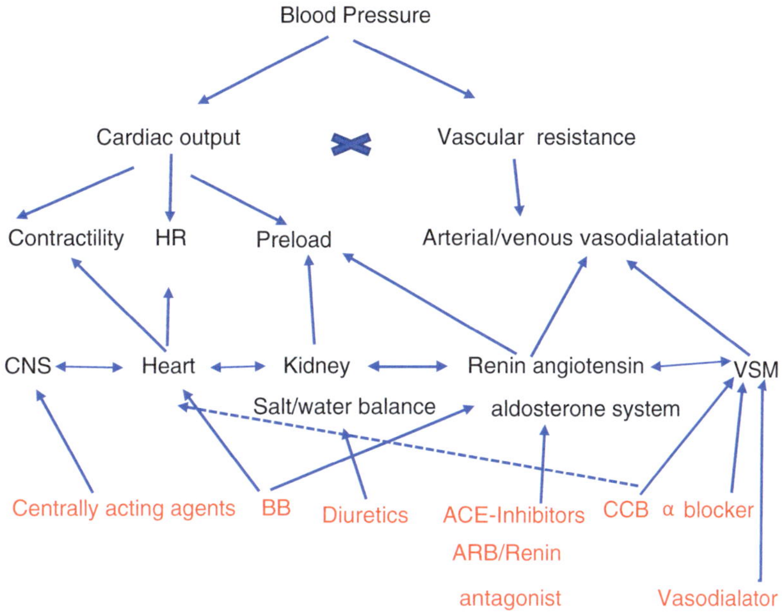

Fig. 21.1 Mechanisms of action of various commonly used antihypertensive agents. Most drugs act on multiple sites to produce their effect. *HR* Heart rate, *VSM* vascular smooth muscle, *ACE* angiotensin converting enzyme, *ARB* angiotensin receptor blocker, *CCB* calcium channel blockers, *BB* beta blockers. Dotted arrows signify varying effect within class

Table 21.2 Classes of antihypertensives

Class	Subclass	Examples
Targeting renin angiotensin system		
	Angiotensin converting enzyme inhibitors	Captopril, Lisinopril, Ramipril
	Angiotensin receptor blockers	Losartan, Valsartan
	Direct Renin Inhibitors	Aliskiren
Adrenoreceptor blockers		
	Beta Blockers	Atenolol, Metoprolol, Propranolol
	Alpha blockers	Doxazosin, Phentolamine, labetalol (mixed)
Calcium channel blockers		
	Phenylalkylamines	Verapamil
	Dihydropyridines	Amlodipine, Nifedipine, Nimodipine
	Benzothiazepines	Diltiazem
Diuretics		
	Thiazides	Hydrochlorothiazide
	Loop	Furosemide, Bumetanide
	Aldosterone agonist	Spironolactone, Amiloride
Vasodilators		Hydralazine, Nitroprusside
Centrally acting agents		Clonidine, Methyldopa
Ganglion blocker		Trimetaphan

varying contractility, heart rate, and preload, while SVR is manipulated by modification of the compliance and reactivity of the arterial and venous system [6]. There is, however, considerable overlap between some of the groups of antihypertensives and their mechanism of action. For example, diuretics affect preload and cause vasodilatation.

The medications available to treat hypertension may be classified based on the mechanism of action or site of action (Table 21.2). Each class of drugs will have multiple drugs with varying structures and pharmacology leading to different therapeutic and side effects [7, 8].

Antihypertensive medications can be broadly categorized into two main categories. First, those drugs that directly or indirectly block the renin-angiotensin system (RAS) (e.g., angiotensin-converting enzyme (ACE) inhibitors, angiotensin receptor blockers (ARBs), direct renin inhibitors (DRIs), and beta-blockers (BBs) to some extent). The second group of drugs acts to decrease intravascular volume by increasing water and sodium excretion or by causing vasodilatation (e.g., diuretics and calcium channel blockers (CCBs)). The second group of drugs increases RAS activity by negative feedback, as a result of which this group of drugs can potentiate the effects of RAS inhibitors.

The appropriate choice of medication to control BP depends on the pathophysiology of acute systemic arterial hypertension (Fig. 21.2). In the neurologically ill patient, there is an increased sympathetic tone with increased SVR making BB and CCB as the drug of choice for controlling an acutely elevated BP. For chronic hypertension, the choice of medication depends on which group of drugs will be effective in controlling BP as well as preventing end-organ damage. As per Indian hypertension guidelines, ACEI and ARBs are the preferred agents in patients aged < 60 years and CCBs and diuretics are preferred in patients above the age of 60 years [7].

21.2.4 RAS Inhibitors

There are three different drug classes that directly act on various points of the RAS pathway. All drugs acting on this pathway have the main goal to reduce the production of angiotensin II or to reduce its receptor binding (Fig. 21.3). Angiotensin II increases arteriolar tone and SVR because of its high affinity for AT1 G protein-coupled receptors (GPCRs). These groups of drugs activate the sympathetic nervous system,

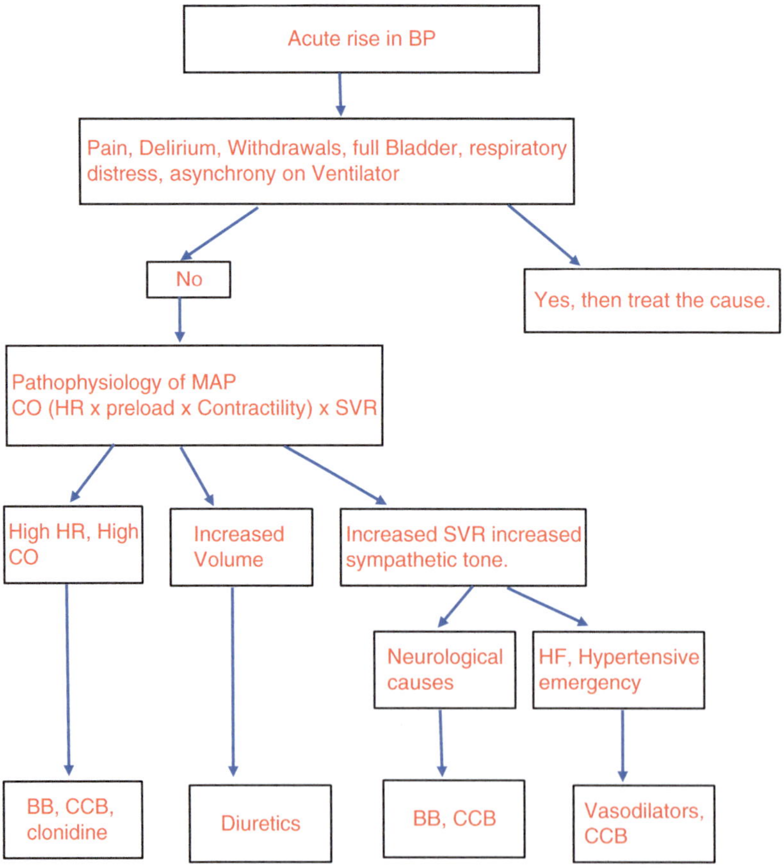

Fig. 21.2 Antihypertensive choice based on pathophysiological disturbance. *HR* Heart rate, *MAP* mean arterial pressure, *CO* cardiac output, *SCR* systemic vascular resistance, *BB* beta blockers, *CCB* calcium channel blockers, *HF* heart failure

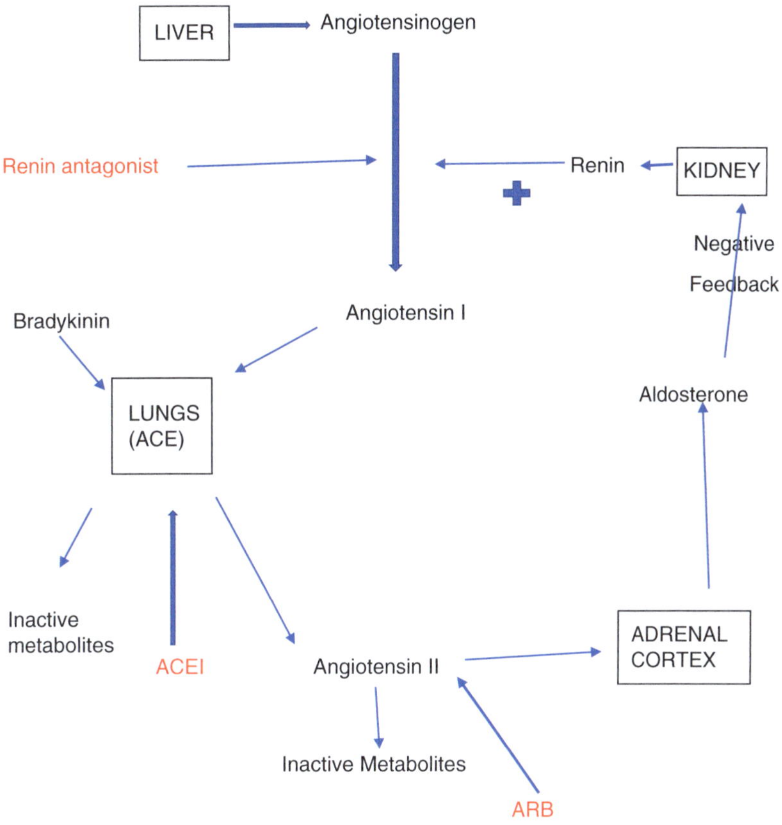

Fig. 21.3 Mechanism of action of drugs acting on the renin angiotensin system (RAS). *ACE* angiotensin converting enzyme, *ACEI* angiotensin converting enzyme inhibitors, *ARB* angiotensin receptor blocker

increase pituitary secretion of ADH and ACTH, and increase the secretion of aldosterone [8]. Drugs that antagonize the RAS pathway cause a reduction in SVR and BP. There is an additive antihypertensive effect due to the decrease in aldosterone production and subsequent reduction in renal sodium and water retention.

21.2.5 Angiotensin-Converting Enzyme (ACE) Inhibitors

ACE inhibitors are the drug of choice for the treatment of hypertension in patients aged < 60 years. ACE inhibitors are also an important treatment for heart failure with reduced ejection fraction, post-myocardial infarction, diabetic nephropathy, and chronic kidney disease. The protective effects of ACEI on the kidneys and heart are not only related to its antihypertensive effects but potentially other effects.

The enzyme ACE is found in the pulmonary vasculature, and its role is in converting angiotensinogen I to angiotensinogen II and decreasing the metabolism of the peptide bradykinin to inactive substances. The decrease in levels of angiotensinogen II results in an overall decrease in the levels of angiotensin and its therapeutic effect as an antihypertensive. The side effect profile of cough is due to the accumulation of bradykinin, whose inactivation is inhibited by ACE. ACEI causes a decrease in renal efferent arteriolar tone, leading to a decrease in glomerular filtration and an acute worsening of renal function, especially in the presence of renal artery stenosis. The other major side effect seen with ACEI is hyperkalemia due to decreased secretion of aldosterone, taste disturbances, skin rash, and rarely agranulocytosis. One of the most feared idiosyncratic reactions with ACEI is angioedema, which can lead to a potential airway emergency due to upper airway obstruction.

ACEIs are contraindicated in pregnancy due to their association with birth defects.

All the ACEIs available are in oral formulation except for enalaprilat, which is available for IV use. There are many drugs in this class of medications. Lisinopril and captopril are active drugs, while enalapril, ramipril, and perindopril are inactive drugs that must be activated by hepatic esterification.

ACEI interacts with medications, especially NSAIDs. NSAIDs cause afferent arteriolar vasoconstriction, thereby acting in tandem with ACEI to worsen renal function. Interactions with diuretics result in hypovolaemia and hyponatremia. Potassium-sparing diuretics and potassium supplements can result in severe hyperkalemia when used concurrently with ACEI. Drugs like lithium and digoxin, which are excreted by the kidneys, will accumulate and can reach toxic levels in the presence of ACEI.

21.2.6 Angiotensin Receptor Blocker (ARB) Drugs

Angiotensin receptor blockers are drugs that target AT_1 G-protein-coupled receptors and thus prevent angiotensin II from exerting its effects. Some of the ARBs like candesartan and telmisartan bind irreversibly, while losartan and valsartan are competitive antagonists. Angiotensin receptor blockage is advantageous as compared to ACE inhibition, as angiotensin II has sources other than the ACE pathway, for example, using enzyme chymase in the kidneys. ARBs do not affect bradykinin metabolism, so the risk of cough and angioedema is much decreased.

21.2.7 Direct Renin Inhibitors

There is only one drug available in this class and not been extensively used so far. Aliskiren is the representative molecule, a piperidine derivative, that inhibits renin directly. Renin is the most upstream in the RAS model, secreted by the juxtaglomerular cells of the kidney, and inhibition of renin reduces the conversion of angiotensinogen to angiotensin I. The renal side effects are the same as that of ACE and ARBs. Diarrhea is a specific side effect of Aliskiren.

21.3 Adrenoceptor Antagonists

21.3.1 Beta-Blockers (BBs)

In neurologically ill patients with an increased sympathetic tone and high heart rate, BBs are one of the preferred drugs for use in neurointensive care units. BBs antagonize the effects of catecholamine. Catecholamine/adrenergic receptors belong to the superfamily of G-protein-coupled receptors (GPCRs). These receptors are of various subtypes such as alpha, beta1, and beta 2. Beta 1 receptors are predominantly located in the heart and kidney and beta 2 in the lungs, blood vessels, and muscle. The antihypertensive effect of BB is due to its effects on multiple pathways. Blocking the beta 1 receptors in the sinoatrial node decreases chronotropy; while blockage of beta 1 receptors in the myocardium reduces contractility, blockage of beta 1 receptors in the kidney decreases renin secretion, and they reduce the overall sympathetic activity.

BBs are classified based on their selectivity of action on beta 1 receptors, i.e., they are cardioselective (metoprolol, esmolol, and atenolol) or non-cardioselective (propranolol and sotalol). Most of the BBs are purely antagonists at the receptor, while some (pindolol and timolol) have some agonist/sympathomimetic action. Some drugs like labetalol have also alpha-blocking effects in addition to being beta-blockers. Some BBs (propranolol and metoprolol) have an effect on the sodium channels and lead to membrane stabilization and act as antiarrhythmics also. The reduction in cardiac output can also be a major adverse effect and should be used carefully in the presence of acute heart failure. Since these drugs are antagonistic at beta 2 receptors also, they can lead to a significant respiratory side effect of bronchospasm, especially in asthmatics. BBs also have significant CNS side effects, and it includes vivid dreams, malaise, and tiredness. Another significant side effect is seen in diabetics where the symptoms of hypoglycemia may be masked due to the sympathetic blocking effects of BBs.

BBs have good oral absorption and bioavailability and are available in IV formulations. Some BBs are lipid-soluble (metoprolol and propranolol), metabolized by the liver, and have shorter half-lives. Some BBs are water-soluble (atenolol) and are excreted unchanged in the urine. Some BBs are metabolized by ester hydrolysis (esmolol), resulting in a very rapid onset of action.

21.3.2 Alpha-Blockers

Alpha-blockers act on the postganglionic alpha-1 GPCR resulting in vascular muscle relaxation, vasodilation, and reduced SVR. Alpha-blockers can again be of the nonselective type (phentolamine and phenoxybenzamine), and these also act on alpha-2 GPCR resulting in the release of norepinephrine and subsequent elevated heart rate and increased cardiac output. Labetalol acts selectively on alpha-1 receptors leading to significant reductions in BP due to its effects on both beta and alpha receptors. Blockade of alpha receptors can lead to orthostatic hypotension with reflex tachycardia. However, an inability to mount a tachycardic response leads to a precipitous fall in BP with alpha-blockers.

21.3.3 Calcium Channel Blockers (CCBs)

These are recommended as first-line therapy for hypertensives above the age of 60 years. They are very commonly used in neurointensive care units, and some of them (nimodipine) have very specific indications in neurocritical care.

CCBs inhibit calcium influx through voltage-sensitive L-type calcium channels in vascular smooth muscle cells inducing arteriolar vasodilation and reducing SVR. The presence of L-type calcium channels in myocardial tissue and inhibition of calcium influx results in reduced contractility. Some CCBs (diltiazem and verapamil) have higher affinity to cardiac tissue leading to decreased contractility and decreased chronotropy. Some CCBs (nifedipine) have a higher affinity to vascular smooth muscles and cause peripheral vasodilatation and reflex tachycardia. Nimodipine preferentially acts on cerebral blood vessels as it is lipophilic and can cross the blood–brain barrier. Proposed mechanisms also include decreased angiographic vasospasm, increased fibrinolytic activity, and enhanced neuroprotection.

Several CCBs are available for use, and they belong to three different chemical groups. Phenylalkylamines, i.e., verapamil, dihydropyridines, i.e., amlodipine and nifedipine, and second generation like nicardipine and clevidipine, and benzothiazepines, i.e., diltiazem. As a result, their pharmacokinetics are different. However, most are orally administered, although their bioavailability is low because of the extensive first-pass effect. I.V. preparations are available for nicardipine, nimodipine, diltiazem, and clevidipine.

The major side effects of CCBS are cardiovascular, which again depends on the agent. Drugs like nifedipine and amlodipine cause reflex tachycardia, disturbance of the peripheral circulation resulting in edema of the feet, flushing, and headache. Rate-limiting agents cause negative inotropy and chronotropy leading to worsening cardiac output and worsening heart failure.

CCBs, especially nimodipine, are commonly used. Neurocritical Care Society guidelines [9] suggest that all patients with aneurysmal subarachnoid hemorrhage should receive oral nimodipine 60 mg every 4 h for 21 days from SAH onset. Nimodipine should start as early as possible or within 96 h of the diagnosis of subarachnoid hemorrhage. The recommended dose for adults is 60 mg (two 30-mg capsules) every 4 h for 21 consecutive days. If the patient is not conscious enough to swallow the nimodipine capsule, a hole can be made in both ends using an 18-gauge needle, and the contents get extracted into a syringe. Then, it can be fed through a nasogastric tube and washed down with 30 ml of normal saline (0.9%). Nimodipine can be given intravenously via a central venous catheter at a starting dose of 1 mg/h (15 mcg/kg per hour, equivalent to 5 ml per hour) for the first 2 h. If the patient tolerates the drug well and has no hypotension, the dose can increase to 2 mg per hour (30 mcg/kg per hour, equivalent to 10 ml per hour) after the first 2 h. The outcome, dosage, and duration of intraventricular administration of nimodipine were assessed in the NEWTON trial [10]. Results of the trial indicated that there was no significant increase in a favorable outcome for intraventricular nimodipine compared with the standard of care.

21.3.4 Diuretics

Not all diuretics are used as antihypertensives. Its predominantly the thiazide (bendroflumethazide and, hydrochlorothiazide) and thiazide like drugs (chlorthalidone and indapamide) that are commonly prescribed as antihypertensives. Thiazides act on the distal convoluted tubule and inhibit sodium, chloride, and water reabsorption resulting in diuresis. Thiazide effects depend on their delivery into the distal tubule, so efficacy is reduced in renal failure. The mechanism of reduction in BP is due to decreased preload due to enhanced water and sodium excretion, and they also cause decreased responsiveness of vascular smooth muscles to vasoactive substances due to their action on calcium-activated potassium channels. This leads to a decrease in SVR and a consequent decrease in BP.

The side effects of thiazides are related to volume loss leading to dehydration and acute kidney injury. Hypokalaemia, hypercalcemia, hyponatremia, and alkalosis are some other side effects seen with thiazides.

The other diuretic group which is used as antihypertensives is the aldosterone antagonists like spironolactone. One needs to be aware of hyperkalemia as a side effect of spironolactone. Loop diuretics are indicated as antihypertensives if there is volume overloaded situation as in chronic kidney disease.

21.3.5 Vasodilators

The mechanism of vasorelaxation in a vascular smooth muscle involves the activation of a kinase that dephosphorylates the light chain of myosin (Fig. 21.4). The dephosphorylation is mediated

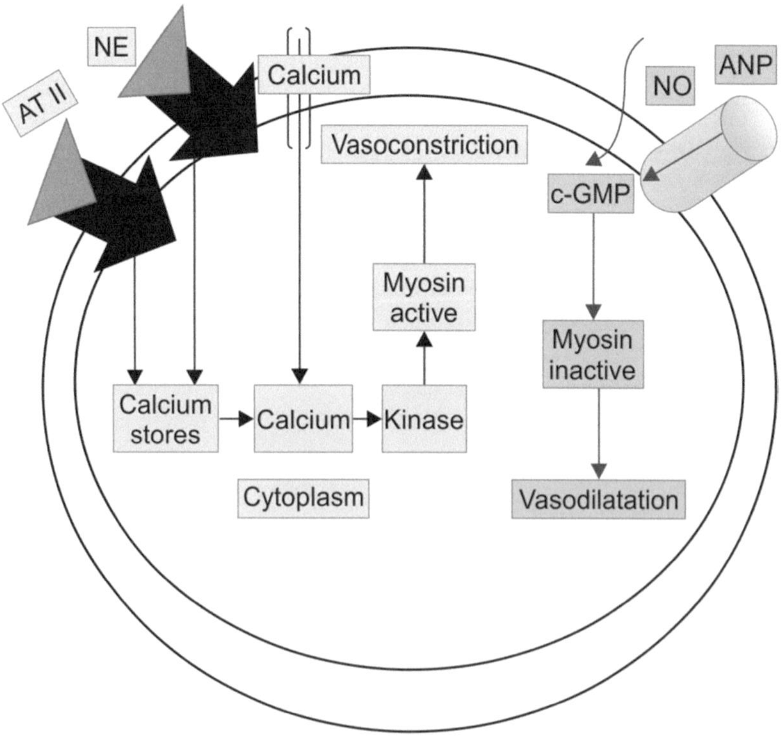

Fig. 21.4 Mechanism of Vasodilatation in vascular smooth muscle: vasodilatation occurs due to the action of nitric oxide (NO) and atrial natriuretic peptide (ANP) releasing cylic-guanosine monophosphate (c-GMP) which activates myosin phosphatase, which dephosphrylates myosin leading to vasodilatation. *AT-II* Angiotensin II, *NE* norepinephrine

by atrial natriuretic peptide and nitric oxide (NO) which through the cyclic guanosine monophosphate (cGMP) pathway activates myosin phosphatase, which is responsible for the dephosphorylation and vasodilatation. Traditionally, vasodilators have been used in the ICU setting for the management of hypertensive emergencies.

Nitroprusside relaxes vascular smooth muscle by producing nitric oxide (NO) and results in significant arteriolar and venous dilatation, resulting in a decreased afterload and preload. However, due to its toxicity related to cyanide formation, its use should be limited in duration and dose. However, the bigger challenge in using nitroprusside in the neurointensive care unit is the side effect of elevated intracranial pressure and decreased cerebral blood flow making it not a favored drug to use for BP control.

Hydralazine: Directly acting vasodilators like hydralazine are not used very commonly as antihypertensives due to their side effect profiles. However, hydralazine is a potent vasodilator and finds its place in treating hypertensive urgency and emergencies. Hydralazine activates adenylate cyclase resulting in increased C-GMP levels.

Hydralazine promotes reflex tachycardia and RAS activation. Other side effects noted with vasodilators include fluid retention, edema, and headaches. Hydralazine can cause the lupus-like syndrome. Hydralazine-induced lupus-like syndrome (HILS) has occurred in up to 10% of patients on doses ≥200 mg for ≥3 months and is reversible upon discontinuation. HILS commonly results in nonadherence or discontinuation and may lead to multi-organ involvement (pericarditis and hepatosplenomegaly), severe malaise/myalgias, acute joint pain and swelling; blood dyscrasias (leukopenia and thrombocytopenia), and positive serologies (antinuclear antibodies, anti-histone antibodies, elevated erythrocyte sedimentation rate). The exact mechanism is unknown and may occur via IL-10 suppression at higher doses of hydralazine.

21.3.6 Centrally Acting Agents

These include clonidine and methyldopa. Clonidine is an alpha 2 adrenoceptor agonist, while methyldopa is a precursor of an alpha 2 adrenoceptor agonist. Their use in the management of hypertension is now limited due to the availability of newer drugs. Dry mouth and sedation are side effects common to both these molecules. Methyldopa has immune side effects and clonidine causes rebound hypertension on sudden stoppage.

21.4 Conclusions

Physicians taking care of neurologically ill patients must be well versed with the therapeutic and side effect profiles of the various drugs available for the treatment of hypertension. This review focused on the pharmacology of the various drugs available to the neurointensivist. Despite the wide armamentarium available, the two main classes of drugs that are commonly used in neurointensive care are BBs and CCBs. The high sympathetic tone and increased SVR make these drugs the go-to drug for the control of BP. Labetalol and nicardipine intravenously are now the drug of choice for most hypertensive emergencies. Since hypertension is a common comorbidity, the continuation of oral medications and their knowledge and side effect profile is also essential.

References

1. Indian Council of Medical Research, Public Health Foundation of India, University of Washington, Institute for Health Metrics and Evaluation. India: Health of the Nation's States: The India State-Level Disease Burden Initiative: Disease Burden Trends in the States of India, 1990 to 2016; 2017
2. International Institute for Population Sciences, National Family Health Survey (NFHS-5), 2019–21. International Institute for Population Sciences (IIPS) and ICF; 2021

3. Deshmukh A, Kumar G, Kumar N, et al. Effect of joint national committee-VII report on hospitalizations for hypertensive emergencies in the United States. Am J Cardiol. 2011;108:1277–82.
4. Katz JN, Gore JM, Amin A, et al. Practice patterns, outcomes, and end organ dysfunction for patients with acute severe hypertension: the studying the treatment of acute hypertension (STAT) registry. Am Heart J. 2009;158:599–606.
5. Standard treatment guidelines of hypertension; MoHFW. https://nhm.gov.in/images/pdf/guidelines/nrhm-guidelines/stg/Hypertension_full.pdf.
6. Salgado DR, Silva E, Vincent JL. Control of hypertension in the critically ill: a pathophysiological approach. Ann Intensive Care. 2013;3(1):17.
7. Peck TE, Hill SA, Williams M. Antihypertensives. In: Pharmacology for anaesthesia and intensive care. 3rd ed. Cambridge: Cambridge University Press; 2008. p. 259–69.
8. Jackson RE, Bellamy MC. Antihypertensive drugs. BJA Educ. 2015;15(6):280–5.
9. Diringer MN, Bleck TP, Claude Hemphill J, Menon D, et al. Neurocritical Care Society. Critical care management of patients following aneurysmal subarachnoid hemorrhage: recommendations from the Neurocritical Care Society's Multidisciplinary Consensus Conference. Neurocrit Care. 2011;15(2):211–40.
10. Macdonald RL, Hänggi D, Ko NU, Darsaut TE, Carlson AP, Wong GK, Etminan N, Mayer SA, Aldrich EF, Diringer MN, Ng D, Strange P, Bleck T, Grubb R, Suarez JI. NEWTON-2 Cisternal (nimodipine microparticles to enhance recovery while reducing toxicity after subarachnoid hemorrhage): a phase 2, multicenter, randomized, open-label safety study of intracisternal EG-1962 in aneurysmal subarachnoid hemorrhage. Neurosurgery. 2020;88(1):E13–26.

22 Hypoglycaemic Drugs

Uma Hariharan, Shagun Bhatia Shah, and Kanwalpreet Sodhi

22.1 Introduction

Hyperglycaemia [1] is a common occurrence in hospitalized patients, and its control is vital for better patient outcome. Raised blood sugar levels can be the result of not only preexisting diabetes mellitus (DM) but also due to steroid therapy, intravenous (IV) fluids, concurrent infections, and stress-induced hyperglycaemia.

Diabetes mellitus [2] is the most common metabolic disorder, and India has the dubious distinction of being the diabetic capital of the world. It affects every system of the body, and the patient has to modify his diet, sleep, and exercise patterns to control the hyperglycaemia and its resultant complications. Besides lifestyle modifications, a cafeteria choice of hypoglycaemic agents is available broadly divisible into two categories: injectable (insulin) and oral hypoglycaemics. The most efficient means of autoantibody and metabolic surveillance are HbA1C (glycosylated hemoglobin) and serum fructosamine levels [3]. These may be combined with polygenic risk screening. Clinicians should aim to achieve an HbA1c level [4] between 7% and 8% in most patients with type 2 diabetes [as per ACP Guidelines]. Use of continuous glucose monitoring (CGM) can help reduce HbA1c and mean glucose levels. Patients admitted in the neurocritical care units comprise a unique subset, with different optimal glycemic targets compared to other critically ill patients. Hyperglycaemia has been associated with worsened outcomes in traumatic brain injury, subarachnoid hemorrhage, spontaneous intracerebral hemorrhage, ischemic stroke, and anoxic brain injury. The underlying mechanisms [5] include free-radical-induced oxidative injury, N-methyl-D-aspartate receptor activation, elevated intracellular calcium, inflammatory and apoptotic pathway activation, and derangement of lactate metabolism-producing acidosis at the tissue level. Hence, vitiation of glycemic control worsens neurological recovery. On the flip side, intensive insulin therapy with target glucose of 80–110 mg/dL (4.4–6.1 mmol/L) significantly increases the risk of iatrogenic hypoglycaemia and enhances mortality among neurocritical care patients. Intermediate glycemic targets (110–180 mg/dL; 6.1–10.0 mmol/L)) are the key to glycemic control in neurocritical care patients. Attempting to maintain lower levels may produce profound neuroglycopenia and secondary brain injury. Enteral/parenteral nutrition must accompany insulin infusions in order to avoid iatrogenic hypoglycaemia.

U. Hariharan (✉)
Department of Department of Critical Care Medicine, Atal Bihari Vajpayee Institute of Medical Sciences and Dr Ram Manohar Lohia Hospital, New Delhi, India

S. B. Shah
Department of Anaesthesia and Critical Care, Rajiv Gandhi Cancer Institute and Research Center, Rohini, New Delhi, India

K. Sodhi
Critical Care Medicine, Deep Hospital, Ludhiana, Punjab, India

H. Prabhakar et al. (eds.), *Principles and Practice of Neurocritical Care*,
https://doi.org/10.1007/978-981-99-8059-8_22

The importance of optimal glycemic control in neurocritical care cannot be overemphasised.

22.2 Classification of Hypoglycaemic Drugs

Hypoglycaemic agents are the drugs used to reduce blood sugar levels in patients with hyperglycaemia and diabetes mellitus. They are used to bring down the levels of fasting and/or postprandial glucose along with reduction of long-term and short-term complications of DM. They are mainly classified [6] on the basis of their utility in either type 1 or type 2 DM, as well as on the basis of their route of administration into oral or parenteral (Fig. 22.1). Some hypoglycaemic agents can be used in both type 1 and type 2 DM, like insulin (subcutaneous/intravenous). Critically ill patients, those with complications and those posted for major surgery or transplant, usually require stricter control of blood sugar levels and are generally controlled with insulin [7]. Neurologic outcomes depend on glycemic control, and insulin forms the mainstay of therapy.

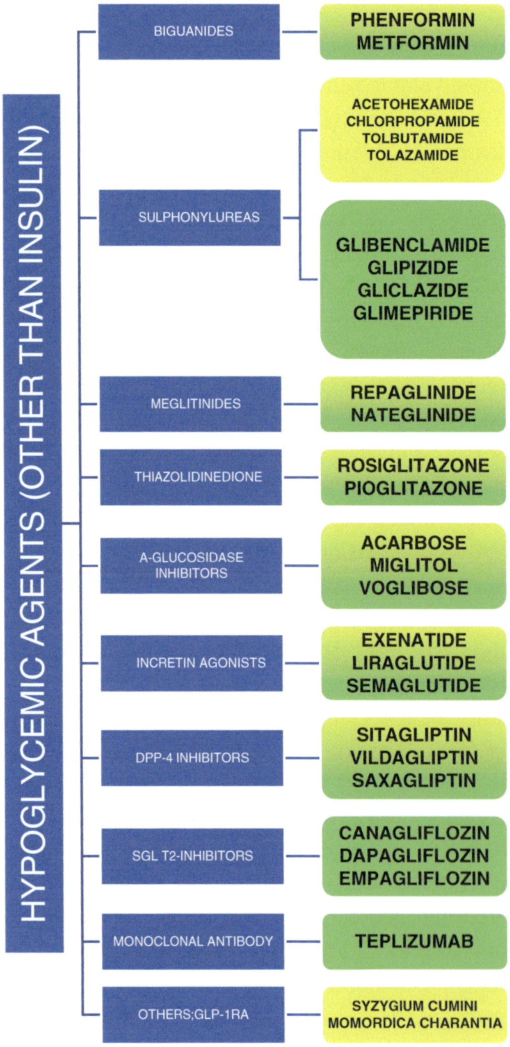

Fig. 22.1 Hypoglycaemic agents (other than insulin)*SGLT2 Inhibitors* sodium glucose cotransporter 2 inhibitors, *GLP-1RA* glucagon-like peptide-1 receptor agonists, *DPP4 inhibitors* dipeptidyl peptidase 4 inhibitors

22.3 Insulin

22.3.1 Chemistry

Human insulin is a peptide hormone [8] secreted by the β-islets of Langerhans in pancreas. It is a small protein (molecular weight of 5808) containing 51 amino acids arranged in two chains (A and B) linked by disulfide bridges, with species differences in the amino acids of both chains. The chief function is to lower blood glucose and promote anabolism. It is also an essential growth factor required for normal metabolism.

22.3.2 Mechanism of Action

Insulin receptors are membrane glycoproteins composed of two alpha-subunits (insulin-binding sites) and two beta-subunits (insulin-stimulated tyrosine-specific protein kinase) which are the signal transduction domains. Insulin action is initiated by binding to these hetero-tetrameric receptors on the cell membrane of the target cells and results in conformational change of the alpha-subunits. This enables adenosine triphosphate (ATP) binding to the beta-subunit's intracellular domain, leading to activation of a tyrosine kinase in the beta-subunit that autophosphorylates the receptor [9]. The phosphorylated receptor further phosphorylates other protein substrates like insulin receptor substrate (IRS) 1 and 2, and thus the insulin signal is propagated through a phosphorylation network involving other intracellular substances. Activation of the signaling pathways is responsible for insulin acting as a powerful regulator of metabolic function, including insulin's action on

Table 22.1 Insulin preparations

Insulin preparations	Onsetof action	Peak action	Effective duration
Insulins lispro	5–15 min	1–1.5 h	3–4 h
Insulin aspart	5–15 min	1–1.5 h	3–4 h
Insulin glulisine	5–15 min	1–1.5 h	3–4 h
Human regular insulin	0.5–1 h	2-3 h	6–8 h
Insulin glargine	0.5–1 h	Flat	@24 h
Insulin degludec	0.5–1.5 h	Flat	>42 h
Insulin detemir	0.5–1 h	Flat	17 h
Human NPH	2–4 h	6–7 h	10–20 h
Novamix 70/30 – 70% NPH, 30% regular	0.5–1 h	Dual peak	10–16 h
Humalog Mix 25%: (75/25) 75% protamine lispro	15 min	Dual peak	10–16 h
Humalog Mix 50% (50/50) 50% protamine lispro	15 min	Dual peak	10–16 h
Novalog Mix 70/30: 70% protamine aspart	15 min	Dual peak	15–18 h

glucose, lipid, and protein metabolism. Defects in insulin signaling have been related to insulin resistance syndromes. The growth-promoting effects of insulin appear to occur through activation of insulin-like growth factors receptors [10].

22.3.3 Types of Insulin

According to the duration of action [11], insulins have been divided into (Table 22.1):

[https://diabetes.org/healthy-living/medication-treatments/insulin-other-injectables/insulin-basics]

Rapid-Acting Insulins

Rapid-acting insulins start their action in 5–15 min and peak in 30 min. The duration of action is 3–5 h. They are generally used before meals and always used along with short-acting or long-acting insulins to control sugar levels throughout the day. All are clear solutions at neutral pH. The short-acting preparations include

*Insulin lispro (Admelog, Humalog, Lyumjev)
*Insulin aspart (Fiasp, NovoLog)
*Insulin glulisine (Apidra)

Short-Acting Insulin

For short acting (regular insulin), the action starts in 30–40 min and peaks in 90–120 min. The duration of action is 6–8 h. Patients take these agents before meals, and it is mandatory to have food within 30 min after its administration so as to avoid hypoglycaemia.

*Regular insulin (Humulin R, Novolin R, Velosulin R)
*Regular insulin inhaled

It is the insulin of choice in ICU settings and during perioperative glucose management, when immediate control of sugars is needed since it can be used as intravenous infusion also. It is particularly useful in the treatment of diabetic ketoacidosis.

Intermediate-Acting Insulins

The action starts in 1–4 h and peak in 4–8 h. It is usually given as twice a day dosing and helps control glucose for 10–12 h.

*NPH insulin (neutral protamine hagedorn) (Humulin N, Novolin N, ReliOn): protamine is a type of protein that slows the action of this insulin.

Long-Acting Insulins

For long-acting insulins, action starts within 1–2 h, and they provide a plateau effect over 12–24 h. Their longer duration of action helps in once-a-day dosing throughout the day. Dosing is usually during nighttime after meals. With no pronounced peak, it works more like physiological pancreatic insulin.

*Insulin glargine (Basaglar, Lantus)
*Insulin detemir (Levemir)
*Insulin degludec (Tresiba)

Ultra-Long Acting Insulin

Reaches the blood stream in 6 h, does not peak, and the effects lasts about 36 h or longer.

*Insulin glargine U-300 (Toujeo)

22.3.4 Insulin Strengths

Current insulin preparations [12] are generated by recombinant DNA technology and all come dissolved or suspended in liquids. Insulins are available in a concentration of U-40, which has 40 units of insulin per milliliter of fluid, U-100, which has 100 units of insulin per milliliter of fluid, and U-500 insulin is available for patients who are extremely insulin-resistant. The most commonly used standard strength is 100 units/mL (U100) and dispensed as 10 mL vials or 0.3 mL cartridges or prefilled disposable pens. Several insulins are also available in the prefilled disposable pen form at higher concentrations: insulin glargine 300 units/mL (U300); insulin degludec 200 units/mL (U200); insulin lispro 200 units/mL (U200); and regular insulin 500 units/mL (U500).

Premixed or combination insulins are fixed components formulations containing a mixture of rapid- or short-acting insulin combined with an intermediate-acting insulin. This eliminates the need to draw insulin from more than one bottle. The commonly available combinations are: Novamix 70/30 with 70% NPH and 30% regular insulin; Novamix 50/50 with 50% NPH and 50% regular insulin; Humalog Mix 50 with 50% Insulin Lispro and 50% Insulin Lispro protamine suspension; Humalog Mix 25 with 25% Insulin Lispro and 75% Insulin Lispro protamine suspension; and Novalog Mix 70/30 with 70% Insulin Aspart protamine and 30% Insulin Aspart. Mixing of NPH and short-acting insulin formulations is a common practice, and this mixing may alter the insulin absorption profile as protamine preparations of its absorption and thereby prolonging the duration of action.

22.3.5 Insulin Administration

Insulin can be administered via subcutaneous, intravenous, and intramuscular routes. The route [13] of administration usually depends on the patient's clinical condition, levels of blood sugars, and the urgency of lowering the blood glucose. For routine domiciliary sugar controls, basal insulin requirements are provided by long-acting insulin formulations which are usually prescribed with short-acting insulin in an attempt to mimic physiologic insulin release with meals. A major shortcoming of current insulin regimens is that injected insulin immediately enters the systemic circulation, while endogenous insulin physiologically is secreted into the portal venous system. Thus, with exogenous insulin administration, liver is exposed to sub-physiologic insulin levels. In addition, no current insulin regimen reproduces the precise insulin secretory pattern of the pancreatic islet. Hence, the most appropriate physiologic regimen entails greater reliance on short-acting insulin with infusions or more frequent insulin injections and stringent glucose monitoring. But critically ill ICU patients need to be on short-acting insulins due to high glycemic variability. Guidelines for managing sugars in critically ill patients in the hospital setting have been issued by the American Diabetes Association with recommended blood sugar targets of 140–180mg/dL for ICU patients [14].

Successful protocols [15] for intravenous insulin administration have established benefits, including ease of implementation, adaptability to varying hospital units, and minimal hypoglycaemia risk. Algorithms designed and standardized to the needs of a multidisciplinary team, including physicians, nurses, pharmacists, nutritionist and cardiologists, and implemented by nursing staff, are becoming a standard of care as they ensure consistency of care with cost-effectiveness. Strategies [16] to address the therapy-associated hypoglycaemia episodes should be set up in advance as a standard component of infusion protocols, to be implemented by a trained multidisciplinary team. Intravenous (IV) route is the usually preferred route in the hospital setting, especially for critically ill patients when immediate and close monitoring of blood glucose levels is needed. IV insulin [17] is used for routine glucose control in ICU patients and in acute emergencies requiring immediate treatment such as diabetic ketoacidosis, hyperosmolar hyperglycaemic state, severe hyperkalemia, beta-blocker toxicity, and calcium channel blocker toxicity. Subcutaneously, insulin can be used in the form of insulin syringes, pens, and pumps. The subcutaneous route [18] is the most widespread route of administration for domiciliary blood glucose management or for clinically stable hospitalized patients on oral diet. It is preferred by most patients for self-administration due to its ease and convenience in administration. Intramuscular insulin use is rarely used in ICU settings. It utilizes concentrated regular insulin.

22.3.6 Insulin Delivery Devices

A variety of devices [19], beyond the routinely used syringes, are available for insulin delivery.

(a) Insulin pens : just like large writing pens. They deliver accurate units of insulin and can help prevent under- and overdosing. They are conveniently prefilled, do not require refrigeration, and are more durable than syringes.
(b) Insulin pumps: The insulin pump is another device available for subcutaneous implantation that works like a natural pancreas. Pumps are computerised or motorized, with glucose monitors available in few models. They deliver insulin before each meal and continuously small amounts of short-acting insulin in the body throughout the day, replacing the need for long-acting insulin.
(c) Jet injection devices: A jet injector holds several doses of insulin. After placing it against the skin, on pressing a button, the insulin is pushed through.
(d) Inhaled insulin: Technosphere insulin-inhalation system (Afrezza) is available as a premeasured inhaler and was first approved by FDA in 2014. It passes through the lungs and into the bloodstream, providing a rapid onset of action within 12 min, peaks by 30 min, and is out of the system in 180 min. As per the pharmacokinetic profile, inhaled insulin has a potential for acute glucose control in ICU patients, but there is paucity of literature. It can be taken by patients with diabetes type 1 and type 2 before meals. Inhaled insulin can cause bronchospasm and cough and should be used cautiously in patients with lung disease or chronic smoker.

22.3.7 Monitoring During Insulin Therapy

Insulin has a low therapeutic index, and regular monitoring of blood glucose levels is required to avoid adverse effects like hypoglycemia, which are a common occurrence in critically ill patients. Monitoring for glucose levels [20] should usually be performed hourly if patient is on IV insulin infusion, so as to adjust the insulin infusion rate accordingly. Otherwise, permeable blood sugar monitoring should be a mandate for ICU patients requiring insulin.

There are no absolute contraindications to insulin therapy, but the dose of insulin needs to be adjusted and effects monitored in following settings:

1. Insulin dosing requires adjustment in patients with renal impairment and liver failure since it is metabolized in the liver and excreted in the urine.
2. Careful monitoring in patients with a history of hypoglycaemic episodes.
3. Insulin should not be given along with drugs causing hypokalaemia, like diuretics; vomiting and diarrhea can cause a hypokalemic state, caution to be exercised while administering insulin.
4. Insulin is contraindicated in patients with cresol sensitivity as insulin preparations contain cresol.

22.3.8 Adverse Effects of Insulin

Adverse effects of insulin may be caused by the drug itself or due to the specific route of administration. Hypoglycaemia [21] is the most common adverse effect of insulin therapy. Some of the symptoms of hypoglycemia include headache, dizziness, palpitations, sweating, abdominal pain, and blurred vision.

The other common adverse effects of insulin therapy [22] include electrolyte disturbances like hypokalemia and allergic reactions in 2% of people. Most allergic reactions are not due to the insulin per se but due to preservatives added to insulin such as zinc, protamine, and meta-cresol, and mostly these are type I hypersensitivity reactions, rarely causing anaphylaxis. The subcutaneous route of administration can lead to pain or lipodystrophy at the injection site [23].

Somogyi effect or Dawn phenomenon [24] is not usually seen in hospitalized patients but are effects of long-acting insulin. Somogyi effect occurs due to insulin causing a hypoglycaemic condition in the body, which activates the antihyperglycemic hormones such as cortisol and adrenaline, resulting in rebound hyperglycemia. This could be the reason, some patients who take insulin at nighttime wake up with high blood sugar levels. This can be corrected by reducing the bedtime insulin dose or changing the timing of insulin dosing. Dawn phenomenon is the presence of high blood glucose levels in the body in the early hours of the day due to inadequate insulin in the body. To correct this phenomenon, the dosing of bedtime insulin needs to be increased so as to keep the blood glucose levels under control throughout the night and early morning hours.

22.3.9 Literature Support for Insulin Use in ICU Patients

Over the years, insulin therapy has been the standard of care for glucose management in ICU patients. Several landmark studies have shown that insulin therapy for adequate glucose control improves acute and long-term outcomes in critically ill adults.

(a) Leuven study by van den Berghe [25] on 1548 surgical ICU patients randomized to intensive insulin therapy (to achieve blood glucose levels of 80–110 mg/dL) or conventional therapy (insulin at blood glucose levels >215 mg/dL to reach 180–200 mg/dL) showed a 42% reduction in ICU mortality at 12 months and overall in-hospital mortality decrease by 34% with intensive insulin therapy ($P < 0.01$). Intensive therapy also reduced morbidity with decrease in episodes of septicemia, red blood cell transfusions, acute renal failure, and critical illness neuropathy.

(b) A later Leuven study [26] of 1200 adult medical ICU patients showed a significantly reduced morbidity ($P = 0.04$) but more frequent hypoglycemia episodes in the intensive treatment group (3.1% versus 18.7% for conventional versus intensive insulin therapy; $P < 0.001$).

(c) A large meta-analysis [27] of 26 trials involving over 13,567 patients, which included the NICE-SUGAR trial, showed that intensive insulin therapy in the ICU setting had no effect on overall risk of 90-day mortality but a sixfold increased risk of severe hypoglycemia, regardless of the type of ICU or the intensity of insulin therapy.

(d) Till date, there is no clear evidence of a clinical benefit of insulin therapy during acute stroke management [28]. In the largest Glucose Insulin in Stroke Trial on 933 patients, stroke patients admitted with hyperglycaemia and randomized to receive 24 h of continuous glucose, potassium and insulin showed no difference in all-cause mortality and functional outcomes as compared to those receiving placebo. Literature has shown strong predictive relationships between glucose variability and mortality in ICU patients.

(e) In a study by Al-Dorzi et al, daytime glucose fluctuation was similar among patients randomized to either intensive or conventional insulin therapy. Regardless of insulin therapy group, patients with wide glycemic fluctuation exhibited a higher mortality (22.2% vs. 8.4%; $P < 0.001$) as compared to those with narrow fluctuation, even after adjusting for patient age, diabetic status, and daily insulin dose [29].

(f) Literature has shown strong predictive relationships between glucose variability [30] and mortality in ICU patients.

22.4 Hypoglycaemic Agents for Type 2 DM

22.4.1 Introduction

Hyperglycemia can be multifactorial in hospitalized patients. Diabetes mellitus (DM) is a complex disease requiring multi-pronged approach for adequate glycemic control, both in the short and long term. Type 2 DM is usually controlled by oral glucose-lowering drugs or oral hypoglycaemic agents (OHA) [31]. They act by affecting one or more of the pathways involved in the pathophysiology of type 2 DM. These agents are ineffective in type 1 DM and are not recommended in critically ill patients of type 2 DM. Hyperglycaemic level and individual patient's glycemic goal should determine the initial choice of therapy. Glycemic management of type 2 DM must follow a combination of lifestyle control, medical nutrition therapy, enhancing physical activity, and oral hypoglycaemic medications. Timely glycemic control reduces glucose toxicity to islet cells and improves outcome. First-line treatment includes integrated lifestyle modifications and the biguanide agent, Metformin. Since type 2 DM is a progressive disorder, ultimately multiple therapeutic agents may be required, including sometimes, insulin.

22.4.2 Mechanism of Action

Hypoglycaemic drugs can be broadly subdivided based on their mechanism of action [32] as follows:

(a) Increase in insulin secretion
(b) Reduce glucose production
(c) Increase insulin sensitivity
(d) Enhance GLP-1 action
(e) Promote urinary excretion of glucose.

The *"octagon pathway"* has been the pathophysiological mechanism [33] underlying development of hyperglycaemia in type 2 DM. These eight mechanisms (either alone or in combination), which have been the targets for action of the hypoglycaemic agents, include the following:

(a) Pancreatic beta cell reduction in insulin secretion
(b) Enhanced secretion of glucagon from pancreatic alpha cells
(c) Elevated liver production of glucose
(d) Brain insulin resistance and dysfunction at neurotransmitter level
(e) Increased lipid breakdown
(f) Enhanced re-absorption of glucose from kidneys
(g) Decreased effect of incretin on small intestine, and
(h) Reduced glucose uptake in peripheral tissues such as skeletal muscle, liver, and adipose tissues.

A patient-centric approach should be used for achieving euglycemia, with due consideration given to factors like drug efficacy, cost, possible side effects, weight gain/loss, presence of comorbid conditions, risk of hypoglycaemia, level of glycemic control, and preferences of the patient. Initiation of drug therapy in type 2 DM should be done when glycemic control is not achieved or if HbA1C rises to 6.5% after 2–3 months of lifestyle interventions. Rise of HbA1C to 7.5% during therapy or the initial HbA1C level >=9% warrants combinations therapy with two or more agents and sometimes insulin. Medical nutrition therapy and exercise must go hand-in-hand with drug treatment for better control of hyperglycaemia and its complications.

The level of hyperglycaemia as per fasting plasma glucose (FPG) levels [34] will determine the therapy/drugs to be used:

(a) Mild hyperglycemia (FPG < 7–11 mmol/L or 126–199 mg/dL): single OHA.
(b) Moderate hyperglycemia (FPG 11.1–13.9 mmol/L or 200–250 mg/dL): more than one OHA or drug combinations.
(c) Severe hyperglycemia (FPG > 13.9 mmol/L or 250 mg/dL): multiple OHA+ insulin.

22.4.3 Types

The following are the major classes [35] of oral hypoglycemic medications used:

(a) Biguanides
(b) Sulphonylureas
(c) Meglitinides
(d) Thiazolidinediones (TZD)
(e) Dipeptidyl peptidase 4 (DPP-4) inhibitors
(f) Sodium-glucose co-transporter (SGLT2) inhibitors
(g) Alpha-glucosidase inhibitors
(h) Miscellaneous agents with glucose-lowering effect: Oral Bromocryptine (Dopamine receptor agonist 0.8 mg tablet) and Colesevelam (bile-acid sequestrant 625 mg tablet).

The following principles may assist therapy of type 2 DM with pharmacological agents [36]:

(a) Biguanides, insulin secretagogues, GLP-1 receptor agonists, and TZDs enhance glycemic control to similar extent (reduction in HbA1C of 1–2%); they are more effective than alpha-glucosidase inhibitors, DPP-4 inhibitors, and SGLT2 inhibitors.
(b) DPP-4 inhibitors, insulin secretagogues, GLP-1 receptor agonists, and alpha-glucosidase inhibitors start to reduce the plasma glucose immediately, in contrast to the delayed (by weeks) glucose-lowering effects of biguanides and TZDs.
(c) All agents may not be effective in every patient of type 2 DM.
(d) Alpha-glucosidase inhibitors, GLP-1 receptor agonists, biguanides, DPP-4 inhibitors, TZDs, and SGLT2 inhibitors do not directly cause hypoglycemia.
(e) In view of progressive nature of type 2 DM, most patients will require more than one class of OHAs or insulin.
(f) Glycemic control is less durable for sulphonylureas compared to metformin or TZDs.
(g) Metformin is recommended by most DM societies as the initial therapy due to its efficacy, known side effect profile, low cost, and promotion of weight loss (Table 22.2).

Table 22.2 Hypoglycaemic agents and their characteristics

S. No.	Class	Drug/agent	Mechanism of action	Hba1c Reduction	Dosage	Adverse effects
1.	Biguanides	Metformin	– Reduce hepatic glucose production – Raised insulin sensitivity – Activate AMP-dependent protein kinases and enter cells through organic cation transporters	1–2%	^Start with oral low dose of 500 mg and increase slowly every 1–2 weeks to maximum dose 2 g	*Gastrointestinal disturbances (nausea, vomiting, metallic taste, diarrhea) *Vitamin B_{12} deficiency *Lactic acidosis (very rare)
2.	Insulin secretagogues	Sulphonylureas *1st generation: Chlorpropamide, Tolazamide, Tolbutamide *2nd generation: Glimipride, Glipizide, Glyburide	– Enhance insulin secretion by stimulating ATP-sensitive K+ channels on beta cells	1–2%	^Start at low dose (taken shortly before meals) as they reduce both fasting and postprandial glucose. ^Glimipride 1–8 mg/day ^Glyburide 1.25 – 20 mg, every 12–24 h	*Hypoglycemia *Weight gain
3.	Insulin Secretagouges	Meglitinides: *Repaglinide, Nateglinide, Mitiglinide	– Increase insulin secretion by interacting with ATP-sensitive Potassium channels in beta cells	1–2%	^Due to short half-life, to be taken orally just before (15 min) meals: 60–120 mg TDS (Nateglinide); 0.5–2 mg (Repaglinide)	*Weight gain *Hypoglycemia in combination with other OHAs
4.	Insulin secretagouges	Incretins [GLP-1 receptor agonist or GLP-1 analogs] *Short-acting: Exenatide, Liraglutide, Lixisenatide (given daily): reduce postprandial glucose *Long-acting: sustained-release Exenatide, Dulaglutide, Lixisenatide, Semaglutide (all given weekly): reduce both fasting and postprandial glucose	– Amplify glucose-stimulated insulin secretion by acting on GLP-1 receptor agonist or enhance endogenous GLP-1 activity – Suppress glucagon – Reduced gastric emptying	0.5–1%	Mostly injectable (subcutaneous) once (0.75–4.5 mg Dulaglutide) or twice weekly; Oral Semaglutide (3–7 mg OD)	*Nausea, vomiting *Diarrhea *Dizziness *Infections *Headache *Pancreatitis *Injection site pruritis, erythema.

(continued)

Table 22.2 (continued)

S. No.	Class	Drug/agent	Mechanism of action	Hba1c Reduction	Dosage	Adverse effects
5.	Dipeptidyl peptidase IV-inhibitors [DPP-4 is a ubiquitous enzyme acting on incretin hormones: GLP1 (glucagon-like peptide 1) and GIP (gastric inhibitory peptide), which maintain glucose homeostasis by increasing insulin secretion and decreasing glucagon secretion. DPP-4 deactivates glucose-dependent insulinotropic polypeptide (GIP) and GLP-1]	Gliptins: FDA-approved agents include Sitagliptin, Saxagliptin, Linagliptin, and Alogliptin	– Act through incretin hormones responsible for glucose homeostasis after oral food intake – Anti-hypertensive, anti-inflammatory, anti-apoptotic, and immunomodulatory effects on heart, kidneys and blood vessels independent of incretin pathway – Decreases hepatic glucose production – Effective in NODAT (new-onset diabetes after transplantation)	0.5–1%	^2nd line agents in type 2 DM ^Monotherapy in patients intolerant or having contraindications to Metformin ^2.5–5 mg once a day oral (Saxagliptin); 25–50 mg OD (Sitagliptin)	*Heart failure *Nasopharyngitis *Hypersensitivity reactions *Pre-cancerous changes in Pancreas
6.	Sodium glucose co-transporter (SGLT) -2 inhibitors	Gliflozins: Canagliflozin, Empagliflozin, Dapagliflozin, Ertugliflozin	– Enhance renal glucose excretion – Act on SGLT-2 proteins expressed in renal proximal convoluted tubules to reduce reabsorption of filtered glucose, decrease renal threshold for glucose – Inhibit SGLT-2-dependent glucose and sodium reabsorption with increase in distal tubular sodium load, inhibiting renin-angiotensin-aldosterone and sympathetic activity	0.5–1%	^100–300mg once daily (Canagliflozin); ^5–10 mg oral once daily (Dapagliflozin) ^10–25 mg Once daily (Empagliflozin) ^5-15 mg once daily (Ertugliflozin)	*Urogenital infections, Dehydration, Hyperkalemia, Respiratory infections, polyuria
7.	Alpha-glucosidase inhibitors	Acarbose, Miglitol, Voglibose	– Reduce carbohydrate breakdown in gut and produce modest postprandial glucose lowering	0.5–0.8%	^Acarbose: 25–100 mg, thrice a day with meals; ^Miglitol: 25–100 mg, thrice a day with meals	*Gastrointestinal intolerance *Flatulence *Raised liver enzymes

22.5 Parenteral Hypoglycaemic Agents

The agents which can be used parenterally [37] for type 2 DM include the following:

(a) GLP-1 (glucagon-like peptide 1) receptor agonists
(b) Amylin agonists
(c) Insulin

The following is a brief description of the parenteral hypoglycaemic agents (apart from insulin):

(a) GLP-1 receptor agonist: It is one of the promising newer agents for the treatment of type 2 DM. These agents act by increasing insulin secretion, delaying gastric emptying, and reducing glucagon secretion. They are used subcutaneously on a daily or weekly basis. They include dulaglutide, exenatide, liraglutide, lixisenatide, and semaglutide (oral formulation also available in a dose of 7–14 mg daily). Dulaglutide is administered as weekly injections of 0.75–4.5 mg. Exenatide, Liraglutide, and Lixisenatide are given as once daily injections. These incretin analogs are advantageous in improving cardiovascular outcomes and aiding weight loss (by early satiety). The major adverse effects include nausea, pancreatitis, and risk of hypoglycemia, especially with insulin. Dose reduction or avoidance is recommended in patients with renal disease, medullary thyroid carcinoma, and with agents reducing gastrointestinal motility. These agents bring about modest reductions in HbA1C to the tune of 0.5–1%.
(b) Amylin agonists: These agents act by slowing the gastric emptying and decreasing glucagon secretion. It causes postprandial reduction in plasma glucose and weight loss. It can be used in both type 1 and type 2 DM. Pramlintide is an amylin analog available as 0.6 mg/mL solution and 15–30 μg pen injector. It is given in the dose of 15–30 μg subcutaneously in type 1 DM and 60–120 μg in type 2 DM, both immediately prior to major meals. It causes 0.25–0.5% reduction in HbA1C. Its major side effects include injection site reactions, nausea/vomiting, loss of appetite, headache, and risk of hypoglycaemia with insulin.

22.6 Advantages and Disadvantages of Hypoglycemics

There are varied advantages and disadvantages [31] of the above-described hypoglycaemic agents, which can be summarized as in Table 22.3 and which needs to be taken into account while formulating the agents to be used in any particular patient.

Table 22.3 Advantages and disadvantages of various oral hypoglycaemic agents

Agent	Advantages	Disadvantages
Biguanides	*Reduce cardiovascular risks (myocardial infarction and coronary deaths); mild weight loss (anorectic effect); cheap and easily available	#Gastrointestinal intolerance needs low-dose introduction and gradual dose escalation; cautious use in patients with renal disease; rare risk of megaloblastic anemia and lactic acidosis
Sulphonylureas	*Inexpensive; most effective in recent-onset type 2 DM with residual endogenous insulin release	#Increased risk of hypoglycaemia especially those with renal disease; weight gain; increased risk of cardiovascular disease #First-generation sulphonylureas are no longer used as they have longer half-lives, greater incidence of hypoglycaemia and more drug interactions
Meglitinides	*Decreases postprandial hyperglycemia; flexible dosing; short duration of action; relatively inexpensive	#Hypoglycaemia; weight gain; need for dose titration and frequent dosing; bBecome ineffective over time due to progressive beta cell loss

(continued)

Table 22.2 (continued)

Agent	Advantages	Disadvantages
Incretin analogs/GLP 1 receptor agonists	*Weight loss; less risk of hypoglycaemia; reduced cardiovascular events	#Cautious use in patients with renal disease, gastric motility-slowing agents, those with medullary thyroid cancer or pancreatic disease
Dipeptidyl peptidase 4 inhibitors	*Modest glucose-lowering effect; low risk of hypoglycaemia; decreases post-prandial lipemia	#Dose reduction required in renal failure; risk of heart failure (degradation of brain natriuretic peptide), pancreatitis, upper respiratory tract infections
SGLT-2 inhibitors	*No hypoglycaemia risk; weight reduction; reduction of blood pressure and cardiovascular risk; reno-protective	#Cautious use in those with renal disease; exacerbates hyperkalemia; predisposes to urogenital infections/genital mycosis, bone fractures and diabetic ketoacidosis
Alpha-glucosidase inhibitors	*Modest postprandial glucose-lowering effects in type 2 DM; adjuvant agents	#Gastrointestinal effects preclude dose escalations; avoid simultaneous treatment with bile acid resins and antacids; should not be given to patients with inflammatory bowel disease, gastroparesis or raised serum creatinine
Thiazolidinediones (TZD)	*Redistribution of fat from central to peripheral locations; raised HDL levels	#Weight gain; ovulation induction leading to pregnancy; fluid retention edema; hepatotoxicity with troglitazone; cardiovascular risk with rosiglitazone; bladder cancer with ioglitazone

22.7 Clinical Implications in Neurocritical Care

Euglycemia is the key toward optimizing patient outcome in neurocritical care. Frequent glucose monitoring, adequate treatment of hyperglycaemia, prevention of hypoglycaemia, management of diabetic complications, and correction of electrolyte abnormalities form the cornerstones of improving patient care and outcomes. Optimal glycemic control is vital to prevent development of secondary brain injury [38]. Risk–benefit ratio must be evaluated for choosing the ideal hypoglycaemic agent in any patient. Assessment of blood sugar levels, ABGs, urine examination, and HbA1C can help in better hyperglycaemia management.

22.8 Future Prospects

Continuous glucose monitoring (CGM) is of immense clinical value in patients on multiple daily insulin injections and continuous subcutaneous/intravenous insulin infusion. CGM is used to suspend insulin infusion when hypoglycaemia is detected until glucose returns to a safe level (low-glucose suspend). Predictive low-glucose suspend provides greater benefits. Closed-loop control with insulin alone or using both insulin and glucagon provides further improvement in quality of glycemic control. A hybrid closed-loop system has recently been approved by the US FDA. Night-scout for remote sharing and monitoring of glucose levels obtained using real-time CGM [39] is a recent advancement which is the forerunner of the open-access artificial pancreas system (OpenAPS).

The quest for an artificial pancreas has moved through several stages [40]:

*Threshold low-glucose suspend of insulin infusion

*Predictive low-glucose suspend of insulin infusion

*The hyperglycaemia/hypoglycaemia minimizer (control to range)

*Hybrid closed-loop systems with user adjustment of pre-meal boluses

*Full closed-loop systems (insulin only)

*Dual-hormone closed-loop systems utilizing insulin and glucagon

A multitude of novel hypoglycaemic agents is a promising addition to our armamentarium. Canagliflozin, dapagliflozin, empagliflozin, and ertugliflozin are FDA-approved sodium-glucose transport protein 2 (SGLT2) inhibitors for managing adult type 2 diabetes mellitus. They act on the SGLT-2 proteins expressed in the renal proximal convoluted tubules to reduce glucose reabsorption, decrease the renal threshold for glucose, and promote urinary glucose excretion. Reduced risk of cardiovascular adverse events in cardiac patients along with reduced end-stage renal disease, CV mortality, hospitalization for heart failure, and increases in serum creatinine in type 2 DM patients with diabetic nephropathy and albuminuria are additional benefits. Prevention is better than treatment. Teplizumab is a monoclonal antibody [41] that modifies T cells in a way that prolongs the pancreas ability to create insulin. The drug is specific to a molecule called CD3, which is the "cognate" component of the T cell. Hence, the onset of IDDM may be pushed away by 5 years. This wonder drug has been approved by FDA in November 2022 and marks the first disease-modifying therapy since the discovery of insulin, a century ago in 1922. Another newer agent, amelexanox [42], an anti-inflammatory agent used in aphthous stomatitis, is under trial for the management of DM. With scientific innovations reaching their zenith, the future of hyperglycaemia management looks promising.

22.9 Conclusions

Relationship between serum glucose concentration and neurological outcomes behaves like a U-shaped curve. Optimal glucose control [43] by judicious use of available hypoglycaemic agents is essential in neurocritical care patients with emphasis on avoiding both hyperglycaemia and hypoglycaemia. Avoidance of bolus insulin with preference for continuous insulin infusion (low doses to begin with, followed by gradual upward titration as per individual requirement) accompanied by meticulous glycemic monitoring is the cornerstone of glycemic control in these patients.

References

1. Godinjak A, Iglica A, Burekovic A, Jusufovic S, Ajanovic A, Tancica I, Kukuljac A. Hyperglycemia in critically ill patients: management and prognosis. Med Arch. 2015;69(3):157–60.
2. Silva-Perez LJ, Benitez-Lopez MA, Varon J, Surani S. Management of critically ill patients with diabetes. World J Diabetes. 2017;8(3):89–96. https://doi.org/10.4239/wjd.v8.i3.89.
3. Nansseu JR, Fokom-Domgue J, Noubiap JJ, Balti EV, Sobngwi E, Kengne AP. Fructosamine measurement for diabetes mellitus diagnosis and monitoring: a systematic review and meta-analysis protocol. BMJ Open. 2015;5(5):e007689. https://doi.org/10.1136/bmjopen-2015-007689.
4. Sherwani SI, Khan HA, Ekhzaimy A, Masood A, Sakharkar MK. Significance of HbA1c test in diagnosis and prognosis of diabetic patients. Biomark Insights. 2016;11:95–104. https://doi.org/10.4137/BMI.S38440.
5. Godoy DA, Di Napoli M, Rabinstein AA. Treating hyperglycemia in neurocritical patients: benefits and perils. Neurocrit Care. 2010;13(3):425–38. https://doi.org/10.1007/s12028-010-9404-8.
6. Chaudhury A, Duvoor C, Reddy Dendi VS, Kraleti S, Chada A, Ravilla R, Marco A, Shekhawat NS, Montales MT, Kuriakose K, Sasapu A, Beebe A, Patil N, Musham CK, Lohani GP, Mirza W. Clinical review of antidiabetic drugs: implications for type 2 diabetes mellitus management. Front Endocrinol (Lausanne). 2017;8:6. https://doi.org/10.3389/fendo.2017.00006.
7. Pasquel FJ, Lansang MC, Dhatariya K, Umpierrez GE. Management of diabetes and hyperglycaemia in the hospital. Lancet Diabetes Endocrinol. 2021;9(3):174–88. https://doi.org/10.1016/S2213-8587(20)30381-8.
8. Weiss M, Steiner DF, Philipson LH. Insulin biosynthesis, secretion, structure, and structure-activity relationships. [Updated 2014 Feb 1]. In: Feingold KR, Anawalt B, Blackman MR, et al., editors. Endotext. South Dartmouth (MA): MDText.com, Inc. p. 2000. Available from: https://www.ncbi.nlm.nih.gov/books/NBK279029/.
9. Kahn CR. The molecular mechanism of insulin action. Annu Rev Med. 1985;36:429–51. https://doi.org/10.1146/annurev.me.36.020185.002241.
10. Posner BI. Insulin signalling: the inside story. Canadian J Diabet. 2017;41(1):108–13.
11. Donner T, Sarkar S. Insulin—pharmacology, therapeutic regimens, and principles of intensive insulin therapy [Updated 2019 Feb 23]. In: Feingold KR, Anawalt B, Blackman MR, et al., editors. Endotext. South Dartmouth (MA): MDText.com, Inc. p. 2000. Available from: https://www.ncbi.nlm.nih.gov/books/NBK278938/.

12. Dashora U, Castro E. Insulin U 100, 200, 300 or 500. Br J Diabetes. 2016;16:10–5. https://doi.org/10.15277/bjd.2016.056.
13. Shah RB, Patel M, Maahs DM, Shah VN. Insulin delivery methods: past, present and future. Int J Pharm Investig. 2016;6(1):1–9. https://doi.org/10.4103/2230-973X.176456.
14. American Diabetes Association Standards of Medical Care in Diabetes—2010. Diabetes Care. 2010;33(Suppl. 1):S11–61.
15. Magee MF. Insulin therapy for intensive glycemic control in hospital patients. Hosp Physician. 2006;38:17–28.
16. Goldberg PA, Siegel MD, Sherwin RS, et al. Implementation of a safe and effective insulin infusion protocol in a medical intensive care unit. Diabetes Care. 2004;27(2):461–7.
17. Pérez A, Ramos A, Carreras G. Insulin therapy in hospitalized patients. Am J Ther. 2020;
18. Bode BW, Braithwaite SS, Steed RD, Davidson PC. Intravenous insulin infusion therapy: indications, methods, and transition to subcutaneous insulin therapy. Endocr Pract. 2004;10(Suppl. 2):71–80.
19. Pisano M. Overview of insulin and non-insulin delivery devices in the treatment of diabetes. P T. 2014;39(12):866–76.
20. Perkins BA, Sherr JL, Mathieu C. Type 1 diabetes glycemic management: insulin therapy, glucose monitoring, and automation. Science. 2021;373(6554):522–7. https://doi.org/10.1126/science.abg4502.
21. Unger J, Parkin C. Hypoglycemia in insulin-treated diabetes: a case for increased vigilance. Postgrad Med. 2011;
22. American Society of Health-System Pharmacists. "Insulin Human". www.drugs.com. [Archived from the original on 22 October 2016. Retrieved 1 January 2017.]
23. Radermecker RP, Piérard GE, Scheen AJ. Lipodystrophy reactions to insulin: effects of continuous insulin infusion and new insulin analogs. Am J Clin Dermatol. 2007;
24. Rybicka M, Krysiak R, Okopień B. The dawn phenomenon and the Somogyi effect—two phenomena of morning hyperglycaemia. Endokrynol Pol. 2011;
25. van den Berghe G, Wouters P, Weekers F, et al. Intensive insulin therapy in critically ill patients. N Engl J Med. 2001;345(19):1359–67.
26. van den Berghe G, Wilmer A, Hermans G, et al. Intensive insulin therapy in the medical ICU. N Engl J Med. 2006;354(5):449–61.
27. Griesdale DE, de Souza RJ, van Dam RM, et al. Intensive insulin therapy and mortality among critically ill patients: a meta-analysis including NICE-SUGAR study data. CMAJ. 2009;180(8):821–7.
28. Gray CS, Hildreth AJ, Sandercock PA, et al. Glucose-potassium-insulin infusions in the management of post-stroke hyperglycaemia: the UK Glucose Insulin in Stroke Trial (GIST-UK). Lancet Neurol. 2007;6(5):397–406.
29. Al-Dorzi HM, Tamim HM, Arabi YM. Glycaemic fluctuation predicts mortality in critically ill patients. Anaesth Intensive Care. 2010;38(4):695–702.
30. Krinsley JS. Glycemic variability: a strong independent predictor of mortality in critically ill patients. Crit Care Med. 2008;36(11):3008–13.
31. Lorenzati B, Zucco C, Miglietta S, Lamberti F, Bruno G. Oral hypoglycemic drugs: pathophysiological basis of their mechanism of action. Pharmaceuticals. 2010;3(9):3005–20. https://doi.org/10.3390/ph3093005.
32. Krentz AJ, Bailey CJ. Oral antidiabetic agents: current role in type 2 diabetes mellitus. Drugs. 2005;65(3):385–411. https://doi.org/10.2165/00003495-200565030-00005.
33. Masharani U, Kroon L. Pancreatic hormones & glucose-lowering drugs. In: Katzung BG, Vanderah TW, editors. Basic & clinical pharmacology. 15th ed. McGraw Hill; 2021. Accessed 21 Feb 2023 https://accessmedicine.mhmedical.com/content.aspx?bookid=2988&sectionid=251128944.
34. Tayek CJ, Cherukuri L, Hamal S, Tayek JA. Importance of fasting blood glucose goals in the management of type 2 diabetes mellitus: a review of the literature and a critical appraisal. J Diabetes Metab Disord Control. 2018;5(4):113–7. https://doi.org/10.15406/jdmdc.2018.05.00148.
35. Powers AC, D'Alessio D. Endocrine pancreas and pharmacotherapy of diabetes mellitus and hypoglycemia. In: Brunton LL, Knollmann BC, editors. Goodman & Gilman's: the pharmacological basis of therapeutics. 14th ed. McGraw Hill; 2023. Accessed 21 Feb 2023. https://hemonc.mhmedical.com/content.aspx?bookid=3191&sectionid=274233574.
36. Ni X, Zhang L, Feng X, Tang L. New hypoglycemic drugs: combination drugs and targets discovery. Front Pharmacol. 2022;13:877797. https://doi.org/10.3389/fphar.2022.877797.
37. Kang H. Current therapeutic agents and anesthetic considerations for diabetes mellitus. Korean Anaesthesiol. 2012;63:195–202. https://doi.org/10.4097/kjae.2012.63.3.195.
38. Fenger A-SW, Olsen MH, Fabritius ML, Riberholt CG, Møller K. Glycaemic control for patients with severe acute brain injury: protocol for a systematic review. Acta Anaesthesiol Scand. 2023;67(2):240–7. https://doi.org/10.1111/aas.14166.
39. Rodbard D. Continuous glucose monitoring: a review of recent studies demonstrating improved glycemic outcomes. Diabetes Technol Ther. 2017;19(S3):S-25.
40. Trevitt S, Simpson S, Wood A. Artificial pancreas device systems for the closed-loop control of Type 1 diabetes: what systems are in development? J Diabetes Sci Technol. 2015:1–10. https://doi.org/10.1177/1932296815617968.

41. Herold KC, Gitelman S, Greenbaum C, Puck J, Hagopian W, Gottlieb P, Sayre P, Bianchine P, Wong E, Seyfert-Margolis V, Bourcier K. Monoclonal antibody. Treatment of patients with new onset Type 1 diabetes with a single course of anti-CD3 mAb Teplizumab preserves insulin production for up to 5 years. Clin Immunol. 2009;132(2):166–73.
42. Dosanjh A, Won CY. Amlexanox: a novel therapeutic for atopic, metabolic, and inflammatory disease. Yale J Biol Med. 2020;93(5):759–63.
43. Bilotta F, Rosa G. Optimal glycemic control in neurocritical care patients. Crit Care. 2012;16(5):1–3.

Vasopressor Drugs

23

Vinay Singhal, Puneet Chopra, and Vikas Sikri

23.1 Introduction

Vasopressors are the agents that increase the vascular tone on administration. On the other hand, inotropes increase the myocardial contractility. Although vasopressors and inotropes have different physiological functions, but in clinical practice these terms are used interchangeably. Many of these pharmacological agents have mixed vasopressor and inotropic effects. These agents are used in critically sick patients with major hemodynamic impairments to a level where there is an imbalance between tissue metabolic needs and tissue blood flow [1]. This imbalance may occur due to poor cardiac output (e.g., cardiogenic shock and hypovolemic shock) or increase tissue demand (e.g., septic shock). These vasopressors and inotropes apart from increasing the cardiac output or tissue blood flow have a diverse range of metabolic effects, which is very important in selecting the agent, its dose, route of administration, and titration.

The objective of this chapter is to understand the basic pharmacokinetics and pharmacodynamics of these vasopressor and inotropes and how best we can use them in neurocritical care practice. A sick patient in neurocritical care may need hemodynamic support either due to septic and cardiogenic shock or may be due to hemodynamic imbalance related to neurological injuries. The term "vasopressor" will be generally used to describe the drugs in this chapter with their spectrum of actions.

23.2 Function of Adrenergic and Dopaminergic Receptors

Endogenous catecholamines (adrenaline, noradrenaline, and dopamine) act as neurotransmitters within the central and the sympathetic division of the autonomic nervous system and hormones in circulating blood. Structural differences in catecholamines result in some differences in adrenergic and dopaminergic receptor affinity and their rates of metabolism. A substitution on the amino group of the catecholamine tail reduces α-receptor affinity but increases β-receptor affinity [2, 3] . Furthermore, affinity for the $\beta_2$receptor is increased by the size of the substituent. The position of hydroxyl groups on the aromatic nucleus also alters adrenoceptor affinity as does hydroxyl substitution on the catecholamine tail. This hydroxyl substitution on the catecholamine tail is the key in determining β_2 affinity.

V. Singhal (✉)
Department of Critical Care & Emergency services, SPS Hospitals, Ludhiana, Punjab, India

P. Chopra
SPS Hospitals, Ludhiana, Punjab, India

V. Sikri
Mohandai Oswal Hospital, Ludhiana, Punjab, India

H. Prabhakar et al. (eds.), *Principles and Practice of Neurocritical Care*,
https://doi.org/10.1007/978-981-99-8059-8_23

Although catecholamine structure can determine the degree of adrenoceptor activation, agonists at specific adrenoceptor subtypes may still generate differing concentrations of second messengers such as cAMP, because of nonselective G-protein coupling [4]. Drug–receptor interactions are also influenced by polymorphisms of adrenoceptor genes [4].

Adrenergic receptors are classified into α-adrenoceptors and β-adrenoceptors and further into respective subtypes (α1,2 & β 1,2,3) [5]. They spread widely throughout the body (Table 23.1), but for their vasopressor and cardiovascular effects, only cardiovascular distribution is discussed here. Adrenoceptor location within the cardiovascular system determines the response to circulating, neuronally released, or administered adrenergic agents [6, 7]. Adrenergic receptors are minimal in the capillaries, but their expression increases if we move away to both the arterioles and venules. Response to the catecholamines also varies across the vascular beds. There is variable response to the vasopressors in splanchnic and skeletal muscle beds (Table 23.2). There is no α2 receptor in the myocardium, although other adrenoceptors are present. β receptors predominantly provide inotropy, while α1 receptors increases the contractility.

There are five subtypes of dopaminergic receptors 5 classed in two groups: D_1 (subtypes DR_1 and DR_5) and D_2 (subtypes DR_2, DR_3 and DR_4). Although dopamine may activate both dopaminergic and adrenoceptors, the other catecholamines do not activate dopaminergic receptors [8]. Dopaminergic receptors in the kidney mediate natriuresis and diuresis [9]. DR1 & DR4 dopaminergic receptors (DR_1 and DR_4) are associated with heart have some inotropic effect. This inotropic effect is less pronounced than β adrenoceptor response [10]. D1 and D2 receptors are found in the blood vessels, and the overall effect of nonselective dopaminergic activation, such as what occurs during low-dose dopamine infusion, is to reduce vascular tone.

Table 23.1 Commonly used vasopressors/inotropes with dose ranges and receptors

Agent	Dose range	Receptor	Effect on hemodynamics	Clinical effects	Adverse effects
Noradrenaline	0.05–1 mcg/kg/min	α1+++, β1++	MAP↑↑, HR ↔ or↓, CO↑	Contractility + Vasoconstriction++	Arrhythmias, ↑Pulmonary vascular resistance, peripheral ischemia
Adrenaline	0.1–1 mcg/kg/min	α1+++, β1+++, β2++	MAP↑↑, HR↑↑, CO↑↑	Contractility + Vasoconstriction++	Ventricular arrhythmias, severe hypertension, cardiac ischemia
Dopamine	Up to 5 mcg/kg/min 5–15 mcg/kg/min >15 mcg/kg/min	D1, D2 D1, D2, β D1, D2, β+, α1+++	CO↑, HR↑ CO↑, HR↑↑ MAP↑, HR↑,CO↓	Vascular resistance ↓ Contractility + Vasoconstriction++	Arrhythmias, increase metabolic rate
Vasopressin	0.01–0.04 units·min^{-1}	V1, oxytocin	MAP↑↑, HR ↔ or ↓,	Vasoconstriction+++	↑Pulmonary vascular resistance, Peripheral ischemia
Dobutamine	2–20 mcg/kg/min	β1++	MAP ↔ or ↓, HR↑↑, CO ↑↑	Contractility ++ Vasoconstriction+	Tachycardia, increased ventricular response rate in AF, ventricular arrhythmias, cardiac ischemia, hypertension, hypotension

Table 23.2 Adrenoceptor distribution

Area	Receptors
Coronary circulation	α_1 and α_2 in large arteries only β present in small and large arteries. $\beta_1 >> \beta_2$
Cerebral circulation	Poor sympathetic innervations α-adrenoceptor expression declines in smaller vessels β-adrenoceptors may mediate vasodilatation
Splanchnic	$\beta2 >> \beta1$
Skeletal and pulmonary	α effects predominate over β in splanchnic circulation
Cutaneous circulation	α_2-adrenoceptors

23.2.1 Norepinephrine (Noradrenaline)

Norepinephrine is a potent α_1 adrenergic agonist with less pronounced effect on β receptor resulting in vasoconstriction, some positive ionotropic action, increased mean blood pressure, and minimal effect on heart rate [11]. Although in higher doses, norepinephrine can result in worsening tachycardia due to β_1 receptor stimulation [12]. As depressed vascular tone is one of the important mechanisms of hypotension in septic shock, norepinephrine should be started early along with fluid resuscitation to restore organ perfusion. Surviving sepsis guidelines recommend using norepinephrine as the first-line agent in septic shock over other vasopressors [13, 14]. The typical dose of norepinephrine infusion is 0.05–1 mcg/kg/min. The use of vasopressors including norepinephrine induces intense vasoconstriction which results in many of the adverse effects, including myocardial ischemia, decreased renal, peripheral, and splanchnic blood flow [11, 12]. A multicenter-randomized trial comparing dopamine versus norepinephrine as initial vasopressor in the management of shock found no difference in mortality between two vasopressors, although norepinephrine was less arrhythmogenic and resulted in lower mortality in subgroup of patients with cardiogenic shock [15].

23.2.2 Epinephrine (Adrenaline)

Epinephrine leads to dose-dependent activation of β_1, β_2, and α_1 adrenergic receptor. Stimulation of β_1 receptor by epinephrine leads to increase in stroke volume and heart rate, while α_1 receptor stimulation causes peripheral vasoconstriction. Epinephrine increases mean arterial pressure by increasing both systemic peripheral resistance and cardiac output [11, 12]. Epinephrine is the drug of choice for anaphylactic shock and during resuscitation of cardiac arrest. The initial recommended dosage for anaphylaxis is 0.5 mg IM (0.5 ml of 1 mg/ml epinephrine) [16]. In septic shock, epinephrine is used as second- or third-line vasopressor and might be useful in refractory septic shock with myocardial dysfunction [14]. The typical dose of epinephrine infusion is 0.1–1 mcg/kg/min. The potential adverse include arrhythmias, impaired splanchnic circulation, and myocardial ischemia. The stimulation of skeletal muscles β_2 adrenergic receptors by epinephrine results in increased aerobic lactate production, which may make it challenging to use serum lactate as a resuscitation marker [11, 12, 17]. A randomized double-blinded trial comparing epinephrine and norepinephrine found no difference in time to achieve target MAP, vasopressor free days, and mortality between two drugs; however, epinephrine use was associated with significant, but transient tachycardia and metabolic side effects [18].

23.2.3 Dobutamine

Dobutamine is a synthetic catecholamine that predominantly stimulates β_1 and β_2 adrenergic receptors resulting in improved myocardial contractility (inotropic action), moderate increase in heart rate with reflex lowering of vascular tone, and peripheral resistance [11, 12]. Dobutamine is commonly used in cardiogenic shock for its positive inotropic action; however, its use may be associated with various side effects including increased risk of myocardial ischemia, tachyarrhythmias and ventricular dysfunction. A meta-analysis assessing the effect of dobutamine for patients with severe heart failure found no mortality benefit [19]. In septic shock patients, use of dobutamine may produce blunted inotropic action and severe vasodilation resulting in lowered mean arterial pressure. There is weak recommendation to consider dobutamine in addition to noradrenaline infusion for septic shock patients who develop cardiac dysfunction with persistent hypoperfusion despite adequate volume status and arterial blood pressure [14].

23.2.4 Vasopressin

Vasopressin is a naturally occurring peptide produced in pituitary gland. Vasopressin has direct action on G protein-coupled vascular (V1) receptors, leading to increase in intracellular calcium and causing vasoconstriction of smooth muscles. The other actions include inhibition of interleukin 1 and decrease vascular endothelial production of nitric oxide, thus inhibiting nitric oxide-mediated vasodilation and further improving shock. Vasopressin being non-adrenergic vasoconstrictor not only restores blood volume and pressure by direct vasoconstrictor effect but also restores serum osmolarity [20, 21]. It does not have any inotropic or chronotropic effect.

The half-life of vasopressin is longer than norepinephrine. Dosing can be titrated in the range of 0.01 U/min to 0.06 U/min. After norepinephrine, vasopressin is an agent of choice for patients requiring second agent in patients with septic shock as highlighted by various international guidelines. It should be started early in refractory shock not responding to norepinephrine. Studies have shown that delayed initiation of vasopressin is associated with significant increase in ICU mortality [22].

The VASST trial [23] (Vasopressin versus Norepinephrine Infusion in Patients with Septic Shock) compared the adjunctive use of vasopressin and nor-epinephrine with norepinephrine alone in patients requiring vasopressors in septic shock. This trial did not demonstrate a mortality benefit from adding vasopressin if mean arterial pressure is adequately maintained with standard vasopressors.

23.3 Exogenous Vasopressors and Inotropes

23.3.1 Dopexamine

Dopexamine is a synthetic structural analog of dopamine and has a greater potency at β_2-adrenoceptors but less active at dopaminergic receptors. Dopexamine's cardiovascular actions include chronotropy, inotropy, and vasodilatation particularly in mesenteric, skeletal, and renal beds [24]. These effects are believed to be due to a combination of direct β_2-adrenoceptor stimulation (vasodilatation and tachycardia), dopaminergic stimulation (decreasing renal and mesenteric vascular resistance), and an increased release of noradrenaline from sympathetic nerve terminals.

23.4 Sympathomimetics

23.4.1 Ephedrine

Ephedrine is a mixed sympathomimetic. It acts indirectly by displacing noradrenaline from vesicles at nerve terminals to cause α-adrenoceptor effects. It exhibits tachyphylaxis with prolonged use due to depletion of noradrenaline. Ephedrine also exhibits mild direct β-adrenoceptor activity [25] with increase in cardiac output of up to 20% due to increase in heart rate and stroke volume. Its use is associated with increase in myocardial oxygen consumption, bronchodilation, respiratory stimulation, mydriasis, and tocolysis

23.4.2 Phenylephrine

Phenylephrine is a selective α_1 adrenoceptor agonist predominantly causing proximal arterial vasoconstriction with terminal arteriolar sparing. It can cause reflex bradycardia with a decrease in cardiac output. It causes pulmonary vasoconstriction and decrease in renal and mesenteric blood flow, which may give cause for concern when used to increase arterial pressure in critically ill patients.

23.4.3 Angiotensin II

Angiotensin II, a naturally occurring hormone of renin-angiotensin system, binds to angiotensin-1 and -2 receptors (AGTR1 and AGTR2) resulting in marked vasoconstriction [26]. A multicenter randomized trial (ATHOS 3 trial) evaluated the role of angiotensin II in patients with refractory vasodilatory shock requiring high-dose vasopressors. Compared to placebo, a significantly greater number of patients in angiotensin II group achieved predefined mean arterial pressure goal within 3 h and had lower requirement of catecholamines. The rates of serious adverse events including tachyarrhythmias and distal ischemia were similar in two groups [27]. Presently, angiotensin II is not recommended as first-line agent in septic shock due to lack of safety profile and limited clinical experience [14].

23.5 Role of Vasopressors in Neurological Conditions

Vasopressors are frequently used along with fluid resuscitation in the setting of acute neurological injury to maintain or augment perfusion to the areas of insult and to prevent further ischemic injury. Despite the existence of various guidelines on the basic principles of blood pressure management and use of vasopressors in neurocritical scenarios, majority of recommendations are based on class III evidence [28].

23.5.1 Subarachnoid Hemorrhage

Delayed cerebral ischemia (DCI) remains the major cause of morbidity and death in aneurysmal SAH and is usually attributed to cerebral vasospasm; however, the exact mechanism is unclear. Earlier, triple H therapy involving hypervolemia, hemodilution, and induced hypertension was used for the management of symptomatic vasospasm. Currently, the practice has shifted from triple H therapy to euvolemia and induced hypertension [29, 30, 31]. Norepinephrine and dopamine are the commonly used vasopressors for induced hypertension as these agents have demonstrated to increase CBF and cerebral oxygenation which may result in improvement of neurological symptoms. The preferred vasopressor is norepinephrine due to its less arrhythmogenic potential and predictable hemodynamic response. Systemic blood pressure should be elevated in stepwise manner in patients with DCI, guided by regular neurological assessments and neuromonitoring evidence of improved perfusion. The initial target systolic blood pressure (SBP) is usually selected between 160 and 180 mmHg, with most centers using a maximum of 220 mmHg for SBP and 140 mmHg for MAP. Patients should be frequently monitored for potential complications of induced hypertension which include myocardial ischemia and pulmonary edema [28, 30, 32].

23.5.2 Traumatic Brain Injury (TBI)

It is important to maintain adequate cerebral perfusion pressure (CPP) in head injury patients to prevent secondary injury and improve neurological outcome. Brain trauma foundation guidelines recommend maintaining systolic blood pressure at ≥100 mmHg for patients with age group of 50–69 years and ≥ 110 mmHg for patients who are younger or older than this age group [33]. Norepinephrine and phenylephrine have been the most common initial agents used for early hemodynamic management following moderate to severe TBI in a multicenter cohort study with no difference in clinical outcome among two vasopressor groups [34]. A recent retrospective review assessing the use of vasopressors in TBI concluded that patients who required vasopressors had more severe TBI and significantly higher overall injury burden. Despite being widely used to increase mean arterial pressure and maintain CPP in TBI patients, the use of norepinephrine is not associated with improved neurological outcomes or survival benefits [35, 36].

23.5.3 Spinal Cord Injury

Acute traumatic spinal cord injury is frequently associated with neurogenic shock characterized by hypotension and bradycardia. It is important to correct hypotension (systolic blood pressure < 90 mmHg) as soon as possible to maintain spinal cord perfusion and avoid secondary ischemic insult. In addition to intravenous volume replacement, vasopressors are routinely used to maintain mean arterial pressure. There is level III recommendation to maintain mean blood pressure between 85 and 90 mmHg for the first 7 days following acute spinal cord injury, which is likely to improve spinal cord perfusion and neurological outcome. Agents with both α and β adrenergic effects such as noradrenaline or dopamine may be better suited to manage spinal cord injury-associated vasoplegia and bradycardia. In the absence of recommended guidelines regarding the use of vasopressors in spinal cord injury, the choice of agent depends on desired pharmacologic activity and institutional preference [37, 38].

23.5.4 Vasopressors in Acute Ischemic Stroke

Hypotension in acute ischemic atroke (AIS) has been traditionally associated with poor neurological outcome. Lot of studies have been conducted, based on the hypothesis, that increasing blood pressure decreases disability and potentially salvaging the ischemic penumbra. Stromnes et al in their recent systematic review of 27 studies concluded that the hypothesis of increasing blood pressure in AIS patients though looks promising on paper but the data is largely inconclusive. In order to identify optimum BP target, more trials are needed in this field [39].

23.6 Sepsis and the Brain

Sepsis is defined as life-threatening organ dysfunction caused by dysregulated host response to infection [40]. Sepsis-associated encephalopathy (SAE) is known identity and is defined as transient and potentially reversible brain dysfunction in a patient of sepsis not caused by neurological cause. SAE is a more frequent problem than commonly thought. It occurs in more than 70% of the patients with sepsis (Fig. 23.1). SAE may present with altered mental status, apathy, anorexia, delirium, and coma. Various cytokines implicated are interleukin(IL)-1 alpha, IL-1 beta, tumor necrotic factor (TNF)-alpha, and IL-6.

Vasopressors are the primary modality in the treatment of septic shock. However, these agents can have alarming effects on cerebral perfusion, thus, worsening/altering neurological function. Altered mental status itself is a poor risk factor

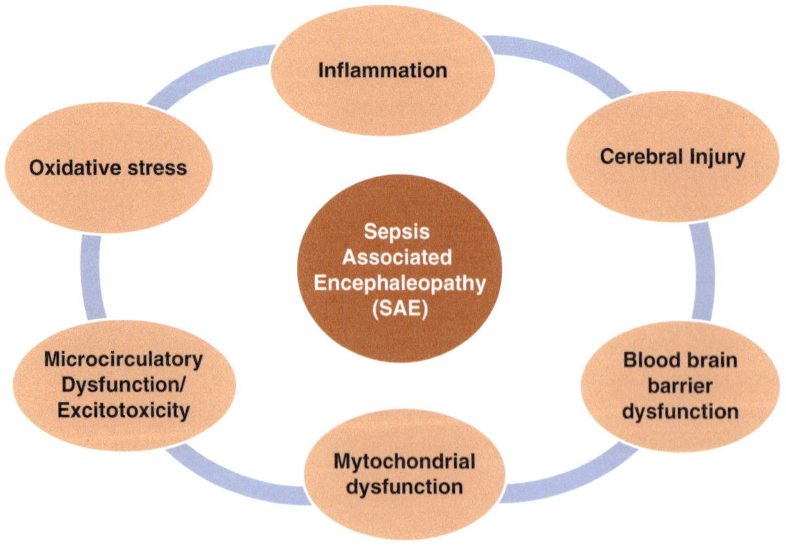

Fig. 23.1 Various mechanisms postulated in the mechanism of SAE

for outcome in patients presenting with infective pathology in emergency [40, 41].

23.7 Conclusion

Despite variability in clinical practice, use of vasopressors and inotropes is extensive in critically sick patients. Their use is to stabilize the patient's hemodynamics, while other resuscitative measures and definitive therapy are being instituted. It is very important to understand the effects and potential toxic effects of various vasopressors and inotropes, to use them in timely manner and with minimal necessary doses. It is also important to continually reevaluate the patient's clinical condition for the relevance of use of selected vasopressor agent.

References

1. Bangash MN, Kong M-L, Pearse RM. Use of inotropes and vasopressor agents in critically ill patients. Br J Pharmacol. 2012;165:2015–33.
2. Henkel JG, Sikand N, Makriyannis A, et al. Synthesis and adrenoceptor affinity of some highly polar beta-substituted catecholamines. J Med Chem. 1981;24:1258–60.
3. Lullman H, Mohr K, Ziegler A, et al. Color Atlas of pharmacology. Stuttgart: Thieme; 2000.
4. Xiao RP, Zhang SJ, Chakir K, et al. Enhanced G(i) signaling selectively negates beta2-adrenergic receptor (AR)–but not beta1-AR-mediated positive inotropic effect in myocytes from failing rat hearts. Circulation. 2003;108:1633–9.
5. Alexander SPH, Mathie A, Peters JA. Guide to Receptors and Channels (GRAC), 5th edition. Br J Pharmacol. 2011;164(Suppl. 1):S1–S324.
6. Brodde OE, Michel MC. Adrenergic and muscarinic receptors in the human heart. Pharmacol Rev. 1999;51:651–90.
7. Guimaraes S, Moura D. Vascular adrenoceptors: an update. Pharmacol Rev. 2001;53:319–56.
8. Missale C, Nash SR, Robinson SW, et al. Dopamine receptors: from structure to function. Physiol Rev. 1998;78:189–225.
9. Lokhandwala MF, Amenta F. Anatomical distribution and function of dopamine receptors in the kidney. FASEB J. 1991;5:3023–30.
10. Wakita Y. Inotropic, chronotropic, and arrhythmogenic effects of dopamine on the isolated working heart of rabbit. J Physiol Sci. 2007;57:147–57.
11. Ammar A, Ammar MA, Tesoro EP. Neuropharmacology in the intensive care unit. Crit Care Clin. 2023;39:171–213.
12. Jentzer JC, Coons JC, Link CB, et al. Pharmacotherapy update on the use of vasopressors and inotropes in the intensive care unit. J Cardiovasc Pharmacol Ther. 2015;20(3):249–60.
13. Hamzaoui O, Scheeren TWL, Teboul JL. Norepinephrine in septic shock: when and how much? Curr Opin Crit Care. 2017;23:342–7.
14. Evans L, Rhodes A, Alhazzani W, et al. Surviving sepsis campaign: international guidelines for management of sepsis and septic shock 2021. Crit Care Med. 2021;49(11):e1063–143.
15. De Backer D, Biston P, Devriendt J, the SOAP II investigators. Comparison of dopamine and norepinephrine in the treatment of shock. N Engl J Med. 2010;362:779–89.
16. Dodd A, Hughes A, Sargant N, et al. Evidence update for the treatment of anaphylaxis. Resuscitation. 2021;163:86–96.
17. Bangash MN, Kong ML, Pearse RM. Use of inotropes and vasopressor agents in critically ill patients. Br J Pharmacol. 2012;165(7):2015–33.
18. Myburgh JA, Higgins A, Jovanovska A, the CAT study investigators. A comparison of epinephrine and norepinephrine in critically ill patients. Intensive Care Med. 2008;34:2226–34.
19. Tacon CL, McCaffrey J, Delaney A. Dobutamine for patients with severe heart failure: a systematic review and meta-analysis of randomized controlled trials. Intensive Care Med. 2012;38:359–67.
20. Hollenberg SM. Vasoactive drugs in circulatory shock. Am J Respir Crit Care Med. 2011;183(7):847–55.
21. Multu GM, Factor P. Role of vasopressin in the management of septic shock. Intensive Care Med. 2004;30(7):1276–91.
22. Sacha GL, Lam SW, Duggal A, et al. Association of catecholamine dose, lactate and shock duration at vasopressin initiation with mortality in patients with septic shock. Crit Care Med. 2021;
23. Russel JA, Walley KR, Singer J, et al. Vasopressin versus norepinephrine infusion in patients with septic shock (VASST Trial). N Engl J Med. 2008;358(9):877–87.
24. Olsen NV, Lund J, Jensen PF, Espersen K, Kanstrup IL, Plum I, Leyssac PP. Dopamine, dobutamine, and dopexamine. A comparison of renal effects in unanesthetized human volunteers. Anesthesiology. 1993 Oct;79(4):685–94.
25. Kobayashi S, Endou M, Sakuraya F, et al. The sympathomimetic actions of l-ephedrine and d-pseudoephedrine: direct receptor activation or norepinephrine release? Anesth Analg. 2003,97:1239–45.
26. Russell JA. Vasopressor therapy in critically ill patients with shock. Intensive Care Med. 2019;45:1503–17.
27. Khanna A, English SW, Wang XS, the ATHOS-3 investigators. Angiotensin II for the treatment of vasodilatory shock. N Engl J Med. 2017;377:419–30.

28. Muzevich KM, Voils SA. Role of vasopressor administration in patients with acute neurologic injury. Neurocrit Care. 2009;11:112–9.
29. Connolly ES Jr, Rabinstein AA, Carhuapoma JR, et al. Guidelines for the management of aneurysmal subarachnoid hemorrhage: a guideline for healthcare professionals from the American Heart Association/American Stroke Association. Stroke. 2012;43(6):1711–37.
30. Smith M, Citerio G. What' s new in subarachnoid hemorrhage. Intensive Care Med. 2015;41:123–6.
31. Muench E, Horn P, Bauhuf C, et al. Effects of hypervolemia and hypertension on regional cerebral blood flow, intracranial pressure, and brain tissue oxygenation after subarachnoid hemorrhage. Crit Care Med. 2007;35:1844–51.
32. Francoeur CL, Mayer SA. Management of delayed cerebral ischemia after subarachnoid hemorrhage. Crit Care. 2016;20:277.
33. Carney N, Totten AM, O'Reilly C, et al. Guidelines for the management of severe traumatic brain injury, 4th edition. Neurosurgery. 2017;80(1):6–15.
34. Toro C, Temkin N, Barber J, TRACK-TBI Investigators. Association of vasopressor choice with clinical and functional outcomes following moderate to severe traumatic brain injury: A TRACK-TBI Study. Neurocrit Care. 2022;36(1):180–91.
35. Dhillon NK, Huang R, Mason R, et al. Vasopressors in traumatic brain injury: quantifying their effect on mortality. Am J Surg. 2020;220(6):1498–502.
36. Lloyd-Donald P, Spencer W, Cheng J, et al. In adult patients with severe traumatic brain injury, does the use of norepinephrine for augmenting cerebral perfusion pressure improve neurological outcome? A systematic review. Injury. 2020;51(10):2129–34.
37. Thomas AX, Riviello JJ Jr, Davila-Williams D, et al. Pharmacologic and acute management of spinal cord injury in adults and children. Curr Treat Options Neurol. 2022;24(7):285–304.
38. Ryken TC, Hurlbert RJ, Hadley MN, et al. The acute cardiopulmonary management of patients with cervical spinal cord injuries. Neurosurgery. 2013;72(Suppl. 2):84–92.
39. Strømsnes TA, Kaugerud Hagen TJ, Ouyang M, et al. Pressor therapy in acute ischaemic stroke: an updated systematic review. Eur Stroke J. 2022 Jun;7(2):99–116.
40. Singer M, Deutschman CS, Seymour CW, et al. The Third International consensus definitions for sepsis and septic shock (Sepsis-3). JAMA. 2016;315(8):801–10.
41. Freund Y, Lemachatti N, Krastinova E, et al. Prognostic accuracy of sepsis-3 criteria for in-hospital mortality among patients with suspected infection presenting to the emergency department. JAMA. 2017;317:301–8.

24 Steroids

Monica S. Tandon, Ankit Sharma,
Rajishth Mittal, and Neha Bhandari

24.1 Introduction

Corticosteroids (CS) have a special place in a neuro-intensivist's armamentarium. Neuroinflammation and cerebral edema play a pivotal role in the development of acute brain injury in several neurological and neurosurgical disorders commonly encountered in a neurointensive care unit (NICU) [1–3] CSs, with their profound anti-inflammatory, immunomodulatory, and neuroprotective effects, confer benefit in these conditions by targeting one or multiple components of the inflammatory or edema-forming processes. These synthetic analogs of natural adrenal hormones are widely used as adjuvants or even as frontline agents across a broad spectrum of neurological disorders, ranging from central nervous system (CNS) infections and brain neoplasms to immune-mediated neurological diseases [1, 3–5]. Their diverse therapeutic potential is also utilized for the management of various non-neurological, critical conditions in the NICU, including critical illness-related corticosteroid insufficiency (CIRCI), airway crises, endocrine failure, anaphylaxis, and organ donor management [6–9]. However, these "multipurpose drugs" are also at times, "double-edged swords," which can cause serious adverse effects, especially when used in high, supraphysiological doses and for a prolonged duration. Hence, a rational and evidence-based approach is crucial for ensuring their optimal utilization in a neurocritical care setting. In the initial sections of this chapter, we describe the fundamental physiological and pharmacological concepts regarding CSs. In subsequent sections, we investigate their efficacy and safety in the management of various critical neurological and non-neurological conditions in an NICU.

M. S. Tandon (✉) · A. Sharma · R. Mittal · N. Bhandari
Department of Anesthesiology and Intensive Care, GB Pant Institute of Postgraduate Medical Education and Research, New Delhi, India

24.2 Fundamental Concepts Regarding CS Therapy in NICU

The main endogenous steroid hormones, cortisol (glucocorticoid) and aldosterone (mineralocorticoid), are synthesized in the adrenal cortex, under directions of the hypothalamic-pituitary-adrenal (HPA) axis; aldosterone's secretion is also regulated by the renin-angiotensin system [2, 6, 7, 9]. Under normal conditions, the hypothalamus secretes corticotrophin-releasing hormone (CRH) and arginine vasopressin, to stimulate the synthesis and release of adrenocorticotrophic hormone (ACTH) from the anterior pituitary. ACTH, in turn, regulates the release of cortisol in a circadian pattern-blood cortisol levels peak in the early morning hours and gradually decline

H. Prabhakar et al. (eds.), *Principles and Practice of Neurocritical Care*,
https://doi.org/10.1007/978-981-99-8059-8_24

during the day. This circulating cortisol itself exerts a subsequent negative feedback effect on the release of CRH and ACTH; this normal HPA axis is essential for normal well-being. Cortisol is present in the circulation in three forms: protein bound—with a high affinity to corticosteroid-binding globulin (CBG; 80–90%) and with a low affinity to albumin (10–15%); "free" or unbound cortisol (5%); and cortisol metabolite (biologically inactive) [9]. It is metabolized primarily in the liver (5 α/β-reductases) and kidneys (11β-hydroxysteroid dehydrogenase- 11β-HSD) [9].

While aldosterone is primarily involved in the regulation of water and electrolyte balance, cortisol's actions include inflammatory and immune response modulation, endocrine function regulation, and widespread homeostatic effects, which pertinently involve the cardiovascular [vasoconstriction, increased myocardial contractility, and blood pressure (BP) due to enhanced responsiveness to catecholamines), metabolic (proteolysis, lipolysis, glycogenolysis, bone, and calcium metabolism) and pulmonary systems (increased sensitivity to bronchodilators) [1, 3, 6, 10–12]. Physiologic CS levels are crucial for normal brain development, neuronal plasticity, and survival [1].

Neuroinflammation is implicated in causing acute brain injury and cerebral edema in several neurological disorders, such as CNS infections, cerebral ischemia, hemorrhage, traumatic brain injury (TBI), spinal cord injury (SCI), and brain neoplasms. It involves a cascade of events, including the recruitment and activation of leukocytes in the CNS, free radical generation, eicosanoid and cytokine release, and nitric oxide synthesis. It is also closely linked with other acute neurodegenerative mechanisms, notably excitotoxicity, oxidative stress, and apoptosis [1]. Cortisol mitigates this CNS damage by virtue of its anti-inflammatory and immunomodulatory effects; however, these effects exhibit a bi-phasic dose–response [10, 11]. Basal cortisol levels upregulate the expression of innate immune components or "danger sensors" and therefore are immuno-stimulatory. In contrast, high concentrations downregulate the expression of these proteins and thereby mitigate inflammation by immunosuppression and decreased proliferation of inflammatory cells. These effects are exerted via genomic as well as non-genomic mechanisms, after binding of the "free" cortisol to the cellular glucocorticoid receptors. In the genomic pathway, the activated glucocorticoid-cytoplasmic glucocorticoid receptor-alpha (GC-GRα) alters gene expression through—direct binding to specific DNA regions (glucocorticoid responsive elements; GREs), tethering [physical interaction with other transcription factors (TFs), without contacting DNA], or composite binding to DNA and protein substrates, in the cell's nucleus [1, 11]. The nongenomic pathway involves the modulation of signaling cascades through interaction with phosphatases and kinases and is important for inhibiting the synthesis of inflammatory cytokines that promote apoptosis [4, 11].

While non-genomic effects are more rapid (within seconds to minutes) than genomic mechanisms (several hours), both pathways, in effect, modulate leukocytes and other cell types during all phases of inflammation and thereby impact both innate and adaptive immunity [1, 4, 6, 8, 10, 11]. During the alarm phase of inflammation, CSs inhibit the release of several proinflammatory mediators from tissue macrophages, mast cells, and stromal cells, including lipid agents, vasoactive amines, and cytokines [interleukins (ILs), interferon-γ, tumor necrosis factor-alpha (TNFα), granulocyte–macrophage colony-stimulating factor, prostaglandin E2 (PGE2) and leukotriene B4 (LTB4)]. This is achieved by dampening signaling pathways downstream of many danger sensors [e.g., cytokine receptors, pattern recognition receptors (PPRs), complement factors, and Fc receptors] and tethering key pro-inflammatory TFs downstream of Toll-like receptors (TLR) signaling [e.g., nuclear factor kappa-light-chain-enhancer of activated B cells (NF-κB), activator protein 1 (AP-1), interferon-regulatory factor 3 (IRF3)] [10, 11]. In the mobilization phase, CSs attenuate leukocyte recruitment to the injured site; and during the resolution phase, they promote the differentiation of alternatively activated 'M2c' macrophages, which clear apoptotic PMNs and secrete anti-inflammatory factors. Since several TLR signaling components are also shared with other signaling pathways, CSs effectively suppress multiple signaling pathways involved in the detection of noxious agents and propagation of inflammatory signals. CSs act on macrophages to inhibit the synthesis of eicosanoids (e.g., prostaglandins, leukotrienes) and thereby suppress vasodilatation, hyper-permeability, and plasma extravasation in inflamed tissues. They also reduce the blood flow to inflammatory sites by inducing the expression of angiotensin-converting enzyme and endothelin, sensitizing endothelial cells to vasoconstrictors, and inhibiting the production of vasodilators (e.g., bradykinin).

In vasogenic edema (VE), hyperpermeability and disruption of the blood brain barrier (BBB) lead to extravasation and accumulation of fluid and albumin in the extracellular brain parenchymal spaces [4, 5]. VE is commonly observed in brain tumors (especially meningiomas, high-grade gliomas, and brain metastases), CNS inflammation (meningitis, abscess), brain trauma, intracranial hemorrhage (ICH), and the secondary phase of cerebral ischemia. In brain neoplasms, angiogenic factors, e.g., vascular endothelial growth factor (VEGF) glutamate and leukotrienes, produced by the host stromal and tumor cells, stimulate the proliferation of leaky tumor blood vessels with absent tight inter-endothelial junctions [5, 13–15]. In acute brain injury, BBB incompetence occurs due to a reversible, excessive release of vascular permeability and inflammatory factors by activated glial cells and an irreversible disruption of inter-endothelial tight junctions by the ischemia-reperfusion injury-induced inflammation and oxidative stress [16]. CSs stabilize the inter-endothelial tight junctions and restore the altered vascular permeability in VE by attenuating the synthesis of inflammatory cytokines through multiple mechanisms, including downregulation of VEGF; upregulation of angiopoietin-1, a BBB-stabilizing factor, occludin and ZO1-tight junction-regulating proteins; nongenomic binding of vascular endothelial-cadherin to capillary endothelium; and cytokine inhibition by binding of NF-kB [4, 5, 16]. They, however, have no role in mitigating cytotoxic edema and may be harmful in patients with brain ischemia [2, 5]. Besides mitigating VE, CSs reduce intracranial pressure (ICP) by decreasing production and enhancing cerebrospinal fluid (CSF) resorption [1]. Their putative neuroprotective mechanisms include inhibition of lipid peroxidation and hydrolysis, reduced intracellular calcium accumulation and neurofilament degradation, maintenance of aerobic metabolism, enhanced synaptic transmission, and augmentation of blood flow in ischemic areas by non-genomic activation of endothelial nitric oxide synthase through the phosphatidylinositol 3-kinase/AKT pathway [1, 17].

Acute stress leads to a marked increase in cortisol synthesis (six to ten times normal, commensurate with stress level) and a loss of its circadian secretory rhythm. These alterations occur due to multidirectional cross-talks between the CRH/ACTH pathways and the autonomic, vasopressinergic, and immune systems, which involve cytokine-induced activation of the noradrenergic—CRH system (additional stimulation of ACTH synthesis), direct adrenal cortical stimulation [binding of neuronal and inflammatory signals, damage-associated molecular patterns (DAMPs), and pathogen-associated molecular patterns (PAMPs) to TLRs in adrenocortical cells]; and adrenal medullary stimulation by paracrine routes [9, 11].

During critical illness (extreme physical stress), the systemic availability of cortisol increases substantially to combat infections, repair tissue damage, prevent shock and organ failure, and ultimately facilitate recovery [10]. This increase is mediated partly through central HPA axis and largely via peripheral driven mechanisms, including increased free cortisol (reduced cortisol-binding affinity, and suppressed cortisol metabolism) and glucocorticoid receptor-driven effects [10]. A state of acute adrenal insufficiency or CIRCI can develop during critical illnesses such as acute respiratory distress syndrome (ARDS), septic shock, and TBI. The circulating cortisol levels are normal or elevated, but the endogenous cortisol effect (intracellular CS -mediated anti-inflammatory activity) becomes insufficient to counterbalance the hyperactive systemic inflammatory response that occurs in response to the noxious stressors of critical illness. Several mechanisms contribute to CIRCI -HPA axis dysregulation, altered cortisol synthesis (damage to neuroendocrine cells, altered CRH/ACTH synthesis), altered cortisol metabolism (reduced plasma cortisol clearance due to suppression of cortisol-metabolizing enzymes in liver and kidney), and tissue resistance to glucocorticoids [inadequate glucocorticoid receptor activity] [9].

24.3 Synthetic CSs

Endogenous cortisol has 21 carbon atoms with a 2-carbon side chain at position 17 and two methyl groups at C-10 and C-13. Minor modifications in its molecular structure create a variety of synthetic glucocorticoid analogs, each with distinct pharmacological properties, including potencies (relative to hydrocortisone), half-lives, and mineralocorticoid activities [11]. Generally, these synthetic CSs are more potent immunoregulators than endogenous cortisol. They also have minimal mineralocorticoid-based side effects because of their lower affinity to mineralocorticoid receptors than endogenous glucocorticoids [11]. Hence, while different CSs have varying potencies of both glucocorticoid and mineralocorticoid effects, the term CSs in practice generally refers to their glucocorticoid effect [6, 7]. Fludrocortisone acetate is an exception, with predominantly mineralocorticoid and minimal glucocorticoid activity. Table 24.1 depicts the comparative glucocorticoid and mineralocorticoid effects, equivalent potencies (relative to hydrocortisone activity), and duration of action of commonly used CSs [6, 7]. The dosages and pertinent considerations regarding their use in various neurological and non-neurological critical conditions in the NICU are enumerated in Table 24.2.

CSs, while useful, are not benign drugs and can cause a wide spectrum of adverse effects, particularly when used in high dosages and for a prolonged duration. Upto 90% of patients who take CSs for more than 8 weeks are highly likely to develop drug-related complications shown in Table 24.3 [18]. Short-term high-dose CS therapy can also cause adverse effects, albeit with a lesser incidence, especially hyperglycemia, hypertension, mental status changes, increased susceptibility to infection, and gastric disturbances. Strategies to mitigate them include vigilant blood glucose monitoring; administration of diuretics; low-dose clonazepam; infection surveillance; and prophylactic use of proton pump inhibitors and H2 antagonists, respectively. Most complications resolve on discontinuing CSs, but some, such as cataract formation and osteoporosis, can persist even after the termination of therapy. Use of the lowest possible CS dose for the shortest duration may help to minimize these complications.

Prolonged exogenous CS administration impairs the HPA axis, and endogenous cortisol release becomes suppressed with an intake of the

Table 24.1 Comparison of systemic corticosteroid preparations

Drug	Equivalent glucocorticoid dose (mg)	Potency relative to hydrocortisone: Relative glucocorticoid potency	Potency relative to hydrocortisone: Relative mineralocorticoid potency	Duration of action (h)
Hydrocortisone[a]	100	1	1	8–12
Cortisone	125	0.8	0.8	8–12
Prednisone	5	4	0.8	12–36
Prednisolone	5	4	0.8	12–36
Methyl prednisolone[a]	4	5	0.5	12–36
Dexamethasone[a]	0.75	30	0	36–54
Fludrocortisone[b]	0	15	150	24–36

[a]IV preparation available
[b]No specific glucocorticoid (anti-inflammatory) action

Table 24.2 Corticosteroid administration related considerations in neuro-intensive care disorders

Central nervous system infections

Bacterial meningitis

- Dexamethasone 10 mg qid i.v., for 4 days
- Initiate dexamethasone empirically with or 20 min before first antibiotic dose. If antibiotic already started, can administer dexamethasone within 4 h of first antibiotic dose
- Discontinue dexamethasone if subsequent diagnosis is not BM or if isolated pathogen is not *H. Influenzae* or S. Pneumoniae
- Caution: Dexamethasone potentially reduces CSF penetration of vancomycin (but not rifampicin)

  Corticosteroid administration should not delay administration of IV antibiotics.

Tubercular meningitis (TBM)

- Grade II or III TBM: Dexamethasone—0.4 mg/kg/day i.v. for first week, then 0.3 mg/kg/day i.v. for second week, then 0.2 mg/kg/day i.v. for third week, then 0.1 mg/kg/per day for fourth week; then oral dexamethasone for 4 weeks, starting at a total of 4 mg per day and decreasing by 1 mg each week
- Grade I TBM: Dexamethasone—0.3 mg/kg/day i.v. for first week, then 0.2 mg/kg/day i.v. for second week; then 0.1 mg/kg/day orally for third week, then a total of 3 mg/day orally, decreasing by 1 mg each week

Brain abscess

- Dexamethasone—Loading dose 10 mg i.v., followed by 4 mg every 6 h
- Discontinue drug once the mass effect and patient's mental status and neurologic manifestations have improved.

Herpes simplex virus encephalitis

- Dexamethasone, 40 mg i.v./day for 4 days

Neurocysticercosis

- Dexamethasone 8 mg, q 8 h; preferably started 2–3 days before anthelmintics; on day 3 decrease dose to 4 mg q 8 h, and on day 6 change to prednisone 0.4 mg/kg/day divided TID.
- In patients with symptoms of intracranial hypertension: Anthelmintic treatment is started after symptoms subside (usually after 3 doses)
- Taper steroids after anthelmintics are discontinued.

Toxoplasma gondii CNS infection

- Dexamethasone 20 mg IV for 7 days

IRIS

- Massive cerebral edema or impending herniation: Methylprednisolone 1 g i.v./day for 3–5 days, followed by gradual tapering dose over 2–3 weeks
- Less severe presentation: Prednisone 1 mg/kg for 5–7 days followed by gradual tapering over 2–3 weeks

Neurological disorders with autoimmune dysregulation

Hyperacute multiple sclerosis

- Methylprednisolone 1 g i.v./day, for 3–5 days ± short taper
- Exclude any acute infection, particularly urinary tract infection, before starting therapy

Manifest/impending myasthenia gravis

- Methylprednisolone 2 g IV/day (HDMP) for 5 days; can repeat up to 3 doses. Follow with prednisolone 100 mg orally/day, gradually tapered by10 mg/day (or 20 mg every other day), while monitoring for recurrence of symptoms, up to a maintenance dose that keeps the patient minimally symptomatic.
- Maintenance dose may be required for years, to avoid relapse
- Avoid abrupt withdrawal in poorly stabilized patients; can lead to recurrent symptoms, even MG crisis.
- HDMP should be administered concurrently with IV immunoglobulin (IVIG)/plasma exchange /Plex), to avoid steroid myopathy; or may be deferred till patient starts improving after IVIG/Plex therapy

Acute demyelinating encephalomyelitis (ADEM), autoimmune Encephalitides (AE), Hashimotos encephalopathy, primary Angiitis of the central nervous system (PACNS)

- Methylprednisolone 1 g i.v./day, for 3–5 days; followed by prednisone 1–2 mg/kg/d orally, gradually tapered over 4–6 weeks, to reduce risk of relapse
- AE: Early, empirical high-dose CS recommended if clinical suspicion of AE, even before availability of antibody tests; conjunctive IVIG may be required in severe acute initial presentations
- ADEM: Repeat pulse of i.v. steroids may be considered if unsatisfactory clinical improvement or early relapse

Central nervous system trauma

Spinal cord injury (SCI)

- Consider methylprednisolone if presentation within 8 h of isolated, nonpenetrating SCI
- Methylprednisolone: Initial bolus of 30 mg/kg i.v. over 15 min, followed 45 min later with continuous infusion of 5.4 mg/kg/h, for 23 h

(continued)

Table 24.3 (continued)

Critical illness-related corticosteroid insufficiency *Refractory septic shock* – Hydrocortisone 50 mg i.v., every 6 h or 200 mg i.v./day as continuous infusion, for refractory shock [systolic BP < 90 mmHg for more than 1 h despite both adequate fluid resuscitation and moderate- to high-dose vasopressor therapy >0.1 µg/kg/min of norepinephrine or equivalent] – Initiate gradual taper when BP is stable, adequate for 12–24 h, without vasopressors; typically, decrease by 10–20 mg over several days to weeks, guided by clinical response, to avoid rebound phenomenon. – Exception: If indication for CS is underlying endocrine disorder, then taper the corticosteroids back to their usual dose *Acute respiratory distress syndrome (ARDS; PaO_2/FiO_2 of < 200)* *Early, moderate ARDS (1–7 days but ideally < 72 h)* – Methylprednisolone. Loading dose 1 mg/kg i.v., followed by infusion 1 mg/kg/day from day 1 to day 14. After 14 days/successful extubation reduce dose to 0.5 mg/kg/day i.v. for 7 days, then 0.25 mg/kg/d for 7 days, and finally 0.125 mg/kg/d for 7 days – If receiving paralytics, delay use until concomitant use of paralytic agents is not required – Discontinue, if no clear physiological or radiological benefit in 3–5 days, *Late persistent ARDS* (by day 7 of ARDS in patients not receiving methylprednisolone for early ARDS/ by day 5–7 of ARDS in patients receiving methylprednisolone for early ARDS) – Methylprednisolone: Loading bolus over 30 min 2 mg/kg i.v., followed by 2 mg/kg/day i.v. infusion for 14 days, then 1 mg/kg/day i.v. infusion for 7 days; then 0.5 mg/kg/day i.v. infusion for 4 days, then 0.25 mg/kg/day i.v. infusion for 3 days, then 0.125 mg/kg/day i.v. for 2 days – If tracheal extubated between days 1 to 14, then patient is advanced to day 15 of drug therapy and tapered according to schedule
Miscellaneous conditions *Postextubation laryngeal edema* – Methylprednisolone: 20 mg IV every 4 h (4 doses), initiated 12 h before extubation and last injection just before extubation OR dexamethasone: 5 mg IV every 6 h (4 doses), initiated 24 h before extubation, with the last injection 24 h before extubation OR hydrocortisone: 4 doses every 6 *Obstructive airway disease* *Asthma exacerbation:* Hydrocortisone 100 mg i.v. every 6 h, for at least 5 days or methyl prednisolone 125 mg i.v., followed by 40–60 mg i.v. every 6–12 h (or equivalent orally). – Consider tapering after 36–48 h, depending on clinical response. *COPD exacerbation:* Methylprednisolone 125 mg i.v. every 6 h for 3 days, then 60 mg daily for 4 days, then 40 mg daily for 4 days, and then 20 mg daily for 4 days. *Anaphylaxis* – Hydrocortisone 1.5–3 mg/kg IV stat dose *Adrenal crisis* – Hydrocortisone 100 mg i.v. stat dose; then 50 mg IV q 6 h and cortisone acetate 75–100 mg IM stat dose, and then 50–75 mg IM q 6 h; duration guided by endocrinologist **Myxoedema coma** – Hydrocortisone 300–400 mg i.v. over 24 h (thyroid replacement may precipitate adrenal crisis); duration guided by endocrinologist **Organ donor optimization** – Methylprednisolone 15 mg/kg i.v. (maximum 1 g), every 24 h
Cerebral salt wasting syndrome – Fludrocortisone 0.1–0.2 mg, i.v. or orally, two times/day, until normalization of serum sodium, and intravascular volume (usually 3–5 days)

Table 24.3 Adverse effects of corticosteroids

Organ system	Adverse effects	Remarks
Gastrointestinal	Gastritis Peptic ulcer disease	– Disputed risk; possibly due to inhibition of gastric-protective prostaglandins, mucus production, and/or bicarbonate secretion – Risk increases significantly, when used in combination with nonsteroidal anti-inflammatory drugs, >3 weeks; or dexamethasone dose >40 mg/day/prednisone>400–1000 mg/day – Histamine H2 antagonists, proton pump inhibitors prescribed to minimize risk, especially with prolonged and/or high dose CS

Table 24.3 (continued)

Organ system	Adverse effects	Remarks
Immune system	Increased susceptibility to opportunistic infection, particularly viral and invasive fungal infections (especially *pneumocystis jerovecii* pneumonitis) with moderate to high CS doses	Consider pneumocystis prophylaxis if >3 mg dexamethasone given for >4 weeks
Metabolic and endocrine	Hyperglycemia Secondary diabetes mellitus Increased insulin resistance in diabetes mellitus HPA axis suppression Secondary hyperparathyroidism Transaminitis, hyperlipidemia Hypokalemic alkalosis	– Dose-dependent hyperglycemia occurs within hours of exposure – Most common cause of drug-induced diabetes mellitus. – Hypoadrenalism (>1 month of use) *Adrenal suppression* occurs after abrupt CS withdrawal Gradual CS tapering advised
Skin, connective tissue musculoskeletal system	– Myopathy – Osteopenia/osteoporosis, fractures – Impaired wound healing – Easy bruising – Avascular necrosis – Acne, hirsutism, Cushingoid appearance	*Myopathy* – Proximal muscle weakness – Likely mechanism: Catabolic effects of CS; induction of glutamine synthetase activity – Develops over several weeks to months; may be faster with higher doses; resolves 3–4 weeks after CS discontinuation – Higher predisposition with fluorinated CSs, e.g., dexamethasone, than nonfluorinated CSs, e.g., hydrocortisone, prednisone – Increased risk with concomitant use of neuromuscular blocking agents *Osteoporosis, fractures, and osteonecrosis:* – *Due to* impaired mineralization of bone matrix; decreased bone formation – Suggested mechanism: direct effect of CS on skeletal muscles; reduced calcium absorption, with secondary hyperparathyroidism and decreased gonadal hormones – Increased risk with use of >5 mg/day of prednisolone (or its equivalent), within 3–6 months of initiation – Consider prophylaxis if duration of therapy > 3 months and a daily dose >7.5 mg prednisone or equivalent – Prevention/treatment: Calcium supplements (1500 mg/day) with vitamin D (800 international units daily) or activated vitamin D (e.g., alfacalcidiol 1 μg/day or calcitriol at 0.5 μg/day). Postmenopausal women: Also give bisphosphonates (etidronate, alendronate, risedronate, or zoledonate) and teriparatide (synthetic parathyroid hormone)
Cardiovascular	Hypertension Fluid retention Peripheral edema	– Mineralocorticoid activity (varies by CS) leads to free water and sodium retention – *Hypertension* – MOST common side effect (20% patients) – Due to abnormal increase in plasma volume by CS – Reversible upon cessation of CS – Diuretics preferred treatment
Neurological and neuropsychiatric	Psychosis Behavioral alterations (agitation, insomnia, irritability, hypomania, anxiety, mood lability) Glaucoma, cataract formation Seizures	*Psychosis*—Typically with use of high doses (>20 mg prednisone/day or equivalent) for prolonged periods – May require antipsychotic treatment Seizures—Rare; occur at high doses in patients with a seizure disorder history

equivalent of 5 mg or more of prednisolone for over 4 weeks [6, 8]. Sudden discontinuation after a prolonged course of CSs can precipitate an Addisonian crisis because of the resulting absolute steroid deficiency; hence, exogenous CSs are never abruptly withdrawn but are gradually tapered to allow recovery of the HPA axis.

24.4 CSs in Critical Neurological/Neurosurgical Disorders

24.4.1 Brain Neoplasms

CSs are the mainstay of symptomatic therapy in patients with brain neoplasms and awaiting definitive therapy but require an emergent NICU admission due to an impending brain herniation [1, 16]. The decrease in peritumoral VE, mass effect, and intracranial hypertension begins within hours, and a clinically dramatic response is usually observed in 70% of patients within 24–72 h of their initiation [1, 4, 19]. Dexamethasone is usually preferred because of its high potency, relative lack of mineralocorticoid activity (reduced risk of worsening of edema due to potential water and sodium retention), long half-life (36–54 h), and possibly a lower index of immunosuppression and cognitive impairment [1, 4–6]. However, since its antiedema, as well as adverse effects, is dose-dependent, it is prudent to individualize the initial dose (based on the severity of edema and clinical presentation) and modify subsequent dosages (based on the clinical response) to use the lowest optimal dose. This practice is especially important with the use of high initial dexamethasone doses (e.g., >8 mg daily), as the proximal myopathy can manifest within weeks at such doses.

24.4.2 CNS Infections

Bacterial Meningitis (BM)

Much of the neurological morbidity in BM is related to the inflammatory cytokines (IL-1, IL-6, TNF α, and matrix metalloproteinases) generated in the subarachnoid space due to complex interactions between the bacterial components and the host inflammatory responses and are further amplified by the antibiotic-induced bacterial lysis [20, 21]. These inflammatory mediators injure the endothelium of the BBB and result in severe neurological complications such as intracranial hypertension, brain herniation, seizures, and cerebral infarction, due to the ensuing VE, cerebrovascular dysautoregulation, brain ischemia, and cytotoxic injury [22–24]. A higher incidence of complications is reported during pneumococcal meningitis as compared to infection with other organisms (e.g., *Neisseria meningitidis*, *Listeria monocytogenes*, *Hemophilus influenzae*, Group B streptococcus); this is most likely due to persistence of potent biologic activity in the debris of the killed *S. pneumoniae* bacteria, which stimulates a stronger host inflammatory response [23].

Substantial evidence from experimental studies, randomized controlled trials (RCTs), and meta-analyses demonstrates that CSs mitigate the inflammatory responses in the CSF and reverse the brain edema in BM (Table 24.4) [21–29]. In a Cochrane review (25 RCTs, 4121 participants), Brower et al. documented an improved neurologic outcome with their use in BM caused by all pathogens and a possible mortality benefit in pneumococcal meningitis (Table 24.4) [29]. Notably, a subgroup analysis in this meta-analysis revealed that these benefits were limited to resource-rich countries, the lack of CS effect in poor resource nations is most probably due to the initial delay in patient presentation, and treatment initiation after the CNS inflammation has already begun and progressed [29–31]. Based on the available evidence, several guidelines strongly recommend early, empiric adjunctive administration of CSs in BM [31–34]. Mortality benefits have been reported in several countries after implementing these guidelines [35–37]. Dexamethasone is usually preferred due to its long half-life and superior penetration into the CSF. Notably, its early administration is critical for blunting the cytokine release that occurs due to antibiotic-induced bacterial lysis; a delayed administration does not reverse the brain edema or intracranial hypertension in the later stages of meningitis [31]. Ideally, it is started with

Table 24.4 Major studies investigating the effect of corticosteroids (CSs) in neurological and non-neurological critical illnesses in the neuro-intensive care unit

Study Author (Reference), Year, *Pathology*	Study design	Major observations
de Gans and van de Beek [22], 2002, *Bacterial Meningitis (BM)*	– Randomized, double-blind, multicenter trial – Adjuvant dexamethasone (DXM) ($n = 157$) versus placebo ($n = 144$), in adults with acute BM	– Reduced mortality and improved outcome with DXM – Beneficial effect observed primarily for pneumococcal meningitis
Brower et al. [25], 2015, *BM*	– Cochrane meta-analysis – 25 studies; 4121 participants; 9 studies in low-income countries and 16 in high-income countries	– Reduced neurological sequelae with adjunctive DXM – Insufficient evidence regarding mortality benefit – Benefits observed mostly in resource rich countries
Thwaites et al. [38], 2004, *Tubercular Meningitis (TBM)*	– Randomized controlled trial (RCT) – 545 patients with TBM ± HIV, randomized to placebo or DXM for 8 weeks	– Significantly decreased mortality with DXM -no benefit of DXM on disability outcome
Prasad et al. [41], 2016, *TBM*	– Cochrane review – 9 RCTs, 1337 participants	– Reduced mortality with CS at 3–18 months follow-up, at all stages of disease – Little or no effect on disabling neurological deficit
Kamei et al. [50], 2005, *Herpes Simplex Virus encephalitis(HSVE)*	– Non-randomized, retrospective study of adjunctive efficacy of CSs with acyclovir in *HSVE* – 45 patients	– Non administration of CSs was an independent predictor of poor patient outcome at 3 months
Cuello-García et al. [55], 2012, *Neurocysticercosis (NCC)*	– Metanalysis of CS versus placebo in NCC – 13 RCTs, 1373 participants	– CSs reduced the rate of seizure recurrence and hastened resolution of lesions at 6–12 months of follow-up
Filippini et al. [66], 2000, *Multiple Sclerosis (MS)*	– Cochrane review; methylprednisolone (MP) or ACTH versus placebo for acute exacerbation of MS – 6 RCTs; 377 participants (199 treatment, 178 placebo) – MP- 4 trials, 140 patients; ACTH-2 trials, 237 patients	– Reduced disease progression within first 5 weeks of treatment with both MP and ACTH – Trend for better efficacy with MP and IV treatment, but no significant difference between short (5 days) and extended (15 days) MP treatment – Insufficient data to reliably estimate MP's effect on prevention of new exacerbations and reduction of long-term disability
Schneider-Gold et al. [70], 2005, *Myasthenia Gravis (MG)*	Cochrane review of efficacy of CSs or ACTH in MG 7 RCTs, 199 participants	Limited evidence suggestive of short-term benefit with CSs in MG compared with placebo
Bracken et al. NASCIS I [84], 1984, *spinal cord injury (SCI)*	Double-blind, RCT of high-dose versus low-dose MP 330 acute SCI patients randomized to either MP 100-mg bolus followed by 25 mg every 6 h or 1000 mg bolus and 250 mg every 6 h for 10 days	No difference in neurologic outcome between the two groups; wound infection more prevalent in high-dose group

(continued)

Table 24.4 (continued)

Study Author (Reference), Year, *Pathology*	Study design	Major observations
Bracken et al. NASCIS II [85], 1990, *Spinal Cord Injury (SCI)*	Randomized, double-blind, placebo-controlled trial (MP vs. naloxone vs. placebo 162 patients with acute SCI received MP 30-mg/kg bolus followed by 5.4 mg/kg/h iv infusion for 23 h	Significant improvement in patients treated with MP 8 h after injury
Bracken et al. NASCIS III [86], 1997, *Spinal Cord Injury (SCI)*	Randomized, double-blind trial (MP 24 h vs. MP 48 h vs. tirilazad) 499 patients with acute SCI randomized to MP or tirilazad	Benefit from 48-h regimen observed in patients treated later (between 3 and 8 h after injury)
Bracken et al. [87], 2004, *Spinal Cord Injury (SCI)*	Meta-analysis of 5 RCTs trials (Cochrane review) Different subgroup analyses performed	Corroborated findings of NASCIS II and III; however, when combined with other (non-NASCIS) trials, no beneficial effect on motor function
Venkatesh et al. adrenal trial [94], 2018, *septic shock*	– Multicenter, placebo-controlled RCT – Low-dose hydrocortisone (200 mg/day) in 3800 sepsis patients on vasopressors and mechanical ventilation	– No statistical difference in 90-day mortality – Significant reduction in median days for resolution of shock, initiation of ventilation and ICU stay, and reduced blood transfusion requirements with CS
Annane et al. CRICS-TRIGGERSEP [95], 2018, *Septic Shock*	– Multicentre, placebo-controlled RCT – 671 intensive care patients with indisputable or probable septic shock for less than 24 h – Hydrocortisone 50 mg IV bolus every 6 h; fludrocortisone 50 mcg tablet once in morning; for 7 days without tapering	– Significant improvement in mortality at 90 days with hydrocortisone and fludrocortisone compared to placebo
Meduri et al. [101], 2018, *ARDS*	Meta-analysis 9 RCTs, 816 patients Low-to-moderate dose prolonged CS in ARDS	CSs reduced time to endotracheal extubation, duration of hospitalization, mechanical ventilation, and mortality
Jesús Villar et al. DEXA ARDS TRIAL [103], 2020, *Adult Respiratory Distress Syndrome (ARDS)*	– Multicenter RCT – 277 patients with moderate to severe ARDS – DXM 20 mg/day for 5 days followed by 10 mg daily for 5 days (stopped at extubation)	– Higher ventilator-free days – Lower mortality in DXM versus control group
Kuriam et al. [105], 2017, *Postextubation airway events*	Cochrane review Effect of prophylactic CSs versus placebo/no treatment on incidence of postextubation airway events 11 trials, 2472 participants	– Reduced incidence of post-extubation airway events with CS as compared with placebo or no treatment
Roberts et al. CRASH Trial [108], 2004, *Traumatic Brain Injury (TBI)*	– Placebo controlled, double-blind RCT – 10,000 TBI patients with GCS of 14 or less, randomized to 48-hr high-dose MP infusion or placebo	– Increased mortality in CS-treated group
Sandercock et al. [110], 2011, *Acute Ischemic Stroke (AIS)*	Cochrane meta-analysis 8 trials; 466 participants CSs with placebo or a control group in patients with acute (presumed or definite) ischemic stroke	No difference in mortality or better functional outcome in survivors between both groups

Table 24.4 (continued)

Study Author (Reference), Year, *Pathology*	Study design	Major observations
Feigin et al. [111], 2005, *Intra-Cranial Hemorrhage (ICH)*	– Meta-analysis of 8 randomized controlled trials (Cochrane review) – 256 randomized patients, on CSs	No evidence of a beneficial or adverse effect of CSs
Hughes [112], 2016, *Guillain-Barré syndrome (GBS)*	– Cochrane review – Effect of CS on recovery and long-term morbidity from GBS – 6 trials; 587 participants	– CS given alone do not significantly hasten recovery or affect the long-term outcome in GBS; – Oral CS may delay recovery

or slightly before the first antibiotic dose; a maximum delay of up to 4 h after initiating antibiotic treatment is permitted by the ESCIM guidelines (expert consensus) [29, 31]. It should be subsequently discontinued if an etiology other than BM is diagnosed or if results indicate that the BM is due to a species other than *H. influenzae* or *S. pneumoniae* (some experts advise continuation of dexamethasone irrespective of the causative bacterium) [31, 34]. Notably, dexamethasone can potentially reduce vancomycin's penetration into the CSF due to decreased inflammation (vancomycin is usually given with a third-generation cephalosporin for treatment of BM); in comparison, it does not affect rifampin's penetration into the CSF.

Tubercular Meningitis (TBM)

The prognosis of TBM, a devastating disease with high mortality and morbidity, is largely linked to the severity of the T-c lymphocytes and TNFα-mediated inflammatory response that develops when TB tubercles (Rich foci) rupture and spill the bacilli and protein into the CSF [30, 38, 39]. The resulting inflammatory adhesive exudates (or caseating granulomas) engulf the structures at the base of the brain and cause severe neurological complications, including intracranial hypertension due to hydrocephalus (CSF outflow obstruction by basal exudates) and cerebral edema (vascular endothelial injury and BBB disruption); necrotizing vasculopathy; obliterative vasculitis induced stroke and cerebral infarction; and coma [38–40].

CSs inhibit the synthesis of inflammatory cytokines in the subarachnoid space, stabilize the BBB, decrease the CSF outflow resistance, and possibly prevent the small-vessel vasculopathy that characteristically affects lenticulostriate and other perforating arteries in TBM. There is strong evidence of a mortality benefit with their adjunctive use in TBM (Table 24.4) [1, 38, 39, 41]. In their Cochrane review of CSs in TBM, Prasad et al. (over nine trials, 1337 participants) reported an almost 25% reduction in mortality at 18 months follow-up across all stages of the disease; their effect on disabling neurologic deficit, however, was less consistent (Table 24.4) [41].

Hence, current guidelines strongly recommend adjunctive CSs as a part of the standard therapy of TBM, regardless of disease severity at presentation; the duration of CS therapy, however, is longer than that required for BM [42, 43].

Tuberculomas, Spinal Cord Tuberculosis

There is insufficient evidence regarding routine adjunctive CS use in patients with tuberculomas without meningitis or in those with spinal cord (SC) tuberculosis. However, they should be administered if cerebral edema is out of proportion to mass effect in the setting of associated altered mental status or focal neurologic deficits or if there is evidence of acute SC compression secondary to vertebral tuberculosis [42, 44].

Brain Abscess

Adjunctive dexamethasone has been shown to reduce the perifocal edema surrounding brain abscesses, with a resultant rapid improvement in the patient's ICP and clinical condition [45–47]. However, the associated reduction in penetration of antibiotics through the BBB and the delay in encapsulation of the suppurative fluid potentially offset its beneficial effects [45]. Hence, its use is limited to patients with prominent focal signs or a cerebral herniation risk due to severe intracranial hypertension (mass effect or significant perifocal edema). It should be tapered off once clinical improvement occurs, especially if there is a concern for resistant strains and decreased antibiotic penetration [1, 45, 47].

Herpes Simplex Encephalitis (HSVE)

The cerebral damage in HSVE, a potentially life-threatening CNS infection with high mortality (20%) and severe neurological disability despite antiviral therapy, primarily results from viral replication and the overzealous host inflammatory response [48]. CSs confer benefits because of their strong immunomodulatory effects but are associated with a potential risk of enhanced viral replication, especially when given early in the course of the disease [49]. Their adjunctive efficacy (in combination with acyclovir) has been reported in several experimental and clinical observations (case reports, retrospective clinical studies), but as yet, there are no randomized controlled trials regarding their role in this condition (Table 24.4) [50–52]. The GACHE study (German Trial on Aciclovir and Corticosteroids in Herpes-simplex-virus-encephalitis), the first prospective multicenter RCT, was prematurely terminated due to lack of recruitment [48]. Currently, the administration of CSs is not a standard of practice; however, they may be considered if there is evidence of severe intracranial hypertension (profound VE, mass effect, and brain shift) [49, 50].

Neurocysticercosis (NCC)

Inflammatory responses dominate the pathophysiology of NCC, a parasitic CNS infection caused by *Taenia solium*. Initiation of antihelminthic therapy can further aggravate these responses and, thereby, the clinical manifestations of NCC. Emergent neuro-intensive care may be required for the management of status epilepticus, stroke (inflammatory occlusive vasculitis at the base of the brain, secondary to arachnoiditis), severe acute intracranial hypertension (due to hydrocephalus, mass effect, or cysticercal encephalitis with diffuse cerebral edema) [53]. Extra-parenchymal NCC (e.g., subarachnoid, intraventricular NCC) is particularly lethal without prompt treatment [54].

In these situations, adjuvant CSs mitigate the perilesional brain edema, and the antihelminth therapy-induced inflammatory responses and combined use of these drugs have demonstrated a reduced incidence of seizures than antiepileptics alone (Table 24.4) [55, 56].

Current guidelines strongly recommend the administration of CSs, prior to the use of antiparasitic drugs, in single-enhancing lesions and viable parenchymal NCC [56]. CSs are also recommended as the primary treatment in cysticercal encephalitis with diffuse cerebral edema, as antiparasitic drugs are avoided because of the risk of worsening cerebral edema [30, 56].

Cerebral Toxoplasmosis, Neurolisteriosis, Cryptococcal Meningitis (CM)

Cerebral toxoplasmosis, the most common cause of expansive brain lesions in HIV-infected patients, causes high mortality and morbidity due to multifocal necrotizing encephalitis [57]. There are no RCTs of adjunctive steroids in this condition; nevertheless, they can be administered if there is evidence of significant mass effect or diffuse brain edema [57, 58]. Adjuvant CSs are, however, not recommended in neurolisteriosis (*L. monocytogenes*) and HIV-associated cryptococcal meningitis (CM) because of evidence of a trend toward increased mortality and adverse events with their use in these conditions [30, 59].

Immune Reconstitution Syndrome (IRIS)

HIV patients who are initiated on antiretroviral therapy (ART) are at risk of developing IRIS, an exaggerated inflammatory reaction to a preexisting infection that was either previously diagnosed and treated (paradoxical IRIS) or was subclinical but has been unmasked due to recovery of the host's immune capacity to mount an inflammatory response (unmasked IRIS) [30, 60]. HIV-related CNS IRIS is commonly observed in TBM, CM, toxoplasmosis, primary CNS lymphoma, HIV encephalitis, and progressive multifocal leukoencephalopathy (PML). Paradoxical TB-related IRIS is also reported in approximately 39% of non-HIV patients who had previously responded to antitubercular therapy [61]. Typically, patients have a paradoxical worsening of the neurological manifestations after an initial period of recovery and may require emergency neuro-care for impending brain herniation due to the development of severe cerebral edema, vasculopathy-related cerebral infarction, severe basilar meningitis, hydrocephalus, or tuberculoma expansion (in CNS TB patients) [30, 62].

CSs play an important role in controlling the hyperactive inflammatory responses in CNS IRIS, as they restore the BBB, reduce T-cell activation, and prevent the influx of inflammatory cells. However, they can aggravate the underlying opportunistic infection and, therefore, should be used cautiously. They are the frontline therapy for controlling inflammation when definitive antimicrobial therapy is not available, e.g., PML, and are given if there is evidence of substantial mass effect due to CNS inflammation; the goal is not to completely obliterate the inflammation but rather to temper the response (cytotoxic T cells are required to control the viral infection) [63]. They are used as adjuvants if definitive antimicrobial therapy is available, e.g., CM, cerebral toxoplasmosis, and should be administered after initiating antimicrobial therapy and optimizing ART [63].

24.4.3 Autoimmune Neurological Disorders

High-dose CSs are widely accepted as first-line therapies for initial emergent or subsequent stabilization of neuro-intensive care patients with autoimmune, inflammatory neurological disorders such as hyperacute multiple sclerosis(MS), myasthenia gravis (MG), steroid-responsive encephalopathies (SRES), acute demyelinating encephalomyelitis (ADEM), and primary angiitis of the central nervous system (PACNS) [3, 64]. Given that B and T cells play a predominant role in the pathogenesis of these disorders, CSs confer benefit by inhibiting B cell proliferation and B cell receptor triggered signaling, plasma cell differentiation, differentiation of naïve T cells into T helper cells, and T cell activation of auto-reactive B cells. Unfortunately, but notably, while they have broad anti-inflammatory and immunosuppressive effects, they possess very little targeted therapy.

MS

Acute episodes of neuro-inflammation checker the early course of most cases of hyperacute MS patients; and the BBB breakdown may occasionally be fulminant enough to cause severe alteration in the level of consciousness, seizures, or intracranial hypertension [64].

Several studies, including Cochrane meta-analyses, reveal that high-dose CSs accelerate remission and limit residual neurological deficits during these exacerbations (Table 24.4) [65–67]. Current guidelines recommend a short course of high-dose glucocorticoids to manage acute MS relapses; a gradual oral corticosteroid taper over the following 2 weeks can be considered in selected patients with a high rebound risk [64, 68]. Notably, CSs do not alter the overall progression of the disease; they are also ineffective in the later stages of the disease because of their largely neurodegenerative pathogenesis [64].

MG

Manifest or impending MG usually necessitates an emergency NICU admission for aggressive management and/or close monitoring of the severe, rapidly progressive respiratory insufficiency and potential airway compromise (ventilatory or bulbar dysfunction). Current guidelines recommend high-dose intravenous CS-pulse therapy, plasmapheresis (PLEX), or intravenous immunoglobulins (IVIG) during these potentially life-threatening situations [69]. CS therapy provides long-term clinical stabilization after the initial effects of the acute therapy with PLEX or IVIg have dissipated [69]. The beneficial effects on motor recovery are observed a few weeks after their initiation. However, a transient worsening of the myesthenic symptoms can occur initially in about 50% of patients (release of immunoglobulins due to lymphocyte lysis; direct effects on the neuromuscular junction [3, 70]. The weakness usually begins within 5 days of starting CSs (range 1–21 days), and in 10% of patients, especially in those with bulbar dysfunction, may be severe enough to lead to a crisis and an imminent need for mechanical ventilation [3, 69]. Hence, concurrent administration of IVIG/PLEx or a delay of CS therapy for a few days until the patient starts improving is recommended to prevent this potential complication [69].

SRE

SREs, such as autoimmune encephalitides (AEs, paraneoplastic or non-paraneoplastic), limbic encephalitis, anti-neutrophil cytoplasmic antibody (ANCA)-associated vasculitis encephalopathy, systemic lupus erythematosus encephalopathy, and primary CNS lymphoma, are typically characterized by diffuse CNS injury that is responsive to steroids or immunosuppressive therapies [3, 71]. In AE, e.g., anti-NMDA receptor (NMDAR) encephalitis, anti-LG1 encephalitis, VGKC antibody encephalitis, Hashimoto's encephalopathy [or steroid-responsive encephalopathy associated with autoimmune thyroiditis (SREAT)], autoantibodies typically trigger damage in the cortical or deep gray matter, and sometimes, in white matter, meninges, or the spinal cord [72]. Development of coma, refractory status epilepticus, severe dysautonomia, respiratory compromise (craniobulbar involvement or medication-induced hypoventilation), or massive brain edema usually necessitate an urgent NICU admission [3, 72]. Likewise, patients with ADEM (or postinfectious encephalomyelitis) frequently require emergent neuro-intensive care to treat the rapidly progressive encephalopathy and multifocal neurologic deficits that develop due to acute inflammatory CNS demyelination [73]. Indications for acute neuro-care in PACNS include the development of severe neurological complications such as stroke, seizures, and rarely intracranial bleeding [74]. There are not many robust RCTs; however, several observational studies and case reports have reported about the substantial efficacy of CSs in these autoimmune neurological disorders [74–77]. In fact, the dramatic improvement observed with early, aggressive use of CSs is sometimes used as a diagnostic criterion for AE [3, 30, 72, 75]. Current treatment guidelines and best practice statements recommend early, empiric high-dose CSs as first-line therapies for these conditions [72, 78–80]. In severe clinical presentations, they are co-administered with intravenous immunoglobulins in AE, cyclophosphamide in PACNS, and acyclovir or antibiotics in ADEM [3, 30, 72, 74, 78–80]. Typically, neurological improvement begins within days, and recovery occurs within a few weeks of their initiation. Notably, CSs can aggravate the psychiatric symptoms associated with AD (e.g., depression, insomnia, agitation, and psychosis) [81].

24.4.4 CNS Trauma

SCI

Methylprednisolone (MP) is the most commonly used yet highly controversial treatment option for SCI. Its neuroprotective efficacy was demonstrated in preclinical studies, wherein it ameliorated the inflammatory changes involved in the pathophysiology of secondary SCI when used in supraphysiological doses, especially within the first 8 h after SCI [1, 2, 82, 83]. These promising results led to three controversial landmark trials—National Acute Spinal Cord Injury Study I, II, and III (NASCIS) (Table 24.4) [84–86]. While the primary outcomes in all three trials were negative, a post hoc analysis revealed a modest improvement in motor recovery in a specific subgroup of patients. A Cochrane review (performed by the lead author of NASCIS trials) also reiterated "high-dose methylprednisolone's (HDMP) efficacy when administered within 8 h of injury." (NASCIS) (Table 24.4) [87]. These results have formed the basis for the widely instituted HDMP protocol for acute SCI. However, these trials have undergone intense scrutiny, and there is moderate skepticism about their validity, given the study design and methodology limitations, incomplete data reporting, inappropriate statistical methodology, and arbitrary subgroup analysis [1, 88, 89]. Moreover, HDMP administration was associated with an increased risk of serious adverse events, such as sepsis, pneumonia, gastrointestinal bleeding, wound infection, pulmonary embolism, and death [1, 90]. Accordingly, several scientific societies concur that HDMP is not a standard of care but may be considered as a treatment option in acute SCI, with complete cognizance of the rather uncertain clinical benefits and the high risk of therapy-induced complications [91, 92].

MP's use in acute SCI has declined in recent times; nevertheless, it is still considered because of the encouraging preclinical results and the limited treatment options available for this devastating condition, especially in acute, isolated nonpenetrating SCI. However, it should be avoided if there are obvious associated risks, such as penetrating SCI, multisystem trauma, especially concomitant moderate to severe TBI, or comorbidities that increase the risk of CS therapy-related complications.

24.5 CS in Critical Non-Neurological Illnesses

24.5.1 CIRCI: Septic Shock, ARDS

CIRCI in TBI, septic shock, BM, and ARDS usually manifests as hemodynamic instability despite adequate fluid resuscitation and fever that does not have an identifiable source of infection and is unresponsive to empiric antimicrobial therapy [8]. Evidence in the literature suggests that the patient outcomes in CIRCI are significantly linked to the extent of elevation of pro-inflammatory cytokines [9]. CSs facilitate a better outcome in patients with septic shock owing to their immunomodulatory effects and ability to increase the cardiovascular tone (enhanced vasoconstrictor responsiveness to exogenous catecholamines, inhibition of cyclo-oxygenase-2 and inducible nitric oxide synthase) and improve the HPA axis dysfunction. Several RCTs (e.g., APROCCHSS, ADRENAL, CRICS-TRIGGERSEP network trials) and meta-analyses reveal a significantly faster shock resolution, higher vasopressor-free days, a shorter duration of mechanical ventilation, hospital, and ICU stay, and possibly lower mortality, with use of low dose CSs in septic shock (Table 24.4) [93–97]. While CS therapy was associated with an increased incidence of hyperglycemia, hypernatremia, and myopathy, no increased risk of superinfection and little or no difference in gastrointestinal bleeding, neuropsychiatric, stroke, or cardiac events were observed in these RCTs [96]. However, the results in patients with sepsis without shock have not been favorable [98]. Based on this data, current guidelines suggest using low-dose corticosteroids (200–300 mg/day) in refractory septic shock but not in sepsis without shock [9, 99]. Hydrocortisone tends to be preferred because of its short duration of action, which allows the HPA axis to recover between doses [8].

Likewise, based on the favorable evidence obtained from several clinical trials and meta-analyses in ARDS, including the DEXA-ARDS trial and a recent individual patient data (IPD) analysis of the largest trials (significantly shorter mechanical ventilation duration, a faster ICU discharge, lower mortality, albeit with a slightly higher risk of hyperglycemia), current guidelines suggest the use of low to moderate doses of MP in early, moderate ARDS (Table 24.4) [9, 100–104]. MP is preferred because of its greater penetration and longer persistence in the lung tissue. However, since CS therapy blunts the febrile response, infection surveillance is recommended to ensure prompt identification and treatment of hospital-acquired infections.

24.5.2 Endocrine Failure

Besides CIRCI, acute, life-threatening adrenal insufficiency can occur due to pathology in any of the three levels of the HPA axis: primary adrenal insufficiency (e.g., adrenal cortex pathology), secondary adrenal failure (e.g., pituitary adenoma, Sheehan's syndrome, and hypopituitarism), and tertiary adrenal failure (e.g., hypothalamic lesion) [6, 7]. Development of cardiovascular collapse, neurological deterioration, and dyselectrolytemia necessitate urgent CS replacement therapy. Adjuvant CSs are also indicated in myxoedema coma patients as they are likely to have a concomitant primary or secondary adrenal insufficiency.

24.5.3 Airway Crisies, Obstructive Airway Disease, Anaphylaxis, Graft Donor Management

CSs have been shown to treat laryngeal edema, prevent the post-extubation stridor, and reduce the re-intubation risk associated with prolonged tracheal intubation in NICU patients or following prolonged cervical spine or prone position surgeries (Table 24.4) [6, 7, 105]. However, they must be administered preemptively, at least 6–24 h before a planned, high-risk tracheal extubation, to allow for an adequate effect [6, 7, 105]. CSs are also effective during acute exacerbations of asthma and chronic obstructive pulmonary disease (COPD); they mitigate the airway inflammation and mucus plugging that complicates bronchospasm not relieved by beta-agonist therapy [6, 7, 106]. CSs also comprise the cornerstone of treatment in anaphylactic reactions in the NICU. They shorten protracted reactions, help prevent a biphasic reaction, and are given after administering adrenaline and intravenous fluids [6, 7]. Further, they are also a part of the standard regimen for organ donor management to suppress the immune response, attenuate the increase in extravascular lung water, and promote hemodynamic stability after brainstem death [6, 7].

24.6 NICU Disorders in Which CSs Are Not Indicated

24.6.1 TBI

Steroids were historically used for TBI management; however, clinical trials did not demonstrate any convincing evidence of clinical benefit, possibly because of the predominance of cytotoxic edema in TBI [107]. In fact, the Corticosteroid Randomisation After Significant Head Injury trial results (CRASH) revealed significantly higher mortality at 2 weeks and 6 months in patients who received MP (Table 24.4) [108]. Hence, current Brain Trauma Foundation guidelines strongly recommend against using CSs for improving the outcome or reducing ICP in severe TBI [109].

24.6.2 Acute Ischemic Stroke (AIS), ICH, Aneurysmal Subarachnoid Hemorrhage (aSAH), Guillian Barre Syndrome (GBS)

Given their anti-inflammatory and immunosuppressive effects, CSs can potentially reduce cerebral edema and intracranial hypertension in patients with AIS, ICH, and aSAH and mitigate the immune-mediated inflammatory polyneuropathy of Guillian Barre Syndrome. Results of clinical studies, however, have been disappointing, and the Cochrane meta-analyses by Sandercock et al. in AIS, Feigin et al. in ICH and a SAH, and Hughes et al. in GBS did not demonstrate any evidence of clinical benefit with their administration in these conditions. AIS (Table 24.4) [110–112]. Hence, CSs are not indicated in these conditions.

24.7 Role of Mineralocorticoids in the NICU

Cerebral salt wasting syndrome (CSWS) is an important cause of hyponatremia in NICU disorders such as AIS, acute encephalitis, TBM, TBI, aSAH, and after intracranial surgeries. The inappropriate natriuresis and volume contraction observed in CSW are primarily attributed to elevated circulating levels of atrial natriuretic peptide (ANP) and brain natriuretic peptide (BNP), which inhibit the release of aldosterone and renin from the adrenal cortex and juxtaglomerular apparatus, respectively [113]. Fludrocortisone, a potent synthetic mineralocorticoid, augments the serum sodium concentration and intravascular volume, by enhancing sodium and water reabsorption in the distal renal tubules [113–115]. Its efficacy in normalizing the serum sodium values has been documented in several case reports of refractory CSWS secondary to intracranial surgery, aSAH, TBM, TBI, and ICH [113–120]. However, adverse effects, such as hypokalemia, hypertension, and pulmonary edema, can occur during prolonged administration of fludrocortisone, which may necessitate its withdrawal [114].

24.8 Conclusions

While CSs have an established adjunctive or frontline efficacy during the management of NICU patients with brain neoplasms, BM, TBM, and immune-mediated neurological disorders, their use in SCI is relatively controversial, and they are not useful in the management of patients with ICH, AIS, aSAH, GBS, and TBI. CSs are also used to manage diverse, non-neurological critical conditions in the NICU, including septic shock, ARDS, airway crises, exacerbation of obstructive airway disease, endocrine failure, anaphylaxis, and organ donor management. Fludrocortisone is indicated for the treatment of refractory hyponatremia due to CSWS. However, given their serious adverse effects, including their ability to suppress endogenous CS release, a rational, evidence-based approach with the use of the lowest possible drug dose for the shortest possible duration and a gradual drug withdrawal is advisable to limit the side effects and allow recovery of the HPA axis.

References

1. Gomes JA, Stevens RD, Lewin JJ 3rd, Mirski MA, Bhardwaj A. Glucocorticoid therapy in neurologic critical care. Crit Care Med. 2005;33(6):1214–24.
2. Samuel S, Nguyen T, Choi A. Pharmacologic characteristics of corticosteroids. J Neurocrit Care. 2017;10(2):53–9.
3. McDaneld LM, Fields JD, Bourdette DN, Bhardwaj A. Immunomodulatory therapies in neurologic critical care. Neurocrit Care. 2010;12(1):132–43.
4. Bebawy JF. Perioperative steroids for peritumoral intracranial edema: a review of mechanisms, efficacy, and side effects. J Neurosurg Anesthesiol. 2012;24(3):173–7.
5. Dietrich J, Rao K, Pastorino S, Kesari S. Corticosteroids in brain cancer patients: benefits and pitfalls. Expert Rev Clin Pharmacol. 2011;4(2):233–42.
6. Young A, Marsh S. Steroid use in critical care. BJA Educ. 2018;18(5):129–34.
7. Abdallah MS, Madi AF, Rana MA. The best use of systemic corticosteroids in the intensive care units, review. J Steroids Hormon Sci. 2015;6(1):149.
8. Pastores SM. Steroids in the acutely ill: evolving recommendations and practice. Cleve Clin J Med. 2022;89(9):505–11.
9. Annane D, Pastores SM, Arlt W, Balk RA, Beishuizen A, et al. Critical illness-related corticosteroid insufficiency (CIRCI): a narrative review from a multispecialty task force of the Society of Critical Care Medicine (SCCM) and the European Society of Intensive Care Medicine (ESICM). Intensive Care Med. 2017;43(12):1781–92.
10. Téblick A, Peeters B, Langouche L, Van den Berghe G. Adrenal function and dysfunction in critically ill patients. Nat Rev Endocrinol. 2019;15(7):417–27.
11. Cain DW, Cidlowski JA. Immune regulation by glucocorticoids. Nat Rev Immunol. 2017;17(4):233–47.
12. Van den Berghe G. Adrenal function/dysfunction in critically ill patients: a concise narrative review of recent novel insights. J Anesth. 2021;35(6):903–10.
13. Carlson MR, Pope WB, Horvath S, Braunstein JG, Nghiemphu P, Tso CL, et al. Relationship between survival and edema in malignant gliomas: role of vascular endothelial growth factor and neuronal pentraxin 2. Clin Cancer Res. 2007;13(9):2592–8.
14. Provias J, Claffey K, delAguila L, Lau N, Feldkamp M, Guha A. Meningiomas: role of vascular endothelial growth factor/vascular permeability factor in angiogenesis and peritumoral edema. Neurosurgery. 1997;40(5):1016–26.
15. Machein MR, Kullmer J, Fiebich BL, Plate KH, Warnke PC. Vascular endothelial growth factor expression, vascular volume, and, capillary permeability in human brain tumors. Neurosurgery. 1999;44(4):732–41.
16. Michinaga S, Koyama Y. Pathogenesis of brain edema and investigation into anti-edema drugs. Int J Mol Sci. 2015;16(5):9949–75.
17. Hall ED. The neuroprotective pharmacology of methylprednisolone. J Neurosurg. 1992;76(1):13–22.
18. Ericson-Neilsen W, Kaye AD. Steroids: pharmacology, complications, and practice delivery issues. Ochsner J. 2014;14(2):203–7.
19. Jessurun CAC, Hulsbergen AFC, Cho LD, Aglio LS, Nandoe Tewarie RDS, Broekman MLD. Evidence-based dexamethasone dosing in malignant brain tumors: what do we really know? J Neuro-Oncol. 2019;144(2):249–64.

20. Van de Beek D, Brouwer M, Hasbun R, Koedel U, Whitney CG, Wijdicks E. Community-acquired bacterial meningitis. Nat Rev Dis Primers. 2016;2:16074.
21. Scheld WM, Koedel U, Nathan B, Pfister HW. Pathophysiology of bacterial meningitis: mechanism(s) of neuronal injury. J Infect Dis. 2002;186(Suppl. 2):S225–33.
22. De Gans J, Van de Beek D. European dexamethasone in adulthood bacterial meningitis study investigators. Dexamethasone in adults with bacterial meningitis. N Engl J Med. 2002;347(20):1549–56.
23. Van de Beek D, de Gans J, Spanjaard L, Weisfelt M, Reitsma JB, Vermeulen M. Clinical features and prognostic factors in adults with bacterial meningitis. N Engl J Med. 2004;351(18):1849–59.
24. Kim KS. Investigating bacterial penetration of the blood-brain barrier for the pathogenesis, prevention, and therapy of bacterial meningitis. ACS Infect Dis. 2020;6(1):34–42.
25. Van Furth AM, Roord JJ, van Furth R. Roles of proinflammatory and anti-inflammatory cytokines in pathophysiology of bacterial meningitis and effect of adjunctive therapy. Infect Immun. 1996;64(12):4883–90.
26. Lutsar I, Friedland IR, Jafri HS, Wubbel L, Ahmed A, Trujillo M, et al. Factors influencing the anti-inflammatory effect of dexamethasone therapy in experimental pneumococcal meningitis. J Antimicrob Chemother. 2003;52(4):651–5.
27. Nguyen TH, Tran TH, Thwaites G, Ly VC, Dinh XS, Ho Dang TN, et al. Dexamethasone in Vietnamese adolescents and adults with bacterial meningitis. N Engl J Med. 2007;357(24):2431–40.
28. Vardakas KZ, Matthaiou DK, Falagas ME. Adjunctive dexamethasone therapy for bacterial meningitis in adults: a meta-analysis of randomized controlled trials. Eur J Neurol. 2009;16(6):662–73.
29. Brouwer MC, McIntyre P, Prasad K, Van de Beek D. Corticosteroids for acute bacterial meningitis. Cochrane Database Syst Rev. 2015;2015(9):CD004405.
30. Gundamraj S, Hasbun R. The use of adjunctive steroids in central nervous infections. Front Cell Infect Microbiol. 2020;10:592017.
31. Van de Beek D, Cabellos C, Dzupova O, Esposito S, Klein M, Kloek AT, et al. ESCMID study Group for Infections of the brain (ESGIB). ESCMID guideline: diagnosis and treatment of acute bacterial meningitis. Clin Microbiol Infect. 2016;22(Suppl. 3):S37–62.
32. McGill F, Heyderman RS, Michael BD, Defres S, Beeching NJ, Borrow R, et al. The UK joint specialist societies guideline on the diagnosis and management of acute meningitis and meningococcal sepsis in immunocompetent adults. J Infect. 2016;72(4):405–38.
33. Tunkel AR, Hartman BJ, Kaplan SL, Kaufman BA, Roos KL, Scheld WM, et al. Practice guidelines for the management of bacterial meningitis. Clin Infect Dis. 2004;39(9):1267–84.
34. Cook AM, Morgan Jones G, Hawryluk GWJ, Mailloux P, McLaughlin D, Papangelou A, et al. Guidelines for the acute treatment of cerebral edema in neurocritical care patients. Neurocrit Care. 2020;32(3):647–66.
35. Hasbun R, Rosenthal N, Balada-Llasat JM, Chung J, Duff S, Bozzette S, et al. Epidemiology of meningitis and encephalitis in the United States, 2011–2014. Clin Infect Dis. 2017;65(3):359–63.
36. Castelblanco RL, Lee M, Hasbun R. Epidemiology of bacterial meningitis in the USA from 1997 to 2010: a population-based observational study. Lancet Infect Dis. 2014;14(9):813–9.
37. Brouwer MC, Heckenberg SG, de Gans J, Spanjaard L, Reitsma JB, van de Beek D. Nationwide implementation of adjunctive dexamethasone therapy for pneumococcal meningitis. Neurology. 2010;75(17):1533–9.
38. Thwaites GE, Nguyen DB, Nguyen HD, Hoang TQ, Do TT, Nguyen TC, et al. Dexamethasone for the treatment of tuberculous meningitis in adolescents and adults. N Engl J Med. 2004;351(17):1741–51.
39. Donald PR, Van Toorn R. Use of corticosteroids in tuberculous meningitis. Lancet. 2016;387(10038):2585–7.
40. Hosoglu S, Geyik MF, Balik I, Aygen B, Erol S, Aygencel TG, et al. Predictors of outcome in patients with tuberculous meningitis. Int J Tuberc Lung Dis. 2002;6(1):64–70.
41. Prasad K, Singh MB, Ryan H. Corticosteroids for managing tuberculous meningitis. Cochrane Database Syst Rev. 2016;4(4):CD002244.
42. Thwaites G, Fisher M, Hemingway C, Scott G, Solomon T, Innes J. British Infection Society. British Infection Society guidelines for the diagnosis and treatment of tuberculosis of the central nervous system in adults and children. J Infect. 2009;59(3):167–87.
43. National Collaborating Centre for chronic conditions (UK), Centre for Clinical Practice at NICE (UK). Tuberculosis: clinical diagnosis and management of tuberculosis, and measures for its prevention and control. London: National Institute for Health and Clinical Excellence (UK); 2011.
44. Prasad K, Singh MB. Corticosteroids for managing tuberculous meningitis. Cochrane Database Syst Rev. 2008;1(1):CD002244.
45. Brouwer MC, van de Beek D. Epidemiology, diagnosis, and treatment of brain abscesses. Curr Opin Infect Dis. 2017;30(1):129–34. https://doi.org/10.1097/QCO.0000000000000334.
46. Simjian T, Muskens IS, Lamba N, Yunusa I, Wong K, Veronneau R, et al. Dexamethasone administration and mortality in patients with brain abscess: a systematic review and meta-analysis. World Neurosurg. 2018;115:257–63.

47. Brouwer MC, Tunkel AR, McKhann GM 2nd, Van de Beek D. Brain abscess. N Engl J Med. 2014;371(5):447–56.
48. Meyding-Lamadé U, Jacobi C, Martinez-Torres F, Lenhard T, Kress B, Kieser M, et al. The German trial on Aciclovir and corticosteroids in herpes-simplex-virus-encephalitis (GACHE): a multicenter, randomized, double-blind, placebo-controlled trial. Neurol Res Pract. 2019;1:26.
49. Ramos-Estebanez C, Lizarraga KJ, Merenda A. A systematic review on the role of adjunctive corticosteroids in herpes simplex virus encephalitis: is timing critical for safety and efficacy? Antivir Ther. 2014;19(2):133–9.
50. Kamei S, Sekizawa T, Shiota H, Mizutani T, Itoyama Y, Takasu T, et al. Evaluation of combination therapy using aciclovir and corticosteroid in adult patients with herpes simplex virus encephalitis. J Neurol Neurosurg Psychiatry. 2005;76(11):1544–9.
51. Mesker AJ, Bon GG, de Gans J, de Kruijk JR. Case report: a pregnant woman with herpes simplex encephalitis successfully treated with dexamethasone. Eur J Obstet Gynecol Reprod Biol. 2011;154:231–2.
52. Maraş Genç H, Uyur Yalçın E, Sayan M, Bayhan A, Öncel S, Arısoy ES, Kara B. Clinical outcomes in children with herpes simplex encephalitis receiving steroid therapy. J Clin Virol. 2016;80:87–92.
53. Abanto J, Blanco D, Saavedra H, Gonzales I, Siu D, Pretell EJ. Cysticercosis working Group in Peru, et al. mortality in parenchymal and subarachnoid neurocysticercosis. Am J Trop Med Hyg. 2021;105(1):176–80.
54. Singhi P. Neurocysticercosis. Ther Adv Neurol Disord. 2011;4(2):67–81.
55. Cuello-García CA, Roldán-Benítez YM, Pérez-Gaxiola G, Villarreal-Careaga J. Corticosteroids for neurocysticercosis: a systematic review and meta-analysis of randomized controlled trials. Int J Infect Dis. 2013;17(8):e583–92.
56. White AC Jr, Coyle CM, Rajshekhar V, Singh G, Hauser WA, Mohanty A, Garcia HH, et al. Diagnosis and treatment of neurocysticercosis: 2017 clinical practice guidelines by the Infectious Diseases Society of America (IDSA) and the American Society of Tropical Medicine and Hygiene (ASTMH). Clin Infect Dis. 2018;66(8):e49–75.
57. Vidal JE. HIV-related cerebral toxoplasmosis revisited: current concepts and controversies of an old disease. J Int Assoc Provid AIDS Care. 2019;18:2325958219867315.
58. Pereira-Chioccola VL, Vidal JE, Su C. Toxoplasma gondii infection and cerebral toxoplasmosis in HIV-infected patients. Future Microbiol. 2009;4(10):1363–79.
59. Beardsley J, Wolbers M, Kibengo FM, Ggayi AB, Kamali A, Cuc NT, et al. Adjunctive dexamethasone in HIV-associated cryptococcal meningitis. N Engl J Med. 2016;374(6):542–54.
60. Murdoch DM, Venter WD, Van Rie A, Feldman C. Immune reconstitution inflammatory syndrome (IRIS): review of common infectious manifestations and treatment options. AIDS Res Ther. 2007;4:9.
61. Singh AK, Malhotra HS, Garg RK, Jain A, Kumar N, Kohli N, et al. Paradoxical reaction in tuberculous meningitis: presentation, predictors and impact on prognosis. BMC Infect Dis. 2016;16:306.
62. El Fane M, Mustapha S, Chakib A, Marhoum EL, Filali K. HIV and immune reconstitution inflammatory syndrome (HIV-IRIS). J Infect Dis Pathog. 2018;1(2):1–8.
63. Bowen L, Nath A, Smith B. CNS immune reconstitution inflammatory syndrome. Handb Clin Neurol. 2018;152:167–76.
64. Bhagavati S. Autoimmune disorders of the nervous system: pathophysiology, clinical features, and therapy. Front Neurol. 2021;12:664664.
65. Milligan NM, Newcombe R, Compston DA. A double-blind controlled trial of high dose methylprednisolone in patients with multiple sclerosis: 1. Clinical effects. J Neurol Neurosurg Psychiatry. 1987;50(5):511–6.
66. Filippini G, Brusaferri F, Sibley WA, Citterio A, Ciucci G, Midgard R, et al. Corticosteroids or ACTH for acute exacerbations in multiple sclerosis. Cochrane Database Syst Rev. 2000;(4):CD001331.
67. Le Page E, Veillard D, Laplaud DA, Hamonic S, Wardi R, Lebrun C, et al. Oral versus intravenous high-dose methylprednisolone for treatment of relapses in patients with multiple sclerosis (COPOUSEP): a randomised, controlled, double-blind, non-inferiority trial. Lancet. 2015;386(9997):974–81.
68. Yamout B, Sahraian M, Bohlega S, Al-Jumah M, Goueider R, Dahdaleh M, et al. Consensus recommendations for the diagnosis and treatment of multiple sclerosis: 2019 revisions to the MENACTRIMS guidelines. Mult Scler Relat Disord. 2020;37:101459.
69. Sanders DB, Wolfe GI, Benatar M, Evoli A, Gilhus NE, Illa I, et al. International consensus guidance for management of myasthenia gravis: executive summary. Neurology. 2016;87(4):419–25.
70. Schneider-Gold C, Gajdos P, Toyka KV, Hohlfeld RR. Corticosteroids for myasthenia gravis. Cochrane Database Syst Rev. 2005;2005(2):CD002828.
71. Tian X, Wang X, Kwan P. Editorial: advances in steroid-responsive encephalopathy. Front Neurol. 2020;11:793.
72. Abboud H, Probasco JC, Irani S, Ances B, Benavides DR, Bradshaw M, et al. Autoimmune encephalitis: proposed best practice recommendations for diagnosis and acute management. J Neurol Neurosurg Psychiatry. 2021;92(7):757 68.
73. Massa S, Fracchiolla A, Neglia C, Argentiero A, Esposito S. Update on acute disseminated encephalomyelitis in children and adolescents. Children (Basel). 2021;8(4):280.
74. Salvarani C, Brown RD Jr, Christianson TJ, Huston J 3rd, Giannini C, Miller DV, et al. Adult primary

central nervous system vasculitis treatment and course: analysis of one hundred sixty-three patients. Arthritis Rheumatol. 2015;67(6):1637–45.
75. Nosadini M, Mohammad SS, Ramanathan S, Brilot F, Dale RC. Immune therapy in autoimmune encephalitis: a systematic review. Expert Rev Neurother. 2015;15(12):1391–419.
76. Pascuzzi RM, Coslett HB, Johns TR. Long-term corticosteroid treatment of myasthenia gravis: report of 116 patients. Ann Neurol. 1984;15(3):291–8.
77. Dalmau J, Lancaster E, Martinez-Hernandez E, Rosenfeld MR, Balice-Gordon R. Clinical experience and laboratory investigations in patients with anti-NMDAR encephalitis. Lancet Neurol. 2011;10(1):63–74.
78. Alexander M, Murthy JM. Acute disseminated encephalomyelitis: treatment guidelines. Ann Indian Acad Neurol. 2011;14(Suppl. 1):S60–4.
79. Tunkel AR, Glaser CA, Bloch KC, Sejvar JJ, Marra CM, Roos KL, et al. The management of encephalitis: clinical practice guidelines by the Infectious Diseases Society of America. Clin Infect Dis. 2008;47(3):303–27.
80. Britton PN, Eastwood K, Paterson B, Durrheim DN, Dale RC, Cheng AC, et al. Consensus guidelines for the investigation and management of encephalitis in adults and children in Australia and New Zealand. Intern Med J. 2015;45(5):563–76.
81. Shin YW, Lee ST, Park KI, Jung KH, Jung KY, Lee SK, et al. Treatment strategies for autoimmune encephalitis. Ther Adv Neurol Disord. 2017;11:1756285617722347.
82. Hansebout RR. Spinal injury and spinal cord bloodflow: the effect of early treatment and local cooling. In: Illis LS, editor. Spinal cord dysfunction: volume II: intervention and treatment. Oxford Press; 1992. p. 58.
83. Lewin MG, Pappius HM, Hansebout RR. Effects of steroids on edema associated with injury of the spinal cord. In: Reulen HJ, Schürmann K, editors. Steroids and brain edema. Berlin, Heidelberg: Springer; 1972. p. 101.
84. Bracken MB, Collins WF, Freeman DF, Shepard MJ, Wagner FW, Silten RM, et al. Efficacy of methylprednisolone in acute spinal cord injury. JAMA. 1984;251(1):45–52.
85. Bracken MB, Shepard MJ, Collins WF, Holford TR, Young W, Baskin DS, et al. A randomized, controlled trial of methylprednisolone or naloxone in the treatment of acute spinal-cord injury. Results of the second national acute spinal cord injury study. N Engl J Med. 1990;322(20):1405–11.
86. Bracken MB, Shepard MJ, Holford TR, Leo-Summers L, Aldrich EF, Fazl M, et al. Administration of methylprednisolone for 24 or 48 h or tirilazad mesylate for 48 h in the treatment of acute spinal cord injury. Results of the third National Acute Spinal Cord Injury Randomized Controlled Trial. National Acute Spinal Cord Injury Study. JAMA. 1997;277(20):1597–604.
87. Bracken MB. Steroids for acute spinal cord injury. Cochrane Database Syst Rev. 2012;1(1):CD001046
88. Short DJ, El Masry WS, Jones PW. High dose methylprednisolone in the management of acute spinal cord injury—a systematic review from a clinical perspective. Spinal Cord. 2000;38(5):273–86.
89. Lee HC, Cho DY, Lee WY, Chuang HC. Pitfalls in treatment of acute cervical spinal cord injury using high-dose methylprednisolone: a retrospect audit of 111 patients. Surg Neurol. 2007;68(Suppl. 1):S37–41.
90. Fehlings MG, Wilson JR, Harrop JS, Kwon BK, Tetreault LA, Arnold PM, et al. Efficacy and safety of methylprednisolone sodium succinate in acute spinal cord injury: a systematic review. Global Spine J. 2017;7(Suppl. 3):116S–37S.
91. Canadian Association of Emergency Physicians. Position statement: Steroids in acute spinal cord injury. www.caep.ca (Accessed on April 19, 2024).
92. Walters BC, Hadley MN, Hurlbert RJ, Aarabi B, Dhall SS, Gelb DE, et al. Guidelines for the management of acute cervical spine and spinal cord injuries: 2013 update. Neurosurgery. 2013;60(Suppl. 1):82–91.
93. Annane D, Buisson CB, Cariou A, Martin C, Misset B, Renault A, APROCCHSS Investigators for the TRIGGERSEP Network, et al. Design and conduct of the activated protein C and corticosteroids for human septic shock (APROCCHSS) trial. Ann Intensive Care. 2016;6(1):43.
94. Venkatesh B, Finfer S, Cohen J, Rajbhandari D, Arabi Y, Bellomo R, ADRENAL Trial Investigators and the Australian–New Zealand Intensive Care Society Clinical Trials Group, et al. Adjunctive glucocorticoid therapy in patients with septic shock. N Engl J Med. 2018;378(9):797–808.
95. Annane D, Renault A, Brun-Buisson C, Megarbane B, Quenot JP, Siami S, et al. Hydrocortisone plus fludrocortisone for adults with septic shock. N Engl J Med. 2018;378(9):809–18.
96. Annane D, Bellissant E, Bollaert PE, Briegel J, Keh D, Kupfer Y, et al. Corticosteroids for treating sepsis in children and adults. Cochrane Database Syst Rev. 2019;12(12):CD002243.
97. Rygård SL, Butler E, Granholm A, Møller MH, Cohen J, Finfer S, et al. Low-dose corticosteroids for adult patients with septic shock: a systematic review with meta-analysis and trial sequential analysis. Intensive Care Med. 2018;44(7):1003–16.
98. Keh D, Trips E, Marx G, Wirtz SP, Abduljawwad E, Bercker S. SepNet–critical care trials group, et al. effect of hydrocortisone on development of shock among patients with severe sepsis: the HYPRESS randomized clinical trial. JAMA. 2016;316(17):1775–85.
99. Evans L, Rhodes A, Alhazzani W, Antonelli M, Coopersmith CM, French C, et al. Executive summary: surviving sepsis campaign: international guidelines for the Management of Sepsis and Septic Shock 2021. Crit Care Med. 2021;49(11):1974–82.

100. Steinberg KP, Hudson LD, Goodman RB, Hough CL, Lanken PN, Hyzy R, National Heart, Lung and Blood Institute Acute Respiratory Distress Syndrome (ARDS) Clinical Trials Network, et al. Efficacy and safety of corticosteroids for persistent acute respiratory distress syndrome. N Engl J Med. 2006;354(16):1671–84.
101. Meduri GU, Bridges L, Shih MC, Marik PE, Siemieniuk RAC, Kocak M. Prolonged glucocorticoid treatment is associated with improved ARDS outcomes: analysis of individual patients' data from four randomized trials and trial-level meta-analysis of the updated literature. Intensive Care Med. 2016;42(5):829–40.
102. Annane D, Sébille V, Bellissant E, Ger-Inf-05 Study Group. Effect of low doses of corticosteroids in septic shock patients with or without early acute respiratory distress syndrome. Crit Care Med. 2006;34(1):22–30.
103. Villar J, Ferrando C, Martínez D, Ambrós A, Muñoz T, Soler JA, Dexamethasone in ARDS Network, et al. Dexamethasone treatment for the acute respiratory distress syndrome: a multicentre, randomised controlled trial. Lancet Respir Med. 2020;8(3):267–76.
104. Chaudhuri D, Sasaki K, Karkar A, Sharif S, Lewis K, Mammen MJ, et al. Corticosteroids in COVID-19 and non-COVID-19 ARDS: a systematic review and meta-analysis. Intensive Care Med. 2021;47(5):521–57.
105. Kuriyama A, Umakoshi N, Sun R. Prophylactic corticosteroids for prevention of postextubation stridor and reintubation in adults: a systematic review and metaanalysis. Chest. 2017;151:1002e10.
106. British Thoracic Society and Scottish Intercollegiate Guidelines Network. SIGN 153: British guideline on the management of asthma: a national clinical guideline.
107. Braakman R, Schouten HJ, Blaauw-van Dishoeck M, Minderhoud JM. Megadose steroids in severe head injury. Results of a prospective double-blind clinical trial. J Neurosurg. 1983;58(3):326–30.
108. Roberts I, Yates D, Sandercock P, Farrell B, Wasserberg J, Lomas G, CRASH Trial Collaborators, et al. Effect of intravenous corticosteroids on death within 14 days in 10008 adults with clinically significant head injury (MRC CRASH trial): randomised placebo-controlled trial. Lancet. 2004;364(9442):1321–8.
109. Carney N, Totten AM, O'Reilly C, Ullman JS, Hawryluk GW, Bell MJ, et al. Guidelines for the management of severe traumatic brain injury, fourth edition. Neurosurgery 2017; 80(1): 6–15.
110. Sandercock PA, Soane T. Corticosteroids for acute ischaemic stroke. Cochrane Database Syst Rev. 2011;2011(9):CD000064.
111. Feigin VL, Anderson N, Rinkel GJ, Algra A, van Gijn J, Bennett DA. Corticosteroids for aneurysmal subarachnoid haemorrhage and primary intracerebral haemorrhage. Cochrane Database Syst Rev. 2005;3:CD004583.
112. Hughes RA, Brassington R, Gunn AA, van Doorn PA. Corticosteroids for Guillain-Barré syndrome. Cochrane Database Syst Rev. 2016;10(10):CD001446.
113. Gurnurkar S, Villacres S, Warner L, Chegondi M. Successful use of fludrocortisone in a child with refractory cerebral salt wasting syndrome: a case report and review of literature. Cureus. 2018;10(10):e3505.
114. Misra UK, Kalita J, Kumar M. Safety and efficacy of fludrocortisone in the treatment of cerebral salt wasting in patients with tuberculous meningitis: a randomized clinical trial. JAMA Neurol. 2018;75(11):1383–91.
115. Yee AH, Burns JD, Wijdicks EF. Cerebral salt wasting: pathophysiology, diagnosis, and treatment. Neurosurg Clin N Am. 2010;21(2):339–52.
116. Choi MJ, Oh YS, Park SJ, Kim JH, Shin JI. Cerebral salt wasting treated with fludrocortisone in a 17-year-old boy. Yonsei Med J. 2012;53(4):859–62.
117. Lee P, Jones GR, Center JR. Successful treatment of adult cerebral salt wasting with fludrocortisone. Arch Intern Med. 2008;168(3):325–6.
118. Momi J, Tang CM, Abcar AC, Kujubu DA, Sim JJ. Hyponatremia-what is cerebral salt wasting? Perm J. 2010;14(2):62–5.
119. Hasan D, Lindsay KW, Wijdicks EF, et al. Effect of fludrocortisone acetate in patients with subarachnoid hemorrhage. Stroke. 1989;20(9):1156–61.
120. Wijdicks EF, Vermeulen M, van Brummelen P, van Gijn J. The effect of fludrocortisone acetate on plasma volume and natriuresis in patients with aneurysmal subarachnoid hemorrhage. Clin Neurol Neurosurg. 1988;90(3):209–14.

Antipsychotic Drugs

25

Sarang Naresh Kshirsagar and Tapas Kumar Sahoo

25.1 Introduction

Antipsychotics, commonly referred to as neuroleptics, is a class of medications used to treat several psychiatric diseases including schizophrenia, bipolar disorder, and other ailments that are similar. They may be used in critical care settings for various reasons, including the treatment of delirium or agitation in critically ill patients. However, the use of antipsychotics in critical care should be carefully considered due to the potential risks and benefits.

Delirium is a common complication in critically ill patients and can lead to poor outcomes, including longer hospital stays and higher mortality rates. Agitation can also be a problem in critically ill patients, especially those who are mechanically ventilated. Antipsychotics may be used to manage agitation, but caution should be taken to avoid over sedation, which can lead to respiratory depression or prolonged mechanical ventilation.

The use of antipsychotic medications in critical care should be carefully evaluated and individualized based on the patient's specific needs and risks. Close monitoring is essential to ensure optimal dosing and to prevent devastating adverse effects.

25.2 Classification

Typical or first-generation antipsychotics (FGAs) and atypical or second-generation antipsychotics (SGAs) are the two primary classes of neuroleptics that can be distinguished pharmacologically.

FGAs prevent the function of dopamine at its receptors in the brain. They include medications like fluphenazine, haloperidol, and chlorpromazine. Usually, FGAs are categorized according to their potency, with high-potency FGAs having a stronger affinity for dopamine receptors and a weaker affinity for other types of receptors in the brain [1–4].

SGAs are also dopamine receptor antagonists, however, have a broader receptor profile than FGAs. They can more effectively treat negative and cognitive symptoms of schizophrenia because they block both dopamine and serotonin receptors in the brain. SGAs include medications including risperidone, clozapine, and olanzapine [5].

Second-generation agents	First-generation agents
Aripiprazole	Chlorpromazine
Asenapine	Fluphenazine
Brexpiprazole	Haloperidol
Cariprazine	Loxapine

S. N. Kshirsagar
Department of Critical Care, University Health Network, Toronto, ON, Canada

T. K. Sahoo (✉)
Department of Critical Care, Medanta Hospital, Ranchi, Jharkhand, India

H. Prabhakar et al. (eds.), *Principles and Practice of Neurocritical Care*,
https://doi.org/10.1007/978-981-99-8059-8_25

Second-generation agents	First-generation agents
Clozapine	Molindone
Iloperidone	Perphenazine
Lumateperone	Pimozide
Lurasidone	Thioridazine
Olanzapine	Thiothixene
Paliperidone	Trifluoperazine
Pimavanserin	
Quetiapine	
Risperidone	
Ziprasidone	

25.3 Mechanism of Action

Neuroleptic drugs have a complicated and poorly known mechanism of action, but dopamine, serotonin, and norepinephrine are among the neurotransmitters thought to be involved.

Their main effect is to stop the brain's dopamine receptors from working. Dopamine activity in the mesolimbic pathway, a reward pathway in the brain linked to psychotic symptoms like delusions and hallucinations, is decreased as a result.

The mechanism of action of first-generation antipsychotic medications is the postsynaptic blockade of dopamine D2 receptors in the brain including the mesolimbic system. There is a stronger relationship between D2 receptor binding and potency and they strongly antagonize D2 receptors in both striatal and cortical areas. Functional brain imaging studies suggest that FGA's need to occupy more than 65% of D2 receptors for their adequate effects. They also block the 5-HT2A, histaminic, muscarinic, and alpha1 receptors in the neurons [6, 7].

High-potency FGAs are required in lower doses. They have lesser sedation and weight gain potential due to their activity on the histamine and muscarinic receptors being low. They have increased risk of extra pyramidal side effects, e.g., haloperidol.

The low-potency FGAs have increased risk for sedation and low risk for EPS as they have increased activity on histamine and muscarinic receptors. They are required in higher doses, e.g., chlorpromazine [8–10].

FGAs are lipophilic and have high affinity for protein and tissue binding, with high volume of distribution. They are metabolized by the cytochrome P450 system.

Second-generation antipsychotics occupy D2 receptors for a short period of time. They rapidly dissociate and allow normal dopamine neurotransmission. They also act on the serotonin receptors mainly 5HT2A and 5HT1A. They have higher binding to serotonin receptors as compared to D2 receptors. These contribute to lower risk of EPS. They have partial agonist or blockade activity on the muscarinic, alpha1, and histamine receptors [11, 12].

Each SGA has a different rate of absorption. They are too metabolized by the cytochrome P450 system and glucuronidation pathway in the liver.

25.3.1 Indication [13–20]

1. Neuroleptics are frequently used to treat the signs and symptoms of schizophrenia, a long-term mental illness that is characterized by a variety of symptoms, including hallucinations, delusions, and distorted thinking.
2. Manic or mixed bouts of bipolar disorder, a mood condition that causes episodes of both mania and sadness, may be treated using neuroleptics.
3. Major depressive disorder: Certain atypical antipsychotics might be used as an adjuvant therapy for major depressive disorder, particularly if previous therapies haven't worked.
4. Neuroleptics may be used to treat severe depression that has psychotic symptoms, such as hallucinations and delusions.
5. Delirium: Patients who are hospitalized, especially the elderly, may have delirium, a state of acute confusion and altered awareness, which can be treated with neuroleptics.
6. Certain neuroleptics may be used to treat the tics brought on by Tourette syndrome, a neurological condition that results in uncontrollable movements and vocalizations.

7. Atypical antipsychotics are frequently used off-label to treat the mood and behavioral symptoms associated with dementia.
8. Severe agitation: Anti psychotics can be used for acute management of severely agitated, hyperactive patients.
9. Borderline personality disorder: Antipsychotics helps in management of symptoms of psychosis and paranoia in such patients.
10. Substance induced psychotic disorder: They can be used for control for severe agitation in patients of substance abuse like alcohol withdrawal.

25.3.2 Side Effects

Antipsychotic medications can have a range of side effects, some of which can be serious requiring ICU admission. The side effects of antipsychotics can vary depending on the specific medication and the individual taking it [21, 22].

Some of the more common side effects include:

1. Anti-Dopaminergic side effects:
   - (a) Extra Pyramidal Symptoms [23].
   - (b) Hyperprolactinemia: increase in the hormone prolactin, which can lead to problems like breast enlargement and milk production in men and women. Change to prolactin sparing antipsychotics and consider lowering dose of the agents. Palipridone, rispridone amongst the second generation and Fluphenazine, Haloperidol, pimozide and thiothixene have the highest propensity [16, 24].
   - (c) NMS(Neuroleptic Malignant Syndrome) [25].
2. Anti-HAM(Histaminic-Adrenergic-Muscarinic) side effects.
   - (a) Anti-Histaminic:
     - (i) Sedation: Can take dose of medication at night before sleep, lower the dose. It is commonly seen with clozapine, olanzapine and quetiapine, chlorpromazine, thioridazine [24].
   - (b) Anti-alpha adrenergic:
     - (i) Orthostatic hypotension: To prevent careful titration of the doses and timings is needed. It is seen commonly with clozapine, Ilopridone, chlorpromazine, and thioridazine. Maintain adequate hydration to prevent hypotension [22].
     - (ii) Cardiac abnormalities: cardiac arrhythmias, QTc prolongation, myocarditis, and sudden death. It is a dose-dependent phenomenon and is more common in thioridazine, i.v. haloperidol and ziprasidone. In high-risk patients, change the antipsychotic agents or discontinue the drug in patients with symptoms. There is no proven effectiveness of checking baseline or post treatment electrocardiography [26–29].
     - (iii) Sexual dysfunction: Decreased libido and erectile dysfunction: Lower the dose, consider phosphodiesterase inhibitors drug [30, 31].
   - (c) Anti-muscarinic: Treatment consists of lowering the agent dose and symptomatic treatment. Clozapine, chlorpromazine, and thioridazine are the most common agents causing symptoms. Limit the use of other anti-cholinergic agents [32].
     - (i) Dry mouth.
     - (ii) Tachycardia.
     - (iii) Urinary Retention.
     - (iv) Blurry vision.
     - (v) Constipation.
   - (d) Obesity/weight gain: Weight gain, which can lead to metabolic problems like diabetes mellitus and high blood pressure. Clozapine and olanzapine have the highest risk. Behavioral changes including diet and exercise. Consider metformin, or switching over to ariprazole, pimavanserin, or ziprasidone. Glucose intolerance is common with clozapine, olanzapine, and quetiapine [33, 34].

(e) Dyslipidemia: Increase in triglyceride levels primarily. Higher risk associated with low-potency FGAs and clozapine, olanzapine, and quetiapine. Such patients should have annual checkup for familial history and measurement of waist circumference; quarterly blood pressure, fasting blood glucose and lipid profile; and monthly weight measurements after initiation of treatment. It is common with clozapine, olanzapine, and quetiapine [35–38].
(f) Ophthalmologic problems.
(g) Dermatological problems.
(h) Liver enzyme elevation.
(i) Seizures: All antipsychotics can lower the seizure threshold. Low-potency FGA's and clozapine have higher risk of seizure potentiation [39].

3. Blood dyscrasias: Neutropenia, leukopenia, and agranulocytosis. Clozapine may cause neutropenia and agranulocytosis, which can lead to fatal infections. Patient require weekly WBC count monitoring for the first 6 months, every 2 weeks for the next 6 months, and monthly afterward [40, 41].

25.3.3 Contraindications

First-generation antipsychotics are contraindicated in the following situations:

1. Cardiac arrhythmias and other severe cardiac disorders.
2. Concomitant with anticholinergic medication as it can lead to EPS.
3. Allergic reaction to previous use of antipsychotics.
4. Concomitant use of opioids, benzodiazepines, or other depressants.
5. History of seizure disorder.

Second-generation antipsychotics

1. FDA Black box warning for a rise in stroke incidence in senior dementia patients [42].
2. Concomitant use with other medications that lengthen the QTc interval.

Common contraindications:

1. first trimester of pregnancy, should only be taken only if the advantages of treatment outweigh the dangers.
2. Avoided during breast feeding because antipsychotics are secreted in breast milk.

Anti-Psychotics Related Problems in ICU

A. Delirium is experienced by 50–80% of mechanically ventilated patients and 20–50% of patients with lower-severity illness, resulting in prolonged hospitalization and duration of mechanical ventilation and increased costs. Long-term effects include increased risk of mortality and long-term cognitive impairment. The 2018 practice guidelines for PADIS has recommended that assessment for delirium should be done at least once per shift in all adult ICU patients regularly [43]. The tools used are.
   1. Confusion Assessment Method for the ICU (CAM-ICU). It is a four-domain assessment [44, 45].

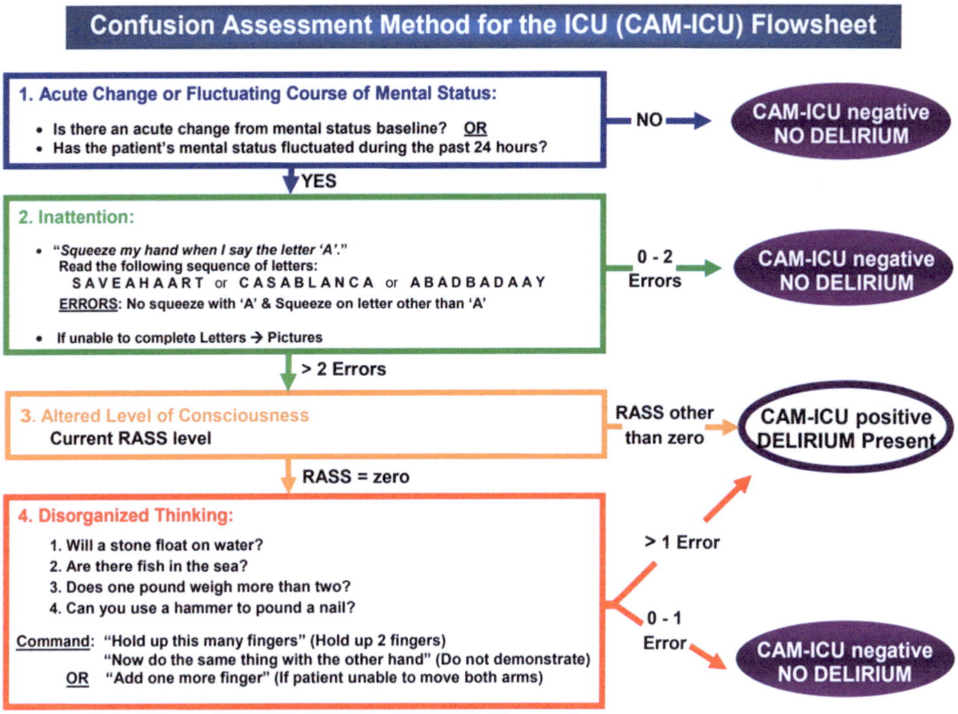

(Copyright © 2002, E. Wesley Ely, MD, MPH and Vanderbilt University, all rights reserved)

2. Intensive Care Delirium Screening Checklist (ICDSC) [46]. Eight items are rated as present = 1 or absent = 0. Score 0 is normal, 1–3 subsyndromal delirium, 4–8 delirium.

They consist of

(a) Altered level of consciousness.
(b) Inattention.
(c) Disorientation.
(d) Hallucination, delusion, or psychosis.
(e) Psychomotor agitation or retardation.
(f) Inappropriate speech or mood.
(g) Sleep-wake cycle disturbance.
(h) Symptom fluctuation.

Both of these scales can be finished in a short amount of time, allowing repeated assessment per day.

B. Extra Pyramidal Symptoms: [23]

Adverse effects	Common drugs causing symptoms	Onset	Symptoms	Treatment
Dystonia's	Fluphenazine, haloperidol, thiothixene	>3 h	Acute muscle stiffness, rigidity, spasm of body parts or eye deviation	Benztropines is the treatment of choice. Can use anti histaminic and benzodiazepines
Pseudo-parkinsonism	Fluphenazine, haloperidol, pimozide, thiothixene	3 days–3 weeks	Shuffling gait, mask facies, drooling, rigidity, and tremors	Lower the dose, use antihistaminic, diphenhydramine, or benztropine
Akathisia	Fluphenazine, haloperidol, pimozide, thiothixene	Usually >3 months	Subjective feeling of restlessness, inability to sit still, constant pacing up and down	Benzodiazepines, consider lowering the dose or changing agent, low-dose beta blockers
Tardive dyskinesia	Fluphenazine, haloperidol, pimozide, thiothixene, Chlorpromazine	Usually >3 years	Involuntary movement of orofacial muscles like tongue protrusion, puckering, chewing, or grimacing. Disappear during sleep.	Stop the offending agent, change to atypical antipsychotics, benzodiazepines, lower the dose of agent

25.4 Neuroleptic Malignant Syndrome

It is a rare, but life threatening, idiosyncratic reaction to neuroleptic medications. Can occur within hours of taking particular medications. It is characterized by high-grade fever (>38 °C), altered mental status, muscular rigidity, autonomic dysfunction, excessive sweating [25, 47].

Common medications causing NMS: antipsychotics like haloperidol, chlorpromazine, thioridazine, clozapine, antiemetic's like metoclopramide, promethazine.

Risk factors include dehydration, agitation, and catatonia. Use of high potency neuroleptics, a rapid increase in the dosage of neuroleptics, and use of long-acting forms of neuroleptics. NMS has no relationship to the duration of treatment [48, 49].

Pathophysiology: The mechanism is commonly thought to depend on decreased levels of dopamine activity due to [50]:

- Blockade of dopamine receptor.
- Genetically reduced function of dopamine receptor D2.
- Sympathoadrenal hyperactivity and autonomic dysfunction.

Diagnosis: Is mostly clinical. Laboratory work may show increased liver enzyme, urine myoglobin, myoglobinemia, and metabolic acidosis.

Complications: Rhabdomyolysis, hyperkalemia, acute kidney injury, seizures rarely death [47].

D/d: serotonin syndrome, malignant hyperthermia.

Treatment: Is mainly supportive. Primary treatment is to stop the offending agent.

(a) Hyperthermia: Dantrolone, cooling blankets, antipyretics, cooled iv fluids.
(b) Agitation: Benzodiazepine.
(c) Anti-dopaminergic effects: give dopamine agonist like bromocriptine, amantadine.

25.5 Conclusion

In conclusion, antipsychotics are used in ICU for multiple reasons like managing delirium, agitation, and other behavioral symptoms in critically ill patients. They can help improve patient outcomes by reducing the risk of adverse events, minimizing the need for physical restraints, and improving overall patient comfort. Given the higher cardiometabolic risk factors and concomitant use of various other medications, the use of antipsychotics in the ICU requires careful consideration and monitoring. It is essential to follow proper dosing guidelines, monitor for drug interactions, and adjust therapy as needed to achieve optimal outcomes. Multidisciplinary collaboration among critical care teams, psychiatrists, and pharmacists can help ensure safe and effective use of antipsychotics in the ICU. Overall, the judicious use of antipsychotics in the ICU can lead to improved patient outcomes and a better quality of care.

References

1. Cussotto S, Clarke G, Dinan TG, Cryan JF. Psychotropics and the microbiome: a chamber of secrets. Psychopharmacology. 2019;236(5):1411–32. https://doi.org/10.1007/s00213-019-5185-8.
2. Drummond N, McCleary L, Freiheit E, et al. Antidepressant and antipsychotic prescribing in primary care for people with dementia. Can Fam Physician. 2018;64(11):e488–97.
3. Jennings AA, Guerin N, Foley T. Development of a tool for monitoring the prescribing of antipsychotic medications to people with dementia in general practice: a modified eDelphi consensus study. Clin Interv Aging. 2018;13:2107–17. https://doi.org/10.2147/CIA.S178216.
4. Faden J, Citrome L. Resistance is not futile: treatment-refractory schizophrenia - overview, evaluation and treatment. Expert Opin Pharmacother. 2019;20(1):11–24. https://doi.org/10.1080/14656566.2018.1543409.
5. Haddad PM, Correll CU. The acute efficacy of antipsychotics in schizophrenia: a review of recent meta-analyses. Ther Adv Psychopharmacol. 2018;8(11):303–18. https://doi.org/10.1177/2045125318781475.
6. Stone JM, Davis JM, Leucht S, Pilowsky LS. Cortical dopamine D2/D3 receptors are a common site of action for antipsychotic drugs—an original patient data meta-analysis of the SPECT and PET in vivo receptor imaging literature. Schizophr Bull. 2009;35(4):789–97. https://doi.org/10.1093/schbul/sbn009.
7. Kapur S, Zipursky R, Jones C, Remington G, Houle S. Relationship between dopamine D(2) occupancy, clinical response, and side effects: a double-blind PET study of first-episode schizophrenia. Am J Psychiatry. 2000;157(4):514–20. https://doi.org/10.1176/appi.ajp.157.4.514.
8. Kotlinska-Lemieszek A, Klepstad P, Haugen DF. Clinically significant drug-drug interactions involving medications used for symptom control in patients with advanced malignant disease: a systematic review. J Pain Symptom Manag. 2019;57(5):989–98. https://doi.org/10.1016/j.jpainsymman.2019.02.006.
9. von Malortie S, Cronqvist E, Ringbäck G, et al. Nya nationella riktlinjer för vård och stöd vid schizofreni—Lyfter fram "återhämtningsperspektivet": Rehabilitering i kombination med läkemedel kan ge bättre livskvalitet [New national guidelines for the treatment of schizophrenia in Sweden]. Lakartidningen. 2019;116:FFPU. Published 2019 Jan 28
10. Taylor DM, Velaga S, Werneke U. Reducing the stigma of long acting injectable antipsychotics—current concepts and future developments [published correction appears in Nord J psychiatry. 2022;76(8):634]. Nord J Psychiatry. 2018;72(Suppl. 1):S36–9. https://doi.org/10.1080/08039488.2018.1525638.
11. Meltzer HY. What's atypical about atypical antipsychotic drugs? Curr Opin Pharmacol. 2004;4(1):53–7. https://doi.org/10.1016/j.coph.2003.09.010.
12. Seeman P. Atypical antipsychotics: mechanism of action. Can J Psychiatr. 2002;47(1):27–38.
13. Bartoli F, Cavaleri D, Callovini T, et al. Comparing 1-year effectiveness and acceptability of once-monthly paliperidone palmitate and aripiprazole monohydrate for schizophrenia spectrum disorders: findings from the STAR network depot study. Psychiatry Res. 2022;309:114405. https://doi.org/10.1016/j.psychres.2022.114405.
14. Leucht S, Corves C, Arbter D, Engel RR, Li C, Davis JM. Second-generation versus first-generation antipsychotic drugs for schizophrenia: a meta-analysis. Lancet. 2009;373(9657):31–41. https://doi.org/10.1016/S0140-6736(08)61764-X.
15. Goikolea JM, Colom F, Torres I, Capapey J, Valentí M, Undurraga J, Grande I, Sanchez-Moreno J, Vieta E. Lower rate of depressive switch following antimanic treatment with second-generation antipsychotics versus haloperidol. J Affect Disord. 2013;144(3):191–8. https://doi.org/10.1016/j.jad.2012.07.038.
16. Taylor D, Paton C, Kapur S, Taylor D. The Maudsley prescribing guidelines in psychiatry. 11th ed. Chichester, West Sussex, UK: Wiley-Blackwell; 2012. 978-0-470-97948-8.
17. Budman CL. The role of atypical antipsychotics for treatment of Tourette's syndrome: an overview. Drugs. 2014;74(11):1177–93. https://doi.org/10.1007/s40265-014-0254-0.
18. Basson R, Gilks T. Women's sexual dysfunction associated with psychiatric disorders and their treatment. Womens Health (Lond). 2018;14:1745506518762664. https://doi.org/10.1177/1745506518762664.
19. Kreys TJ, Phan SV. A literature review of quetiapine for generalized anxiety disorder. Pharmacotherapy. 2015;35(2):175–88. https://doi.org/10.1002/phar.1529.
20. Chokhawala K, Stevens L. Antipsychotic medications [updated 2023 Feb 26]. In: StatPearls. Treasure Island, FL: StatPearls Publishing; 2023. Available from: https://www.ncbi.nlm.nih.gov/books/NBK519503/.

21. Muench J, Hamer AM. Adverse effects of antipsychotic medications. Am Fam Physician. 2010;81(5):617–22.
22. Haddad PM, Sharma SG. Adverse effects of atypical antipsychotics: differential risk and clinical implications. CNS Drugs. 2007;21(11):911–36. https://doi.org/10.2165/00023210-200721110-00004.
23. Carbon M, Kane JM, Leucht S, Correll CU. Tardive dyskinesia risk with first- and second-generation antipsychotics in comparative randomized controlled trials: a meta-analysis. World Psychiatry. 2018;17(3):330–40. https://doi.org/10.1002/wps.20579.
24. Leucht S, Cipriani A, Spineli L, et al. Comparative efficacy and tolerability of 15 antipsychotic drugs in schizophrenia: a multiple-treatments meta-analysis [published correction appears in lancet. 2013;382(9896):940]. Lancet. 2013;382(9896):951–62. https://doi.org/10.1016/S0140-6736(13)60733-3.
25. Ware MR, Feller DB, Hall KL. Neuroleptic malignant syndrome: diagnosis and management. Prim Care Companion CNS Disord. 2018;20(1):17r02185. https://doi.org/10.4088/PCC.17r02185.
26. Kritharides L, Chow V, Lambert TJ. Cardiovascular disease in patients with schizophrenia. Med J Aust. 2017;206(2):91–5. https://doi.org/10.5694/mja16.00650.
27. Sarvaiya N, Lapitskaya Y, Dima L, Manu P. Clozapine-associated pulmonary embolism: a high-mortality, dose-independent and early-onset adverse effect. Am J Ther. 2018;25(4):e434–8. https://doi.org/10.1097/MJT.0000000000000806.
28. Kutcher S, Brooks SJ, Gardner DM, et al. Expert Canadian consensus suggestions on the rational, clinical use of ziprasidone in the treatment of schizophrenia and related psychotic disorders. Neuropsychiatr Dis Treat. 2005;1(2):89–108. https://doi.org/10.2147/nedt.1.2.89.61042.
29. Roden DM. Drug-induced prolongation of the QT interval. N Engl J Med. 2004;350(10):1013–22. https://doi.org/10.1056/NEJMra032426.
30. Picchioni MM, Murray RM. Schizophrenia. BMJ. 2007;335(7610):91–5. https://doi.org/10.1136/bmj.39227.616447.BE.
31. Adam RL, Sidi H, Midin M, Zakaria H, Das S, Mat KC. The role of atypical antipsychotics in sexuality: road to recovery in schizophrenia. Curr Drug Targets. 2018;19(12):1402–11. https://doi.org/10.2174/1389450118666170502130126.
32. Lieberman JA 3rd. Managing anticholinergic side effects [published correction appears in prim care companion J Clin psychiatry. 2012;14(1):PCC.12lcx01362]. Prim Care Companion J Clin Psychiatry. 2004;6(Suppl. 2):20–3.
33. Barry SJ, Gaughan TM, Hunter R. Schizophrenia. BMJ Clin Evid. 2012;2012:1007. Published 2012 Jun 28
34. Koller EA, Doraiswamy PM. Olanzapine-associated diabetes mellitus. Pharmacotherapy. 2002;22(7):841–52. https://doi.org/10.1592/phco.22.11.841.33629.
35. Koro CE, Meyer JM. Atypical antipsychotic therapy and hyperlipidemia: a review. Essent Psychopharmacol. 2005;6(3):148–57.
36. Melkersson K, Dahl ML. Adverse metabolic effects associated with atypical antipsychotics. Drugs. 2004;64(7):701–23.
37. Meyer JM, Koro CE. The effects of antipsychotic therapy on serum lipids: a comprehensive review. Schizophr Res. 2004;70(1):1–17.
38. Newcomer JW. Metabolic considerations in the use of antipsychotic medications. J Clin Psychiatry. 2007;68(Suppl. 1):20–7.
39. Pacia SV, Devinsky O. Clozapine-related seizures: experience with 5,629 patients. Neurology. 1994;44(12):2247–9.
40. De Berardis D, Rapini G, Olivieri L, et al. Safety of antipsychotics for the treatment of schizophrenia: a focus on the adverse effects of clozapine. Ther Adv Drug Saf. 2018;9(5):237–56. https://doi.org/10.1177/2042098618756261.
41. Legge SE, Walters JT. Genetics of clozapine-associated neutropenia: recent advances, challenges and future perspective. Pharmacogenomics. 2019;20(4):279–90. https://doi.org/10.2217/pgs-2018-0188.
42. Maust DT, Kim HM, Seyfried LS, et al. Antipsychotics, other psychotropics, and the risk of death in patients with dementia: number needed to harm. JAMA Psychiatry. 2015;72(5):438–45. https://doi.org/10.1001/jamapsychiatry.2014.3018.
43. Devlin JW, Skrobik Y, Gélinas C, et al. Clinical practice guidelines for the prevention and management of pain, agitation/sedation, delirium, immobility, and sleep disruption in adult patients in the ICU. Crit Care Med. 2018;46(9):e825–73. https://doi.org/10.1097/CCM.0000000000003299.
44. Ely EW, Margolin R, Francis J, et al. Evaluation of delirium in critically ill patients: validation of the confusion assessment method for the intensive care unit (CAM-ICU). Crit Care Med. 2001;29(7):1370–9. https://doi.org/10.1097/00003246-200107000-00012.
45. Ely EW, Inouye SK, Bernard GR, et al. Delirium in mechanically ventilated patients: validity and reliability of the confusion assessment method for the intensive care unit (CAM-ICU). JAMA. 2001;286(21):2703–10. https://doi.org/10.1001/jama.286.21.2703.
46. Bergeron N, Dubois MJ, Dumont M, Dial S, Skrobik Y. Intensive care delirium screening checklist: evaluation of a new screening tool. Intensive Care Med. 2001;27(5):859–64. https://doi.org/10.1007/s001340100909.
47. Berman BD. Neuroleptic malignant syndrome: a review for neurohospitalists. Neurohospitalist. 2011;1(1):41–7. https://doi.org/10.1177/1941875210386491.
48. Strawn JR, Keck PE Jr, Caroff SN. Neuroleptic malignant syndrome. Am J Psychiatry. 2007;164(6):870–6. https://doi.org/10.1176/ajp.2007.164.6.870.

49. Buckley PF, Hutchinson M. Neuroleptic malignant syndrome. J Neurol Neurosurg Psychiatry. 1995;58(3):271–3. https://doi.org/10.1136/jnnp.58.3.271.
50. Mihara K, Kondo T, Suzuki A, et al. Relationship between functional dopamine D2 and D3 receptors gene polymorphisms and neuroleptic malignant syndrome. Am J Med Genet B Neuropsychiatr Genet. 2003;117B(1):57–60. https://doi.org/10.1002/ajmg.b.10025.

Anticoagulants Antiplatelets and Antifibrinolytics

26

Jayanth R. Seshan

26.1 Introduction

Hemostasis, the complex process of maintenance of blood flow under normal physiological conditions, depends on the collective interaction of the vascular endothelium, platelets, and the coagulation factors. Inhibitors of coagulation and fibrinolysis (clot dissolution) also play an equally important role in establishing hemostasis by balancing the prothrombotic and antithrombotic mechanisms [1]. Coagulopathy is described by the loss of equilibrium between hemostatic and fibrinolytic processes and leads to excessive bleeding, uninhibited thrombosis, or manifest as abnormal coagulation profile on testing [2]. This chapter aims to provide an overview of the major pharmacological agents affecting the hemostatic mechanisms—antiplatelets, anticoagulants and antifibrinolytics—the knowledge of which is essential in the management of patients with coagulopathy in the neurocritical care setting.

26.2 Physiology of Hemostasis

The classical description of hemostasis is with the involvement of platelets, the clotting cascade—extrinsic and intrinsic pathway, and fibrinolysis where the former two components are responsible for thrombus formation to prevent hemorrhage and the latter being a limiting mechanism for the same [3, 4]. Recently, the cell-based model of hemostasis has been recognized due to failure of the classical model in explaining the hemostatic mechanisms in vivo. The current understanding is that coagulation is a combination of three different processes—**initiation, amplification, and propagation—**not necessarily occurring as a cascade.

Briefly, any vascular injury causes the release of tissue factor into circulation and initiates the clotting process with other factors. A small amount of thrombin generated amplifies the process of coagulation by activation of platelets. Propagation occurs through the activation of clotting factors on the surface of the tissue factor bearing cells and platelets leading to generation of more thrombin which in turn leads to conversion of fibrinogen into fibrin and ultimately resulting in formation of a stable clot along with the platelet plug [5] (Fig. 26.1).

Once hemostasis is achieved, the fibrin clot is cleared by the process of fibrinolysis carried out by activation of plasminogen into plasmin. This conversion is mediated by the tissue plasminogen activator (t-PA) and to a certain extent by the urokinase-type plasminogen activator (u-PAI), which are released following tissue injury and endothelial damage [6, 7].

J. R. Seshan (✉)
Division of Neuroanaesthesiology and Neurocritical Care, Department of Anaesthesiology, JIPMER, Puducherry, Puducherry, India

H. Prabhakar et al. (eds.), *Principles and Practice of Neurocritical Care*,
https://doi.org/10.1007/978-981-99-8059-8_26

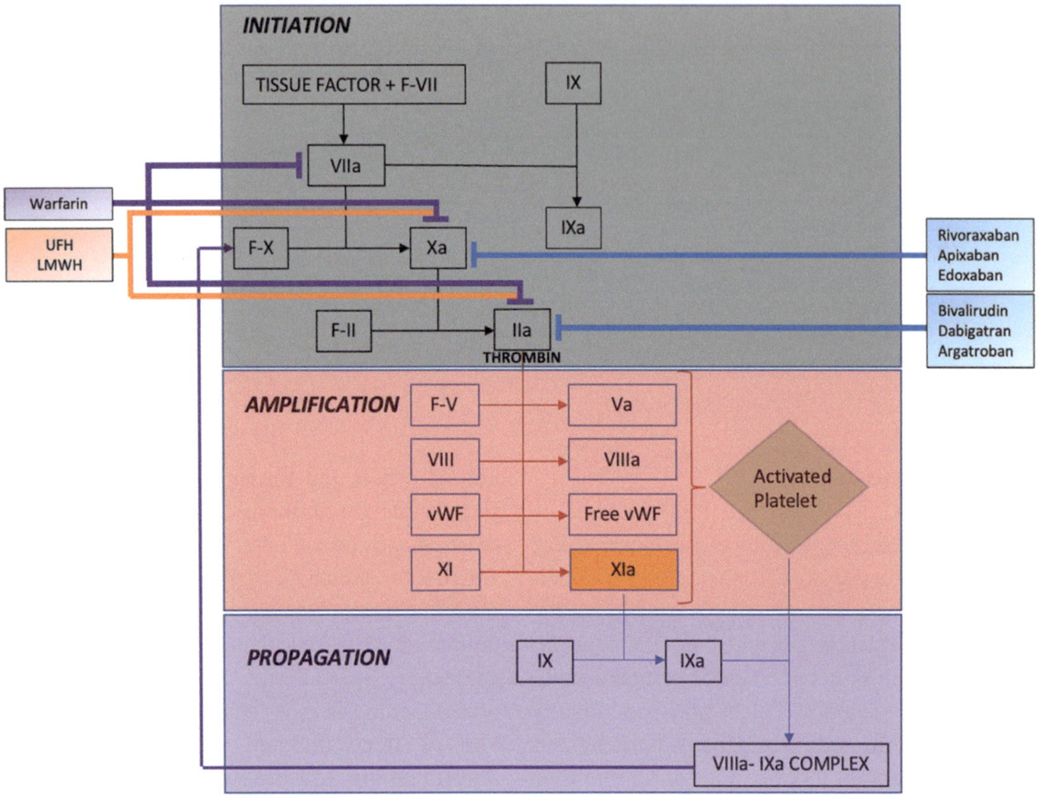

Fig. 26.1 Schematic representation of the cell-based model of the coagulation pathway. Also represented are the anticoagulant drugs acting through different mechanisms. *UFH* unfractionated heparin, *LMWH* low molecular weight heparin

26.3 Anticoagulants

Anticoagulants are indicated in the treatment of a variety of neurological conditions in the intensive care unit like cardioembolic strokes, deep vein thrombosis and pulmonary embolism, cerebral venous sinus thrombosis, and ischemic strokes due to carotid or vertebral artery dissection. They also have an important role in prevention of stroke due to atrial fibrillation or in the setting of mechanical heart valves. The knowledge of management of anticoagulation, that is either initiation or reversal is paramount in ICU practice. This chapter (i) outlines the limitations of oral and parenteral anticoagulants, (ii) describes the advantages of newer drugs, (iii) reviews the pharmacology and side effects of these agents, and (iv) mentions on reversal of anticoagulation. The reader is advised to refer to the guidelines on reversal of antithrombotics in intracranial hemorrhage for a more detailed review [8].

The various anticoagulants used in the neurocritical care practice are given in Fig. 26.2.

26.3.1 Unfractionated Heparin (UFH)

Heparin is a sulfated polysaccharide polymer containing alternating D-glucuronic acid and N-acetyl-D-glucosamine moieties. It is an acidic molecule with a mean molecular weight of 15–20 kDa.

Mechanism of Action

Heparin acts by inhibiting thrombin by binding to antithrombin III and inducing a conformational change. This binding leads to enhancement of its inhibition properties, including factor X and

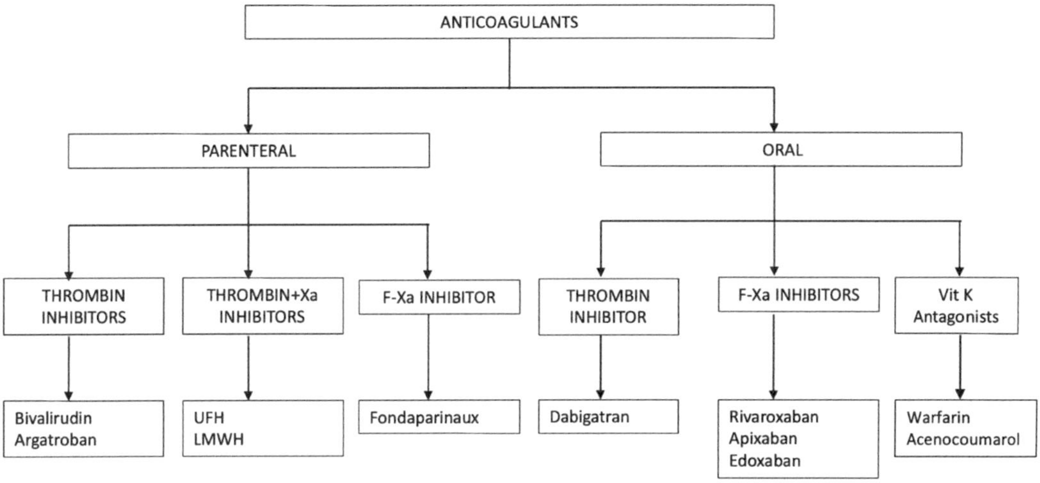

Fig. 26.2 Classification of Anti-coagulants

thrombin. Binding of factor Xa causes reduced conversion of prothrombin to thrombin. This in turn reduces conversion from fibrinogen to fibrin.

Route of Administration
Subcutaneous or intravenous.

Pharmacologic Properties
It has an immediate onset of action on intravenous administration, and on subcutaneous administration, there is a delay of 1–2 h. It is mainly confined to the intravascular compartment. It is metabolized by the reticuloendothelial cells and a very small amount of intact heparin is excreted in urine. The plasma half-life ($t_{1/2}$) depends on the dose administered. As dose increases the heparin kinetics changes from zero to first order.

Adverse Effects
The most common adverse event is bleeding. It is also associated with other side effects like heparin-induced thrombocytopenia (HIT), hyperkalemia (suppresses aldostcrone synthesis), and in some cases, anaphylaxis and hepatitis.

Alternative anticoagulants such as bivalirudin, argatroban, or fondaparinux should be administered to patients with HIT.

Monitoring Test
aPTT (1.5–2.5 × baseline).

Neurocritical Care Indications
Thromboprophylaxis prophylaxis and treatment of cardioembolic stroke associated with AF, prevention of thrombosis associated with endovascular procedures, treatment of carotid/vertebral artery dissection leading to stroke.

Contraindications
Hypersensitivity, patients with severe thrombocytopenia, or history of HIT in the past, uncontrolled bleeding.

Interactions
To be used with caution in patients on other antithrombotic medications.

Nonsteroidal anti-inflammatory drugs may enhance the anticoagulant effect of heparin.

Concurrent angiotensin receptor blocker administration may add to the hyperkalemic effect.

Reversal Agent
Protamine sulfate (1mg for every 100U of heparin administered).

26.3.2 Low-Molecular-Weight Heparins (LMWH)

Low-molecular-weight heparins (LMWH) are fragments of UFH with comparatively less antithrombin activity than UFH but have advantages compared to UFH. These agents can be given without the need for close monitoring of coagulation parameters, and they have a better bioavailability compared to UFH. Moreover, the risk of HIT is lower with LMWH [9].

Mechanism of Action

LMWH binds to antithrombin and accelerates the rate at which it inhibits clotting factors (factor Xa and thrombin).

Route of Administration

Subcutaneous or intravenous.

Therapeutic Dose

Enoxaparin 1 mg/kg every 12 h.

Pharmacologic Properties

The volume of distribution is 4.3 L. The peak effect is seen at 3–5 h when it is given subcutaneously. It is metabolized by the liver by desulfation and is mainly excreted in urine. LMWH is to be used with caution in patients who have chronic renal disease (with a creatinine clearance of <30 ml/min) with dose modification.

The indications, contraindications, and drug interactions are similar to those of UFH.

LMWH needs to be used with caution in patients >60 years of age and creatinine clearance of <30 ml/min.

Reversal Agent

Protamine sulfate.

Monitoring Test

Antifactor-Xa assay.

26.3.3 Fondaparinaux

It is a synthetic pentasaccharide chemically related to LMWH, with similar mechanism of action as LMWH. It binds to antithrombin and accelerates the rate at which it inhibits and inactivates factor Xa. It is employed in the management of HIT. No specific antidote to reverse the bleeding caused by fondaparinaux. Activated prothrombin complex concentrates (aPCC) or recombinant factor VIIa (rVIIa) may be employed (Table 26.1).

26.3.4 Warfarin

Warfarin is a synthetic 3-substituted derivative of 4-hydroxycoumarin and is employed routinely in clinical practice as an oral anticoagulant. It is a racemic mixture of S- and R-warfarin; S-Warfarin is three- to fivefold more potent than R-warfarin.

Mechanism of Action

It is an inhibitor of Vitamin K epoxide reductase enzyme and inhibits gamma-carboxylation of anticoagulant proteins like factors II, VII, IX, and X along with proteins C and S.

Route of Administration

Oral.

Pharmacologic Properties

It is nearly 99% protein bound and metabolized by liver via CYP2C9 enzyme. It is completely absorbed, and the half-life is nearly 40 h. Maximum plasma concentration of warfarin is reached between 2 and 6 h of intake.

Table 26.1 gives comparison between UFH, LMWH, and fondaparinaux

Properties	UFH	LMWH	Fondaparinaux
Molecular weight (Da)	15,000	5000	1500
Target	Xa = thrombin	Xa > thrombin	Xa
Half-life (h)	1	4	17
Renal route of excretion	Yes	No	No
Reversal with protamine	Complete	Partial	None

Dosing and Administration

About 5 mg orally once a day may be employed as starting dose and titrated based on INR. Dose needs to be reduced in individuals with liver function abnormalities, congestive heart failure, and older age. Also, due precaution is to be taken of diet and other drugs with warfarin administration. It is usually administered along with heparin overlap in treating venous thromboembolism.

Monitoring Test

INR test; target between 2 and 3 for most indications, while for prosthetic heart valves, INR needs to be maintained between 2.5 and 3.5.

Adverse Effects

Hemorrhage, skin necrosis, purple toe syndrome (from rapid depletion of clotting factors), and vascular calcification.

Indications of Warfarin in Neurocritical Care Setting

Prevention and treatment of cardioembolic strokes, cerebral venous sinus thrombosis (CVST).

26.3.5 Novel Oral Anticoagulants (NOAC)

The novel anticoagulant drugs used in clinical practice are rivaroxaban, apixaban, edoxaban, and dabigatran. These drugs have shown to be efficacious in the prevention and management of CES due to nonvalvular AF and venous thromboembolism. They are classified as direct thrombin inhibitors (dabigatran) and Factor Xa inhibitors (apixaban, rivaroxaban, and edoxaban). The NOACs have an efficacy similar to warfarin. They are easy to administer as they can be given in fixed doses, need no bridging or routine coagulation monitoring, and are safer compared to warfarin as the incidence of intracerebral hemorrhage is low. These agents have less food and drug interactions as well [10].

In contrast to warfarin, the NOACs directly inhibit a single clotting enzyme. They have a rapid onset of action such that peak plasma levels are achieved 1–4 h after oral administration. These agents are eliminated renally and the extent of renal clearance varies; ≈80% of absorbed dabigatran is cleared unchanged by the kidneys, whereas 50%, 33%, and 27% of absorbed edoxaban, rivaroxaban, and apixaban, respectively, are cleared unchanged via the renal route. Therefore, these agents may accumulate in patients with renal impairment and may contribute to potential bleeding risk. NOACs should be used with caution in those with a creatinine clearance <30 ml/min and are contraindicated if the creatinine clearance is <15 ml/min.

Dabigatran Etexilate

Dabigatran etexilate is a prodrug of dabigatran and competitively and reversibly inhibits the active site of thrombin, exerting its anticoagulant effect.

Pharmacologic Properties

The oral bioavailability is 6%; it is rapidly metabolized by esterases to dabigatran on oral administration. The plasma levels of dabigatran peak 2 h after administration. Dabigatran has a half-life of 14–17 h, which permits once- or twice-daily administration, and almost 80% is excreted unchanged via the renal route. Co-administration of P-glycoprotein inhibitors can lead to increased plasma levels of dabigatran and may increase the risk of bleeding. Verapamil, dronedarone, quinidine, ketoconazole, and clarithromycin can increase dabigatran concentrations, while rifampicin may decrease the concentration.

Dose

One hundred and fifty milligram twice daily for prevention and treatment of stroke and systemic embolism in patients with non-valvular AF. It is also used for the treatment and prevention of DVT-PE.

Contraindications

Active bleeding, hypersensitivity to dabigatran, patients with prosthetic heart valves.

Adverse Effects

Bleeding, especially the risk of GI bleeding, is higher with dabigatran; also dyspepsia and gastritis may be associated with its use.

Reversal

Activated charcoal can be given orally immediately to prevent further absorption.

Idarucizumab is the specific reversal agent, which is a monoclonal antibody fragment (Fab) that binds specifically to the thrombin binding site of dabigatran with very high affinity [11]. If unavailable, prothrombin complex concentrates (PCC) or fresh frozen plasma (FFP) may be administered to arrest bleeding.

Rivaroxaban

Rivaroxaban is a reversible and selective factor Xa inhibitor. Rivaroxaban inhibits free and clot-associated factor Xa, leading to reduced thrombin formation, causing decreased platelet aggregation.

Pharmacologic Properties

It is rapidly absorbed and reaches peak plasma concentration in 2–4 h. Bioavailability of the 10 mg dose is >80%. Peak onset of action in 3 h and a plasma $t_{1/2}$ of 7–11 h. It is metabolized by liver and excreted predominantly by kidneys.

Dose

Twenty milligram once a day.

Contraindications

Active bleeding, hypersensitivity.

Reversal

If ingested within 2 h, administer activated charcoal. *Andexanet alfa* is the pharmacological reversal agent that binds and sequesters the F-Xa inhibitors [12]. Dose depends on the amount and time of the ingestion of rivaroxaban. PCC may be considered when andexanet alfa is unavailable. Andexanet alfa can cause heparin resistance and in patients who require bridging with heparin, caution must be exercised with use of this reversal agent [13].

Apixaban

Apixaban is a highly selective and reversible FXa inhibitor. It is given at a dose of 5 mg twice daily in treatment of CES due to NVAF.

Pharmacologic Properties

It is absorbed in the stomach and small intestine, and the bioavailability is about 50%. Peak onset of action is 3 h, with a $t_{1/2}$ of 12 h. It is about 87% bound to plasma proteins and mainly undergoes o-demethylation and hydroxylation to metabolites. It is metabolized by CYP3A4. 27% of apixaban is renally excreted and the rest is eliminated via feces.

Apixaban as a result of FXa inhibition prolongs clotting tests such as prothrombin time (PT), INR, and activated partial thromboplastin time (aPTT).

Contraindications are similar to the other NOACs.

Interactions

Plasma apixaban levels are reduced by potent inducers of both P-glycoprotein and CYP3A4, like carbamazepine, phenytoin and rifampicin, and increased by potent inhibitors, such as dronedarone, ketoconazole, itraconazole, ritonavir, clarithromycin, erythromycin, and cyclosporin.

Side Effects

Hemorrhage, increased gamma glutamyl transferase levels, nausea, and hepatitis.

Antidote

Andexanet alfa. Hemodialysis has no effect as NOACs are highly bound to plasma proteins.

26.4 Antifibrinolytics

Fibrinolysis is a physiological process in the hemostatic mechanism where excess fibrin deposited in the site of vascular injury is cleared by activated plasminogen, thus preventing the formation of fibrin degradation products and D-dimers. Physiologically, plasminogen is activated by the serine proteases—tissue plasminogen activator (tPA) and urinary plasminogen activator. Plasminogen acts by binding to lysine residues in the interacting molecules. Inhibition of the fibrinolytic system by either inhibiting the serine proteases or by the use of lysine analogs is a targeted mechanism to reduce bleeding in several situations like cardiac, hepatic, and neurosurgeries and in obstetric hemorrhage [14]. This section describes the drugs in this category—aprotinin, tranexamic acid, and epsilon amino caproic acid (EACA) and their implications in the neurocritical care setting.

26.4.1 Aprotinin

Aprotinin is a polypeptide nonspecific serine protease inhibitor extracted from bovine lung.

Mechanism of Action

Aprotinin inhibits plasmin and its attachment to the fibrin polymer. It also acts on trypsin, kallikrein, urokinase, and thrombin; hence, it also affects the coagulation pathway by interfering with factor XII, the renin-angiotensin system, and neutrophil activation (at doses higher than that required for plasmin inhibition).

Dose and Route of Administration

Intravenous. Loading dose of 20,00,000 KIU (kallikrein international units) followed by an infusion of 250,000–500,000 KIU [15].

Pharmacokinetics

Aprotinin has a plasma distribution half-life of 0.3–0.7 h. It is highly protein bound (80%). It undergoes rapid metabolism by renal lysosomal activity and higher doses may lead to nephrotoxicity [16].

Clinical Indications

Cardiopulmonary bypass (CPB). Currently, other antifibrinolytic agents with safer side effect profile have rendered the use of aprotinin obsolete.

Adverse Effects

Hypersensitivity reactions.

Precautions

Administer a test dose to test for hypersensitivity.

26.4.2 Tranexamic Acid

Tranexamic acid (TxA) is a synthetic lysine analog.

Mechanism of Action

TxA acts by competitive inhibition of the lysine receptor on plasminogen. By binding to this receptor, attachment of plasminogen to the fibrin matrix is prevented, thus inhibiting fibrinolysis. The action is reversible.

Dose and Route of Administration

Available in oral and intravenous formulations. Commonly used i.v. dose or the low-dose regimen comprises of loading with 10–15 mg/kg (usually 1gm) followed by a continuous infusion of 1 mg/kg/h.

Pharmacokinetics

After an intravenous dose, plasma concentration of more than 10 mcg/ml (minimum required for effective antifibrinolytic action) is achieved in about an hour and remains for up to 6 h. TxA has relatively low plasma protein binding. Highest tissue concentrations are found in the liver, lungs, and kidney. It easily crosses the blood brain barrier (BBB) and the placenta. The drug has an elimination half-life of 2.3 h and is primarily excreted unchanged in urine. Bioavailability after an oral dose is around 33% [17].

Clinical Indications

Tranexamic acid has been majorly used in the perioperative setting in the context of major bleeding. Loading dose is begin prior to incision and infusion continued up to the end of the procedure. Oral route is utilized in menorrhagia. Management of hemophilia is one of the FDA-approved indications for the use of this drug.

Adverse Effects

1. All antifibrinolytic agents have the inherent risk of promoting thrombosis by inhibiting breakdown of the formed clot. This theoretically leads to increased risk of vascular occlusive events like myocardial infarction, stroke, deep venous thrombosis, and pulmonary embolism. But such risks are relatively rare with the use of TxA and have been associated with higher doses and use in patients with a baseline hypercoagulable state. The incidence of vascular complications is 1–5% [18, 19].
2. Seizures (1–3%) [20, 21]. TxA has been found to be structurally analogous to glycine, an inhibitory neurotransmitter. By competitively binding to glycine receptors, CNS excitation is promoted and is postulated as the mechanism behind seizures as an adverse effect of TxA. The hypothesis is supported by the relative BBB permeability to this drug as well. Higher doses and renal function are risk factors for seizures.
3. Hypotension from rapid iv administration. Maximum rate of infusion is 100 mg/min.

Precautions

Dose adjustments in renal failure are required as the drug is primarily excreted unchanged in urine. Tranexamic acid in pregnancy is classified as category B and no adverse effects are proven in human studies. Though TxA may be transmitted via breast milk, the concentrations are much lower and hence can be given safely in breastfeeding women.

Contraindications

Renal failure, intracranial bleeding, and documented allergy to TxA.

26.4.3 Epsilon Amino Caproic Acid

Epsilon aminocaproic acid (EACA) was introduced prior to TxA as an antifibrinolytic agent. Also a synthetic lysine analog, it has a similar mechanism of action to TxA.

Dose and Route of Administration

Oral and intravenous formulations of EACA are available for use. Intravenously, EACA is primarily used in CPB with a loading dose of 100 mg/kg followed infusion of 30 mg/kg/h.

Pharmacokinetics

Based on in vitro studies, the therapeutic plasma concentration required for antifibrinolytic activity was found to be 130 mcg/ml, and a loading dose of EACA produces a peak plasma concentration of around 150 mg/100 ml (1500 mcg/ml). The drug has a biological half-life of 77 min. EACA is extensively distributed through the intra and extra vascular spaces and tissues with a volume of distribution of around 30 L/kg. EACA is primarily excreted unchanged in urine. Filtration by the kidneys results in 65% of the drug being recovered, requiring 24 h for drug elimination. EACA is less potent compared to tranexamic acid.

Side Effects

Side effects and complications are similar to that of tranexamic acid. Rare complications include muscle necrosis, myoglobinuria, and rhabdomyolysis.

26.4.4 Monitoring Antifibrinolytics

Neither of the lysine analogs produce any effect on coagulation system and hence parameters like prothrombin time (PT), activated partial thromboplastin time (aPTT), nor platelet counts are affected. Clinically, patients receiving these drugs are monitored for signs of bleeding. With high concentrations of TxA, thrombin time (TT) may be elevated, but monitoring for TT is not utilized routinely.

26.4.5 Antifibrinolytics in Neurocritical Care

The lysine analogs—tranexamic acid and EACA—are in use currently, and the major indication is the management of severe bleeding, especially in the perioperative setting. In neurologically ill patients, the major use of TxA is in the prevention of rebleeding in aneurysmal subarachnoid hemorrhage and in traumatic brain injury (TBI).

Traumatic Brain Injury

The CRASH-2 (Clinical Randomization of an Antifibrinolytic in Significant Hemorrhage) trial was the earliest randomized controlled trial (RCT) that evaluated the use of TxA in trauma to study the effect on mortality. The trial demonstrated a significant reduction in mortality [14.5% vs 16%, RR, 0.91 (CI 0.85–0.97)] *if administered within the first hour of injury and if administered beyond 3 h, there was an increased risk of mortality* [22–24]. Based on a subgroup analysis (TBI patients), which showed a nonsignificant decrease in hemorrhage growth, the CRASH-3 trial was proposed.

This multicenter RCT evaluating the efficacy of TxA in reducing mortality in isolated TBI did not demonstrate any difference in 28-day mortality with TxA or placebo [18.5% vs 19.8%, RR 0.94 (0.86–1.02)]. But, a subgroup analysis of patients with mild to moderate head injury revealed a mortality benefit with administration of TxA within 3 h of injury. The trial also reaffirmed the safety of this drug by noting similar incidence of thrombotic complications and seizures in either group [25].

Currently, tranexamic acid in a dose of 1 g loading (administered within 3 h) followed by 1 g over 8 h is indicated in patients with mild to moderate head injury with mortality benefits.

Spontaneous Intracranial Hemorrhage (ICH)

Limitation of hematoma expansion has been the major target in the management of patients with spontaneous ICH. Though the focus-based on recommendations has been on optimal blood pressure, few studies have come up evaluating the role of TxA.

The tranexamic acid for hyperacute primary intracerebral hemorrhage-2 (TICH-2), a double-blind RCT compared the effects of TxA administered within 8 h of symptom onset with placebo on hematoma expansion. Though there was smaller expansion of hematoma, there was no significant difference in the functional outcome or mortality at 90 days. Only patients with initial hematoma volume of 30–60 ml had better outcomes in the study [OR 0.66 (CI 0.44–0.98)] [26].

The Spot Sign and Tranexamic Acid on Preventing ICH-Growth-AUStralasia study (STOP-AUST) RCT involved the use of TxA in adult patients with spontaneous ICH with a positive spot sign within 4.5 h of symptom onset and 1 h of CT angiography. There were no differences in the incidence of hematoma expansion, mortality, and functional outcome at 90 days or the incidence of thrombo-embolic phenomena in the study [27]. The results of the TRAIGE (Tranexamic acid for Acute Intracerebral Hemorrhage Growth Based on Imaging Assessment) trial were also similar to the previous study (Liu). Meta-analysis of RCTs revealed a significantly lower rate of hematoma expansion with TxA but did not identify any outcome benefit [28].

These results indicate that tranexamic acid may be used to decrease the hematoma expansion but without any significant benefit in mortality rates.

Aneurysmal Subarachnoid Hemorrhage (SAH)

The role of tranexamic acid in preventing rebleeding after an SAH has been studied extensively considering the plausible mechanism of rebleeding being the fibrinolysis of the established clot. Historically, multiple evidences in the use of TxA suggested no significant role in prevention of rebleeding [29, 30]. But this was prior to the results of the International Cooperative Study on the Timing of Aneurysm Surgery which favored early obliteration [31].

The Ultra-Early Tranexamic Acid After Subarachnoid Hemorrhage (ULTRA) RCT studied the use of 1gm loading dose of TxA followed by infusion of 1 every 8 h for up to 24 h in SAH patients before 24 h of symptom onset. The incidence of clinical outcomes, mortality, and complications were similar when compared with placebo [32].

A more recent meta-analysis of 13 RCTs did not recommend the routine use of TxA in SAH due to lack of benefit on clinical outcomes [33].

Available evidence suggests that TxA may be used as a short-term measure in the early phase after an SAH to reduce the risk of rebleeding but without any significant effects on outcome.

26.5 Antiplatelet Agents

Antiplatelet agents are the mainstay of treatment for atherosclerotic vascular disease—stroke, coronary artery disease (CAD), and peripheral vascular disease. They can be broadly classified as oral and parenteral agents. They can also be classified by the mechanism of their action. Prior to discussing the pharmacology, it is essential to briefly understand the role of platelets in the hemostatic process.

26.5.1 Role of Platelets

Essential for the initial response after a vascular injury in the formation of a clot, platelets exert their role through four main steps—activation, adhesion, aggregation, and secretion [34]. Activation takes place through numerous agonists like collagen, thromboxanes, and ADP, activating the intracellular pathways. These pathways are accomplished through second messengers—cyclic adenosine monophosphate (cAMP) and cyclic guanine monophosphate (cGMP). Stimulation of cyclo-oxygenase (COX) pathway leads to the formation of thromboxane A_2, which is responsible for further activation through platelet membrane receptors and also platelet aggregation. Conformational changes on the platelet membrane maximize the surface area for the next step which is platelet adhesion. Von-willebrand factor (vWF) plays a major role here. Cross-linking of glycoprotein receptors (GPIIb/IIIa) results in platelet aggregation and formation of platelet-fibrinogen bridges. Positive feedback of this mechanism is facilitated by the release of procoagulant substances from the secretory granules within the platelets—ADP, thromboxane A_2, serotonin, fibrinogen, etc.

Antiplatelet agents target these pathways and receptors and are explained below (Fig. 26.3).

26.5.2 Aspirin

Aspirin was the first antiplatelet medication introduced and still continues to be the most common antiplatelet in use. It is a nonsteroidal

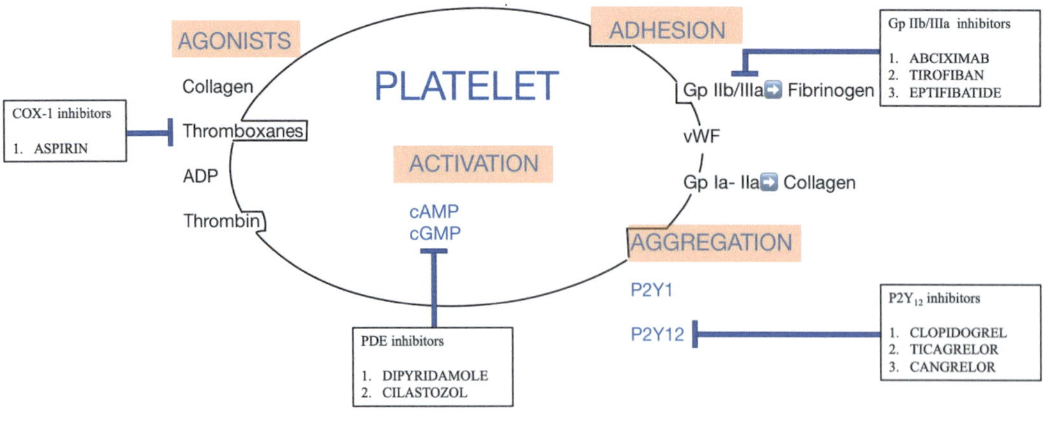

Fig. 26.3 Classification of anti-platelet agents and their mechanism of actionPlatelet activity occurs through agonistic action through collagen, thromboxane, ADP and thrombin. Activation takes place through intracellular second messengers cAMP and cGMP. Adhesion to fibrinogen and collagen takes place through glycoprotein receptors. Aggregation of platelets is facilitated by the platelet receptors $P2Y_{12}$ and $P2Y_1$

anti-inflammatory drug (NSAID) with antiplatelet actions.

Chemical Properties

The chemical formula of aspirin or acetylsalicylic acid is $C_9H_8O_4$. It has a molecular weight of 180.16 g/mol.

Mechanism of Action

Aspirin acts by irreversible inhibition of the cyclo-oxygenase (COX), the enzyme responsible for the conversion of arachidonic acid into prostaglandin H_2 (PGH_2). PGH_2 is rapidly converted into active prostanoids like thromboxane A_2 and PGI_2. Thromboxane is a potent agonist of platelet activation, and hence its inhibition effectively produces antiplatelet activity. COX has 2 isoforms (COX-1 and COX-2). Low-dose aspirin effectively inhibits COX-1, while COX-2 mediated PGI2 actions including regulation of blood pressure and renal functions are preserved [35, 36]. The irreversible inhibition of COX means that the antiplatelet activity lasts until the time the platelets are regenerated (7–10 days).

Dose and Route of Administration

Aspirin is usually administered orally in doses of 75–325 mg/day. Rectal suppositories are available if oral intake is not possible (300 mg). Irreversible COX inhibition permits for once daily dosing. Chewable formulation is available (81 mg) for use as monotherapy in the secondary prevention of stroke. Loading dose of 325 mg is given at presentation for acute coronary syndrome (ACS) and cerebrovascular accident (CVA).

Pharmacokinetics

The drug is rapidly and completely absorbed when given orally. Aspirin is highly protein bound (albumin) and has a volume of distribution of 0.1–0.2 L/kg. Following administration, peak plasma concentration and antiplatelet action are observed as early as 30 min and 1 h respectively. The half-life is 3 h (300 mg dose). Aspirin is metabolized by esterases in the gastrointestinal (GI) mucosa, red blood cells (RBC), and synovial fluid into salicylate which then is conjugated with glycine by the liver to form salicyluric and glucuronic acid, and excreted in urine.

Pharmacodynamics

Aspirin, apart from exhibiting antiplatelet activity, is also used for its analgesic, antipyretic, anti-inflammatory, and antirheumatic agent mainly due to its inhibitory effects on prostaglandins. It appears to act on the hypothalamus to exert its antipyretic actions by suppression of PGE_2 [37].

Indications

Common indications for aspirin use includes fever, temporary relief of pain, and control of inflammation in conditions like rheumatoid arthritis, systemic lupus erythematosus (SLE). The antiplatelet activity is utilized in angina pectoris, ischemic stroke and transient ischemic attack (TIA), myocardial infarction, and cardiovascular risk reduction.

Side Effects

Gastrointestinal (GI) side effects are common with GI ulcer in up to one-third of patients. Dyspepsia, nausea and vomiting, and epigastric distress may be observed. Upper GI bleeding due to GI erosion is seen with high doses along with the possibility of pancytopenia [38]. Hypersensitivity reactions manifest as rash to angioedema or even anaphylaxis. Central nervous system side effects include hearing loss and tinnitus (3–4 g/day), Reye syndrome, and intracerebral hemorrhage.

Precautions

Administer with food to minimize GI side effects, although the rate of absorption maybe reduced. Supplement with proton pump inhibitors and exercise caution while administering aspirin in patients with gastritis. Avoid concurrent use with other NSAIDs to prevent the risk of salicylate toxicity and avoid use in hepatic failure.

26.5.3 Clopidogrel

Clopidogrel is a thienopyridine prodrug that undergoes biotransformation into an active thiol metabolite.

Mechanism of Action

Clopidogrel acts by irreversible inhibition of the platelet receptor $P2Y_{12}$. This receptor, upon activation by ADP, functions by inhibition of adenylyl cyclase to lower the levels of cAMP and reduces the cAMP-dependent platelet-activation inhibition. Inhibition of this $P2Y_{12}$ results in reduced platelet activation.

Dose and Route of Administration

Clopidogrel is administered orally. Loading dose of 300 mg is given orally for TIA and minor stroke. Co-loading of aspirin and clopidogrel is given prior to certain neurointerventional procedures like carotid artery stenting.

Pharmacokinetics

The drug is well absorbed orally and has 50% bioavailability. Onset of action occurs within 2 h following a loading dose and after 24 h in cases of maintenance doses (75 mg). It is 98% protein bound and undergoes ester-mediated hydrolysis in the liver to form an active thiol (through the cytochrome P450-mediated pathway—CYP2C19) and an inactive carboxylic acid derivative. The elimination half-life ($T_{1/2}$) of the active metabolite is 30 min, and the drug is excreted in both urine and feces.

Clinical Indications

The food and drug administration (FDA) approved indications for the use of clopidogrel are secondary prevention of stroke and MI, peripheral arterial disease, and ACS. It is often used as a part of dual antiplatelet therapy (along with aspirin) in neurointerventional procedures for the prevention of procedure-related thrombi.

Side Effects and Contraindications

Diarrhea and rash are possible side effects with comparatively lesser GI issues than with aspirin. Bleeding, neutropenia, and thrombocytopenia are the major complications, and active bleeding is an essential contraindication to the use of clopidogrel. Thrombotic thrombocytopenic purpura is a rare but significant complication reported.

Drug Interactions and Precautions

Concurrent administration with Omeprazole (an inhibitor of CYP2C19) may lead to reduced effects of this drug. Clopidogrel resistance or treatment failure maybe observed in patients with genetic deficiency of CYP2C19, and alternate therapies should be considered.

26.5.4 Prasugrel

Mechanism of Action

A thienopyridine derivative similar to clopidogrel, prasugrel also acts by inhibition of $P2Y_{12}$ receptor and prevents the activation of the GPIIb/IIIa complex, with a higher potency.

Pharmacokinetics

Orally administered, the prodrug is metabolized into its active component (R-138727) in the liver by CYP3A4 and -2B6 enzymes. The higher potency (10–100 times more than clopidogrel) is attributed to a more efficient conversion of the prodrug into the active metabolite. Bioavailability after oral dose, loading dose of 60 mg followed by 10 mg daily, is higher than clopidogrel (80%) and excretion takes place by both urine (70%) and feces.

Uses

Currently, it is used in ACS patients undergoing percutaneous coronary interventions (PCI) to reduce the rate of stent thrombosis.

Adverse Effects

The risk of bleeding complications is generally higher with the use of this drug, and its use in the neurocritical care setting is limited due to the risk of intracerebral hemorrhage [39].

Contraindications

It is contraindicated in patients with active bleeding disorders or with prior TIA or stroke. Dose reduction is required in elderly (>75 years) and those weighing <60 kg to minimize the risk of bleeding.

26.6 ADP Receptor Antagonists

26.6.1 Ticagrelor

Ticagrelor is an adenosine triphosphate analog used as an antiplatelet drug in myocardial ischemia and in patients with stroke or TIA.

Mechanism of Action

Ticagrelor acts by reversible inhibition of the P2Y12 platelet receptor by noncompetitive binding. Prevention of ADP-mediated activation of the GPIIb/IIIa receptor complex occurs which prevents platelet aggregation.

Dose and Route of Administration

The drug is administered orally with a bioavailability of 36%. A loading dose of 180 mg is administered usually followed by 90 mg twice daily. When used in conjunction with aspirin, the dose of aspirin should not exceed 100 mg as higher doses tend to reduce the effectiveness of the former.

Pharmacokinetics

After oral administration, the drug undergoes metabolism in the liver by CYP3A4 and eliminated by feces and urine. Peak effect of action usually occurs in 2–4 h.

Indications

Currently, ticagrelor is used in ACS undergoing PCI to reduce the rate of stent thrombosis. It is also preferred in patients not tolerating aspirin.

Contraindications

Active bleeding.

Side Effects

Bleeding, dyspnea, bradycardia, ECG abnormalities, and increased serum creatinine and uric acid levels are the common side effects observed and require monitoring.

Drug Interactions

Efficacy of this drug may be affected by co-administration of both CYP3A4 inhibitors (ketoconazole and ritonavir) and enzyme inducers (rifampicin, phenytoin, and carbamazepine) and should be avoided.

26.6.2 Cangrelor

Also an ADP receptor antagonist, cangrelor acts similar to ticagrelor by reversible inhibition of platelet function. It is short-acting, available in intravenous formulation, and has the potential to be used in the periprocedural period during endovascular interventions for acute myocardial ischemia and stroke.

Mechanism of Action

Dose-dependent inhibition $P2Y_{12}$ receptors blocking platelet activation and aggregation.

Dose

Loading dose of 15–30 mcg/kg followed by infusion of 0.025–4 mcg/kg/min for 2 h [40].

Pharmacokinetics

After intravenous administration, the drug follows linear pharmacokinetics with a short half-life of 3–6 min. It rapidly undergoes dephosphorylation by nucleotidases in the circulation producing an active metabolite (AR-C69712XX), which is less potent than the parent drug and multiple inactive products. The metabolites are predominantly excreted by bile.

Pharmacodynamics

Bolus dose (30 mcg/kg) of cangrelor results in significant platelet inactivation within 2 min. After cessation of the dose, platelet function returns rapidly to baseline (60–90 min) [41]. Hence, it is imperative to start an oral antiplatelet drug (clopidogrel or prasugrel) immediately to within 30 min of cessation of cangrelor infusion [42].

Side Effects

As with other high potency antiplatelet agents, bleeding is the major side effect. Others include transient elevation of hepatic enzymes and bleeding from injection sites.

26.7 Phosphodiesterase Inhibitors

Phosphodiesterases (PDE) are enzymes that catalyze the hydrolysis of cAMP and CGMP, which are important intracellular signaling pathways regulating the platelet activity. Multiple isoforms of PDE are present in platelets (PDE-2, 3, 5). Inhibition of this enzyme results in increase in the inhibitory intracellular messengers and hence, antiplatelet activity.

26.7.1 Dipyridamole

Introduced initially as a coronary vasodilator, this drug has also been found to inhibit platelet aggregation.

Mechanism of Action

Dipyridamole inhibits both PDE-3 and PDE-5. By increasing the cAMP and cGMP levels, it promotes the inhibition of platelet aggregation. Other possible mechanisms include antioxidant activity by scavenging free radicals that inactivate COX, hence increasing PGI_2 synthesis (vasodilator).

Dose

Two hundred milligram orally twice daily.

Pharmacokinetics

The drug has a variable absorption and metabolized into glucuronide in the liver and excreted in bile. It is highly protein bound.

Side Effects

Headache is the most common side effect of chronic use of dipyridamole [43]. Vasodilation and tachycardia can occur with high doses. Bleeding is also a major side effect.

26.7.2 Cilostazol

Cilostazol, a quinolone derivative, is a reversible inhibitor of the PDE-3 enzyme with antiplatelet and vasodilator activity. It is mainly indicated in the management of patients with intermittent claudication [44].

Dose and Route of Administration

The drug is available as tablets for oral intake. 100 mg twice daily is the recommended dose for claudication and off-label use for secondary prevention of stroke or TIA.

Pharmacokinetics

Well-absorbed orally, cilastazol is metabolized by CYP3A4 into active metabolites and excreted primarily in urine.

Pharmacodynamics

Antiplatelet activity occurs by PDE-3 inhibition. Similar mechanism is responsible for vasodilatory activity resulting in tachycardia and hypotension.

Indications

FDA-approved indication for cilastazol use is intermittent claudication. Off-label use as third line agent for secondary prevention of stroke/TIA is also indicated [45].

Adverse Effects

Headache, palpitations, transient increase in heart rate, and diarrhea are common complications. Thrombocytopenia and leucopenia are reported rarely (Woo).

26.8 Glycoprotein (GP) IIb/IIIa Inhibitors

GP IIb/IIIa provides cross-linking of adjacent platelets (platelet aggregation) by binding to fibrinogen or vWF. Inhibitors of this complex form the newer generation of effective antiplatelet medications aimed at managing ongoing thrombosis.

26.8.1 Abciximab

Abciximab is a chimeric monoclonal antibody (human-murine) Fab (fragment antigen binding) fragment.

Mechanism of Action

Abciximab blocks the GPIIb/IIIa receptor platelet complex, which is the ultimate step in platelet aggregation during hemostasis. It also inhibits monocyte adhesion and cell adhesion by blocking Mac-1 and the vitronectin receptors, respectively.

Dose and Route

It is available only as intravenous formulation, administered as a loading dose of 0.25 mg/kg followed by continuous infusion of 0.125 mcg/kg/min (10 mcg/min) for 12–24 h for sustained antiplatelet activity.

Pharmacokinetics

Following a bolus dose, up to 80% of the GPIIb/IIIa receptors are blocked within 10 min. Peak plasma concentration is achieved in 30 min. The half-life is 30 min [46]. The drug is cleared by the reticuloendothelial system followed by renal excretion.

Clinical Indications

Abciximab is used in PCI with a loading dose beginning 10–60 min before the procedure followed by a continuous infusion for 12 h. It is also used in unstable angina or non-ST segment elevation MI (NSTEMI) with planned PCI within 24 h. It is the treatment of choice for rescue of acute thrombus formation in neurointerventional procedures. Rescue therapy may be provided by wither intravenous or intra-arterial route.

Contraindications

There are several contraindications for the use of abciximab.

1. Hypersensitivity to the drug or its components.
2. Recent or active internal hemorrhage.
3. Recent trauma or major surgery (<6 weeks).
4. History of CVA within 2 years.
5. Use of oral anticoagulation <7 days (unless INR <1.2).
6. Thrombocytopenia (<1,00,000 cells/mm^3).
7. Intracranial pathologies—tumor, arteriovenous malformation (AVM), or aneurysm.
8. Uncontrolled hypertension.
9. Vasculitis.

Side Effects

The major side effect of abciximab is bleeding. Thrombocytopenia and hypersensitivity/ anaphylaxis are also reported. Risk of adverse effects is enhanced with combining abciximab with other antiplatelet medications.

Monitoring

PT/INR, aPTT, and platelet count.

Management of Toxicity

Despite a short half-life, the platelet-bound drug remains in circulation and exerts antiplatelet activity for up to 24–48 h, hence enhancing the toxicity. Stop the infusion immediately and consider platelet transfusion to address thrombocytopenia. There is no specific antidote.

26.8.2 Eptifibatide

Mechanism of Action

A protein found in the snake venom, eptifibatide acts by binding to the beta-subunit of the GPIIb/IIIa receptor and competitively inhibits the receptor from binding with fibrinogen, Vwf, and prothrombin, thus inhibiting platelet aggregation.

Dose and Route of Administration

Intravenous. Loading dose 180 mcg/kg (90–250 mcg/kg) followed by continuous infusion of 2 mcg/kg/min for up to 72 h.

Pharmacokinetics

Following a loading dose, rapid onset of action is achieved (within 15 min), and steady-state plasma concentrations are achieved within 4–6 h with the infusion. The drug has low plasma protein binding (25%). The drug is excreted in urine mainly unmetabolized along with other polar metabolites. Advantages over other drugs of this class are the rapid reversibility upon termination of the infusion.

Indications
Patients with ACS undergoing PCI.

Adverse Effects
Bleeding, thrombocytopenia.

Contraindications
Similar to abciximab. Renal failure (creatinine >4 mg/dl) is a major contraindication.

26.8.3 Tirofiban

Mechanism of Action
Tirofiban is a reversible and competitive inhibitor of the GPIIb/IIIa platelet complex with a higher affinity than eptifibatide.

Dose
25 mcg/kg intravenous loading dose over 3–5 min followed by 0.15 mcg/kg/min for up to 18 h.

Pharmacokinetics
Loading dose results in 90% antiplatelet activity within 10 min. The half-life is 1.5–2 h. Metabolism is negligible, and excretion occurs through both urine and feces. The drug undergoes rapid elimination with restoration of hemostatic function within 3–4 h of termination of infusion.

Indications, contraindications, and adverse effects are similar to other drugs belonging to this class.

26.8.4 Monitoring Antiplatelet Agents

Bleeding time has been used conventionally as the monitor for platelet function by assessing the ability to form a plug. Currently, the role of using this parameter has been contested due to its possible inaccuracy [47, 48]. Newer technologies for platelet function assessment include light transmittance aggregometry, VerifyNow analyzer, impedance aggregometry, and platelet function assay (PFA-100) analyzer. Though point-of-care thromboelastography (TEG) is preferred for rapid assessment of hemostasis in a patient with suspected coagulation abnormality with ongoing bleeding, optical/light platelet aggregometry is currently considered as the gold standard for platelet function.

Commonly, results are obtained specific for the agents used and are quantified as reactivity units (eg: $P2Y_{12}$ reactivity units or PRU for Clopidogrel) or as percentage (%) of inhibition. Accepted values for optimal actions are >295 PRU or > 72–74% inhibition. These values obtained from studies have shown high sensitivity and specificity for drug action [49, 50].

26.8.5 Antiplatelets in Neurocritical Care

Aspirin is the most commonly used agent in the neurocritical care unit, in the management of patients with ischemic stroke, to prevent recurrence. But there are other acute indications for antiplatelet agents like carotid artery recanalization and stenting where peri-procedurally, intravenous agents are used, for rapid onset and potent action.

Stroke
Major role of antiplatelet drugs is in the patients with TIA, for the prevention of a future stroke (the risk being highest in the initial 3 months of the event). Earlier studies evaluated the role of antiplatelet monotherapy and established their safety and efficacy in the secondary prevention of stroke [51–54]. More recent studies on the role of dual antiplatelet therapy (DAPT) have led to the recent guidelines adapting their usage in stroke due to various causes [55–59].

Summary of recommendations for the use of antiplatelet agents in stroke:

1. For noncardioembolic stroke or high-risk TIA, DAPT with aspirin (50–325 mg/day) and clopidogrel (75 mg daily) or ticagrelor (in cases of clopidogrel resistance) should begin within 24 h and continued for 3–4 weeks and later followed by monotherapy (Ia recommendation).

2. In cases of large artery atherosclerosis as the cause of stroke, monotherapy with aspirin (50–70% stenosis) or DAPT with aspirin and clopidogrel (70–99% occlusion) is recommended and may be continued for up to 90 days. (IIa).
3. The use of aspirin, clopidogrel, or aspirin-dipyridamole is recommended for prolonged durations in cases of extracranial carotid or vertebral artery stenosis to prevent recurrent strokes (Ia).

Spontaneous Intracerebral Hemorrhage

In the neurocritical care setting, it is important that the intensivist is aware of the implications of prior antiplatelet medication history of the patient and decide upon restarting the medication after a point where the risk of thrombotic complications might be more life-threatening. Two major recent studies, the VISTA-ICH and the RESTART, have provided data to suggest that the resumption of antiplatelets did not result in significant rebleeding. Although the ideal time to restart aspirin is still unknown, the above studies mention a median duration of 7 days (up to 39 days) after the ictus [60, 61].

The current guidelines state that in patients with spontaneous ICH, resumption of antiplatelet therapy, if indicated, may be considered reasonably for the prevention of thromboembolic complications [62] (IIb).

Subarachnoid Hemorrhage

Delayed cerebral ischemia (DCI), one of the dreaded complications of aneurysmal subarachnoid hemorrhage, is associated with multiple causative factors and increased platelet activity and release of thromboxanes are among them. Aspirin has been studied as one of the management modalities for DCI, but results are conflicting [63–65]. Current evidence suggests no role or even a possible negative impact with the use of aspirin in SAH. But in patients undergoing endovascular embolization and hence requiring periprocedural antiplatelet treatment, the incidence of DCI is lower.

Current guidelines do not support the use of aspirin in SAH for the prevention or management of DCI.

Periprocedural Antiplatelets in Neuroendovascular Interventions

Numerous neurointerventional procedures, carried outstenting of cervical and intracranial carotid arteries, embolization, and flow diverter placements for cerebral aneurysms, require periprocedural antiplatelet cover to reduce the risk of thrombosis. They are also used as rescue agents in patients who develop a thrombus during or after the procedure. Both oral and intravenous agents are in use.

1. Aspirin is generally begun 3–5 days prior to the procedure.
2. Clopidogrel: initiated concurrently with aspirin or as monotherapy. The risk of resistance has resulted in alternatives to be considered.
3. Ticagrelor: 180 mg per day. Started 2–3 days prior to procedure, or even the night before, results in good antiplatelet activity peri procedurally.
4. Gp IIb/IIIa inhibitors: intravenous infusion at the start of the procedure and continued for 12–18 h and later bridged with oral antiplatelet agents provide ideal action for prevention of thrombus formation.

26.8.6 Resistance to Antiplatelet Therapy

Antiplatelet resistance may be categorized as clinical or laboratory. Clinical resistance generally refers to the inability to prevent thrombotic complications despite the optimal use of this class of drugs. Laboratory resistance is defined differently with different drugs as either a failure to reduce thromboxane A_2 after COX enzyme inhibition (aspirin) or an inability to reduce platelet aggregation by $P2Y_{12}$ receptor inhibition (thienopyridines). The prevalence of resistance to aspirin and clopidogrel varies from 5–65% to 30–45%, respectively.

Poor drug compliance is considered to be the major mechanism behind resistance. Other important factors include poor bioavailability, tachyphylaxis due to long-term use, concurrent administration with other NSAIDs (aspirin), and genetic polymorphisms (CYP2C19 receptor and clopidogrel).

Management includes the use of enteric coated formulations to increase bioavailability, use of platelet function testing to document resistance, and the use of alternatives to clopidogrel like ticagrelor [66].

26.9 Summary

Aspirin remains the mainstay of secondary prevention of ischemic stroke. Dual antiplatelets are indicated in vascular stenting but should not be used indefinitely. Low-molecular-weight heparin is currently in use in the ICU for prevention and management of venous thrombosis. Reversal of anticoagulants must be undertaken promptly in accordance with the guidelines. Among the antifibrinolytics, tranexamic acid has been the agent of choice in the neurological setting due to its relatively safer profile. Recent trials of tranexamic acid in head trauma have demonstrated its acceptability in moderate head injury when administered early.

26.10 Conclusion

With increasing incidence of vascular diseases, the use of antiplatelets and anticoagulants is on the rise which has resulted in a greater number of patients with neurological complications due to their intake. Knowledge of the pharmacology of these agents is essential in the management of reversal of such agents in case of hemorrhagic complications. Similarly, antiplatelets and antifibrinolytics have found more role in the management of brain ischemia. This chapter has attempted to summarize the current role of antiplatelets, anticoagulants, and anti-fibrinolytics in the neurocritical care setting.

References

1. Zaidi A, Green L. Physiology of haemostasis. Anaesth Intensive Care Med. 2019;20(3):152–8.
2. Salem AM, Roh D, Kitagawa RS, Choi HA, Chang TR. Assessment and management of coagulopathy in neurocritical care. J Neurocrit Care. 2019;12(1):9–19.
3. Mackman N, Tilley RE, Key NS. Role of the extrinsic pathway of blood coagulation in hemostasis and thrombosis. Arterioscler Thromb Vasc Biol. 2007;27(8):1687–93.
4. Gailani D, Renné T. Intrinsic pathway of coagulation and arterial thrombosis. Arterioscler Thromb Vasc Biol. 2007;27(12):2507–13.
5. Hoffman M, Monroe DM. A cell-based model of hemostasis. Thromb Haemost. 2001;85(6):958–65.
6. Sierra C, Moreno M, García-Ruiz JC. The physiology of hemostasis. Blood Coagul Fibrinolysis. 2022;33:S1.
7. Collen D. On the regulation and control of fibrinolysis. Thromb Haemost. 1980;43(02):077–89.
8. Frontera JA, Lewin JJ, Rabinstein AA, Aisiku IP, Alexandrov AW, Cook AM, et al. Guideline for reversal of Antithrombotics in intracranial hemorrhage: a statement for healthcare professionals from the Neurocritical care society and Society of Critical Care Medicine. Neurocrit Care. 2016;24(1):6–46.
9. Babin JL, Traylor KL, Witt DM. Laboratory monitoring of low-molecular-weight heparin and Fondaparinux. Semin Thromb Hemost. 2017;43(3):261–9.
10. Chen A, Stecker EA, Warden BA. Direct oral anticoagulant use: a practical guide to common clinical challenges. J Am Heart Assoc. 2020;9(13):e017559.
11. Pollack CV, Reilly PA, van Ryn J, Eikelboom JW, Glund S, Bernstein RA, et al. Idarucizumab for dabigatran reversal—full cohort analysis. N Engl J Med. 2017;377(5):431–41.
12. Siegal DM, Curnutte JT, Connolly SJ, Lu G, Conley PB, Wiens BL, et al. Andexanet alfa for the reversal of factor Xa inhibitor activity. N Engl J Med. 2015;373(25):2413–24.
13. Müther M, Schwindt W, Mesters RM, Minnerup J, Stracke P, Holling M, et al. Andexanet-alfa-associated heparin resistance in the context of hemorrhagic stroke. Neurocrit Care. 2022;37(2):372–6.
14. Ortmann E, Besser MW, Klein AA. Antifibrinolytic agents in current anaesthetic practice. Br J Anaesth. 2013;111(4):549–63.
15. Royston D, Bidstrup BP, Taylor KM, Sapsford RN. Effect of aprotinin on need for blood transfusion after repeat open-heart surgery. Lancet. 1987;2(8571):1289–91.
16. Székely A, Lex DJ, Merkely B. Aprotinin: pharmacological benefits and safety concerns. In: Landoni G, Ruggeri L, Zangrillo A, editors. Reducing mortality in the perioperative period. Cham: Springer International Publishing; 2014. p. 125–30. https://doi.org/10.1007/978-3-319-02186-7_16.

17. Michalets E, Harris L. Chapter 44: Antifibrinolytics: pharmacologic profile and clinical utilization. In: Topaz O, editor. Cardiovascular thrombus. Academic Press; 2018. p. 615–49. Available from: https://www.sciencedirect.com/science/article/pii/B9780128126158000442.
18. Roberts I, Prieto-Merino D, Manno D. Mechanism of action of tranexamic acid in bleeding trauma patients: an exploratory analysis of data from the CRASH-2 trial. Crit Care. 2014;18(6):685.
19. Sigaut S, Tremey B, Ouattara A, Couturier R, Taberlet C, Grassin-Delyle S, et al. Comparison of two doses of tranexamic acid in adults undergoing cardiac surgery with cardiopulmonary bypass. Anesthesiology. 2014;120(3):590–600.
20. Lin Z, Xiaoyi Z. Tranexamic acid-associated seizures: a meta-analysis. Seizure. 2016;36:70–3.
21. Kalavrouziotis D, Voisine P, Mohammadi S, Dionne S, Dagenais F. High-dose tranexamic acid is an independent predictor of early seizure after cardiopulmonary bypass. Ann Thorac Surg. 2012;93(1):148–54.
22. Perel P, Al-Shahi Salman R, Kawahara T, Morris Z, Prieto-Merino D, Roberts I, et al. CRASH-2 (Clinical Randomisation of an Antifibrinolytic in Significant Haemorrhage) intracranial bleeding study: the effect of tranexamic acid in traumatic brain injury—a nested randomised, placebo-controlled trial. Health Technol Assess. 2012;16(13):iii–xii. 1–54
23. CRASH-2 Collaborators, Roberts I, Shakur H, Afolabi A, Brohi K, Coats T, et al. The importance of early treatment with tranexamic acid in bleeding trauma patients: an exploratory analysis of the CRASH-2 randomised controlled trial. Lancet. 2011;377(9771):1096–101. 1101.e1–2
24. CRASH-2 Trial Collaborators, Shakur H, Roberts I, Bautista R, Caballero J, Coats T, et al. Effects of tranexamic acid on death, vascular occlusive events, and blood transfusion in trauma patients with significant haemorrhage (CRASH-2): a randomised, placebo-controlled trial. Lancet. 2010;376(9734):23–32.
25. CRASH-3 Trial Collaborators. Effects of tranexamic acid on death, disability, vascular occlusive events and other morbidities in patients with acute traumatic brain injury (CRASH-3): a randomised, placebo-controlled trial. Lancet. 2019;394(10210):1713–23.
26. Sprigg N, Flaherty K, Appleton JP, Al-Shahi Salman R, Bereczki D, Beridze M, et al. Tranexamic acid for hyperacute primary IntraCerebral Haemorrhage (TICH-2): an international randomised, placebo-controlled, phase 3 superiority trial. Lancet. 2018;391(10135):2107–15.
27. Meretoja A, Yassi N, Wu TY, Churilov L, Sibolt G, Jeng JS, et al. Tranexamic acid in patients with intracerebral haemorrhage (STOP-AUST): a multicentre, randomised, placebo-controlled, phase 2 trial. Lancet Neurol. 2020;19(12):980–7.
28. Ovesen C, Jakobsen JC, Gluud C, Steiner T, Law Z, Flaherty K, et al. Tranexamic acid for prevention of hematoma expansion in intracerebral hemorrhage patients with or without spot sign. Stroke. 2021;52(8):2629–36.
29. Roos Y. Antifibrinolytic treatment in subarachnoid hemorrhage: a randomized placebo-controlled trial. STAR Study Group. Neurology. 2000;54(1):77–82.
30. Baharoglu MI, Germans MR, Rinkel GJ, Algra A, Vermeulen M, van Gijn J, et al. Antifibrinolytic therapy for aneurysmal subarachnoid haemorrhage. Cochrane Database Syst Rev. 2013:8. https://doi.org/10.1002/14651858.CD001245.pub2/full.
31. Haley EC, Kassell NF, Torner JC. The international cooperative study on the timing of aneurysm surgery. The North American experience. Stroke. 1992;23(2):205–14.
32. Post R, Germans MR, Tjerkstra MA, Vergouwen MDI, Jellema K, Koot RW, et al. Ultra-early tranexamic acid after subarachnoid haemorrhage (ULTRA): a randomised controlled trial. Lancet. 2021;397(10269):112–8.
33. Shi M, Yang C, Chen ZH, Xiao LF, Zhao WY. Efficacy and safety of tranexamic acid in aneurysmal subarachnoid hemorrhage: a systematic review and meta-analysis of randomized controlled trials. Front Surg. 2021;8:790149.
34. Ramalingam G, Jones N, Besser M. Platelets for anaesthetists—Part 1: Physiology and pathology. BJA Educ. 2016;16(4):134–9.
35. Patrono C, Baigent C, Hirsh J, Roth G. Antiplatelet drugs: American College of Chest Physicians evidence-based clinical practice guidelines, 8th edition. Chest. 2008;133(Suppl. 6):199S–233S.
36. Hansson L, Zanchetti A, Carruthers SG, Dahlöf B, Elmfeldt D, Julius S, et al. Effects of intensive blood-pressure lowering and low-dose aspirin in patients with hypertension: principal results of the hypertension optimal treatment (HOT) randomised trial. HOT Study Group. Lancet. 1998;351(9118):1755–62.
37. Aronoff DM, Neilson EG. Antipyretics: mechanisms of action and clinical use in fever suppression. Am J Med. 2001;111(4):304–15.
38. Wijnja L, Snijder JAM, Nieweg HO. Acetylsalicylic acid as a cause of pancytopenia from bone-marrow damage. Lancet. 1966;288(7467):768–70.
39. Wiviott SD, Braunwald E, McCabe CH, Montalescot G, Ruzyllo W, Gottlieb S, et al. Prasugrel versus clopidogrel in patients with acute coronary syndromes. N Engl J Med. 2007;357(20):2001–15.
40. Waite LH, Phan YL, Spinler SA. Cangrelor: a novel intravenous antiplatelet agent with a questionable future. Pharmacotherapy. 2014;34(10):1061–76.
41. Akers WS, Oh JJ, Oestreich JH, Ferraris S, Wethington M, Steinhubl SR. Pharmacokinetics and pharmacodynamics of a bolus and infusion of cangrelor: a direct, parenteral P2Y12 receptor antagonist. J Clin Pharmacol. 2010;50(1):27–35.
42. De Luca L, Steg PG, Bhatt DL, Capodanno D, Angiolillo DJ. Cangrelor: clinical data, contemporary use, and future perspectives. J Am Heart Assoc. 2021;10(13):e022125.

43. Gresele P, Momi S, Falcinelli E. Anti-platelet therapy: phosphodiesterase inhibitors. Br J Clin Pharmacol. 2011;72(4):634–46.
44. Sobel M, Verhaeghe R. Antithrombotic therapy for peripheral artery occlusive disease: American College of Chest Physicians Evidence-Based Clinical Practice Guidelines, 8th edition. Chest. 2008;133(Suppl. 6):815S–43S.
45. Niu PP, Guo ZN, Jin H, Xing YQ, Yang Y. Antiplatelet regimens in the long-term secondary prevention of transient ischaemic attack and ischaemic stroke: an updated network meta-analysis. BMJ Open. 2016;6(3):e009013.
46. Faulds D, Sorkin EM. Abciximab (c7E3 Fab). Drugs. 1994;48(4):583–98.
47. Hayward CPM. How I investigate for bleeding disorders. Int J Lab Hematol. 2018;40(S1):6–14.
48. Peterson P, Hayes TE, Arkin CF, Bovill EG, Fairweather RB, Rock WA Jr, et al. The preoperative bleeding time test lacks clinical benefit: College of American Pathologists' and American Society of Clinical Pathologists' position article. Arch Surg. 1998;133(2):134–9.
49. Ospel JM, Brouwer P, Dorn F, Arthur A, Jensen ME, Nogueira R, et al. Antiplatelet management for stent-assisted coiling and flow diversion of ruptured intracranial aneurysms: a DELPHI consensus statement. AJNR Am J Neuroradiol. 2020;41(10):1856–62.
50. Kim KS, Fraser JF, Grupke S, Cook AM. Management of antiplatelet therapy in patients undergoing neuroendovascular procedures. J Neurosurg. 2017;129(4):890–905.
51. Sacco RL, Diener HC, Yusuf S, Cotton D, Ounpuu S, Lawton WA, et al. Aspirin and extended-release dipyridamole versus clopidogrel for recurrent stroke. N Engl J Med. 2008;359(12):1238–51.
52. The international stroke Trial (IST). A randomised trial of aspirin, subcutaneous heparin, both, or neither among 19435 patients with acute ischaemic stroke. International stroke Trial collaborative group. Lancet. 1997;349(9065):1569–81.
53. Johnston SC, Amarenco P, Albers GW, Denison H, Easton JD, Evans SR, et al. Ticagrelor versus aspirin in acute stroke or transient ischemic attack. N Engl J Med. 2016;375(1):35–43.
54. Shinohara Y, Katayama Y, Uchiyama S, Yamaguchi T, Handa S, Matsuoka K, et al. Cilostazol for prevention of secondary stroke (CSPS 2): an aspirin-controlled, double-blind, randomised non-inferiority trial. Lancet Neurol. 2010;9(10):959–68.
55. Kleindorfer DO, Towfighi A, Chaturvedi S, Cockroft KM, Gutierrez J, Lombardi-Hill D, et al. 2021 guideline for the prevention of stroke in patients with stroke and transient ischemic attack: a guideline from the American Heart Association/American Stroke Association. Stroke. 2021;52(7):e364–467.
56. Wang Y, Wang Y, Zhao X, Liu L, Wang D, Wang C, et al. Clopidogrel with aspirin in acute minor stroke or transient ischemic attack. N Engl J Med. 2013;369(1):11–9.
57. Wang Y, Meng X, Wang A, Xie X, Pan Y, Johnston SC, et al. Ticagrelor versus clopidogrel in CYP2C19 loss-of-function carriers with stroke or TIA. N Engl J Med. 2021;385(27):2520–30.
58. Johnston SC, Amarenco P, Denison H, Evans SR, Himmelmann A, James S, et al. Ticagrelor and aspirin or aspirin alone in acute ischemic stroke or TIA. N Engl J Med. 2020;383(3):207–17.
59. Johnston SC, Easton JD, Farrant M, Barsan W, Conwit RA, Elm JJ, et al. Clopidogrel and aspirin in acute ischemic stroke and high-risk TIA. N Engl J Med. 2018;379(3):215–25.
60. Murthy SB, Biffi A, Falcone GJ, Sansing LH, Torres Lopez V, Navi BB, et al. Antiplatelet therapy after spontaneous intracerebral hemorrhage and functional outcomes. Stroke. 2019;50(11):3057–63.
61. Al-Shahi Salman R, Dennis MS, Sandercock PAG, Sudlow CLM, Wardlaw JM, Whiteley WN, et al. Effects of antiplatelet therapy after stroke caused by intracerebral hemorrhage: extended follow-up of the RESTART randomized clinical trial. JAMA Neurol. 2021;78(10):1179–86.
62. Greenberg SM, Ziai WC, Cordonnier C, Dowlatshahi D, Francis B, Goldstein JN, et al. 2022 guideline for the management of patients with spontaneous intracerebral hemorrhage: a guideline from the American Heart Association/American Stroke Association. Stroke. 2022;53(7):e282–361.
63. Phan K, Moore JM, Griessenauer CJ, Ogilvy CS, Thomas AJ. Aspirin and risk of subarachnoid hemorrhage. Stroke. 2017;48(5):1210–7.
64. Ewbank F, Birks J, Gaastra B, Hall S, Galea I, Bulters D. Aspirin and subarachnoid Haemorrhage in the UK biobank. Transl Stroke Res. 2022;14:490. https://doi.org/10.1007/s12975-022-01060-1.
65. Cagnazzo F, Derraz I, Lefevre PH, Gascou G, Dargazanli C, Riquelme C, et al. Antiplatelet therapy in patients with aneurysmal SAH: impact on delayed cerebral ischemia and clinical outcome. A meta-analysis. AJNR Am J Neuroradiol. 2019;40(7):1201–6.
66. Krishnan K, Nguyen TN, Appleton JP, Law ZK, Caulfied M, Cabrera CP, et al. Antiplatelet resistance: a review of concepts, mechanisms, and implications for management in acute ischemic stroke and transient ischemic attack. Stroke: Vasc Intervent Neurol. 3(3):e000576.

Osmotherapy

27

Rajeeb Kumar Mishra

27.1 Introduction

Cerebral edema is a nonspecific pathological swelling of the brain that may develop in a focal or diffuse pattern after any type of neurological injury [1]. In other words, cerebral edema is abnormal accumulation of excessive fluid in the intracellular or extracellular spaces [1]. Cerebral edema can be seen as a consequence of several acute brain injury (ABI) such as traumatic brain injury (TBI), subarachnoid haemorrhage (SAH), edema associated with intracranial space occupying lesions, and with acute ischemic strokes. Cerebral edema is classically divided into four major categories; vasogenic edema, cytotoxic edema, interstitial edema, and osmotic edema [2]. Prompt diagnosis and management of cerebral edema should be done as it is associated with significant morbidity and mortality. If not effectively managed it can lead to rise in intracranial pressure (ICP) with appalling consequences. Osmotherapy remains one of the mainstay of medical management of cerebral edema along with temporary hyperventilation, metabolic suppression, cerebrospinal fluid diversion, and decompressive craniectomy in the neurocritical care units [1, 3]. Several osmotherapeutic agents such as mannitol, hypertonic saline (HTS), and several hypertonic sodium solutions, e.g., sodium bicarbonate, lactate are used in neurocritical care to reduce the brain bulk. Different agents have distinct pharmacokinetics and pharmacodynamics, which should be understood to effectively manage the clinical situations. The focus of the chapter is to inform the readers about the subtle differences in the characteristics of the osmotic agents, which are practically useful in deciding the right agent for the management of an acute life-threatening condition such as cerebral edema in neurocritical care.

27.2 Principles Behind the Use of Osmotherapy

Normally, serum osmolality is 280–290 mOsm/L, which is predominantly determined by serum sodium concentration [Na^+]. The calculated serum osmolarity formula is as follows:

R. K. Mishra (✉)
Department of Neuroanaesthesia and Neurocritical Care, NIMHANS, Bengaluru, Karnataka, India

H. Prabhakar et al. (eds.), *Principles and Practice of Neurocritical Care*,
https://doi.org/10.1007/978-981-99-8059-8_27

$$\text{Serum osmolality}(\text{mOsm}/\text{L}) = 2\left[\text{Na}^{+} + \text{K} + (\text{mEq}/\text{L})\right] + \left[\text{plasma glucose}(\text{mg}/\text{dL})\right]/18 + \left[\text{BUN}(\text{mg}/\text{dL})\right]/2.8$$

where BUN is blood urea nitrogen.

The goal of osmotherapy is to create an osmotic gradient between the intravascular compartment and brain to cause movement of extracellular and intracellular water into the vascular compartment. This decreases total brain water content leading to reduction in intracranial volume. In order to achieve the required osmotic effect, the serum osmolality should be above the normal osmolality. After mannitol administration, the target osmolality is up to 320 mOsm/L [4]. There are other factors that can influence the effectiveness of a given osmotic agents. The blood brain barrier (BBB) integrity is such a factor. These osmotic agents are effective in regions of brain where BBB is intact. Moreover, an ideal osmotic agent is one which is inert, relative non-toxic, and completely impermeable to the brain. This leads to the concept of reflection coefficient of an agent. The relative impermeability of these agents with respect to the BBB is described as reflection coefficient (σ). A value of σ equal to zero indicates that the molecule is freely permeable to the BBB, while a σ value of one suggests complete impermeability. The reflection coefficients for mannitol and HTS are 0.9 and 1.0, respectively; whereas that of glycerol is 0.47. Compounds with σ approaching 1 are more ideal osmotic agents as they are more entirely excluded by the BBB and, thus, less likely to demonstrate "rebound" cerebral edema and elevations in ICP during withdrawal of therapy.

27.3 What Are the Options?

Several osmotic agents are available that can be used in the neurocritical care units. Agents such as different concentrations of intravenous (IV) mannitol, hypertonic saline, 8.4% sodium bicarbonate [5], sodium lactate [6], and glycerol are used. The commonly used concentrations of mannitol are 10% and 20%, while HTS is available in 3%, 5%, 7.5%, and 23.4% concentration. Osmolarity of 20% mannitol is 1098 mOsm/L, whereas that of 3% HTS is 1026 mOsm/L. The osmolar load is as high as 8008 mOsm/L with 23.4% HTS. Clinically, 5 mL/kg of 20% (1 g/kg) of mannitol is equiosmolar to 5 mL/kg of 3% HTS [7].

27.3.1 Pharmacology of the Agents

This section of the chapter deals with brief pharmacology of the osmotic agents, which are useful clinically.

Mannitol

Mannitol is an alcohol derivative of sugar mannose, with a molecular weight of 182 Da. The usual dose range of 20% mannitol is 0.25–1 g/kg with a target serum osmolality upto 320 mOsm/L [4]. Often mannitol is given IV over 30 min to prevent occurrence of hypotension after rapid administration. The onset of action is 4–5 min, and peak effect is seen in 30–45 min. The main mechanism of action is movement of intracellular water from intracellular and extracellular space to the intravascular space along the osmotic gradient across the intact BBB. Other attributed mechanism could be the reduction in CSF secretion by mannitol.

The hemodynamic response is often triphasic: transient, delayed, and late. Transient hypotensive response is noted within 1–2 min of rapid IV mannitol administration due to a reduction in peripheral vascular resistance and thus hypotension. Hence, the dose should be instituted over 30 min. Mannitol then transiently increases cardiac index (CI), cerebral blood flow (CBF), cerebral blood volume (CBV), and ICP. Half an hour after, the blood volume returns to normal and cardiac index drops further drops owing to peripheral vasodilation and pooling. Mannitol-related diuresis is partly due to increased osmotic load in the proximal convoluted tubules and loop of Henle after filtration, hampering water reabsorption from the lumen, and partly due to increase in glomerular filtration rate by rise in renal blood flow and reducing the urine concentring ability of renal medulla. Other important extraosmotic mechanisms associated with mannitol are reduction in blood viscosity, red blood cell rigidity, leading to improved blood rheology [4], which enhances the cerebral micro perfusion. It also possesses free-radical scavenging properties, which can be neuroprotectant. Therapeutic effectiveness of mannitol may decrease due to rebound increases in ICP ($\sigma = 0.9$).

Hypertonic Saline

Hypertonic saline (HTS) is a crystalloid fluid, composed of sodium chloride (NaCl) dissolved in water with a significantly higher [Na^+] and higher osmolality as compared to plasma. HTS has a σ of 1.0, which implies the permeability across BBB is low, thus theoretically a superior osmotic agent. HTS in various concentrations imparts different osmotic load, and thus primarily this compound exerts its effect by the water movement across the osmotic gradient. After a bolus dose of HTS, the ICP reduces, with augmented intravascular volume, central venous pressure, and CO, without causing diuresis. This advantage of HTS over mannitol is an important consideration while managing hemodynamically unstable patients with cerebral edema. Additionally, it has theoretical benefit of restoring resting cell membrane potential, modulation of inflammation [8]. The adverse effects noted are rebound increase in ICP, hyperchloremic acidosis, renal impairment [8]. Children undergoing continuous HTS infusion and having sustained elevations (72 h) of serum sodium levels of more than 170 meq/L had more episodes of renal dysfunction, anemia, neutropenia, thrombocytopenia, and acute respiratory distress syndrome as compared to sodium levels below this threshold [9]. HTS can cause a precipitous rise in serum [Na^+] raising concern for central pontine myelinolysis. As a plasma expander, it possess theoretical risk of volume overload. The usual dose of 3% HTS for treating increased ICP and cerebral edema is 2–5 mL/kg over 10–20 min.[8] For continuous infusion, the recommended dose of 3% HTS is 0.1–1 mL/kg/h.

Sodium Bicarbonate

Sodium bicarbonate has been widely utilized to treat systemic metabolic acidosis. The adverse effect of hyperchloremic acidosis with the use of HTS prompted researchers to investigate sodium bicarbonate instead of HTS. It is demonstrated that 85 mL of 8.4% sodium bicarbonate provides a comparable solute load (170 mOsm) and sodium load (85 mmol) to 100 mL 5% saline (171 mOsm and 85.5 mmol sodium) [10]. And the osmolarity of 8.4% sodium bicarbonate is 2000 mOsm/L, which is equivalent to the 5.8% saline [11]. Several clinical studies have shown encouraging results with treatment with sodium bicarbonate and without the incidence of hyperchloremic acidosis [5, 10]. One study concluded that in adult TBI patients, 85 mL of sodium bicarbonate over 30 min can cause reduction in ICP equivalent to HTS [5]. The important concern in the use of IV sodium bicarbonate is the rise in partial pressure of carbon dioxide, which can be monitored during IV infusion of the agent, and if required, transient hyperventilation can help to reduce the carbon dioxide burden.

Hypertonic Sodium Lactate

Another important compound for management of cerebral edema is hypertonic sodium lactate (HSL). Lactate is a source of energy to injured brain specially in the hypermetabolic stages of the injury. Besides an alternate energy source the HSL in half molar solution is an osmotic agent [12]. The osmolarity of sodium lactate is 1020 mOsm/L. Authors of an randomised controlled trial have concluded that equiosmolar and isovolumetric dose of HSL as compared to 20% mannitol is superior in controlling the ICP [6]. Similarly in patients with mild traumatic brain injury, the cognition was well preserved at 24 h, 30, and 90 days post-surgery, when they were treated with HSL as compared to group treated with HTS [13].

Glycerol

Glycerol is a hyperosmotic natural alcohol and acts as a laxative. Its intravenous formulation (10% glycerol) has been tried for management of acute cerebral edema associated with stroke. Glycerol can significantly reduce ICP [14]. A dose of 0.4–0.5 g of glycerol per kilogram body weight can cause the desired ICP effect [15]. Glycerol has a low reflection coefficient ($\sigma = 0.47$) readily moves across the BBB into the brain. Hence, the rebound effect of an increase in ICP after repeated administration is observed with glycerol. In a study, authors found out that a brief rise in ICP at 40 min after glycerol is withdrawn [14]. The same group of authors did not observe any changes in cerebral lactate, pyruvate, and glutamate concentrations measured by cerebral microdialysis after glycerol administration, which implies glycerol had little improvement in cerebral ischemia markers [14]. Apart from the osmotic effect, glycerol can be an alternate source of energy, can increase regional cerebral blood flow, and reduce focal edema. Intravenous glycerol can only cause hemolysis, which can be reduced by the addition of fructose to glycerol [15].

27.4 Practical Pearls

27.4.1 Indications

Evidence in Different Pathologies

The neurocritical care has laid down practice guidelines in conjunction with the use of osmotic agents, which can be followed to manage different etiologies of neurological insult admitted to neurocritical care units [1]. The guideline evaluates the role of mannitol and HTS in the initial management of cerebral edema of several etiologies such as TBI, SAH, acute ischemic, and haemorrhagic stroke. In this chapter, we are summarizing the recommendations provided in the guidelines.

In patients with TBI with cerebral edema, the authors conditionally recommend with low-quality evidence to use of HTS over mannitol for the initial management of cerebral edema. However, the brain trauma foundation (BTF) fourth edition do not recommend any particular hyperosmolar agents over other for clinical improvement. They suggest using mannitol, while cautioning for the hypotension [3]. While formulating the BTF guidelines in 2016, the available literature was not sufficient enough to recommend HTS over mannitol. However, while writing the guidelines in the neurocritical care, the panel found evidence albeit low quality to recommend HTS over mannitol for initial management of cerebral edema. The panel also felt that the accepted advantages of HTS over mannitol for fluid resuscitation and cerebral perfusion justify the recommendation [1]. All the available hypertonic sodium solutions (chloride, lactate, or bicarbonate) are effective in reducing ICP [1].

In patients with SAH, the panel suggests using symptom-based bolus dosing of hypertonic sodium solutions rather than sodium target-based dosing to effectively manage cerebral edema. The overall quality of this evidence is low. There is insufficient data to support HTS can improve neurological outcome in these patients [1].

For patients of acute ischemic stroke and intracerebral bleed, the panel suggests using either hypertonic solutions or mannitol for the initial management of ICP or cerebral edema in patients (conditional recommendation, low-quality evidence) [1]. There is insufficient evidence to recommend either hypertonic saline or mannitol for improving neurological outcomes in patients with acute ischemic stroke.

27.4.2 Routes of Administration (Peripheral vs Central)

Hyperosmolar agents can cause phlebitis and ischemic injury if extravasated from a peripheral venous site. Hence, traditionally, central venous line is the preferred route of administration. However, recently growing number of evidence supports the use of peripheral venous lines for administration of 3% HTS specially in emergency situations to initiate therapy where central venous access is not available. In such situations, it is prudent to take a large peripheral venous access to administer HTS [16]. Sodium bicarbonate (8.4%) should be given in a central vein, but in emergency it can be given via a peripheral vein [11]. Phlebitis of the infused vein always remains a practical concern if peripheral venous route is used.

27.4.3 Combination of Therapy (Mannitol and HTS)

At times, neurointensivists use a combined regimen of IV boluses of HTS and mannitol alternatively to aggressively treat cerebral edema. However, concerns are raised the combination therapy can increase the risk of acute renal injury. In a randomized controlled trial, investigators concluded that combining mannitol to the HTS did not pose increase renal dysfunction as compared to HTS alone [17].

27.4.4 How Long to Be Given

Longer use of hyperosmolar agents beyond 24–48 h remains largely unknown [18]. In the event of prolonged administration of these agents, brain gradually adapts to osmotic derangement by modifying brain-cell osmolar content. It gradually compensates for the plasma osmolar imbalance by generating osmotically active molecules called a "idiogenic osmoles," which are organic by-products such as polyols, amino acids, and triethylamines [19]. This highlights the importance of gradual weaning from the osmotherapy after therapeutic intervention. If abruptly discontinued, rebound increase in brain water leading to increase in ICP can occur [20].

27.4.5 Hyperosmolar Agents and Acute Kidney Injury

Mannitol is reno-protective, however, osmotic diuresis leading to dehydration, and pre-existing renal function can lead to further renal damage. The incidence of acute renal failure varies from 0.5% to 35% [21]. In a study, the authors found out that mannitol is an independent risk factor for development of acute kidney injury (AKI) after TBI [21]. Mannitol can lead to swelling of the proximal tubular cells, a condition called as "osmotic nephrosis" [21]. The guidelines suggest to use osmolar gap over serum osmolarity thresholds during treatment with mannitol to monitor for the risk of AKI [1]. Osmolar gap is the difference between measured and calculated osmolarity. In patients with mannitol therapy, it should not exceed 20 mOsm/kg [22]. The osmolar gap correlates with serum mannitol concentration, which is associated with renal toxicity.

In the guidelines for the osmotherapy in neurocritical care units, the panel of authors suggest to avoid severe hypernatremia and hyperchloremia in patients receiving HTS and other hyperosmolar sodium solutions [1]. These elevated serum sodium and chloride are the risk factors for development of AKI. They authors suggest an upper serum sodium concentration range of 155–160 mEq/L, and a serum chloride concentration range of 110–115 mEq/L may be reasonable to decrease the risk of AKI [1].

27.5 Conclusion

Till date, the available evidence and guidelines are of low-quality evidence when it comes to the use of osmotic agents in the neurocritical care units. The recommendations provided by the guidelines are of conditional recommendations. There is lack of clarity whether appropriate management with osmotherapy leads to good long-term neurological outcome. However, initial management is required to treat the cerebral edema and improve intracranial hemodynamic. The goals of management involve maintaining desired serum osmolality and to simultaneously prevent significant rise in serum sodium concentration. The duration of osmotherapy is largely unknown; however, the risk of rebound increase in ICP remains high after sudden withdrawal following with prolonged administration. Finally, one should also keep a tab on the adverse effects of osmotherapy which are preventable with judicious use of the agents.

References

1. Cook AM, Morgan Jones G, Hawryluk GWJ, et al. Guidelines for the acute treatment of cerebral edema in neurocritical care patients. Neurocrit Care. 2020;32(3):647–66. https://doi.org/10.1007/s12028-020-00959-7.
2. Dalby T, Wohl E, Dinsmore M, Unger Z, Chowdhury T, Venkatraghavan L. Pathophysiology of cerebral edema: a comprehensive review. J Neuroanaesth Crit Care. 2020;08:08. https://doi.org/10.1055/s-0040-1721165.
3. Carney N, Totten AM, O'Reilly C, et al. Guidelines for the management of severe traumatic brain injury, fourth edition. Neurosurgery. 2017;80(1):6–15. https://doi.org/10.1227/NEU.0000000000001432.
4. Bruder NJ, Ravussin P, Schoettker P. Supratentorial masses: anesthetic condsiderations. In: Cottrell JE, Patel P, editors. Cottrell and Patel's neuroanesthesia. 6th ed. Elsevier; 2020. p. 189–208.
5. Bourdeaux CP, Brown JM. Randomized controlled trial comparing the effect of 8.4% sodium bicarbonate and 5% sodium chloride on raised intracranial pressure after traumatic brain injury. Neurocrit Care. 2011;15(1):42–5. https://doi.org/10.1007/s12028-011-9512-0.
6. Ichai C, Armando G, Orban JC, et al. Sodium lactate versus mannitol in the treatment of intracranial hypertensive episodes in severe traumatic brain-injured patients. Intensive Care Med. 2009;35(3):471–9. https://doi.org/10.1007/s00134-008-1283-5.
7. Rozet I, Tontisirin N, Muangman S, et al. Effect of equiosmolar solutions of mannitol versus hypertonic saline on intraoperative brain relaxation and electrolyte balance. Anesthesiology. 2007;107(5):697–704. https://doi.org/10.1097/01.anes.0000286980.92759.94.
8. Kochanek PM, Tasker RC, Carney N, et al. Guidelines for the management of pediatric severe traumatic brain injury, third edition: update of the brain trauma foundation guidelines, executive summary. Neurosurgery. 2019;84(6):1169–78. https://doi.org/10.1093/neuros/nyz051.
9. Gonda DD, Meltzer HS, Crawford JR, et al. Complications associated with prolonged hypertonic saline therapy in children with elevated intracranial pressure. Pediatr Crit Care Med. 2013;14(6) https://journals.lww.com/pccmjournal/Fulltext/2013/07000/Complications_Associated_With_Prolonged_Hypertonic.7.aspx
10. Bourdeaux C, Brown J. Sodium bicarbonate lowers intracranial pressure after traumatic brain injury. Neurocrit Care. 2010;13(1):24–8. https://doi.org/10.1007/s12028-010-9368-8.
11. Bithal PK. Sodium bicarbonate is knocking at the door of neurocritical care unit: should we allow its entry? J Neuroanaesth Crit Care. 2018;05(02):75–6. https://doi.org/10.1055/s-0038-1660961.
12. Bajamal AH, Apriawan T, Ranuh IGMAR, Servadei F, Faris M, al Fauzi A. Comparison of half-molar sodium lactate and mannitol to treat brain edema in severe traumatic brain injury: a systematic review. Chin J Traumatol. 2021;24(6):344–9. https://doi.org/10.1016/j.cjtee.2021.07.005.
13. Bisri T, Utomo BA, Fuadi I. Exogenous lactate infusion improved neurocognitive function of patients with mild traumatic brain injury. Asian J Neurosurg. 2016;11(2):151–9. https://doi.org/10.4103/1793-5482.145375.
14. Berger C, Sakowitz OW, Kiening KL, Schwab S. Neurochemical monitoring of glycerol therapy in patients with ischemic brain edema. Stroke. 2005;36(2):e4–6. https://doi.org/10.1161/01.STR.0000151328.70519.e9.
15. Sakamaki M, Igarashi H, Nishiyama Y, et al. Effect of glycerol on ischemic cerebral edema assessed by magnetic resonance imaging. J Neurol Sci. 2003;209(1):69–74. https://doi.org/10.1016/S0022-510X(02)00465-3.
16. Metheny NA, Moritz ML. Administration of 3% sodium chloride via a peripheral vein: a literature review. J Infusion Nurs. 2021;44(2):94. https://journals.lww.com/journalofinfusionnursing/Fulltext/2021/03000/Administration_of_3__Sodium_Chloride_Via_a.4.aspx
17. Narayan SW, Castelino R, Hammond N, Patanwala AE. Effect of mannitol plus hypertonic saline combination versus hypertonic saline monotherapy on acute kidney injury after traumatic brain injury. J Crit Care. 2020;57:220–4. https://doi.org/10.1016/j.jcrc.2020.03.006.
18. Vagnerova K, Rusa R. Fluid management during craniotomy. In: Cottrell JE, Patel P, editors. Cottrell and Patel's neuroanesthesia. 6th ed. Elsevier; 2017. p. 152–65.
19. Ichai C, Fenouil E, Grimaud D. Osmolality and brain. Ann Fr Anesth Reanim. 1994;13(1):68–79. https://doi.org/10.1016/S0750-7658(94)80189-4.
20. Boone MD, Oren-Grinberg A, Robinson TM, Chen CC, Kasper EM. Mannitol or hypertonic saline in the setting of traumatic brain injury: what have we

learned? Surg Neurol Int. 2015;6:177. https://doi.org/10.4103/2152-7806.170248.
21. Fang L, You H, Chen B, et al. Mannitol is an independent risk factor of acute kidney injury after cerebral trauma: a case–control study. Ren Fail. 2010;32(6):673–9. https://doi.org/10.3109/0886022X.2010.486492.
22. García-Morales EJ, Cariappa R, Parvin CA, Scott MG, Diringer MN. Osmole gap in neurologic-neurosurgical intensive care unit: its normal value, calculation, and relationship with mannitol serum concentrations. Crit Care Med. 2004;32(4):986. https://journals.lww.com/ccmjournal/Fulltext/2004/04000/Osmole_gap_in_neurologic_neurosurgical_intensive.15.aspx

Part V

Systemic Neurocritical Care

Cardiac Problems in Neurocritical Care

28

Sethuraman Manikandan and Ajayprasad Hrishi

28.1 Introduction

Managing patients in the neurocritical care unit is very challenging as compared to patients in other intensive care units (ICU). Patients admitted with acute neurological conditions can develop other organ dysfunctions which needs great attention. Among those, cardiopulmonary dysfunction is more common occurring up to 70–80% in neurocritical patients [1]. These complications may be present at admission or during the course of ICU stay. The importance of these organ dysfunction is that they influence the management, outcomes of the brain injury, increase the costs of care, and hospital stay [2]. It is estimated that over 1.5 million people die of neurocardiogenic interactions [3] However, unlike other critical care units, the cardiopulmonary complications are modifiable if timely intervened. Hence, prompt recognition and management can reduce these complications. This chapter gives the various cardiopulmonary complications that can occur in acute neurological conditions with an aim to recognize and provide concepts in the management.

28.2 Pathophysiology of Cardiac Injury in Brain Injury

The brain controls the heart by connections involving central and peripheral autonomic network of sympathetic and parasympathetic system, which is also called as *Brain-Heart Axis*. Various areas in the cerebral cortex like insula, pre frontal cortex, amygdala, paraventricular, dorsomedial nuclei of hypothalamus, stria nucleus, as well as brain stem via nucleus tractus solitorius and dorsal nuclei of vagus (parasympathetic outflow) periaqueductal gray matter, rostral ventrolateral medulla; and rostral ventromedial medulla (preganglionic sympathetic fibers) (Fig. 28.1) In the peripheral autonomic network, the para sympathetic cholinergic innervation via vagus is to the conduction system and the noradrenergic sympathetic innervation is to the atria and to ventricles. The apex of the heart is very low in innervation, and the base has rich innervations. There is also intrinsic network of innervation in the heart, which is under the control of extrinsic autonomic output from brain. Acute brain injury can result in the following pattern of cardiac involvement;

S. Manikandan (✉) · A. Hrishi
Division of Neuroanaesthesiology and Neurocritical Care, Department of Anaesthesiology, Sree Chitra Tirunal Institute for Medical Sciences and Technology (SCTIMST), Trivandrum, Kerala, India

H. Prabhakar et al. (eds.), *Principles and Practice of Neurocritical Care*,
https://doi.org/10.1007/978-981-99-8059-8_28

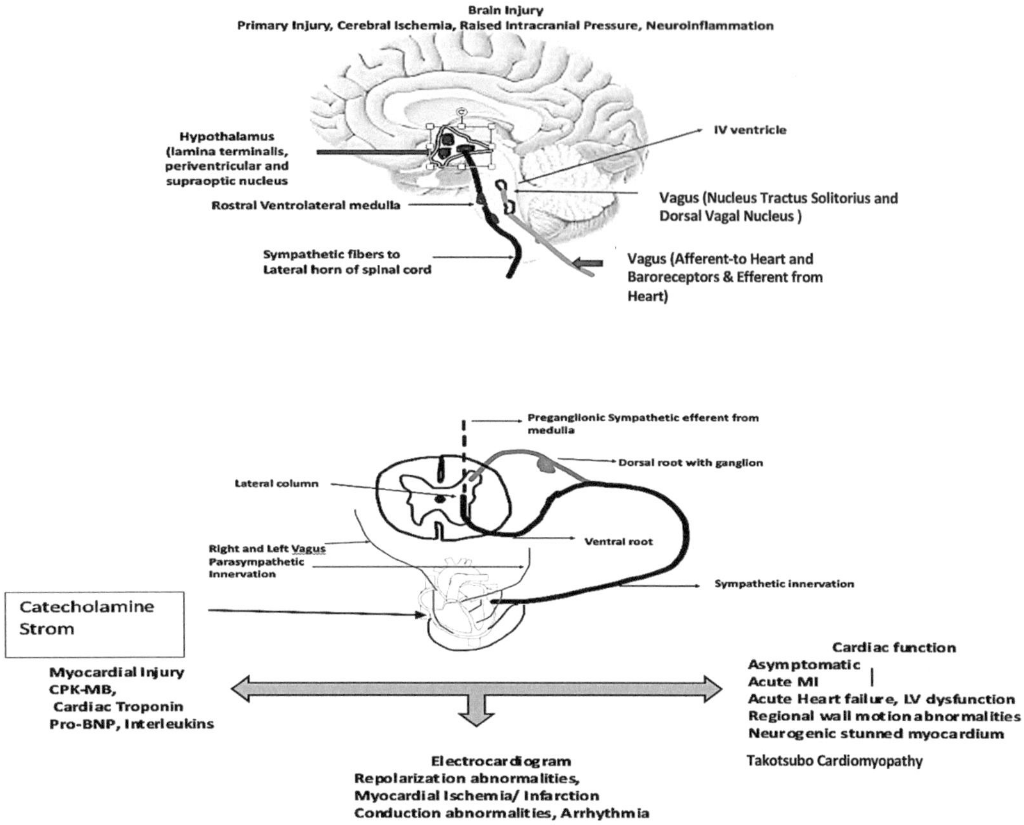

Fig. 28.1 Illustrating the central and peripheral autonomic innervations of the brain–heart axis(CPK-MB-myocardial specific creatinine phosphokinase, Pro-BNP-pro brain natriuretic peptide)

28.2.1 Neurogenic Stunned Myocardium (NSM)

Neurogenic stunned myocardium is a form of reversible left ventricular dysfunction presenting with features like acute myocardial infarction due to the sudden sympathetic storm. The inciting cause is acute ischemia, injury, raised ICP, and neuroinflammation. The brain areas subserving central autonomic network like medulla, hypothalamus, insular cortex, and amygdala is affected, which leads to excess release of catecholamines from nor adrenergic nerve endings (preganglionic) and from adrenal medulla. The sudden surge in norepinephrine and epinephrine levels causes myocardial damage. The pathogenesis is thought to be coronary vasospasm, micro thrombosis, excessive calcium entry into myocytes, severe ventricular myocytes contraction, myocardial injury, and contraction band necrosis. The damaged cardiac muscle release biomarkers of injury like cardiac specific Troponin (cTnI). The resultant myocardial dysfunction and heart failure lead to elevation of N terminal pro-brain natriuretic peptide (NT Pro BNP). The features of NSM are ECG changes of ST segment elevation, T wave inversion, Q wave, echocardiography shows low ejection fraction, regional wall motion abnormalities which is non-specific of a coronary artery territory, basal and mid hypokinesia, poor radial and circumferential strain in speckle tracking echo, and increased cTnI and NT-pro BNP levels [4].

28.2.2 Stress Cardiomyopathy

Stress cardiomyopathy also called as Takotsubo cardiomyopathy or broken heart syndrome occurs due to brain injury and is less common compared to NSM. The pathogenesis is similar to NSM, but the echocardiography shows apical ballooning with preserved basal segments contraction. Clinically, the patients can present with features of ST segment elevation acute MI. The ratio of NT-Pro BNP/cTnI is higher in stress cardiomyopathy, whereas it is revere in acute MI. There are no specific guidelines in management. In majority of cases, the condition is self-limiting; however, in severe forms where the patient present with acute heart failure, the management includes provision of hemodynamic support, using inotropes using drugs like levosimendan, adequate oxygenation, beta blockers to reduce the stress, diuretics, and in extreme cases intra-aortic balloon counter pulsation for maintaining circulation [5].

28.2.3 Neurogenic Pulmonary Edema (NPE)

NPE is a life-threatening condition that can occur in a wide variety of conditions with incidence between 8% and 25%. The excess and acute sympathetic discharge caused by acute brain damage leads to systemic and pulmonary vasoconstriction thereby cause increase in systemic arterial, pulmonary arterial pressure, enhanced venous return, interstitial edema, and alveolar hemorrhages [6]. NPE occurs as early as 30 min of initial brain insult and can persist up to 72 h. Severity can be assessed by degree of hypoxia, PaO_2/FiO_2 ratio. Management of the condition is mainly supportive like lung protective ventilation, hemodynamic support, and diuretics. Use of alpha-adrenergic blockers like phentolamine has been tried. NPE can occur along with stress cardiomyopathy. NPE is associated with increased mortality in acute brain injury [7].

28.3 Cardiac Complications in Traumatic Brain Injury (TBI)

Traumatic brain injuries by road traffic accidents are a leading cause of death worldwide in the 5–29 years age group. It is projected that over three million death and 7.4 million disability will occur by 2030 worldwide due to RTA [8]. Management of TBI is one of the most difficult challenge of neurocritical care due to the intensity of monitoring and interventions required. The association of severe cardiac dysfunction in TBI was well-recognized 50 years ago [9]. The research on the effects of raised intracranial pressure on the autonomic dysfunction in head injuries and the brain–heart interaction also started in similar times [10].

The cardiac dysfunction occurs within minutes following TBI as shown in an in an animal model, where the TBI caused fall in mean arterial pressure, cerebral prefusion pressure (CPP), and elevated ICP. Echocardiography showed features of left ventricular (LV) dysfunction [11]. The systolic dysfunction occurs early and becomes normalized in a week in isolated adult moderate to severe TBI. Those who had systolic dysfunction presented with early hypertension and tachycardia followed by excessive hypotension over the first day [12, 13].

ECG changes of repolarization abnormalities (QTc prolongation, ST segment changes, T wave changes) were seen in 53% of TBI patients, and these abnormalities make the victims vulnerable for tachyarrhythmias, atrial fibrillation, etc. Elevation of cardiac-specific troponin (cTn I) occurred very early (in 3–5 h) in 31% of patients, signifying underlying myocardial injury and the levels returned to baseline in a week in most patients. Higher serum values of cTnI (12–14 ng/dL) have been correlated with mortality in TBI. If persistent elevation of cTnI beyond 1 week is seen in patients, it can be due to underlying heart disease, sepsis, etc. In addition, other biomarkers like NT pro-BNP levels also are elevated that occur after 2–3 days. The levels correlate with degree of raised ICP, hyponatremia, cerebral edema, and size of brain lesions [14]. Studies have shown that there is higher levels of circulating catecholamine like norepinephrine, epinephrine in blood in TBI, and the levels correlated with severity of injury, mechanical ventilation, and mortality. Severe myocardial injury in TBI can lead to neurogenic stunned myocardium or Takotsubo disease. The greater the head abbreviated injury scoring (AIS), and severe the TBI (poor Glasgow coma scale-GCS score), greater the incidence and severe is the myocardial dysfunction [15].

Studies have shown that cardiac dysfunction in TBI is associated with high mortality. To assess the presence and severity of cardiac dysfunction, a Neurogenic Cardiac Injury Score (NCIS) is devised with the following points;

(a) Elevated cardiac troponin (marker of myocardial injury) = 1 point.
(b) Altered cardiac function by echocardiography(representing the severity of cardiac injury) = 1 point.
(c) Systemic hypotension (effect of myocardial damage) = 1 point.

NCIS value varies between 0 and 3. It was noted that higher the score, greater the mortality in TBI (odds ratio 8.3; confidence interval 95%) [16].

28.3.1 Cardiac Complications in Acute Ischemic Stroke (AIS)

Stroke is second leading cause of with incidence of death worldwide with occurrence of 13 million new cases annually [17]. The etiology can be varied from cryptogenic to sequalae of heart diseases like atrial fibrillation, aggressive and ultra-early/ early-intensive interventions like intravenous thrombolysis and mechanical thrombectomy are employed to manage AIS patients to reduce the ischemic area and re perfuse the brain. Patients presenting with AIS may have associated systemic complications, which will affect the outcomes and need aggressive therapy [18]. The involvement of heart in AIS is a well-known phenomenon. In an early retrospective study, 28% of patients with AIS had low ejection fraction (<50%), ischemic changes in ECG, and elevated cardiac troponin levels. Those who had cardiac dysfunction had higher mortality [19]. In a recent large study of 1999 patients with AIS, elevated cardiac troponin was seen at admission in 20% of AIS patients and was associated with echocardiographic abnormalities. Those who had elevated cTn had increased mortality at 1- and 3-year following AIS [20]. Moreover, an association was found between elevated cardiac troponin levels at admission and large vessel occlusion (LVO) in AIS patients. These patients needed mechanical thrombectomy [21]. This association of very high biomarkers could be due to the fact LVO can cause large areas of brain ischemia, which in turn causes severe sympathetic mediated cardiac dysfunction and a more severe cardiac dysfunction. It may also be noted that periprocedural management for mechanical thrombectomy needs to address both the brain and heart dysfunction.

Recently, the pattern of involvement of heart in AIS is specifically termed as "Stroke heart Syndrome (SHS)" [3]. The importance in recognition of this syndrome is due to the fact that an estimated one million die due to these complications post stroke Five post stroke subtypes of cardiac involvement have been identified;

1. Acute myocardial injury characterized by elevated biomarker(cTn), which may be ischemic or non- ischemic origin and are asymptomatic.
2. Acute myocardial infarction (AMI) caused by coronary vasospasm or coronary supply demand mismatch, coronary artery disease.
3. Acute heart failure or left ventricular dysfunction, heart failure (HF), and Takotsubo syndrome.
4. ECG changes, cardiac arrhythmias including post-stroke atrial fibrillation (AF);
5. Neurogenic sudden cardiac death.

The postulated mechanisms of cardiac injury include local and systemic inflammation, autonomic dysregulation, excessive circulating catecholamines, which affects the myocardial structural and functional damage.

Post stroke AMI due to coronary artery disease can complicate the ICU course with a reported incidence of 1.6%. However, management of this condition is challenging, and optimum treatments such as percutaneous coronary interventions and antithrombotic agents are not adequately administered as these interventions carries high risk of bleeding complications [22].

28.3.2 Cardiac Complications in Subarachnoid Hemorrhage (SAH)

Nontraumatic subarachnoid hemorrhage is usually caused by rupture of intracranial aneurysms. Myocardial necrosis induced by excess catecholamines and features of abnormal ECG and mortality is a well-recognized entity following aneurysmal SAH and beta blocker therapy was shown to reduce the mortality for the same [23].

Overall, the cardiac dysfunction was seen in more than 50% of SAH. The incidence of ECG changes is reported to be as high as 65%, and stress cardiomyopathy in 15% was associated with adverse outcomes in SAH [24]. In another meta-analysis, RWMA was seen in 22% and elevated cTnI and high proBNP/cTnI in 37% of SAH. The LV dysfunction and the biomarker levels were thought to normalize within 10–14 days of ictus onset in majority of cases without long term sequlae. However, there are recent literature shows that in 17% of SAH patients, the cardiac dysfunction (low EF < 50% and diastolic dysfunction) persisted on follow-up echocardiographic analysis at 90 days [25].

In the ECG, QTc prolongation was associated with delayed cerebral ischemia and NPE, whereas ST depression was correlated to death [26]. Moreover, abnormal rhythm as high as 90% and severe arrhythmias like ventricular tachyarrhythmias in 40% were noted in acute phase of SAH [27]. Cardiac electrophysiological balance index (ICEB) is considered to be better than ECG alone in identifying the risk of arrhythmias. The indices, QT/QRS duration, and QTc/QRS were increased in SAH and found to correlate with Fisher grade [28].

Considering that early surgery/intervention is needed for aneurysmal SAH and high incidence of cardiac injury, the perioperative and intensive care management needs to be aggressive addressing to the needs of heart as well as brain. The key to successful management is to assess the severity, type of cardiac injury, and maintain hemodynamic stability and optimum cerebral perfusion pressure as there are no guidelines exists in managing this complex scenario.

28.3.3 Cardiac Complications in Intracerebral Hemorrhage (ICH)

Intracerebral hemorrhage (ICH) is a devastating acute condition with high mortality and morbidity. ICH can cause sudden increase in intracranial pressure, disrupts the neurons, and tracks leading to various neurological deficits and altered sensorium. ICH has been associated with various cardiovascular events. ICH patients have history of hypertension, and in acute stage, the blood pressure can be very high which is also an important risk factor for ICH size increase. Aggressive management of blood pressure and its beneficial effects on cardiovascular and cerebrovascular adverse events have been evaluated [29]. In the post hoc analysis of Antihypertensive Treatment of Acute Cerebral Hemorrhage-II Trial (ATACH-2), comparing aggressive reduction in SBP to 110–130 mmHg in patients with SBP of >20 mmHg vs <200 mmHg, showed neurological deficits were higher in the former group without hemotaoma size reduction, disability, and mortality benefits [30]. However, another post hoc analysis of ATACH-2 in patients with moderate to severe ICH has shown hematoma expansion is reduced in patients where aggressive BP reduction was achieved [31]. A pooled analysis of INTERACT-2 (Intensive Blood Pressure Reduction in Acute Cerebral Hemorrhage Trial –2), and ATACH-2 trial noted that there is a J-shaped relationship between the BP reductions and poor functional outcome assesses by modified Rankin Scale. A modest reduction (approx.

60 mmHg) in BP from initial high BP in first 24 h is associated with better functional outcome compared to aggressive reduction of >70 mmHg or no BP reduction [32].

Very limited literature is available on cardiovascular issue in acute ICH. Severe adverse in hospital cardiac complications in acute ICH patients was found to be 4.1%. These include acute heart failure (AHF), serious cardiac arrhythmias like ventricular tachycardia, ventricular fibrillation, and new onset atrial fibrillation (AF). History of severe hypertension with ECG changes of LVH was seen in ICH patients, whereas prior MI, old or new onset AF, hyperglycemia were risk factors for severe adverse cardiovascular events. ICH patients may be associated with higher incidence of other ECG changes like tachycardia, PR interval prolongation, QTc prolongation, QRS changes, bundle branch block. Cardiac-specific troponin levels also were found to be higher in ICH with cardiovascular changes. The cardiac vascular complications are treatable and were not found to be major cause of death in ICH. The major cause of death in ICH was found to be due to brain herniation.

Patients who had history of ICH have been associated with long-term major adverse cardiovascular complications (MACE), recurrent ICH, and ischemic stroke. In a large study, it was noted that patients with history of ICH had higher incidence of MACE (4.2 vs 1.35) compared to controls [33]. Patients with ICH also found to have labile hypertension, and the fluctuations were associated with adverse cardiovascular complications. It is now being recognized that patients with ICH need to be managed aggressively blood pressure control, prevention of adverse evets with statins, and antiplatelet drugs. A recent study found that those patients who have systolic blood pressure of <120 mmHg post ICH had reduced cardiovascular adverse events compare to those with BP targets of <130 mmHg [34].

28.4 Cardiac Complications in Spinal Cord Injury

Acute spinal cord injury (SCI) can occur due to trauma, vascular, infectious, and demyelinating diseases. Among these traumatic spinal cord injury is very common and usually affects the young. Since spinal cord carries sympathetic innervations (preganglionic sympathetic fibers) to the heart and blood vessels, injury can lead to loss of sympathetic innervation distal to injury and unopposed parasympathetic activity. This can cause autonomic dysregulation of the heart and blood vessels. The degree to which it is affected depends on the site and severity of the SCI [35]. Injury from upper cervical to T1 cord can cause complete loss of sympathetic innervation, lesions from T1 to T6 can lead to maintenance of some sympathetic functions, whereas lesions below T7 have only minimal effect t of sympathetic supply.

Immediately following SCI, there is a phase of "Neurogenic shock" characterized by severe hypotension and bradycardia which when in severe form can lead to asystole. Neurogenic shock can occur due to either primary or secondary SCI. This period last for days and even up to 5 weeks [36]. Both systolic and diastolic hypotension, orthostatic hypotension can be seen in acute phase. Neurogenic shock must be differentiated from hypovolemic/hemorrhagic shock and cardiogenic shock. Management consists of aggressive fluid resuscitation, use of inotropes (if both hypotension and bradycardia is present), or vasopressors (if only hypotension). If the low heart rate is unresponsive to pharmacotherapy, temporary cardiac pacing may be required. Autonomic dysreflexia (AD) is another cardiovascular complication seen in SCI. It is characterized by elevation of systolic blood pressure > 20%, changes in heart rate, to noxious and non-noxious stimuli along with features sweating, piloerection, facial, skin flushing with symptoms of headache, stuffy nose, and visual disturbances. Sometimes, AD can be severe leading to arrhythmias. Though AD is seen in chronic phase, it was seen in 5.7% of acute SCI [37].

In a large meta-analysis, Alexandra et al. found that patients with SCI had smaller left ventricular volumes (end diastolic and end systolic volume, stroke volume) low LV mass, preserved ejection fraction, diastolic dysfunction in echocardiography even at rest [38]. This can lead to long-term cardiovascular complications.

28.5 Cardiac Complications in Potential Brain Death Organ Donors

Brain death is an end stage of brain structural damage associated with cessation of brain stem functions. Those suspected brain as well as confirmed brain death victims pose special challenges in their management. Cardiac dysfunction occurs in various stages of evolution of brain death. It is noted initial period is characterized by excess parasympathetic activity manifesting as bradycardia and hypotension. As the intracranial pressure raises to dangerous levels, herniation of brain stem occurs. There is severe brain stem ischemia, leading to excess sympathetic output form the brain stem centers causing "Catecholomine strom." This is manifested by severe hypertension (sometimes SBP in excess of 250 mmHg) and tachyarrhythmias including VF. This storm also causes excessive systemic and pulmonary vascular resistance, neurogenic pulmonary edema, myocardial ischemia, and various organ damage. Once the brain death occurred, there is loss of autonomic function, circulating catecholamines, leading to bradycardia and hypotension [39]. Cardiac arrest is the most frequent sequlae of brain death and loss of potential organ donor. Maintenance of cardiovascular function is important requisites in managing these patients.

A protocol-based hemodynamic approach has been shown to reduce the incidence of cardiac arrest in these patients [40].

The goal-directed therapy also commonly termed as VIP (ventilation, infusion, and pumping) consists of maintenance of;

(a) Ventilation: Maintenance of $PaO_2 > 100$ mmHg, adapting lung protective ventilation, reduce systemic inflammation with steroids.
(b) Infusion: Maintenance of intravascular volume by goal-directed fluid therapy and intense hemodynamic monitoring, managing diuresis to maintain urine output of 100 mL/h and to treat diabetes insipidus with vasopressin or desmopressin.
(c) Pumping and Pressure: Maintenance of cardiac contractility with use of inotropes/vasopressors to maintain normal cardiac output, mean arterial pressure > 65 mmHg, systolic blood pressure > 100 mmHg.

Additional goals include maintenance of normothermia, blood sugar levels<180 mg/dL, serum sodium <150 mEq/dL, and maintenance of protocols 12–24 h [41].

28.6 Cardiac Complications in Epilepsy

Epilepsy is one of the common neurological disorder seen in general population. Acute emergencies can occur in epilepsy patients as seen in trauma from sudden falls, status epilepticus, loss of consciousness, and hypoxia. Association of cardiac dysfunction in epilepsy patients has been of interest to researchers in the recent years [42]. In patients with chronic epilepsy, systemic hypertension, and myocardial fibrosis have been demonstrated. Presence of risk factors like smoking, diabetes mellitus, and age can increase the severity of cardiac dysfunction. Coronary artery disease has also been reported. Preictal or baseline tachycardia and absence of heart rate variability (HRV) have been found in these patients at risk of cardiac arrythmias, and they are due to autonomic imbalance at the level of insular cortex [43]. Ictal bradycardia and asystole are seen in temporal lobe epilepsy, whereas ictal tachycardia and tachyarrhythmias are seen in generalized seizure.

Patients with refractory status epilepticus (RSE) usually require mechanical ventilation along with prolonged use of anesthetic agents. A high incidence (up to two-thirds) of cardiac dysfunction in these patients as evaluated by cardiac enzymes. Various cardiac abnormalities that are prevalent include left ventricular dysfunction of varying severity including Takotsubo cardiomyopathy. ECG changes include repolarization abnormalities, T wave inversion (37%), nonspecific ST-T changes (37%), less incidence of ST elevation and ST depression, sinus tachycardia, and sinus bradycardia [44]. Arrythmias can be also seen like atrial tachycardia, atrial fibrillation, atrioventricular conduction blocks, and extreme cases ventricular fibrillation.

The presence of cardiac dysfunction has been shown to increase the mortality in RSE. Hence, intense cardiovascular evaluation is needed in patients with seizures admitted to neuro critical care with ECG and cardiac enzyme levels followed by echocardiogram. Besides specific management of RSE, recognizing and treating systemic factors like metabolic, electrolyte imbalances, intravascular fluids, fever, sepsis, drug interactions of anaesthetic agents (as many antiepileptics affect the cardiac conduction), appropriate use of inotropes/vasopressors are needed in caring these RSE patients.

28.7 Cardiac Dysfunction in Guillain Barre Syndrome (GBS)

Guillain Barre syndrome (GBS) is an autoimmune disorder and most common cause of acute flaccid paralysis. The onset of the disease occurs few days post viral infection. The presentation and severity of the disease can be varied. Patients with GBS usually need neurointensive care admission, long-term mechanical ventilation depending upon severity, subtypes, and response to therapy. Cardiac and hemodynamic issues are common in ICU with up to 70% of GBS patients have involvement of autonomic fibers in the acute stage. Sympathetic hyperactivity is more common compared to parasympathetic activity. The denervation hypesensitivity of the heart and blood vessels, increasing levels of circulating catecholamines, and carotid sinus dysfunction are important mechanisms of cardiac dysfunction [45]. These are exaggerated by intravascular volume shifts, medications affecting the autonomic function, position changes painful procedures, etc. commonly seen in ICU care. In a retrospective analysis of GBS patients requiring intensive care, autonomic dysfunction was found in 16%, and it was associated with mortality [46]. Hence, it is important to identify and manage these cardiovascular complications in GBS (Table 28.1).

28.8 Cardiac Complications in Myasthenia Gravis (MG)

Myasthenia gravis (MG) is autoimmune disorder needing neurocritical care admission for respiratory failure, myasthenic, or cholinergic crisis. MG is a disorder characterized by the muscle weakness due to autoantibodies to the acetylcholine receptors at the NM junction. These patients

Table 28.1 Showing cardiovascular abnormalities in GB syndrome [47]

Category	Hemodynamic changes	Remarks
Heart rate	Sinus tachycardia	Most common
	Sinus bradycardia	Less common, precipitated by procedures like tracheal suction, eye ball pressure, carotid sinus dysfunction. May be associated with AV conduction abnormalities and may require temporary pacemaker
	Atrial and ventricular tachyarrhythmias	Less common. May require medications like esmolol, labetalol
Blood pressure	Hypotension, hypertension	Labile BP fluctuations are common due to autonomic dysfunction. If mean arterial pressure > 125 mmHg, treatment is warranted. Use of titratable, short-acting agents like SNP may be of choice
Myocardial involvement	Myocarditis (post infectious	Associated with tachycardia. Cardiac enzyme levels will help in diagnosis.
	LV dysfunction	Varying severity from low EF to neurogenic stunned myocardium due to catecholamine injury has been reported. Management is usually symptomatic
	Acute coronary syndrome (ACS)	ACS with involvement of posterior wall MI has been reported in elderly in undiagnosed GB syndrome. ECG changes (ST elevation/depression) cardiac enzyme levels and ECHO for RWMA will help in diagnosis
	Electrocardiogram changes	Besides rhythm disturbances, tall T waves, QT prolongation, U waves are seen in GBS patients

are treated with anti-choline-esterase medications along with steroids and immunosuppressive agent. In crisis, the management consists of mechanical ventilation, plasmapheresis, or immunoglobulin use. Cardiovascular and hemodynamic issues have occurred in ICU management.

MG may be associated with cardiac abnormalities. 16% of the MG patients had myocardial involvement specific to MG characterized by focal myocarditis, myocardial edema, and dysfunction. These may be immune mediated (immune myocarditis), and MRI is useful in identifying the condition. The clinical presentation frequently occurs in thymoma patient and mostly are arrythmias. Rarely, MG crisis may be associated with Takotsubo or reverse Takotsubo cardiomyopathy [48].

Patients administered anti-choline esterase medications can have bradycardia especially it is more prominent in cholinergic crisis where it is associated with sialorrhea, inability to cough, etc. A case of acute coronary spasm leading to myocardial ischemia due to pyridostigmine has been reported in a young onset MG [49].

28.9 Cardiac Issues in Neuromuscular Disorders (NMD)

Neuromuscular diseases are broad group of disease involving the muscle, neuromuscular junction, or the nerve. The clinical presentation is usually muscle weakness with or without sensory involvement. The etiology of the disease is varied from genetic, congenital, inflammatory, infectious, nutritional, autoimmune, electrolytes imbalance, drugs, and toxins, etc. Patients with NMD can be associated with neurological emergency to ICU with either acute neuromuscular paralysis or gradual worsening of the muscle weakness leading to end-stage disease. The emergency can be either acute respiratory distress or cardiovascular dysfunction.

The patients belonging to various genetic or congenital NMD may have cardiac abnormalities. The cardiac abnormalities can be broadly

(a) Cardiomyopathy (Dilated/Hypertrophic): Duchenne, Becker muscular dystrophy, Limb gridle muscular dystrophy (LGMD), NMD associated with mitochondrial dysfunction like Friedreich ataxia, Barth syndrome, myofibrillar myopathies.
(b) Conduction abnormalities and arrhythmias: Muscle dystrophy like Emery-Dreifuss, certain subtypes of LGMD (LGMDB1, LGMD2E) myopathies like Nemaline rod myopathy.

The presentation and severity of cardiac manifestations may not be parallel with NMD severity. Hence, caution must be exercised during their evaluation and management. It is recommended to evaluate for cardiac status using ECG, imaging studies like echocardiography, ambulatory ECGs in specific interval to know the progression of the condition. It is also recommended that cardiac evaluation be done before anesthesia or major procedures. (Level 1 recommendation) [50].

28.10 Management of Cardiac Complications in Neurocritical Care

There are no guidelines, literature on the exact management of the patients with cardiac complications with acute brain injury. The general principle of neurocritical care in maintaining the adequate cerebral perfusion pressure, cerebral oxygenation, control and treatment of raised ICP, systemic hemodynamics, avoidance of factors that aggravates the brain injury needs to be aggressively undertaken. In majority of the cases, the cardiac dysfunction improves within hours to days especially when the insult to brain is treated. The principle of managing those with cardiac complications include;

(a) Recognizing the presence of cardiac dysfunction using serial investigations; at the time of admission (3–5 h of acute insult), thereafter till 1 week; ECG, echocardiogram, chest radiography, and biomarkers of myocardial injury. If persistent abnormalities noted, then distinguish with structural cardiac abnormality or other causes.

(b) Distinguishing the benign changes from severe forms of cardiac injury like low ejection fraction (<50%), regional wall motion abnormalities (RWMA), neurogenic stunned myocardium, Takotsubo cardiomyopathy, cardiogenic shock, neurogenic pulmonary edema, QTc prolongation, and severe arrhythmias.

(c) Rule out neurogenic cause from cardiac causes like acute myocardial infarction from coronary artery diseases.

(d) Management of the neurocritical care of these patients must involve the guidelines of VIPPS (ventilation, infusion, pumping and perfusion) along with pharmacological support and specificities) [40].

(e) Role of pharmacotherapy with beta blockers to reduce the injury in select stable patient has been suggested, but there is not strong evidence for routine use [15].

(f) Since the neurogenic-induced myocardial injury is caused by high catecholamines or sympathetic activity, use of phosphodiesterase inhibitors like milrinone or calcium sensitizer like levosimendan can be the choice for hemodynamic support. In extreme cases, intra-aortic balloon pump use may be needed.

Key Points

- A high percentage of patients admitted with acute neurological problems in neurocritical care can present with or will have hemodynamic instability or features of cardiac dysfunction.
- An acute brain/spinal cord injury is associated with severe stress caused by trauma, cerebral ischemia, raised intracranial pressure (ICP), altered brain functions, neuroinflammation, and increased circulating catecholamines.
- The above pathological process causes the autonomic dysfunction (AD) causing myocardial damage which occurs within minutes to hours of neuronal damage.
- The damage can be asymptomatic or associated hemodynamic perturbations with electrocardiographic (ECG), echocardiographic changes affecting the structure and function of the heart/ blood vessels .
- Biomarker analysis of specific for myocardial injury can help in assessing the time course and severity of injury.
- The moderate to severe myocardial injury is found to be an important cause of morbidity and mortality in an acute brain injured patient. Underlying intrinsic cardiac problems needs to be differentiated which can be challenging.
- Early recognition and aggressive management may mitigate the damage to the patients.

References

1. Zygun DA, Doig CJ, Gupta AK, Whiting G, Nicholas C, Shepherd E, Conway-Smith C, Menon DK. Non-neurological organ dysfunction in neurocritical care. J Crit Care. 2003;18:238–44. https://doi.org/10.1016/j.jcrc.2003.10.007.
2. Zygun D. Non-neurological organ dysfunction in neurocritical care: impact on outcome and etiological considerations. Curr Opin Crit Care. 2005;11:139–43. https://doi.org/10.1097/01.ccx.0000155356.86241.c0.
3. Sposato LA, Hilz MJ, Aspberg S, Murthy SB, Bahit MC, Hsieh CY, Sheppard MN, Scheitz JF, World Stroke Organisation Brain & Heart Task Force. Post-stroke cardiovascular complications and neurogenic cardiac injury: JACC state-of-the-art review. J Am Coll Cardiol. 2020;76:2768–85. https://doi.org/10.1016/j.jacc.2020.10.009.
4. Kerro A, Woods T, Chang JJ. Neurogenic stunned myocardium in subarachnoid hemorrhage. J Crit Care. 2017;38:27–34. https://doi.org/10.1016/j.jcrc.2016.10.010.
5. Matta AG, Carrié D. Epidemiology, pathophysiology, diagnosis, and principles of management of Takotsubo cardiomyopathy: a review. Med Sci Monit. 2023;6(29):e939020. https://doi.org/10.12659/MSM.939020.
6. Šedý J, Kuneš J, Zicha J. Pathogenetic mechanisms of neurogenic pulmonary edema. J Neurotrauma. 2015;32:1135–45. https://doi.org/10.1089/neu.2014.3609.
7. Davison DL, Terek M, Chawla LS. Neurogenic pulmonary edema. Crit Care. 2012;16:212. https://doi.org/10.1186/cc11226.
8. Symons J, Howard E, Sweeny K, Kumnick M, Sheehan P. Reduced road traffic injuries for young people: a preliminary investment analysis. J Adolesc Health. 2019;65:S34–43.

9. Julkunen H, Kataja J, Lahdensuu M, Rokkanen P. Electrocardiographic changes in severely injured patients treated at the intensive care unit. Analysis of 328 consecutive cases. Ann Chir Gynaecol Fenn. 1972;61:107–11.
10. Lowensohn RI, Weiss M, Hon EH. Heart-rate variability in brain-damaged adults. Lancet. 1977;19:626–8. https://doi.org/10.1016/s0140-6736(77)92060-8.
11. Adedipe A, John AS, Krishnamoorthy V, Wang X, Steck DT, Ferreira R, White N, Stern S. Left ventricular function in the initial period after severe traumatic brain injury in swine. Neurocrit Care. 2022;37:200–8. https://doi.org/10.1007/s12028-022-01468-5.
12. Krishnamoorthy V, Rowhani-Rahbar A, Gibbons EF, Rivara FP, Temkin NR, Pontius C, Luk K, Graves M, Lozier D, Chaikittisilpa N, Kiatchai T, Vavilala MS. Early systolic dysfunction following traumatic brain injury: a cohort study. Crit Care Med. 2017;45:1028–36. https://doi.org/10.1097/CCM.0000000000002404.
13. Krishnamoorthy V, Rowhani-Rahbar A, Chaikittisilpa N, Gibbons EF, Rivara FP, Temkin NR, Quistberg A, Vavilala MS. Association of early hemodynamic profile and the development of systolic dysfunction following traumatic brain injury. Neurocrit Care. 2017;26:379–87. https://doi.org/10.1007/s12028-016-0335-x.
14. Wu X, Sha H, Sun Y, Gao L, Liu H, Yuan Q, Zhang T, Zhu J, Zhou L, Hu J. N-terminal pro-B-type natriuretic peptide in patients with isolated traumatic brain injury: a prospective cohort study. J Trauma. 2011;71:820–5.; discussion 825. https://doi.org/10.1097/TA.0b013e3182277b69.
15. El-Menyar A, Goyal A, Latifi R, Al-Thani H, Frishman W. Brain-heart interactions in traumatic brain injury. Cardiol Rev. 2017;25:279–88. https://doi.org/10.1097/CRD.0000000000000167.
16. Hasanin A, Kamal A, Amin S, Zakaria D, El Sayed R, Mahmoud K, Mukhtar A. Incidence and outcome of cardiac injury in patients with severe head trauma. Scand J Trauma Resusc Emerg Med. 2016;24:58. https://doi.org/10.1186/s13049-016-0246-z. Erratum in: Scand J Trauma Resusc Emerg Med. 2016;24:79. PMID: 27121183; PMCID: PMC4848772
17. Saini V, Guada L, Yavagal DR. Global epidemiology of stroke and access to acute ischemic stroke interventions. Neurology. 2021;97(20 Suppl. 2):S6–S16. https://doi.org/10.1212/WNL.0000000000012781.
18. Wu F, Liu Z, Zhou L, Ye D, Zhu Y, Huang K, Weng Y, Xiong X, Zhan R, Shen J. Systemic immune responses after ischemic stroke: from the center to the periphery. Front Immunol. 2022;20(13):911661. https://doi.org/10.3389/fimmu.2022.911661.
19. Wira CR 3rd, Rivers E, Martinez-Capolino C, Silver B, Iyer G, Sherwin R, Lewandowski C. Cardiac complications in acute ischemic stroke. West J Emerg Med. 2011;12:414–20. https://doi.org/10.5811/westjem.2011.2.1765.
20. Wrigley P, Khoury J, Eckerle B, Alwell K, Moomaw CJ, Woo D, Flaherty ML, Rios DL, la Rosa F, Mackey J, Adeoye O, Martini S, Ferioli S, Kissela BM, Kleindorfer DO. Prevalence of positive troponin and echocardiogram findings and association with mortality in acute ischemic stroke. Stroke. 2017;48:1226–32. https://doi.org/10.1161/STROKEAHA.116.014561.
21. Chang A, Ricci B, Grory BM, Cutting S, Burton T, Dakay K, Jayaraman M, Merkler A, Reznik M, Lerario MP, Song C, Kamel H, Elkind MSV, Furie K, Yaghi S. Cardiac biomarkers predict large vessel occlusion in patients with ischemic stroke. J Stroke Cerebrovasc Dis. 2019;28:1726–31. https://doi.org/10.1016/j.jstrokecerebrovasdis.2019.02.013.
22. Suzuki T, Kataoka Y, Shiozawa M, Morris K, Kiyoshige E, Nishimura K, Murai K, Sawada K, Iwai T, Matama H, Honda S, Fujino M, Yoneda S, Takagi K, Otsuka F, Asaumi Y, Koga M, Ihara M, Toyoda K, Tsujita K, Noguchi T. Heart-brain team approach of acute myocardial infarction complicating acute stroke: characteristics of guideline-recommended coronary revascularization and antithrombotic therapy and cardiovascular and bleeding outcomes. J Am Heart Assoc. 2023;12:e027156. https://doi.org/10.1161/JAHA.122.027156.
23. Neil-Dwyer G, Walter P, Cruickshank JM, Doshi B, O'Gorman P. Effect of propranolol and phentolamine on myocardial necrosis after subarachnoid haemorrhage. Br Med J. 1978;2:990–2. https://doi.org/10.1136/bmj.2.6143.990.
24. Norberg E, Odenstedt-Herges H, Rydenhag B, Oras J. Impact of acute cardiac complications after subarachnoid hemorrhage on long-term mortality and cardiovascular events. Neurocrit Care. 2018;29:404–12. https://doi.org/10.1007/s12028-018-0558-0.
25. Lång M, Jakob SM, Takala R, Lyngbakken MN, Turpeinen A, Omland T, Merz TM, Wiegand J, Grönlund J, Rahi M, Valtonen M, Koivisto T, Røsjø H, Bendel S. The prevalence of cardiac complications and their impact on outcomes in patients with non-traumatic subarachnoid hemorrhage. Sci Rep. 2022;12:20109. https://doi.org/10.1038/s41598-022-24675-8.
26. Zhang L, Qi S. Electrocardiographic abnormalities predict adverse clinical outcomes in patients with subarachnoid hemorrhage. J Stroke Cerebrovasc Dis. 2016;25:2653–9. https://doi.org/10.1016/j.jstrokecerebrovasdis.2016.07.011.
27. Andreoli A, di Pasquale G, Pinelli G, Grazi P, Tognetti F, Testa C. Subarachnoid hemorrhage: frequency and severity of cardiac arrhythmias. A survey of 70 cases studied in the acute phase. Stroke. 1987;18:558–64. https://doi.org/10.1161/01.str.18.3.558.
28. Yücetas SC, Kaya H, Kafadar S, Kafadar H, Tibilli H, Akcay A. Evaluation of index of cardiac-electrophysiological balance in patients with subarachnoid hemorrhage. BMC Cardiovasc Disord. 2022;22:477. https://doi.org/10.1186/s12872-022-02924-y.
29. Putaala J, Lehto M, Meretoja A, Silvennoinen K, Curtze S, Kääriäinen J, Koivunen RJ, Kaste M, Tatlisumak T, Strbian D. In-hospital cardiac compli-

cations after intracerebral hemorrhage. Int J Stroke. 2014;9:741–6. https://doi.org/10.1111/ijs.12180.
30. Qureshi AI, Huang W, Lobanova I, Barsan WG, Hanley DF, Hsu CY, Lin CL, Silbergleit R, Steiner T, Suarez JI, Toyoda K, Yamamoto H, for ATACH-II trial investigators. Outcomes of intensive systolic blood pressure reduction in patients with intracerebral hemorrhage and excessively high initial systolic blood pressure: post hoc analysis of a randomized clinical trial. JAMA Neurol. 2020;77:1355–65. https://doi.org/10.1001/jamaneurol.2020.3075.
31. Qureshi AI, Foster LD, Lobanova I, Huang W, Suarez JI. Intensive blood pressure lowering in patients with moderate to severe grade acute cerebral hemorrhage: post hoc analysis of antihypertensive treatment of acute cerebral hemorrhage (ATACH)-2 trial. Cerebrovasc Dis. 2020;49:244–52. https://doi.org/10.1159/000506358.
32. Wang X, Di Tanna GL, Moullaali TJ, Martin RH, Shipes VB, Robinson TG, Chalmers J, Suarez JI, Qureshi AI, Palesch YY, Anderson CS. J-shape relation of blood pressure reduction and outcome in acute intracerebral hemorrhage: a pooled analysis of INTERACT2 and ATACH-II individual participant data. Int J Stroke. 2022;17:1129–36. https://doi.org/10.1177/17474930211064076.
33. Gaist D, Hald SM, García Rodríguez LA, Clausen A, Möller S, Hallas J, Al-Shahi SR. Association of prior intracerebral hemorrhage with major adverse cardiovascular events. JAMA Netw Open. 2022;5:e2234215. https://doi.org/10.1001/jamanetworkopen.2022.34215.
34. Teo KC, Keins S, Abramson JR, Leung WCY, Leung IYH, Wong YK, Yeung C, Kourkoulis C, Warren AD, Chan KH, Cheung RTF, Ho SL, Gurol ME, Viswanathan A, Greenberg SM, Anderson CD, Lau KK, Rosand J, Biffi A. Blood pressure control targets and risk of cardiovascular and cerebrovascular events after intracerebral hemorrhage. Stroke. 2023;54:78–86. https://doi.org/10.1161/STROKEAHA.122.039709.
35. Furlan JC, Fehlings MG. Cardiovascular complications after acute spinal cord injury: pathophysiology, diagnosis, and management. Neurosurg Focus. 2008;25(5):E13. https://doi.org/10.3171/FOC.2008.25.11.E13.
36. Krassioukov A, Claydon VE. The clinical problems in cardiovascular control following spinal cord injury: an overview. Prog Brain Res. 2006;152:223–9. https://doi.org/10.1016/S0079-6123(05)52014-4.
37. Krassioukov AV, Furlan JC, Fehlings MG. Autonomic dysreflexia in acute spinal cord injury: an under-recognized clinical entity. J Neurotrauma. 2003;20:707–16. https://doi.org/10.1089/089771503767869944.
38. Williams AM, Gee CM, Voss C, West CR. Cardiac consequences of spinal cord injury: systematic review and meta-analysis. Heart. 2019;105:217–25. https://doi.org/10.1136/heartjnl-2018-313585.
39. Yoshikawa MH, Rabelo NN, Welling LC, Telles JPM, Figueiredo EG. Brain death and management of the potential donor. Neurol Sci. 2021;42:3541–52. https://doi.org/10.1007/s10072-021-05360-6.
40. Westphal GA, Coll E, de Souza RL, Wagner S, Montemezzo A, Cani de Souza FC, Torres G, Halla S, Carnin TC, Machado MC, Berbigier E, Busetto F, Bittencourt I, Gerent K, de Souza BS, Tassinari M, de Andrade J. Positive impact of a clinical goal-directed protocol on reducing cardiac arrests during potential brain-dead donor maintenance. Crit Care. 2016;20:323. https://doi.org/10.1186/s13054-016-1484-1.
41. Westphal GA. A simple bedside approach to therapeutic goals achievement during the management of deceased organ donors—an adapted version of the "VIP" approach. Clin Transpl. 2016;30:138–44. https://doi.org/10.1111/ctr.12667.
42. Hawkes MA, Hocker SE. Systemic complications following status epilepticus. Curr Neurol Neurosci Rep. 2018;18:7. https://doi.org/10.1007/s11910-018-0815-9.
43. Tahsili-Fahadan P, Geocadin RG. Heart–brain axis. Circ Res. 2017;120:559–72. https://doi.org/10.1161/circresaha.116.308446.
44. Hocker S, Prasad A, Rabinstein AA. Cardiac injury in refractory status epilepticus. Epilepsia. 2013;54:518–22. https://doi.org/10.1111/epi.12017.
45. Pfeiffer G, Schiller B, Kruse J, Netzer J. Indicators of dysautonomia in severe Guillain-Barré syndrome. J Neurol. 1999;246:1015–22. https://doi.org/10.1007/s004150050506.
46. Netto AB, Taly AB, Kulkarni GB, Uma Maheshwara Rao GS, Rao S. Prognosis of patients with Guillain-Barré syndrome requiring mechanical ventilation. Neurol India. 2011;59 Hofstad H, ohm OJ, Mørk SJ, Aarli JA. Heart disease in myasthenia gravis. Acta Neurol Scand 1984;70(3):176–184. doi: https://doi.org/10.1111/j.1600-0404.1984.tb00817.x:707-11. doi: 10.4103/0028-3886.86545.
47. Mukerji S, Aloka F, Farooq MU, Kassab MY, Abela GS. Cardiovascular complications of the Guillain-Barré syndrome. Am J Cardiol. 2009;104:1452–5. https://doi.org/10.1016/j.amjcard.2009.06.069.
48. Youssef S, Adam I, Chablani M, Taleyratne D. A myasthenic crisis of broken hearts (reverse takotsubo): case report and review of literature. J R Coll Physicians Edinb. 2022;52:27–9. https://doi.org/10.1177/14782715221088913.
49. Chuapakdee O, Layangkool T, Theerasuwipakorn N. Pyridostigmine-induced coronary artery spasm in early-onset myasthenia gravis: a case presentation and review of the literature. BMJ Case Rep. 2022;15(9):e249819. https://doi.org/10.1136/bcr-2022-249819.

50. Feingold B, Mahle WT, Auerbach S, Clemens P, Domenighetti AA, Jefferies JL, Judge DP, Lal AK, Markham LW, Parks WJ, Tsuda T, Wang PJ, Yoo SJ, American Heart Association Pediatric Heart Failure Committee of the Council on Cardiovascular Disease in the Young; Council on Clinical Cardiology; Council on Cardiovascular Radiology and Intervention; Council on Functional Genomics and Translational Biology; and Stroke Council. Management of cardiac involvement associated with neuromuscular diseases: a Scientific Statement From the American Heart Association. Circulation. 2017;136:e200–31. https://doi.org/10.1161/CIR.0000000000000526.

29 Respiratory Problems in Neurocritical Care

Shalini Nair

29.1 Introduction

This chapter deals with the respiratory problems in patients treated in neurocritical care facility. The respiratory or breathing issues may be due to neurological diseases per se or may be following neurotrauma or neurosurgical procedures.

29.2 Neurological Diseases

(a) Neuromuscular diseases:

Most of neuromuscular diseases cause gradual reduction in inspiratory muscle strength. This results in ineffective alveolar ventilation and inspiratory muscle weakness, resulting in inadequate clearance of airway secretion [1]. These changes lead to chronic respiratory insufficiency and potentially life-threatening problems. It may also cause acute worsening of gradual deterioration in the wake of aspiration or a superimposed respiratory tract infection. Aspiration is seen commonly from bulbar muscle weakness (facial, oropharyngeal, and laryngeal muscles) affecting the speech, swallowing, and clearance of airway secretions. Drooling is an indicator of a severe swallowing impairment [1].

Since mobility affects early in the disease, complaints of dyspnea come up late in the disease progression. Early lung and respiratory muscle function monitoring are the best prognostic indicators and serial spirometric values help monitor progress of the disease [2]. Arterial blood gases at this stage of respiratory failure will reveal only a subtle drop in the PO_2. Hypercapnia is a late sign of neuromuscular respiratory insufficiency. Among various electrophysiological features, a drop in vital capacity (VC) between the supine and the semi-recumbent positions of 30% or greater is generally associated with severe diaphragmatic weakness [3]. Carrié et al. used diaphragmatic ultrasound study to rapidly identify impaired respiratory function. They used a threshold of maximum end expiratory diaphragmatic excursion of 5.5 cm as defined by an FVC $\leq$ 50% of predicted values, to attain a 100% sensitivity [4].

Figure 29.1 represents diaphragmatic palsy in a patient of Myasthenia Gravis with impending respiratory failure.

(b) Stroke:

The various abnormalities in respiration that may manifest in a patient with stroke are tabulated in Table 29.1. The respiratory pattern varies based on the neural structure involved.

S. Nair (✉)
Christian Medical College Vellore,
Vellore, Tamil Nadu, India
e-mail: drsahalininair@cmcvellore.ac.in

H. Prabhakar et al. (eds.), *Principles and Practice of Neurocritical Care*,
https://doi.org/10.1007/978-981-99-8059-8_29

Types of respiratory abnormalities seen in stroke:

- Automatic respiration: Patient is able to voluntarily alter respiration to maintain homeostasis like in acid base abnormalities or hypoxemia. However, when not awake or in sleep, central apnea develops due to sudden reduction in tidal volume and rate of respiration.
- Primary central neurogenic hyperventilation: A rapid rate with normal pattern of breathing characterises this hyperventilation that persists despite respiratory alkalosis, normal oxygenation, and without any parenchymal or airway respiratory pathology.
- Ataxic breathing: An irregular pattern of respiration with varying rate and depth of respiration is followed by a period of apnea.
- Cheyne-Stokes breathing: A smooth waxing and waning of rate and depth of respiration is observed with intervening periods of apnea.

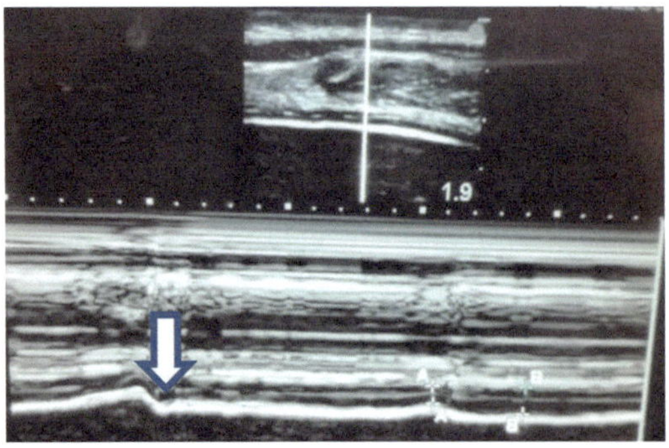

Fig. 29.1 Downward excursion of diaphragm (indicated by arrow) suggesting diaphragmatic palsy on ultrasound

- Respiratory apraxia: The involuntary breathing is maintained without any anomaly. However, any voluntary/ volitional alteration of respiration as in coughing, singing, crying, etc. is not possible. Respiratory variation to maintain eucapnia and involuntary sneeze or cough is maintained.
- Limbic respiration: Changes in respiration in accordance to emotions like laughing, crying, etc. are preserved, but voluntary control of breathing is lost.

(c) Subarachnoid hemorrhage (SAH):

There could be respiratory concerns primarily from the disease or secondarily due to infection from aspiration or ventilation.

- Respiratory problems from SAH:

  Friedman et al. encountered 22% respiratory complications in 305 aneurysmal SAH over 8 years [5]. The disease per se (theories related to brain–lung interaction follows in subsequent sections) can lead to neurogenic pulmonary edema, cardiogenic pulmonary edema, acute respiratory distress syndrome (ARDS),
- Respiratory problems secondarily associated with SAH:
  - Pneumonia:

    Low consciousness associated with severe grade SAH may cause aspiration.

    Ventilator-associated pneumonia in SAH patients on ventilator.

    The consequences of pulmonary complications have been found to be worse with higher incidence of symptomatic vasospasm. However, they have been correlated to only short-term poorer outcome at one year alone [5, 6].

Table 29.1 Pattern of respiration in various types of stroke

Type of respiration	Frequency	Voluntary control	Involuntary control	Cerebral area involved
Automatic	Normal	Present	Absent	Cervical spine
Central Hyperventilation	Increased	Present	Present	Brainstem
Apneustic	Normal	Absent	Present	Pons
Cheyne-Stokes	Normal increased	Absent	Present	Brainstem
Respiratory Apraxia	Normal	Absent	Present	Cortical
Limbic	Normal	Absent	Present	Base of pons

(d) Brainstem and cervical tumors: Lesions involving anterior pathways including reticulospinal tracts lead to loss of automatic control of respiration, but maintains normal voluntary respiration and sudden nocturnal death from apnea. Involvement of dorsolateral corticospinal tracts may lead to automatic respiration, where metabolic requirements are met by maintaining ventilation mediated by acid base and oxygenation demands.

29.3 Neurosurgical Procedures

(a) Anterior cervical spine procedures:

By causing swelling of retropharyngeal soft tissue, airway may be compromised (Fig. 29.2).

Thomas et al. [7] have studied prevertebral soft tissue swelling that may threaten the airway. It was worst for patients undergoing cervical corpectomy, mainly in the first 3 days after surgery. Those undergoing three-level central corpectomy, or having inclusion of C4 in the central corpectomy, have a greater degree of postsurgical soft tissue swelling and have a higher risk of postoperative airway obstruction [7].

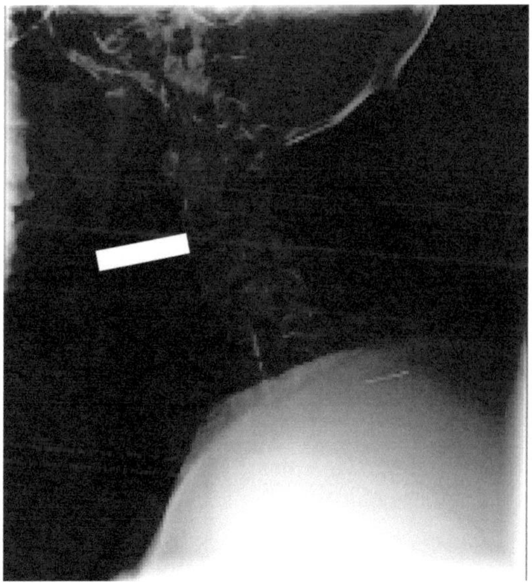

Fig. 29.2 Depicts widened retropharyngeal soft tissue shadow on fourth postoperative day following cervical spine procedure

b. High cervical procedures:

Damage to higher cervical segments can result in dysfunction of the diaphragm (phrenic nerve has C3–5 root value). This is more prone to occur in surgeries for atlanto-axial dislocation (AAD). The respiratory involvement could be from direct compression of neural tissue (poor drive) or due to weak respiratory muscles (poor effort) [8]. Marutirao et al. suggested that surgical outcome also depends on unexplored factors including preoperative respiratory reserve, body mass index, adequate preoperative respiratory optimization, postoperative intensive care protocol and physiotherapy [9]. Analyzing their protocol of preoperative respiratory optimization with incentive spirometry, chest physiotherapy, assessment of pulmonary function, and postoperative arterial blood gas analysis, Marutirao et al. found that patients having moderate to severe primary or mixed acid-base disorder have a probability of reintubation or delayed extubation. Physiological compensations of these patients crumble in situations of severe metabolic acidosis with a base deficit of more than −9 or even with mild mixed-acid base disorders [9].

(c) Thoracic spine procedures:

Anterior approaches to thoracic spine surgeries have traditionally been thought to have more pulmonary complications. Xu et al. [10] found chest tube insertions to be more common with anterior approach, while the duration of chest tube placement and incidence of pleural effusion were higher with combined approach compared to anterior or posterior approaches. A recent systematic analysis concluded that there is insufficient data to determine the risk of pulmonary complications following anterior, posterior, or lateral approaches to the thoracic spine [11].

(d) Posterior fossa surgeries:

Patients undergoing posterior fossa surgeries are at a higher risk for respiratory complications due to central respiratory dysfunction, mechanical obstruction, and neuromuscular dysfunction [12]. Hooda et al. documented respiratory complications in 12.1% patients following elective surgeries for posterior fossa tumors [13]. The various factors found to be correlating with respiratory complications were grouped as patient related like American society of Anaesthesiologist's grade III, preoperative status like lower cranial nerve involvement, surgical factors as duration of surgery, blood loss and need for massive transfusion, and finally, postoperative factors such as lower level of consciousness, lower cranial nerve involvement, need for blood transfusion, need for tracheostomy, longer duration of mechanical ventilation, and longer ICU (intensive care unit) stay [13].

29.4 Neurotrauma

- Diaphragmatic dysfunction.

  Inadequate breathing may be the result of direct injury to phrenic nerve (Fig. 29.3).
- Respiratory problems from spinal injury: Physiologic changes in respiration from spinal cord injury relate to level of injury and extent of neurologic impairment. The American Spinal Injury Association (ASIA) [14] grade assesses the strength of involved muscles and stratifies the severity of involvement. The changes involve muscle strength of respiratory muscles, neural control of respiration, altered chest wall compliance, and airflow limitation and bronchial hyperresponsiveness. The consequent respiratory complications include paradoxical chest wall movement, low tidal volumes, increased volume of upper respiratory tract secretions, and an ineffective cough. These changes modulate during various phases of injury. In the acute phase, there is sudden loss of muscle tone. As injury progresses, there may be functional descent of the neurologic injury level due to resolving inflammation, enhanced recruitment of accessory ventilatory muscles, retraining of deconditioned muscles, and the evolution from flaccid to spastic paralysis [15].

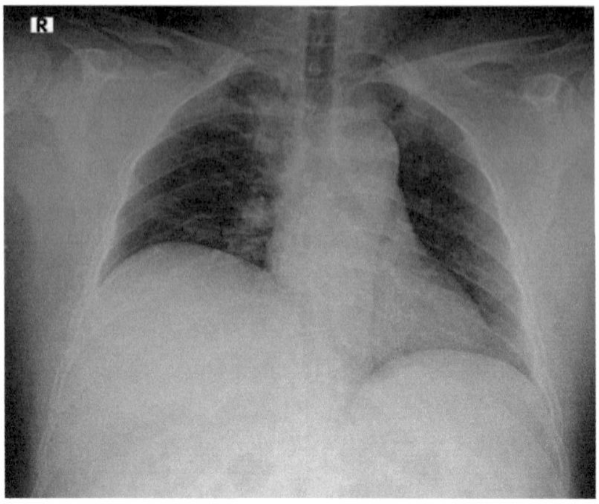

Fig. 29.3 Diaphragmatic palsy following polytrauma involving right phrenic nerve

- Aspiration pneumonia due to inability to maintain airway in view of low sensorium in head injuries.

29.5 Brain–lung Cross Talk

Pulmonary complications can also occur in patients requiring neurocritical care due to factors not directly affecting respiratory centers or the respiratory apparatus. These are usually consequence of aspiration, ventilator dependence, neurogenic pulmonary oedema, and acute respiratory distress syndrome (ARDS). Neurologically critical patients are more vulnerable to aspiration and ventilator-associated pneumonia. This could be by virtue of the low Glasgow coma scale score and need for prolonged ventilation and sedation. Acute brain injury also leads to immunosuppression, which could predispose to pulmonary infection [16]. An abrupt sympathetic storm from raised ICP could cascade a severe systemic vasoconstriction and shift of blood from systemic to pulmonary circulation. This results in pulmonary edema [17, 18] (Fig. 29.4). Development of ARDS in brain injured patients can have two

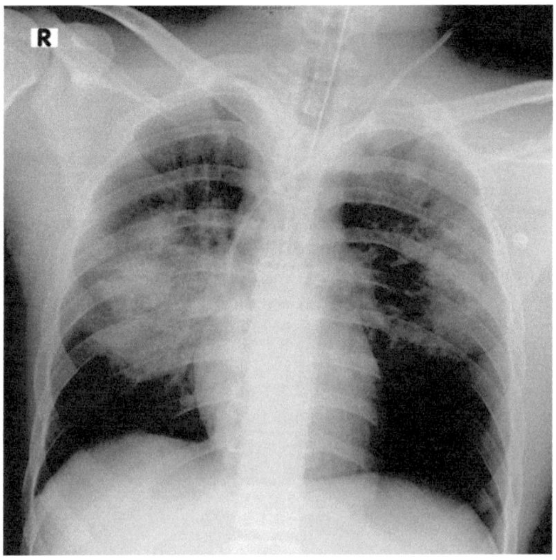

Fig. 29.4 Neurogenic pulmonary edema following traumatic brain injury

peaks at 2–3 or 7–8 days after initiation of mechanical ventilation [19].

The various theories advocated for development of acute lung injury in a brain injured patient include:

- Blast theory: A transient increase in intravascular pressure due to adrenergic storm following acute brain injury accompanied with intravascular pressure damages to the alveolo-capillary membrane [20].
- Pulmonary venule adrenergic hypersensitivity theory: Isolated pulmonary vasoconstriction results from catecholamine storm of acute brain injury [21].
- Double hit theory: A transient increase in release of proinflammatory markers is seen immediately after acute brain injury. This is followed by a second peak arising from a systemic immune suppression [22].

Thus, lung, though a silent bystander, seems an organ of collateral damage in acute brain damage very often. Depending on the pathophysiology of pulmonary involvement, the resulting extent of damage can be predicted, and management tailored with better precision.

References

1. Ambrosino N, Carpenè N, Gherardi M. Chronic respiratory care for neuromuscular diseases in adults. Eur Respir J. 2009;34:444–51.
2. Toussaint M, Steens M, Soudon P. Lung function accurately predicts hypercapnia in patients with Duchenne muscular dystrophy. Chest. 2007;131:368–75.
3. Fromageot C, Lofaso F, Annane D, et al. Supine fall in lung volumes in the assessment of diaphragmatic weakness in neuromuscular disorders. Arch Phys Med Rehabil. 2001;82:123–8.
4. Carrié C, Bonnardel E, Vally R, Revel P, Marthan R. Vital capacity impairment due to neuromuscular disease and its correlation with diaphragmatic ultrasound: a preliminary study. Ultrasound Med Biol. 2016;42(1):143–9.
5. Friedman JA, Pichelmann MA, Piepgras DG, McIver JI, Toussaint LG 3rd, McClelland RL, Nichols DA, Meyer FB, Atkinson JL, Wijdicks EF. Pulmonary complications of aneurysmal subarachnoid hemorrhage. Neurosurgery. 2003;52:1025–31.
6. Cavallo C, Safavi-Abbasi S, Kalani MYS, Gandhi S, Sun H, Oppenlander ME, Zabramski JM, Nakaji P, Lawton MT, Spetzler RF. Pulmonary complications after spontaneous aneurysmal subarachnoid hemorrhage: experience from Barrow Neurological Institute. World Neurosurg. 2018;119:e366–73.
7. Thomas SG, Joseph V, Rajshekhar V. Temporal progression and spatial distribution of "normal" prevertebral soft tissue swelling following central corpectomy for cervical spondylotic myelopathy. Neurol India. 2012;60:217–23.
8. Uppar AM, Vilanilam GC. Respiratory dysfunction in craniovertebral junction pathology: a pulmonary function test correlation. J Spinal Surg. 2017;4:164–70.
9. Marutirao R, Singh S, Shamshery C, Sardhara J, Mishra P, Mehrotra A, et al. Impact of postoperative ABG analysis and ICU weaning protocol in surgical outcome of Atlanto-axial dislocation: it's not the towering sail, but the unseen wind that moves the ship. Neurol India. 2022;70:1540–7.
10. Xu R, Garcés-Ambrossi GL, McGirt MJ, Witham TF, Wolinsky JP, Bydon A, et al. Thoracic vertebrectomy and spinal reconstruction via anterior, posterior, or combined approaches: clinical outcomes in 91 consecutive patients with metastatic spinal tumors. J Neurosurg Spine. 2009;11:272–84.
11. Gabel BC, Schnell EC, Dettori JR, Jeyamohan S, Oskouian R. Pulmonary complications following thoracic spinal surgery: a systematic review. Global Spine J. 2016;6:296–303.
12. Howard R, Mahoney A, Thurlow AC. Respiratory obstruction after posterior fossa surgery. Anaesthesia. 1990;45:222–4.
13. Hooda B, Chouhan RS, Rath GP, Lamsal R, Bithal PK. Incidence and predictors of postoperative pulmo-

nary complications in patients undergoing craniotomy and excision of posterior fossa tumor. J Anaesthesiol Clin Pharmacol. 2019;35:254.
14. ASIA and ISCoS International Standards Committee. The 2019 revision of the International Standards for Neurological Classification of Spinal Cord Injury (ISNCSCI)-What's new? Spinal Cord. 2019;57: 815–7.
15. McMichan JC, Michel L, Westbrook PR. Pulmonary dysfunction following traumatic quadriplegia. recognition, prevention, and treatment. JAMA. 1980;243:528.
16. Robba C, et al. Mechanical ventilation in patients with acute ischaemic stroke: from pathophysiology to clinical practice. Crit Care. 2019;23:388.
17. Davison DL, Terek M, Chawla LS. Neurogenic pulmonary edema. Crit Care. 2012;16:212.
18. Zhao J, et al. Neurogenic pulmonary edema following acute stroke: the progress and perspective. Biomed Pharmacother. 2020;130:110478.
19. Piek J, Chesnut RM, Marshall LF, van Berkum-Clark M, Klauber MR, Blunt BA, et al. Extracranial complications of severe head injury. J Neurosurg. 1992;77:901–7.
20. Theodore J, Robin ED. Pathogenesis of neurogenic pulmonary oedema. Lancet. 1975;2:749–51.
21. Keegan MT, Lanier WL. Pulmonary edema after resection of a fourth ventricle tumor: possible evidence for a medulla-mediated mechanism. Mayo Clin Proc. 1999;74:264–8.
22. Chang L, et al. Cocaine-and amphetamine-regulated transcript modulates peripheral immunity and protects against brain injury in experimental stroke. Brain Behav Immun. 2011;25:260–9.

Renal Problems in Neurocritical Care

30

Nidhi Gupta

30.1 Introduction

The brain and kidney share an intimate relationship at anatomical and physiological levels, both in health and diseased states. The two organs work in an integrated way to maintain normal blood pressure and tonicity via sodium and water homeostasis. Both are highly vascular structures with high oxygen demands and share the functional characteristics of blood flow autoregulation. Hence, an injured brain has the potential to disrupt normal renal functioning, leading to an acute derangement in its function, termed broadly as acute kidney injury (AKI). AKI, in turn, is a multisystemic disease associated with multitude of extrarenal complications, with high morbidity and mortality in critically ill patients [1, 2]. The successful management of neurocritically ill patients with renal problems, thus, mandate a multi-disciplinary approach.

In this chapter, we address the common renal problems encountered in neurocritically ill patients and their optimal management strategies.

N. Gupta (✉)
Neuroanesthesia, Indraprastha Apollo Hospitals, New Delhi, Delhi, India

30.2 Defining Acute Kidney Injury

Existing literature is plagued with inconsistencies in the definition of AKI, leading to incomparable data regarding the incidence and its associated consequences in critically ill [3].

Over the years, numerous definitions have been proposed by different working groups on AKI, based on changes in the glomerular filtration rate (GFR) or serum creatinine (SCr) levels, or the urinary output (UO) over time. The most referred definitions include the risk, injury, failure, loss of kidney function and end-stage kidney disease (RIFLE) definition, Acute Kidney Injury Network (AKIN) and the Kidney Disease Improving Global Outcome (KDIGO) criteria published in 2012 [4].

The 2012 KDIGO guideline defined AKI as an abrupt decrease in kidney function occurring over 7 days or fewer, as evident by any increase in SCr by at least 0.3 mg/dL (26.5 μmol/L) within 48 h, or by 1.5 times the baseline SCr value within 7 days, or any reduction in UO to 0.5 mL/kg/h for at least 6 h [4]. AKI can be further classified into three different stages of severity based on an increasing trend in SCr and/or worsening oliguria. The repeated measurements, however, may be influenced by the ongoing treatments in neurointensive care unit (NICU) and are prone for inconsistencies. Thus, defining AKI solely on basis of SCr and/or UO measurements lacks the potential for early prediction of AKI [3]. This

H. Prabhakar et al. (eds.), *Principles and Practice of Neurocritical Care*,
https://doi.org/10.1007/978-981-99-8059-8_30

may lead to missed or delayed diagnosis with its consequent effect on patients' prognosis.

The new KDIGO AKI guidelines are expected to be published in near future based on the conclusions from the KDIGO 2019 Controversies Conference on Acute Kidney Injury and the 2020 Consensus Conference on Harmonizing Acute and Chronic Kidney Disease Definitions and Classification. The proposed modification of KDIGO AKI definition by Ostermann and colleagues [5] attempts to incorporate the presence of structural biomarkers in addition to the functional SCr and UO criteria, to better predict the severity and persistence of AKI (Table 30.1).

30.3 Burden of AKI in Neurocritically Ill Patients

AKI is common in critically ill patients, with an incidence ranging dramatically from 0.7% to 77.7%, owing to different diagnostic criteria, patient population and timing of diagnosis [3, 6, 7]. The incidence of AKI in neurocritical patients ranges from 11.6% to 23.5%, with 1% and 2% requiring renal replacement therapy (RRT) [8, 9]. The overall prognosis in this subset of patients, however, remains poor consequent to complex interactions between an injured brain and kidney and prolonged course of stay in NICU. The extent of underlying neurological injury, advanced age, and comorbidities are the commonly implicated predisposing risk factors in the majority of studies, with preexisting chronic kidney disease (CKD) being the strongest independent risk factor (Table 30.2). In addition, AKI itself is an independent predictor of prolonged use of mechanical ventilation, cerebral edema, and mortality in neurocritically ill [9].

Approximately 10–12% patients with isolated traumatic brain injury (TBI) patients develop AKI during the course of their NICU stay, though severe AKI is rare (2–3% of cases, as defined by KDIGO criteria). Nonetheless, AKI is associated with an increase in in-hospital mortality (adjusted odds ratio 2.2), increased length of hospital stay, need for tracheostomy and poor neurologic outcomes at 6 months [10–13]. AKI sets in early after admission to ICU, with a median onset of 2 days. Some of the common predisposing risk factors include preinjury comorbidities like renal dysfunction, insulin-dependent diabetes, severity of TBI, rhabdomyolysis, and administration of osmotic therapy.

In aneurysmal subarachnoid hemorrhage (SAH) patients, AKI develops in approximately 10% of patients, with severe AKI occurring in approximately 3% [14, 15]. AKI

Table 30.1 New proposed KDIGO definition and classification of acute kidney injury based on damage biomarker assessment

KDIGO AKI staging	KDIGO SCr criteria	KDIGO UO criteria	Damage biomarker	New proposed KDIGO AKI staging
	No change or ↑ SCr < 0.3 mg/dL	No decrease	Biomarker positive	1S
1	↑ SCr ≥ 0.3 mg/dL in 48 h or ↑SCr × 1.5–1.9 times the baseline within 7 days	<0.5 mL/kg/h × 6–12 h	Biomarker negative	1A
			Biomarker positive	1B
2	↑ SCr × 2–2.9 times the baseline	<0.5 mL/kg/h × >12 h	Biomarker negative	2A
			Biomarker positive	2B
3	↑ SCr × 3 times the baseline or ↑ SCr ≥ 4 mg/dL or Need for RRT	<0.3 mL/kg/h × 24 h or Anuria × 12 h	Biomarker negative	3A
			Biomarker positive	3B

SCr serum creatinine, *UO* urine output, *RRT* renal replacement therapy

Table 30.2 Risk factors for acute kidney injury in neurocritically ill patients

AKI risk factors in TBI	AKI risk factors in SAH	AKI risk factors in AIS	AKI risk factors in sICH
– Baseline impaired renal function – Advanced age – Insulin-dependent diabetes – Severity of neurological injury (GCS score/ pupillary abnormalities) – Hyperadrenergic state – Presence of extracranial injuries – H emodynamic instability – Hypovolemia – Sepsis – Osmotic nephrosis – Nephrotoxic medications[a] – Rhabdomyolysis – Trauma-associated coagulopathy – Early transfusion of packed red-blood-cell concentrates – Abdominal compartment syndrome	– Baseline impaired renal function – Advanced age – Pre-existing hypertension – Severity of aneurysmal bleed – Hypertonic saline induced hypernatremia and hyperchloremia – Osmotic nephrosis – Clinical vasospasm – Sepsis – Nephrotoxic medications[a] – Iodinated contrast agents	– Baseline impaired renal function – Advanced age – Pre-existing hypertension – Renal hypoperfusion secondary to therapeutic blood pressure lowering. – Proteinuria – NIHSS score – Sepsis – Nephrotoxic medications[a] – Iodinated contrast agents	– Baseline impaired renal function – Advanced age – Pre-exiting diabetes – APACHE-II score – Total amount of mannitol use – Renal hypoperfusion secondary to therapeutic blood pressure lowering. – Patients receiving higher doses of nicardipine. – Infections – Hypernatremia – Metabolic acidosis – Elevated serum creatine kinase – Hyperuricaemia – Proteinuria – Use of colloids and diuretics. – Nephrotoxic medications[a]

[a] Nephrotoxic medications—nonsteroidal anti-inflammatory drugs, renin-angiotensin-aldosterone system inhibitors, calcineurin inhibitors (cyclosporine, tacrolimus), antimicrobials (vancomycin, aminoglycosides, β-lactams-penicillin, first-generation cephalosporins and carbapenems, fluoroquinolones—ciprofloxacin, colistin, trimethoprim-sulfamethoxazole), antiepileptics (levetiracetam, phenytoin), acyclovir, proton-pump-inhibitors, H_2-antagonists, intravenous immunoglobulins

TBI traumatic brain injury, *SAH* subarachnoid hemorrhage, *AIS* acute ischemic stroke, *sICH* spontaneous intracranial hemorrhage, *GCS* Glasgow Coma scale, *NIHSS* High National Institutes of Health Stroke Scale, *APACHE* Acute Physiology, Age and Chronic Health Evaluation

developing early during ICU admission is associated with the severity of aneurysmal bleed and/or clinical vasospasm, and prexisting hypertension, and/or renal dysfunction [14–16]. In a multivariable analysis, increased SCr levels on admission (>1.0 mg/dL), poor-grade SAH, age over 65 years, and delayed cerebral ischemia (DCI) were found to be independently associated with an unfavorable outcome [17]. An unresolved renal dysfunction remains the strongest independent predictor of mortality in this cohort.

The occurrence rate of AKI in acute ischemic stroke (AIS) patients is comparatively low, at around 3.5%, but is associated with worse neurological outcomes and nearly threefold increase in mortality [18, 19]. Patients with preexisting hypertension and preexisting renal disease are at a higher risk of developing AKI. The AKI risk did not increase in AIS patients who underwent either CT angiogram or those who received endovascular treatment [18].

In patients with spontaneous intracerebral hemorrhage (ICH), the incidence of AKI ranges from 8% to 21% and is associated with poor neurologic outcome and higher mortality with increasing severity of AKI [20, 21]. High APACHE II score, diabetes, higher baseline SCr, high doses of mannitol, and use of higher doses of blood pressure lowering medications (e.g., nicardipine) are the common independent AKI risk factors in this patient population.

30.4 Pathophysiology of AKI in Neurocritically Ill Patients

The pathophysiology of AKI in neurocritically ill patients is complex and multifactorial (Fig. 30.1).

30.4.1 Brain–Kidney Organ Crosstalk

The two most prominent pathways that perpetuate AKI in neurocritically ill involve the activation of the inflammatory and the neuroendocrine cascade [22]. The altered drug metabolism secondary to renal hyperfiltration, electrolyte and acid–base disturbances, sepsis, distant effects of uremic toxins (acute uremic encephalopathy), neurotransmitter derangement, and hippocampal transcriptional dysregulation may further perpetuate this bidirectional organ damage.

Preclinical evidence has revealed that presence of acute cerebral damage may make the kidney vulnerable for tubular dysfunction (the so called "subclinical AKI"), by promoting a proinflammatory phenotype, alteration of mitochondrial biogenesis and function, and apoptotic death in tubular epithelial cells [23]. Secondary to disruption of blood brain barrier, severe brain injury induces a generalized neuroinflammatory response, which may further be aggravated by episodes of ischemia-reperfusion injury. Consequently, a high circulating levels of systemic leukocytes, proinflammatory cytokines [tumor necrosis factor (TNF)-α, and interleukin (IL)-1β, IL-6, and IL-18], chemokines, and initiation of complement cascade may lead to the renal tubular epithelium damage, which is a hallmark of ischemic and nephrotoxic AKI [24].

Another important pathway is the activation of sympathetic autonomic nervous system releasing systemic catecholamines (epinephrine and norepinephrine), that compromises renal perfusion by preferential vasoconstriction of the afferent renal vasculature and an increased sodium reabsorption. Activation of the reno-cerebral sympathetic reflex by ischemia-reperfusion injury, is a novel pathway discovered that interlinks intra-renal and cerebral (but not the

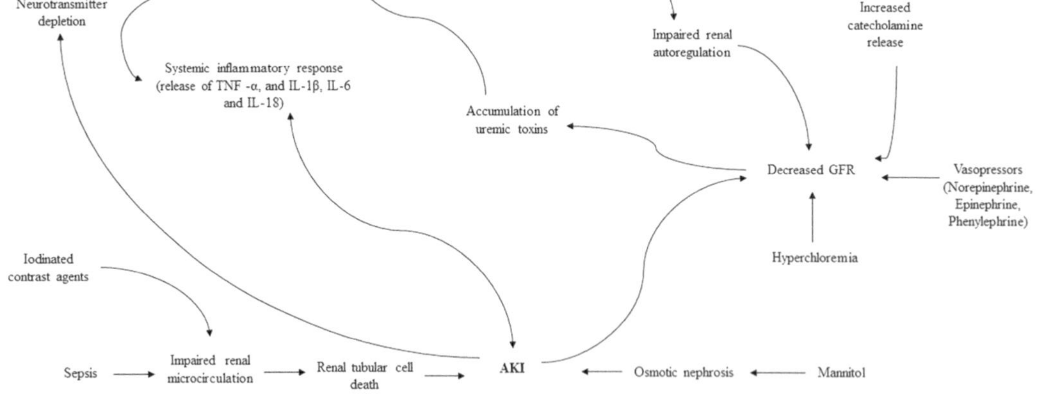

Fig. 30.1 Pathophysiological mechanisms of acute kidney injury in neurocritically ill patients*ABI* acute brain injury, *TBI* traumatic brain injury, *SAH* subarachnoid hemorrhage, *AIS* acute ischemic stroke, *sICH* spontaneous intracranial haemorrhage, *GFR* glomerular filtration rate, *AKI* acute kidney injury

circulating) renin-angiotensin system (RAS) and promotes brain inflammation and worsening of AKI [25].

AKI, in turn, predisposes to an augmented state of systemic inflammation and oxidative stress secondary to altered metabolism and increased production of proinflammatory cytokines and chemokines, reactive oxygen and nitrogen species and nitic oxide. Hence, an increased concentration of systemic inflammatory markers and disruption of normal immunological barriers of brain primarily contribute to progressive and bilateral organ damage, the term described as the "brain-kidney crosstalk" [1, 2, 22].

30.4.2 Osmo-Diuretics in AKI

Being a highly effective osmotic diuretic, mannitol has been traditionally used for perioperative renal protection in patients undergoing major vascular and cardiac surgery. The renoprotective effects are attributable to its promotion of excretion of toxic substances, renal vasodilatation secondary to release of prostaglandins and free radical scavenging. However, in NICU settings, mannitol has been implicated in the genesis of AKI secondary to osmotic nephropathy and renal vasoconstriction in large doses. *Osmotic nephrosis* is a phenomenon wherein osmotically active agents enter the renal proximal tubular cells by means of pinocytosis, leading to increased vacuolization and swelling. In addition, the prolonged hyperosmolar state activates the tubuloglomerular feedback (TGF), which results in decrease in intrarenal microcirculatory flow, ultimately reducing the GFR [26].

Hypertonic saline (HTS) is another commonly administered hyperosmolar agent in neurocritically ill patients and is also used for hyponatremia correction. It is postulated to result in hyperchloremic metabolic acidosis, which is implicated in the pathophysiological consequences such as coagulopathy, hypotension, and AKI. In addition, hyperchloremia may raise the overall renal interstitial chloride concentration, including the glomerular mesangium, leading to afferent arteriolar vasoconstriction. This may result in decreased renal blood flow (RBF) and a fall in GFR, independent of chloride-mediated changes in TGF [27]. In a retrospective cohort study of AKI in NICU, Ramírez-Guerreroa et al. reported a change in chloride levels greater than 4 mmol/L at 48 h (OR 2.44) as a risk factor for developing AKI in the first 14 days of hospitalization in neurocritical patients [9]. However, in another study, Yamane et al. observed that it is the duration of hyperchloremia, rather than the highest chloride level or the duration of HTS infusion, that is independently associated with AKI in ABI patients [28].

To evaluate the harmful renal effects of hyperchloremia per se, the post hoc analysis of the COBI trial did not find any association between the cumulative chloride load (which was significantly higher in intervention group receiving 20% HS infusion compared to control group) and the occurrence of AKI in patients with moderate to severe TBI during their NICU stay [29]. Hypernatremia has also been documented as a significant risk factor for developing early AKI, both in TBI and SAH patents. In a retrospective study, for each 1 mEq/L increase in the daily serum sodium, the hazard of developing AKI was found to increase by 5.4% (95% CI, 1.4–9.7), during HTS therapy in SAH patients [30].

Overall, the current literature suggests that the early use of mannitol, but not HTS, is independently associated with an increase in the risk of AKI, which is dose dependent. Till further randomized control trials (RCTs) prove otherwise [awaiting results of sugar or salt ("SOS") trial], HTS may be considered a safer option than mannitol for the treatment of intracranial hypertension (ICHT) in neurocritically ill patients at high risk for AKI. To minimize the risk of renal injury after hyperosmolar therapy for cerebral edema in neurocritically ill, the 2020 Neurocritical Care Society guidelines recommend an upper serum sodium range of 155-160 mEq/L and a serum chloride range of 110–115 mEq/L in patients receiving hypertonic sodium solutions [31]. When using mannitol, measuring serum mannitol concentration is the most effective method of assessing the AKI risk. However, the laboratory measurement is not easily available.

Thus, monitoring serum osmolality and osmolar gap may be of help, with both being surrogates of the serum mannitol concentration. It is ideal to maintain serum osmolarity of < 320 mOsm/kg or an osmolar gap of 20–55 mOsm/kg to minimize the risk of mannitol associated renal dysfunction.

30.4.3 Loop Diuretics in AKI

Furosemide reduces kidney's oxygen consumption by inhibiting the $Na^{+}/K^{+}/Cl^{2-}$ cotransporter present in the tubular epithelial cells in the thick ascending loop of Henle. It may also increase RBF secondary to reduced degradation of renal vasodilator prostaglandin E2 by inhibiting prostaglandin dehydrogenase. These effects, in theory, explain the potential protective effects of furosemide against renal ischemia.

However, the clinical evidence concerning any beneficial effect of loop diuretics in AKI is ambiguous at present. A meta-analysis of 20 RCTs have indicated that furosemide has no impact on either mortality or the need for RRT in AKI, though a small beneficial effect is found in patient with contrast-induced AKI (CI-AKI) when used in conjunction with matched hydration strategy [32]. On the contrary, Zhao et al. showed an improved short-term survival and recovery of renal function in critically ill AKI patients after furosemide administration [33].

The ongoing debate of furosemide use and survival benefit in AKI still exists and needs more well-designed research. Until then, the current ISCCM and KDIGO Guidelines on AKI do not recommend furosemide use in AKI, except in the setting of fluid overload [4, 34]. Metabolic alkalosis and electrolyte abnormalities, including hypokalemia, are the common side effects of loop diuretics.

30.4.4 Vasopressors in AKI

Catecholamine infusions in critically ill patients have been shown to trigger renal vasoconstriction. Norepinephrine (an a1-, a2-, b1-, and b3-receptor agonist) is the most commonly used catecholamines with regard to AKI in septic shock (a form of vasodilatory shock). It exerts its vasopressor activity via a1 adrenergic stimulation causing arterial and venous vasoconstriction. It is known to increase RBF, GFR, and sodium filtration and reabsorption, with no effect on urine flow or renal vascular resistance. However, it predisposes the already vulnerable renal medulla to ischemia by significantly reducing medullary perfusion and oxygenation, which is independent of RBF and cortical perfusion. Hence, it is currently being increasingly implicated in the pathogenesis of AKI in ICU patients [35–37].

Renal effects of vasopressin differ considerably from that of norepinephrine. While norepinephrine constricts both the afferent and efferent arterioles, vasopressin exerts its vasoconstrictor properties mainly on the efferent arteriole, resulting in increase in glomerular renal perfusion pressure and thus higher glomerular filtration, without exacerbating renal medullary ischemia and hypoxia [36]. It also augments intravascular volume through stimulation of V2 receptors in the renal collecting ducts, causing free water retention.

Angiotensin II, part of RAS axis, is the newest vasopressor available with possible renoprotective effects [38]. It mostly interacts with AT1 receptors, located in the kidneys, heart, pituitary, adrenal glands, and endothelium of vascular smooth muscle. It increases mean arterial pressures through direct simulation of the sympathetic nervous system, release of calcium from the sarcoplasmic reticulum of smooth muscle cells, enhancement of catecholamine and vasopressin secretion, and release of aldosterone and cortisol which increase salt and water retention by the kidneys. Like vasopressin, it increases glomerular efferent arteriolar tone more than the afferent tone, thus improving glomerular perfusion.

Dopamine (dopamine, $\alpha 1$ and $\beta 1$ receptor agonist) induces intrarenal vasodilation through dopamine receptors at low doses (0.5–3.0 mcg/kg/min) and increase RBF by augmenting cardiac output at intermediate doses (3.0–10.0 mcg/kg/min. However, at higher doses, the systemic a-1 receptor-mediated vasoconstriction compromises RBF. The reno-protective effect of low-dose dopamine has not been replicated in clinical studies [39]. Furthermore, dopamine has been found to be associated with higher incidence of arrythmias, infection, and mortality compared to norepinephrine, and is thus no longer recommended in septic hypotensive patients at risk of AKI.

30.5 Diagnosis of AKI IN Neurocritically Ill Patients

An initial detailed history and clinical evaluation followed by diagnostic testing allow us to delineate the main etiology behind the renal insult.

30.5.1 History and Clinical Evaluation

A history of prior comorbidities, use of osmotic diuretics, iodinated contrast exposure, chronic use of over the- counter herbal medications or recreational drugs and recent surgery or hospitalization needs to be elicited from the patient or family. The clinical examination is focussed on careful assessment of patient's haemodynamics, intravascular volume status, signs of infection, sepsis and nutritional assessment. The intravascular volume deficit may be inferred by assessing fluid responsiveness in mechanically ventilated critically ill patients [40].

30.5.2 Diagnostic Testing

The gold standard methods for GFR determination, such as inulin or iohexol clearance, are labor intensive and not feasible in acute clinical conditions. Traditionally, SCr and UO are used as functional biomarkers for the diagnosis of AKI. Both are deemed readily available at the bedside, reproducible, and essential for diagnosis as well as staging the severity of AKI. However, they have diagnostic limitations, with limited sensitivity and specificity for AKI.

In recent years, several new biomarkers have been investigated for their role in diagnosis and prognostication of AKI. Considering the fact that most cases of AKI have an earlier renal tubular damage than any evidence of decreased GFR, it has been found that damage biomarkers detect AKI earlier than using functional markers alone. The expert committee of the recent ADQI meeting recommends that along with clinical profile, a combination of damage and functional biomarkers should be used to diagnose and evaluate individual cases of AKI (Table 30.3) [5]. In addition, the combined use of both biomarkers may help to optimize the dosing and duration of treatment with potential nephrotoxic drugs and thus prevent AKI.

Functional Biomarkers

Urine output: Oliguria lasting for more than 12 h (KDIGO stage 2 or 3) has major AKI diagnostic implications and is associated with higher 90-day mortality, irrespective of SCr elevations [7]. Hence, measuring UO should always be included in ICU studies, which otherwise underestimate AKI incidence. However, measuring hourly UO has technical limitations and is affected by certain concomitant factors in neurocritically ill patients, such as volume diuresis, presence of disorders of water homeostasis (most prominently DI) and the administration of vasopressors, osmotic diuretics and contrast agents. The implementation of electronic flow measurement devices (e.g., RenalSense Clarity RMS device) with real-time UO monitoring may facilitate early identification of AKI in critically ill [41, 42]. They may also help to significantly lower cumulative fluid volume in critically ill ICU patients.

Serum creatinine: SCr is the most commonly accepted surrogate marker of GFR in clinical use. It is, however, a late biomarker for kidney injury as it may take 48 h or more to reach equilibrium after a stepwise reduction in GFR and the levels increase only after approximately 50% loss of renal function [4]. Moreover, the values are affected by many potentially confounding nonrenal factors including body composition, diet, certain medications which compete reversibly for

Table 30.3 Diagnostic tests for acute kidney injury

AKI biomarker/ functional tests	Mechanism	Clinical application	Comments
Functional biomarkers			
Oligouria	Detects decrease in RBF and/or a decline in renal perfusion pressure	Easily available biomarker Identify AKI in patients without any elevation of SCr levels Time frame to reach AKI diagnosis by the UO criterion is shorter than by SCr criterion	Relatively complex and cumbersome KDIGO criteria Requires – Hourly UO monitoring – Presence of an indwelling catheter – Documentation within precise time frames (6, 12, and 24 h) – Correct estimation or documentation of patients' body weight Affected by other factors including volume status, osmotic diuretics, vasopressors, ICA, disorders of water homeostasis
Serum Creatinine	Endogenously produced end product of creatine phosphate derived from muscle creatine Freely filtered through the glomeruli Actively secreted by proximal tubular cells Half-life of 4 h	Criterion for AKI diagnosis Universally available and easily tested marker of GFR Correlates inversely with GFR Degree of elevation is directly related to AKI severity and need for RRT	Late biomarker of AKI. Increases 24–48 h after an initial insult, when >50% nephrons are lost Lacks specificity Levels are modified by gender, diet (protein intake), decreased muscle mass (elderly, debilitated patients, prolonged ICU admission), medications, and volume status Not validated in non-steady-state settings (during RRT, acute heart failure, sepsis, hypovolemia, and obstruction) Overestimates actual GFR by around 10–20%, due to active tubular secretion
Cystatin-C	LMW protein that functions as a cysteine protease inhibitor Produced by all nucleated cells and eliminated by glomerular filtration, without reabsorption or secretion Half-life of 1.5 h	Surrogate marker of eGFR Shorter half-life than SCr, changes in plasma levels occur earlier, and plateau sooner after an abrupt change in GFR Can be detected 12–24 h after injury and peaks at 24–48 h, when >50% nephrons are lost Earlier detection of AKI prior to renal functional decline Not affected by age, sex, muscle bulk, diet, or inflammation	Levels influenced by albuminuria , thyroid dysfunction, and high-dose glucocorticoid therapy Costly Still not recommended for AKI diagnosis

(continued)

Table 30.3 (continued)

AKI biomarker/ functional tests	Mechanism	Clinical application	Comments
Proenkephalin-A	Precursor molecule of the endogenous polypeptide family Widely expressed in adrenal medulla, nervous system, immune system, and renal tissue Not protein bound in plasma Freely and exclusively filtered by glomeruli Half-life of 2-5 min	Suggested as an accurate and precise surrogate marker for eGFR and AKI detection Very short half-life Promising tool in both early AKI and mortality prediction Strong correlation with changes in GFR: Baseline values above 84.8 pmol/mL—optimal cutoffs for AKI detection. Values > 105.7 pmol/mL—independently predicts worse outcome	Promising as a functional biomarker in AKI and other non-steady-state conditions, including myocardial infarction, heart failure, sepsis
Damage/stress biomarkers			
NGAL	Pervasive 21–25 kD iron-carrying protein of the lipocalin subfamily 3 different types include: – monomeric 25 kDa glycoprotein produced by neutrophils and epithelial tissues, including tubular cells – homodimeric 45 kDa protein produced by neutrophils; and – heterodimeric 135 kDa protein produced by tubular cells Released in plasma and urine from renal tubular cells under any stress condition as well as from neutrophils during inflammation	Earlier detection of AKI Detectable 3 h after tubular injury and peaks after 6–12 h persists up to 5 days Strong association with eGFR, cystatin C, and SCr Can be used as screening tool to predict high risk for AKI in neurocritically ill	May be elevated in CKD, urinary tract infection and conditions of systemic inflammation and malignancies Cutoff unclear Available for clinical use in Europe only
Interleukin-18	Regulates innate and adaptive immunity	Levels rise 6 h after ischemic injury and peaks at 12–18 h	Levels may be high in inflammation, sepsis, and heart failure Lack of suitable cutoff level
KIM-1	Transmembrane glycoprotein produced by proximal tubular cell Involved in tubular regeneration and mediates the phagocytosis of apoptotic cells Released into urine after tubular damage	Earlier prediction of AKI Can be detected 12–24 h post-injury and peaks after 2–3 days	Tubular KIM-1 expression affected by ischemia, sepsis, iodinated contrast media May be elevated in chronic proteinuria and inflammatory diseases

(continued)

Table 30.3 (continued)

AKI biomarker/ functional tests	Mechanism	Clinical application	Comments
L-FABP	14 kDa intracellular lipid chaperone Freely filtered and reabsorbed in proximal tubule Excreted in urine after proximal tubular cell damage	Prediction of AKI	Preexisting CKD, early diabetic nephropathy, polycystic kidney disease, and idiopathic focal glomerulosclerosis potentially influence urinary L-FABP levels Available for clinical use in Japan only
Urinary IGFBP7 and TIMP-2	Cell cycle arrest biomarkers Released during renal tubular cell ischemia or inflammation	Earlier detection AKI stage 2 or 3 within 12-h Levels rise 4 h after tubular injury and peaks at 12 h following which they normalize rapidly in the absence of persistent insult Validated for early AKI risk prediction in critically ill adults Can be used for predicting recovery Cutoffs: • 0.3 (ng/mL)2/1000—progressive AKI High sensitivity and negative predictive value • 2 (ng/mL)2/1000—major adverse kidney events (death, the need of RRT, or persistent renal dysfunction) High specificity and moderate positive predictive values	May be elevated in presence of proteinuria (>3000 mg/dL) and bilirubinuria—invalidate the result Commercially available as NephroCheck® FDA approved for use in the United States and available in several European countries Currently, under evaluation for routine clinical use
Furosemide stress test	UO is measured 2 h after one-time dose of IV furosemide (1.0 mg/kg for loop diuretic naïve patients and 1.5 mg/kg if loop diuretics were used during the previous 7 days) and appropriate fluid resuscitation. FST responsive: >200 mL UO FST Nonresponsive: <200 mL UO	Predicting AKI progression Predicting the initiation of RRT in severe AKI	Not to be done in hypovolemic patients

RBF renal blood flow, *AKI* acute kidney injury, *UO* urine output, *SCr* serum creatinine, *KDIGO* kidney disease improving global outcomes, *ICA* iodinated contrast agents, *eGFR* estimated glomerular filtration rate, *RRT* renal replacement therapy, *ICU* intensive care unit, *LMW* low-molecular-weight, *NGAL* neutrophil gelatinase-associated lipocalin, *CKD* chronic kidney disease, *KIM-1* kidney injury molecule-1, *L-FABP* liver-type fatty acid binding, *IGFBP7* insulin-like growth factor-binding protein 7, *TIMP-2* tissue inhibitor of metalloproteinase-2, *FST* furosemide stress test

secretion (including trimethoprim, cimetidine, and tyrosine kinase inhibitors), diuretics, and volume status. Hence, under non-steady state conditions, typical in AKI, changes in SCr values do not accurately represent real-time changes in GFR. Also, due to loss of lean body mass in critically ill, SCr values are known to undergo slow decreases during prolonged ICU stays.

Plasma cystatin C and proenkephalin-A: The alternative kidney functional biomarkers, including plasma cystatin C and proenkephalin-A, are more specific than SCr and can detect AKI early. Cystatin C is created at a comparatively steady rate, released into the plasma, and 99% of it is filtered by glomeruli, making it a useful biomarker of impaired kidney function. However, neither of them have been recommended for routine clinical use as of now [34].

Damage and Stress Biomarkers

Tubular cell proteins, such as kidney injury molecule-1 (KIM-1), neutrophil gelatinase-associated lipocalin (NGAL), and monocyte chemoattractant protein-1 (MCP-1) appear early in urine after tubular injury. Hence, they can be measured to help detect AKI many hours prior to SCr elevation. Glomerular injury can be detected by measuring biomarkers of glomerular injury in urine, such as immunoglobulin G, nephrin, podocalyxin, podocin, transferrin, Netrin-1, and pyruvate kinase M2.

Urinary and plasma NGAL: Urinary and plasma NGAL appears to be an independent predictor of outcome and severity of AKI occuring in multiple disease settings (including CI-AKI), and irrespective of age [43]. It can be detected in the plasma as early as 2 -3 h after an initial insult, reaches its highest point at around 6 h, and then remain high for up to 5 days before starting to decline. High urinary NGAL can be used to predict AKI, discriminate intrinsic AKI from pre-renal AKI, predict renal non-recovery, in-hospital mortality, long-term CKD progression, ESRD, and mortality [44]. NGAL, both filtered and tubule derived, MCP-1, and IL-18 also increase with inflammation and cytokine release.

TIMP-2 and IGFBP7: G1 cell cycle arrest biomarkers, including Tissue inhibitor of metalloproteinase-2 (TIMP-2) and Insulin-like growth factor-binding protein 7 (IGFBP7), suggest a transient early phase of renal injury [45]. This biomarker is FDA approved for prediction of rapid progression of AKI to more severe stages and is commercially available as 'NephroCheck'. At present, it is one of the most promising biomarker which can reliably predict all cause-AKI and has an excellent potential for implementation in clinical decision- making algorithms.

Inflammatory Markers: Generalized markers of inflammation and damage may also increase in plasma and urine, including IL-6, soluble triggering receptor expressed on myeloid cells-1, Liver-Type Fatty Acid Binding Protein, and KIM-1.

Overall, these novel biomarkers provide useful information for assessing the initial insult and thus directing timely management and disease prognostication. However, many are still in the developmental phase and the rest lacks evidence for their cost-effectiveness in improving the clinical outcomes of AKI patients [46]. Future studies need to ascertain the validity of single versus combination of biomarkers and certain other non-kidney biomarkers (e.g., procalcitonin, natriuretic peptide, troponin) to identify high-risk patients in specific patient populations, such as neurocritically ill.

Additional Tests

Biochemical measurements performed to differentiate between pre-renal and renal causes of AKI such as blood urea nitrogen (BUN), BUN/SCr ratio, urine-specific gravity, urine sodium, fractional excretion of sodium and fractional excretion of urea, lack accuracy and consistency to diagnose AKI in critically ill and thus have limited role in NICU patients [34]. "Furosemide stress test" is a tubular stress test which assesses lack of response to a furosemide challenge as a clinical assessment of tubular function. It is basically a standardized form of "trial of Lasix" in patients with mild AKI. In recent years, there has been increasing interest in using FST in predicting the progression of AKI and guide timely initiation of RRT in critically ill AKI patients [47].

Contrast-enhanced ultrasonography (CEUS) of renal vasculature provides quantitative assessment of the alterations in renal microcirculatory blood flow occurring before SCr changes [48]. This can help in the early diagnosis and individualized hemodynamic therapy targeting improved renal microcirculation, thus avoiding progression of AKI to severe stages.

Large scale clinical studies are needed to further validate the technique and CEUS quantitative parameters in patients at a high risk of developing AKI.

30.6 Management of AKI in Neurocritically Ill Patients

Managing AKI in neurocritically ill patients involves multidisciplinary approach with the involvement of neurointensivists, nephrologists, and nutritionists. Being a multifactorial systemic disease, AKI lacks specific treatment. Hence, preventive therapy and good supportive care remains the mainstay of management [49].

30.6.1 AKI Risk-Prediction

For preventive strategies to be effective in avoiding the irreversible kidney damage, it is of utmost importance that they are instated timely in high-risk patients. To date, multiple methods have been devised for AKI risk prediction in critically ill including prediction scores and models, Renal Angina Index, and renal functional and damage biomarkers [5, 50–52].

An AKI prediction nomogram specific for neurosurgical intensive care unit patients was developed by An et al. using ten specified risk factors, including the Glasgow Coma Scale (GCS) classification and its coefficient of variation; past history of hypertension and coronary disease; pneumonia and heart failure in the first 7 days of hospitalization; and use of furosemide, torsemide, dopamine, and noradrenaline, with a tested good predictive performance for AKI [50]. Recently, Wang et al. compared the predictive accuracy of classic machine learning based algorithm (composed of glucose, cystatin C, serum uric acid, and chloride) with the conventional logistic regression-based predictive model (composed of glucose, serum creatinine, cystatin C, serum uric acid, and fresh frozen plasma transfusions) for AKI in patients with TBI [52]. Authors found that though the logistic regression model had a higher sensitivity (1.000), the machine learning based decision tree model had a higher specificity (0.821) for predicting AKI in patients with TBI and is convenient to use by physicians. Among damage biomarkers, NGAL and NephroCheck (TIMP-2 and IGFBP7) have shown the most promising results by allowing the physicians to predict AKI, thereby adjusting the treatment strategies to avoid its occurrence [45, 46]. In severe TBI patients, an early increase in the level of urinary NGAL has been used as a sensitive screening tool for AKI immediately after the injury [53]. Studies have also explored the potential of serum biomarkers including magnesium, procalcitonin, uric acid, Cystatin C, and lactate levels in predicting AKI in TBI patients [54–58].

30.6.2 Minimizing Secondary Injury

Considering the fact that AKI further perpetuates ABI and vice versa, measures should be taken to avoid secondary injury to the brain and kidney and other organs. Early institution of RRT and use of antioxidants, anti-inflammatory, and repair agents have been investigated to minimize the distant organ effects of AKI [59]. Another important step is to identify and remove the cause of AKI as early as possible, such as urinary tract infection or obstructive nephropathy.

30.6.3 Management Strategies

Guidelines recommend a bundle of different supportive measures including close monitoring of SCr and urine output, optimization of volume status, maintenance of adequate MAP, consideration of functional haemodynamic monitoring, early detection and management of sepsis, discontinuation or avoidance of nephrotoxic drugs, avoiding high tidal volume ventilation, and achieving euglycemia with minimal variability in plasma blood glucose levels, in patients at high risk for AKI [4, 34]. When evaluated individually, haemodynamic optimization and discontinuing nephrotoxic medications appear to be of greater significance than avoiding hyperglycemia or ICA in reducing the AKI burden [53].

Hemodynamic Management

In the presence of an impaired autoregulatory capacity, both hypovolemia and hypervolemia, and hypertension as well as hypotension, have the potential to adversely affect the cerebral and renal outcomes in neurocritically ill patients with AKI. Liberal use of vasopressors to maintain BP goals, but without adequate fluid administration is associated with an added insult to already compromised renal perfusion. These patients thus need a tight-rope balance of fluid therapy and inotropic/vasopressor support to optimize clinical outcomes.

Fluid management: A goal-directed fluid therapy (GDFT) aimed at dynamic preload is optimal to avoid the extremes of hypovolemia and volume overload. GDFT employs early adequate fluid resuscitation and the combined effect of vasopressors, to improve renal perfusion and oxygenation in patients who are "volume responsive" [60].

The literature exploring the effect of GDFT in preventing AKI in neurologically injured patients is sparse. GDFT was found to be associated with a lower incidence of hypotension, anemia, coagulopathy, and hyperglycemia; the known risk factors for AKI, along with a lower incidence of resistant ICHT in patients with moderate to severe TBI [61]. In SAH patients, Anetsberger et al. demonstrated lower incidence of DCI (13% vs. 32%) as well as AKI (2% vs. 6%, defined using AKIN criteria) in patients given GDFT (focusing on normovolemia and, in the presence of vasospasm, induced hypertension) compared to standard therapy [62].

Fluid overload can be managed with either diuretics or RRT, depending on the patient's clinical condition. REVERSE-AKI trial have shown that in patients with early AKI, a restrictive fluid therapy (after initial fluid resuscitation in combination with diuretics) resulted in lower cumulative fluid balance along with a lower risk of worsening renal function and need for RRT [63]. Positive fluid balance is independently associated with worse renal outcomes and increased mortality in patients diagnosed with early onset AKI [64]. However, the clinical advantage of fluid restriction in NICU patients cannot be generalized. Hence, an individualized fluid strategy based on functional indices appears optimal to minimize the risk of AKI and improve the neurological outcomes in neurocritically ill patients.

Fluid choice: The ideal fluid for volume resuscitation in AKI is still to be determined. In debate of colloid versus crystalloid, experts worldwide recommend crystalloids over colloid as a resuscitation fluid of choice in patients with injured brain, or septic AKI, with a lower incidence of AKI and RRT [4, 34, 65]. Thus, isotonic crystalloids are the preferred fluids for volume resuscitation in the absence of hemorrhagic shock. Use of albumin for resuscitation in patients with severe TBI is associated with increased intracranial pressure (ICP) and thus should be avoided [66].

Large volume resuscitation with isotonic normal saline (NS) may lead to hyperchloremic metabolic acidosis causing vasoconstriction of the afferent arteriole and reduced glomerular blood flow, thereby increasing the risk of AKI [67]. Compared to NS, balance crystalloids contain substrates for bicarbonate generation and consequently a lower chloride content, thus reducing the risk of hyperchloremic acidosis and associated kidney injury.

However, the recent large RCTs do not find significant difference in between NS and balance crystalloids in terms of risk of severe AKI, need for RRT or mortality, though some suggest modest reduction in early damage biomarkers with use of balance crystalloids in critically ill patients and mortality benefits in subpopulation with sepsis [65, 68–70]. Furthermore, balance crystalloids are associated with higher mortality in patients with an injured brain, owing to their hypotonicity and increase in cerebral edema [71, 72]. Hence, in the light of available evidence, NS may be preferred volume resuscitation in neurocritically ill patients at risk of AKI, with possible exception of patients with sepsis or septic shock.

Vasopressor therapy: Experts on AKI recommend a mean arterial pressure (MAP) of 65 mmHg for optimal perfusion of kidneys in sepsis [65]. The optimal MAP targets in patients with ABI vary with underlying pathology and course of treatment. Vasopressor therapy is often indicated in neurocritically ill patients with AKI to support cerebral and kidney perfusion. Chronic hypertensives have higher MAP targets secondary to the rightward shift of both cerebral and renal autoregulatory curves. Consequently, utmost caution is advised to set the treatment goals in sICH patients undergoing therapeutic blood pressure reduction to limit hematoma expansion so as not to compromise renal perfusion. Patients undergoing RRT often require larger doses of vasopressors because of their rapid clearance from circulation. Hence, for a targeted population of patients with ABI and AKI, the best strategy is to individualize the MAP goals, guided by dynamic status of cerebral autoregulation and renal parameters (urine output and lactate levels) [73].

The best choice of vasopressor agent to increase MAP in brain-injured patients with AKI is not yet certain. The 2012 KDIGO guidelines does not recommend either norepinephrine or vasopressin as superior to another in preventing AKI [4]. Guidelines on AKI recommend norepinephrine as the preferred vasopressor in adults with septic shock and AKI [34]. However, recent studies have questioned the practice, with some suggesting possible harmful effects of norepinephrine on renal circulation, thus possibly exacerbating AKI [37].

Phenylephrine and norepinephrine are the most commonly used vasopressors in ABI. Norepinephrine is preferred as the first-line agent in the management of hypotension in patients with ABI by the European Society of Intensive Care Medicine [74]. However, in US hospitals, phenylephrine (60.6%) is the most used vasopressor in patients with severe TBI, while use of norepinephrine (10.8%) is found to be associated with an increased risk of in-hospital mortality [75]. The TRACK-TBI study found equivocal results, with no better clinical or functional outcomes with norepinephrine compared to phenylephrine in moderate-to-severe TBI cases [76]. Thus, there is minimal clinical evidence at present to support the use of norepinephrine over phenylephrine in neurocritically ill patients to improve neurological outcomes or reduce mortality [77]. Phenylephrine, being a pure α-1 agonist, is not preferred in AKI secondary to concerns related to intense vasoconstriction mediated reduction in RBF and oxygen delivery [78].

Vasopressin infusion has been shown to improve cerebral perfusion pressure (CPP) in TBI and SAH patients, without increase in cerebral edema, despite theoretical concerns for associated hyponatremia [79, 80]. Furthermore, vasopressin is the only non-catecholamine vasopressor recommended in the septic patients unresponsive to norepinephrine. However, despite preclinical evidence of more sustained improvement in renal function with vasopressin compared to nor-epinephrine, the clinical evidence in its favour is poor at present [36]. Meta-analysis of vasopressin use in patients with septic shock has revealed that though vasopressin administration was associated with less use of RRT, it was not robust to sensitivity analysis [81].

Angiotensin II was approved by FDA in 2017 for adults with septic or other distributive shock. Post hoc analysis of the ATHOS-3 trial found higher incidence of renal recovery and mortality benefits with Angiotensin-II in the subset of the critically ill patients with vasodilatory shock and AKI requiring RRT [82]. However, in TBI patients, the upregulation of angiotensin type 1 receptors of local RAS has been implicated in the angiotensin II-mediated neurodegeneration, secondary to release of proinflammatory cytokines, oxidative stress, vasoconstriction, and cell death [83]. No data exists regarding the use of angiotensin II for vasopressor therapy in ABI patients.

To conclude, the choice of ideal vasopressor in neurocritically ill patients with AKI rests in between norepinephrine and vasopressin (with the role of norepinephrine being superseded by vasopressin) depending upon local-institutional choice. Future cerebral and renal outcome-based clinical trials exploring the role of vasopressor in this subset of patients are urgently needed.

Nephrotoxic Drug Management

All potential nephrotoxic agents should be stopped or best avoided in patients at high risk for AKI (enumerated in Table 30.2). However, if considered indispensable, such medications should be administered under close monitoring and after discussion with nephrologists and clinical pharmacologists. The altered drug pharmacokinetics of renally excreted medications with augmented renal clearance (such as levetiracetam) should also be taken into consideration in neurocritical patients [84]. Clinicians should ideally opt for an individualized drug dosing using drug serum concentration and measured creatinine clearance to guide drug dose adjustments.

Ventilatory Management

The crosstalk between the lung and kidney in the critically ill, involving hemodynamic, immuno-inflammatory, and neuro-hormonal mechanisms, may account for an increased incidence of AKI during invasive mechanical ventilation. Experts recommend lung protective ventilation (with low tidal volumes and optimal positive end expiratory pressures as determined by patients' oxygenation and lung compliance), conservative fluid management and early recognition and treatment of pulmonary infections to reduce the incidence of AKI in high-risk patients [85].

However, this strategy of lung protective ventilation and conservative fluid management may hamper the CPP in brain-injured patients and predispose to significant additional injury [86]. Overall, clinicians at present have limited means to identify the optimal ventilator strategy for each specific patient. Beqiri et al. have suggested that baseline ICP, brain compensatory reserve, and mechanical power can be used to formulate personalized ventilatory settings in high-risk neurocritically ill patients [87].

Anemia Management

Though preventing anemia is a desirable goal to maximize renal as well as cerebral oxygen supply, there are no clear guidelines regarding blood transfusion to optimize patients' hemoglobin levels. Blood transfusion in critically ill patients is fraught with numerous adverse effects, including an increased risk of AKI. Use of erythropoietin was found to have no effect on the need for blood transfusion, renal recovery, or mortality in AKI patients with anaemia [88]. Further studies are needed to ascertain other means of optimizing patients' hemoglobin levels in neurocritically ill patients at high risk for AKI. A large prospective multicenter randomized interventional trial is underway (ClinicalTrials.gov NCT02968654), evaluating the impact of two different transfusion strategies (liberal vs restrictive) on neurological outcomes and extra-cerebral organ dysfunction (including AKI), in patients with ABI.

Glycemic Control

Dysglycemias and glycemic variability are known risk factors for the onset and progression of both AKI and ABI. An improved glycemic control may thus reduce the risk of AKI in patients with an injured brain [89]. While the KDIGO guidelines recommend insulin therapy targeting plasma glucose 110–149 mg/dL, the recent IJCCM guidelines accept the blood glucose target of 180 mg/dL as beneficial in patients at risk of AKI [4, 34]. The optimal recommended plasma glucose levels in brain-injured patients are targeted at a higher range of 140–180 mg/dL, to avoid hypoglycemia.

Until further research on optimal blood sugar levels in neurocritically ill patients with or at-risk for AKI, an individualized glycemic control, targeting mean blood glucose levels between 140 and 180 mg/dL appears to be most appropriate.

Nutritional Support

AKI patients are prone for malnutrition secondary to the effects of critical illness, hypermetabolic state with hypertriglyceridemia and hyperglycemia, increased protein breakdown, uremia, fluid retention, and the ongoing loss of nutrients during CRRT. An early assessment of nutritional requirements and adequate supplementation is therefore essential to improve outcomes in AKI.

Guidelines recommend calorie intake up to 25–30 kcal/kg/day in AKI patients, with a high protein intake of up to 1.7 g/kg/day (1.3–1.7 g/kg/day) in patients either without RRT and on CRRT [4, 34]. In patients receiving intermittent RRT, a lower protein intake of 1–1.5 g/kg/day is suggested. Early enteral (oral or nasogastric) nutrition within 48 h is preferred in critically ill patients whenever possible to help maintain gut integrity and prevent bacterial translocation [4, 34, 90].

A high proportion of neurocritically ill patients have protein hypercatabolism, requiring high-protein intake (reaching up to 1.5–2 g/kg/day) [90]. Studies have shown that an early enteral nutrition and an optimal nitrogen balance (zero or positive) with high protein intake may lead to improved outcomes in neurocritically ill patients [90–92].

High-protein diets (2.0–2.5 g/kg/day of protein) with early supplemental parenteral nutrition or supplemental high-dose glutamine have been linked with adverse effects including increased ureagenesis, hypertonic dehydration, development of AKI, and potentially increased requirement for RRT [93]. Kim et al. showed that in neurocritically ill patients, a zero to positive nitrogen balance achieved with high protein intake (mean, 1.94 g/kg/day) was associated with better functional outcome, lesser neurological worsening, and lower in-hospital mortality, with no new development of AKI [92]. However, these results cannot be extrapolated to patients with AKI as patients with oliguria and on RRT were excluded from the retrospective cohort.

Overall, there is paucity of good clinical data concerning protein targets in critically ill patient including those with ABI and AKI. The nutritional goals should, therefore, be individualized depending upon underlying illness, disease severity, preexisting nutritional status, and type of RRT.

30.7 Contrast-Induced Acute Kidney Injury

In the current critical care era, presence of AKI post ICA administration remains an enigma, with many believing its existence in true "causal" manner to be a rare entity. The ambiguity regarding this entity includes multiple nomenclatures over the years, with varying definitions, including "Contrast Induced Nephropathy", CI-AKI, post-contrast AKI and the recently proposed contrast-associated AKI (CA-AKI).

CI-AKI is a specific term that describes a causal relationship between the contrast-media and the development of AKI secondary to the exposure of ICAs and in absence of other predisposing factors. KDIGO defines CI-AKI as $\geq$50% increase in creatinine from baseline within 7 days of exposure, or a $\geq$0.3 mg/dl increase within 48 hours, or urine output reduced to $\leq$0.5 ml/kg/hour for at least 6 hours [4].

The terms CA-AKI suggest a correlative rather than causative diagnosis, defining as AKI within 48 h of an intravenous or intra-arterial administration of ICA, with no definite causal link in between the two. Risk factors unique to neurocritical patient population includes use of mannitol, poor initial GCS, proteinuria, high NIHSS in stroke, prolonged carotid sinus reflex during carotid procedures, and administration of large volume of ICA (>250 mL) during embolization procedures [94, 95].

30.7.1 Incidence in Neurocritically Ill

The real incidence of CI-AKI is extremely difficult to retrieve from literature considering the lack of consensus definition and data derived from uncontrolled studies. Kim et al. observed 9.46% incidence of CI-AKI (defined, using RIFLE criteria) after elective neurointerventional procedures including diagnostic angiography and endovascular surgery [96]. In contrast, contrast-enhanced computed tomography (CECT) scans, CT angiogram, and CT perfusion studies are not associated with an increased risk of CI-AKI.

30.7.2 Pathogenesis

Though not completely understood, the pathogenesis of CI-AKI is multifactorial with cumulative effects of hypoxic as well as toxic renal epithelial cell damage including renal hemodynamic changes with afferent arteriolar vasoconstriction, decreased RBF, renal oxidative stress, medullary hypoxia with impaired microcirculation; and direct tubular epithelial cell toxicity (osmotic nephrosis, cellular apoptosis).

30.7.3 Periprocedural Management

The existing controversy revolving around its existence and role (if any) in worsening patients' prognosis has resulted in a multitude of guidelines, plagued by inconsistencies, published by various medical bodies. More than 10 guidelines have been published between 2018 and 2024, concerning ICA use in patients with kidney disease, including the latest guidelines from American College of Radiology, published in 2023 [97, 98]. The updated guidelines from KDIGO are soon to follow. Typically, CI-AKI typically have a self-limiting natural course, with SCr levels returning to baseline within 7 to 10 days of supportive care in the postexposure period. To date, no long term permanent renal dysfunction may be attributed to CI-AKI per se. Nonetheless, risk mitigation is paramount as no therapy exists once the renal damage sets in and even if not evident in post ICA exposure renal investigations, it may predispose the patients to future risk by decreasing the renal functioning reserve. Recently Zhong et al. systematically appraised the existing guidelines on intravenous ICA use in patients with kidney disease and highlighted the points with maximum consensus and disagreement amongst them [97]. Maximum consensus exists on defining the high-risk cases based on eGFR measurements, supporting the use of iso-osmolar or low-osmolar agents over high-osmolar agents, and the beneficial effect of hydration therapy in mitigating the risk associated with ICA administration (Table 30.4).

Identifying high-risk patients: Patients at high CI-AKI risk includes those with preexisting AKI, underlying Stage IV and Stage V CKD (eGFR ≤30 mL/min/1.73m2), given large doses of ICAs (>70 ml) or high osmolality contrast agents. No definite causal relationship has been identified

Table 30.4 Measures to mitigate the risk of contrast-induced acute kidney injury

Recommended therapies	Supported with good evidence: *1. Hydration:* *– Volume expansion for patients with eGFR ≤ 30 mL/min/1.73 m2.* *– IV hydration with 0.9% NS or 1.26% sodium bicarbonate. No sufficient evidence of superiority of one over other* *– Functional hemodynamic monitoring or forced diuresis protocol in patients with poor cardiac reserve.* *2. Rationale use of ICA* *– Choice of contrast: Use iso-osmolar or low-osmolar contrast agents*
	Needs further evaluation: *1. Route of hydration: Oral versus intravenous route of hydration.* *2. Hydration protocols: Timing, volume, speed.* *3. Dose of contrast: Minimum dosing necessary for diagnostic efficacy versus standard diagnostic dosing.* *– For IV administration, appropriate doses for high-quality imaging should be used in all patients.* *– For Intra-arterial ICA, a pragmatic approach is recommended to obtain the best results.* *4. Repeat Contrast study: 24 h versus 48 h versus 72 h time-interval.* *– Avoid repeated exposure within 24–48 h in high-risk cases, if feasible.* *– No such limitation in life threatening critical situations*
Therapies not recommended or supported by evidence-based medicine	• N-acetylcysteine • Diuretics • Renal replacement therapy • Statins (used mostly in the setting of coronary angiography and percutaneous coronary interventions; use of statins for the sole purpose of prophylaxis is not recommended.) • Other pharmacological agents, including mannitol, theophylline, prostaglandin E1, nicorandil, ascorbic acid, allopurinol, alphatocopherol, fenoldopam, natriuretic peptides, and trimetazidine.

eGFR estimated Glomerular filtration rate, *IV* Intravenous, *NS* normal saline, *ICA* iodinated contrast agent with route or frequency of administration of ICA, though some suggest a higher risk with intraarterial versus IV administration [97, 98]. In the absence of validated prediction models, it is recommended to consider the risk-benefit ratio of a contrast-based study in these high-risk patients on an individual-case basis. New biomarkers are being evaluated for CI-AKI risk prediction, including the urinary dickkopf-3 (DKK3) (a stress-induced renal tubular epithelium–derived glycoprotein), uNGAL, sNGAL and serum cystatin C [99].

Maintaining adequate hydration: Most guidelines recommend post exposure IV hydration therapy to enhance washout of contrast through the kidney as the mainstay strategy to prevent CI-AKI. [Zhao et al] However, the protocols including timing, volume and speed are highly variable. In general, normal saline is the preferred fluid over IV 1.26% sodium bicarbonate, given its easy availability and the result of the large, well conducted PRESERVE trial showing equivalent efficacy [100]. To avoid the harmful effects of volume loading, use of individualized hemodynamic monitoring and matched hydration with forced diuresis protocols have been advised in patients with poor cardiac reserves. In a recent propensity matched score study, Yan et al. revealed no beneficial effect of IV hydration before and after IV administration of ICA in preventing PC-AKI in patients with eGFR <30mL/min/1.73 m2 [101]. Thus, in the presence of conflicting results, further studies seem prudent exploring the effect of prophylactic hydration after IV as well as intraarterial contrast exposure in the high-risk neurocritical patients. Till further evidence, hydration protocol should be best decided by the neurointensivist and nephrologist on an individual case basis.

Rationale ICA administration: Non-ionic and low-osmolar as well as iso-osmolar ICA are universally recommended and easily available. Though no guideline recommends a specific type, recent studies have revealed a significant reduction in major adverse renal and cardiovascular events with isoosmolar iodixanol versus low-osmolar contrast media [102, 103]. Likewise, no clear recommendations have been given regarding the optimal frequency of ICA administration. However, it is recommended to avoid repeat contrast exposure within 24-48 hours duration in high-risk cases, provided there is no delay in establishing a critical diagnosis [97, 98]. Considering the dosage, guidelines do not recommend withholding adequate ICA administration at the expense of good quality imaging. Hence, neurocritically ill patients should not be denied any neurodiagnostic and therapeutic neurointerventional procedures based on unfounded fears of renal damage.

30.8 Gadolinium-Based Contrast Agents and Nephrotoxicity

Gadolinium, a rare heavy metal, is used as a contrast media agent for contrast enhanced MRI (CE-MRI) and MR angiography, which are frequently performed in neurocritically ill patients. Gadolinium-based contrast agents (GBCA) have been implicated in the genesis of nephrotoxicity and a potentially debilitating fibrotic condition called nephrogenic systemic fibrosis (NSF).

When present as a free ionic compound, gadolinium is highly toxic in humans. It competes with bivalent calcium and magnesium ions, thus interfering with their biologic functions. Furthermore, at physiologic pH, ionic gadolinium tends to precipitate in brain, kidney, liver, spleen, and bones, causing intense inflammation ultimately leading to fibrosis.

Patients with AKI, stages 4 or 5 CKD, or on RRT are at greater risk of NSF, particularly with old Group I GBCM [104]. The standard doses of Group II GBCA (currently in use) are associated with a very low, if any, incidence of NSF or nephrotoxicity and does not mandate prior kidney function screening. The experts from the American College of Radiology and the National Kidney Foundation states that considering the very low incidence of NSF with group II GBCA, the potential harms of delaying or withholding GBCA MRI in a patient with AKI or eGFR < 30 mL/min per 1.73 m^2 is likely to outweigh the risk in most clinical situations [105].

30.9 Renal Replacement Therapies in Neurocritically Ill Patients

RRT is often indicated in patients with stage 3 AKI to correct acidosis, remove inflammatory mediators, and help ultrafiltrate the excess fluid in oliguric AKI. Traditional RRT indications in critically ill patients include severe hyperkaliemia (K+ >6.0 mmol/L) or rapidly rising serum potassium (K^+) levels, severe acidemia (pH < 7.1–7.2), metabolic acidosis (HCO_3^- < 12–15 mmol/L), and fluid overload. RRT may frequently be indicated in known end-stage renal disease (ESRD) patients presenting with a neurological emergency.

RRT causes unique changes in the intracranial physiology secondary to de novo or an increase of existing vasogenic cerebral edema, referred to as "*Dialysis associated Neurovascular Injury*" (or *Dialysis Disequilibrium Syndrome* in ESRD patients) (Fig. 30.2). It is a rare but well-known and potentially fatal complication of RRT, specifically in NICU patients with exhausted cerebral reserves. Hence, an understanding of the different types of RRT techniques and their modifications for safe application in neurocritically ill patients are of paramount importance to neurointensivists.

30.9.1 Techniques

RRT aims to remove nitrogenous waste and maintain acid–base and water balance in the body, via the principles of diffusion, convection, ultrafiltration, and sometimes adsorption. Various RRT techniques are available based on one or on the combination of the above principles. In general, intermittent hemodialysis (IHD) and continuous renal replacement therapy (CRRT) are the most prescribed extracorporeal RRT techniques in critically ill patients (Table 30.5).

The 2012 KDIGO AKI guidelines recommend using CRRT, rather than intermittent RRT, for AKI patients with ABI or other causes of increased ICP or generalized brain edema" [4]. Among all RRT techniques, convective CVVH modality is considered most efficient for patients with ABI as it allows a gradual reduction in the concentration of uremic toxins and fluids, thus avoiding sudden changes in serum osmolality and maintains hemodynamic stability [106–108].

Sustained low-efficiency dialysis (SLED) is a hybrid RRT modality, which uses conventional hemodialysis machines but for longer durations than typical IHD sessions (6–12 h vs. 3–4 h for IHD) and with lower blood flows. The level of evidence regarding SLED in neurocritically ill patients is still limited [108]. Compared to CRRT, it may be advantageous in terms of reduced costs and flexibility of treatment and avoiding prolonged immobilization of patients with no difference in acute hemodynamic effects or mortality.

30.9.2 Mechanism of Worsening Cerebral Edema

RRT or dialysis causes rapid clearance of plasma solutes and toxins (predominantly urea) from systemic circulation than intracranial compartment. This creates an osmotic gradient between the two compartments causing ingress of water from hypo-osmolal plasma to brain in a "reverse urea effect." In addition, paradoxical intracellular acidosis is created secondary to bicarbonate-buffers derived carbon-dioxide crossing the cellular membranes. This further leads to neuronal swelling and cerebral edema. The magnitude of increase in ICP is independent of dialysis modality, but peaks earlier with IHD technique compared to CRRT in brain-injured patients and correlates positively to pre RRT plasma urea levels [109].

Hemodynamic instability is a common complication of all RRT modalities in critically ill AKI patients, though more frequent with IHD than CRRT treatments. It may compromise cerebral as well as renal perfusion in patients with altered cerebral and renal autoregulation. Thus, neurocritically ill patients are at an increased risk of worsening vasogenic and cytotoxic cerebral edema leading to fatal cerebral herniations and poor renal recovery as well. In a systematic review, Parsons et al. have revealed a high inci-

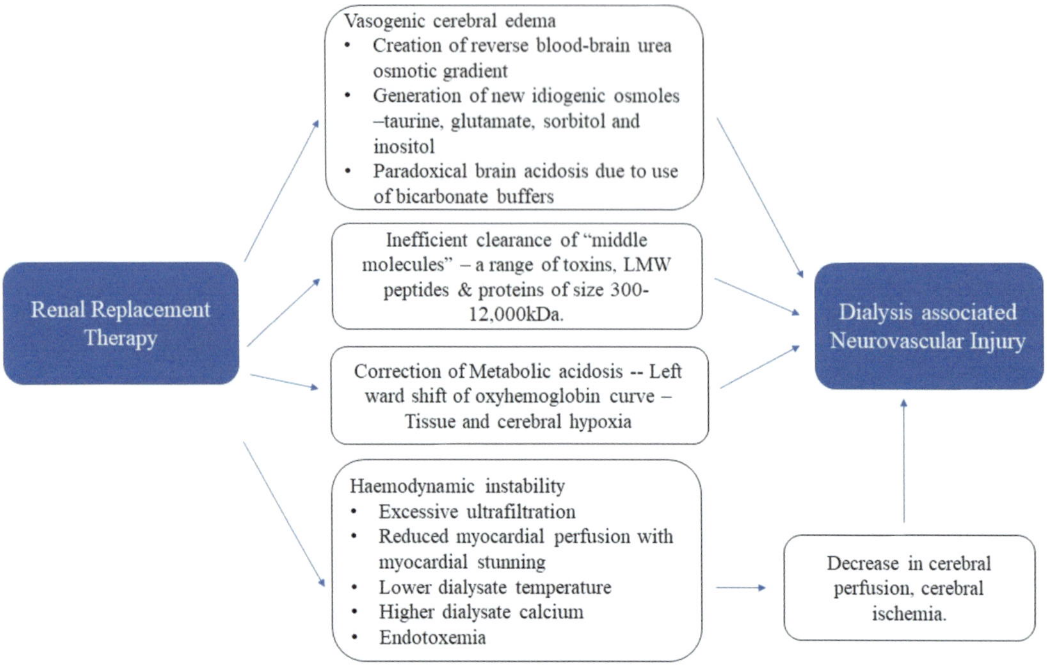

Fig. 30.2 Pathophysiological mechanisms of dialysis associated neurovascular injury in patients undergoing renal replacement therapy

dence (up to 60%) of potentially life-threatening ICHT in neurosurgical patients during RRT, with mortality rates as high as 65% [110]. When comparing the RRT techniques, authors found greater ICP increase (73% vs. 37.5%, $P = 0.01$) and higher mortality (75% vs. 39.1%, $P = 0.01$) with IHD than CRRT technique.

30.9.3 Timing of Initiation of RRT

Clinical trials have been ambiguous in determining the best time for initiating RRT in critically ill patients. While the STARRT-AKI trial concluded against the accelerated use of RRT prior to developing standard RRT initiation criteria, the AKIKI-2 trial showed that a more-delayed RRT was associated with a trend toward poor outcome [111, 112]. Hence, the right time to initiate RRT, in neurocritically ill patients is still a matter of research. Experts consider use of stress tests such as damage biomarkers (including urinary NGAL, IL18, or the NephroCheck) and FST to predict the initiation of CRRT in critically ill AKI patients [47].

30.9.4 Treatment Modifications in Neurocritically Ill

CRRT (or SLED, depending on availability) is the preferred modality in hemodynamically unstable and neurocritically ill patients. However, high cost of CRRT limits its use, particularly in resource limited setting [113]. Hence, IHD may also need to be considered for brain-injured patients with AKI. Efforts should be taken to prevent and effectively manage hemodynamic instability associated with RRT, in particular IHD, in critically ill (Table 30.6).

Slow ultrafiltration: For patients presenting with diuretic-refractory volume overload as primary indication for RRT, isolated slow ultrafiltration may be considered for fluid removal, followed by brief session of IHD to maintain plasma urea concentration. This technique does

Table 30.5 Renal replacement therapies in neurocritically ill patients

	IHD	CRRT
Indications	• Considered in patients with a minimal brain injury without significant vasogenic edema or midline shift • May be done in patients with raised ICP in the event of nonavailability of CRRT with certain modifications	• Recommended by KDIGO in patients with ABI or other causes of increased ICP • Hemodynamically unstable patients
Principle based on	Diffusion	CVVH:Convection CVVHD:Diffusion CVVHDF: Both diffusion and convection
Anticoagulation	*With anticoagulation:* • Systemic anticoagulation (UFH or LMWH). LMWH: – Usual first choice for systemic anticoagulation – Single-dose convenience – Lower risk of bleeding and HIT – More reliable response UFH – Increased risk of bleeding and HIT compared to LMWH *Without anticoagulation:* • By using heparin-coated filters, saline flush, shorter sessions, and higher blood flows	*With anticoagulation:* • Systemic anticoagulation with UFH (use of LMWH is limited) • Regional citrate anticoagulation – Recommended in KDIGO-AKI guidelines in absence of other systemic causes for anticoagulation – Citrate concentration in the circuit must range between 4 and 6 mmol/L to achieve an ionic calcium concentration <0.4 mmol/L. – No risk of HIT – Lower risk of bleeding. – May cause citrate accumulation with high anion gap metabolic acidosis, hypocalcemia, and hypomagnesemia. *Without anticoagulation:* • By using methods reducing filtration fraction (reducing net ultrafiltrate, increase blood flow)
Advantages	• Highly efficient—In patients with severe acute electrolyte disturbances, may rapidly restore serum calcium and/or potassium concentrations. • More practical • Cost-effective • Eliminates the need for systemic anticoagulation • Reduced risk of bleeding. • Shorter duration sessions allow intermittent examinations and mobilization. • Dialysate sodium can be modified and higher sodium concentrations may be used in patients with TBI	• Maintains hemodynamic stability. • Reduces the risk of cerebral edema: less efficient clearance of solutes prevents sudden changes in serum osmolality. • Fine fluid control • Less complicated technically for ICU staff

(continued)

Table 30.5 (continued)

	IHD	CRRT
Disadvantages	• Higher risk of inducing cerebral edema. • Hemodynamic instability with rapid fluid removal • More complicated to operate. • Need dedicated dialysis staff	• High risk of clotting if no anticoagulation is prescribed • Citrate accumulation if RCA is used • Limits out of bed mobilization • Labor-intensive—needs constant supervision • Costly • Hypophosphatemia • CRRT solutions have prefixed low sodium concentration

IHD intermittent haemodialysis, *CRRT* continuous renal replacement therapy, *ABI* acute brain injury, *ICP* intracranial pressure, *CVVH* continuous slow ultrafiltration continuous venovenous hemofiltration, *CVVHD* continuous venovenous hemodialysis diffusion, *CVVHDF* continuous venovenous hemodiafiltration, *UFH* unfractionated heparin, *LMWH* low molecular weight heparin, *HIT* heparin induced thrombocytopenia, *RCA* regional citrate anticoagulation

Table 30.6 Steps for preventing hemodynamic instability during renal replacement therapy

• Fluid removal rate: Set fluid removal goals to avoid or reduce net positive fluid balance.
• Longer treatment times: allow lower ultrafiltration rates with same ultrafiltration goals and sufficient time for plasma refiling thereby preventing intravascular hypovolemia.
– Minimum 4 h treatment time for IHD, slightly longer session time for SLED.
• Graded flow rates for more gradual reduction in plasma osmolality: Allows less fluid shift with better plasma refilling.
– For IHD: Blood flow rate of ≤200 mL/min and dialysate flow rate of ≤300 mL/min
– For CRRT: Total effluent rate of 20–25 mL/kg/h. Do not reduce the blood flow rate <150–200 mL/min to prevent clotting risk.
• Use of higher dialysate sodium concentration (≥145 mmol/L) for intermittent RRT techniques (IHD and SLED): Minimizes osmolar shifts, avoid hypovolemia.
• Use of higher dialysate calcium concentration (1.5 or 1.75 mmol/L)) for intermittent RRT techniques (IHD and SLED): Maintains vascular tone, increases myocardial contractility, and decreases arrhythmia risk.
• Use of cooled dialysate: Causes catecholamine release, which causes peripheral vasoconstriction and an increase in heart rate inotropy
– 0.5 °C less than the patient's temperature, to a minimum of 35.0–35.5 °C.
• Use a bicarbonate-based buffer instead of lactate based.
– Bicarbonate-based dialysate causes lower serum lactate levels and less hemodynamic instability.

IHD intermittent hemodialysis, *SLED* sustained low-efficiency dialysis, *CRRT* continuous renal replacement therapy, *RRT* renal replacement therapy

not affect the serum osmolality, reducing the risk of cerebral edema.

CRRT modifications: For CRRT dosing, the KDIGO group recommends a EFV of 30–35 mL/kg/h to achieve the effective dose of 20–25 mL/kg/h (regardless of the modality and form of pre or post filter fluid replacement) [4]. The use of acetate-free replacement solution is recommended as it allows rapid control of metabolic acidosis and uremia.

An important consideration during CRRT is the use of anticoagulation to maintain adequate patency of the extracorporeal circuit and the performance of the filter. Both ABI and AKI induce strong systemic inflammatory response, thus creating a prothrombotic state. At the same time, systemic anticoagulation with unfractionated heparin (UFH) or low molecular weight heparin (LMWH) should be avoided in ABI patients due to their inherent increased risk of bleeding. KDIGO guidelines recommends regional citrate anticoagulation (RCA), rather than no anticoagulation, during CRRT in a patient with high risk of bleeding and without contraindications for citrate [4]. For patients presenting with concomitant contraindications to citrate (i.e., liver failure and shock with skeletal muscle hypoperfusion), anticoagulation-free CRRT is advised.

Current evidence reveals that compared with anticoagulation-free protocol, RAC-based protocol results in longer filter lifespan and better azotemic control without increasing new bleeding episodes in patients with increased bleeding risk, and thus appears safe in this subset of critically ill patients [114, 115]. An impaired citrate metabolism or an inadequate amount of buffer during CRRT may lead to acid–base and electrolyte disturbances, predominantly metabolic acidosis, hypocalcemia, and hypomagnesemia, which can further compromise hemodynamic stability. Since citrate binds to ionized calcium and removes it from circulation, the total calcium/ionized calcium ratio should be measured daily. A ratio of >2.5 suggests citrate accumulation risk and treatment must be stopped.

Maintaining sodium balance is another critical element while prescribing CRRT in neurocritically ill, considering the prefixed sodium (136–140 mmol/L) in CRRT replacement solutions. Higher dialysate sodium concentration (≥145 mmol/L) is recommended to maintain hemodynamic stability and to counteract the "reverse urea effect." In patients presenting with chronic hyponatremia and undergoing CRRT, hypertonic (3%) saline infusion may be administered either as a separate infusion or as post-filter replacement fluid to increase serum sodium. The increase should however, be gradual (daily rate of increase of 4–6 mEq/L), to prevent the risk of osmotic demyelination. Hypophosphatemia and hypomagnesemia are another common electrolyte abnormality during CRRT, which needs to be managed through proper supplementation in replacement fluids.

IHD modifications: Coagulation-free IHD is a feasible option in patents at high risk of intracranial bleeding and preexiting vascular access, provided certain technical modifications are made to minimize osmotic gradients (reduced blood and dialysate flow rates, small surface area dialyzer membranes, slow urea removal rate with reduction ratio of 0.4, and shorter, frequent treatment sessions) and hemodynamic instability (discussed in Table 30.6) [115, 116].

Anticoagulant-free circuits alone or with heparin-precoated dialyzers or dialysate containing low levels of citrate can be used. Sodium modeling by deliberately changing the sodium concentration in dialysate during the course of IHD has been shown to reduce the incidence of intradialytic hypotension in ESRD patients undergoing chronic hemodialysis, but it has little to no effect among AKI patients receiving IHD [117]. HTS or mannitol administration may help to control the decrease in plasmatic osmolality, thus maintaining the therapeutic hyperosmolar state and hemodynamic stability [118]. Albumin or mannitol should be avoided in the presence of sepsis as the leaky vessels are unable to retain these compounds in intravascular space.

It may be prudent to slightly delay initiating IHD it in the first 72 h of an expanding hematoma or worsening cerebral edema, though treatment decisions need to be individualized. Continuous ICP monitoring may help in early diagnosis of raised ICP during IHD and clinical decision-making in neurocritically ill patients with severe AKI and poor neurological status. CSF diversion, via external ventricular drain or less invasive lumbar CSF drainage (after excluding obstructive hydrocephalus), has also been mentioned as one of the strategies to manage refractory ICHT during IHD in patients with existing intracranial injuries [119].

30.10 Future Directives

In recent years, various machine learning approaches have been devised for prediction of AKI in neurologically injured patients [120]. Modern machine learning tools and technological advancements may lead to improved prediction, detection, and individualized management decisions and outcome assessment in critically ill patients with AKI. The application of artificial intelligence for early prediction of AKI is, however, still in its nascent stage and needs further research and external validation for widespread use [121].

With the growing role of precision medicine in modern critical care, the genomic studies have provided greater insights into the molecular mechanisms of AKI and ABI. This may enable us to find the treatment targets for precision medicine in the highly variable, unstable, neurocritically ill patient with AKI. The Kidney Precision Medicine Project is designed to create a reference kidney atlas, based on results obtained from kidney biopsies of participants with CKD or AKI to determine the treatment targets for novel therapies and preventive strategies [122]. The advent of mesenchymal stem cell treatments and other emerging pharmaceutical strategies could also help the intensivists to better treat AKI in this subset of neurocritically ill patients with few management options available at present [59].

References

1. Pesonen A, Ben-Hamouda N, Schneider A. Acute kidney injury after brain injury: does it exist? Minerva Anestesiol. 2021;87:823–7.
2. Li X, Yuan F, Zhou L. Organ crosstalk in acute kidney injury: evidence and mechanisms. J Clin Med. 2022;11(22):6637.
3. Honore PM, Redant S, Kaefer K, Barreto Gutierrez L, Kugener L, Attou R, Gallerani A, De Bels D. Acute kidney injury definition in traumatic brain injury patients only based on serum creatinine criteria and not together with urine output criteria: are we missing some acute kidney injury patients? Crit Care Med. 2021;49(5):e553–4.
4. Kidney Disease: Improving Global Outcomes (KDIGO) Acute Kidney Injury Work Group. KDIGO Clinical Practice Guideline for acute kidney injury. Kidney Int. 2012;2:1–138.
5. Ostermann M, Zarbock A, Goldstein S, Kashani K, Macedo E, Murugan R, et al. Recommendations on acute kidney injury biomarkers from the acute disease quality initiative consensus conference: a consensus statement. JAMA Netw Open. 2020;3(10):e2019209.
6. Koeze J, Keus F, Dieperink W, et al. Incidence, timing and outcome of AKI in critically ill patients varies with the definition used and the addition of urine output criteria. BMC Nephrol. 2017;18:70.
7. Bianchi NA, Stavart LL, Altarelli M, Kelevina T, Faouzi M, Schneider AG. Association of oliguria with acute kidney injury diagnosis, severity assessment, and mortality among patients with critical illness. JAMA Netw Open. 2021;4(11):e2133094.
8. Büttner S, Stadler A, Mayer C, et al. Incidence, risk factors, and outcome of acute kidney injury in neurocritical care. J Intensive Care Med. 2020;35:338–46.
9. Ramírez-Guerrero G, Lucero C, Villagrán-Cortés F, Hauway E, Torres-Cifuentes V, Baghetti-Hernández R, Vera-Calzaretta A, Ronco C, Garay O. Acute kidney injury in neurocritical patients: a retrospective cohort study. Int Urol Nephrol. 2023;
10. Robba C, Banzato E, Rebora P, Iaquaniello C, Huang CY, Wiegers EJA, et al. Collaborative European NeuroTrauma Effectiveness Research in Traumatic Brain Injury (CENTER-TBI) ICU Participants and Investigators. Acute Kidney Injury in Traumatic Brain Injury Patients: Results From the Collaborative European NeuroTrauma Effectiveness Research in Traumatic Brain Injury Study. Crit Care Med. 2021;49(1):112–26.
11. Luu D, Komisarow J, Mills BM, Vavilala MS, Laskowitz DT, Mathew J, et al. Association of severe acute kidney injury with mortality and healthcare utilization following isolated traumatic brain injury. Neurocrit Care. 2021;35(2):434–40.
12. Skrifvars MB, Bailey M, Moore E, Mårtensson J, French C, Presneill J, et al. A post hoc analysis of osmotherapy use in the erythropoietin in traumatic brain injury study—associations with acute kidney injury and mortality. Crit Care Med. 2021;49(4):E394–403.
13. Barea-Mendoza JA, Chico-Fernández M, Quintana-Díaz M, Serviá-Goixart L, Fernández-Cuervo A, Bringas-Bollada M, et al. Neurointensive Care and Trauma Working Group of the Spanish Society of Intensive Care Medicine (SEMICYUC). Traumatic brain injury and acute kidney injury-outcomes and associated risk factors. J Clin Med. 2022;11(23):7216.
14. Tujjar O, Belloni I, Hougardy JM, Scolletta S, Vincent JL, Creteur J, Taccone FS. Acute kidney injury after subarachnoid hemorrhage. J Neurosurg Anesthesiol. 2017;29(2):140–9.
15. Xiao Y, Wan J, Zhang Y, Wang X, Zhou H, Lai H, Chong W, Hai Y, Lunsford LD, You C, Yu S, Fang F. Association between acute kidney injury and long-term mortality in patients with aneurysmal subarachnoid hemorrhage: a retrospective study. Front Neurol. 2022;13:864193.
16. Guillemin L, Goronflot T, Desal H, Rozec B, Lakhal K. Early Acute kidney injury in patients with non-traumatic subarachnoid hemorrhage who undergo catheter angiography: incidence, associated risk factors and impact on outcome. J Stroke Cerebrovasc Dis. 2022;31(7):106488.
17. Lampmann T, Hadjiathanasiou A, Asoglu H, Wach J, Kern T, Vatter H, Güresir E. Early serum creatinine levels after aneurysmal subarachnoid hemorrhage predict functional neurological outcome after 6 months. J Clin Med. 2022;11:4753.
18. Qureshi AI, Aslam H, Zafar W, Huang W, Lobanova I, Naqvi SH, Malhotra K, Arora N, Chandrasekaran PN, Siddiq F, French BR, Gomez CR. Acute kidney injury in acute ischemic stroke patients in clinical trials. Crit Care Med. 2020;48(9):1334–9.
19. Nagaraja N, Farooqui A, Ballur Narayana Reddy V, Shukla AM. Kidney impairment and outcomes in acute ischaemic stroke. Intern Med J. 2022; https://doi.org/10.1111/imj.15852.
20. Qureshi AI, Huang W, Lobanova I, Hanley DF, Hsu CY, Malhotra K, Steiner T, Suarez JI, Toyoda K, Yamamoto H. Antihypertensive Treatment of Cerebral Hemorrhage 2 Trial Investigators. Systolic blood pressure reduction and acute kidney injury in intracerebral hemorrhage. Stroke. 2020;51(10):3030–8.

21. Dai H, Ding F, Ma J, Zhao S. Risk factors for acute kidney injury after intracranial hemorrhage. Neuro Endocrinol Lett. 2022;43(5):257–64.
22. Gupta N. Brain and kidney crosstalk. In: Brain and kidney crosstalk; 2020. p. 89–117.
23. Civiletti F, Assenzio B, Mazzeo AT, Medica D, Giaretta F, Deambrosis I, Fanelli V, Ranieri VM, Cantaluppi V, Mascia L. Acute tubular injury is associated with severe traumatic brain injury: in vitro study on human tubular epithelial cells. Sci Rep. 2019;9(1):6090.
24. Jassam YN, Izzy S, Whalen M, McGavern DB, El Khoury J. Neuroimmunology of traumatic brain injury: time for a paradigm shift. Neuron. 2017;95(6):1246–65.
25. Cao W, Li A, Li J, et al. Reno-cerebral reflex activates the renin angiotensin system, promoting oxidative stress and renal damage after ischemia-reperfusion injury. Antioxid Redox Signal. 2017;27(7):415–32.
26. Dabrowski W, Siwicka-Gieroba D, Robba C, Bielacz M, Sołek-Pastuszka J, Kotfis K, Bohatyrewicz R, Jaroszyński A, Malbrain MLNG, Badenes R. Potentially detrimental effects of hyperosmolality in patients treated for traumatic brain injury. J Clin Med. 2021;10(18):4141.
27. Rein JL, Coca SG. "I don't get no respect": the role of chloride in acute kidney injury. Am J Physiol Renal Physiol. 2019;316(3):F587–605.
28. Yamane DP, Maghami S, Graham A, Vaziri K, Davison D. Association of hyperchloremia and acute kidney injury in patients with traumatic brain injury. J Intensive Care Med. 2022;37(1):128–33.
29. Huet O, Chapalain X, Vermeersch V, Moyer JD, Lasocki S, Cohen B, Dahyot-Fizelier C, Chalard K, Seguin P, Hourmant Y, Asehnoune K, Roquilly A, Atlanrea Study Group and the Société Française d'Anesthésie Réanimation (SFAR) Research Network. Impact of continuous hypertonic (NaCl 20%) saline solution on renal outcomes after traumatic brain injury (TBI): a post hoc analysis of the COBI trial. Crit Care. 2023;27(1):42.
30. Kumar AB, Shi Y, Shotwell MS, Richards J, Ehrenfeld JM. Hypernatremia is a significant risk factor for acute kidney injury after subarachnoid hemorrhage: a retrospective analysis. Neurocrit Care. 2015;22(2):184–91.
31. Cook AM, Morgan Jones G, Hawryluk GWJ, Mailloux P, McLaughlin D, Papangelou A, Samuel S, Tokumaru S, Venkatasubramanian C, Zacko C, Zimmermann LL, Hirsch K, Shutter L. Guidelines for the Acute Treatment of Cerebral Edema in Neurocritical Care Patients. Neurocrit Care. 2020;32(3):647-66.
32. Krzych ŁJ, Czempik PF. Impact of furosemide on mortality and the requirement for renal replacement therapy in acute kidney injury: a systematic review and meta-analysis of randomised trials. Ann Intensive Care. 2019;9(1):85.
33. Zhao GJ, Xu C, Ying JC, Lü WB, Hong GL, Li MF, Wu B, Yao YM, Lu ZQ. Association between furosemide administration and outcomes in critically ill patients with acute kidney injury. Crit Care. 2020;24(1):75.
34. Mishra RC, Sodhi K, Prakash KC, Tyagi N, Chanchalani G, Annigeri RA, Govil D, Savio RD, Subbarayan B, Arora N, Chatterjee R, Chacko J, Khasne RW, Chakravarthi RM, George N, Ahmed A, Javeri Y, Chhallani AK, Khanikar RG, Margabandhu S, Lopa AJ, Chaudhry D, Samavedam S, Kar A, Dixit SB, Gopal P. ISCCM guidelines on acute kidney injury and renal replacement therapy. Indian J Crit Care Med. 2022;26(Suppl 2):S13–42.
35. Gordon AC, Mason AJ, Thirunavukkarasu N, Perkins GD, Cecconi M, Cepkova M, Pogson DG, Aya HD, Anjum A, Frazier GJ, Santhakumaran S, Ashby D, Brett SJ. VANISH Investigators. Effect of early vasopressin vs norepinephrine on kidney failure in patients with septic shock: the VANISH randomized clinical trial. JAMA. 2016;316(5):509–18.
36. Okazaki N, Iguchi N, Evans RG, Hood SG, Bellomo R, May CN, Lankadeva YR. Beneficial effects of vasopressin compared with norepinephrine on renal perfusion, oxygenation, and function in experimental septic acute kidney injury. Crit Care Med. 2020;48(10):e951–8.
37. Al-Husinat L, Alsabbah A, Hmaid AA, Athamneh R, Adwan M, Hourani MN, Almakhadmeh S, Modanat ZJA, Ismail MIA, Varrassi G. Norepinephrine may exacerbate septic acute kidney injury: a narrative review. J Clin Med. 2023;12(4):1373.
38. Busse LW, Ostermann M. Vasopressor therapy and blood pressure management in the setting of acute kidney injury. Semin Nephrol. 2019;39(5):462–72.
39. De Backer D, Aldecoa C, Njimi H, Vincent JL. Dopamine versus norepinephrine in the treatment of septic shock: a meta-analysis*. Crit Care Med. 2012;40(3):725–30.
40. Alvarado Sánchez JI, Caicedo Ruiz JD, Diaztagle Fernández JJ, Amaya Zuñiga WF, Ospina-Tascón GA, Cruz Martínez LE. Predictors of fluid responsiveness in critically ill patients mechanically ventilated at low tidal volumes: systematic review and meta-analysis. Ann Intensive Care. 2021;11(1):28.
41. Willner D, Goldman A, Azran H, Stern T, Kirshenbom D, Rosenthal G. Early identification of acute kidney injury in the ICU with real-time urine output monitoring: a clinical investigation. BMC Nephrol. 2021;22(1):293.
42. Murad O, Orjuela Cruz DF, Goldman A, Stern T, van Heerden PV. Improving awareness of kidney function through electronic urine output monitoring: a comparative study. BMC Nephrol. 2022;23(1):412.
43. Marakala V. Neutrophil gelatinase associated lipocalin (NGAL) in kidney injury—a systematic review. Clin Chim Acta. 2022;536:135–41.
44. McMahon BA, Galligan M, Redahan L, Martin T, Meaney E, Cotter EJ, Murphy N, Hannon C, Doran P, Marsh B, et al. Biomarker predictors of adverse acute kidney injury outcomes in critically ill patients:

the Dublin Acute Biomarker Group Evaluation Study. Am J Nephrol. 2019;50:19–28.
45. Huang F, Zeng Y, Lv L, Chen Y, Yan Y, Luo L, Pan R, Jiang J, Wei X. Predictive value of urinary cell cycle arrest biomarkers for all cause-acute kidney injury: a meta-analysis. Sci Rep. 2023;13(1):6037.
46. Brazzelli M, Aucott L, Aceves-Martins M, Robertson C, Jacobsen E, Imamura M, Poobalan A, Manson P, Scotland G, Kaye C, Sawhney S, Boyers D. Biomarkers for assessing acute kidney injury for people who are being considered for admission to critical care: a systematic review and cost-effectiveness analysis. Health Technol Assess. 2022 Jan;26(7):1-286
47. Zhang K, Zhang H, Zhao C, Hu Z, Shang J, Chen Y, Huo Y, Zhao C, Li B, Guo S. Hebei Key Laboratory of Critical Disease Mechanism and Intervention. The furosemide stress test predicts the timing of continuous renal replacement therapy initiation in critically ill patients with acute kidney injury: a double-blind prospective intervention cohort study. Eur J Med Res. 2023;28(1):149.
48. Li Y, Chen L, Feng L, Li M. Contrast-Enhanced Ultrasonography for Acute Kidney Injury: A Systematic Review and Meta-Analysis. Ultrasound Med Biol. 2023 Sep;49(9):1930-9.
49. Ramírez-Guerrero G, Baghetti-Hernández R, Ronco C. Acute kidney injury at the neurocritical care unit. Neurocrit Care. 2022;36(2):640–9.
50. An S, Luo H, Wang J, Gong Z, Tian Y, Liu X, Ma J, Jiang R. An acute kidney injury prediction nomogram based on neurosurgical intensive care unit profiles. Ann Transl Med. 2020;8(5):194.
51. Ortiz-Soriano V, Kabir S, Claure-Del Granado R, Stromberg A, Toto RD, Moe OW, Goldstein SL, Neyra JA. Assessment of a modified renal angina index for AKI prediction in critically ill adults. Nephrol Dial Transplant. 2022;37(5):895–903.
52. Wang R, Zhang J, He M, Xu J. Classification and Regression Tree Predictive Model for Acute Kidney Injury in Traumatic Brain Injury Patients. Ther Clin Risk Manag. 2024 Feb 22;20:139-49.
53. Li N, Zhao WG, Xu FL, Zhang WF, Gu WT. Neutrophil gelatinase-associated lipocalin as an early marker of acute kidney injury in patients with traumatic brain injury. J Nephrol. 2013;26(6):1083–8.
54. Liu Z, Wang R, He M, Kang Y. Hypomagnesemia Is Associated with the Acute Kidney Injury in Traumatic Brain Injury Patients: A Pilot Study. Brain Sci. 2023 Mar 31;13(4):593.
55. Wang R, He M, Ou XF, Xie XQ, Kang Y. Serum procalcitonin level predicts acute kidney injury after traumatic brain injury. World Neurosurg. 2020;141:e112–7.
56. Wang RR, He M, Ou XF, Xie XQ, Kang Y. The predictive value of serum uric acid on acute kidney injury following traumatic brain injury. Biomed Res Int. 2020;2020:2874369.
57. Wang RR, He M, Gui X, Kang Y. A nomogram based on serum cystatin C for predicting acute kidney injury in patients with traumatic brain injury. Ren Fail. 2021;43(1):206–15.
58. Wang R, Wang S, Zhang J, He M, Xu J. Serum Lactate level in early stage is associated with acute kidney injury in traumatic brain injury patients. Front Surg. 2022;8:761166.
59. Xu Y, Zou P, Cao X. Advances in pharmacotherapy for acute kidney injury. Expert Opin Pharmacother. 2022;23(6):713–26.
60. Zhao CC, Ye Y, Li ZQ, Wu XH, Zhao C, Hu ZJ. Effect of goal-directed fluid therapy on renal function in critically ill patients: a systematic review and meta-analysis. Ren Fail. 2022;44(1):777–89.
61. Merck LH, Yeatts SD, Silbergleit R, Manley GT, Pauls Q, Palesch Y, et al. The effect of goal-directed therapy on patient morbidity and mortality after traumatic brain injury: results from the progesterone for the treatment of traumatic brain injury III clinical trial. Crit Care Med. 2019;47(5):623–31.
62. Anetsberger A, Gempt J, Blobner M, Ringel F, Bogdanski R, Heim M, et al. Impact of goal-directed therapy on delayed ischemia after aneurysmal subarachnoid hemorrhage: randomized controlled trial. Stroke. 2020;51(8):2287–96.
63. Vaara ST, Ostermann M, Bitker L, Schneider A, Poli E, Hoste E, et al. REVERSE-AKI study team. Restrictive fluid management versus usual care in acute kidney injury (REVERSE-AKI): a pilot randomized controlled feasibility trial. Intensive Care Med. 2021;47(6):665–73.
64. Martos-Benítez FD, Burgos-Aragüez D, García-Mesa L, Orama-Requejo V, Cárdenas-González RC, Michelena-Piedra JC, Izquierdo-Castañeda J, Sánchez-de-la-Rosa E, Corrales-González O. Fluid balance, biomarkers of renal function and mortality in critically ill patients with AKI diagnosed before, or within 24 h of intensive care unit admission: a prospective study. J Nephrol. 2024 Jan 8. Epub ahead of print.
65. Evans L, Rhodes A, Alhazzani W, Antonelli M, Coopersmith CM, French C, et al. Surviving sepsis campaign: international guidelines for management of sepsis and septic shock 2021. Intensive Care Med. 2021;47(11):1181–247.
66. Cooper DJ, Myburgh J, Heritier S, Finfer S, Bellomo R, Billot L, Murray L, Vallance S, SAFE-TBI Investigators, Australian and New Zealand Intensive Care Society Clinical Trials Group. Albumin resuscitation for traumatic brain injury: is intracranial hypertension the cause of increased mortality? J Neurotrauma. 2013;30(7):512–8.
67. Haines RW, Kirwan CJ, Prowle JR. Managing chloride and bicarbonate in the prevention and treatment of acute kidney injury. Semin Nephrol. 2019;39(5):473–83.
68. Funke BE, Jackson KE, Self WH, Collins SP, Saunders CT, Wang L, et al. SMART Investigators; Pragmatic Critical Care Research Group. Effect of

balanced crystalloids versus saline on urinary biomarkers of acute kidney injury in critically ill adults. BMC Nephrol. 2021;22(1):54.
69. Finfer S, Micallef S, Hammond N, Navarra L, Bellomo R, Billot L, PLUS Study Investigators and the Australian New Zealand Intensive Care Society Clinical Trials Group, et al. Balanced multielectrolyte solution versus saline in critically Ill adults. N Engl J Med. 2022;386(9):815–26.
70. Wang P, Huang Y, Li J, Cao D, Chen B, Chen Z, Li J, Wang R, Liu L. Balanced crystalloid solutions versus normal saline in intensive care units: a systematic review and meta-analysis. Int Urol Nephrol. 2023;
71. Lombardo S, Smith MC, Semler MW, Wang L, Dear ML, Lindsell CJ, Freundlich RE, Guillamondegui OD, Self WH, Rice TW, Isotonic Solutions and Major Adverse Renal Events Trial (SMART) Investigators and Vanderbilt Learning Healthcare System Platform Investigators. Balanced crystalloid versus saline in adults with traumatic brain injury: secondary analysis of a clinical trial. J Neurotrauma. 2022;39(17-18):1159–67.
72. Zampieri FG, Machado FR, Biondi RS, Freitas FGR, Veiga VC, Figueiredo RC, et al. Effect of Intravenous fluid treatment with a balanced solution vs 0.9% saline solution on mortality in critically ill patients: the BaSICS randomized clinical trial. JAMA. 2021;326(9):818–29.
73. De Vlieger G, Meyfroidt G. Kidney dysfunction after traumatic brain injury: pathophysiology and general management. Neurocrit Care. 2023;38(2):504–16.
74. Messina A, Villa F, Lionetti G, Galarza L, Meyfroidt G, van der Jagt M, Monnet X, Pelosi P, Cecconi M, Robba C. Hemodynamic management of acute brain injury caused by cerebrovascular diseases: a survey of the European Society of Intensive Care Medicine. Intensive Care Med Exp. 2022;10(1):42.
75. Toro C, Ohnuma T, Komisarow J, Vavilala MS, Laskowitz DT, James ML, Mathew JP, Hernandez AF, Goldstein BA, Sampson JH, Krishnamoorthy V. Early vasopressor utilization strategies and outcomes in critically Ill patients with severe traumatic brain injury. Anesth Analg. 2022;135(6):1245–52.
76. Toro C, Temkin N, Barber J, Manley G, Jain S, Ohnuma T, Komisarow J, Foreman B, Korley FK, Vavilala MS, Laskowitz DT, Mathew JP, Hernandez A, Sampson J, James ML, Goldstein BA, Markowitz AJ, Krishnamoorthy V, TRACK-TBI Investigators. Association of vasopressor choice with clinical and functional outcomes following moderate to severe traumatic brain injury: A TRACK-TBI Study. Neurocrit Care. 2022;36(1):180–91.
77. Lloyd-Donald P, Spencer W, Cheng J, Romero L, Jithoo R, Udy A, Fitzgerald MC. In adult patients with severe traumatic brain injury, does the use of norepinephrine for augmenting cerebral perfusion pressure improve neurological outcome? A systematic review. Injury. 2020;51(10):2129–34.
78. Khanna AK, Saha AK, Segal S. Association of the exclusive use of intraoperative phenylephrine for treatment of hypotension with the risk of acute kidney injury after noncardiac surgery. Anaesth Crit Care Pain Med. 2023;42(5):101224.
79. Allen CJ, Subhawong TK, Hanna MM, Chelala L, Bullock MR, Schulman CI, Proctor KG. Does vasopressin exacerbate cerebral edema in patients with severe traumatic brain injury? Am Surg. 2018;84(1):43–50.
80. Elgebaly AS, Abd El Ghafar MS, Fathy SM, Shaddad MN. Vasopressin continuous infusion improves intracranial pressure and patient outcomes after surgical clipping or endovascular coiling of cerebral aneurysm. Anesth Essays Res. 2019;13(3):528–34.
81. Huang H, Wu C, Shen Q, Xu H, Fang Y, Mao W. The effect of early vasopressin use on patients with septic shock: a systematic review and meta-analysis. Am J Emerg Med. 2021;48:203–8.
82. Tumlin JA, Murugan R, Deane AM, Ostermann M, Busse LW, Ham KR, et al. Angiotensin II for the Treatment of High-Output Shock 3 (ATHOS-3) Investigators. Outcomes in patients with vasodilatory shock and renal replacement therapy treated with intravenous Angiotensin II. Crit Care Med. 2018;46(6):949–57.
83. Mirzahosseini G, Ismael S, Ahmed HA, Ishrat T. Manifestation of renin angiotensin system modulation in traumatic brain injury. Metab Brain Dis. 2021;36(6):1079–86.
84. Cook AM, Hall K, Kolpek JH, Morbitzer KA, Jordan JD, Rhoney DH. Enhanced renal clearance impacts levetiracetam concentrations in patients with traumatic brain injury with and without augmented renal clearance. BMC Neurol. 2024;24(1):12.
85. Joannidis M, Forni LG, Klein SJ, Honore PM, Kashani K, Ostermann M, et al. Lung-kidney interactions in critically ill patients: consensus report of the Acute Disease Quality Initiative (ADQI) 21 Workgroup. Intensive Care Med. 2020;46(4):654–72.
86. Taran S, Cho SM, Stevens RD. Mechanical ventilation in patients with traumatic brain injury: is it so different? Neurocrit Care. 2023;38(1):178–91.
87. Beqiri E, Smielewski P, Guérin C, Czosnyka M, Robba C, Bjertnæs L, Frisvold SK. Neurological and respiratory effects of lung protective ventilation in acute brain injury patients without lung injury: brain vent, a single centre randomized interventional study. Crit Care. 2023;27(1):115.
88. Aoun M, Sleilaty G, Boueri C, et al. Erythropoietin in Acute Kidney Injury (EAKI): a pragmatic randomized clinical trial. BMC Nephrol. 2022;23:100.
89. Xu Y, Surapaneni A, Alkas J, Evans M, Shin JI, Selvin E, Chang A, Grams ME, Carrero JJ. Glycemic control and the risk of acute kidney injury in patients with Type 2 diabetes and chronic kidney disease: parallel population-based cohort studies in U.S. and Swedish Routine Care. Diabetes Care. 2020;43(12):2975–82.

90. Singer P, Blaser AR, Berger MM, Alhazzani W, Calder PC, Casaer MP, et al. ESPEN guideline on clinical nutrition in the intensive care unit. Clin Nutr. 2019;38(1):48–79.
91. Choi YK, Kim HJ, Ahn J, Ryu JA. Impact of early nutrition and feeding route on clinical outcomes of neurocritically ill patients. PLoS One. 2023;18(3):e0283593.
92. Kim TJ, Park SH, Jeong HB, Ha EJ, Cho WS, Kang HS, Kim JE, Ko SB. Optimizing nitrogen balance is associated with better outcomes in neurocritically Ill patients. Nutrients. 2020;12(10):3137.
93. Gunst J, Vanhorebeek I, Casaer MP, Hermans G, Wouters PJ, Dubois J, Claes K, Schetz M, Van den Berghe G. Impact of early parenteral nutrition on metabolism and kidney injury. J Am Soc Nephrol. 2013;24(6):995–1005.
94. Kato T, Sakai H, Tsujimoto M, Nishimura Y. Prolonged carotid sinus reflex is a risk factor for contrast-induced nephropathy following carotid artery stenting. Am J Neuroradiol 2011;32(3):441–5
95. Lee HG, Kim WK, Yeon JY, et al. Contrast induced acute kidney injury after coil embolization for aneurysmal subarachnoid hemorrhage. Yonsei Med J 2018;59(1):107–112
96. Kim H, Jo K. Laboratory Predictors of Contrast-Induced Nephropathy After Neurointervention: A Prospective 3-Year Observational Study. World Neurosurg. 2020 Mar;135:e77-e82
97. Zhong J, Chen L, Xing Y, et al. Just give the contrast? Appraisal of guidelines on intravenous iodinated contrast media use in patients with kidney disease. Insights Imaging. 2024;15(1):77
98. https://www.acr.org/-/media/ACR/Files/Clinical-Resources/Contrast_Media.pdf. Accessed 20.04.2024.
99. Lareyre F, Raffort J. Biomarkers of contrast-induced nephropathy after non-cardiac vascular procedures: an underexplored area. Angiology 2022; 73(3): 193-4
100. Partovi S, Trischman T, Kang PS. Lessons learned from the PRESERVE trial. Br J Radiol. 2018 Jul;91(1087):20180092.
101. Yan P, Duan SB, Luo XQ, Zhang NY, Deng YH. Effects of intravenous hydration in preventing post-contrast acute kidney injury in patients with eGFR<30 ml/min/1.73m2. Eur Radiol. 2023;33(12):9434-43.
102. Amin AP, Prasad A, Ryan MP, Gunnarsson C, Brilakis ES. Association of iso-osmolar vs low-osmolar contrast media with major adverse renal or cardiovascular events in patients at high risk for acute kidney injury undergoing endovascular abdominal aortic aneurysm repair. J Invasive Cardiol 2021; 33(8): E640-E646
103. Prasad A, Amin AP, Ryan MP, Gunnarsson C, Brilakis ES. Use of iso-osmolar contrast media during endovascular revascularization is associated with a lower incidence of major adverse renal, cardiac, or limb events. Catheter Cardiovasc Interv 2022; 99(4): 1335-42
104. Attari H, Cao Y, Elmholdt TR, Zhao Y, Prince MR. A systematic review of 639 patients with biopsy-confirmed nephrogenic systemic fibrosis. Radiology. 2019;292(2):376–86.
105. Weinreb JC, Rodby RA, Yee J, Wang CL, Fine D, McDonald RJ, Perazella MA, Dillman JR, Davenport MS. Use of intravenous gadolinium-based contrast media in patients with kidney disease: consensus statements from the American College of Radiology and the National Kidney Foundation. Radiology. 2021;298(1):28–35.
106. Gaudry S, Grolleau F, Barbar S, Martin-Lefevre L, Pons B, Boulet É, et al. Continuous renal replacement therapy versus intermittent hemodialysis as first modality for renal replacement therapy in severe acute kidney injury: a secondary analysis of AKIKI and IDEAL-ICU studies. Crit Care. 2022;26(1):1–10.
107. Osgood M, Muehlschlegel S. POINT: Should continuous venovenous hemofiltration always be the preferred mode of renal replacement therapy for the patient with acute brain injury? Yes. Chest. 2017;152:1109–11.
108. Wu VC, Huang TM, Shiao CC, Lai CF, Tsai PR, Wang WJ, et al. The hemodynamic effects during sustained low-efficiency dialysis versus continuous veno-venous hemofiltration for uremic patients with brain hemorrhage: a crossover study. J Neurosurg. 2013;119(5):1288–95.
109. Lund A, Damholt MB, Wiis J, Kelsen J, Strange DG, Møller K. Intracranial pressure during hemodialysis in patients with acute brain injury. Acta Anaesthesiol Scand. 2019;63(4):493–9.
110. Parsons AD, Sanscrainte C, Leone A, Griepp DW, Rahme R. Dialysis disequilibrium syndrome and intracranial pressure fluctuations in neurosurgical patients undergoing renal replacement therapy: systematic review and pooled analysis. World Neurosurg. 2023;170:2–6.
111. STARRT-AKI Investigators, Canadian Critical Care Trials Group, Australian and New Zealand Intensive Care Society Clinical Trials Group, United Kingdom Critical Care Research Group, Canadian Nephrology Trials Network, Irish Critical Care Trials Group, Bagshaw SM, Wald R, Adhikari NKJ, Bellomo R, da Costa BR, Dreyfuss D, et al. Timing of initiation of renal-replacement therapy in acute kidney injury. N Engl J Med. 2020;383(3):240–51.
112. Gaudry S, Hajage D, Martin-Lefevre L, Lebbah S, Louis G, Moschietto S, et al. Comparison of two delayed strategies for renal replacement therapy initiation for severe acute kidney injury (AKIKI 2): a multicentre, open-label, randomised, controlled trial. Lancet. 2021;397(10281):1293–300.
113. Sodhi K, Phillips A, Mishra RC, Tyagi N, Dixit SB, Chaudhary D, et al. Renal replacement therapy practices in India: a nationwide survey. Indian J Crit Care Med. 2020;24(9):823–31.

114. Zhang W, Bai M, Yu Y, Chen X, Zhao L, Chen X. Continuous renal replacement therapy without anticoagulation in critically ill patients at high risk of bleeding: a systematic review and meta-analysis. Semin Dial. 2021;34(3):196–208.
115. Ghoshal S, Parikh A. Dialysis-associated neurovascular injury (DANI) in acute brain injury: practical considerations for intermittent dialysis in the neuro-ICU. Clin J Am Soc Nephrol. 2021;16(7):1110–2.
116. Gupta N, Aggarwal S, Singhal V. Neuroanesthesia and coexisting renal problems. In: Prabhakar H, Singhal V, Gupta N, editors. Co-existing diseases and neuroanesthesia. Springer; 2019.
117. Lynch KE, Ghassemi F, Flythe JE, Feng M, Ghassemi M, Celi LA, Brunelli SM. Sodium modelling to reduce intradialytic hypotension during haemodialysis for acute kidney injury in the intensive care unit. Nephrology (Carlton). 2016;21(10):870–7.
118. Mc Causland FR, Claggett B, Sabbisetti VS, Jarolim P, Waikar SS. Hypertonic mannitol for the prevention of intradialytic hypotension: a randomized controlled trial. Am J Kidney Dis. 2019;74(4):483–90.
119. Hong CS, Wang K, Falcone GJ. The CSF diversion via lumbar drainage to treat dialysis disequilibrium syndrome in the critically Ill neurological patient. Neurocrit Care. 2020;33(1):312–6.
120. Peng C, Yang F, Li L, Peng L, Yu J, Wang P, Jin Z. A machine learning approach for the prediction of severe acute kidney injury following traumatic brain injury. Neurocrit Care. 2023;38(2):335–44.
121. Bajaj T, Koyner JL. Artificial intelligence in acute kidney injury prediction. Adv Chronic Kidney Dis. 2022;29(5):450–60.
122. de Boer IH, Alpers CE, Azeloglu EU, Balis UGJ, Barasch JM, Barisoni L, Kidney Precision Medicine Project, et al. Rationale and design of the Kidney Precision Medicine Project. Kidney Int. 2021;99(3):498–510.

31 Endocrine Dysfunction in Acute Brain Injury

Katarzyna Prus, Başak Akça, and Federico Bilotta

31.1 Introduction

Endocrine dysfunction is a common event among patients presenting with acute brain injury (ABI) [1]. In the course of traumatic brain injury (TBI), subarachnoid hemorrhage (SAH), intracranial hemorrhage (ICH), or acute ischemic stroke (AIS), various mechanisms can cause disruptions to multiple neuroendocrine axes [2].

In the course of ABI, patients may demonstrate severe disruptions to the hypothalamus, pituitary, and peripheral endocrine glands. Symptoms may be nonspecific and remain unidentified in comatose or mechanically ventilated patients [3]. Endocrine dysfunctions may significantly impact patients' recovery; therefore, a proper diagnostic and therapeutic approach is essential for an improved future outcome.

This chapter will report basic elements of the physiology of the brain–endocrine axis, characteristics of neuroendocrine dysfunction following ABI, and clinical aspects of these disorders, which are essential in neurocritical patient management.

K. Prus
Department of Neurology,
Medical University of Lublin, Lubin, Poland

B. Akça
Department of Anesthesiology and Reanimation,
Hacettepe University, Ankara, Turkey

F. Bilotta (✉)
Department of Anesthesiology,
Intensive Care and Pain Management, "Sapienza"
University of Rome, Rome, Italy
e-mail: federico.bilotta@uniroma1.it

31.2 Physiology of the Brain–Endocrine Axis

Neurons, endocrine cells, as well as non-endocrine tissues producing neurotransmitters and hormones form the neuroendocrine system. The hypothalamus, pituitary gland, and its connections to the extra hypothalamic regions compose a complex net of axes, which regulate human physiological and behavioral states (Table 31.1).

The hypothalamic–pituitary–adrenal axis (HPA) is responsible for the regulation of multiple physiological processes including stress and immune response, energy metabolism, autonomic nervous system, and neuropsychiatric function. The key elements of HPA are the paraventricular nucleus of the hypothalamus, the anterior lobe of the pituitary gland, and the adrenal cortex. Disruptions to the HPA axis can result in acute complications as well as chronic alterations in neurotransmission throughout the central nervous system and hormonal synthesis in the periphery [4].

The hypothalamic–neurohypophyseal system consists of the paraventricular nucleus and supraoptic nucleus of the thalamus, the posterior part

H. Prabhakar et al. (eds.), *Principles and Practice of Neurocritical Care*,
https://doi.org/10.1007/978-981-99-8059-8_31

of the pituitary gland, and a collection of axonal projections [5]. Its main function is associated with the secretion of oxytocin and vasopressin into the systemic circulation. Posterior pituitary hormones are responsible for reproductive functions and social bonding as well as regulation of water balance and blood pressure.

Hypothalamic–pituitary–gonadal axis (HPG) is the system connecting the hypothalamus, the anterior part of the pituitary, and the gonads. Its function is essential in the development process as well as the regulation of reproductive and immune systems [6].

The hypothalamic–pituitary–thyroid axis (HPT) consists of the connections between the hypothalamus, pituitary, and thyroid. Its function is associated with metabolism and stress response regulation [7].

The pineal gland is responsible for sleep modulation and both circadian and seasonal cycle control. It is located in the epithalamus, and it is one of the brain circumventricular organs with a profuse blood flow and highly permeable capillaries [8].

All of the elements of the neuroendocrine system may be affected in the course of ABI resulting in acute systemic complications as well as delayed, chronic dysfunctions.

31.3 Endocrine Dysfunction in Traumatic Brain Injury

Traumatic brain injury with all its consequences remains the major cause of mortality and morbidity in the younger population [9]. Advances in the management of TBI in neuro-intensive care units provided improved survival rates with a higher demand for prolonged treatment and rehabilitation [10].

Endocrine dysfunctions following TBI may strongly affect patients' future prognosis, functional outcome, and quality of life (QoL) [1]. Research states that one-third of patients with blunt traumatic brain injury will eventually develop at least one type of anterior pituitary dysfunction [11]. The epidemiological data regarding posterior pituitary disorders in the course of TBI are inconsistent and range between 2.9 and 51%, depending on the type of testing and cut-off values [12, 13]. A strong correlation is reported between subacute HPA suppression and poor prognosis after TBI [14].

Several mechanisms are proposed as a possible cause of endocrine pathologies following TBI. The most widely reported are increased intracranial pressure (ICP) related to brain edema, shearing force applied to intracranial structures due to high-energy trauma, and consequences of hypoxia [15]. It has been suggested that autoimmunity also may play a significant role in the process, especially during the subacute and chronic phases. Higher rates of post-traumatic endocrine dysfunction have been described in patients positive for anti-hypothalamic and anti-pituitary antibodies in a follow-up period of 5 years. Another major contributor to post-injury impairment is maladaptive neuroinflammation with a central role in microglia [16]. Chronic microglial-mediated inflammation has been proven to contribute to motor deficits, cognitive disorders, and neurodegeneration in numerous experimental TBI models [17, 18]. Another point is that microglia may remain reactive years after brain injury, which correlates with slower cognitive processing and poor functional outcome [19].

Symptoms of endocrine disorders can differ depending on the phase of the disease. Acute pituitary dysfunction might result in adrenal insufficiency (AI) or diabetes insipidus (DI), which can cause hemodynamic instability and transient derangements in fluid balance. In some cases, however, a permanent anterior pituitary dysfunction may last throughout the chronic period causing long-term complications [9].

The symptoms associated with dysfunction of the HPA axis after TBI are especially significant, due to its regulative function in the secretion of glucocorticoids (GCs), insulin, and growth hormone (GH) [20]. Under standard conditions, the cortisol level in trauma survivors is expected to increase immediately, as a result of stress, with a further gradual decline to normal within the next few days [21]. Glucocorticoid levels are correlated positively with the severity of the injury. Abnormally low levels of cortisol indicate an interrupted functioning of the HPA axis, associated with the high risk of developing AI and its possible catastrophic consequences. This complication is most common during the acute phase, and data regarding AI in TBI patients suggest that a predominance of patients recover soon after [22]. Clinical presentation of AI, especially during the acute phase of TBI, may be blurred by the overall critical state of the TBI patients as well as overlapping complications, such as cardiac dysfunction or sepsis. Early diagnosis is often difficult but crucial for proper therapeutic management.

Suppression of the hypothalamic–pituitary–gonadal axis is an adaptive response of the organism against stressors [22]. There seems to be a significant positive correlation between acute serum testosterone levels and GCS scores on admission, indicating a strong correlation with the severity of brain trauma [23]. Another factor that can cause gonadal suppression, both in the acute and chronic phases of TBI, is hyperprolactinemia [23, 24]. However, the typical symptoms of hypogonadism such as amenorrhoea in women or erectile dysfunction in men are usually diagnosed in the late phase and do not significantly affect management in the critical period.

TBI is one of the main causes of posterior pituitary dysfunction; therefore, the management of dysnatremias should be a part of the "immediate routine" protocols in TBI [9]. Acute traumatic injury may cause harm to the hypothalamic neurons secreting anti-diuretic hormone (ADH) or posterior pituitary cells resulting in DI. Sodium level alterations occur more often in the acute phase of TBI and rarely persist into the chronic period [11]. The type of dysnatremia may depend on the site of the injury. Data state that lesions affecting the hypothalamus are more often associated with DI or inappropriate secretion of antidiuretic hormone (SIADH) [22]. The most common electrolyte disturbance following TBI is hyponatremia (Na $<$135 mEq/lt). Both retrospective and prospective studies indicate that 10–15% of patients will develop severe hyponatremia (Na$<$ 130 mEq/lt) in the course of TBI [12, 13].

DI is seen mostly during the acute phase of TBI [13], and it affects between 21.6 and 26% of patients. The first clinical symptom is polyuria, with subsequent hypovolemia and hypernatremia. It occurs because of inappropriate fluid intake and decompensation of the fluid balance since most of the TBI survivors can not express thirst, due to neurologic impairment [12]. When suspecting DI, it is necessary to exclude other possible iatrogenic causes of hypernatremia such as excessive administration of hyperosmolar solutions or forced diuresis, as soon as possible [25].

Growth hormone deficiency (GHD) is one of the most frequently diagnosed endocrine dysfunctions after TBI [24]. In the course of moderate and severe trauma, 15–20% of the survivors experience severe GHD [26]. GH is essential for maintaining a proper lipid profile and glucose metabolism and plays a major role in neuroplasticity [27]. GHD is a relevant factor of cognitive impairment following TBI, especially affecting deficits in attention and memory [28]. Research state that patients with GHD exhibit decreased level of cerebral glucose metabolism in cortical areas associated with intellectual function and memory [29].

Hypothyroidism due to brain trauma and steroid use during trauma treatment is another common neuroendocrine dysfunction reported in this group of patients. A prevalence rate of 7% was revealed in a meta-analysis among the adults following TBI [30]. Symptoms associated with hypothyroidism are common but not specific. Asthenia, cognitive impairment, and lethargy may be an indication for further diagnostics. Hypothyroidism might also affect information processing and short-term memory during the chronic phase [9].

Identifying post-traumatic hypopituitarism (PTHP) is crucial both in the acute and chronic phases, in order to ensure the proper management of a possible catastrophic situation in a timely manner. Most of the hormonal fluctuations appear to be an acute adaptive response to high-energy trauma and, therefore, are predominantly of a transient character [23].

In case of suspected AI, it is advised to perform a serial assessment of morning cortisol levels. Results below 300 nmol/l indicate a high probability of acute adrenocorticotropic hormone

(ACTH) deficiency and the need for glucocorticoid substitution. Symptoms suggestive of AI may include hypoglycemia, low sodium level, hypotension, or unexpected slow recovery [26].

In the presence of symptomatic cranial DI (hypernatremia and hypotonic polyuria) or SIADH (euvolemic hyponatremia), hormonal blood tests should be performed with the consideration of hormone replacement (Table 31.2).

There is no confirmed indication to treat acute GH, thyroid, or gonadotropic hormone deficiencies during the acute phase of TBI. Interpretation of the results during this period remains difficult, and there is no need for early assessment of these hormonal axes. The diagnostics of the acute pituitary dysfunction should, therefore, be focused on ACTH deficiency, due to its association with morbidity and mortality in TBI patients. In acute settings, dynamic tests can turn out inappropriate or unreliable.

Patients with mild TBI should be clinically evaluated for endocrine dysfunction, but there is no indication for routine screening for pituitary dysfunction unless symptoms of hypopituitarism are present. Features increasing the risk of PTHP are basal skull fracture, advanced age, diffuse axonal injury, and prolonged stay in the ICU [28].

Screening for PTHP in patients who experienced moderate to severe TBI at 3–6 months is highly recommended [31]. Testing should include renal-thyroid function, cortisol, and gonadal hormone assessment. If any abnormality is detected, the patient should be referred to an endocrinologist for further diagnostics. Healthcare providers should be aware of the possibility of PTHP in TBI patients and plan follow-up visits accordingly. If hormonal deficiency is confirmed, a replacement therapy should be implemented with reassessment at 12 months.

31.4 Endocrine Dysfunction Following Acute Stroke

Research states that patients after ischemic and hemorrhagic stroke have a significantly increased risk of developing endocrine dysfunctions [32]. Hormonal alterations in the course of stroke can present as metabolic, immune, cognitive, and behavioral disorders and may severely impact the future outcome of stroke patients.

Neuroendocrine changes following AIS and ICH may represent both adaptive and deleterious functions. They are predominantly based on activation of the HPA axis and excessive sympathetic response. Researchers suggest that alterations of the HPA function, increased levels of catecholamines and natriuretic peptides, as well as low insulin growth factor (IGF-1) and melatonin concentration, are strongly associated with future prognosis in stroke patients [33].

Epidemiology data reveal that anterior pituitary deficiency may occur in 19% of patients after AIS [34]. Secondary AI is reported as the most clinically significant hormonal disorder and has been identified in up to 31% of stroke cases [35]. Approximately, 12% of AIS survivors may exhibit GH deficiency, and only a small group is affected by gonadal axis alterations.

Extensive brain ischemia strongly affects neuroendocrine and immune homeostasis [32]. During the acute phase of stroke, disorders in pituitary hormone secretion might be a part of the adaptive response to brain injury. Immunosuppression mediated by GCs is an attempt to limit the overwhelming inflammation in the brain tissue and reduce the autoimmune reactions against neuroantigens [36]. Hyperactivation of the HPA axis stimulates adrenal glands while enhancing brain damage and causing systemic complications. It was proven that stroke patients with high cortisol levels are prone to acute cardiac sequelae, such as severe arrhythmias, myocardial ischemia, or myogenic fibrous degeneration [37]. Furthermore, a cortisol level surge is associated with an elevated post-stroke infection rate, which results in higher mortality and worse functional outcomes [38].

Hyper-activation of the HPA axis may have additional long-term consequences. It has been associated with delayed cognitive and behavioral impairment [39]. Increased HPA activity results in altered expression of GC receptors. This may lead to functional and morphological changes in stress-sensitive areas of the CNS, such as the limbic system and hippocampus [40]. The

Development of post-stroke depressive disorder (PSDD) is probably associated with chronic inflammation and hyper-activation of the sympathoadrenal medullary system. Researchers suggest that cortisol and pro-inflammatory cytokines surge following stroke plays an essential role in the pathogenesis of PSDD. Patients presenting high cortisol levels following stroke should be monitored for cognitive impairment and mood disorders

Insufficient GH secretion results in low IGF-I levels, which are confirmed to be associated with worse neurological outcomes and high mortality in stroke patients. GHD triggers dyslipidemia and alterations in glycemic control, which can add up to overall metabolic dysfunctions following stroke. Data suggest that IGF-I levels increase during rehabilitation treatment, which may indicate its potential neuroprotective role [41].

Hyperglycemia is a common disorder in the course of AIS and ICH as well as in non-diabetics [42]. It is estimated that around 30% of patients with no previous history of diabetes can present with hyperglycemia during the acute period. Impaired glucose metabolism results most probably from extensive sympathetic signaling, which reduces insulin release from the pancreas. It can be associated with an acute stress response and reflects an underlying diabetes. In a large group of stroke patients, hyperglycemia may continue into the chronic period and result in the final diagnosis of diabetes mellitus (DM). Hyperglycemia is correlated with a larger size of the ischemic lesion and results in worse functional outcomes. It was proven that post-load hyperglycemia—an indicator of abnormal glucose metabolism—may additionally be a risk factor for cardiovascular complications in the course of stroke [43].

In more than half of AIS patients, triiodothyronine (T3) decreases immediately after onset, irrespective of pre-existing thyroid dysfunctions. Research proved that low levels of T3 and the presence of thyroid autoantibodies are an indicator of poor functional outcomes after IS [37]. It was also confirmed that patients with hypothyroidism are less likely to achieve favorable outcomes in NIHSS as well as mRS measures [42]. Thyroid disorders may be caused by enhanced inflammatory response and GCs hyperstimulation. Low level of T3 with TSH in the normal range usually reflects dysfunction of the HPT axis with inhibition of thyroxine to T3 conversion due to acute stress [44].

There is information on the disruptive impact of AIS on the production of melatonin and circadian rhythms, even when ischemic lesions do not directly affect the pineal gland [37]. Stroke causes immediate changes in melatonin secretion, including its timing and rhythm [42]. Furthermore, disturbances to melatonin secretion might be important considering its neuroprotective, anti-inflammatory, and anti-oxidative role [45]. Despite recent encouraging results of clinical trials on the potential therapeutic effect of melatonin in stroke, no treatment recommendations were made in this area.

Findings suggest that alterations in hypothalamic ADH secretion following stroke may affect the severity and outcome of the cerebral injury. At present, only a limited amount of studies on ADH in stroke patients have been carried out [46]. Water balance and sodium level disorders may have a severe impact on stroke patient recovery. They may present as the syndrome of SIADH, cerebral salt wasting (CSW), and DI [47].

Recent research confirms that CSW is the most common cause of hyponatremia in stroke patients, whereas only a small percentage of cases can be attributed to SIADH [37]. Correct diagnosis of the exact source of water balance and electrolyte disorders is crucial for further treatment decisions, as the therapeutic strategies for CSW, SIADH, and DI differ significantly [35].

Immediate management of pituitary deficiency in AIS is mainly supportive. The most urgent intervention is needed in the case of ACTH deficiency, due to possible acute AI and cardiovascular collapse. In the case of suspected HPA axis insufficiency, basal morning cortisol should be tested at all times, especially, when clinical symptoms of AI are present. Hydrocortisone replacement should be administered immediately in hemodynamically unstable patients [42]. There are no specified recommendations for strict monitoring, routine diagnostics, and treatment of other pituitary axes. Specific laboratory tests should be based on observed symptoms (Table 31.2).

Guidelines for the management of AIS patients recommend maintaining blood glucose concentration (BGC) between 140 and 180 mg/dL, especially in the first 24 h after the onset [48]. That usually involves intensive insulin therapy and close monitoring of BGC. Randomized trials (SHINE), however, did not prove that intensive blood glucose control (between 80 and 130 mg/dL) in the acute stroke period is associated with a better prognosis. At the same time, it may pose an elevated risk of hypoglycemia in the course of intensive insulin therapy [49].

Diagnosis of water balance and sodium level disorders can be difficult in sedated, neurocritical patients receiving intravenous fluid therapy. Urine volume exceeding 3 l/day without glycosuria should suggest the possible diagnosis of DI [50].

Thyroid hormone replacement is advised only in cases of confirmed, clinical insufficiency. There are no indications to substitute treatment in patients demonstrating isolated TSH level increase [51].

31.5 Endocrine Dysfunction in Aneurysmal SAH

Neuroendocrine dysfunctions may cause metabolic disturbances during the acute and subacute periods of aSAH [52] as well as contribute to decreased cognition and low QoL following the event. Hypopituitarism after SAH may affect at least one of the hormonal axis in around 55% of patients [53].

Endocrine disturbances may be caused by aneurysm-induced direct gland compression, ischemia during the acute phase, increased ICP, or intervention-related injuries [54]. Autopsy findings in SAH patients revealed ischemic necrosis as well as hemorrhagic transformation in the hypothalamus, probably secondary to the obstructed venous drainage. The presence of extravasated blood is also a trigger for a pro-inflammatory cascade, which results in various complications.

AI and water balance disorders are the most common endocrine complications following aSAH. Hormonal disorders manifesting during the acute phase of SAH need special attention, due to possible devastating consequences.

Hypocortisolemia following aSAH is common, especially during the acute phase. It may lead to severe, immediate complications and, therefore, increase mortality rates [55]. During the acute period, diagnosis of adrenal insufficiency is critical. Due to direct life risk, aSAH patients should be routinely evaluated for signs and symptoms of hypocortisolism such as hyponatremia, hypotension, and hypoglycemia (Table 31.2). Daily serum cortisol assessment is advised in the first days after the onset [56]. It is important to notice that total serum cortisol levels can be affected by accompanying chronic diseases, medications, and acute complications (e.g., respiratory failure or sepsis). Therefore, defining a cortisol cut-off value diagnostic for AI in the course, one SAH may pose a challenge. At the same time, empirical GC administration without confirmed acute HPA dysfunction may be ineffective or even harmful [57]. Low levels of cortisol may also result in chronic complications. Hypocortisolemia was proven to be associated with a high risk of depressive disorders and lower QoL scores in SAH survivors.

Hypothalamic–pituitary and adrenal dysfunction following SAH have also been correlated with poor neurological outcomes and increased mortality. A surge in catecholamine levels in the hyper-acute phase of aSAH is reported to be associated with a higher complication rate; however, the data are not consistent [52]. Research states that long-term dysregulation of neurohormonal axes may develop; nevertheless, it appears to be less frequent than in the acute phase.

Sodium level disturbances strongly affect a patient's neurologic state and functional outcome. Hyponatremia is a common complication following aSAH present in around 30% of patients [58]. Mechanisms responsible for low sodium levels are mostly related to SIADH and CSW. Hyponatremia was proved to be associated with longer hospitalization but not with higher mortality [59]. Hypernatremia, on the other hand, appears to be more predictive of worse outcomes [60]. Its cause in the course of aSAH is usually iatrogenic—due to the widespread use of mannitol and hypertonic saline. It may also result from secondary pituitary–hypothalamic ischemia resulting in DI with hypertonic hypovolemia and excessive diuresis [1].

Deficiencies in other hypopituitary axes do not play a significant role in the acute period following SAH. Furthermore, since there is no evidence for improved outcomes of the treatment of gonadal, somatotropin, and thyroid axes disorders in the acute phase of aSAH, hormonal assessment in these areas is not recommended. At the same time it is worth noticing that in the chronic period, GH deficiency contributes to low QoL and late cognitive complications. Typical symptoms of GH deficiency may include fatigue, attention impairment, and memory problems [61]. Somatotrophs are the predominant pituitary cells and, together with gonadotrophs, remain most vulnerable to SAH consequences. Some researchers claim that the somatotropic axis is the one most affected during post-SAH hypophysial deficiency, and this fact may be associated with pituitary gland volume loss. During the chronic period, clinical symptoms suggesting hypopituitarism (impaired sexual function, oligomenorrhea/amenorrhea, weight loss, hyponatremia, hypotension, hypo-and hyperglycemia, or polydipsia) should imply further diagnostics [52]. An endocrine follow-up is advised up to 1 year following aSAH to assess less common, new-onset dysfunctions.

31.6 Summary

- Monitoring for endocrine dysfunction and timely hormonal replacement may be lifesaving in ABI patients.
- Assessment of neuroendocrine function in the acute period of ABI is critical, especially in patients demonstrating symptoms of adrenal crisis or severe fluid balance and electrolyte disorders.
- Symptoms of other hormonal disorders (GHD, hypothyroidism, gonadal axis dysfunction) are usually late-onset complications; however, their presence can strongly affect patients' QoL and future outcomes.
- Follow-up assessment on 3, 6, and 12 months from the onset should be considered in selected ABI patients demonstrating endocrine deficiency symptoms. In case of inappropriate laboratory results of basic hormonal tests, endocrinologist referral is advised.
- Current research concentrates on the prognostic value of endocrine disorders. Specific recommendations for diagnostic and therapeutic work-up designed for ABI patients are still missing.

Appendix

Table 31.1 Symptoms of hypophyseal hormonal deficiencies

Deficient hormone	Symptoms
GH	• Decreased muscle mass and muscle strength • Visceral obesity • Fatigue • Impaired cognitive functions • Atherosclerosis • Dyslipidemia • Decrease in quality of life
Gonadotropins	• Libido loss, impaired sexual function, infertility • Women: Oligo-amenorrhea • Men: Loss of pubic/ truncal hair • Weight changes • Decreased muscle mass • Osteoporosis
ACTH	• Acute phase; circulatory collapse, fever, shock, weakness • Chronic phase: Fatigue, anorexia, weight loss, hyponatremia, hypotension, hypoglycemia
TSH	• Cognitive impairment • Newly onset arrhythmias • Hypotension • Fatigue • Hair loss, dry skin, cold intolerance • Weight gain
ADH	• Polydipsia • Polyuria • Decreased urine osmolality • Hypernatremia

GH growth hormone, *ACTH* adrenocorticotropic hormone, *TSH* thyrotropic hormone, *ADH* anti-diuretic hormone

Table 31.2 Diagnostic and therapeutic work-up in ABI patients

Hormonal deficiency type	Symptoms	Diagnostics	Indication for treatment	Treatment strategy
AI Acute phase	• Circulatory collapse • Fever • Shock • Weakness • Hypotension • Hypoglycemia • Hyponatremia	Early morning cortisol serum level assessment Stimulation tests are not advised during the acute stage	• Morning cortisol <200 nmol/l • 200–500 nmol/l in the presence of features suggestive of adrenal insufficiency	In case of adrenal crisis: • 100 mg HC bolus • 200 mg/day continuous iv infusion or iv boli (50 mg every 6 h) • 1000 mL 0.9%NaCl in the first hour • Clinical assessment, CVP, IBP monitoring

Table 31.2 (continued)

Hormonal deficiency type	Symptoms	Diagnostics	Indication for treatment	Treatment strategy
AI Chronic phase	• Fatigue • Anorexia • Weight loss • Hypotension • Hypoglycemia • Hyponatremia	Referral to endocrinologist Basal cortisol level ACTH stimulation Test Glucagon stimulation test (GST)	• Basal cortisol level > 18 μg/dL is accepted as normal and < 3 μg/ dL as abnormal. Between these levels, dynamic assessment is required • Low dose (1 μg) ACTH test is a sensitive test and a peak cortisol level < 18 μg/dL is accepted as insufficient	• 15–20 mg/day of hydrocortisone (tailored to patients age and body weight)
GHD	• Fatigue • Low energy level • Decline in cognitive function	Serum IGF-1 Glucagon stimulation test (GST) Insulin tolerance test (ITT)	A peak GH level ≤ 3 μg/L during ITT or ≤ 1.1 μg/L during GST are accepted as GHD	• GH replacement may be considered in selected patients
Glycemic disorders	• Hyperglycemia • Hypoglycemia • High infection rate	BGC FBG GTT HbA1C	Blood glucose >180 mg/dL	• BGC target of 140–180 mg/dL • Subcutaneous insulin / IV insulin infusion protocol
CSW	• Hypovolemic hyponatremia • Hypotension • High HR • More common in stroke patients than SIADH	Plasma and urine osmolarity Spot urinary sodium	• Plasma osmolarity <270 mOsm/kg • Urine osmolarity >100 mOsm/kg • Pot urinary sodium >> > 30 mmol/l • Low CVP • Elevated BNP?	• IV fluids administration sodium supplementation, normal saline • Fludrocortisone
SIADH	• Euvolemic hyponatremia in the absence of GCs deficiency and hypothyroidism	Plasma and urine osmolarity Spot urinary sodium	• Plasma osmolarity <270 mOsm/kg • Urine osmolarity >100 mOsm/kg • Spot urinary sodium >40 mmol/L	• Fluid restriction, hypertonic saline (0.25–0.5 mL/kg per hour), or urea (second line) • Tolvaptan
DI	• Polyuria • Dilute urine • Increased thirst • Hypovolemia • Dehydration • Electrolyte imbalances	• Urine osmolarity and urine output assessment	• > 3 L of dilute urine (<300 mOsm/kg) in 24 h (>50 mL/kg) • Plasma sodium >145 mmol/L	• Adequate fluid replacement + ADH analog (desmopressin) • Dosing should be adjusted due to hourly urine output and plasma sodium level

(continued)

Table 31.2 (continued)

Hormonal deficiency type	Symptoms	Diagnostics	Indication for treatment	Treatment strategy
Thyroid disorders	• Hypotension • Newly onset arrhythmias • Fatigue • Cognitive impairment • lethargy	TSH FT3 FT4	• Combination of freeT4, T3, and TSH levels is adequate for the evaluation of the integrity of thyroid axis • Low free T4 in the presence of inappropriately normal or low TSH should be accepted as secondary hypothyroidism	• subclinical hypothyroidism was proven to have a neuroprotective role and does not need supplementation

AI adrenal insufficiency, *CVP* central venous pressure, *IBP* invasive blood pressure, *HC* hydrocortisone *GHD* growth hormone deficiency, *GH* growth hormone, *BGC* blood glucose concentration, *FBG* fasting blood glucose, *HbA1C*—glycated hemoglobin, *CSW* cerebral salt wasting, *SIADH*—inappropriate secretion of antidiuretic hormone, *DI* diabetes inisipidus, *TSH* thyrotropic hormone, *T3* triiodothyronine, *T4* thyroxine.

References

1. Garrahy A, Sherlock M, Thompson CJ. Management of endocrine disease: neuroendocrine surveillance and management of neurosurgical patients. Eur J Endocrinol. 2017;176(5):217–33.
2. Scranton RA, Baskin DS. Impaired pituitary axes following traumatic brain injury. J Clin Med. 2015;4(7):1463–79.
3. Mahajan C, Prabhakar H, Bilotta F. Endocrine dysfunction after traumatic brain injury: an ignored clinical syndrome? Neurocrit Care. 2023;10:1007.
4. Sheng JA, Bales NJ, Myers SA, et al. The hypothalamic-pituitary-adrenal axis: development, programming actions of hormones, and maternal-fetal interactions. Front Behav Neurosci. 2021;14:601939.
5. Malenka RC, Nestler EJ, Hyman SE. Chapter 5: excitatory and inhibitory amino acids. In: Sydor A, Brown RY, editors. Molecular neuropharmacology: a foundation for clinical neuroscience. 2nd ed. New York: McGraw-Hill Medical; 2009. pp. 246, 248–259.
6. Charlton H. Hypothalamic control of anterior pituitary function: a history. J Neuroendocrinol. 2008;20(6):641–6.
7. Dietrich JW, Landgrafe G, Fotiadou EH. TSH and thyrotropic agonists: key actors in thyroid homeostasis. J Thyroid Res. 2012;2012:351864.
8. Gross PM, Weindl A. Peering through the windows of the brain. J Cereb Blood Flow Metab. 1987;7(6):663–72.
9. Caputo M, Mele C, Prodam F, Marzullo P, Aimaretti G. Clinical picture and the treatment of TBI-induced hypopituitarism. Pituitary. 2019;22(3):261–9.
10. Ma VY, Chan L, Carruthers KJ. Incidence, prevalence, costs, and impact on disability of common conditions requiring rehabilitation in the United States: stroke, spinal cord injury, traumatic brain injury, multiple sclerosis, osteoarthritis, rheumatoid arthritis, limb loss, and back pain. Arch Phys Med Rehabil. 2014;95(5):986–95.
11. Lauzier F, Turgeon AF, Boutin A, et al. Clinical outcomes, predictors, and prevalence of anterior pituitary disorders following traumatic brain injury: a systematic review. Crit Care Med. 2014;42(3):712–21.
12. Agha A, Thornton E, O'Kelly P, Tormey W, Phillips J, Thompson CJ. Posterior pituitary dysfunction after traumatic brain injury. J Clin Endocrinol Metab. 2004;89(12):5987–92.
13. Capatina C, Paluzzi A, Mitchell R, Karavitaki N. Diabetes insipidus after traumatic brain injury. J Clin Med. 2015;4(7):1448–62.
14. Tanriverdi F, De Bellis A, Ulutabanca H, et al. A five year prospective investigation of anterior pituitary function after traumatic brain injury: is hypopituitarism long-term after head trauma associated with autoimmunity? J Neurotrauma. 2013;30(16):1426–33.
15. Yang WH, Chen PC, Wang TC, Kuo TY, Cheng CY, Yang YH. Endocrine dysfunction following traumatic brain injury: a 5-year follow-up nationwide-based study. Sci Rep. 2016;6:32987.
16. DiSabato DJ, Quan N, Godbout JP. Neuroinflammation: the devil is in the details. J Neurochem. 2016;139(2):136–53.
17. Leach JB, Szeto GL, Wu J, Stoica BA, Faden AI, Loane DJ. Microglial depletion with CSF1R inhibitor during chronic phase of experimental traumatic brain injury reduces neurodegeneration and neurological deficits. J Neurosci. 2020;40(14):2960–74.
18. Kokiko-Cochran ON, Saber M, Puntambekar S, et al. Traumatic brain injury in hTau model mice: enhanced acute macrophage response and altered long-term recovery. J Neurotrauma. 2018;35(1):73–84.

19. Johnson VE, Stewart JE, Begbie FD, Trojanowski JQ, Smith DH, Stewart W. Inflammation and white matter degeneration persist for years after a single traumatic brain injury. Brain. 2013;136(1):28–42.
20. Tapp ZM, Godbout JP, Kokiko-Cochran ON. A tilted axis: maladaptive inflammation and HPA axis dysfunction contribute to consequences of TBI. Front Neurol. 2019;10:345.
21. Dalwadi PP, Bhagwat NM, Tayde PS, Joshi AS, Varthakavi PK. Pituitary dysfunction in traumatic brain injury: is evaluation in the acute phase worthwhile? Indian J Endocrinol Metab. 2017;21(1):80–4.
22. Hannon MJ, Sherlock M, Thompson CJ. Pituitary dysfunction following traumatic brain injury or subarachnoid haemorrhage—in "endocrine Management in the Intensive Care Unit". Best Pract Res Clin Endocrinol Metab. 2011;25(5):783–98.
23. Agha A, Thompson CJ. High risk of hypogonadism after traumatic brain injury: clinical implications. Pituitary. 2005;8(3–4):245–9.
24. Cuesta M, Hannon MJ, Crowley RK, et al. Symptoms of gonadal dysfunction are more predictive of hypopituitarism than nonspecific symptoms in screening for pituitary dysfunction following moderate or severe traumatic brain injury. Clin Endocrinol. 2016;84(1):92–8.
25. Adrogué HJ, Madias NE. Hypernatremia. N Engl J Med. 2000;342(20):1493–9.
26. Ghigo E, Masel B, Aimaretti G, et al. Consensus guidelines on screening for hypopituitarism following traumatic brain injury. Brain Inj. 2005;19(9):711–24.
27. Gray S, Bilski T, Dieudonne B, Saeed S. Hypopituitarism after traumatic brain injury. Cureus. 2019;11(3):4163.
28. Gilis-Januszewska A, Kluczyński Ł, Hubalewska-Dydejczyk A. Traumatic brain injuries induced pituitary dysfunction: a call for algorithms. Endocr Connect. 2020;9(5):112–23.
29. Park KD, Lim OK, Yoo CJ, et al. Voxel-based statistical analysis of brain metabolism in patients with growth hormone deficiency after traumatic brain injury. Brain Inj. 2016;30(4):407–13.
30. Garmendia Madariaga A, Santos Palacios S, Guillén-Grima F, Galofré JC. The incidence and prevalence of thyroid dysfunction in Europe: a meta-analysis. J Clin Endocrinol Metab. 2014;99(3):923–31.
31. Tan CL, Alavi SA, Baldeweg SE, et al. The screening and management of pituitary dysfunction following traumatic brain injury in adults: British Neurotrauma group guidance. J Neurol Neurosurg Psychiatry. 2017;88(11):971–81.
32. Wang F, Luo MY, Zhou L, et al. Endocrine dysfunction following stroke. J Neuroimmune Pharmacol. 2021;16(2):425–36.
33. El Husseini N, Laskowitz DT. The role of neuroendocrine pathways in prognosis after stroke. Expert Rev Neurother. 2014;14(2):217–32.
34. Bondanelli M, Ambrosio MR, Zatelli MC, Basaglia N, Degli Uberti EC. Prevalence of hypopituitarism in patients with cerebrovascular diseases. J Endocrinol Investig. 2008;31(9):16–20.
35. Robba C, Battaglini D, Samary CS, et al. Ischaemic stroke-induced distal organ damage: pathophysiology and new therapeutic strategies. Intensive Care Med Exp. 2020;8(1):23.
36. Shi K, Wood K, Shi F, et al. Stroke-induced immunosuppression and poststroke infection. Stroke Vasc Neurol. 2018;3(1):34.
37. Neidert S, Katan M, Schuetz P, et al. Anterior pituitary axis hormones and outcome in acute ischaemic stroke. J Intern Med. 2011;269(4):420–32.
38. Barugh AJ, Gray P, Shenkin SD, MacLullich AM, Mead GE. Cortisol levels and the severity and outcomes of acute stroke: a systematic review. J Neurol. 2014;261(3):533–45.
39. Gulyaeva NV, Onufriev MV, Moiseeva YV. Ischemic stroke, glucocorticoids, and remote hippocampal damage: a translational outlook and implications for modeling. Front Neurosci. 2021;15:781964.
40. Zhanina MY, Druzhkova TA, Yakovlev AA, Vladimirova EE, Freiman SV, Eremina NN, Guekht AB, Gulyaeva NV. Development of post-stroke cognitive and depressive disturbances: associations with neurohumoral indices. Curr Issues Mol Biol. 2022;44(12):6290–305.
41. Sanchez-Bezanilla S, Åberg ND, Crock P, et al. Growth hormone promotes motor function after experimental stroke and enhances recovery-promoting mechanisms within the peri-infarct area. Int J Mol Sci. 2020;21(2):606.
42. Balch MHH, Nimjee SM, Rink C, Hannawi Y. Beyond the brain: the systemic pathophysiological response to acute ischemic stroke. J Stroke. 2020;22(2):159–72.
43. Lau LH, Lew J, Borschmann K, Thijs V, Ekinci EI. Prevalence of diabetes and its effects on stroke outcomes: a meta-analysis and literature review. J Diabetes Investig. 2019;10(3):780–92.
44. Zhang Y, Meyer MA. Clinical analysis on alteration of thyroid hormones in the serum of patients with acute ischemic stroke. Stroke Res Treat. 2010;2010:2906784.
45. Sadanandan N, Cozene B, Cho J, Park YJ, Saft M, Gonzales-Portillo B, Borlongan CV. Melatonin-a potent therapeutic for stroke and stroke-related dementia. Antioxidants (Basel). 2020;9(8):672.
46. Franceschini R, Tenconi GL, Zoppoli F, Barreca T. Endocrine abnormalities and outcome of ischaemic stroke. Biomed Pharmacother. 2001;55(8):458–65.
47. Liamis G, Barkas F, Megapanou E, et al. Hyponatremia in acute stroke patients: pathophysiology, clinical significance, and management options. Eur Neurol. 2019;82(1–3):32–40.
48. Fuentes B, Ntaios G, Putaala J, et al. European stroke organisation (ESO) guidelines on glycaemia management in acute stroke. Eur Stroke J. 2018;3(1):5–21.
49. Johnston KC, Bruno A, Pauls Q, et al. Intensive vs standard treatment of hyperglycemia and functional outcome in patients with acute ischemic

stroke: the SHINE randomized clinical trial. JAMA. 2019;322(4):326–35.
50. Kerr DE, Wenham T, Newell-Price J. Endocrine problems in the critically ill 2: endocrine emergencies. BJA Educ. 2017;1(11):377–82.
51. Calissendorff J, Falhammar H. To treat or not to treat subclinical hypothyroidism, what is the evidence? Medicina (Kaunas). 2020;56(1):40.
52. Karaca Z, Hacioglu A, Kelestimur F. Neuroendocrine changes after aneurysmal subarachnoid haemorrhage. Pituitary. 2019;22(3):305–21.
53. Tanriverdi F, Ulutabanca H, Unluhizarci K, Selcuklu A, Casanueva FF, Kelestimur F. Three years prospective investigation of anterior pituitary function after traumatic brain injury: a pilot study. Clin Endocrinol. 2008;68(4):573–9.
54. Aimaretti G, Ambrosio MR, Di Somma C, et al. Residual pituitary function after brain injury-induced hypopituitarism: a prospective 12-month study. J Clin Endocrinol Metab. 2005;90(11):6085–92.
55. Ioachimescu AG, Barrow DL. Subarachnoid Hemorrhage and the pituitary. World Neurosurg. 2015;83(6):1026–8.
56. Karamouzis I, Pagano L, Prodam F, et al. Clinical and diagnostic approach to patients with hypopituitarism due to traumatic brain injury (TBI), subarachnoid hemorrhage (SAH), and ischemic stroke (IS). Endocrine. 2016;52(3):441–50.
57. Vespa P. Participants in the international multidisciplinary consensus conference on the critical care management of subarachnoid hemorrhage. SAH pituitary adrenal dysfunction. Neurocrit Care. 2011;15(2):365–8.
58. Hannon MJ, Behan LA, O'Brien MM, et al. Hyponatremia following mild/moderate subarachnoid hemorrhage is due to SIAD and glucocorticoid deficiency and not cerebral salt wasting. J Clin Endocrinol Metab. 2014;99(1):291–8.
59. Connolly ES Jr, Rabinstein AA, Carhuapoma JR, et al. Guidelines for the management of aneurysmal subarachnoid hemorrhage: a guideline for healthcare professionals from the American Heart Association/American Stroke Association. Stroke. 2012;43(6):1711–37.
60. D'Souza S. Aneurysmal subarachnoid hemorrhage. J Neurosurg Anesthesiol. 2015;27(3):222–40.
61. Khajeh L, Blijdorp K, Heijenbrok-Kal MH, et al. Pituitary dysfunction after aneurysmal subarachnoid haemorrhage: course and clinical predictors—the HIPS study. J Neurol Neurosurg Psychiatry. 2015;86(8):905–10.

Myopathies in Neurocritical Care

32

Sangeetha R. Palaniswamy, Ajay Prasad Hrishi, and Manikandan Sethuraman

32.1 Introduction

Myopathy in critical care occurs frequently and is often underdiagnosed, posing a serious clinical concern in the intensive care unit (ICU). It is a constellation of the clinical variants of muscular weakness, which develops secondary to long-standing critical illness. The spectrum of etiologies leading to upper and lower motor neuron paralysis resulting in muscular dysfunction in the ICU is described in Table 32.1. Intensive care unit-acquired weakness (ICUAW) is a blanket term that encompasses these variants. This is characterized by acute onset neuromuscular dysfunction with no plausible etiology apart from the critical illness per se, has an intensity greater than that resulting from prolonged immobilization, and is typically associated with multiorgan failure [1].

Table 32.1 Spectrum of etiologies leading to upper and lower motor neuron paralysis resulting in muscular dysfunction in the ICU

The primary site of origin	Disease
Brain	Acute stroke: ischemic, hemorrhagic, or subarachnoid hemorrhage, intracranial mass, meningitis/encephalitis, ypoglycemia/hyperglycemia, and postictal Todd's paresis Hemiplegic migraine and metabolic infarcts (e.g., MELAS)
Spinal cord	Transverse myelitis Spinal cord infarction/compression
Anterior horn cell	Amyotrophic lateral sclerosis, West Nile virus, and Polio
Peripheral nerve	Guillain-Barre syndrome, vasculitic neuropathy, toxin-induced nerve compression syndromes, and acute diabetic lumbosacral radiculoplexus neuropathy
Neuromuscular junction	Myasthenia gravis, Lambert-Eaton myasthenic syndrome, botulism, tick bite, and organophosphate toxicity
Muscle	Acute myopathy, rhabdomyolysis, and myositis

S. R. Palaniswamy
Department of Neuroanaesthesia and Neurocritical Care, National Institute of Mental Health and Neurosciences, Bengaluru, Karnataka, India
e-mail: sangeetharp@nimhans.ac.in

A. P. Hrishi (✉) · M. Sethuraman
Fellowship in Neuroanesthesia and Neurocritical Care, Oxford University Hospitals, Oxford, UK

Department of Anaesthesiology, Sree Chitra Tirunal Institute for Medical Sciences and Technology, Trivandrum, Kerala, India
e-mail: drajay@sctimst.ac.in; kanmanis@sctimst.ac.in

H. Prabhakar et al. (eds.), *Principles and Practice of Neurocritical Care*,
https://doi.org/10.1007/978-981-99-8059-8_32

The common predispositions are systemic sepsis, prolonged mobility restriction, uncontrolled hyperglycemia, and indiscriminate use of glucocorticoids or neuromuscular blocking drugs [2]. The typical presentation of these disorders is characterized by generalized, symmetrical, skeletal muscle weakness that selectively affects the limb (proximal more than distal) and respiratory muscles, with characteristic sparing of the ocular and facial muscles [3, 4]. Here, the muscle tone is invariably reduced with either normal or reduced deep tendon reflexes [5]. There may be associated diaphragmatic dysfunction that clinically manifests more frequently than limb muscle paresis [6].

32.2 Epidemiology and Risk Factors

A systematic review of 31 studies reported the prevalence of ICUAW to be as high as 43% [7] across varied ICU patient populations, risk factors, and diagnostic assessment methods [8–11]. The modifiable and non-modifiable risk factors for the development of ICUAW are listed in Fig. 32.1.

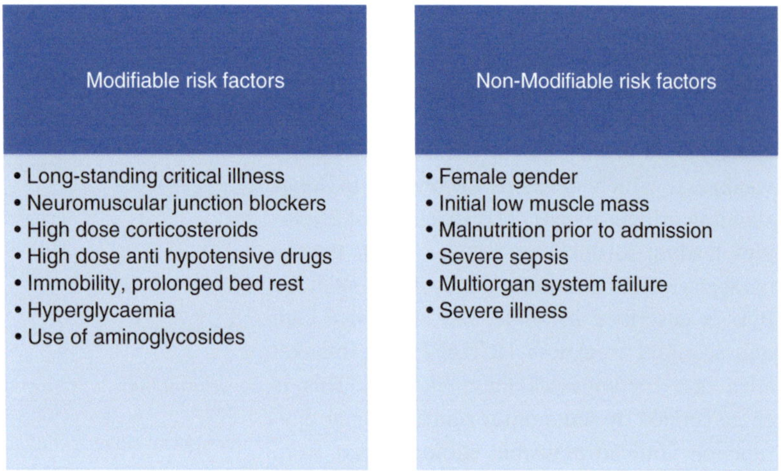

Fig. 32.1 Modifiable and non-modifiable risk factors for the development of ICUAW

32.3 Pathophysiology

The underlying pathophysiological process culminating in ICUAW in susceptible patients is complex and multifactorial. Both structural and functional aberrations in muscle homeostasis culminate in the paresis and paralysis of skeletal muscles among susceptible critically ill patients (Fig. 32.2).

Prolonged immobilization, denervation [12], and a predominance of catabolic state [13] in the critically ill leads to disuse atrophy of skeletal muscles, which vitiates further movement restriction and muscle weakness. Moreover, systemic homeostatic perturbations trigger multiple microcirculatory changes, including vasodilatation and enhanced permeability of myogenic blood vessels. This results in a stormy infiltration of the muscles with inflammatory cells, leucocytes, and cytokines (tumor necrosis factor-alpha and interleukin 1), leading to edema of the involved muscles. Furthermore, myocytic cells get converted to adipose or fibrotic tissue, further aggravating muscle dysfunction [14]. Muscle atrophy is compounded by an imbalanced protein turnover and accelerated protein breakdown by an activated proteolytic (ubiquitin–proteasome) enzyme system in the background of reduced protein synthesis [15].

32.3.1 Functional Aberrations in the Involved Muscle

The myocytic inflammation, leucocytic infiltration, and muscle edema following systemic inflammatory response (SIRS) results in hypoperfusion and impaired oxygen delivery to the myocytes. Impairment of autophagy activation further complicates this condition. This precedes multiple cellular and organelle dysfunctions, among which the most critical insult occurs secondary to a disrupted mitochondrial respiratory chain. The dysregulated mitochondrial energy production can affect the adjacent neuronal tissue through abnormal membrane depolarization and axonal degeneration. This results in the inactivation of the Na^+ channels contributing to a brief and reversible hypo-excitability or in-excitability of muscle and nerve membranes in these patients [16].

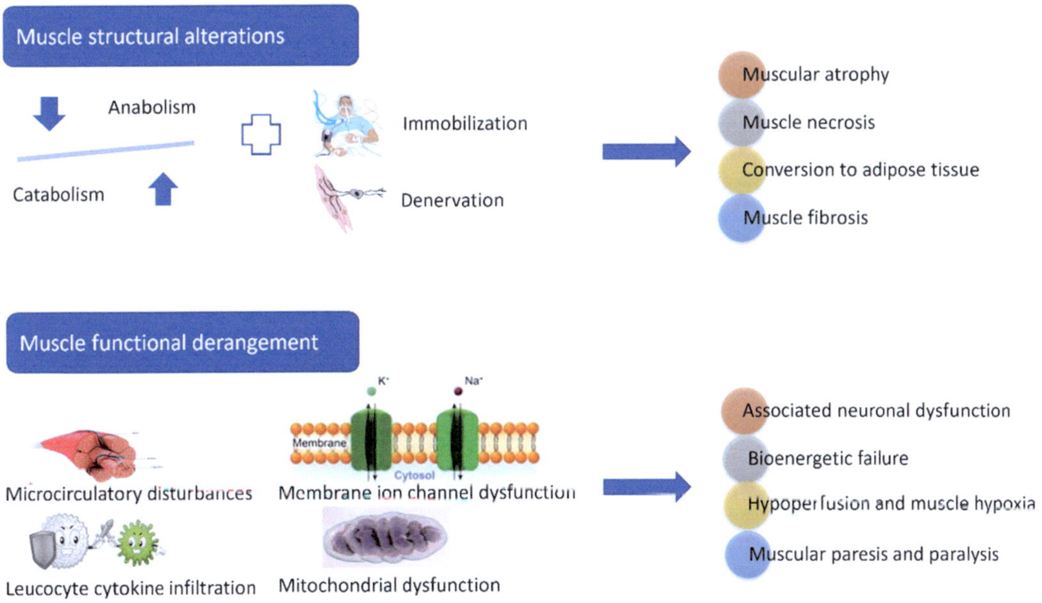

Fig. 32.2 Structural changes in the affected muscle of a patient with ICUAW

32.4 Classification of ICUAW

The broad categorization of ICUAW based on the primary site of disease origin is as follows:

1. Critical illness polyneuropathy
2. Critical illness myopathy
   (a) Diffuse non-necrotizing cachectic myopathy
   (b) Acute necrotizing myopathy of intensive care
3. Critical illness neuromyopathy

The characteristic clinical presentations and neurophysiological findings aid in the differentiation of these subtypes, thereby guiding the appropriate management.

32.5 Clinical Presentation

Critical illness polyneuropathy (CIP) is an acute onset of sensorimotor axonal neuropathy (occasionally a pure motor neuropathy) that may primarily present as failure to wean from mechanical ventilation. It is characterized by severe distal flaccid weakness, reduced or absent reflexes, and marked muscle wasting. The prevalence is around 60% in patients with prolonged ICU stay, among whom 80% have associated systemic inflammatory response syndrome and multi-organ failure [17].

Critical illness myopathy (CIM) is an acute primary myopathy causing weakness and paralysis in critically ill patients. The synonyms for this condition are myopathy with selective loss of thick filaments (myosin), acute quadriplegic myopathy, acute illness myopathy, acute myopathy of intensive care, and rapidly evolving myopathy with myosin-deficient fibers. As with CIP, CIM usually manifests as difficulty weaning from mechanical ventilation. The clinical features of CIM include predominantly proximal muscle weakness, facial and neck muscle weakness, and reduced reflexes. Blood creatine kinase levels are raised in 50% of cases. Although neurophysiological studies may be helpful in cooperative patients, they are neither sensitive nor specific in patients who are noncooperative or have reduced sensorium. Large cumulative steroid doses exceeding 10-gram hydrocortisone over 1–2 weeks and prolonged administration of neuromuscular antagonists for 3–5 days are the commonly implicated risk factors in causing CIM [18].

Diffuse non-necrotizing cachectic myopathy variant of CIM presents with muscle wasting and associated proximal or generalized weakness. It is associated with prolonged ICU admission, sedation, or paralysis, causing muscle disuse and poor nutrition with protein catabolism. Creatine kinase levels and electromyography (EMG) are normal, and the biopsy shows type 2 fiber atrophy and neurogenic atrophy [19]. Acute necrotizing myopathy of the intensive care variant of CIM is a rare myopathy that may be a form of rhabdomyolysis. It is commonly associated with administering neuromuscular blocking agents with or without corticosteroid therapy. It may also occur after infective or metabolic insults. Serum creatine kinase is usually markedly elevated, and myoglobinuria is common. Muscle biopsy reveals patchy or widespread fiber necrosis with vasculitic infarction within the muscle. Recovery of muscle power is often poor [20].

CIP is characterized by a more distal than proximal limb muscle weakness, sensory changes, and limited muscle atrophy. On the other hand, CIM presents with a more proximal than distal limb muscle weakness, sensory preservation, and muscle atrophy, depending on the duration of the critical illness. The key features for a reliable comparison and differentiation between the commonly observed variants, namely CIP and CIM, are depicted in Table 32.2 [21].

CINM is indicative of a combined polyneuropathy with myopathy. Patients with CINM present with overlapping symptoms and may have predominant symptoms of either condition elaborated above [22].

Table 32.2 The characteristics between critical illness polyneuropathy and critical illness myopathy

Critical illness polyneuropathy	Critical illness myopathy
Common features	
Limb weakness is present	Limb weakness is present
Difficulty in weaning from mechanical ventilatory support with the exclusion of cardiac and pulmonary causes	Difficulty in weaning from mechanical ventilatory support with the exclusion of cardiac and pulmonary causes
Differentiating features	
Critically ill (sepsis and multi-organ failure)	Not required; typically exposed to a variable combination of neuromuscular blocking agents and corticosteroids in the setting of sepsis and multi-organ failure
Electrophysiological evidence of 1. Axonal sensorimotor neuropathy	Electrophysiological evidence of 1. Preserved sensory response (>80% of the lower limit of normal) 2. Reduced motor responses (compound muscle action potential <80% lower limit than normal) 3. Normal repetitive nerve stimulation, and EMG with short-duration, low-amplitude motor unit potential with early full or normal recruitment of motor unit action potentials 4. Muscle inexcitability with direct muscle stimulation
Other causes of acute neuropathy should be excluded, for example, porphyria, acute massive intoxications of heavy metals, and vasculitis	Muscle biopsy consistent with myopathy and myosin loss

32.6 Evaluation and Diagnosis

32.6.1 Functional Assessment

Volitional Functional Testing for Peripheral Muscle Assessment

(a) Functional measurements of *Peripheral muscle*

These tests require the patients to be awake, cooperative, and capable of performing the measurements. Tables 32.3 and 32.4 show the detailed assessment method of the Medical Research Council (MRC) sum score.

This system of scoring uses 5 to denote the normal strength. Each of these six muscle movements is elicited and evaluated for their strength bilaterally, adding to a total of 5 × 12 = 60. Diagnostic thresholds for significant weakness:< 48/60 and severe weakness: < 36/60. This is a reliable, valid, gold standard non-invasive bedside testing for the overall estimation of motor function [23–25].

This simplified system of scoring denotes 3 as the normal strength. Each of these six muscle movements is elicited and evaluated for their strength bilaterally, adding to a total of 3 ×12 = 36. A significant weakness is

Table 32.3 MRC sum score—6 categories

Scoring	Bilateral scoring of muscle groups
0: No contraction	Shoulder abduction
1: Contraction without movement	Elbow flexion
2: Movement, gravity eliminated	Wrist extension
3: Movement against gravity	Hip flexion
4: Movement against resistance	Knee extension
5: Normal muscle force	Foot dorsiflexion

Table 32.4 MRC sum score—4 categories

Scoring	Bilateral scoring of muscle groups
0: paralysis	Shoulder abduction
1: > 50% loss of strength	Elbow flexion
2: < 50% loss of strength	Wrist extension
3: normal strength	Hip flexion
-	Knee extension
-	Foot dorsiflexion

diagnosed when the score is <24/36 and remains to be validated. This is a non-invasive, bedside testing, with good inter-observer reliability and accuracy in diagnosing muscle weakness between grades than a 6-grade score requiring further validation [26]. A limitation of the MRC score is its applicability in immobile patients due to orthopedic or other injury that precludes muscle testing. In these cases, the corresponding contralateral muscle score is substituted to derive the MRC score.

(b) *Hand-held dynamometry*

This is a quick, easy, gold standard non-invasive bedside testing with a high inter-observer reliability [3, 25, 27]. The quadriceps force and handgrip strength are assessed here. Diagnosis of weakness is made when < 11 kg for men and < 7 kg for women.

(c) *Scored physical function in intensive care test (PFIT-s)*

This test evaluates the patient's functional abilities on a 0–3 based on shoulder flexion strength, knee extension strength, sit-to-stand assistance, and step cadence [28].

(d) *Functional status score for the ICU*

This estimates the functional abilities to perform activities like rolling, transfer from spine to sit, sitting at the edge of the bed, moving from sitting to standing, and walking on a score ranging from 0–7 with 0: not able to perform and 7: complete independence [29].

Volitional Functional Testing for Respiratory Muscles

Functional assessments require the patients to be awake, cooperative, and capable of performing the measurements.

(a) *Maximal inspiratory and expiratory pressure*

This helps to determine both the inspiratory and expiratory muscle strength and global respiratory muscle strength. While high values exclude respiratory weakness, low values can predict the prolonged duration of mechanical ventilation and greater incidence of mortality [30, 31].

(b) *Transdiaphragmatic pressure*

The measurements of maximal transdiaphragmatic pressure following inspiration against a closed glottis (Pdimax), transdiaphragmatic pressure upon twitch phrenic nerve stimulation (Pdi,tw), and the endotracheal tube pressure upon phrenic nerve stimulation (Pet,tw) are invasive techniques for respiratory muscle assessment using gastric and esophageal balloons. While high values exclude respiratory weakness, a Pdimax < 60 cm H_2O signals diaphragm strength weakness [32, 33].

Non-Volitional Functional Testing for Respiratory Muscles

These maneuvers are invasive and require magnetic stimulation with considerable technical difficulty.

(a) *Transdiaphragmatic pressure in response to bilateral twitch phrenic nerve stimulation*

This invasive method requires magnetic stimulation and is one of the most objective tests for predicting mechanical ventilation duration and mortality (better than maximum inspiratory pressure). This technique involves magnetic stimulation of the phrenic nerve and elicitation of diaphragmatic muscle CMAP responses through placing an esophageal catheter with electrodes or transcutaneous direct needle placement inserted under the costal margin behind the eighth, ninth, or tenth rib cartilage. Diaphragmatic weakness is diagnosed with a Pdi,tw < 10 cm H_2O [32–34].

(b) *Endotracheal tube pressure in response to bilateral phrenic nerve stimulation during airway occlusion*

An in-line valve is placed along the ventilator circuit and is closed intermittently to perform airway occlusion. The endotracheal tube pressure following bilateral phrenic nerve stimulation during airway occlusion is measured. Diaphragm strength weakness is diagnosed with a Pet,tw < 11 cm H_2O [4, 35].

(c) *Airway occlusion pressure (P0.1)*

This a simple, non-invasive measure to monitor the neuro-muscular activation of the respiratory system. This is the negative airway pressure generated during the first 100 ms after initiating an inspiratory effort against a closed respiratory circuit [36]. In healthy subjects, P0.1 varies between 0.5 and 1.5 cm H_2O [37]. Greater values suggest an increased work of breathing [37].

(d) *Amplitude of the electrical activity of the diaphragm (EAdi)*

The placement of an esophageal catheter with electrodes facilitates the recording of EAdi. Here, the ratio of actual EAdi to maximum EAdi estimates the patient's breathing effort. Maximum EAdi(max EAdi) can be defined as the peak activity observed during a 20-s inspiratory occlusion. if EAdi/max EAdi is very low, it suggests poor diaphragm loading and a possibility of diaphragm atrophy [31].

32.6.2 Imaging

1. Peripheral muscle
   (a) Ultrasonography: It allows quantitative and qualitative evaluation of muscle area and thickness, central tendon thickness, muscle vascularization, fasciculations, and the presence of any subcutaneous edema/ intramuscular fluid/ fat infiltration or intramuscular fibrous tissue. It can also detect muscle necrosis and fasciitis, which accompany more advanced stages of ICUAW [38, 39].
   (b) Computed tomography (CT) and Magnetic resonance imaging (MRI) detect infiltration of muscle by adipose tissue and fat-free skeletal muscle.
   (c) Bioelectrical impedance, dual-energy X-ray absorptiometry, and neutron activation analysis aid in the analysis of the body composition [40].
2. Respiratory muscle
   (a) Chest X-rays provide information about the diaphragm position at the bedside [31, 33].
   (b) Ultrasonography helps in the assessment of the diaphragmatic thickening fraction. The 3.5–5 MHz phased array probe is placed along the right or left midclavicular line under the costal margin, directed cranially, medially, and dorsally. The two-dimensional B mode is used to identify the zone of apposition. The M-mode is then used to define the range of diaphragmatic movements. The normal movement during expiration is away from the probe and hence recorded as a positive peak. The magnitude of normal excursion ranges from 16 to 18 mm during quiet breathing and 50–70 mm during deep breathing. Diaphragmatic weakness is diagnosed with < 11 mm, and the degree of the diaphragmatic excursion is considered abnormal if <20%. This simple bedside repeatable assessment guides the prediction of the weaning outcome [31–33, 41].

The normal mean diaphragmatic thickness (MDT) ranges between 1.7 and 2 millimeters (mm) when measured in the zone of apposition. The diaphragmatic thickness fraction (TF) is calculated using the formula TF = thickness at end inspiration − thickness at end-expiration/thickness at end-expiration [39]. In healthy individuals, TF ranges between 24.5% and 53.2% during normal breathing. A decline of 6% per day of mechanical ventilation is noted in these patients when measured in the zone of apposition owing to disuse atrophy [42].

3. *Electrodiagnostic and tissue biopsy testing of peripheral muscle*

   This panel of workup entails the performance of single or complete nerve conduction studies (NCS), needle electromyography (EMG), and direct neuromuscular electrical stimulation (EMS).

32.7 Diagnostic Criteria for ICUAW Based on Electrodiagnostic Testing [43]

1. Compound muscle action potential (CMAP) amplitudes <80% of the lower limit of normal amplitude in >2 nerves
2. Sensory nerve action potential (SNAP) amplitudes <80% of the lower limit of normal amplitude in >2 nerves
3. Normal or near normal nerve conduction velocities (NCV)
4. The absence of a decremental response to repetitive nerve stimulation

The results of these tests act as key differentiators between CIP and CIM, as tabulated in Table 32.5.

Patients with ICUAW require prolonged respiratory support. Apart from rapid and effective SIRS management, no specific CIP prophylaxis or treatment exists. High-dose IVIg has failed to show benefit, but excellent glycemic control might minimize the risk of developing CIP. Patients may also benefit from strict potassium control, including early renal replacement therapy in those with elevated serum potassium secondary to renal failure. As axonal hypoxia appears to be an important etiological factor for CIP, providing optimal oxygenation and perfusion must be important [44].

Myopathy treatment (due to CIP, CIM, and CINM) is targeted toward aggressive management of the primary and co-existing medical con-

Table 32.5 Key differences between CIP, CIM, and CINM

Investigation	CIP	CIM	CINM
Creatine kinase	Normal or mildly elevated	Elevated in the majority (usually ≤10 000 IU/L)	Normal or elevated
Cerebrospinal fluid	Normal cell counts; normal or slightly elevated protein levels (<0.8 g/L)	Cerebrospinal fluid Normal cell counts; normal or slightly elevated	normal or slightly elevated protein levels (<0.8 g/L)
Nerve conduction studies	Reduced CMAP amplitudes, reduced SNAP amplitudes, and normal conduction velocities and latencies	Reduced CMAP amplitudes; normal SNAP amplitudes; and normal conduction velocities and latencies	Reduced CMAP amplitudes; reduced SNAP amplitudes; and normal
Electromygraphy	Spontaneous fibrillation potentials and sharp waves; ±long duration, high-amplitude polyphasic MUPs (reinnervation)	Spontaneous fibrillation potentials and sharp waves; short duration, low-amplitude MUPs with early recruitment	Features of both CIP and CIM
Direct muscle stimulation	Nerve: muscle ratio <0.5; normal direct muscle CMAP amplitude	Nerve: muscle ratio ≥0.5; reduced direct muscle CMAP amplitude	Variable depending on the relative components of CIP and CIM
Muscle biopsy	Features of denervation and reinnervation: small angulated muscle fibers; target and targetoid fibers; group fiber atrophy; and fiber type regrouping	Cachectic myopathy with myofibrillar degeneration; thick filament myopathy with a selective loss of myosin filaments; and necrotizing myopathy with muscle fiber necrosis	Both features of CIP and CIM
Nerve biopsy	Normal, or motor and sensory nerve axonal degeneration	Normal	Normal, or motor and sensory nerve axonal degeneration

ditions and prevention of associated complications such as pressure ulceration and venous thrombosis. In addition, judicious use of sedation, muscle relaxants, and early mobilization of critically ill patients may benefit the prevention or mitigation of neuromuscular weakness.

32.8 Preventive and Therapeutic Interventions for ICUAW

A recent Cochrane review outlines some preventative measures for developing ICUAW with potential short- and long-term repercussions. These include but are not limited to the following feasible bedside practices [44].

(a) Adequate nutrition
(b) Electrolyte replacement
(c) Strict glucose control
(d) Early mobilization and rehabilitation
(e) Daily scrutiny and prompt de-escalation of steroids, sedatives, and NMJ blockade
(f) Early attempts at weaning from mechanical ventilation
(g) Regular limb physiotherapy while still critically ill
(h) Neuromuscular electrical stimulation (EMS)

32.8.1 Role of Pharmacological Interventions

(a) Levosimendan, a calcium channel sensitizer used as a cardiac inotrope, enhances the binding of calcium to troponin and improves the contractile efficiency of the muscle fibers. The administration of levosimendan improved neuro-mechanical efficiency by > 20% and prevented contractile fatigue during a diaphragm-loading task in healthy subjects. Studies should be undertaken to evaluate the effects of levosimendan on respiratory muscle function in difficult-to-wean patients [45].
(b) Antioxidants, namely selenium, zinc, beta carotene, vitamin E, vitamin C, and glutamine, have been tried, but no study has specifically evaluated the effect of antioxidants on respiratory muscle function.
(c) Anabolic hormones like growth hormone (GH), insulin-like growth factor-1 (IF-I), insulin, and the anabolic steroid testosterone and its analogs have been used to enhance skeletal muscle mass. However, the safety and efficacy of anabolic steroids in ICU patients with respiratory muscle weakness have not been evaluated [46].
(d) Nandrolone and high-caloric feeding significantly improved inspiratory muscle strength.

32.8.2 Role of Physiotherapy in ICUAW

Respiratory Muscle Training
Inspiratory Muscle Strength Training (IMST) by spontaneous breathing using a nonlinear resistor that increases respiratory workload has improved whole-body exercise performance. Training consisted of providing an inspiratory load of 30% maximum inspiratory pressure for 5 min, BD × 7 days a week. In studies conducted in the ICU, the maximum inspiratory pressure was significantly increased. Further research will be able to guide the optimal training protocol and appropriate timing for the initiation of IMST [47].

Physical Training
(a) Joint mobilization and muscle training regimes to increase muscle strength, minimize atrophy, and improve muscle mass and function during ICU stay when the patient is on a ventilator and post-ICU rehabilitation when the patient is weaned [48].
(b) A review by Nobuto Nakanishi et al. shows that there exists progressive muscle atrophy in critically ill patients, and physical therapy, electrical muscle stimulation, muscle protective ventilator settings, and glucose control can help prevent atrophy and preserve muscle mass [49].
(c) A systematic review and meta-analysis suggest that early rehabilitation in the ICU reduces the incidence of developing ICUAW [50]. Physical training for patients with

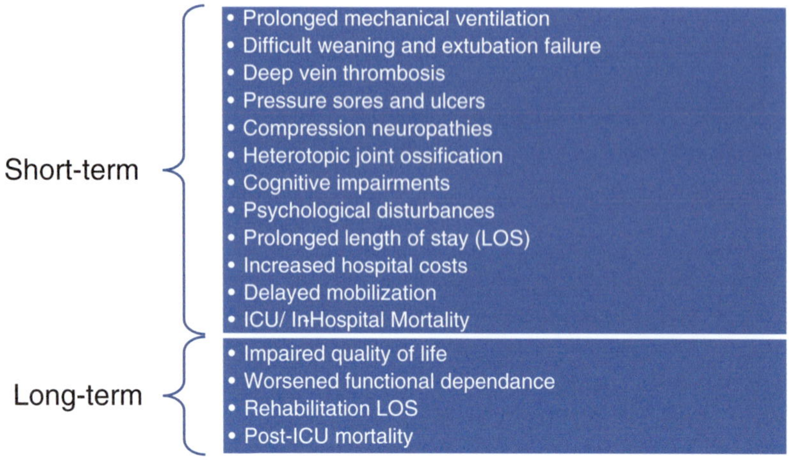

Fig. 32.3 The short-term and long-term consequences in patients with ICUAW

ICUAW during admission includes passive range of motion sessions, passive cycling, and electrical muscle stimulation (EMS).

32.8.3 Prognosis

CIP is usually self-limiting, and the overall prognosis is influenced by the severity of the underlying critical illness, which accounts for most of the CIP-related mortality. The outcome is associated with the severity of sepsis, the extent and severity of neuropathy, time spent in the ICU, and the presence of hyperglycemia, hyperosmolality, and hypoalbuminemia. Recovery is relatively rapid and complete when CIP is mild or moderate; however, severe polyneuropathy results in high mortality and limited recovery in survivors. Follow-up studies show that persisting residual clinically relevant motor and sensory deficits are common in survivors with CIP. This leads to chronic weakness, fatigue, and difficulty with mobilization [51]. The outcome of CIM is better than CIP or CINM, and most patients fully recover unless paralysis has been severe and prolonged.

In-hospital mortality is estimated to be approximately 45% in patients diagnosed with ICUAW, with a further 20% mortality within 1 year following ICU discharge. Most survivors of ICUAW demonstrate improvement in clinical and electrophysiological findings over time. However, complete functional recovery occurs in only 68% of the patients, with persistent severe disability in nearly 28% [52].

32.8.4 Complications

The course of ICUAW can negatively impact the short-term and long-term consequences in the affected patients, as elaborated in Fig. 32.3.

32.9 Management

32.9.1 Rehabilitation During the ICU Stay

A broad range of rehabilitation strategies are under the current research lens that includes phased physical and mobilization therapy (passive and active limb movements, transferring, sitting, and standing to walk), occupational therapy (training and practice in performing activities of daily living (e.g., grooming and washing), cycle ergometry, electrical muscle stimulation, and self-help rehabilitation manuals [53]. These have demonstrated some benefits in short-term outcomes (increased ventilator-free days, reduced length of stay in the ICU and hospital, increased return to independent functional status, and improved quality of life) [54]. However, these strategies require validation through extensive prospective studies. While, currently, there is no clear consensus regarding

Patient-related barriers	Hemodynamic instability	*Solutions to patient-related barriers*	Pain management before mobilization
	Deep sedation		Regular assessment, lighter sedation and antipsychotic medications
	Pain, agitation and delirium		Patient education and encouragement
	Patient denial, lacking motivation		Portable devices, secure lines, drains, and interdisciplinary teamwork
Structural barriers	Limited staff	*Solutions to structural barriers*	Additional staff, independent mobility team
	Lack of protocols and limited guidelines		Develop protocols, safety criteria
	Limited equipment		Training for appropriate use of equipment, financial, and the cost analysis model of economic benefit
Cultural barriers	Lack of mobilization culture	*Solutions to cultural barriers*	Promotion of mobility programs
	Early mobilization, not a priority		Interprofessional education
Process-related barriers	Dearth of coordination and planning	*Solutions to process-related barriers*	Regular screening of patients, interprofessional coordination, and planning
	Risks for mobility providers		Training, appropriate equipment, and mobility team

Fig. 32.4 The various challenges with solutions to facilitate mobilization

optimal management, the available clinical research echoes a central tenet of ICU care through the minimization of inactivity and early commencement of rehabilitation processes within the ICU [55].

32.9.2 Barriers to Successful Mobilization

With mobilization as an essential intervention for successfully managing patients with ICUAW, one must be familiar with the common challenges and be equipped with an appropriate plan to circumvent them [56]. Figure 32.4 illustrates the various challenges with possible solutions to facilitate mobilization.

32.9.3 Safety Concerns During Mobilization

Significant tachycardia, postural hypotension, tachypnea, oxygen desaturation, unplanned extubation, discomfort, agitation, dislodgement of devices, and falls are among the various adverse events that can complicate patient mobilization as summarized in a systematic review [56]. According to the expert consensus by Hodgson et al., the presence of endotracheal intubation was not a contraindication to early mobilization. A fraction of inspired oxygen less than 0.6 with a peripheral oxygen saturation above 90% and a respiratory rate less than 30 breaths/min were considered safe criteria for in and out-of-bed mobilization in the absence of other contraindications [57].

32.9.4 Newer Horizons in Rehabilitation

(a) *Neuromuscular electrical stimulation (NMES)*

NMES deconditions and reverses muscle weakness when applied to areas around the muscle fibers and at the neuromuscular junction. The contractions generated prevent muscle atrophy, improve blood circulation, and alleviate the effects of prolonged immobility without overburdening the cardiovascular system [58]. These effects may persist for up to 4–6 weeks after the treatment completion [59, 60]. NMES is demonstrated for its efficacy in preserving critically ill patients' muscle thickness at the chest and abdomen [61].

(b) *Artificial intelligence in rehabilitation (robotics and virtual reality-assisted physiotherapy)*

Conventional physiotherapy has an undisputable role in the management of patients with ICUAW. Efforts are underway to explore the various possibilities for clinically useful adjuncts to this technique. The ever-expanding clinical applicability of artificial intelligence has recently established its utility in critically ill patients through robotics and virtual reality [62]. These substitutional electromedical devices provide an assisted, repetitive, and intensive task-oriented rehabilitation essential for maximizing functional recovery despite a severe motor deficit [63–65]. Furthermore, these advances provide tremendous sensorimotor information for carrying out complex ecological tasks in a safe and controllable environment, mimicking a real-world setting [66, 67]. The feasibility and applicability of robot-assisted early mobilization to facilitate the early mobilization of critically ill patients in the ICU is the focus of contemporary studies [68]. Its role in influencing patient outcomes remains to be conclusively established through large-volume trials.

(c) *Cycle ergometry*

The role of early mobilization using in-bed passive cycling has been demonstrated to facilitate the improvement of peripheral limb muscle strength in mechanically ventilated patients without significant changes in the mechanical ventilation duration and length of hospital stay [69].

32.9.5 Rehabilitation and Care after ICU Discharge

Following hospital discharge, the continuation of physical rehabilitation therapy of a patient with ICUAW includes muscle strength training, aerobic sessions, such as walking, arm-leg cycling exercises, and functional therapies with self-help manuals and programs.

32.10 Summary and Conclusion

Myopathy in neurocritical care often develops in critically ill patients during their ICU stay. Adequate awareness, careful vigilance, appropriate workup, and prompt diagnosis are key to the early detection and proper management of this preventable yet devastating condition. A lower threshold for suspicion in vulnerable patients with concomitant sepsis, multiorgan failure, and systemic inflammatory response syndrome should trigger the preventive strategies discussed above. Judicious use of sedatives, neuromuscular blockade, adequate nutrition, adequate glycemic control, and early mobilization must be emphasized in managing these patients.

References

1. Hermans G, Berghe GV. Clinical review: intensive care unit acquired weakness. Crit Care. 2015;19:274–82.
2. Wang W, Xu C, Ma X, Zhang X, Xie P. Intensive care unit-acquired weakness: a review of recent progress with a look toward the future. Front Med (Lausanne). 2020;7:559789.
3. Latronico N, Herridge M, Hopkins RO, et al. The ICM research agenda on intensive care unit-acquired weakness. Intensive Care Med. 2017;43(9):1270–81. https://doi.org/10.1007/s00134-017-4757-5.
4. Piva S, Fagoni N, Latronico N. Intensive care unit-acquired weakness: unanswered questions and targets for future research. F1000Res 8. 2019;8:508.
5. Vanhorebeek I, Latronico N, Van den Berghe G. ICU-acquired weakness. Intensive Care Med. 2020;46(4):637–53. https://doi.org/10.1007/s00134-020-05944-4.
6. Dres M, Dubé BP, Mayaux J, et al. Coexistence and impact of limb muscle and diaphragm weakness at time of liberation from mechanical ventilation in medical intensive care unit patients. Am J Respir Crit Care Med. 2017;195(1):57–66. https://doi.org/10.1164/rccm.201602-0367OC.
7. Fan E, Cheek F, Chlan L, et al. An official American Thoracic Society Clinical Practice guideline: the diagnosis of intensive care unit-acquired weakness in adults. Am J Respir Crit Care Med. 2014;190(12):1437–46. https://doi.org/10.1164/rccm.201411-2011ST.
8. Parry SM, Puthucheary ZA. The impact of extended bed rest on the musculoskeletal system in the critical care environment. Extrem Physiol Med. 2015;4:16. Published 2015 Oct 9. https://doi.org/10.1186/s13728-015-0036-7.

9. Thabet Mahmoud A, Tawfik MAM, Abd El Naby SA, Abo El Fotoh WMM, Saleh NY, Abd El Hady NMS. Neurophysiological study of critical illness polyneuropathy and myopathy in mechanically ventilated children; additional aspects in pediatric critical illness comorbidities. Eur J Neurol. 2018;25(7):991–e76. https://doi.org/10.1111/ene.13649.
10. De Jonghe B, Sharshar T, Lefaucheur JP, et al. Paresis acquired in the intensive care unit: a prospective multicenter study. JAMA. 2002;288(22):2859–67. https://doi.org/10.1001/jama.288.22.2859.
11. Hanna JS. Sarcopenia and critical illness: a deadly combination in the elderly. J Parenter Enteral Nutr. 2015;39:273–81.
12. Puthucheary ZA, Rawal J, McPhail M, et al. Acute skeletal muscle wasting in critical illness [published correction appears in JAMA. 2014 Feb 12;311(6):625. Padhke, Rahul [corrected to Phadke, Rahul]]. JAMA. 2013;310(15):1591–600. https://doi.org/10.1001/jama.2013.278481.
13. Plant PJ, Bain JR, Correa JE, Woo M, Batt J. Absence of caspase-3 protects against denervation-induced skeletal muscle atrophy. J Appl Physiol. 2009;107:224–34. https://doi.org/10.1152/japplphysiol.90932.2008.
14. Derde S, Hermans G, Derese I, Güiza F, Hedström Y, Wouters PJ, Bruyninckx F, D'Hoore A, Larsson L, Van den Berghe G, Vanhorebeek I. Muscle atrophy and preferential loss of myosin in prolonged critically ill patients. Crit Care Med. 2012;40:79–89.
15. Batt J, Herridge M, Dos Santos C. Mechanism of ICU-acquired weakness: skeletal muscle loss in critical illness. Intensive Care Med. 2017;43:1844–6. https://doi.org/10.1007/s00134-017-4758-4.
16. Friedrich O, Reid MB, Van den Berghe G, Vanhorebeek I, Hermans G, Rich MM, Larsson L. The sick and the weak: neuropathies/myopathies in the critically ill. Physiol Rev. 2015;95:1025–109.
17. Bolton CF. Neuromuscular manifestations of critical illness. Muscle Nerve. 2005;32:140–63.
18. Appleton R, Kinsella J. Intensive care unit-acquired weakness. Contin Educ Anaesth Crit Care Pain. 2012;12(2):62–6. https://doi.org/10.1093/bjaceaccp/mkr057.
19. Chawla J. Stepwise approach to myopathy in systemic disease. Front Neurol. 2011;2:49. https://doi.org/10.3389/fneur.2011.00049.
20. Chawla J, Gruener G. Management of critical illness polyneuropathy and myopathy. Neurol Clin. 2010;28:961–77. https://doi.org/10.1016/j.ncl.2010.03.027.
21. Shepherd S, Batra A, Lerner DP. Review of critical illness myopathy and neuropathy. Neurohospitalist. 2017;7(1):41. https://doi.org/10.1177/1941874416663279.
22. Park S-H, Jeong Y-J, Kim N-H. Critical illness neuromyopathy. Ann Clin Neurophysiol. 2020;22(2):61–6.
23. Stevens RD, Marshall SA, Cornblath DR, Hoke A, Needham DM, de Jonghe B, Ali NA, Sharshar T. A framework for diagnosing and classifying intensive care unit-acquired weakness. Crit Care Med. 2009;37:S299–308.
24. Vanpee G, Hermans G, Segers J, Gosselink R. Assessment of limb muscle strength in critically ill patients: a systematic review. Crit Care Med. 2014;42:701–11.
25. Kelmenson DA, Quan D, Moss M. What is the diagnostic accuracy of single nerve conduction studies and muscle ultrasound to identify critical illness polyneuromyopathy: a prospective cohort study. Crit Care. 2018;22:342.
26. Parry SM, Berney S, Granger CL, Dunlop DL, Murphy L, El-Ansary D, Koopman R, Denehy L. A new two-tier strength assessment approach to the diagnosis of weakness in intensive care: an observational study. Crit Care. 2015;19:52.
27. Roberson AR, Starkweather A, Grossman C, Acevedo E, Salyer J. Influence of muscle strength on early mobility in critically ill adult patients: systematic literature review. Heart Lung. 2018;47:1–9.
28. Denehy L, de Morton NA, Skinner EH, Edbrooke L, Haines K, Warrillow S, Berney S. A physical function test for use in the intensive care unit: validity, responsiveness, and predictive utility of the physical function ICU test (scored). Phys Ther. 2013;93:1636–45.
29. Huang M, Chan KS, Zanni JM, Parry SM, Neto SG, Neto JA, da Silva VZ, Kho ME, Needham DM. Functional Status Score for the ICU: an international clinimetric analysis of validity, responsiveness, and minimal important difference. Crit Care Med. 2016;44:e1155–64.
30. Supinski GS, Westgate P, Callahan LA. Correlation of maximal inspiratory pressure to transdiaphragmatic twitch pressure in intensive care unit patients. Crit Care. 2016;20:77.
31. Doorduin J, van Hees HW, van der Hoeven JG, Heunks LM. Monitoring of the respiratory muscles in the critically ill. Am J Respir Crit Care Med. 2013;187:20–7.
32. Dres M, Goligher EC, Heunks LMA, Brochard LJ. Critical illness associated diaphragm weakness. Intensive Care Med. 2017;43:1441–52.
33. Qian Z, Yang M, Li L, Chen Y. Ultrasound assessment of diaphragmatic dysfunction as a predictor of weaning outcome from mechanical ventilation: a systematic review and meta-analysis. BMJ Open. 2018;8:e021189.
34. Parry SM, Granger CL, Berney S, Jones J, Beach L, El-Ansary D, Koopman R, Denehy L. Assessment of impairment and activity limitations in the critically ill: a systematic review of measurement instruments and their clinimetric properties. Intensive Care Med. 2015;41:744–62.
35. Casaer MP, Mesotten D, Hermans G, Wouters PJ, Schetz M, Meyfroidt G, Van Cromphaut S, Ingels C, Meersseman P, Muller J, Vlasselaers D, Debaveye Y, Desmet L, Dubois J, Van Assche A, Vanderheyden S, Wilmer A, Van den Berghe G. Early versus late parenteral nutrition in critically ill adults. N Engl J Med. 2011;365:506–17.

36. Kuhlen R, Mohnhaupt R, Slama K, et al. Validation and clinical application of a continuous P0.1 measurement using standard respiratory equipment. Technol Health Care. 1996;4(4):415–24.
37. Telias I, Damiani F, Brochard L. The airway occlusion pressure ($P_{0.1}$) to monitor respiratory drive during mechanical ventilation: increasing awareness of a not-so-new problem. Intensive Care Med. 2018;44(9):1532–5. https://doi.org/10.1007/s00134-018-5045-8.
38. Hernández-Socorro CR, Saavedra P, López-Fernández JC, Ruiz-Santana S. Assessment of muscle wasting in long-stay ICU patients using a new ultrasound protocol. Nutrients. 2018;10:E1849.
39. Witteveen E, Sommers J, Wieske L, Doorduin J, van Alfen N, Schultz MJ, van Schaik IN, Horn J, Verhamme C. Diagnostic accuracy of quantitative neuromuscular ultrasound for the diagnosis of intensive care unit-acquired weakness: a cross-sectional observational study. Ann Intensive Care. 2017;7:40.
40. Joskova V, Patkova A, Havel E, Najpaverova S, Uramova D, Kovarik M, Zadak Z, Hronek M. Critical evaluation of muscle mass loss as a prognostic marker of morbidity in critically ill patients and methods for its determination. J Rehabil Med. 2018;50:696–704.
41. Matamis D, Soilemezi E, Tsagourias M, et al. Sonographic evaluation of the diaphragm in critically ill patients. Technique and clinical applications. Intensive Care Med. 2013;39(5):801–10. https://doi.org/10.1007/s00134-013-2823-1.
42. Zambon M, Greco M, Bocchino S, Cabrini L, Beccaria PF, Zangrillo A. Assessment of diaphragmatic dysfunction in the critically ill patient with ultrasound: a systematic review. Intensive Care Med. 2017;43(1):29–38. https://doi.org/10.1007/s00134-016-4524-z.
43. Judemann K, Lunz D, Zausig YA, Graf BM, Zink W. Intensive care unit-acquired weakness in the critically ill: critical illnesspolyneuropathy and critical illness myopathy. Der Anaesthetist. 2011;60(10):887–901. (https://www.ncbi.nlm.nih.gov/pubmed/22006117)
44. Hermans G, De Jonghe B, Bruyninckx F, Van den Berghe G. Interventions for preventing critical illness polyneuropathy and critical illness myopathy. Cochrane Database Syst Rev. 2009:CD006832. https://doi.org/10.1002/14651858.CD006832.pub2.
45. Roesthuis L, van der Hoeven H, Sinderby C, et al. Effects of levosimendan on respiratory muscle function in patients weaning from mechanical ventilation. Intensive Care Med. 2019;45(10):1372–81. https://doi.org/10.1007/s00134-019-05767-y.
46. Schellekens WJ, van Hees HW, Doorduin J, Roesthuis LH, Scheffer GJ, van der Hoeven JG, Heunks LM. Strategies to optimize respiratory muscle function in ICU patients. Crit Care. 2016;20:103.
47. Bezerra AL, Anderlini A, de Andrade FMD, Figueiroa JN, Lemos A. Inspiratory muscle training and physical training for reducing neuromuscular dysfunction in critically ill adults in intensive care units. Cochrane Database Syst Rev. 2017;2017(5):CD009970. Published 2017 May 30. https://doi.org/10.1002/14651858.CD009970.pub2.
48. Hodgson CL, Stiller K, Needham DM, et al. Expert consensus and recommendations on safety criteria for active mobilization of mechanically ventilated critically ill adults. Crit Care. 2014;18(6):658. https://doi.org/10.1186/s13054-014-0658-y.
49. Nakanishi N, Takashima T, Oto J. Muscle atrophy in critically ill patients: a review of its cause, evaluation, and prevention. J Med Invest. 2020;67(1.2):1–10. (https://pub med.ncbi.nlm.nih.gov/32378591/)
50. Anekwe DE, Biswas S, Bussières A, Spahija J. Early rehabilitation reduces the likelihood of developing intensive care unit-acquired weakness: a systematic review and meta-analysis. Physiotherapy. 2020;107:1–10. https://doi.org/10.1016/j.physio.2019.12.004.
51. Batt J, Herridge MS, Dos Santos CC. From skeletal muscle weakness to functional outcomes following critical illness: a translational biology perspective. Thorax. 2019;74:1091–8.
52. Latronico N, Shehu I, Seghelini E. Neuromuscular sequelae of critical illness. Curr Opin Crit Care. 2005;11:381–90.
53. Morris PE, Goad A, Thompson C, et al. Early intensive care unit mobility therapy in the treatment of acute respiratory failure. Crit Care Med. 2008;36:2238–43.
54. Eggmann S, Luder G, Verra ML, Irincheeva I, Bastiaenen CH, Jakob SM. Functional ability and quality of life in critical illness survivors with intensive care unit acquired weakness: a secondary analysis of a randomised controlled trial. PLoS One. 2020;15(3):e0229725. (https://www.ncbi.nlm.nih.gov/pmc/articles/PMC7056321/)
55. Huebner L, Schroeder I, Kraft E, et al. Early mobilization in the intensive care unit-Are robot-assisted systems the future? Anaesthesiologie. 2022;71(10):795–800. https://doi.org/10.1007/s00101-022-01130-x.
56. Alaparthi GK, Gatty A, Samuel SR, Amaravadi SK. Effectiveness, safety, and barriers to early mobilization in the intensive care unit. Crit Care Res Prac. 2020:7840743. https://doi.org/10.1155/2020/7840743.
57. Conceição TMAD, Gonzáles AI, Figueiredo FCXS, Vieira DSR, Bündchen DC. Safety criteria to start early mobilization in intensive care units. Systematic review. Critérios de segurança para iniciar a mobilização precoce em unidades de terapia intensiva. Revisão sistemática Rev Bras Ter Intensiva. 2017;29(4):509–19. https://doi.org/10.5935/0103-507X.20170076.
58. Santos LJ, Dall' Acqua AM, Sachetti A, et al. Use of electrical neuromuscular stimulation to preserve the morphology of abdominal and chest muscles of critical patients: randomized clinical trial. Intensive Care Med Exp. 2015;3(Suppl 1):A552. https://doi.org/10.1186/2197-425X-3-S1-A552.
59. Hodgson CL, Tipping CJ. Physiotherapy management of intensive care unit-acquired weakness. J

Physiother. 2017;63(1):4–10. (https://www.sciencedirect.com/scien ce/article/pii/S183695531630090X)
60. Falavigna LF, Silva MG, Freitas AL, et al. Effects of electrical muscle stimulation early in the quadriceps and tibialis anterior muscle of critically ill patients. Physiother Theory Pract. 2014;30(4):223–8. https://doi.org/10.3109/09593985.2013.869773.
61. Kho ME, Truong AD, Brower RG, et al. Neuromuscular electrical stimulation for intensive care unit-acquired weakness: protocol and methodological implications for a randomized, sham-controlled, phase II trial. Phys Ther. 2012;92(12):1564–79. https://doi.org/10.2522/ptj.20110437.
62. Dall' Acqua AM, Sachetti A, Santos LJ, et al. Use of neuromuscular electrical stimulation to preserve the thickness of abdominal and chest muscles of critically ill patients: a randomized clinical trial. J Rehabil Med. 2017;49(1):40–8. https://doi.org/10.2340/16501977-2168.
63. Chillura A, Bramanti A, Tartamella F, et al. Advances in the rehabilitation of intensive care unit acquired weakness: a case report on the promising use of robotics and virtual reality coupled to physiotherapy. Medicine (Baltimore). 2020;99(28):e20939. https://doi.org/10.1097/MD.0000000000020939.
64. Dobkin BH. Strategies for stroke rehabilitation. Lancet Neurol. 2004;3:528–36.
65. Krakauer JW. Motor learning: its relevance to stroke recovery and neurorehabilitation. Curr Opin Neurol. 2006;19:84–90.
66. Burdea G. Virtual rehabilitation—benefits and challenges. Methods Inf Med. 2003;42:519–23.
67. Maggio MG, Maresca G, De Luca R, et al. The growing use of virtual reality in cognitive rehabilitation: fact, fake or vision? A scoping review. J Natl Med Assoc. 2019;111:457–63.
68. Fluet GG, Deutsch JE. Virtual reality for sensorimotor rehabilitation post-stroke: the promise and current state of the field. Curr Phys Med Rehabil Rep. 2013;1:9–20.
69. Machado ADS, Pires-Neto RC, Carvalho MTX, Soares JC, Cardoso DM, Albuquerque IM. Effects that passive cycling exercise have on muscle strength, duration of mechanical ventilation, and length of hospital stay in critically ill patients: a randomized clinical trial. J Bras Pneumol. 2017;43(2):134–9. https://doi.org/10.1590/S1806-37562016000000170.

Gastrointestinal Problems in Neurocritical Care

33

Aleksandr Solodov

In the pathogenesis of acute cerebral injury, the state of the gastrointestinal tract is of great importance. The formation of concomitant systemic disorders significantly worsens the course and prognosis of patients with initially isolated acute cerebral injury. Up to 50% of patients with brain lesions have gastrointestinal (GI) complications [1]. Adverse effects include gastrointestinal dysfunction, which can manifest itself as functional disorders of internal organs, limiting the absorption of nutrients, increasing intestinal permeability, provoking translocation of bacterial flora, and developing infectious complications. Frequent complications of the critical condition are erosive gastritis, "stress ulcers" of the upper gastrointestinal tract, and gastroduodenal bleeding (Table 33.1). Intensive therapy of critical conditions with active use of antibacterial drugs and gastroprotectors increases the risk of antibiotic-associated lesions of the large intestine in the patient. A frequent complication is reactive pancreatitis, which, in patients in critical condition, may be masked and have no clinical manifestations. Special attention is paid to the state of the intestinal microbiota and ways to restore it.

A. Solodov (✉)
Federal State Budgetary Educational Institution of Higher Education "Russian University of Medicine" of the Ministry of Health of the Russian Federation, Moscow, Russian Federation

Table 33.1 Gastrointestinal disorders in patients with acute cerebral injury

Erosions and ulcers of the stomach and duodenum
Gastroduodenal bleeding
Increased intestinal permeability and translocation of intestinal flora
Gastrointestinal motility disorders
Systemic immune reactions in gastrointestinal lesions
Gut microbiota disorder
Antibiotic-associated diarrhea

33.1 Introduction

The GI tract plays a more significant role in the body than just providing digestion. The key importance of this system has been demonstrated in the development of pathological conditions. Acute cerebral injury (ACI) in stroke or traumatic brain injury (TBI) triggers an innate and adaptive immune response, which is implemented locally in the affected brain tissues and also has systemic manifestations through specialized pattern recognition receptors. The gastrointestinal tract is the main "immune" organ, having the largest composition of immune cells (up to 70% of the human immune system) and macrophages in the body. The lesion of the stomach and intestines in critical condition, in addition to the direct impact on digestion, has a negative impact on the body's defense against infectious agents. Excessive response of the immune system to the lesion of

H. Prabhakar et al. (eds.), *Principles and Practice of Neurocritical Care*,
https://doi.org/10.1007/978-981-99-8059-8_33

internal organs initiates pathophysiological mechanisms of systemic damage. Primary intestinal inflammation and a pronounced immune response are involved in pathophysiological processes provoking stroke, which can be used as an additional therapeutic target in the prevention and treatment of ACI.

GI occurs mostly during the first week after the onset of the disease or injury, so immediately after admission to the clinic, it is necessary to take measures for their prevention and timely treatment. The leading trigger mechanism of GI system lesions in ACI is tissue hypoperfusion and microcirculatory disorders, which lead to the weakening of upper GI mucosa protection, impaired motor function, and permeability of the intestinal wall. Joint functioning of the brain and gastrointestinal system is carried out through humoral and neurogenic regulation. Activation of the immune system and an inflammatory response in response to cerebral damage leads to damage to the "peripheral" internal organs, which may significantly worsen the patient's condition. The brain–GI system has bidirectional interaction pathways through which neuroinflammation and neurodegenerative processes affect both organs. Gut dysautonomia and systemic inflammation, due to cerebral damage, contribute to the development of secondary GI dysfunction, including motility dysfunction and increased intestinal mucosal permeability. There are changes in the microbiota of the system, resident and recruited immune cells are activated, and the concentration of microbial products and inflammatory mediators increases. Changes in the microbiota are often found in neurodegenerative diseases [2]. The feedback between the GI tract and the brain is equally important since sensory information from the gut lumen coordinates functions in different regions of the gut. Secondary inflammatory processes in the gut prolong systemic inflammation, which can aggravate the consequences of primary cerebral damage, leading to functional and cognitive deficits [3, 4]. The high importance for the body of the connection between the brain and the GI tract may become an effective therapeutic target for improving the treatment outcomes of patients with ACI. Currently, the most promising methods are those for the correction of systemic inflammation, dysautonomia, and GI dysbiosis.

33.2 Erosive Gastritis and Duodenitis

Frequent systemic complications in patients in critical condition are "stress" erosions and ulcers of the upper gastrointestinal tract. The neurogenic basis in the formation of such ulcers was first revealed by Rokitansky in 1841 when examining patients with brain tumors and severe cachexia [5]. Cushing, in 1932, reported the results of the surgical treatment of 11 patients with similar complications [6]. He suggested a hypothesis about the leading role of parasympathetic centers and their connection with vagus nuclei in gastric lesions. The leading pathogenetic importance of the vagus nerve in the formation of mucosal erosions/ulcers has now been proven, but the process of "stress lesion" of the GIT is multifactorial and represents an imbalance between protective and destructive factors affecting the gastric mucosa. The main protective elements against "stress ulcers" are considered to be a thin layer of mucus and glycoprotein matrix, which is a physical barrier to the penetration of hydrogen ions and pepsin. Mucus forms a surface-thin gel layer (about 0.6 mm thick) in which bicarbonates are concentrated. The alkaline environment neutralizes the acid and protects the mucosa from the damaging effects of pepsin and hydrochloric acid. The amount and thickness of the mucus layer depend on normal gastric juice secretion. Damaging factors directly affecting the gastric mucosa include gastric hydrochloric acid, pepsin, and bile. Hypoperfusion of internal organs in critical condition indirectly damages gastrointestinal tissues. Additional factors of internal organ damage are reperfusion changes. When microcirculation is restored after a long period of hypoperfusion, inflammatory mediators enter the tissues in large quantities, which trigger the processes of hyperemia, increased inflammatory response, and cell death. Gastric juice proteolytic enzymes increase mucosal damage. Many critically ill patients with ACI have reflux of bile acid salts, which further compromises protective barriers and increases damage to the gastric mucosa. Erosive damage of the upper gastrointestinal tract reaches its peak manifestations as early as 3–5 days after the cerebral catastrophe.

One of the most life-threatening complications is **Gastroduodenal Bleeding**, which can occur during the first 4 weeks after the disease onset [7]. The greatest number of symptomatic bleeding from the upper gastrointestinal tract occurs in the first 4–10 days. The incidence of gastrointestinal bleeding (GIB) after stroke is 1.5–7.8 [8]. Bleeding, depending on its duration and severity, can lead to severe anemia, hemodynamic instability, deterioration of the patient's condition, and an increase in the number of infectious complications. The duration of stay in the ICU of patients with GIB is 8 days longer compared to patients who had no clinical or laboratory manifestations of bleeding [9].

In critical condition, patients are predisposed to the formation of deep gastric ulcers and GIB, regardless of the presence of ulcer history. The high incidence of bleeding is due to the serious condition of patients as well as the consequences of active treatment, including surgery and intensive care. Up to 14 independent risk factors of GIB associated with upper GI stress ulcers are distinguished (Table 33.2) [11]. For patients with ACI, high risks are associated with respiratory failure requiring ALV for more than 48 h, severe head or spinal cord trauma, use of anticoagulants, surgery lasting more than 4 h, and the use of high-dose corticosteroids (equivalent to a hydrocortisone dose > 250 mg/day). Glucocorticoids can have a dual effect on the gastric mucosa, providing both physiological protection and provoking ulcer formation by inhibiting the secretion of gastric mucus, epithelial proliferation, and prostaglandin biosynthesis, as well as synchronous dysregulation of glucose homeostasis. Active use of proton pump inhibitors can predispose patients to peptic ulcer disease [12]. All of the above risk factors are cumulative. In patients with craniocerebral trauma, the degree of risk of GIB correlates with the severity of the trauma, regardless of the presence or absence of other factors [13].

Table 33.2 Risk factors for gastrointestinal bleeding in critical patients with acute brain injury [10]

Risk factors for bleeding associated with stress ulcers
Respiratory failure requires artificial lung ventilation for more than 48 h.
Coagulopathy (international normalized ratio greater than 1.5 or platelet count less than 50,000 thrombocytes/μL)
Acute renal failure
Acute liver failure
Sepsis
Arterial hypotension
Severe craniocerebral or spinal cord injury
History of an episode of GI tracts
Use of anticoagulants
High gastric acidity (low pH of gastric contents)
Thermal lesions over 35% of the body surface
Surgical intervention lasting more than 4 h
High-dose corticosteroid administration (>250 mg/day hydrocortisone or equivalent steroid dose)
Acute lung injury

Among patients with stroke, the highest incidence of GIB is observed in wakefulness depression to coma, the development of syndrome of inappropriate antidiuretic hormone secretion (SIDH), infectious complications, including central nervous system involvement, prolonged episodes of arterial hypotension, and pH < 4 gastric juice [10, 14]. An independent risk factor is age over 60 years. It is assumed that patients with ischemic stroke have an additional risk of bleeding due to continuous administration of anticoagulants and disaggregants [15]. Such patients require monitoring of blood plasma coagulological properties. In some cases, the high risk of GIB influences the choice of treatment strategy of a patient with stroke, for example, reduction of antiplatelet or anticoagulant therapy. Predictors of GIB in patients with hemorrhagic stroke may include large intracranial hematoma size, infectious complications, and a low Glasgow Coma Scale score [16].

Prevention and treatment of stress-induced gastric mucosal **damage** are aimed at preventing clinically significant GIB. There are pharmacological and therapeutic options for correction. The key point is to reduce destructive factors of mucosal damage. The main efforts are aimed at reducing the acidity of gastric juice. Among gastroprotectors, the most commonly used are proton pump inhibitors (PPIs), which have a fairly safe, pronounced, and long-lasting effect on gastric juice production. PPIs can also stimulate the blood supply of the gastric mucosa, improve local microcirculation, accelerate regeneration and repair of the mucosa, and additionally control bleeding. Histamine receptor antagonists (ranitidine) have not been shown to be effective in preventing GIB in ICU patients and may increase the risk of pneumonia. Antacids rapidly and prolongedly increase gastric pH. In critically ill patients, administration of such drugs may be limited because of difficulty in delivery through a gastric tube. Large doses and increased frequency of administration increase the risk of adverse effects of antacids, including diarrhea, constipation, metabolic alkalosis, and water-electrolyte disturbances. Excessive use of gastroprotectors with a significant increase in the pH of gastric juice reduces the protective properties of the acidic environment of the stomach, which may cause additional contamination and translocation of pathogens with increased risk of infectious complications against immunosuppression in patients in critical condition.

To date, the role of *Helicobacter pylori* in the pathogenesis of stress-induced gastrointestinal mucosal damage is not clear. Unjustified prophylactic antibacterial therapy against *H. pylori* can lead to the formation of resistance of pathogens to antibiotics (e.g., the emergence of methicillin-resistant strains of *Staphylococcus aureus* (MRSA)), with an increase in the frequency of infectious complications, as well as the development of antibiotic-associated colitis. The best way to prevent erosive lesions is considered to be effective enteral tube feeding of critically ill patients.

The timing and duration of prophylactic therapy for stress ulcers are individual. Decrease or cancellation of gastroprotectors is most often performed when resuming oral feeding or when transferring a patient from the ICU to a specialized department.

33.3 Increased Intestinal Permeability and Bacterial Translocation

The intestinal mucosa functions as a physical and immunological protective barrier. The main elements of the barrier are the outer layer of mucus with commensal intestinal microbiota, antimicrobial proteins and molecules of secretory immunoglobulin A (sIgA), the central unicellular layer with specialized epithelial cells, and the inner intrinsic lamina of the mucosa, which contains blood and lymphatic vessels, nerve endings, and innate and adaptive immune cells, such as T- and B-lymphocytes, macrophages, and dendritic cells [17].

The intestinal barrier of a healthy person is very dynamic and responds to both internal and exogenous stimuli (e.g., cytokines, bacteria, and food factors). Meanwhile, the intraluminal side of the barrier is contaminated with a wide range of intestinal microbes, while the basolateral side remains virtually sterile. The critical condition can weaken or destabilize the integrity of the intestinal epithelium. Dense contacts between mucosal epithelial cells play an important role in maintaining the barrier function of the intestine. They act as adhesive and mechanical mediators, preserving barrier function but not sealing the paracellular space. Dysfunction of the mucosal barrier can occur early in a critical condition, participating in pathophysiological processes that determine the severity of the patient's condition. The most serious complication is the translocation of microorganisms and the development of systemic infectious complications. GIT barrier homeostasis is regulated by a complex interaction between epithelial, immune, and glial cells [18].

The GIT is innervated by the parasympathetic and sympathetic autonomic nervous systems as well as the intrinsic enteric nervous system integrated into the intestinal wall. The afferents of these systems are located throughout the intestine, including the surface of the mucosa, and the fibers project to the nuclei of the posterior roots (vagus nerve) or terminate in the spinal cord (spinal nuclei) [19]. Information from the intestine is also transmitted by visceral afferents, which are connected with the autonomic nervous system. Visceral afferents can be sensitized by intestinal inflammation and activated by increased levels of inflammatory mediators. Gut dysautonomia is associated with worse outcomes and increased mortality in patients with ACI [20].

The vagus nerve innervates almost the entire length of the intestine from the esophagus to the middle of the colon and plays a key role in coordinating functions between the various parts of the intestine. Although stimulation of the parasympathetic nerves has both excitatory and inhibitory effects on secretomotor bowel function, the vagus nerve consists of 80–90% of afferent fibers. The information transmitted from the gut to the CNS is crucial for the organization of reflex activity during food intake. The vagus nerve can also respond to nociceptive signals. In cerebral damage, vagus nerve afferents provide modulation of CNS function by inflammatory mediators, microbiota, and microbial products [4].

Sympathetic nerves make up half of the afferent fibers. Spinal afferents primarily transmit nociceptive information from the GI tract and are activated during inflammation and intestinal damage. Stimulation of sympathetic nerves is involved in the regulation of blood flow in the intestine and, as a rule, inhibits the secretomotor function of the GI tract. Increased sympathetic activity in response to brain damage causes a "sympathetic storm" [21]. Massive release of catecholamines can contribute to GIT motility impairment, leading to gastroparesis and food intolerance.

Cerebral damage is characterized by an imbalance of signals emanating from the brain, which provokes dysautonomy of the "brain–gut" system and leads to GIT dysfunction. A noninvasive marker reflecting the tone of the autonomic nervous system is heart rate variability. This parameter is used to determine the balance of sympathetic and vagus nerve tone. A high heart rate frequency reproduces the basal tone of the vagus nerve, and a low heart rate is associated with the sympathetic component. The correlation of these frequencies is considered a clinical indicator of target organ regulation by the autonomic nervous system. In cerebral damage, there is a decrease in heart rate variability, indicating the dominance of the sympathetic nervous system [22]. Pharmacological drugs have been suggested for the correction of intestinal dysautonomia in traumatic brain injury victims [23].

The vagus nerve determines the response of the intestinal mucosa to injury and inflammation. The vagus anti-inflammatory pathway involves efferent activation of the enteric nervous system near resident macrophages in the intestine or spleen. The cholinergic reflex leads to inhibition of proinflammatory cytokine release [24]. Direct electrical stimulation or pharmacological modulation of the vagus nerve is used to eliminate intestinal dysautonomia [4].

The enteric nervous system consists of more than 20 subtypes of neurons located in two main ganglia: the musculo-intestinal, extending from the esophagus to the anus, and the submucosal, located mainly in the small and large intestine. This system independently integrates internal information from the intestinal lumen with external signals from parasympathetic and sympathetic nerves. The bilateral connection between the central and enteric nervous systems is the basis of the brain–gut axis of interaction. Both systems use identical neurotransmitters, such as acetylcholine and norepinephrine, which cause acute and chronic dysfunction after brain injury [25]. The enteric nervous system enables the GIT to maintain many of its functions independently of external regulation by the central nervous system. The main component of the enteric nervous system is intestinal glial cells (IGC), the number of which exceeds the number of neurons by more than four times [26]. IGCs resemble brain astrocytes in morphology and expression of common markers [4]. The location of the mucosal IGC population affects neuroepithelial interactions, and mucosal IGC S-nitrosoglutathione production directly affects epithelial permeability. Stimulation of the vagus nerve activates α7-nicotin receptors on the IGC and improves intestinal barrier integrity after severe trauma [27]. The enteric nervous system is responsible for the control of motility and transit of the small intestine. Enteral sensory neurons are important for retropulsive reflexes, such as vomiting in the small intestine, as well as for propulsive contractions and abundant fluid secretion in the large intestine. Small intestinal secretomotor neurons regulate fluid movement and electrolyte secretion between the intestinal lumen and the interstitial tissues of the body. In the large intestine, the ENS is able to reproduce the defecation reflex with lumbosacral stimulation independently of central regulation [28].

Barrier homeostasis is maintained through a complex interaction between epithelial cells, immune cells, and intestinal glial cells [18]. Intestinal mucus is an important component of the barrier because its close association with intestinal epithelial cells provides a physical barrier to limit direct contact with pathogenic microbiota or other harmful agents [29]. When using the lactulose/mannitol absorption ratio to assess intestinal permeability in patients with brain injury, impaired barrier function was observed as early as 4 days after injury and correlated with injury severity and long-term prognosis of disease outcome [30]. An increase in circulating microbial products and proinflammatory cytokines released from activated intestinal and systemic immune cells in response to infection leads to increased permeability of the blood–brain barrier. Penetration of circulating immune cells and mediators into brain tissue activates microglia and causes neuroinflammation. A weakened cell-mediated immune response against a background of a critical condition may contribute to a high incidence of infections in patients with ACI [31].

Brain injury induces region-specific reactive gliosis in the intestine, which may be part of a local neuroprotective response to mucosal barrier function impairment and may also contribute to long-term secondary effects in the intestine [32]. Increased intestinal permeability plays a key role in the pathogenesis of Crohn's disease, gluten disease, and diabetes mellitus [33]. Adverse disease outcomes in patients with ACI result from translocation of bacteria causing a systemic inflammatory response and sepsis, followed by multiple organ failure [34].

33.4 Gastrointestinal Motility Disorders

Gastrointestinal motility disorders of varying severity are detected in patients with ACI. Motility changes include gastroesophageal reflux associated with decreased tone of the lower esophageal sphincter and delayed gastric emptying. Isolated gastroparesis is the most common in patients with severe traumatic brain injury. Gastroparesis is considered to be delayed gastric emptying in the absence of mechanical obstruction. The incidence of gastroparesis reaches 45–50% of cases and correlates with the severity of injury and the presence of intracranial hypertension. Delayed gastroparesis is typical for the first 2 weeks after injury with subsequent recovery of motility. The leading cause of gastroparesis in brain injury is thought to be impaired neuroregulation of the stomach by the brain. Other factors contributing to its occurrence are inflammation, sepsis, severe water–electrolyte disorders, hyperglycemia, use of opioids, furosemide, antacids, and corticosteroids, and renal and hepatic dysfunction. In severe gastroparesis patients in critical condition, gastric tube feeding is not effective. In these situations, double-lumen probes are inserted into the small intestine for artificial feeding and evacuation of "pathological" gastric contents through the proximal opening in the probe. Gastric motility is restored as the damaged brain tissue recovers and the patient's level of alertness increases. Pharmacological stimulation of gastrointestinal motility will not be effective in most cases and is not recommended for routine use.

33.5 Systemic Immune Reactions in Lesions of the Gastrointestinal System

In ACI, the hypothalamic–pituitary–adrenal system and sympathetic autonomic nervous system are activated in response to a stressful situation for the body, which leads to increased release of glucocorticoids and catecholamines [4, 35]. Massive release of endogenous hormones is proportional to the severity of brain damage and determines the severity of clinical manifestations in response to a critical condition [36]. The systemic response is aimed at early compensation for the negative consequences of cerebral damage. Prolonged body response to stress is associated with numerous negative effects, including GI motility disorder, arterial hypertension, and heart failure. Prolonged exposure is associated with internal organ damage leading to multiple organ failure.

In addition to the release of catecholamines, brain tissue damage induces a systemic immune response in which immune mediators of inflammation (cytokines and chemokines) are released into the bloodstream. Laboratory signs of systemic inflammation may persist for several months after a brain injury [37, 38]. The concentration of cytokines in the bloodstream in the acute period after trauma correlates with the severity of cognitive impairment. Negative effects of ACI in the form of cognitive impairment have been observed in patients with high concentrations of IL-1β, TNF-α, sIL-6R, RANTES, and MIP-1β [39].

33.6 Microbiota Disorder

The gastrointestinal tract contains complex bacterial communities (microbiota) that jointly perform a wide range of functions [40]. The human intestinal microbiota contains approximately 1000 bacterial species, dominated by four types: Firmicutes, Bacteroidetes, Proteobacteria, and Actinobacteria, representing over 95% of the resident bacteria in healthy adults. A balanced gut microbiota enhances the body's defense against infection by fine-tuning the local and systemic immune system, suppressing intestinal pathogens, and maintaining the integrity of the epithelial barrier. The microbiota of critically ill patients is constantly subjected to aggression by factors resulting from the disease and iatrogenic effects of intensive care. As a result, almost all patients in the intensive care unit have severe disorders of the gut microbiota (dysbiosis) [41, 42]. Dysbiosis is associated with ventilator-associated pneumonia as well as an increase in recurrent infections [43].

The gut microbiota interacts with the central nervous system through neural, vascular, and lymphatic pathways as part of a bidirectional brain–gut system. The most direct and rapid route through which the intestinal microbiota can affect brain function is the vagus nerve [44]. Microbial products bind to vagus nerve receptors in the intestinal mucosa, providing information about changes in the composition and pathogenicity of the microbiota. The brain regulates ENS activity by influencing the composition and diversity of the gut microbiota as well as modulating gut peristalsis, transit, barrier integrity, and intraluminal secretion of factors that determine microbial gene expression and function [45, 46]. Abnormal intestinal peristalsis causes changes in the microbiota, closing the vicious circle between dysbacteriosis and motility disorders [47]. The microbiome is extremely sensitive to changes in diet [48]. In this regard, critically ill patients receiving artificial nutrition have acute changes in the microbiome as a result of food intolerance and motility disorders. In the remote period of the disease, patients with brain injury have persisted changes in eating behavior, including anorexia as well as hyperphagia, with a high risk of obesity [49].

Patients in critical condition have significant gut microbiota disorders characterized by loss of diversity, depletion of commensal bacteria, and dominance of pathogenic microbes, such as *Enterococcus*, *Staphylococcus*, and *Enterobacteriaceae* [40]. Such disorders contribute to the excessive growth of viruses and opportunistic fungal microorganisms. The formation of dysbiosis in patients in the intensive care unit is facilitated by impaired GI motility, changes in acidity in the intestinal lumen, increased production of catecholamines, treatment with antibiotics, proton pump inhibitors, opioids, and artificial nutrition.

Overgrowth of commensal microbes with pathogenic potential is associated with adverse clinical outcomes. Excessive numbers of Gram-negative bacteria are associated with the development of bloodstream infections [50]. The dominance of *Enterococcus* in the gut microbiota may be associated with a 19% increase in the probability of death [51]. Microbiota disorders, due to uncontrolled use of antibiotics or diseases associated with dysbiosis, increase the risk of septic conditions. Administration of high-risk antibiotics for colitis (e.g., III–IV generation cephalosporins or fluoroquinolones) has been associated with a 1.65-fold increased risk of severe sepsis within 90 days of discharge [52]. The beneficial effects of the restored microbiome, in addition to the positive effects on the GI tract, extend beyond the gut through the production of immunomodulatory metabolites [53].

The use of probiotics to correct dysbiosis is aimed at enhancing or restoring the intestinal microbiota for both preventive and therapeutic purposes. Other strategies for modulating the microbiome include the use of pre/synbiotics, probiotics, fecal microbiota transplantation, and the use of antibacterial drugs. Pretreatment with *Lactobacillus acidophilus* or *Clostridium butyricum* attenuates the neurological effects, neuroinflammation, and neuropathology caused by brain injury [54]. Despite the theoretical benefits, the routine use of drugs that modulate the gut microbiota in ICU patients is not currently recommended. The limitation of the use of pro- and prebiotics is due to the lack of information on the effects of these agents in the context of weakened state and reduced immunity in patients in critical condition. In the PROPATRIA study, in which patients with predicted severe acute pancreatitis received enteric probiotics or placebo, treatment with probiotics resulted in higher mortality (16%, 24 of 152 patients) compared with placebo (6%, 9 of 144 patients). These results were presumably due to intestinal ischemia and translocation of intestinal bacteria into the bloodstream with the formation of multiple organ failure [55]. It remains unclear whether the probiotics used correspond to the functions of the human commensal microbiota. In addition, the intestinal microbiota is only one of many factors regulating the systemic immune response. Nevertheless, the selection of drugs beneficial to the gut microbiota remains one of the most promising methods of correcting dysbiosis. Another direction of therapy is the prevention of microbiota destruction by antibiotics with special antidotes, which can specifically mitigate the side effects of antibiotics on commensal bacteria [56].

33.7 Antibiotic-Associated Diarrhea

Antibiotic-associated diarrhea (AAD) is a syndrome of intestinal flora disruption caused by taking antibiotics that cannot be explained by other causes, and diarrhea is the main symptom. Diarrhea is diagnosed when three or more episodes of watery or liquid stools occur per day for two consecutive days or more. Among critically ill patients, the incidence of diarrhea is 14–36% and varies depending on the type of antibiotic used and the characteristics of the population. AAD can occur within hours of starting antibiotic therapy and persist for up to 6–8 weeks after discontinuation [57]. A characteristic morphological sign of the disease is the appearance of a large number of pseudomembranes consisting of fibrin, mucus, necrotized epithelial cells, and leukocytes, determined in the watery stool, which may also present with pus and blood. Clinical symptoms of AAD include leukocytosis, hyperthermia, abdominal pain and bloating, toxic enlargement of the colon, and, in severe cases, multiple organ dysfunction [58].

The main pathophysiological cause of the disease is an imbalance of the intestinal microflora. Antibiotic-sensitive bacteria are killed or suppressed, and drug-resistant microorganisms multiply, disrupting the intestinal flora and causing enteritis and diarrhea. AAD is mainly caused by *Clostridium difficile* (CD), *Klebsiella* sp., and *Staphylococcus aureus* as well as by some fungi and viruses. The most common pathogen is *Clostridium difficile*. The development of *Clostridium difficile*-associated forms of intestinal damage does not depend on the dose of the prescribed drug, and the disease may occur both after the first antibiotic administration and several weeks after therapy withdrawal. Initial treatment proves ineffective in more than 20% of patients with AAD, and relapse occurs in 40–60%

of patients [59]. A special category is patients in the intensive care unit, with a high risk of infectious complications, who have a need to prescribe antibiotics. Adequate selection of drugs and careful monitoring of antibiotic therapy is necessary. The development of antibiotic-associated colitis significantly worsens the condition of critically ill patients. In this regard, prevention of AAD is of paramount importance.

Three groups of factors determine the risk of AAD in adults: factors characterizing the patient (age, condition, and comorbidities), destructive factors (exposure to antibiotics or other medications), and increased exposure to *C. difficile* spores on the patient (prolonged hospital stay) [60]. Complications of antibiotic-associated colitis include marked water–electrolyte disorders, arterial hypotension, dehydration, exudative enteropathy, intestinal perforation and peritonitis, and toxic megacolon.

The increase in the incidence of AAD is associated with the active use of antibiotics, especially broad-spectrum drugs. The high risk of antibiotic-associated colitis is accompanied by the use of III-IV fourth-generation cephalosporins, carbapenems, and fluoroquinolones. When two or more antibiotics are combined, the probability of AAD increases significantly [61]. *Clostridium difficile* produces enterotoxin A and cytotoxin B, the laboratory diagnosis of which allows a more accurate diagnosis of AAD. Ultrasound examination reveals bloated loops and thickening of the colon wall to 0.5 mm or more.

Methods for prevention and treatment of AAD include the withdrawal of systemic antibacterial therapy, the prescription of drugs against *C. difficile* (metronidazole, vancomycin, or fidaxomicin), the use of probiotics, the correction of artificial nutrition, and diet. If it is necessary to continue antibiotic therapy, the choice of drug is made depending on the minimal risk of AAD. Vancomycin is prescribed for moderate to severe antibiotic-associated colitis. Intraintestinal administration of the drug is effective. Of more than 20 types of probiotics, only a few have been shown to be effective [60]. The heterogeneity of the results of various studies does not allow us to formulate an objective conclusion, despite the fact that many specialists recognize the validity of probiotic use in AAD. The method of passive immunization with monoclonal antibodies and vaccines against *C. difficile* refers to promising but experimental ways to treat AAD. A diet with restriction of large amounts of carbohydrates is recommended. In severe intestinal insufficiency, it is necessary to consider the possibility of a temporary transition to parenteral nutritional mixtures. Oral and intravenous rehydration, fluid replenishment, correction of electrolyte balance, and enterosorbents are prescribed [62]. Enterosorbents should be continued until stool normalization on average for 10–12 days.

References

1. Wen SW, Wong CH. An unexplored brain-gut microbiota axis in stroke. Gut Microbes. 2017;8:601–6.
2. Carabotti M, et al. The gut-brain axis: interactions between enteric microbiota, central and enteric nervous systems. Ann Gastroenterol. 2015;28(2):203–9.
3. Glynn H, Möller SP, Wilding H, Apputhurai P, Moore G, Knowles SR. Prevalence and impact of post-traumatic stress disorder in gastrointestinal conditions: a systematic review. Dig Dis Sci. 2021;66(12):4109–19. https://doi.org/10.1007/s10620-020-06798-y.
4. Hanscom M, Loane DJ, Shea-Donohue T. Brain-gut axis dysfunction in the pathogenesis of traumatic brain injury. J Clin Invest. 2021;131(12):e143777. https://doi.org/10.1172/JCI143777.
5. Rokitansky C. Handbuch der pathologischen Anatomie, vol. 3. Wien: Braunmueller und Seidel; 1842. p. 197.
6. Cushing H. Peptic ulcer and the interbrain. Surg Obst. 1932;55:1–34.
7. Wang J, Zhang J, Ye Y, Xu Q, Li Y, Feng S, Xiong X, Jian Z, Gu L. Peripheral organ injury after stroke. Front Immunol. 2022;13:901209. https://doi.org/10.3389/fimmu.2022.901209.
8. Hsu HL, Lin YH, Huang YC, Weng HH, Lee M, Huang WY, et al. Gastrointestinal hemorrhage after acute ischemic stroke and its risk factors in Asians. Eur Neurol. 2009;62(4):212–8. https://doi.org/10.1159/000229018.
9. Cook DJ, Griffith LE, Walter SD, et al. The attributable mortality and length of intensive care unit stay of clinically important gastrointestinal bleeding in critically ill patients. Crit Care. 2001;5:368–75.
10. Schirmer CM, Kornbluth J, Heilman CB, Bhardwaj A. Gastrointestinal prophylaxis in neurocritical care. Neurocrit Care. 2012;16(1):184–93. https://doi.org/10.1007/s12028-011-9580-1.

11. Quenot JP, Thiery N, Barbar S. When should stress ulcer prophylaxis be used in the ICU? Curr Opin Crit Care. 2009;15(2):139–43.
12. Shi S, Klotz U. Proton pump inhibitors: an update of their clinical use and pharmacokinetics. Eur J Clin Pharmacol. 2008;64(10):935–51.
13. Liu B, Liu S, Yin A, Siddiqi J. Risks and benefits of stress ulcer prophylaxis in adult neurocritical care patients: a systematic review and meta-analysis of randomized controlled trials. Crit Care. 2015;19:409. https://doi.org/10.1186/s13054-015-1107-2.
14. Yang JX, Han YJ, Yang MM, Gao CH, Cao J. Risk factors and predictors of acute gastrointestinal injury in stroke patients. Clin Neurol Neurosurg. 2022;225:107566. https://doi.org/10.1016/j.clineuro.2022.107566.
15. Chou YF, Weng WC, Huang WY. Association between gastrointestinal bleeding and 3-year mortality in patients with acute, first-ever ischemic stroke. J Clin Neurosci. 2017;44:289–93. https://doi.org/10.1016/j.jocn.2017.06.068.
16. Barletta JF, Mangram AJ, Sucher JF, Zach V. Stress ulcer prophylaxis in neurocritical care. Neurocrit Care. 2018;29(3):344–57. https://doi.org/10.1007/s12028-017-0447-y.
17. Vancamelbeke M, Vermeire S. The intestinal barrier: a fundamental role in health and disease. Expert Rev Gastroenterol Hepatol. 2017;11(9):821–34. https://doi.org/10.1080/17474124.2017.1343143.
18. Sharkey KA. Emerging roles for enteric glia in gastrointestinal disorders. J Clin Invest. 2015;125(3):918–25. https://doi.org/10.1172/JCI76303.
19. Robinson DR, Gebhart GF. Inside information: the unique features of visceral sensation. Mol Interv. 2008;8(5):242–53. https://doi.org/10.1124/mi.8.5.9.
20. Baguley IJ, et al. The incidence of dysautonomia and its relationship with autonomic arousal following traumatic brain injury. Brain Inj. 2007;21(11):1175–81. https://doi.org/10.1080/02699050701687375.
21. Esterov D, Greenwald B. Autonomic dysfunction after mild traumatic brain injury. Brain Sci. 2017;7(12):100. https://doi.org/10.3390/brainsci7080100.
22. Conder RL, Conder AA. Heart rate variability interventions for concussion and rehabilitation. Front Psychol. 2014;5:890.
23. Ammar MA, Hussein NS. Using propranolol in traumatic brain injury to reduce sympathetic storm phenomenon: a prospective randomized clinical trial. Saudi J Anaesth. 2018;12(4):514–20.
24. Cailotto C, et al. Neuro-anatomical evidence indicating indirect modulation of macrophages by vagal efferents in the intestine but not in the spleen. PLoS One. 2014;9(1):e87785. https://doi.org/10.1371/journal.pone.0087785.
25. Shin SS, Dixon CE. Alterations in cholinergic pathways and therapeutic strategies targeting cholinergic system after traumatic brain injury. J Neurotrauma. 2015;32(19):1429–40. https://doi.org/10.1089/neu.2014.3445.
26. Gulbransen BD, Sharkey KA. Novel functional roles for enteric glia in the gastrointestinal tract. Nat Rev Gastroenterol Hepatol. 2012;9(11):625–32. https://doi.org/10.1038/nrgastro.2012.138.
27. Costantini TW, et al. Vagal nerve stimulation protects against burn-induced intestinal injury through activation of enteric glia cells. Am J Physiol Gastrointest Liver Physiol. 2010;299(6):G1308–18. https://doi.org/10.1152/ajpgi.00156.2010.
28. Panther EJ, Dodd W, Clark A, Lucke-Wold B. Gastrointestinal microbiome and neurologic injury. Biomedicines. 2022;10(2):500. https://doi.org/10.3390/biomedicines10020500.
29. McGuckin MA, et al. Mucin dynamics and enteric pathogens. Nat Rev Microbiol. 2011;9(4):265–78. https://doi.org/10.1038/nrmicro2538.
30. Faries PL, et al. Intestinal permeability correlates with severity of injury in trauma patients. J Trauma. 1998;44(6):1031–5. https://doi.org/10.1097/00005373-199806000-00016.
31. Esnault P, et al. Early-onset ventilator-associated pneumonia in patients with severe traumatic brain injury: incidence, risk factors, and consequences in cerebral oxygenation and outcome. Neurocrit Care. 2017;27(2):187–98. https://doi.org/10.1007/s12028-017-0397-4.
32. Ma EL, et al. Bidirectional brain-gut interactions and chronic pathological changes after traumatic brain injury in mice. Brain Behav Immun. 2017;66:56–69. https://doi.org/10.1016/j.bbi.2017.06.018.
33. Bischoff SC, Barbara G, Buurman W, Ockhuizen T, Schulzke JD, Serino M, Tilg H, Watson A, Wells JM. Intestinal permeability—new target for disease prevention and therapy. BMC Gastroenterol. 2014;14:19. https://doi.org/10.1186/1471-230X-14-19.
34. Katzenberger RJ, Ganetzky B, Wassarman DA. The gut reaction to traumatic brain injury. Fly (Austin). 2015;9(2):68–74. https://doi.org/10.1080/19336934.2015.1085623.
35. McDonald SJ, et al. Beyond the brain: peripheral interactions after traumatic brain injury. J Neurotrauma. 2020;37(5):770–81. https://doi.org/10.1089/neu.2019.6885.
36. Schroeppel TJ, et al. Beta-adrenergic blockade for attenuation of catecholamine surge after traumatic brain injury: a randomized pilot trial. Trauma Surg Acute Care Open. 2019;4(1):e000307. https://doi.org/10.1136/tsaco-2019-000307.
37. Kumar RG, et al. Chronic inflammation after severe traumatic brain injury: characterization and associations with outcome at 6 and 12 months postinjury. J Head Trauma Rehabil. 2015;30(6):369–81. https://doi.org/10.1097/HTR.0000000000000067.
38. Zhang W, et al. Systemic inflammatory response syndrome in Sepsis-3: a retrospective study. BMC Infect Dis. 2019;19(1):139. https://doi.org/10.1186/s12879-019-3790-0.
39. Milleville KA, et al. Early chronic systemic inflammation and associations with cognitive performance

after moderate to severe TBI. Brain Behav Immun. 2021;11(3):100185. https://doi.org/10.1016/j.bbih.2020.100185.
40. Schuurman AR, Kullberg RFJ, Wiersinga WJ. Probiotics in the intensive care unit. Antibiotics. 2022;11:217. https://doi.org/10.3390/antibiotics11020217.
41. Dickson RP. The microbiome and critical illness. Lancet Respir Med. 2016;4:59–72.
42. Lankelma JM, van Vught LA, Belzer C, Schultz MJ, van der Poll T, de Vos WM, Wiersinga WJ. Critically ill patients demonstrate large interpersonal variation in intestinal microbiota dysregulation: a pilot study. Intensive Care Med. 2017;43:59–68.
43. Adelman MW, Woodworth MH, Langelier C, Busch LM, Kempker JA, Kraft CS, Martin GS. The gut microbiome's role in the development, maintenance, and outcomes of sepsis. Crit Care. 2020;24:278.
44. Ma Q, et al. Impact of microbiota on central nervous system and neurological diseases: the gut-brain axis. J Neuroinflammation. 2019;16(1):53. https://doi.org/10.1186/s12974-019-1434-3.
45. Lyte JM, et al. Gut-brain axis serotonergic responses to acute stress exposure are microbiome-dependent. Neurogastroenterol Motil. 2020;32(11):e13881.
46. Martin CR, et al. the brain-gut-microbiome axis. Cell Mol Gastroenterol Hepatol. 2018;6(2):133–48. https://doi.org/10.1016/j.jcmgh.2018.04.003.
47. Halfvarson J, et al. Dynamics of the human gut microbiome in inflammatory bowel disease. Nat Microbiol. 2017;2(5):1–7.
48. David LA, et al. Diet rapidly and reproducibly alters the human gut microbiome. Nature. 2014;505(7484):559–63. https://doi.org/10.1038/nature12820.
49. McGlennon TW, et al. Bypassing TBI: metabolic surgery and the link between obesity and traumatic brain injury—a review. Obes Surg. 2020;30(12):4704–14. https://doi.org/10.1007/s11695-020-05065-3.
50. Stoma I, Littmann ER, Peled JU, Giralt S, van den Brink MRM, Pamer EG, Taur Y. Compositional flux within the intestinal microbiota and risk for bloodstream infection with gram-negative bacteria. Clin Infect Dis. 2020;73:e4627–35.
51. Freedberg DE, Zhou MJ, Cohen ME, Annavajhala MK, Khan S, Moscoso DI, Brooks C, Whittier S, Chong DH, Uhlemann AC, et al. Pathogen colonization of the gastrointestinal microbiome at intensive care unit admission and risk for subsequent death or infection. Intensive Care Med. 2018;44:1203–11.
52. Baggs J, Jernigan JA, Laufer Halpin A, Epstein L, Hatfield KM, McDonald LC. Risk of subsequent sepsis within 90 days after a hospital stay by type of antibiotic exposure. Clin Infect Dis. 2018;66:1004–12.
53. Sencio V, Barthelemy A, Tavares LP, Machado MG, Soulard D, Cuinat C, Queiroz-Junior CM, Noordine ML, Salomé-Desnoulez S, Deryuter L, et al. Gut dysbiosis during influenza contributes to pulmonary pneumococcal superinfection through altered short-chain fatty acid production. Cell Rep. 2020;30:2934–47.
54. Ma Y, et al. Lactobacillus acidophilus exerts neuroprotective effects in mice with traumatic brain injury. J Nutr. 2019;149(9):1543–52. https://doi.org/10.1093/jn/nxz105.
55. Bongaerts GP, Severijnen RS. A reassessment of the PROPATRIA study and its implications for probiotic therapy. Nat Biotechnol. 2016;34:55–63.
56. Maier L, Goemans CV, Wirbel J, Kuhn M, Eberl C, Pruteanu M, Müller P, Garcia-Santamarina S, Cacace E, Zhang B, et al. Unravelling the collateral damage of antibiotics on gut bacteria. Nature. 2021;599:120–4.
57. Kopacz K, Phadtare S. Probiotics for the prevention of antibiotic-associated diarrhea. Healthcare. 2022;10(8):1450. https://doi.org/10.3390/healthcare10081450.
58. Litao G, Jingjing S, Yu L, Lei Z, Xiaona H, Zhijing Z. Risk factors for antibiotic-associated diarrhea in critically ill patients. Med Sci Monit. 2018;24:5000–7. https://doi.org/10.12659/MSM.911308.
59. Shen NT, Maw A, Tmanova LL, et al. Timely use of probiotics in hospitalized adults prevents Clostridium difficile infection: a systematic review with meta-regression analysis. Gastroenterology. 2017;152:1889–900.
60. McFarland LV, Ozen M, Dinleyici EC, Goh S. Comparison of pediatric and adult antibiotic-associated diarrhea and Clostridium difficile infections. World J Gastroenterol. 2016;22(11):3078–104. https://doi.org/10.3748/wjg.v22.i11.3078.
61. Rodríguez-Varón A, Muñoz OM, Pulido-Arenas J, et al. Antibiotic-associated diarrhea: clinical characteristics and the presence of Clostridium difficile. Rev Gastroenterol Mex. 2017;82(2):129–33.
62. Zhou H, Xu Q, Liu Y, Guo LT. Risk factors, incidence, and morbidity associated with antibiotic-associated diarrhea in intensive care unit patients receiving antibiotic monotherapy. World J Clin Cases. 2020;8(10):1908–15. https://doi.org/10.12998/wjcc.v8.i10.1908.

34 Role of Clinical Neuropsychology

Ashima Nehra, Rhythm Makkar, Ruchita Hazrati, and Gunjan Singh

34.1 Introduction

The brain and behavior are interlinked. This relationship of mind has two components, which include awareness and emotions. Awareness (verbal) + emotions (nonverbal) = leads to action [1]. Clinical neuropsychology/neuropsychology is a para-clinical/non-medical discipline of psychological science, which has a role in the continuum of care (CoC) model, while the primary role in a medical setup is of a clinician/medical doctor who is a primary source of contact for such patients. Since clinical neuropsychology/neuropsychology is a para-medical/non-medical discipline; hence, the importance of training with regular teaching in psychology with the knowledge of theories and systems and regular practical training cannot be undermined. It focuses on the behavior associated with an injured brain (emotions and awareness) as well as changes in cognitive processing and affective responses. Injured brains are functionally less efficient. Neuropsychological psycho-diagnostics includes clinical history taking + complete psychometric assessment, which includes selection, administration, scoring, and interpretation of test results [2] + clinical observation [3]; hence, a typical assessment is not just psychometrics. Qualified and regularly trained neuropsychologists conduct psychological testing, assessment, and evaluation endeavors to select (a) assessment tools that demonstrate sufficient validity and evidence for their uses, sufficient score reliability, and sound psychometric properties and (b) measures that are fair and appropriate for the evaluation purpose, population, setting, and context at hand [2].

Hence, psychology has a key role in the continuum of care (CoC) model but not a primary role. The basic assumption is that a focal lesion may lead to an impairment of function, e.g., impairment in cognitive functions. As you are aware, every neural tissue has a specific function, and any interruption in this complex functional network may lead to problems, e.g., learning and memory are complex. The functions are associated with different areas of the brain. These can be measured by appropriate tests, hence the importance of neuropsychological psycho-diagnostics [3]. For example, in the higher brain center, for the cortex of the frontal lobe, the whole brain operates, which is presumed to have higher mental processes and critical areas. Clinical neuropsychologists can attempt localization. This effort can be futile without assessment of higher-level skills, learning, long-term memory, orbitofrontal functions/personality assessment, etc. [1] Hence, the importance of cognitive functions and non-cognitive functions is observed, both of which are

A. Nehra (✉) · R. Makkar · R. Hazrati
Clinical Neuropsychology, Cardiothoracic and Neurosciences Centre, All India Institute of Medical Sciences, New Delhi, India

G. Singh
Department of Neurology, Cardiothoracic and Neurosciences Centre, All India Institute of Medical Sciences, New Delhi, Delhi, India

H. Prabhakar et al. (eds.), *Principles and Practice of Neurocritical Care*,
https://doi.org/10.1007/978-981-99-8059-8_34

interlinked. If a person is not motivated, he will not perform well in tests. Hence, regular training is important to elicit the best results from the patient. All of these depend upon some of the basic building blocks. The functions impaired due to lesions of the brain are attentional processes, regulatory functions, psychomotor functions, i.e., thinking, abstraction, problem-solving, learning & memory function, visuospatial & integrative functions, speech, specific skills, and personality & emotional responses. Neuropsychological psycho-diagnostics can also provide syndrome analysis by comparison with the performance of other normal subjects or an inferred understanding of the level of premorbid functioning, to demonstrate the deficit & to independently elicit the deficit, and elicit the deficit with simple testing procedures [1]. An instrument called AIIMS Comprehensive Neuropsychological Battery based upon Luria's functional approach had been suggested to be a useful investigatory procedure in the detection, lateralization, and localization of discrete brain lesions that are typically seen in a neurological setting. On the question of the accuracy of the diagnosis, the battery can identify brain dysfunction in neurological patients with a success rate of more than 80%. Furthermore, whenever the patient is diagnosed as having a brain dysfunction, the battery can identify a right/left/diffuse brain damage with over 90% success rate. Once the patient's brain dysfunction is lateralized either to the right/left side of the brain, the validation and cross-validation data suggested neuropsychological localization (in one of the eight anatomically determined divisions of the brain such as left frontal, left sensorimotor, left patient occipital, left temporal, right frontal, right sensorimotor, right parietal occipital, and right temporal) with 95% success rate. Besides the usefulness of the battery in neuropsychological localization, there are implications for its application in neuropsychological rehabilitation in so far as one gets clear-cut neuropsychological profiles in areas like speech, memory, intelligence, reading, writing, arithmetic, motor, tactile, and visual functions indicating remaining skills in the neurologically impaired individuals [4]. But for the same, the importance of "*Reason for Referral*" by clinicians and their provisional diagnosis is important. To ascertain a provisional diagnosis, the clinicians run various tests. It is important for them to carry out quick screening tools (Bed Side/O.P.D. Set up). Such screening tools will help clinicians know about some neurocognitive functions. They may further consider sharing the results of the same along with their provisional diagnosis while referring patients for neuropsychological psycho-diagnostics as well as the specific question, i.e., "*Reason for Referral*," which they would have formulated by their history taking and administration of screening tools (which are validated against full neuropsychological psycho-diagnostics) (Tables 34.1, 34.2 and 34.3).

To understand the neuropsychological psycho-diagnostics for neurological patients and their management during neuro-critical care (NCC) further, let us understand the What, Why, How, and Whom of neuropsychological psycho-diagnostics.

34.2 What

Cognition includes all processes involved in attention, perception, acquiring, comprehending, and responding to information or stimulus from within as well as in the environment. Cognitive

Table 34.1 Reasons for referral: some neuropsychological profile signs [1]

• Disorientation	• Episodic amnesia
• Absence of attention	• Axial amnesia
• Distractibility	• Apraxia
• Confusion	• Constructional apraxia
• Apathy	• Aphasia—expressive
• Akinesia	• Aphasia—receptive
• Emotional lability	• Conduction aphasia
• Personality change	• Nominal aphasia
• Lack of initiative	• Visual agnosia
• Disinhibition	• Finger agnosia
• Indifferent	• Prosopagnosia
• Impulsiveness	• Astereognosis
• Irritability/violence	• Left-right orientation
• Perseveration	• Dyscalculia
• Incontinence	• Route finding difficulty
• Semantic amnesia	• Dysgraphia
• Neglect of half	• Semantic speech impaired

Table 34.2 Some of the uses of neuropsychological psycho-diagnostic (NP)/assessment

1.	Used in the process of Clinical History Taking + Psychometric Assessment + Clinical Observation for clinical diagnosis (following the CoC model)
2.	Used for predicting cognitive decline even before structural changes are seen
3.	Used to monitor the course and outcome of treatment
4.	Used in deciding neurosurgical strategies (especially before elective surgeries)
5.	Used for devising neuropsychological rehabilitation
6.	Assist with timely management of the progression of degenerative conditions.
7.	Used for predicting patient's return to normalcy
8.	Used for judgment of fitness
9.	Used in forensic psychology for certification purposes

dysfunction may be understood as the impairment of these functional abilities. While some cognitive dysfunctions are reversible or improve with rehabilitative techniques, some may worsen over time. This may impact other domains of the patient's life. These deficits may not be clinically apparent. The adequate working of these cognitive domains is assessed by various psycho-diagnostic tests.

Studying cognition is important in neurological conditions as in such conditions, the patients are at the highest risk of nervous system injuries. In mild traumatic brain injury (mTBI), dysfunction is seen across the domains of attention, memory, executive functioning, and processing speed. Mood symptoms like depression, anxiety, and irritability also persist. It is also associated with cognitive deficits in verbal learning and memory [5]. Disruption of these domains causes additional disturbances in communication, activities of daily living, and quality of life of patients as well as caregivers [6].

Table 34.3 Neuropsychological psycho-diagnostics/ assessment and steps

1.	Review of the history of the present illness for clinical diagnosis
2.	Interview the patient whenever possible and collate collected information to elicit details of onset, course, and degree & nature of cognitive & personality changes
3.	Interview the patient wherever possible and collate information to elicit a profile of premorbid functions
4.	Choice of tests
5.	Tests of handedness
6.	Neuropsychological testing (psychometric testing)
7.	Clinical observation while testing (personal and family)
8.	Interpretation and report writing (correlating the test results, history information, and observation based on the "reason for referral")

The clinical role of neuropsychology in epilepsy is to identify the impact of the disease through its relationship with different factors like age of onset of epilepsy, etiology, type of seizure, and biopsychosocial and cognitive factors. Quality of life (QoL) is an important core component of quality of care in epilepsy, which is assessed by diverse personality and cognitive measures [6]. Neuropsychology focuses on the neuroplasticity mechanisms and the clinical symptoms of cognitive disruption caused by the same [7]. Functional recovery in epilepsy patients is highly attributed to the reorganization processes in the damaged brain, wherein neuropsychological components, such as cognitive retraining hold immense importance [8]. Researchers emphasize the need for multidisciplinary care for the patient, as also supported in the Sneh Bhargava Commission. According to Santhosh et al. [9], all epilepsy surgery centers should have advanced technologies like MRI, SPECT, and PET as well as multidisciplinary teams with neurologists, neurosurgeons, neuroradiologists, psychologists, psychiatrists, and medical social workers in a country like India.

Frequent interictal epileptic activity, recurrent or prolonged seizures, and anti-epileptic drugs may lead to cognitive decline [10]. Poststroke cognitive decline (PSCG) was found to have commonly developed within 3 months of the onset of stroke with varying levels of severity [11]. According to a study, infarction in cerebral arteries could lead to neglect, visual-spatial failures, language disorders, aphasia, mutism, ideational apraxia, right/left confusion, amnesia, and associative visual agnosia, deficits in planning, initiation, monitoring, concentration, and flexibility, sensory loss, impaired arousal, attention, motivation, and executive functioning, memory, or impaired problem solving, attention, memory [12].

34.3 Why

The association between cognitive performance and accomplishments in everyday functioning is one of the most robust correlations in mental/brain health research. This relationship has been recognized for over three decades and replicated across multiple neurological disorders [13].

The most important clinical implication of what we know about cognition and functioning is that individuals with neurological disorders are least likely to have functional deficits when their current cognitive abilities are consistent with their pre-illness functioning. Multiple studies of TBI have demonstrated that recovery of cognitive functioning predicts recovery of everyday functioning much more accurately than measures of the "severity" of the injury [5]. The domains of executive functioning and processing speed may be some of the most crucial measures to indicate functional normality.

Assessment of cognitive changes in progressive degenerative conditions necessitates a methodology distinct from that required for the initial diagnosis of dementia or the evaluation of recovery following TBI. Comparing the patients at different levels of illness duration (and progressive course) enables the clinician to study the pattern of progression in the worsening or improvement of cognitive impairments. This is especially required for pediatric NCC units, wherein longitudinal assessments should be conducted to study the impact of the illness on the cognitive abilities of the patient, and the impact of treatment on the development of other undesirable conditions, such as the use of anesthesia and the probability of developing learning difficulties [14]. Numerous studies have been conducted studying pre- and post-operative neurocognitive factors exhibiting the importance of longitudinal studies and long-term impact in cardiology critical care, and similar studies may be undertaken for NCC [15].

Given below is a brief description of the CoC Model and the types of responsibilities of different psychology support services/para-clinical services that can be provided:

- **Preventive** aspects should include prevention through careful identification of the problem by conducting epidemiological research and by identifying stages where the problems are occurring, thus helping in providing holistic psychological care (counseling and behavioral modification).
- In the **promotive** aspect that includes supporting or actively encouraging, counseling, psycho-educating, and developing a psychosocial model to deal with the idiosyncrasies, e.g., of each neurological condition; the conservative approach using auto-suggestions/meditation/breathing exercises/stress management teams/visualization programs.
- The **curative** medical aspect that becomes functional while the patient is undergoing treatment (either clinical or surgical) and ideally should, e.g., include all neuropsychological standards of care as a part of the core aspect (e.g., treatment of dementia, stroke, epilepsy, head injury, and movement-related disorders,); for pediatric cases besides other, there may be a need to identifying POCD (post-operative cognitive decline) and long-term follow-up of children so that they do not develop scholastic backwardness due to the medical-health condition because these could lead to disability.
- **Rehabilitative Services:** A medical doctor may further refer the patient for different rehabilitative services to other support staff, while he may continue the medical treatment of the patient. Out of many types of rehabilitative services (which the doctor may consider following his final diagnosis), one such service could be a psychological service, e.g., for neurological conditions; neuropsychological services may be needed and provide appropriate psychological intervention/rehabilitation.
- **Palliative Care Services**: These are end-of-life care services. Patients may require psychological services like counseling, supportive therapy, and guidance (e.g., identifying issues that need to be addressed immediately, e.g., focusing on personal issues–finances/registering a will.
- **Disability Assessment:** Psychological disability assessment needs to be done after the medical doctor is of the opinion that all possible treatment options (CoC) have been attempted. Now the patient needs to be con-

sidered for disability under the Chronic Neurological Conditions Act, 2016; assessment of malingering including the percentage of disability following objective measures and not subject measures. This is needed to reduce the financial burden on the government.

A review of the global burden of neurological disease reveals that neurological disorders remain a public health concern (PHC) [16, 17]. Neuropsychological assessment and evaluation provide a thorough clinical presentation of the associated cognitive symptoms, premorbid patient characteristics, and psychosocial history that may be important for the case. According to Prince [11], if neuropsychological psychodiagnostics is done shortly after mTBI, the multidisciplinary team can be informed about any important factors that may interfere with proper recovery, and interventions could be developed to handle the same. Cognitive and psychosocial rehabilitation as well as psychoeducation are provided to the patients and caregivers. The Mental Health Atlas-2017 of the World Health Organization (WHO) [17] compiled data on neurological disorders in various countries and addressed the mental health issues related to said disorders. This further validates the need and importance of the role of clinical neuropsychology in the modern era.

A multi-disciplinary team works together as a part of the Continuum of care *(CoC), a* model where the primary source of contact is a medical doctor, i.e., a neurologist/neurosurgeon for a neurological condition. The patients are referred to different disciplines, such as neuropsychology, a para-clinical service, as the need is felt with a specific reason for the referral, such as clinical neuropsychology for objective psycho-diagnostic assessment to be done and shared back with the primary source of contact of the patient. It is increasingly important for MBBS and MD students to be trained in formulating "reason for referrals" in their medical education to effectively follow the systematic procedure of preoperative assessment and evaluation to elicit the best outcome. Figure 34.1 highlights the role of

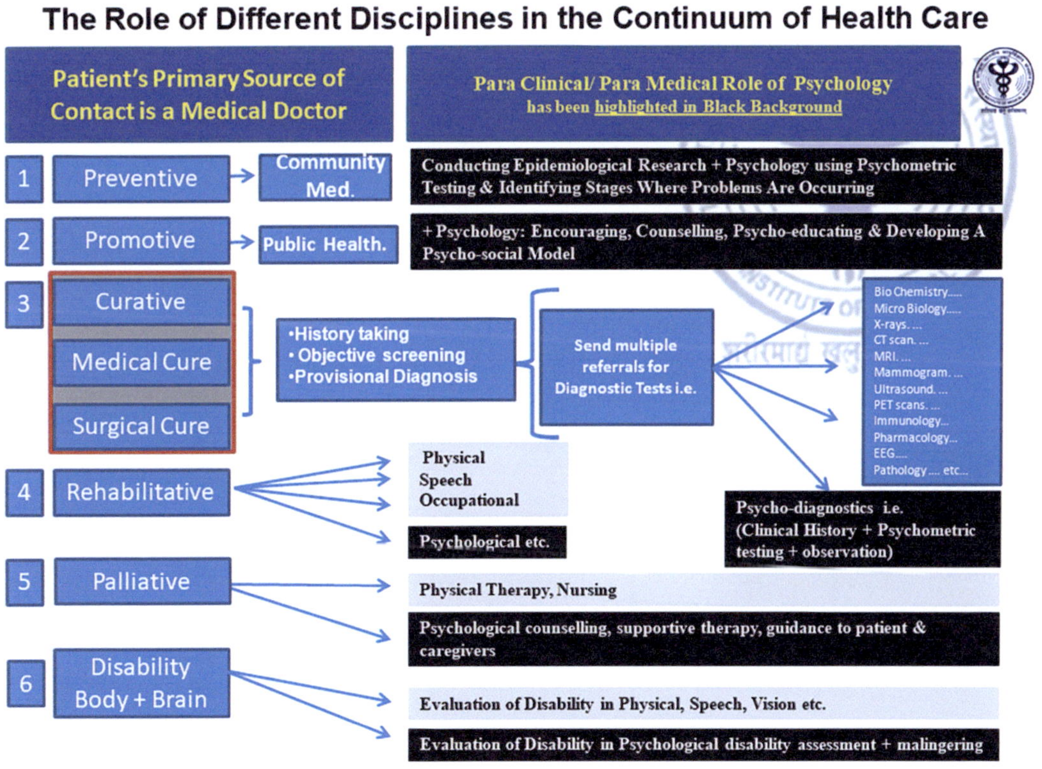

Fig. 34.1 The role of different disciplines in the continuum of health care

neuropsychology among other disciplines in the health care process.

It is also important to note here that patients and caregivers often feel confused and helpless when admitted urgently due to critical cases. They have apprehensions/concerns about what is happening, and how the treatment will be panned out. The role of rapport formation and briefing is critical here for the patient/caregiver to be able to give timely informed consent. Often, they present low insight into the disease and could require assistance with awareness and decision-making, which a clinical neuropsychologist is trained at. Information about the procedure must be provided to the patient based on their level of education and understanding, and document the same. There should be coordination between the medical and para-clinical teams to streamline the process. If the patient is conscious and responding, their informed consent should be taken. The decision to opt for an invasive vs conservative procedure is often shadowed by the caregiver's convenience or financial condition. The patient may even give biased responses or consent in the presence of a caretaker. It is thus important for psychologically and practically trained personnel to be present in the team to facilitate this.

34.4 How

Neuropsychological psycho-diagnostics include (i) clinical history taking, (ii) psychometric assessment, and (iii) clinical observation (Refer to Fig. 34.2). Each neural tissue has a specific function. Any interruption in this complex functional network may lead to problems, r.g., learning and memory issues are complex and may be affected by any disturbance in the neural network. The functions are associated with different areas of the brain. These can be measured by appropriate tests, hence the importance of neuropsychological psycho-diagnostics used by clinical neuropsychologists [an acceptable term by the Houston Conference Guidelines; clinical neuropsychology is a specialty formally recognized by the American Psychological Association (APA) and the Canadian Psychological Association (CPA)]. Clinical neuropsychologists attempt localization but the same may become futile without assessment of higher-level skills, learning, long-term memory, orbitofrontal functions/personality assessment, etc. This highlights the importance of cognitive functions and non-cognitive functions and their inter-linkage, for example, if a person is not motivated, he will not perform well in tests.

Cognitive functioning is evaluated using a performance-based procedure called neuropsychological psycho-diagnostic. Psycho-diagnostics is employed to investigate the cognitive effects of brain injury, brain disease, and severe mental illness. The specific applications of neuropsychological psycho-diagnostic are the collection of diagnostic information, differential diagnostic information, evaluation of treatment response, and prediction of functional potential and functional recovery.

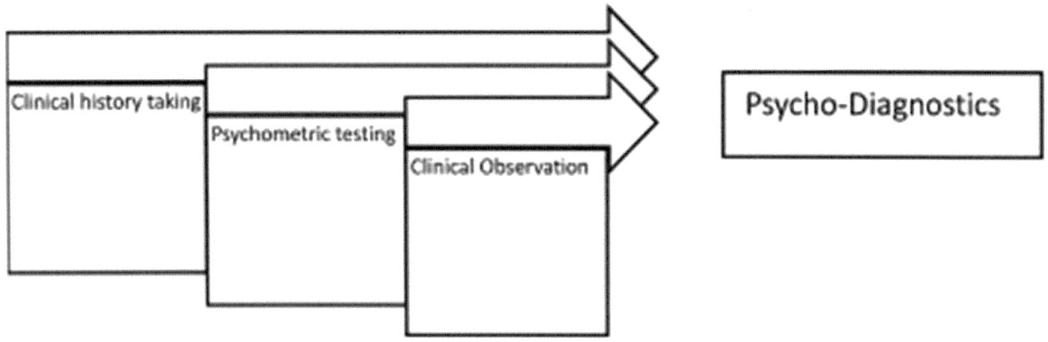

Fig. 34.2 What is psycho-diagnostics

Neuropsychological psycho-diagnostic is indicated when a disease or injury has the potential to impair cognitive functioning. These conditions include diseases or injuries that have a direct effect on cognition (such as degenerative dementias or traumatic brain injuries) as well as instances in which the treatment for a disease influences cognitive functioning, such as chemotherapy. Due to the complexity of neurological disorders, there are chances of altering non-cognitive factors, such as induced mood or motivational changes that may have secondary effects on cognitive functioning. As these secondary effects can result in cognitive changes that are just as real as those induced by a brain injury, a contemporary comprehensive neuropsychological evaluation must include an evaluation of other factors that may be contributing to cognitive impairment.

Neuropsychological psycho-diagnostics is the normatively informed application of performance-based cognitive skill evaluations [5]. The score obtained is compared to norms for age, education, and sex. It includes a clinical and psychometric testing procedure to objectively measure the effects of neurological conditions on cognition, behavioral, vocational, social, and emotional functioning. Typically, neuropsychological psycho-diagnostic is conducted using a battery approach that includes tests of multiple cognitive ability domains and multiple tests per domain, which are selected based on the condition, age, and co-morbidities of the testee. As depicted in Fig. 34.3, the battery approach can be a fixed approach or a flexible approach. These ability domains include memory, focus, processing speed, reasoning, judgment, problem-solving, spatial, and linguistic functions. The trained psychologist/neuropsychologist is to choose between a fixed and flexible approach while choosing these tests. A fixed approach is one wherein a neuropsychological battery is used, all tests need to be administered without omitting as per feasibility or requirement, such as NIMHANS Neuropsychological Battery by Dr. Mukunandan (1996) [1], NIMHANS Neuropsychological battery by Dr. Rao [18], AIIMS Comprehensive Neuropsychological battery by Dr. Surya Gupta (2000), or PGI Battery for Brain Dysfunction by Dr. Pershad and Verma [19]. Practically trained personnel will be able to choose the correct tests using a flexible system to fulfill the requirement based on the reason for referral. Commonly, these assessments may be administered alongside other vital screenings in neuro-critical care units. These screenings may be undertaken by professionals who see the patients' bedside. This not only demonstrates the current cognitive status and non-cognitive factors but also enables tracking the level of cognitive stability, impairment, or improvement following a surgical procedure, medication, or post-discharge. An A-B-A approach is followed for interventions, where possible, i.e., "A" pre-assessment or baseline neuropsychological assessment (best suited for persons undergoing elective procedures after formal consent, followed by the "B" intervention and an "A" post-assessment.

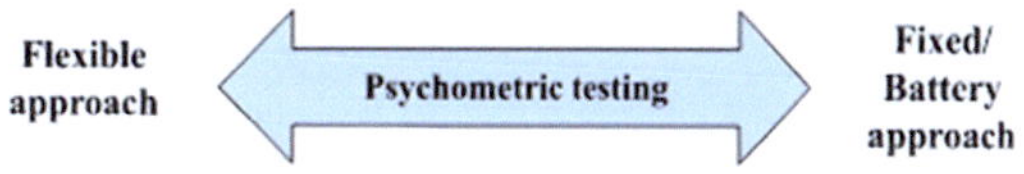

Fig. 34.3 Dichotomy in psychometric testing

Provided that the patient is conscious, alert, awake, and oriented, which may be ensured by screening such as the mini-mental status examination (MMSE), neuropsychological assessments may be used to detect dementia or other memory issues, provide a differential diagnosis, evaluate functional capacity, and assist with timely management of progression of degenerative conditions. These may also assist in the evaluation of functional recovery and evaluation of treatment response. It is important to note that the role of psycho-diagnostics in a clinical setting becomes limited if pre-morbid functioning screening is not done.

Given below is a list of screening tools that can be used by the clinicians (neuro critical care / NCC team in this case) for a quick assessment to formulate a provisional diagnosis and prepare a "Reason for Referral" for sending patients for psycho-diagnostics (Table 34.4).

The neuropsychological psycho-diagnostic provides both general and specific information regarding current cognitive performance levels.

Table 34.4 Useful screenings for NCC units

The table shows a list of screening tools that can be used by a neurocritical team. (The qualifications to administer the same needs to be checked for each of these screening tools.)

Domain	Screening tool	Time is taken (min)
Cognitive	Mini Mental Status Examination (MMSE) [20]	10
	Hindi Mental Status Examination (HMSE) [21]	10
	Montreal Cognitive Assessment (MoCA) [22]	5
	Dementia Assessment Rapid Test (DART) [23]	15
	Neuropsychological Evaluation Screening Tool (NEST) [24]	10
Functional status	Glasgow Outcome Scale (GOS)/ EGOS [25]	5
	Dementia Rating Scale (DRS) [26]	10
	Early Assessment Self Inventory (EASI) [27]	5
	Barthel Index [28]	10
	Functional Independence Measure (FIM) [29]	15
	36-Item and 12-Item Short-Form Health Survey (SF-36/SF-12) [30]	20
	World Health Organization Quality of Life (WHOQOL)/ WHO-BREF [31]	20

The average or composite score across multiple ability domains provides a comprehensive measure of a person's cognitive functioning at the present time. These global scores prove to be the most prevalent indices used to predict real-world functional milestones and to evaluate functioning in conditions where multiple ability domains are affected, such as in traumatic brain injury.

However, it is also essential to be able to make judgments regarding specific deficits across ability domains to be evaluated. For example, a person who has suffered a focal stroke or brain injury may have limited cognitive deficits, with most of their abilities remaining unchanged. When determining the presence of a specific cognitive deficit, such as amnesia, or a broader condition, such as dementia, it is crucial to be able to precisely identify a "differential deficit." [5] In order to distinguish normal variation between ability domains from neuropsychological deficits, it is necessary to consider several distinct factors. This mandates the neuropsychological psycho-diagnostic to be administered and interpreted by a full-time, trained neuropsychologist/ psychologist.

Multiple factors influence intra-individual variation across cognitive ability domains. These include the reliability of the measurements, the normative standards for the measurements, and the individual's level of performance [5]. The discrepancies between ability areas that can be interpreted as genuinely distinct depend on whether the normative standards for the tests were developed using a single sample (i.e., co-normed) or independently. Due to their co-norming on a single sample, meaningful differences between subtests on intelligence tests such as the Wechsler Adult Intelligence scales are smaller than differences between tests that were devised wholly independently of one another. With the same goals in mind, normative comprehensive standards for extended neuropsychological assessment batteries have also been developed. Lastly, performance extremes, both high and low, result in increased evident disparities between ability areas. At the extremes of the distribution, lesser absolute score differences result in larger normative differences.

34.5 Three Stages of Neuropsychological Psycho-diagnostics

34.5.1 Clinical Interview

The trained clinical neuropsychologist asks questions regarding the current condition and symptoms, history of the patient and family's illness, pre-morbid and post-morbid abilities and their impact on their day-to-day lives, and other trivial psycho-social factors. They also interview the caregivers to get a holistic view of the lives of the patients. According to Nehra [13], social, emo-

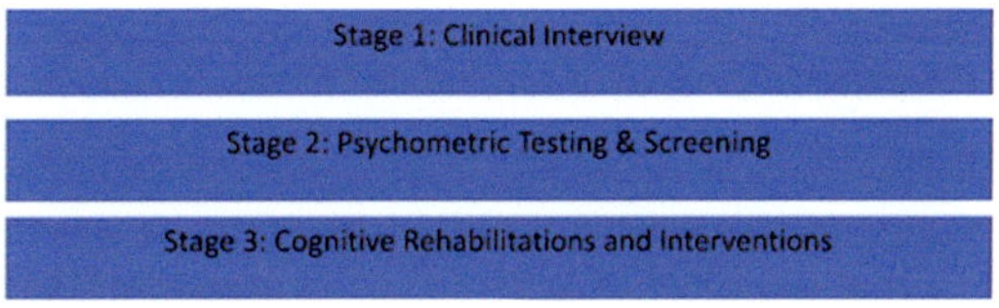

Fig. 34.4 Stages of neuropsychological psycho-diagnostics

tional, personal, family, and vocational factors greatly affect the long-term prognosis of diseases and could lead to heightened psychological stress. Additionally, cognitive, emotional, and somatic symptoms are also taken into account. This information can help identify patients at greater risk of delayed recovery. Recommendations are made in order to prevent any complications that could arise due to such factors that usually go unaddressed/unnoticed. For example, research shows that psychological distress increases the likelihood of mild traumatic brain injury (mTBI) progressing to persistent PCS, and factors like marital status, unemployment, education, disability, and recreational setbacks may lead to a poorer prognosis post-PCS [32]. The earlier neuropsychological evaluation is done post-mTBI, the sooner the medical doctors can be informed of any factors interfering with recovery. Interventions can then be developed timely to prevent the worsening of said factors (Fig. 34.4).

Example. The clinical interview includes [33] (*Assessment Tools for Alzheimer's and Other Dementias as per Indian Setting*):

(1) Socio-demographic details
(2) Major issues (including source and reason for referral)
(3) Family history
(4) Personal and social history
(5) Substance use/dependence
(6) Medical history
(7) Premorbid personality
(8) Neuropsychiatric history
(9) History of present illness
(10) Examinations
(11) Laboratory evaluations

34.5.2 Psychometric Testing

According to the American Psychological Association (APA) [2], psychologists who use psycho-diagnostics strive to maintain their own competence in terms of selecting, using, interpreting, integrating, and communicating their findings; use tests that have sound psychometric properties; are mindful of their potential negative consequences on the patient; and use multiple and reliable clinical information as well as culture fair practices.

Clinical Neuropsychologists use comprehensive neuropsychological batteries that consist of various affected cognitive domains (chosen based on the screening and the reason for referral). For example, patients with mTBI are assessed on usually affected areas like attention, processing speed, executive functioning, and memory [32]. Testing also incorporates self-report measures that probe emotional and somatic symptoms. Patients can also be asked to rank their complaints on a scale of most to least concerning. The gathered information is synthesized to get a holistic view of the etiology of the patient's present complaints.

Qualified professionals can identify which tests to administer at times of urgency for a more brief and focused approach. Trained neuropsychologists know the strengths and weaknesses of all psychometric tests being used and hence can identify the patterns of deficits across the tests since impairment in one domain may not be sufficient to declare a diagnosis.

At times of neurocritical care, it is impractical to administer thorough neuropsychological batteries of assessment. According to Chopra et al. [24], assessment tools should be easy to use, have a short application time, be reliable and valid, and be able to discriminate between cognitive impact and impaired patients. Screening for cognitive deficits becomes increasingly relevant as the incidence of neurological and psychiatric illnesses rises. The authors of the study also explained that numerous screening tests exist but their merit has been questionable, leaving only a few credible ones in the industry [33]. One such Indian screening test is NEST, which was developed with three major objectives: (i) for brief cognitive assessment by clinicians, (ii) for large-scale community screenings, and (iii) for guided and detailed assessment across cognitive abilities. It measures immediate recall, verbal fluency, abstraction, temporal sequencing/executive functioning, visual-constructional ability, and delayed recall. The test can be used on various neurological, neurosurgical, psychiatric, and other medical conditions to screen for cognitive impairment.

34.5.3 Cognitive Rehabilitation and Interventions

Clinical Neuropsychologists address the interplay of cognitive, emotional, and somatic factors in the patients' lives. Additional data regarding their education, disability level, familial situation, financial status, standard of living, mood, motivation, recreational setbacks, and personality are also taken into account while developing effective interventions. Cognitive rehabilitation targets the affected domains identified after evaluation. Clinical Neuropsychologists must first, with psycho-diagnostics, address what is to be rehabilitated and then plan an appropriate goal and strategy. Regular assessments must be done at different time points during this to ensure the success of the rehabilitation model. These neurocognitive interventions and training are provided to help patients regain some level of functioning in their affected cognitive domains like memory, executive functioning, and response inhibition among many others. Interventions could be psycho-educative in nature and involve behavioral, emotional, and social intervention strategies; for example, reassurance and education regarding expectations of recovery, guidance regarding rest, and gradual resumption of daily activities. It is found that brief neuropsychological evolutions done early in the period post-admission may be beneficial. A personalized plan of action is devised for both the patient and the caregiver to follow. Compensatory strategies are taught for optimal functioning as possible to develop and maintain basic life skills. External strategies are also suggested, e.g., keeping a diary to note things and keeping reminders in place.

We anticipate that trained and qualified neuropsychological psychodiagnostics will continue to be utilized, despite advances in imaging technology, because it is well known that the presence of significant brain changes can be associated with nearly normal cognitive functioning, whereas individuals with no lesions detectable on imaging can have significant cognitive and functional limitations.

Neuropsychological psycho-diagnostics require the patient to perform on certain dimensions, actively participate in the procedure, and be fully present. It is thus imperative that the patient should not be under the influence of sedatives at the time of the cognitive evaluation. Psychometric tests should be chosen keeping in consideration factors such as handedness, visual and verbal ability, and cultural, as well as educational backgrounds. An important factor relevant to neuropsychological testing in NCC units is time constraints. Full-fledged psycho-diagnostics may take up to several hours, limiting the feasibility of the procedure altogether. In such scenarios, screenings of various dimensions such as memory, executive functioning, anxiety, or depression may be performed. Commonly employed screenings in India that the authors deem feasible for use in NCC are MMSE [20]/ Hindi Mental Status Examination (HMSE) [21], Montreal Cognitive Assessment (MoCA) [22], Dementia Assessment by Rapid Test (DART) [23], Neuropsychological Evaluation Screening Tool (NEST) [24], and Preliminary Aphasia Screening Test (PAST) [34] among others. There are a few issues to consider when interpreting the results, these include performance changes due to random variation and practice effects, as well as the fact that some cognitive measures are more susceptible to these effects than others, thereby limiting their usefulness as outcome measures. Interpretation of the results on these tests is a training-based skill and must only be done by trained and qualified neuropsychologists to have the best outcome and avoid assessment bias and under or over-generalization of results, cognitive overload, an impaired performance due to lack of motivation and other associated factors, and best ways to overcome these biases for the best outcome. Post-discharge, a full neuropsychological assessment should be planned for a better diagnosis.

34.6 Whom

At times of post-acute phases of neurocritical care, it is less feasible to administer a thorough neuropsychological battery or refer the patient for psycho-diagnostic. Hence, a more brief and focused approach should be taken for evaluation, answering the specific question of the clinician/reason for referral. For the same, experienced neuropsychologists and efficient systematic processes of evaluation should be in place. This would ensure the right information is elicited in the best way possible, with proper pauses and non-verbal cues such as expressions. Cognitive screening tests should be developed for all neuro-critical conditions and situations. These help in recognizing patients who would need further comprehensive assessment.

Since most of the medical tests are machine-driven, there is less chance of error since the accuracy of medical tests is dependent more upon the equipment and less on the person evaluating it. The same is not true for psycho-diagnostics. It is primarily driven by the evaluator wherein; their clinical expertise and experience play a major role in understanding the patient accurately. According to APA [2], psychologists seek to consider the unique issues that may arise when test instruments and assessment approaches designed for specific populations are used with diverse populations. This underlines the importance of competence building/ training of evaluators for performing important psychological assessments [4].

While many of today's medical tests are accurate, the occurrence of false negatives or positives is a well-known fact to clinicians. The same applies to psychological tests/evaluations. The expertise of psychologists is required to understand the patient's feelings of pain, fear, anxiety, and tendency of malingering, neuro-cognitive, and behavioral issues, which are co-morbid throughout the course of illness and often exacerbate the patient's condition. These issues are obligatory to be addressed and are prerequisites for the successful eradication of any psychological illness/concern. The role of psychology in the medical field encompasses diagnosis, breaking bad news, intervention, support, resilience, rehabilitation, return to normalcy, accepting a new normal, and so on and so forth. If psychological aspects are evaluated by untrained persons, it may give false negative or false positive results, which may have an adverse impact on the medical conditions of the patients.

34.7 Conclusion

This chapter discussed the role of neuropsychology in the continuum of care of neuro-critical patients. While the primary role in the multidisciplinary team remains that of the medical doctor, the para-clinical field of clinical neuropsychology requires a specific "reason for referral," which will help them in providing the psycho-diagnostic report, relevant information for predicting functionality and recovery and developing general awareness, insight, and decision-making capacity in the patient. This will also be helpful in obtaining consent from the patient. It will also provide information on insight into the patient, and curative and rehabilitative services to the neuro-critical team for accurately devising the case plan and eliciting the best outcome. There are some implications for the subject matter at hand, which need to be worked on in the future. First, more brief, specific, and focused screening tests should additionally be developed for neuro-critical conditions and situations. For the same, experienced neuropsychologists along with efficient systematic processes of evaluation should be in place with the team. Second, a concept of a multidisciplinary NCC-consent team needs to be conceived for cases where the patient has some level of insight but requires decision-making assistance while giving informed consent. This would ensure efficient and ethical services for the best outcome.

References

1. Mukundan CR. NIMHANS Neuropsychological battery: test description, instruction, clinical data and interpretation. In: Proceedings of national workshop in clinical neuropsychology. Bangalore, India; 1996.
2. American Psychological Association, APA Task Force on Psychological Assessment and Evaluation Guidelines; 2020. APA guidelines for psychological assessment and evaluation. Retrieved from https://www.apa.org/about/policy/guidelines-psychological-assessment-evaluation.pdf
3. Verma SK, Nehra A. Psycho-diagnostics. Psychiatry Today. 1997;1(2):81–4.
4. Talwar S, Gupta A, Nehra A, Makhija N, Kapoor PM, Sreenivas V, Choudhary SK, Airan B. Bidirectional superior cavopulmonary anastomosis with or without cardiopulmonary bypass: a randomized study. J Cardiac Surg. 2017;32(6):376–81. https://doi.org/10.1111/jocs.13149.
5. Harvey PD. Clinical applications of neuropsychological assessment. Dialog Clin Neurosci. 2012;14(1):91–9. https://doi.org/10.31887/dcns.2012.14.1/pharvey.
6. Hermann BP. Quality of life in epilepsy. J Epilepsy. 1992;5(3):153–65. Available from: https://www.sciencedirect.com/science/article/pii/S0896697405801343
7. Armstrong CL, Morrow LA, editors. Handbook of medical neuropsychology: applications of cognitive neuroscience. Cham: Springer International Publishing; 2019.
8. Chaudhary K, Kumaran SS, Chandra SP, Wadhawan AN, Tripathi M. Mapping of cognitive functions in chronic intractable epilepsy: role of fMRI. Indian J Radiol Imaging. 2014;24(1):51–6. https://doi.org/10.4103/0971-3026.130694.
9. Santhosh NS, Sinha S, Satishchandra P. Epilepsy: Indian perspective. Ann Indian Acad Neurol. 2014;17(Suppl. 1):S3–11. https://doi.org/10.4103/0972-2327.128643.
10. Novak A, Vizjak K, Rakusa M. Cognitive impairment in people with epilepsy. J Clin Med. 2022;11(1):267. https://doi.org/10.3390/jcm11010267.
11. Chaurasia RN, Sharma J, Pathak A, Mishra VN, Joshi D. Poststroke cognitive decline: a longitudinal study from a tertiary care center. J Neurosci Rural Pract. 2019;10(3):459–64. https://doi.org/10.1055/s-0039-1697872.
12. Al-Qazzaz N, Ali S, Ahmad SA, Islam S, Mohamad K. Cognitive impairment and memory dysfunction after a stroke diagnosis: a post-stroke memory assessment. Neuropsychiatr Dis Treat. 2014:1677. https://doi.org/10.2147/ndt.s67184.
13. Nehra A, Tripathi M, Srivastava MVP. Neuropsychological disability: a hidden epidemic of neurological conditions. Neurol India. 2020;68(1):154–8. https://doi.org/10.4103/0028-3886.279709.
14. Slomine BS, Silverstein FS, Christensen JR, Page K, Holubkov R, Dean JM, et al. Neuropsychological outcomes of children 1 year after pediatric cardiac arrest: Secondary analysis of 2 randomized clinical trials: secondary analysis of 2 randomized clinical trials. JAMA Neurol. 2018;75(12):1502–10. https://doi.org/10.1001/jamaneurol.2018.2628.
15. Kidambi BR, Purohit V, Bajpai S, Nehra A, Karthikeyan G. Is the use of high-intensity atorvastatin associated with memory impairment? Indian Heart J. 2022;74(1):66–8. https://doi.org/10.1016/j.ihj.2021.12.006.
16. Nehra A. Role of neuropsychology in continuum of health care in neurological conditions. Neurol India. 2019;67(2):404–9. https://doi.org/10.4103/0028-3886.258013.
17. Mental Health Atlas 2017. Geneva: World Health Organization; 2018. Licence: CC BY-NC-SA 3.0 IGO.
18. Kar BR, Rao SL, Chandramouli BA, Thennarasu K, Satishchandra P. Neuropsychological lateralization of brain dysfunction in children with mesial temporal sclerosis: a presurgical evaluation. J Child Neurol. 2010;25(6):705–14. https://doi.org/10.1177/0883073810363998.
19. Pershad D, Verma SK. Handbook of PGI battery of brain dysfunction (PGI-BBD). Agra: National Psychological Corporation; 1990.
20. Folstein MF, Folstein SE, McHugh PR. "Mini-mental state". A practical method for grading the cognitive state of patients for the clinician. J Psychiatr Res. 1975;12(3):189–98. https://doi.org/10.1016/0022-3956(75)90026-6.
21. Tiwari SC, Tripathi RK, Kumar A. Applicability of the mini mental state examination (MMSE) and the Hindi mental state examination (HMSE) to the urban elderly in India: a pilot study. Int Psychogeratr. 2009;21(1):123–8. https://doi.org/10.1017/S1041610208007916.
22. Nasreddine ZS, Phillips NA, Bédirian V, Charbonneau S, Whitehead V, Collin I, Cummings JL, Chertkow H. The Montreal Cognitive Assessment, MoCA: a brief screening tool for mild cognitive impairment. J Am Geriatr Soc. 2005;53(4):695–9. https://doi.org/10.1111/j.1532-5415.2005.53221.x. Erratum in: J Am Geriatr Soc. 2019 Sep;67(9):1991
23. Swati B, Sreenivas V, Manjari T, Ashima N. Dementia assessment by rapid test (DART): An Indian screening tool for dementia. J Alzheimers Dis Parkinsonism. 2015 (3) (PDF) Dementia Assessment by Rapid Test (DART): An Indian Screening Tool for Dementia. Available from: https://www.researchgate.net/publication/290211871_Dementia_Assessment_by_Rapid_Test_DART_An_Indian_Screening_Tool_for_Dementia [accessed Apr 21 2023].

24. Chopra S, Kaur H, Pandey RM, Nehra A. Development of neuropsychological evaluation screening tool: an education-free cognitive screening instrument. Neurol India. 2018;66(2):391–9. https://doi.org/10.4103/0028-3886.227304.
25. McMillan T, Wilson L, Ponsford J, Levin H, Teasdale G, Bond M. The Glasgow outcome scale—40 years of application and refinement. Nat Rev Neurol. 2016;12(8):477–85. https://doi.org/10.1038/nrneurol.2016.89.
26. Mattis S. Dementia rating scale. Professional manual. Odessa: Psychological Assessment Resources; 1988.
27. Horn L, Cohen CI, Teresi J. The EASI: a self-administered screening test for cognitive impairment in the elderly. J Am Geriatr Soc. 1989;37(9):848–55. https://doi.org/10.1111/j.1532-5415.1989.tb02265.x.
28. Lee YC, Chen SS, Koh CL, Hsueh IP, Yao KP, Hsieh CL. Development of two Barthel index-based supplementary scales for patients with stroke. PLoS One. 2014;9(10):e110494. https://doi.org/10.1371/journal.pone.0110494.
29. Dickson HG, Köhler F. Functional independence measure (FIM). Scand J Rehabil Med. 1999;31(1):63–4. https://doi.org/10.1080/003655099444740.
30. Ware JE, Kosinski M, Dewey JE, et al. SF-36 health survey: manual and interpretation guide. Lincoln: Quality Metric Inc.; 2000.
31. Development of the World Health Organization. WHOQOL-BREF quality of life assessment. The WHOQOL Group. Psychol Med. 1998;28(3):551–8. https://doi.org/10.1017/s0033291798006667.
32. Prince C, Bruhns ME. Evaluation and treatment of mild traumatic brain injury: the role of neuropsychology. Brain Sci. 2017;7(8):105. https://doi.org/10.3390/brainsci7080105.
33. Nehra A. Assessment tools for Alzheimer's and other dementias as per indian setting. In: Tripathi M, editor. Dementia decoded. Kontentworx; 2014. p. 255–92.
34. Kaur H, Nehra A, Chopra S, Bhatia R. Aphasia screening test; 2020 [Unpublished manuscript].

Part VI

Supportive Neurocritical Care

35 Mechanical Ventilation in Traumatic/Acute Brain Injury

Kapil G Zirpe and Sushma Gurav

35.1 Introduction

Neurocritical care covers a variety of patients, among them are majority of patients with acute brain injury (ABI) defined as acute cerebral disorder secondary to traumatic brain injury (TBI), acute ischemic stroke (AIS), intracranial hemorrhage (ICH), or subarachnoid hemorrhage (SAH) [1, 2]. Primary brain injury is the main factor in determining morbidity and mortality in these patients, but medical complications do occur frequently, with respiratory dysfunction being the commonest cause [3]. Associated risk factors further complicate acute respiratory distress syndrome which has been associated with poor outcomes. About 30% of cases of ABI are associated with acute lung injury (ALI), and occurrence of acute respiratory distress syndrome (ARDS) is observed [4, 5]. Raised intracranial pressure (ICP) was defined as >20 mmHg when invasive monitoring was done, or as clinical or radiological signs of intracranial hypertension are seen [2, 6]. ABI patients often require invasive ventilation or other forms of respiratory support during their admission period in intensive care. Due to the scarcity of proper evidence-based studies, there is a lack of clarity about guidelines on intubation in ABI ventilation, ventilator liberation, extubation, and tracheostomy in ABI patients.

Acute respiratory distress syndrome (ARDS) is characterized by a heterogeneous inflammatory process of the lung, causing edema, disruption of alveolar endothelial and epithelial linings, leading to hypoxia and decreased compliance. Thus, it is defined as acute onset of pulmonary edema, within a week of the clinical brunt, development of bilateral radiographic opacities on chest imaging, and a PaO_2/FiO_2 ratio of <300 mmHg overt cardiac etiology is ruled out. Based on the degree of hypoxemia, ARDS is classified into three categories: mild (200 mmHg > $PaO_2/FIO_2 \leq$ 300 mmHg), moderate (100 mmHg < $PaO_2/FIO_2 \leq$ 200 mmHg), and severe ($PaO_2/FIO_2 \leq$ 100 mmHg) [7].

The main goal of mechanical ventilation (MV) is to provide oxygenation and modulate cerebral hemodynamics through the control of arterial carbon dioxide tension. But along with this hemodynamics, MV exerts harmful effects on the brain due to complex interactions occurring between intrathoracic, central venous and intracranial compartments. Changes in the partial pressure of carbon dioxide ($PaCO_2$) and oxygen affect cerebral perfusion pressure and cause secondary injury [1]. This interaction acts as a hurdle in managing brain-injured patients with ARDS by lung protective ventilation. The efficacy of rescue therapies such as prone positioning, alveolar recruitment maneuvers (ARMs), and extracorpo-

K. G. Zirpe · S. Gurav (✉)
Neuro Trauma Intensive Care Unit, Grant Medical Foundation, Ruby Hall Clinic,
Pune, Maharashtra, India

H. Prabhakar et al. (eds.), *Principles and Practice of Neurocritical Care*,
https://doi.org/10.1007/978-981-99-8059-8_35

real membrane oxygenation (ECMO) in acute brain injury with ARDS is not established.

35.2 Epidemiology and Risk Factors of ARDS in Acute Brain Injury

Incidence of ARDS/ALI in neurocritical care ranged from 10 to 35% [4, 8]. Hoesch et al. have shown that there is a strong association between loss of cough or gag reflexes and development of ARDS in patients with ABI [9]. Loss of these protective reflexes increases the risk of aspiration. Loss of lower brain stem function is an important factor that can independently cause acute lung injury [9].

Traumatic brain injury and acute stroke patients are widely being studied for the association of ARDS. Apart from above-mentioned risk factors, polytrauma leads to pulmonary contusions and hemorrhagic shock requiring massive transfusion of blood products, use of vasoactive agents, history of drug abuse, and hypertension [10]. Severe head injury which is defined by GCS and radiological findings has been associated with ARDS. TBI patients who develop ARDS have higher mortality and have lower functional outcomes defined by the Glasgow Outcome Scale >4 (23 vs. 34% $p = 0.02$), compared with those without ARDS [11].

The prevalence of ARDS in stroke varies widely depending on the type of stroke and the level of availability of the health care system. Thus, the prevalence of ARDS varies from 4% in acute ischemic stroke to 27% in intracerebral bleed and 15% in aneurysmal subarachnoid patients [10, 12]. Elmer also documented that the use of high tidal volume (TV) (>8 mL/kg) was strongly associated with the development of ARDS in mechanically ventilated ICH patients [12].

35.2.1 Milestone of MV in Neurologically Diseased Patients

In 1952, during the poliomyelitis epidemic in Copenhagen, Dr. Lassen, chief physician and incharge of poliomyelitis cases, took the help of anesthesiologist, Dr. Björn Ibsen, in the management of 12-year-old polio patient. The patient was tracheostomized, sedated, and manually ventilated. She survived this polio battle; thus became the first neurological diseased patient requiring mechanical ventilation (MV) [13, 14].

35.3 Pathophysiology of Lung Injury in Acute Brain Injury: Brain Lung Cross Talk

There are multiple theories about the mechanism of injury to the lung shortly after brain injury. The "blast injury" is a widely accepted theory for lung injury after brain damage. Sympathetic storm occurs post-brain injury leading to an increase in intravascular pressure followed by disruption of the alveolocapillary membrane. This theory is attributed either to hydrostatic forces (supported by a low pulmonary/plasma protein ratio) or to high-permeability mechanisms. This catecholamine surge causesincreased extravascular lung water causing neurogenic pulmonary edema [15].

A systemic inflammatory response after brain injury plays an important role in causing lung injury. After a brain injury, there is increased intracranial production and release of proinflammatory mediators in microglia and astrocytes. These mediators leak into systemic circulation via the disrupted blood-brain barrier and reach various organs. These inflammatory mediators and cytokine together can cause pulmonary tissue damage [16].

Another hypothesis is that severe brain damage may induce lung injury through the modulation of neurokinins (substance P and neurokinin A). Neurokinins cause bronchoconstriction mucosal edema, increased vascular permeability, and pulmonary edema, leading to lung injury. Increased respiratory system flow resistance (Rmin, rs) could be due to bronchoconstriction [17].

One more concept is that acute brain injury leads to impairment of the parasympathetic nervous system and the immunoregulatory function of the vagus. This causes loss of the protective

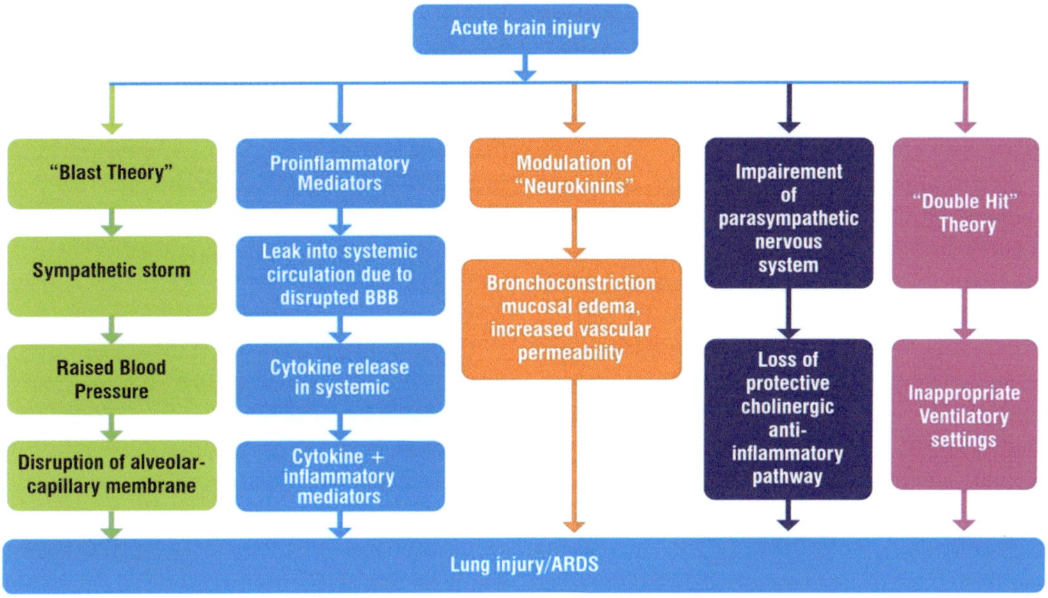

Fig. 35.1 Pathophysiology of acute lung injury in acute brain injury brain-lung cross talk

cholinergic anti-inflammatory pathway. This can cause acute lung injury in acute brain injury patients. In "double hit" theory inappropriate ventilator settings will escalate the injury caused by "first hit"-inflammatory mediators, sympathetic storm or direct injury to lung [3, 18]. See Fig. 35.1 for the pathophysiology of brain and lung cross talk in ABI.

Thus, brain-lung interaction in brain injury patients seems to be fragile, so mechanical ventilator management in this situation is a challenge.

35.4 Ventilatory Strategies

The ventilatory strategy for any patient requiring mechanical ventilation aims at maintaining adequate oxygenation and avoiding hypercapnia. The control of carbon dioxide protects the intracranial pressure and cerebral blood flow and thus prevent secondary brain injury. While achieving this, we need to prevent ventilator-induced lung injuries (VILI). Intense hypocapnia should be avoided, as this may compromise cerebral blood flow and aggravate hypoperfusion. At the same time, high tidal volumes to maintain mild hypocapnia ($PaCO_2$—30 to 35 mmHg) for the treatment of raised intracranial pressure may trigger the pulmonary and systemic inflammatory response in patients with ARDS [19]. This deleterious effect can be seen even in patients without ARDS. As stated in the "double hit" theory, inappropriate ventilator settings would escalate the injury caused by "first hit"-inflammatory mediators, sympathetic storm, or direct injury to the lung in brain injury patients [18].

Elmer et al. showed that in mechanically ventilated patients with intracerebral hemorrhage, high tidal volume causes VILI which further leads to ARDS. The probable reasons put forth are high mechanical stretch with consequent alveolar distention, alveolar epithelial and vascular endothelial disruption and inflammation may have led to the exacerbation of lung injury and ARDS in acute brain injury patients [12].

Quilez has stated in his study that MV promoted brain activation and highlighted the cross talking mechanism between the lungs and the brain [20]. He further found that brain activation was seen more in patients ventilated with high tidal volume. The pathogenic mechanism of lung stretch induced hippocampal apoptosis. Lopez in his study put forth the pathogenic mechanism of lung stretch-induced hippocampal apoptosis as a result of type 2 dopamine receptor activation in response to vagal signaling. Hence, the importance of selection of appropriate ventilatory settings in the management of acute lung injury with acute brain injury.

Koutsoukou carried out a study about the application of positive end-expiratory pressure (PEEP) in brain injury patients without acute lung injury [21]. Application of moderate levels of PEEP for 5 days prevented lung damage in these patients. In his study, Korovesi ventilated acute brain injury patients with no apparent lung injury, with zero positive end-expiratory pressure (ZEEP) [22]. He observed that these patients exhibited early and sustained increases of circulating inflammatory indices as compared with patients on 8 cmH_2O of PEEP. The reasons put forth were the application of PEEP prevents end-expiratory collapse and maintains alveoli recruited. In acute brain injury patients, damage to pneumocytes II causes abnormal surfactant production. This along with the release of inflammatory mediators may increase peripheral airway closure and atelectasis. Opening and closing of these atelectatic airways during the respiratory cycle generates shear stresses, causing damage to peripheral airways. Thus, PEEP protects against "low volume" injury, that is the lung damage attributable to cyclic airway closure [22].

Studies about the effects of PEEP on ICP and cerebral perfusion pressure have conflicting results; hence, application of PEEP in ventilating head-injured patients is considered controversial. PEEP helps in improving oxygenation [23] but on the other hand increases mean intrathoracic pressure and therefore might increase ICP by reducing venous drainage. Raised intrathoracic pressure causes a decrease in mean arterial pressure and, in turn, may decrease cerebral blood flow in patients with compromised cerebral autoregulation. In an animal study, Luce et al. published that the effect of PEEP on ICP was obvious if PEEP applied was more than ICP [24]. McGuire et al. documented that PEEP up to 15 cmH_2O did not affect central nervous system if baseline ICP values were more than PEEP set on a ventilator [25]. Huynch et al. have shown that increases in PEEP up to 15 cmH_2O by an increment of 5 cmH_2O reduced ICP and improved cerebral perfusion pressure [26]. Doblar et al. showed that euvolemia prevented a drop in mean arterial pressure and cerebral perfusion pressure [27].

Clinical studies about the influence of respiratory system mechanics on the transmission of PEEP to intracranial pressure are contradictory. Lima et al. documented that the PEEP effect on ICP was not clinically observed. In patients with hemorrhagic stroke and normal respiratory system compliance, PEEP up to 14 cmH2O significantly increased ICP but had no effect on cerebral perfusion pressure [28].

Optimal ventilator strategies in the management of acute respiratory failure associated with brain injury are not well established. An international survey was carried out by the European Society of Intensive Care Medicine (ESICM) on the VENTILO-VENTILatOry strategies in patients with severe traumatic brain injury [29]. An electronic questionnaire, including 38 items and 3 different clinical scenarios, was drafted. This questionnaire was available on the European Society of Intensive Care Medicine (ESICM) website between November 2018 and March 2019. The three case scenarios included arterial partial pressure of oxygen (PaO_2)/inspired fraction of oxygen (FiO_2) > 300 (scenario 1), 150–300 (scenario 2), and <150 (scenario 3). About 687 responses were recorded, and maximum were intensivists and anesthesiologists. The data collected revealed the ventilatory setting commonly preferred: tidal volume (TV) was 6–8 mL/kg of predicted body weight (PBW) in scenarios 1–2 and 4–6 mL/kg/PBW in scenario 3. The common level of highest positive end-expiratory pressure (PEEP) used was 15 cmH_2O in patients with a $PaO_2/FiO_2 \leq 300$ without intracranial

Table 35.1 Lung protective ventilator settings and goals (adapted from www.ardsnet.org)

Basic settings	1. Calculate predicted body weight (PBW) of patient Male: 50 + 2.3 (height in inches—60) Female: 45 + 2.3 (height in inches—60) 2. Initial tidal volume: 8 mL/kg 3. Set PEEP (positive end-expiratory pressure): 5 cmH_2O 4. Set FiO_2 to accept SaO_2: 88–95% 5. Reduce tidal volume 1 mL/kg every 2 h till we reach 6 mL/kg
Monitoring of plateau pressure	When tidal volume = 6 mL/kg achieved, measure Ppl If Ppl > 30 cmH_2O reduce tidal volume 1 mL/kg increments until tidal volume + 4 mL/kg or Ppl < 30 cmH_2O achieved
Monitoring pH	1. Arterial blood gas analysis: look for respiratory acidosis 2. Look for pH: If pH = 7.15–7.30 increase respiratory rate until pH > 7.30 or respiratory rate = 35 3. If pH < 7.15, increase the respiratory rate to 35, if respiratory rate is already 35, increase tidal volume 1 mL/kg increments until pH > 7.15
Lung protective optimal settings	Tidal volume, V_T: 6 mL/kg, Ppl ≤ 30 cmH_2O, pH = 7.30–7.45, SpO_2–88-95%

hypertension and 10 cmH_2O in patients with intracranial hypertension. The accepted carbon dioxide target was 36–40 mmHg, whereas the PaO_2 target was 81–100 mmHg in all the three scenarios.

The lung protective MV (LPMV) is now a proven effective method in reducing complications and side effects in ARDS patients (see Table 35.1).

Evidence-based recommendations on best clinical practices for mechanical ventilation in patients with ABI are considered sequentially right from the need for intubation to liberation. These points are depicted in Fig. 35.2.

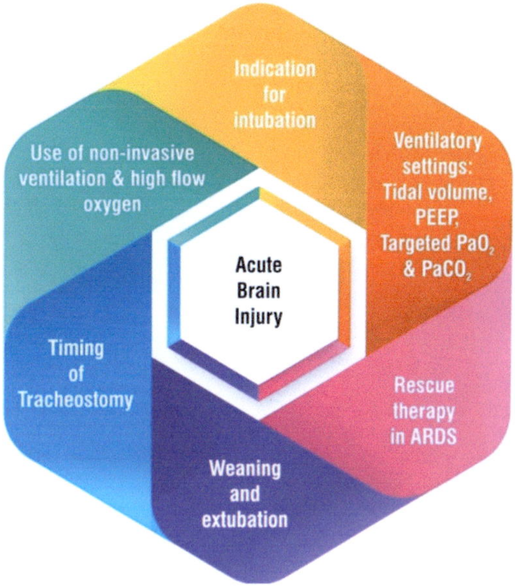

Fig. 35.2 Points to be considered in mechanical ventilation in acute brain injury

35.5 Putting It All Together from Intubation to Extubation and Finally Indications for Tracheostomy [2]

No robust recommendation can be made but consensus recommendations are put fourth regarding the indications of intubation, ventilator strategy, tracheostomy, rescue therapies, and weaning from the ventilator.

1. **What Are the Indications for Endotracheal Intubation in Patients with ABI?**

   The factors that contribute to the decision to intubate in ABI are specifically related to neurological, respiratory, circulatory failure, and general factors. The recommendations for endotracheal intubations are guided by factors such as level of consciousness, severe agitation, loss of airway protective reflexes, and significant raised ICP (see Fig. 35.3).

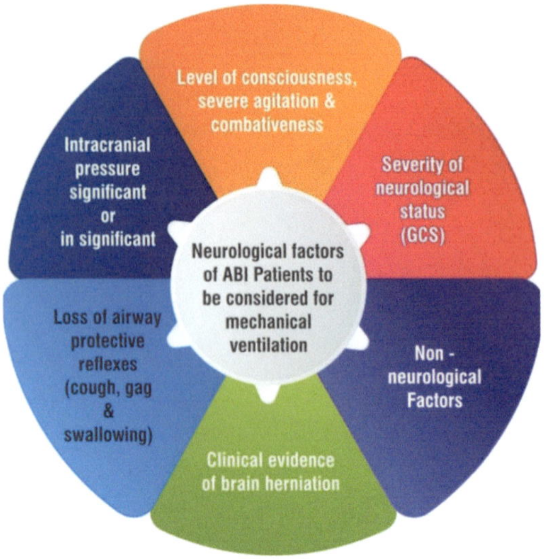

Fig. 35.3 Neurological factors of patient with acute brain injury to be considered for mechanical ventilation

Intubation is recommended in the following:

(a) Patient who are comatose (Glass Coma Scale [GCS] ≤ 8)
(b) Loss of airway protective reflexes (cough reflex, gag, and swallowing)
(c) An increased intracranial pressure (>20 mmHg or radiological or clinical signs of raised intracranial pressure)
(d) Patients with ABI who have clinical evidence of brain herniation
(e) Patients with ABI who have nonneurological indications for intubation
(f) Patients with ABI who have severe agitation and combativeness

2. **Can We Use Noninvasive Respiratory Support in Patients with ABI?**

There was no firm recommendation found on the use of noninvasive ventilation for hypercapnic or mixed hypercapnic/hypoxemic respiratory insufficiency in acute brain-injured patients with TBI.

3. **What Are the Specific Mechanical Ventilation Settings** in Patients with ABI?

Specific ventilator settings [tidal volume and positive end-expiratory pressure (PEEP)] that would benefit patients with ABI depend on whether the patient has ARDS or whether patient has significantly raised ICP (see Table 35.2).

(a) **Category A:** ABI without ARDS who do not have clinically significant ICP elevation: The patient should be ventilated similar to patients without brain injury.
(b) **Category B**: ABI without ARDS who have clinically significant ICP elevation that is PEEP-insensitive (patients who do not experience ICP elevation after an increase of PEEP): This patient should be ventilated with the same level of PEEP that is used as in patients without ABI.
(c) **Category C**: ABI and ARDS who do not have clinically significant intracranial pressure (ICP) elevation: This patient needs to be ventilated with a lung protective setting.
(d) **Category D**: ABI with ARDS clinically significant raised ICP consensus is unable to provide recommendations regarding lung protective ventilation.

4. **What Are the Target Values of Partial Pressure of Oxygen (PaO_2) and Partial Pressure of Carbon Dioxide ($PaCO_2$) in Patients with ABI?**

We should aim for normoxia as hypoxemia and hyperoxia may have an unfavorable effect on clinical outcomes. The optimal goal for PaO_2 in patients with ABI who do not have clinically significant ICP elevation or have clinically significant ICP elevation is 80–120 mmHg.

For patients with ABI with brain herniation or management of TBI patients who have increased intracranial pressure, hyperventilation is a therapeutic option or bridge before surgery. In patients with ABI without significant increased ICP, we should aim for a normal range of $PaCO_2$ values (35–45 mmHg).

5. **What Are the Criteria for Ventilator Weaning and Extubation in Patients with ABI?**

For weaning in patients with ABI, the neurological status and course of disease should be taken into account.

The important factors to be considered before extubation in a patient with ABI are

Table 35.2 Recommendations for ventilation in patients with acute brain injury (ABI)

1. Category	ABI who do not have clinically significant ICP elevation	ABI who have clinically significant ICP elevation that is PEEP-insensitive	ABI who have clinically significant ICP elevation that is PEEP-sensitive	ABI and ARDS who do not have clinically significant ICP elevation	ABI + ARDS & clinically significant ICP elevation
2. Ventilatory strategy	Lung protective ventilation	Unable to provide a recommendation	No recommendation	Lung protective ventilation	Unable to provide a recommendation
PEEP	Same level of PEEP should be used as in patients without brain injury	Same level of PEEP should be used as in patients without ABI			
Strength of recommendation	Strong recommendation	Strong recommendation		Strong recommendation	No recommendation
PaO_2	The optimal target range of 80–120 mmHg accepted				
$PaCO_2$ *level*		35–45 mmHg	Hyperventilation as a bridge to surgery		
Rescue interventions: (a) Recruitment maneuver, ECMO, ECCOR (b) Prone (c) Muscle relaxant				(a) Unable to provide recommendation (b) Can give prone (c) short-term treatment	(a) Unable to provide recommendation (b) No recommendation – Short-term treatment
Extubation criteria	Points to consider: Clinical trajectory of the underlying neurological condition, – the level of consciousness, – the presence of airway protective reflexes, and – factors relevant to the extubation of nonneurological patients – No specific GCS threshold to be considered in the decision to extubate mechanically ventilated acute brain-injured patients				
Weaning	Points to consider: Same as above				
Indications for tracheostomy in patients with ABI and optimal timing of tracheostomy	Points to consider: 1. Failed one or several trials of extubation 2. Persistently reduced level of consciousness Timing of tracheostomy: unable to provide a recommendation				

expected clinical illness outcome, neurological condition (GCS), the level of consciousness, the presence of airway protective reflexes (cough, gag, swallowing), and factors relevant to the extubation of nonneurological patients.

6. **What Are the Indications for and Optimal Timing of Tracheostomy in Patients with ABI**?

   The decision to perform tracheostomy should be one or more failed attempts of extubation trials and depressed neurological responsiveness. Regarding timing of tracheostomy in these patients, no optimal timing is being recommended.

7. **Are Rescue Interventions to Support Severe Respiratory Failure Effective and Safe in Patients with ABI**?

   Prone Positioning

   Prone position can be considered in patients with ABI and moderate ARDS (PaO_2/FiO_2 < 150), without significant raised ICP. Here, benefits of improving oxygenation to brain and favorable effect on ARDS lung with its outcome are weighed against the risk of complications in ABI patients.

   Alveolar Recruitment Maneuver

   No studies are found specifically for assessing muscle relaxants as recruitment maneuvers or as rescue techniques for ventilation of ABI patients with ARDS. Laurent Papazian in his multicenter, double-blind trial on patients undergoing mechanical ventilation for severe acute respiratory distress syndrome (ARDS) concluded that early administration of a neuromuscular blocking agent improved the adjusted 90-day survival and increased the time off the ventilator without increasing muscle weakness.

   Thus short-term treatment with neuromuscular blockers, combined with appropriate sedation, may be considered in mechanically ventilated patients who have concurrent ABI and severe ARDS.

   No recommendations are put forth about the role of ECMO and extracorporeal CO2 removal (ECCO2R) in ABI with severe respiratory failure patients.

35.6 Conclusion

Neuroprotection and prevention of secondary brain injury are the main principles in neurointensive care. ARDS is the most common nonneurologic organ dysfunction in severe acute brain injury patients. Cross talk between the brain and lung is the culprit for acute lung injury. Protecting the lungs while protecting the brain is the mission of modern neurointensive care. Lung protective ventilation is effective in patients of ABI with ARDS. ICP level needs to be considered before adjusting PEEP. Targeted PaO_2 is 80–120 mmHg and normocapnia is recommended.

References

1. Borsellino B, Schultz MJ, de Abreu MG, Robba C, Bilotta FF. Mechanical ventilation in neurocritical care patients: a systematic literature review. Expert Rev Respir Med. 2016;10(10):1123–32.
2. Robba C, Poole D, McNett M, Asehnoune K, Bösel J, Bruder N, et al. Mechanical ventilation in patients with acute brain injury: recommendations of the European Society of Intensive Care Medicine consensus. Intensive Care Med. 2020;46:2397–410.
3. Koutsoukou A, Katsiari M, Orfanos SE, Kotanidou A, Daganou M, Kyriakopoulou M, et al. Respiratory mechanics in brain injury: a review. World J Crit Care Med. 2016;5(1):65–73.
4. Holland MC, Mackersie RC, Morabito D, et al. The development of acute lung injury is associated with worse neurologic outcome in patients with severe traumatic brain injury. J Trauma. 2003;55(1):106–11.
5. Kahn JM, Caldwell EC, Deem S, et al. Acute lung injury in patients with subarachnoid hemorrhage: incidence, risk factors, and outcome. Crit Care Med. 2006;34(1):196–202.
6. de Moraes FM, Silv GS. Noninvasive intracranial pressure monitoring methods: a critical review. Arq Neuropsiquiatr. 2021;79(5):437–46.
7. Gorman EA, O'Kane CM, McAuley DF. Acute respiratory distress syndrome in adults: diagnosis, outcomes, long-term sequelae, and management. Lancet. 2022;400(10358):1157–70.
8. Ziaka M, Exadaktylo A. Brain–lung interactions and mechanical ventilation in patients with isolated brain injury. Crit Care. 2021;25:358.
9. Hoesch RE, Lin E, Young M, Gottesman RF, Altaweel L, Nyquist PA, et al. Acute lung injury in critical neurological illness. Crit Care Med. 2012;40:587–93.
10. Humayun M, Premraj L, Shah V, Cho S-M. Mechanical ventilation in acute brain injury patients with acute

respiratory distress syndrome. Front Med (Lausanne). 2022;9:99988.
11. Fan TH, Huang M, Gedansky A, Price C, Robba C, Hernandez AV, et al. Prevalence and outcome of acute respiratory distress syndrome in traumatic brain injury: a systematic review and meta-analysis. Lung. 2021;199:603–10.
12. Elmer J, Hou P, Wilcox SR, Chang Y, Schreiber H, Okechukwu I, et al. Acute respiratory distress syndrome after spontaneous intracerebral hemorrhage. Crit Care Med. 2013;41:1992–2001.
13. Bruni A, Garofalo E, Pelaia C, Longhini F, Navales P. Mechanical ventilation in brain injured patients: seeing the forest for the trees. Intensive Care Med. 2017;43:957–70.
14. Lassen HC. A preliminary report on the 1952 epidemic of poliomyelitis in Copenhagen with special reference to the treatment of acute respiratory insufficiency. Lancet. 1953;1:37–41.
15. Theodore J, Robin ED. Pathogenesis of neurogenic pulmonary oedema. Lancet. 1975;2:749–51. [PMID: 52777].
16. Ott L, McClain CJ, Gillespie M, Young B. Cytokines and metabolic dysfunction after severe head injury. J Neurotrauma. 1994;11:447–72. [PMID: 7861440].
17. Campos MM, Calixto JB. Neurokinin mediation of edema and inflammation. Neuropeptides. 2000;34:314–22.
18. Mascia L. Acute lung injury in patients with severe brain injury: a double hit model. Neurocrit Care. 2009;11:417–26.
19. Ranieri VM, Suter PM, Tortorella C, De Tullio R, Dayer JM, Brienza A, et al. Effect of mechanical ventilation on inflammatory mediators in patients with acute respiratory distress syndrome. JAMA. 1999;282:54–61.
20. Quilez ME, Fuster G, Villar J, Flores C, Martí-Sistac O, Blanch L, López-Aguilar J. Injurious mechanical ventilation affects neuronal activation in ventilated rats. Crit Care. 2011;15:R124.
21. Koutsoukou A, Perraki H, Raftopoulou A, Koulouris N, Sotiropoulou C, Kotanidou A, et al. Respiratory mechanics in brain-damaged patients. Intensive Care Med. 2006;32:1947–54.
22. Korovesi I, Papadomichelakis E, Orfanos SE, GiamarellosBourboulis EJ, Livaditi O, Pelekanou A, et al. Exhaled breath condensate in mechanically ventilated brain-injured patients with no lung injury or sepsis. Anesthesiology. 2011;114:1118–29.
23. Miller JD, Sweet RC, Narayan R, Becker DP. Early insults to the injured brain. JAMA. 1978;240:439–42.
24. Luce JM, Huseby JS, Kirk W, Butler J. A starling resistor regulates cerebral venous outflow in dogs. J Appl Physiol Respir Environ Exerc Physiol. 1982;53:1496–503.
25. McGuire G, Crossley D, Richards J, Wong D. Effects of varying levels of positive end-expiratory pressure on intracranial pressure and cerebral perfusion pressure. Crit Care Med. 1997;25:1059–62.
26. Huynh T, Messer M, Sing RF, Miles W, Jacobs DG, Thomason MH. Positive end-expiratory pressure alters intracranial and cerebral perfusion pressure in severe traumatic brain injury. J Trauma. 2002;53:488–92; discussion 492–493.
27. Doblar DD, Santiago TV, Kahn AU, Edelman NH. The effect of positive end-expiratory pressure ventilation (PEEP) on cerebral blood flow and cerebrospinal fluid pressure in goats. Anesthesiology. 1981;55:244–50.
28. Lima WA, Campelo AR, Gomes RL, Brandão DC. The impact of positive end-expiratory pressure on cerebral perfusion pressure in adult patients with hemorrhagic stroke. Rev Bras Ter Intensiva. 2011;23:291–6.
29. Picetti E, Pelosi P, Taccone FS, Citerio G, Mancebo J, Robba C. VENTILatOry strategies in patients with severe traumatic brain injury: the VENTILO Survey of the European Society of Intensive Care Medicine (ESICM). Crit Care. 2020;24:158.
30. Papazian L, Forel JM, Gacouin A, et al. Neuromuscular blockers in early acute respiratory distress syndrome. N Engl J Med. 2010;363(12):1107–16.

Fluid Management in Neurocritical Care

36

Khalid Khatib

36.1 Introduction

Even though fluid management comprises part of the routine care of critically ill patients, it has profound implications in the neurocritically ill patients. Fluids (type, quantity, and tonicity) have an effect on the state of health and the response to the illness of the injured brain. The injudicious use of fluids in the neurocritical care (NCC) unit leads to complications and secondary injury to the brain in these patients. Various guidelines regarding fluid management in different neurocritical disease states are in use. The overriding principle in almost all guidelines is maintaining euvolemia. Not only is hypovolemia deleterious, but even hypervolemia is dangerous. The factors governing the complex relationship between brain tissue, fluids, and electrolytes and how they are used for the clinical benefit of the patient will ultimately decide the end result.

36.2 Pathophysiology

The various factors affecting fluid balance in patients with brain injury are summarized in Table 36.1. These patients are also likely to develop central endocrine abnormalities and the use of hyperosmolar or other drug therapies will lead to sodium (Na) and water disturbances. These two factors will further enhance the difficulty in fluid management.

Table 36.1 Factors affecting fluid balance in the brain-injured patient

Fluid factors	Patient-dependent factors
Quantity/Volume	State of blood brain barrier
Components/Type	Volume and circulation of CSF
Tonicity	Presence of inflammation
	Autoregulation
	Venous obstruction
	State of systemic circulation

36.2.1 Tonicity of Administered Fluids

Plasma, CSF, and brain interstitial fluid are normally in a state of osmolar equilibrium. The administration of hypotonic fluid leads to a cerebral shift of water as the blood brain barrier (BBB) is permeable to water. But, autoregulation of the cerebral circulation will prevent large shifts of water and consequent cerebral edema. However, an injured/disrupted BBB is unable to do this efficiently. Hence, the infusion of hypotonic saline in brain-injured patients may lead to cerebral edema.

Administration of hypertonic fluids will lead to a shift of water out of neurons and resultant

K. Khatib (✉)
Department of Medicine, SKN Medical College, Pune, Maharashtra, India

H. Prabhakar et al. (eds.), *Principles and Practice of Neurocritical Care*,
https://doi.org/10.1007/978-981-99-8059-8_36

shrinkage of neurons and also a shift of water to the intravascular compartment.

36.2.2 Cerebral Edema

Cerebral edema may be due to the swelling of neurons and astrocytes (cellular edema). It occurs as a result of Na and water moving into the cell following injury disrupting the mitochondrial function. Damage to the BBB will lead to the movement of water and albumin through the vascular endothelial cells. A combination of the two is called ionic edema.

36.2.3 Autoregulation

The ability of cerebral circulation to respond to hypotension and/or hypovolemia by causing vasodilation and respond to hypervolemia by vasoconstriction in an attempt to keep constant the cerebral perfusion pressure is lost when the brain suffers injury. The perfusion of the brain is then excessively dependent on changes in the fluid and electrolyte status.

36.3 Fluid Management in NCC: Quantity of Maintenance Fluids: How Much to Give?

Fluid balance should be used as the criterion to guide the quantity of maintenance fluids in a brain-injured patient. Multiple studies have demonstrated that patients with subarachnoid hemorrhage (SAH), who receive higher fluid intake, have more cardiovascular abnormalities as well as more delayed neurological events (ischemia and infarcts) [1–3]. A review of various studies that looked at fluid management in NCC found the mean fluid administered per day to be about 3–5 L/day [4]. Patients with SAH who have positive fluid balance were found to have more cerebral vasospasm, longer length of stay in hospital, and worse neuro-outcomes [3, 5]. In a trial in which prophylactic hypervolemia was used to prevent vascular complications, in patients who underwent clipping of aneurysm following rupture leading to SAH, it was found that it did not improve cerebral blood flow nor did it improve outcomes. In a randomized controlled trial (RCT) to determine the effect of hypervolemia in patients with SAH undergoing clipping for a ruptured aneurysm, patients had fluid intake ranging from 3.7 to 4.5 L/day. There was no increase in cerebral blood flow in the patients treated with hypervolemia [6]. A RCT evaluating the role of triple-H therapy in patients suffering SAH, triple-H therapy resulted in more fluid administration (4–5 vs 3 L/day), more adverse events (bleeding episodes, cardiac arrhythmias, congestive cardiac failure, and extradural hematomas), but no improvement in clinical and neurological outcomes [7].

Patients with SAH who have associated hypovolemia are at increased risk of delayed cerebral ischemia (DCI), which is associated with poor neurological and clinical outcomes [8–10].

Studies in traumatic brain injury (TBI) patients regarding fluid intake, fluid balances, and their effects on clinical outcomes are very few, and the topic requires further research [11].

36.4 Type of Maintenance Fluids: Which Fluids to Give?

Isotonic crystalloids are the preferred fluid of choice in NCC. These should form the mainstay of fluid therapy in patients with SAH, TBI, and acute ischemic stroke (AIS) [12–14].

Colloids should be avoided in patients with SAH. In a propensity score matching study in patients with SAH, patients receiving colloids (whether plasma or dextran or starch or albumin was used) were found to have worse outcomes (NIHSS score) after 6 weeks as compared to patients receiving crystalloids [15]. In another study on 160 patients of aneurysmal SAH, the total daily dose of colloids was associated with worse delayed (>6 months) neurological outcomes, while the use of crystalloids had the opposite effect [16]. A study of colloids in patients with severe TBI did not find any association between the use of colloids and mortality in these patients [17].

Among crystalloids, though there are some trials showing minor (decreased hypochloremia, Na, osmolarity) advantages in favor of balanced crystalloids, there is no hard evidence to favor the use of balanced crystalloids over standard crystalloids [18]. A double-blind RCT conducted in patients with TBI, who received a 48 h infusion of sodium lactate or NS, found better ICP and Na control and improved fluid balance in patients who received sodium lactate [19].

Hypertonic fluids should not be used for either resuscitation or maintenance. RCTs comparing the use of hypertonic saline (7.5%) versus crystalloids or colloids failed to show any advantage of the use of hypertonic fluids in this setting [20, 21].

Controversy exists regarding the use of albumin in NCC. Evidence for benefit and harm exists in patients with TBI. A multicentric RCT using a high dose of 25% albumin found no advantage of the use of albumin versus normal saline (NS) in patients with acute ischemic stroke (AIS) [13]. An observational single center study found evidence of better outcomes in patients given high-dose albumin in patients with acute ischemic stroke [14]. The SAFE study found more mortality in TBI patients given a low dose of 4% albumin when compared with NS [22]. Two studies with low-quality evidence had found better neurological outcomes in patients with SAH who received high dose albumin when compared with patients who received crystalloids [23, 24].

36.5 Fluid Administration Based on Assessment of Circulation

One would ideally like to base the fluid management strategy in patients in NCC on the blood volume and circulatory status of the individual patient. However, it is not possible to assess the volume status accurately and easily at the bedside without the availability of sophisticated equipment. In patients with SAH, it is possible to guide fluid administration based on transpulmonary thermodilution [25]. In SAH patients, CO monitoring guided fluid therapy may help to improve cerebral oxygenation, but not all studies have shown this correlation [26, 27]. Such correlation has also not been shown in patients with TBI [28]. Ultrasound-guided inferior vena cava distensibility-guided fluid therapy in SAH patients may be used with promising results [29].

Hemodynamic monitoring using a multimodal approach should be used routinely in patients with NCC. This should take into account goals depending on cerebral oxygenation and perfusion pressure. These approaches may include invasive (arterial line, central venous line) or noninvasive techniques to assess fluid volume. Advanced hemodynamic monitoring (echocardiography, TPT) may be used in selected hemodynamic unstable patients depending upon availability and local expertise.

36.6 Conclusions

Fluid therapy in NCC should target euvolemia. Patients will have adverse effects if they are hypo or hypervolemic. Both these states may have detrimental effects on the injured brain. However, the way to achieve euvolemia in clinical practice is difficult even with the use of hemodynamic monitoring. There is lack of adequate evidence regarding optimal fluid therapy practice in various patients in NCC (SAH, TBI, AIS, etc.). Further pragmatic studies are required.

References

1. Mutoh T, Kazumata K, Ishikawa T, Terasaka S. Performance of bedside transpulmonary thermodilution monitoring for goal-directed hemodynamic management after subarachnoid hemorrhage. Stroke. 2009;40(7):2368–74.
2. Martini RP, Deem S, Brown M, Souter MJ, Yanez ND, Daniel S, et al. The association between fluid balance and outcomes after subarachnoid hemorrhage. Neurocrit Care. 2012;17(2):191–8.
3. Gura M, Elmaci I, Cerci A, Sagiroglu E, Coskun KK. Haemodynamic augmentation in the treatment of vasospasm in aneurysmal subarachnoid hemorrhage. Turk Neurosurg. 2012;22(4):435–40.
4. van der Jagt M. Fluid management of the neurological patient. Crit Care. 2016;20:126.
5. Kissoon NR, Mandrekar JN, Fugate JE, Lanzino G, Wijdicks EF, Rabinstein AA. Positive fluid bal-

ance is associated with poor outcomes in subarachnoid hemorrhage. J Stroke Cerebrovasc Dis. 2015;24(10):2245–51.
6. Lennihan L, Mayer SA, Fink ME, Beckford A, Paik MC, Zhang H, et al. Effect of hypervolemic therapy on cerebral blood flow after subarachnoid hemorrhage: a randomized controlled trial. Stroke. 2000;31(2):383–91.
7. Egge A, Waterloo K, Sjoholm H, Solberg T, Ingebrigtsen T, Romner B. Prophylactic hyperdynamic postoperative fluid therapy after aneurismal subarachnoid hemorrhage: a clinical, prospective, randomized, controlled study. Neurosurgery. 2001;49(3):593–605.
8. Solomon RA, Post KD, McMurtry JG. Depression of circulating blood volume in patients after subarachnoid hemorrhage: implications for the management of symptomatic vasospasm. Neurosurgery. 1984;15:354–61.
9. Kasuya H, Onda H, Yoneyama T, Sasaki T, Hori T. Bedside monitoring of circulating blood volume after subarachnoid hemorrhage. Stroke. 2003;34:956–60.
10. van Gijn J, Kerr RS, Rinkel GJ. Subarachnoid haemorrhage. Lancet. 2007;369:306–18.
11. Schmoker JD, Shackford SR, Wald SL, Pietropaoli JA. An analysis of the relationship between fluid and sodium administration and intracranial pressure after head injury. J Trauma. 1992;33(3):476–81.
12. Wright WL. Sodium and fluid management in acute brain injury. Curr Neurol Neurosci Rep. 2012;12(4):466–73.
13. Ginsberg MD, Palesch YY, Hill MD, Martin RH, Moy CS, Barsan WG, Waldman BD, Tamariz D, Ryckborst KJ, ALIAS and Neurological Emergencies Treatment Trials (NETT) Investigators. High-dose albumin treatment for acute ischaemic stroke (ALIAS) part 2: a randomised, double-blind, phase 3, placebo-controlled trial. Lancet Neurol. 2013;12(11):1049–58.
14. Palesch YY, Hill MD, Ryckborst KJ, Tamariz D, Ginsberg MD. The ALIAS Pilot Trial: a dose-escalation and safety study of albumin therapy for acute ischemic stroke—II: neurologic outcome and efficacy analysis. Stroke. 2006;37(8): 2107–14.
15. Ibrahim GM, Macdonald RL. The effects of fluid balance and colloid administration on outcomes in patients with aneurysmal subarachnoid hemorrhage: a propensity score-matched analysis. Neurocrit Care. 2013;19(2):140–9.
16. Tseng MY, Hutchinson PJ, Kirkpatrick PJ. Effects of fluid therapy following aneurysmal subarachnoid haemorrhage: a prospective clinical study. Br J Neurosurg. 2008;22(2):257–68.
17. Sekhon MS, Dhingra VK, Sekhon IS, Henderson WR, McLean N, Griesdale DE. The safety of synthetic colloid in critically ill patients with severe traumatic brain injuries. J Crit Care. 2011;26(4):357–62.
18. Oddo M, Poole D, Helbok R, Meyfroidt G, Stocchetti N, Bouzat P, et al. Fluid therapy in neurointensive care patients: ESICM consensus and clinical practice recommendations. Intensive Care Med. 2018;44(4):449–63.
19. Ichai C, Payen JF, Orban JC, Quintard H, Roth H, Legrand R, Francony G, Leverve XM. Half-molar sodium lactate infusion to prevent intracranial hypertensive episodes in severe traumatic brain injured patients: a randomized controlled trial. Intensive Care Med. 2013;39(8):1413–22.
20. Cooper DJ, Myles PS, McDermott FT, Murray LJ, Laidlaw J, Cooper G, et al.; HTS Study Investigators. Prehospital hypertonic saline resuscitation of patients with hypotension and severe traumatic brain injury: a randomized controlled trial. JAMA. 2004;291(11):1350–1357.
21. Baker AJ, Rhind SG, Morrison LJ, Black S, Crnko NT, Shek PN, et al. Resuscitation with hypertonic saline-dextran reduces serum biomarker levels and correlates with outcome in severe traumatic brain injury patients. J Neurotrauma. 2009;26(8):1227–40.
22. SAFE Study Investigators, Australian and New Zealand Intensive Care Society Clinical Trials Group, Australian Red Cross Blood Service, George Institute for International Health, Myburgh J, Cooper DJ, Finfer S, Bellomo R, Norton R, et al. Saline or albumin for fluid resuscitation in patients with traumatic brain injury. N Engl J Med. 2007;357(9):874–84.
23. Kuwabara K, Fushimi K, Matsuda S, Ishikawa KB, Horiguchi H, Fujimori K. Association of early post-procedure hemodynamic management with the outcomes of subarachnoid hemorrhage patients. J Neurol. 2013;260(3):820–31.
24. Suarez JI, Shannon L, Zaidat OO, Suri MF, Singh G, Lynch G, Selman WR. Effect of human albumin administration on clinical outcome and hospital cost in patients with subarachnoid hemorrhage. J Neurosurg. 2004;100(4):585–90.
25. Taccone FS, Citerio G, Participants in the International Multi-disciplinary Consensus Conference on Multimodality Monitoring. Advanced monitoring of systemic hemodynamics in critically ill patients with acute brain injury. Neurocrit Care. 2014;21(2):S38–63.
26. Kurtz P, Helbok R, Ko SB, Claassen J, Schmidt JM, Fernandez L, et al. Fluid responsiveness and brain tissue oxygen augmentation after subarachnoid hemorrhage. Neurocrit Care. 2014;20(2):247–54.
27. Muench E, Horn P, Bauhuf C, Roth H, Philipps M, Hermann P, et al. Effects of hypervolemia and hypertension on regional cerebral blood flow, intracranial pressure, and brain tissue oxygenation after subarachnoid hemorrhage. Crit Care Med. 2007;35(8):1844–51; quiz 1852.
28. Bouma GJ, Muizelaar JP. Relationship between cardiac output and cerebral blood flow in patients with intact and with impaired autoregulation. J Neurosurg. 1990;73(3):368–74.
29. Moretti R, Pizzi B. Inferior vena cava distensibility as a predictor of fluid responsiveness in patients with subarachnoid hemorrhage. Neurocrit Care. 2010;13(1):3–9.

Nutrition in Neurocritical Care 37

Khalid Khatib and Subhal B. Dixit

37.1 Introduction

Medical nutrition therapy (MNT) should be thought of in all critically ill patients staying in the ICU for more than 48 h. This is especially true for patients in neurocritical ICUs. These ICUs comprise brain-injured patients [traumatic brain injury (TBI)], patients with cerebrovascular accidents (acute ischemic and hemorrhagic stroke, and subarachnoid hemorrhage), spinal cord injuries, or patients with nerve or muscle diseases. There is a paucity of research and evidence about the use of MNT in these sub-classes of patients, and at times, recommendations are made as extrapolation of evidence from general critically ill patients.

Some general rules of critical care nutrition applicable to all critically ill patients should be kept in mind. Validated nutrition assessment tools should be used to assess the risk of malnutrition in all patients in neurocritical ICU. Oral diet is preferable to EN/PN in patients who can do so. In patients in whom this is not possible, EN is preferable to PN. If both oral intake and EN are not possible, PN may be started within 3–7 days (ESPEN guidelines) or after 7 days (ASPEN guidelines) [1, 2]. In patients who are exhibiting features of severe malnutrition and in whom EN is contraindicated, PN may be started instead of not providing any nutrition [1].

37.2 Nutritional Assessment in Patients Admitted to Neurocritical ICUs

This comprises two steps: (1) screening of patients for risk of developing malnutrition during their stay in the neurocritical ICU. (2) Assessment of current nutritional status of the patient.

Screening of Patients for Malnutrition Risk: It should be assessed within the first 48 h of hospitalization. Patients in the neurocritical ICU are more at risk of developing malnutrition during their stay in the ICU as these patients may have a background of dementia (affecting volitional food intake), difficulty swallowing due to various neurologic or muscular causes, and altered levels of consciousness [3]. Also nil by mouth status for investigations or procedures, stopping or delaying feeds for other reasons, and hypercatabolism due to illness also contribute to this risk.

This may be done using any of the following scores/tools: (a) nutrition risk in the critically ill (NUTRIC) score, (b) mini nutritional assessment (MNA), (c) malnutrition universal screening tool

K. Khatib
Department of Medicine, SKN Medical College, Pune, Maharashtra, India

S. B. Dixit (✉)
Department of Critical Care, Sanjeevan and MJM Hospital, Pune, Maharashtra, India

H. Prabhakar et al. (eds.), *Principles and Practice of Neurocritical Care*,
https://doi.org/10.1007/978-981-99-8059-8_37

(MUST), (d) short nutritional assessment questionnaire (SNAQ), (e) nutritional risk screening-2002 (NRS-2002)], and (f) radiological tools include ultrasonography of quadriceps muscle (to measure muscle mass and changes during course of illness) and CT scan analysis of skeletal muscle density.

Patients are at high nutrition risk if the NUTRIC score is ≤5 or the NRS score is >3. MNA score value of 0–7 points denotes malnourished individuals at the start of the illness, while a score of 8–11 points denotes individuals at risk of malnutrition.

Assessment of Current Nutritional Status of the Patient: A nutritional assessment is done to identify patients who will benefit from MNT. The factors to be kept in mind when conducting nutritional assessment are given in Table 37.1.

Nutrition can be assessed by various tools used in combination as no single tool gives the best assessment (see Table 37.2).

Table 37.1 Factors to be considered when undertaking nutritional assessment

Factors	Remarks
Presence of co-morbidities	Especially diabetes, hypertension, renal, or liver failure as they will have an impact on patient nutrition and also impact the type and quantity of nutrition therapy provided to the patient
Abnormal GI function, presence of any dysphagia	Dysphagia may be due to CVA or oropharyngeal muscle or nerve etiology. GI function may be affected by autonomic nervous dysfunction
Alteration in body composition (muscle loss, presence of edema)	
Serum protein, albumin, prealbumin	Not very reliable as they may increase in acute illnesses due to their function as acute phase reactants
Presence of serum ketones	As an indicator of starvation when they are present in the absence of hyperglycemia

Table 37.2 Tools used for assessment of nutrition in critically ill patients

Tools	Calculation	Comments
Anthropometry		Simple and inexpensive, can be performed at the patient's bedside
Percentage weight loss	[(Usual body weight – actual body weight)/Actual body weight)] × 100	Significant if >5%, 7.5%, and 10% at 1, 3, and 6 months, respectively
Body mass index (BMI)	Weight in kg/(height in m)^2	BMI < 20 is associated with high mortality
Skin fold thickness (SFT)	Measured at the biceps, triceps, subscapular region, and iliac crest. It is calculated as the mean of at least three measurements	Measured using skin fold calipers
Mid arm circumference (MAC)	Measured at the midpoint of the line joining acromion and olecranon processes	Measured in non-dominant upper limb
Subjective global assessment (SGA)	Takes into account the following points—anorexia, functional capacity, GI symptoms, weight loss over 6 months, and visual assessment of subcutaneous fat and muscle mass	Patients classified as well as nourished and moderately or severely malnourished. Correlates well with prognosis
Biochemistry: serum albumin/prealbumin	Measured using bromcresol green, cellulose acetate electro-phoresis, or sodium sulfite precipitation/biuret methods	Simple, widely available. Lower values are associated with poor prognosis. However, it is an unreliable indicator of nutritional status as its value depends on many variables
Others (X-ray absorptiometry, bioelectrical impedance, and near-infrared)		Not widely and easily available

37.3 Estimation of Nutritional Requirements

Energy Requirement: Brain-injured patients are in a hypercatabolic state, just as other critically ill patients. Increased secretion of glucocorticoids, catecholamines, and glucagon are responsible for this. Metabolic demand varies depending on the stage and type of critical illness. The resting energy expenditure (REE) may be about double the usual requirement in 75% of patients with TBI. This enhanced REE may last for 2–4 weeks [3–5]. The REE in patients with AIS depends on the type of stroke but has wide variations. In addition, in patients with SAH, raised REE may lead to more incidence of vasospasm. As in other types of critical illness, REE in patients in neurocritical ICU will also depend on the treatment process that the patient undergoes (drugs like sedatives and benzodiazepines, targeted temperature management) [6, 7]. There are various methods used to calculate REE. However, the gold standard method to estimate energy requirements in critically ill patients is indirect calorimetry (IC) [7]. Other modalities to calculate the energy requirements of patients are the use of simplistic formulas and predictive equations (see Table 37.3).

Protein Requirement: The other metabolic abnormality in neuro-critically ill patients is skeletal protein catabolism. Along with reduced provision of nutrition (either due to reduced delivery or absorption), this results in negative nitrogen balance (NNB). This has been shown to last for weeks in patients with TBI and increases the morbidity and 1-month, 3-month, and one-year mortality in such patients [8, 9]. These patients also develop more hospital-acquired infections, and neurologic outcomes may worsen [10]. NNB is seen in almost half of all patients with AIS leading to malnutrition, which is observed in about 16% of patients on admission to NCC and increasing to 26% within a week [11, 12]. Protein requirement is in the range of 1.2–2.0 g/kg/day, with higher disease severity and malnutrition requiring the upper dosage [13].

Whichever modality is used to evaluate the patient's nutritional status, the key is repeated frequent measurements and an integrated nutritional team leading to a wholesome assessment of the patient's nutritional assessment.

Table 37.3 Tools for calculating energy requirements in NCC patients

Tools	Remarks
(a) Indirect calorimetry	
Principle	Measures consumed O_2 and CO_2 in the lungs and helps to measure current resting energy expenditure, which is then extrapolated over 24 h
Advantages	Considered Gold standard Non-invasive Provides real-time information
Limitations	Costly and labor-intensive Needs specialized staff calculations affected in mechanically ventilated patients with high pressures and FiO_2, and those undergoing RRT and ECMO
(b) Predictive equations	
Harris-Benedict equation: Formula *Males:* [13.7516 × W (kg)] + [5.003 × H (cm)] − [6.755 × age (y)] *Females:* 655.0955 + [9.5643 × W (kg) + [1.8496 × height (cm)] − [4.6756 × age (y)]	May require multiplying with a stress factor in certain situations
Others: Ireta Jones or Penn State	
(c) Simplistic formulas	25–30 kcal/kg/day

37.4 Initiation and Monitoring of Nutrition

Patients at high risk of malnutrition (or already found to be malnourished on admission to NCC) and who are unable to meet their nutritional needs orally should be started on enteral nutrition. This decision needs to be taken without wasting much time. Early enteral nutrition is the one where enteral nutrition is started within 24–48 h of admission to the NCC unit. Once enteral nutrition is tolerated, the goal is to advance nutrition toward 80% of target (estimated or calculated) energy and protein requirements [13]. This needs to be achieved over the next 7–10 days. Enteral nutrition is the preferred route as it helps to maintain gut integrity and gut immune function.

For those patients who are not able to meet their energy and protein requirements (<60%) through enteral nutrition, the further course of action will depend on their baseline nutritional status. For those patients with adequate premorbid nutritional status, parenteral nutrition (PN) may be thought of only if inadequate enteral nutrition lasts for 7–10 days. Supplemental PN should not be started earlier in these patients as it has been found to be harmful in these patients [13]. For those with inadequate premorbid nutrition status and at high risk for malnutrition or those already severely malnourished prior to hospitalization, supplemental parenteral nutrition may be started early if an oral or enteral route is not able to provide adequate nutrition.

One of the important principles of nutrition delivery in critically ill patients including NCC patients is to prevent overfeeding. Overfeeding critically ill patients in the first week of critical illness has been found to be hazardous and actually increases mortality and should be avoided at all costs [1, 2, 13–15]. Hence patients receiving MNT should be frequently monitored with repeated IC measurements or when calculating energy and protein requirements using predictive or simplistic equations.

The practice of measurement of gastric residual volumes (GRV) to determine whether the next feed may be administered to the patient should be discouraged. There was no correlation found between the amount of GRV and the incidence of complications (ventilator-associated pneumonia, aspiration) [1, 2]. Hemodynamically unstable patients with ongoing vasopressor therapy should be monitored for gut ischemia and feeding intolerance. This is manifested by abdominal distension, decreased peristaltic sounds, or constipation. If any of the symptoms of gut ischemia/feeding intolerance are found, EN should be withheld till such time the condition improves. EN may be restarted gradually once the condition of the gut stabilizes. PN may be started during such intervals.

37.5 Special Nutritional Considerations in NCC

Ketogenic Diets: These diets are rich in proteins and lipids and poor in carbohydrates and lead to alterations in metabolism, including reduction in glycolysis and increase in free fatty acid production and associated production of ketones. There are also changes in neurotransmitter synthesis, release, and mechanism of action [16, 17]. It has been shown to reduce cerebral edema and to change cerebral metabolism following TBI in animal studies [18]. In human studies, ketogenic diets reduce the frequency (almost by half) of seizure episodes in both adults and children [19, 20]. Adjuvant therapy of seizures has been found to be as safe and as efficacious as medication and even reduces episodes of status epilepticus, even super refractory status epilepticus [12, 20, 21].

Cerebral Microdialysis: It is a semicontinuous, invasive, bedside brain monitoring modality that studies cerebral metabolism and allows for real-time information on cerebral substrates like pyruvate, lactate, and glucose. The lactate /pyruvate (L/P) ratio and glucose levels are monitored among other metabolites. Post-acute brain injury, diminished CMD glucose levels, or elevated L/P ratio > 25 is associated with increased mortality [22]. Few studies have described the use of CMD in SAH and TBI patients [23]. In a study of SAH patients, when CMD showed low glucose levels, the provision of EN increased the levels of CMD glucose [22]. However, there are no studies to date showing the effect of the use of such neurologic monitoring on morbidity and mortality in NCC patients.

Immunonutrition: Nutrients (amino acids like glutamine and arginine, n-3 fatty acids, vitamins like vitamin C, and other micronutrients like zinc and selenium) used with the intention of modifying the immune system are used in NCC. Glutamine and arginine are conditionally essential amino acids and act as fuel for the cells during metabolic stress. n-3 Fatty acids (Eicosapentaenoic acids and docosahexaenoic acid) supplementation leads to reduced inflammatory cytokine response and reduced secondary cell injury. Vitamins reduce oxidative cellular injury. As these nutrients have low toxicity, they are attractive as supplements.

In a small study of glutamine and probiotics supplemented to brain-injured patients, it was found to reduce ICU length of stay and rate of infections [24]. Guidelines recommend the use of immune-modulating supplementation in patients with TBI based on this weak evidence [13]. Vitamins D, C, and E are associated with improved survival and neurological outcomes in patients with TBI and AIS [25, 26].

37.6 Conclusions

Nutrition support is important for long-term health as well as during critical illness, especially neurocritical illness. Macronutrient supply and micronutrient supplementation may be used to improve patient outcomes depending on the underlying neurological disease. Current research has revealed some potential beneficial effects of MNT in patients in NCC. However, there is a lot of data lacking on the different mechanisms of actions of MNT in neurologic disease. There is a definite need for pragmatic large randomized control trials to answer questions regarding the benefit of MNT in neurocritically ill patients.

References

1. Singer P, Blaser AR, Berger MM, Waleed Alhazzani W, Calder PC, Casaer MP, et al. ESPEN guideline on clinical nutrition in the intensive care unit. Clin Nutr. 2019;38:48–79.
2. Compher C, Bingham AL, McCall M, Patel J, Rice TW, Braunschweig C, et al. Guidelines for the provision of nutrition support therapy in the adult critically ill patient: the American Society for Parenteral and Enteral Nutrition. J Parenter Enter Nutr. 2022;46:12–41.
3. Chapple LS, Deane AM, Heyland DK, Lange K, Kranz AJ, Williams LT, et al. Energy and protein deficits throughout hospitalization in patients admitted with a traumatic brain injury. Clin Nutr. 2016;35(6):1315–22.
4. Foley N, Marshall S, Pikul J, Salter K, Teasell R. Hypermetabolism following moderate to severe traumatic acute brain injury: a systematic review. J Neurotrauma. 2008;25(12):1415–31.
5. Dickerson RN. Nitrogen balance and protein requirements for critically ill older patients. Nutrients. 2016;8(4):226.
6. Kurtz P, Rocha EEM. Nutrition therapy, glucose control, and brain metabolism in traumatic brain injury: a multimodal monitoring approach. Front Neurosci. 2020;14:190.
7. Delsoglio M, Achamrah N, Berger MM, Pichard C. Indirect calorimetry in clinical practice. J Clin Med. 2019;8(9):1387.
8. Abdelmalik PA, Dempsey S, Ziai W. Nutritional and bioenergetic considerations in critically ill patients with acute neurological injury. Neurocrit Care. 2017;27(2):276–86.
9. Quintard H, Ichai C. Nutritional and metabolic supplementation for the injured brain: an update. Curr Opin Crit Care. 2019;25(2):126–31.
10. Oddo M, Vespa P, Menon DK. Boosting the injured brain with supplemental energy fuels. Intensive Care Med. 2019;45(6):872–5.
11. Achanta LB, Rowlands BD, Thomas DS, Housley GD, Rae CD. β-Hydroxybutyrate boosts mitochondrial and neuronal metabolism but is not preferred over glucose under activated conditions. Neurochem Res. 2017;42(6):1710–23.
12. Cervenka MC, Hocker S, Koenig M, Bar B, Henry-Barron B, Kossoff EH, et al. Phase I/II multicenter ketogenic diet study for adult superrefractory status epilepticus. Neurology. 2017;88(10):938–43.
13. McClave SA, Taylor BE, Martindale R, Warren MM, Johnson DR, Braunschweig C, et al. Guidelines for the provision and assessment of nutrition support therapy in the adult critically ill patient: Society of Critical Care Medicine (SCCM) and American Society for Parenteral and Enteral Nutrition (ASPEN). J Parenter Enter Nutr. 2016;40(2):159–211.
14. Braunschweig CL, Freels S, Sheean PM, Peterson SJ, Perez SG, McKeever L, et al. Role of timing and dose of energy received in patients with acute lung injury on mortality in the intensive nutrition in acute lung injury trial (INTACT): a post hoc analysis. Am J Clin Nutr. 2017;105(2):411–6.
15. Peterson SJ, Lateef OB, Freels S, McKeever L, Fantuzzi G, Braunschweig CA. Early exposure to recommended calorie delivery in the intensive care unit is associated with increased mortality in patients with acute respiratory distress syndrome. JPEN J Parenter Enteral Nutr. 2018;42(4):739–47.
16. Klein P, Tyrlikova I, Mathews GC. Dietary treatment in adults with refractory epilepsy: a review. Neurology. 2014;83(21):1978–85.

17. Rho JM. How does the ketogenic diet induce antiseizure effects? Neurosci Lett. 2017;637:4–10.
18. Greene AE, Todorova MT, McGowan R, Seyfried TN. Caloric restriction inhibits seizure susceptibility in epileptic EL mice by reducing blood glucose. Epilepsia. 2001;42(11):1371–8.
19. Martin K, Jackson CF, Levy RG, Cooper PN. Ketogenic diet and other dietary treatments for epilepsy. Cochrane Database Syst Rev. 2016;2:CD001903.
20. Ye F, Li XJ, Jiang WL, Sun HB, Liu J. Efficacy of and patient compliance with a ketogenic diet in adults with intractable epilepsy: a meta-analysis. J Clin Neurol. 2015;11(1):26–31.
21. Mahmoud SH, Ho-Huang E, Buhler J. Systematic review of ketogenic diet use in adult patients with status epilepticus. Epilepsia Open. 2020;5(1):10–21.
22. Kofler M, Schiefecker AJ, Beer R, Gaasch M, Rhomberg P, Stover J, et al. Enteral nutrition increases interstitial brain glucose levels in poor-grade subarachnoid hemorrhage patients. J Cereb Blood Flow Metab. 2018;38(3):518–27.
23. Glenn TC, Martin NA, Horning MA, McArthur DL, Hovda DA, Vespa P, et al. Lactate: brain fuel in human traumatic brain injury: a comparison with normal healthy control subjects. J Neurotrauma. 2015;32(11):820–32.
24. de Arruda ISF, de Aguilar-Nascimento JE. Benefits of early enteral nutrition with glutamine and probiotics in brain injury patients. Clin Sci (Lond). 2004;106(3):287–92.
25. Razmkon A, Sadidi A, Sherafat-Kazemzadeh E, Mehrafshan A, Jamali M, Malekpour B, et al. Administration of vitamin C and vitamin E in severe head injury: a randomized double-blind controlled trial. Clin Neurosurg. 2011;58:133–7.
26. Gupta A, Prabhakar S, Modi M, Bhadada SK, Kalaivani M, Lal V, et al. Effect of Vitamin D and calcium supplementation on ischaemic stroke outcome: a randomized controlled open-label trial. Int J Clin Pract. 2016;70(9):764–70.

Fever in Neurocritical Care

38

Sharmili Sinha, Saurabh Debnath,
and Vivek Gupta

38.1 Introduction

Fever is a common occurrence in patients admitted to the neuro-intensive care unit (NICU). This can be due to a variety of causes, including both infectious and non-infectious causes [1]. Infectious causes of fever in the NICU may include bacterial, viral or fungal infections, while non-infectious causes may include inflammation, injury to the central nervous system or unwanted effects of medications. The management of fever in the NICU requires a thorough understanding of the underlying causes and the potential complications that can arise. This includes the need for prompt diagnosis and treatment of the underlying condition, as well as close monitoring of the patient's vital signs and neurological status. Additionally, the use of antipyretic medications and other interventions to control fever or its antecedent cause may be necessary to prevent the development of serious complications. In this topic, we will discuss the causes, diagnosis and management of fever in patients in the NICU, including both infectious and non-infectious causes.

S. Sinha (✉)
Apollo Hospitals, Bhubaneswar, Odisha, India

S. Debnath
Critical Care Medicine, B.P.Poddar Hospital and Medical Research Ltd., Kolkata, India

V. Gupta
Hero DMC Heart Institute, Ludhiana, India

38.2 What Is Fever? Why Is It Harmful for Neurological Disease-Affected Patients?

Fever, also known as pyrexia, is a physiological response characterized by an elevation of the body's temperature above its normal range. The normal body temperature varies depending on the individual and the method of measurement, but it is generally considered to be between 36.5 and 37.5 °C [2]. A fever is typically defined as a body temperature greater than 38 °C when taken orally, or greater than 38.3 °C when taken rectally. The primary function of a fever is to help the body fight off infections or other causes of inflammation by making it less hospitable to harmful microorganisms and by increasing the production of white blood cells and other immune cells [3].

The pathophysiological mechanism of fever is closely related to the hypothalamus, a small region in the brain that acts as the body's thermostat. The hypothalamus maintains a "set point" for body temperature, which is normally set at around 37 °C. When the body is exposed to an infection or other cause of inflammation, the hypothalamus increases this set point, leading to an increase in the body's temperature [4]. This increase in temperature is brought about by a variety of mechanisms, including the release of pyrogenic cytokines from immune cells, which stimulate the hypothalamus to release substances called prostaglandins that promote fever. Additionally, the hypothalamus also influences the production of

H. Prabhakar et al. (eds.), *Principles and Practice of Neurocritical Care*,
https://doi.org/10.1007/978-981-99-8059-8_38

heat by increasing the activity of the muscles and by constricting blood vessels in the skin, which reduces heat loss from the body [5].

Fever can be classified into four grades: low-grade fever, moderate-grade fever, high-grade fever and hyperpyrexia (Table 38.1). A low-grade fever is defined as a body temperature between 38.1 and 39 °C, moderate-grade fever is between 39.1 and 40 °C, high-grade fever is between 40.1 and 41 °C and hyperpyrexia is a fever above 41.1 °C [6]. The grading of fever can be useful in determining the appropriate management and treatment of the underlying cause, as well as assessing the severity of the fever.

Fever can be detrimental for neurological patients for several reasons (Fig. 38.1).

[CMRO2:Cerebral Metabolic Rate of Oxygen; CBF:Cerebral Blood Flow] First, fever can lead to increased intracranial pressure, which can be dangerous for patients with head injuries, brain tumours or other conditions that affect the brain. This increased pressure can lead to brain tissue damage, and can also increase the risk of seizures or herniation.

Second, fever can lead to dehydration and electrolyte imbalances, which have implications for neurological patients. Dehydration can lead to decreased blood flow to the brain, which can affect brain function and increase the risk of complications. Electrolyte imbalances can also affect brain function and can increase the risk of seizures.

Third, fever can lead to increased metabolic demand, which can intensify the risk of decreased oxygen delivery to the injured brain. This increased metabolic demand can lead to further brain damage and worsen the neurological outcome.

Fourth, fever can also increase the risk of infections and precipitate cardiovascular instability like tachycardia and arrhythmias especially in patients with multiple co-morbid conditions like coronary artery diseases, hypertension and diabetes mellitus.

Finally, fever adds general discomfort and distress, which has an impact on the patient's well-being and ability to recover [7].

Table 38.1 Classification of fever

Classification of fever	
Normal temperature	37–380 °C
Low grade fever	38.1–390 °C
Moderate grade fever	39.1–400 °C
High grade fever	40.1–410 °C
Hyperpyrexia	>41.10 °C

38.3 Why Treat a Fever?

It is often prudent to have a low threshold for treating a rise in body temperature in neuro-intensive care. This is because fever can be particularly detrimental for neurological patients, as outlined above. Moreover, a small increase in body temperature can quickly escalate and become dangerous for these patients, who may already be at a higher risk of complications due to their underlying condition. Therefore, it is important to closely monitor body temperature and take prompt action if a fever is detected. This may include administer-

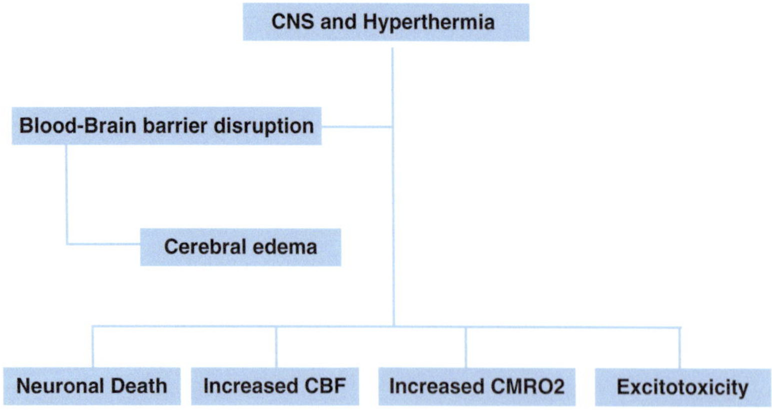

Fig. 38.1 Effects of hyperthermia on Central Nervous System. *CMRO2* Cerebral Metabolic Rate of Oxygen, *CBF* Cerebral Blood Flow

ing antipyretic medications, providing cooling measures, and identifying and treating the underlying cause of the fever. By having a low threshold for treating a rise in body temperature, healthcare providers can help to minimize potential complications and promote recovery in neurological patients [8]. Thus, fever is considered to be a serious occurrence, especially in the neuro-intensive care patient population.

38.4 Pathophysiology of Fever in Neuro ICU

The fever response is brought about by a variety of mechanisms, including the release of pyrogenic cytokines from immune cells, which stimulate the hypothalamus to release substances called prostaglandins that promote fever. Prostaglandins are hormone-like substances that are produced by many cells in the body, including immune cells and cells in the hypothalamus. These substances act on the hypothalamus to increase the body's temperature set point, which leads to an increase in the body's temperature. Additionally, the hypothalamus also influences the production of heat by increasing the activity of the muscles and by constricting blood vessels in the skin, which reduces heat loss from the body [5].

During fever, the body's internal homeostasis is affected, as the body's temperature is not within its normal range. This could affect the normal functioning of enzymes and other biological molecules that are temperature-sensitive. The body's metabolism increases to generate heat and the body's immune system is activated to fight off the infection. Fever also causes a decrease in appetite and an increase in the heart rate, which can cause an increase in the oxygen demand [9].

The effects of fever can be beneficial, as it helps to fight off the infection, but it can also be detrimental if the fever is too high or if it lasts for a prolonged period. High fever can lead to dehydration, electrolyte imbalances and increased metabolic demand, which can lead to further damage to the body. Therefore, it is important to monitor and control fever to minimize the potential complications [9].

38.5 Manifestations of Fever on the Brain

Fever can have several detrimental effects on the brain, particularly if the fever is too high or if it lasts for a prolonged period. One of the most dangerous effects of high fever is increased intracranial pressure, which can be dangerous for patients with head injuries, brain tumours or other conditions that affect the brain. This increased pressure can lead to brain tissue damage, and can also increase the risk of seizures. In severe cases, increased intracranial pressure can lead to cerebral herniation, which is a life-threatening condition that occurs when the brain tissue is squeezed and displaced from its normal position within the skull. This can cause severe brain damage or even death if not treated promptly [10].

Cerebral herniation is a medical emergency that requires immediate treatment, which may include medications to reduce the pressure inside the skull, or surgery to remove the pressure by removing part of the skull or brain tissue. It is therefore important to closely monitor body temperature and take prompt action if a fever is detected in neurological patients to minimize the potential complications, including cerebral herniation.

Fever can also lead to increased blood flow to the brain (cerebral blood flow, CBF), which can affect brain function and increase the risk of complications. Electrolyte imbalances can also affect brain function and can increase the risk of seizures.

Fever can also lead to increased metabolic demand, which can be problematic for neurological patients who may already have decreased oxygen delivery to the brain. This increased metabolic demand can lead to further brain damage and worsen the neurological outcome [11].

38.6 Causes of Fever in Neuro ICU

The aetiologies of fever can be due to infectious and non-infectious causes (Figs. 38.2 and 38.3).

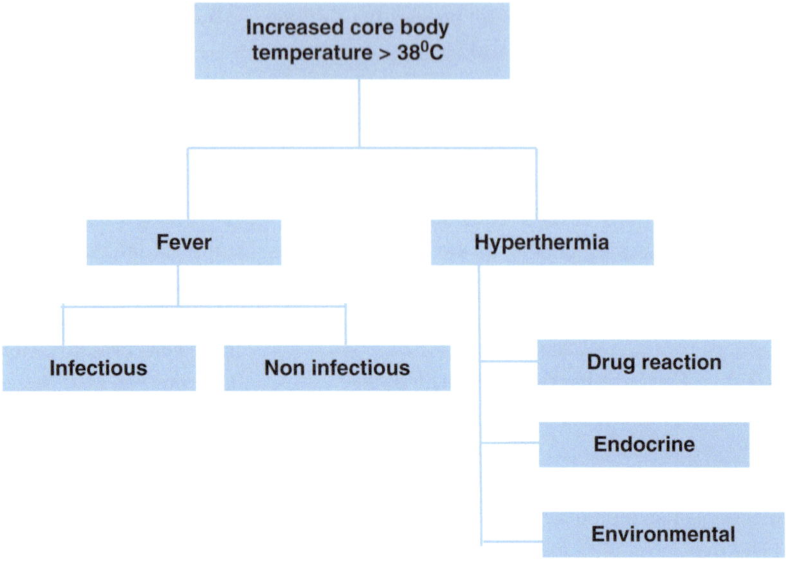

Fig. 38.2 Etiology of Fever

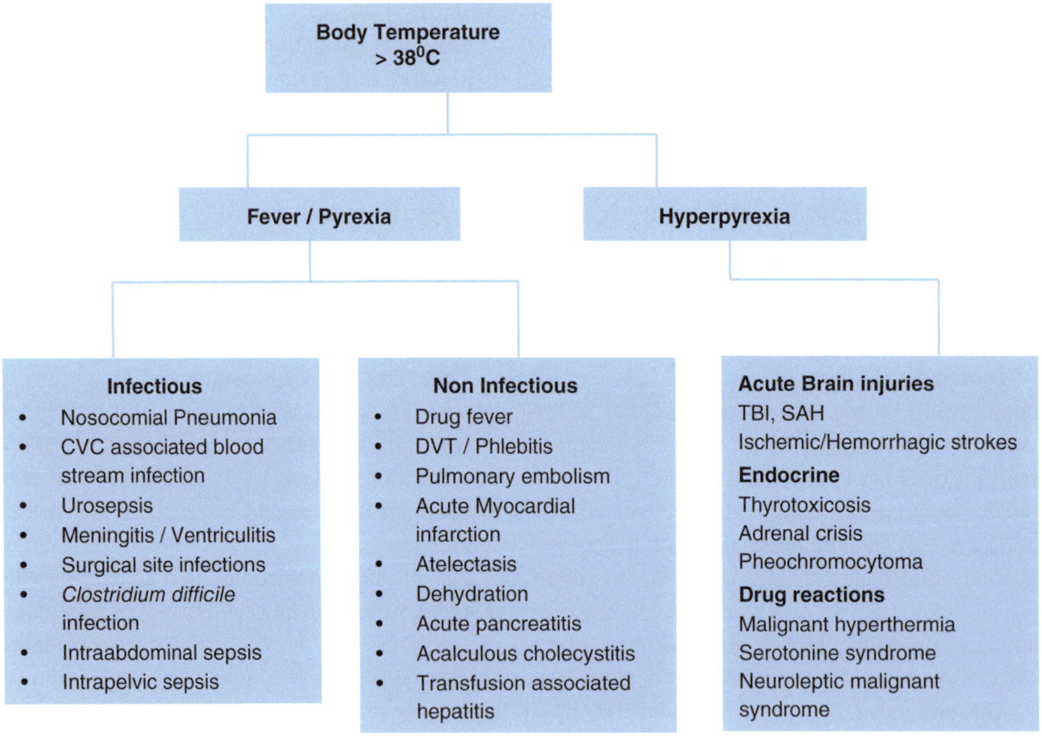

Fig. 38.3 Differential diagnosis of fever in neuro-intensive care unit

38.6.1 Infectious

In neuro-intensive care units, common infectious causes of fever include meningitis, brain abscess and ventriculitis. Other potential causes include urinary tract infections, pneumonia and bloodstream infections.

In addition to the infectious causes of fever mentioned above, hospital-acquired infections (HAI), such as Ventilator-Associated Pneumonia (VAP), Central Line-Associated Bloodstream Infections (CLABSI), Catheter-Associated Urinary Tract Infections (CAUTI), *Clostridium difficile* (*C. difficile*) infection and trophic ulcer infections can also be cause of fever in neuro-intensive care units. These infections are more common in patients who are critically ill and require prolonged hospitalization, invasive procedures and the use of devices such as ventilators, central venous catheters and urinary catheters. It is important for healthcare providers to be aware of these potential infections and to implement appropriate infection prevention and control measures to reduce the risk of these infections [12].

38.6.2 Non-infectious

Common non-infectious causes of fever in neuro-intensive care units include:

Inflammation: Inflammation in the brain or spinal cord (such as from a traumatic injury or a stroke) can cause fever.

Neoplasms: Brain tumours or metastatic tumours to the brain can cause fever as a result of the body's immune response to the tumour.

Drug reactions: Certain medications, such as antibiotics and anticonvulsants like penicillin, cephalosporin and phenytoin, can cause fever as a side effect (drug fever).

Blood clot: Deep vein thrombosis (DVT) and pulmonary embolism (PE) can cause fever.

Metabolic disorders: Some metabolic disorders, such as hyperthyroidism and hyperparathyroidism, can cause fever as a symptom.

Autoimmune disorders: Certain autoimmune disorders, such as lupus and sarcoidosis, can cause fever.

Transfusion reaction: Transfusion reaction can cause fever as a reaction to the transfused blood product [13].

38.6.3 Hyperthermia Syndromes in Neuro-intensive Care

Hyperthermia is a condition in which the body's temperature is elevated above 41 °C. Hyperthermia syndromes are a group of conditions that are characterized by high-grade fever, musculoskeletal and neurocognitive manifestations and are caused by various underlying mechanisms.

Neuroleptic malignant syndrome (NMS) is a rare but serious complication that can occur as a result of treatment with certain antipsychotic medications (most common with haloperidol, chlorpromazine, trifluoperazine, fluphenazine and prochlorperazine). It is characterized by symptoms such as fever, muscle rigidity and confusion. Other symptoms can include changes in mental status, autonomic instability (such as high blood pressure or irregular heart rate) and laboratory evidence of muscle injury. NMS is a medical emergency that requires immediate treatment. Treatment typically involves discontinuation of the offending medication and supportive care to maintain vital organ function. Medications such as dantrolene and bromocriptine may also be used to reduce muscle rigidity and fever. With prompt recognition and treatment, the prognosis for NMS is generally good. However, if not treated in a timely manner, NMS can be fatal [14].

Serotonin syndrome is a potentially life-threatening condition that can occur as a result of an excessive amount of serotonin in the body. Serotonin is a chemical messenger that plays a role in regulating mood, sleep and other bodily functions. Serotonin syndrome typically occurs as a result of the use of certain medications, such as antidepressants, painkillers and illegal drugs, which increase the levels of serotonin in the body (most common with fluoxetine, paroxetine, escitalopram and sertraline). Symptoms of serotonin syndrome can include agitation, confusion, muscle rigidity, changes in heart rate, fever and sweating, among others.

The diagnosis of serotonin syndrome is often made based on the presence of characteristic symptoms and a history of exposure to serotonergic medications. Treatment for serotonin syndrome typically involves removing the offending medication and providing supportive care to manage symptoms. Medications such as cyproheptadine, benzodiazepines and chlorpromazine may be used to reduce muscle rigidity and agitation. In severe cases, intensive care may be required.

It's important to note that serotonin syndrome can be caused by interactions between different medications, so it is crucial to review all medications, including over-the-counter medications and supplements when starting a new medication. With prompt recognition and treatment, the prognosis for serotonin syndrome is generally good, but if not treated in a timely manner, it can be fatal [15].

Malignant catatonia is a rare but potentially fatal condition characterized by muscle rigidity, altered mental status and autonomic instability including fever. It is a subtype of catatonia, a state of motor dysfunction characterized by muscle rigidity, immobility and other abnormal movements. Malignant catatonia is considered a medical emergency that requires prompt recognition and treatment.

The cause of malignant catatonia is often associated with medical or psychiatric conditions, such as infections, brain injury or schizophrenia. It can also be caused by certain medications, such as neuroleptics. The diagnosis of malignant catatonia is often made based on the presence of characteristic symptoms and a history of exposure to known risk factors.

Treatment for malignant catatonia typically involves the use of benzodiazepines, such as lorazepam, to reduce muscle rigidity and agitation. Electroconvulsive therapy (ECT) may also be used in some cases. In addition, the underlying cause should be identified and treated. Supportive care, such as maintaining hydration and electrolyte balance, is also important.

The prognosis for malignant catatonia is generally good with prompt recognition and treatment, but if not treated in a timely manner, it can be fatal. It is important to be aware of the symptoms of malignant catatonia and to seek medical attention immediately if they occur [16].

Parkinsonism-hyperpyrexia syndrome (PHS) is a rare but potentially fatal complication that can occur in patients with Parkinson's disease or other Parkinsonian disorders who are being treated with antipsychotic medications. PHS is characterized by symptoms such as fever, muscle rigidity and confusion, as well as changes in heart rate and blood pressure. The exact cause of PHS is not well understood, but it is thought to be related to the use of antipsychotic medications that block dopamine receptors in the brain.

The diagnosis of PHS is often made based on the presence of characteristic symptoms and a history of exposure to antipsychotic medications. Treatment for PHS typically involves the discontinuation of the offending medication, as well as supportive care to maintain vital organ function. Medications such as dantrolene, bromocriptine and amantadine may also be used to reduce muscle rigidity and fever [17].

PHS is a medical emergency that requires prompt recognition and treatment. If not treated in a timely manner, it can be fatal. Therefore, it is important to be aware of the symptoms of PHS and to seek medical attention immediately if they occur. It is also important to review all medications, including over-the-counter medications and supplements when starting a new medication.

Drug fever is a condition characterized by fever as a side effect of certain medications. It is a non-infectious cause of fever and it is caused by a drug-induced immune response. The fever is usually low grade and the symptoms usually occur within hours to days after starting the offending medication.

Drug fever can be caused by a wide range of medications, including antibiotics, antipsychotics, anti-inflammatory drugs and others. Some examples of drugs that can cause drug fever include sulphonamide, penicillin and NSAID. The diagnosis of drug fever is often made based on the presence of fever and a history of recent medication use.

Treatment for drug fever typically involves discontinuation of the offending medication and supportive care to manage symptoms. Medications such as acetaminophen or ibuprofen can be used to reduce fever and discomfort. In some cases, an alternative medication may be prescribed [13].

Drug fever is generally a benign condition and it usually resolves once the medication is discontinued. However, it is important to be aware of the symptoms and to consider the diagnosis if they occur after starting a new medication. Nevertheless, it remains a challenge to suspect and establish a drug as a cause of fever especially in a critically ill patient in a neuro-intensive care unit who has high probabilities of other non-infectious and infectious aetiologies. Therefore, many times, drug fever becomes a diagnosis of exclusion.

Figure 38.3 entails the common causes of all categories of fever in the neuro intensive care unit.

38.7 Investigations and Treatment

Several laboratory tests can be used to diagnose and evaluate fever, these include:

Blood cultures: to detect bacterial infection.

CSF analysis: Analysis of cerebrospinal fluid (CSF) can reveal the presence of infection or inflammation in the central nervous system. This includes measuring the white blood cell count, protein and glucose levels in the CSF.

PCR: Polymerase chain reaction (PCR) can be used to detect the presence of specific viruses or bacteria or fungi in the CSF.

Serological tests: such as ELISA, western blot or immunofluorescence assay can be used to detect antibodies against certain viruses or bacteria in the blood.

Imaging studies: CT scan or MRI of the brain can help in identifying brain abscesses, tumour or other structural changes in the brain.

Electroencephalogram (EEG): it is used to detect abnormal brain activity which can help in certain cases of encephalitis.

It is important to note that these tests are not specific to central fever (fever with a CNS pathology) and they may be used along with clinical examination and other tests to arrive at a definitive diagnosis.

There are several general inflammatory markers that can be used to evaluate a patient with central fever. Some of these include:

Erythrocyte sedimentation rate (ESR): Elevated ESR levels can indicate inflammation in the body.

C-reactive protein (CRP): Elevated CRP levels can also indicate inflammation in the body.

Procalcitonin (PCT): Elevated PCT levels can indicate systemic bacterial infection, it is particularly useful to differentiate between viral and bacterial meningitis or encephalitis. However, in certain cases of localized inflammation, PCT levels may not rise despite the presence of florid symptoms of CNS infection.

White blood cell count (WBC): An elevated WBC count can indicate an infection or inflammation. A high neutrophil count may suggest a bacterial infection while a high lymphocyte count may suggest a viral infection.

These markers can provide important information about the presence and severity of inflammation or infection; however, they should be interpreted in conjunction with the patient's clinical presentation and other laboratory results [5, 18, 19].

The treatment of central fever depends on the underlying cause. Both pharmacological and non-pharmacological measures are applied as necessary (Fig. 38.4). However, some common pharmacological treatments include:

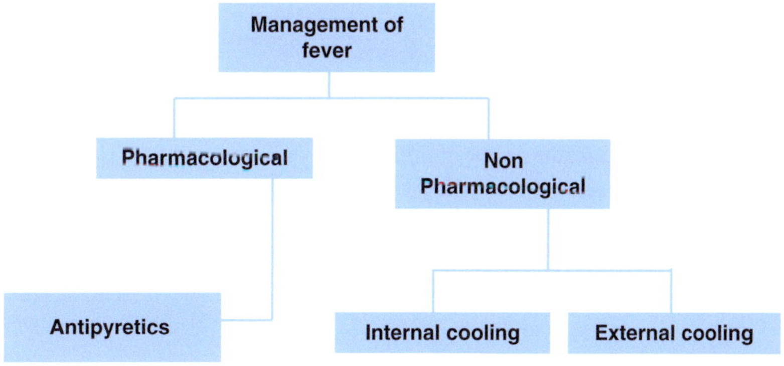

Fig. 38.4 Management options of fever

Antipyretics: Paracetamol is commonly used in higher doses. Sometimes a non-steroidal agent is necessary to control recurring high temperatures.

Antibiotics: used to treat bacterial infections such as meningitis.

Antiviral drugs: used to treat viral infections such as encephalitis.

Steroids: used to reduce inflammation and swelling in the brain and spinal cord.

Analgesics: used to relieve pain and fever.

Anticonvulsants: used to control seizures.

Immunomodulatory therapy: used to modulate the body's immune response in certain cases like autoimmune encephalitis [20, 21].

It is important to note that the treatment should be tailored to the specific cause and should be administered under the supervision of a specialist in neuro-intensive care in consultation with an infectious disease specialist as necessary.

Nonpharmacological measures:

There are several non-pharmacological ways to manage fever, which include:

Rest: Getting enough rest and sleep can help the body cope with stress and raise metabolic demands.

Hydration: Drinking plenty of fluids can help prevent dehydration and promote sweating, which can help bring down a fever.

Cool compresses: Applying cool compresses to the forehead, wrists or armpits can help lower body temperature [22].

Light clothing: Dressing in light clothing can help dissipate heat and keep the body cool.

Sponging: A lukewarm water sponge bath can help lower a fever by promoting sweating.

Internal cooling measures: Like cold saline intravenous infusion, ice-water gastric lavage and urinary bladder continuous irrigation with ice-cold saline can be employed [23].

Other measures:

Changing lines/catheters or draining localized collections as feasible if suspected to be a source of fever.

Actively searching for occult infection/inflammation like thrombophlebitis, sinusitis, otitis or cellulitis.

38.8 Conclusion

In conclusion, fever is a serious issue for neurological patients in the neuro-intensive care setting. The high fever can cause secondary injury to the brain and worsen the patient's outcome. The goal of fever management in neuro-intensive care is to keep the patient's body temperature within a normal range. Therefore, it is imperative to have a low threshold and proactive approach in the management of fever in these patients. Non-pharmacological measures, including external and internal cooling methods, can be effective in treating fever in the neuro-intensive care setting. However, it is important to use these measures with caution and under close medical supervision, as they can have potential side effects or complications. A thorough assessment of the patient's condition, along with monitoring of vital signs, is necessary to ensure that the fever management strategy is safe and effective. It is necessary to address the underlying cause of the fever by performing an active search and targeted treatment for all possible infective and non-infective causes. This may involve starting antibiotics in case of an infection, or other treatments as appropriate for non-infective causes such as neoplastic fever, drug fever or autoimmune fever.

References

1. Laupland KB, Shahpori R, Kirkpatrick AW, Ross T, Gregson DB, Stelfox HT. Occurrence and outcome of fever in critically ill adults. Crit Care Med. 2008;36(5):1531–5.
2. Mackowiak PA, Wasserman SS, Levine MM. A critical appraisal of 98.6 degrees F, the upper limit of the normal body temperature, and other legacies of Carl Reinhold August Wunderlich. JAMA. 1992;268(12):1578–80.
3. Rincon F, Hunter K, Schorr C, Dellinger RP, Zanotti-Cavazzoni S. The epidemiology of spontaneous fever and hypothermia on admission of brain injury patients to intensive care units: a multicenter cohort study. J Neurosurg. 2014;121(4):950–60.
4. Zawadzka M, Szmuda M, Mazurkiewicz-Bełdzińska M. Thermoregulation disorders of central origin: how

to diagnose and treat. Anaesthesiol Intensive Ther. 2017;49:227–34.
5. Dimopoulos G, Falagas ME. Approach to the febrile patient in the ICU. Infect Dis Clin N Am. 2009;23:471–84.
6. Circiumaru B, Baldock G, Cohen J. A prospective study of fever in the intensive care unit. Intensive Care Med. 1999;25(7):668–73.
7. Commichau C, Scarmeas N, Mayer SA. Risk factors for fever in the neurologic intensive care unit. Neurology. 2003;60(5):837–41.
8. Ntaios G, Dziedzic T, Michel P, Papavasileiou V, Petersson J, Staykov D, et al. European Stroke Organisation (ESO) guidelines for the management of temperature in patients with acute ischemic stroke. Int J Stroke. 2015;10:941–9.
9. Greer DM, Funk SE, Reaven NL, Ouzounelli M, Uman GC. Impact of fever on outcome in patients with stroke and neurologic injury: a comprehensive meta-analysis. Stroke. 2008;39(11):3029–35.
10. Meier K, Lee K. Neurogenic fever: review of pathophysiology, evaluation and management. J Intensive Care Med. 2017;32(2):124–9.
11. Badjatia N. Fever control in the neuro-ICU: why, who, and when? Curr Opin Crit Care. 2009;15(2):79–82.
12. Schwarz S, Häfner K, Aschoff A, Schwab S. Incidence and prognostic significance of fever following intracerebral hemorrhage. Neurology. 2000;54:354–61.
13. Rabinstein AA, Sandhu K. Noninfectious fever in the neurological intensive care unit: incidence, causes and predictors. J Neurol Neurosurg Psychiatry. 2007;78:1278–80.
14. Pelonero AL, Levenson JL, Pandurangi AK. Neuroleptic malignant syndrome: a review. Psychiatr Serv. 1998;49(9):1163–72.
15. Dunkley EJC, Isbister GK, Sibbritt D, Dawson AH, Whyte IM. The Hunter serotonin toxicity criteria: simple and accurate diagnostic decision rules for serotonin toxicity. QJM. 2003;96(9):635–42.
16. Luchini F, Medda P, Mariani MG, Mauri M, Toni C, Perugi G. Electroconvulsive therapy in catatonic patients: efficacy and predictors of response. World J Psychiatry. 2015;5(2):182–92.
17. Newman EJ, Grosset DG, Kennedy PGE. The parkinsonism-hyperpyrexia syndrome. Neurocrit Care. 2009;10(1):136–40.
18. Egi M, Morita K. Fever in nonneurological critically ill patients: a systematic review of observational studies. J Crit Care. 2012;27:428–33.
19. Marik PE. Fever in the ICU. Chest. 2000;117(3):855–69.
20. Gaieski DF, Mikkelsen ME, Band RA, et al. Impact of time to antibiotics on survival in patients with severe sepsis or septic shock in whom early goal-directed therapy was initiated in the emergency department. Crit Care Med. 2010;38(4):1045–53.
21. Dippel DWJ, van Breda EJ, van der Worp HB, et al.; PISA-Investigators. Effect of paracetamol (acetaminophen) and ibuprofen on body temperature in acute ischemic stroke PISA, a phase II double-blind, randomized, placebo-controlled trial [ISRCTN98608690]. BMC Cardiovasc Disord. 2003;3:2.
22. Schortgen F, Clabault K, Katsahian S, et al. Fever control using external cooling in septic shock: a randomized controlled trial. Am J Respir Crit Care Med. 2012;185(10):1088–95.
23. Fink EL, Kochanek PM, Clark RSB, Bell MJ. Fever control and application of hypothermia using intravenous cold saline. Pediatr Crit Care Med. 2012;13(1):80–4.

Sepsis in Neurocritical Care

39

Konstantin A. Popugaev and Sergey S. Petrikov

39.1 Introduction

Sepsis is one of the most actual problems of medicine and healthcare systems. In Russia, sepsis is diagnosed in almost one million people each year [1]. A comparable level of sepsis development is typical for Europe and the United States [2, 3]. An unfavorable epidemiological feature of sepsis is an increase in its frequency and severity during the last decades [4, 5]. One of the greatest epidemiological problems is the absence of exact number of cases with sepsis worldwide due to diagnostic difficulties and issues, related to the interpretation of sepsis criteria. A rough assessment of the occurrence of sepsis worldwide is 31.5 million cases annually, and 5.3 million deaths are associated with sepsis [4, 6, 7]. Obviously, sepsis is a typical issue of intensive care, since multiple organ dysfunction syndrome is the essence of sepsis.

Sepsis is a common complication in neurocritical care patients. Sepsis and septic shock develop in 3.6% and 1.3% appropriately of cases after elective cranial surgery and in 0.9% and 0.3% appropriately of cases after elective spinal surgery [8]. Some cohorts of patients after elective neurosurgery have a greater risk of infectious complications. For example, postoperative sepsis develops in almost 3% of cases after skull base neurosurgery [9]. Incidence of sepsis in patients with intracerebral hemorrhage (ICH) ranges from 1 to 4%, in patients with ischemic stroke—from 12 to 13%, patients with aneurismal subarachnoid hemorrhage (aSAH)—from 33% to 50%, and in patients with traumatic brain injury—from 55 to 75% [10–19]. Neurocritical care settings are unique, because, on the one hand, brain injury predisposes to the development of sepsis, and, on the other hand, sepsis itself leads to brain damage. The chapter is dedicated to this issue.

39.2 Definitions

There were three definitions of sepsis. In the Sepsis 2 definition, created in 2001, the leading role played the concept of systemic inflammatory response syndrome (SIRS) [20]. SIRS consists of four criteria: hypothermia (<36 °C) or fever (>38 °C); tachycardia (>90 beats per minute); tachypnea (>20 breaths per minute); and leukopenia (<4000/mcL) or leukocytosis (>12,000/mcL) [20]. Complications of SIRS are a multiple organ dysfunction syndrome, including shock. Causes of SIRS can be both infectious and noninfectious [21]. A combination of SIRS and a source of infection was interpreted as sepsis. Along with this, brain damage due to aneurysmal aSAH, ICH, severe traumatic brain injury, and other pathological conditions can be a cause of noninfectious SIRS [22, 23], which is one of the

K. A. Popugaev (✉) · S. S. Petrikov
Regional Vascular Centre of Sklifosovsky Research Institute of Emergency Medicine, Moscow, Russia
e-mail: Petrikovss@sklif.mos.ru

H. Prabhakar et al. (eds.), *Principles and Practice of Neurocritical Care*,
https://doi.org/10.1007/978-981-99-8059-8_39

main sources of diagnostic difficulties in neurocritical care settings. From a formal point of view, some therapeutic options, routinely used in neurocritical care patients for neuroprotection, or for other specific neurocritical care purposes, can be mistakenly interpreted in the light of sepsis conceptions. For example, the usage of norepinephrine in patients with aSAH as a maneuver for blood pressure management in the treatment of cerebral vasospasm has nothing to do with the septic condition. By definition, such a clinical situation cannot be interpreted as sepsis despite the development of SIRS or elevation of SOFA scoring, because the cause of these phenomena is a brain injury. However, misdiagnosis of sepsis instead of noninfectious SIRS is typical for neurocritical care settings [24, 25].

The third definition, approved by the international critical care community in 2016, interprets sepsis as a "life-threatening organ dysfunction due to a dysregulated host response to infection" [25]. In the Sepsis 3 definition, the key role for the diagnosis of sepsis belongs to the Sequential Organ Failure Assessment (SOFA) scale [25]. Sepsis 3 definition implies the presence of a source of infection and an increase in the SOFA by two points. Severe brain damage commonly leads to organ dysfunction and, accordingly, to such an increase in the SOFA, which can be mistakenly regarded as a criterion for sepsis [26–30]. Thus, the currently existing criteria for sepsis in both Sepsis 2 and Sepsis 3 definitions complicate and confuse the diagnosis of sepsis in neurocritical care patients.

Some groups dedicated their investigations for looking for more reliable diagnostic criteria for sepsis in neurocritical care. For example, Centner FS and colleagues, who have been investigating different diagnostic criteria, showed that the so-called modified SOFA scale, which is presented in Table 39.1, allows to improve diagnosis of sepsis and to clarify outcomes in neurocritical care patients with sepsis [31]. In comparison with SIRS or SOFA, the usage of modified SOFA had some advantages [31]. Obviously, the data presented by Centner FS and colleagues are of high importance for neurocritical care, but further studies should be performed.

Table 39.1 Alternative sepsis criteria to detect an organ dysfunction caused by a dysregulated host response to infection

Organ system	Criteria for organ dysfunction
Cardiovascular	Sepsis-induced hypotension (SBP <90 mmHg or MAP <70 mmHg) or new necessity of norepinephrine to reach MAP ≥70 mmHg or increase of norepinephrine ≥1.5 times baseline (if norepinephrine was used previously to induce hypertension to treat delayed cerebral injury)
Renal	Urine-output <0.5 mL/kg/h for ≥6 h; increase in serum creatinine ≥1.5 times baseline
Respiration	$p_aO_2/FiO_2 < 250$ in the absence of pneumonia, or $p_aO_2/FiO_2 < 200$ if pneumonia is present (pneumonia according to CDC criteria)
Liver	Bilirubin >2 mg/dL
Coagulation	Platelet count <100,000/μL or coagulation abnormalities (INR > 1.5)
CNS	Septic encephalopathy (confusion or agitation)
Gastrointestinal	Ileus or gut ischemia

CNS central nervous system, *FiO2* fraction of inspired oxygen, *INR* international normalized ratio, *MAP* mean arterial pressure, p_aO_2 partial pressure of arterial oxygen, *SBP* systolic blood pressure

39.3 Primary Brain Injury and Secondary Sepsis

It is generally accepted that brain injury leads to the development of infection, or, at least, increases the risk of infection, which can progress to sepsis. Urinary tract infection (UTI), pneumonia, and central nervous system (CNS) infection are the most frequent sources of infection in neurocritical care patients [22, 32–34]. The pathogenesis of CNS infection is mainly caused by loss of isolation of the brain from the environment, which makes brain injury an understandable mechanism for the development of CNS infection. UTI, which developed in 24–27% of neurocritical patients, rarely leads to sepsis [34]. Another situation is pneumonia, developed in 16–20% of neurocritical patients [22, 32, 33]. Pneumonia is the most frequent source of sepsis in neurocritical care patients. More severe brain injury leads to more severe pneumonia, which, in turn, typically leads to sepsis [10, 12, 19, 35–38], which is extremely interesting and important dependence and deserves attention and discussion.

More severe aSAH and more severe aSAH-associated cerebral vasospasm more often lead to more severe pneumonia [35]. In turn, the more severe the pneumonia means the higher the risk of sepsis and unfavorable outcome. For example, mortality in aSAH is 52.5% for septic patients and 16% for non-septic patients [22]. There are several explanations for the greater risk of pneumonia and sepsis in neurocritical care patients, especially in patients with aSAH: decreased level of consciousness, dysphagia and aspiration, decreased clearance of sputum, mechanical ventilation, immobilization, and many others. However, one of the most significant risk factors for the development of infectious complications, in general, and, in particular, pneumonia and sepsis in neurocritical care patients is immunodepression [35].

Immunodepression has been previously described in the broad spectrum of neurocritical care pathology: ischemic stroke, aSAH, ICH, severe traumatic brain injury, and complicated postoperative period of elective neurosurgery [39, 40]. Most experts in this field consider that hypothalamic-pituitary-adrenal axis damage due to very different mechanisms is the keystone and leads to complex neurohumoral stress pathways and autonomic imbalance (dysautonomia) and eventually to the inhibition of immune function or immunodepression [35].

Brain ischemia in patients with stroke leads to stroke-associated immunodepression [39, 41]. Localization of brain damage after stroke plays a great role in the development of stroke-associated immunodepression. Lesions of the insula and anterior part of the cortex in the territory of blood supplement of the middle cerebral artery lead to immunodepression, infection, sepsis, and worsening outcomes [42, 43]. Immunodepression develops due to a decrease in the secretion of interferon-gamma production by lymphocytes [44]. Stroke-associated immunodepression can lead to the development of pneumonia after only 2–3 days after stroke, even in patients without such significant risk factors, such as dysphagia. For understanding the significance of the problem of stroke-associated immunodepression, it is important to keep in mind that this phenomenon can be persistent and affect the course of the disease, at least, during the entire period of the patient's hospitalization.

The phenomenon of aSAH-associated immunodepression has been previously described. aSAH-induced damage of the hypothalamic-pituitary-adrenal axis leads to a rapid and significant decrease of T-cell counts, reduction in the secretion of interferon-gamma by lymphocytes, the release of tumor necrosis factor by monocytes, and surface expression of antigen-DR by leukocytes [35]. Another important possible cause of aSAH-associated immunodepression is the usage of catecholamines, which is a frequent therapeutic option in the treatment of neurocritical care patients with aSAH [44]. Such immunological disturbances develop very early after aSAH. After 24 h after aSAH, these changes are registered. Thus, aSAH-immunodepression is an important pathogenetic mechanism for the development of infection and sepsis in this group of neurocritical care patients.

ICH-associated immunodepression is realized by lymphopenia, which is not only a marker of ICH-associated immunodepression, but that is a cornerstone immunological phenomenon for both pathogenesis and outcomes of ICH [39]. Lymphopenia at admission in patients with ICH is a commonly accepted significant prognostic marker of unfavorable outcome [39, 45]. Male sex is associated with worse outcomes in patients with ICH due to the increased rate of infectious and septic complications [46–50]. Such association can be explained by differences in immunological response, depending on sex [39]. The mechanisms of this phenomenon consist in the peculiarities of the influence of male sex steroids and the expression of X-chromosome gene [51–53].

Lymphopenia is caused by apoptosis of lymphocytes due to acute secretion of stress mediators, and the severity of lymphopenia significantly correlates with the patient's condition, level of consciousness, and severity of infectious complications [44, 54, 55]. Also, it is considered that migration of lymphocytes to the hematoma and to the area of the brain, around the hematoma, leads to such severe complications, as hematoma enlargement, intraventricular bleeding, and brain edema.

Normal levels of lymphocytes might have protective effects against infection in patients with ICH [45]. In contrast, immunological therapy, directed to reduce lymphocyte count, enhances inflammation and increases the risk of infection and sepsis [56–59]. Lymphocyte activation in the acute phase of inflammation hypothetically can be protective, and such conception was suggested at Harvard University [45]. Obviously, the regulation of immunological response to ICH is extremely complex, and this conception requires further thorough research.

Patients with complicated postoperative period after elective neurosurgery is a special cohort of neurocritical care patients. On the one hand, neurocritical care specialists typically face in their routine clinical practice with acute vascular or traumatic cerebral catastrophes. However, on the other hand, elective neurosurgery is a rapidly developing area of neurosciences, and thousands of patients around the world undergo neurosurgical operations annually. In this regard, neurocritical care specialists face with such patients more and more frequently.

The principle difference of patients after elective neurosurgery from other groups of neurocritical care patients in light of immunodepression is routine usage of glucocorticosteroids and perioperative damage of certain anatomical areas of the brain due to tumor growth and operation. The majority of neurosurgical patients with brain or spinal tumors receive glucocorticosteroids perioperatively. There is some evidence that showed a decreased risk of development of immunodepression due to glucocorticosteroids [44, 60]. On the other hand, perioperative damage of diencephalon, insula, another important anatomical structures, or regulated autonomic functions leads to the development of immunodepression [42]. Thus, immunodepression can develop in neurocritical care patients after elective surgery; however, this cohort, unlike other groups of neurocritical care patients, has such a significant factor, preventing the development of immunodepression, as the use of steroids.

39.4 Primary Sepsis and Secondary Brain Injury

Sepsis is a systemic pathology. Any patient without preexisting damage to the central nervous system (CNS) can develop acute cerebral dysfunction due to sepsis. There are several important damaging factors that affect the brain in patients with sepsis: blood-brain barrier (BBB) impairment with or without microglial activation, sympathoadrenal surge, mitochondrial dysfunction, and apoptosis [61–65]. The first concept of sepsis-associated brain injury appeared in the early 2000s, and this phenomenon then was called "sepsis-associated delirium" [66]. The authors of this concept are Wesley Ely and colleagues, who have been creating the concept of delirium during that time period. The concept of sepsis-associated delirium was only a part of this general concept, which was a significant step in the understanding of the matter of brain injury due to sepsis. However, it soon became clear that the term sepsis-associated delirium does not unite the entire spectrum of all possible clinical conditions of brain injury, developing due to sepsis. In 2003, Wilson and Young created the term "septic encephalopathy," which implied the following definition: diffuse, possible also multifocal disturbance of cerebral function as a consequence of the systemic inflammatory response triggered by the contact of the host with potent pathogenic microbes [67]. The term septic encephalopathy has been successfully used until the present.

Sepsis can lead to different types of brain injury (Fig. 39.1). First of all, sepsis-associated brain injury should be divided into infectious and noninfectious. Infectious sepsis-associated brain injury develops due to BBB impairment and pathogen penetration from the blood into the brain. That is a hematogenic way of CNS infection. The problem of CNS infection is beyond the scope of the topic of this chapter.

Noninfectious sepsis-associated brain injury should be divided into focal and generalized (Fig. 39.1). Sepsis itself and different treatment options predispose to the development of stroke or ICH. For example, atrial fibrillation, frequently developed during sepsis, can be a cause of thromboembolic stroke in patients with sepsis [68]. Septic-induced coagulopathy and thrombocytopenia, commonly developed during sepsis in combination with anticoagulant usage, can be a cause of ICH [69]. Thus, stroke and ICH are causes of focal noninfectious sepsis-associated brain injury. It should be kept in mind that multifocal brain injury is hypothetically possible [69]. However, such type of brain injury, in fact, has signs of focal injury with several localizations at the same time. For example, thromboembolic stroke in the areas of different cerebral arteries leads to multifocal brain injury.

From the Confusion Assessment Method in Intensive Care Unit (CAM-ICU), delirium is considered a combination of consciousness alteration and attention impairment or disorganized thinking [70]. In accordance with the CAM-ICU, delirium can be hyperactive, hypoactive, or mixed [71]. The majority of septic patients meet these criteria, or in other words, the majority of septic patients have delirium. In most cases, septic delirium is hypoactive [71]. Two principle issues are extremely actual for patients with sepsis-associated delirium. First is the global lack of routine screening for delirium in septic patients. Second is an absolute predominance of the hypoactive type of delirium. Both these facts hamper to detect delirium in critical care patients with sepsis [72].

Early detection of delirium and its timely correction in critical care patients might be a separate and important avenue in the treatment septic neurocritical care patients. Obviously, hypoactive delirium, as the predominant type of delirium in neurocritical care, requirement of sedation, and primary brain injury in the neurocritical care cohort are objective causes of difficulties in the verification of delirium. Another important issue that deserves attention is the much lesser effectiveness of the treatment of

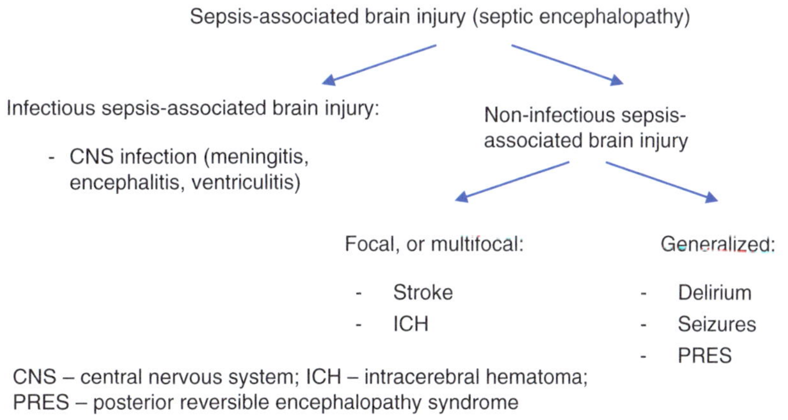

Fig. 39.1 Structure of sepsis-associated brain injury (septic encephalopathy). *CNS* central nervous system, *ICH* intracerebral hematoma, *PRES* posterior reversible encephalopathy syndrome

hypoactive delirium compared with hyperactive or mixed delirium. Any type of delirium requires prompt pharmacological and non-pharmacological correction [71, 72].

In a population of critically ill patients, seizures appear in 8–34% [73, 74]. Seizures in this population are usually nonconvulsive, and the rate of their verification depends on the practice of usage of EEG monitoring [62]. Sepsis is one of the most significant risk factors for the development of seizures and status epilepticus in the cohort of critical care patients [75]. The basic pathophysiological mechanism of seizures in septic patients is an imbalance between N-methyl-D-aspartate (NMDA) and γ-amino-butyric-acid (GABA) [76, 77]. Many other pathophysiological mechanisms of seizures, such as interleukins and cytokines surge, vascular permeability, BBB disruption, activation of excitotoxicity pathways, and neuroinflammation, ultimately create conditions for the realization of an imbalance between NMDA and GABA, which leads to seizures. Commonly seizures in critical care patients, especially, in those, who are sedated, are underdiagnosed. Timely verification of seizures with their subsequent immediate and effective correction can be considered one of the most important areas of treatment of patients with noninfectious sepsis-associated brain injury.

Posterior reversible encephalopathy syndrome (PRES) was first described by Hinchey and coauthors in 1996 [78]. The main manifestation of the PRES is cortico-subcortical damage of different brain areas, predominantly occipital lobes. There is a plethora of different pathologies, during which PRES can develop [79, 80]. The baseline pathophysiological mechanism, leading to the development of PRES, is a combination of cerebral autoregulation impairment, immunological disturbances, and hemodynamic instability with episodes of arterial hypertension [78–80]. The appearance of such a combination is very possible during sepsis. Typical for sepsis pathophysiological links, repeatedly mentioned and discussed above, can easily lead to the combination of cerebral autoregulation impairment, immunological disturbances, hemodynamic instability, and eventually PRES. In this regard, it is necessary to focus on this important issue. It is not completely clear, why the same, in fact, mechanisms in some patients lead to seizures and in others to PRES. It is possible that in some septic patients the cause of seizures is precisely PRES. Further investigations, dedicated to this problem, are extremely warrantable.

The spectrum of clinical symptoms of PRES is wide, including headache, confusion, different types of consciousness alterations, visual disturbances, seizures, and motor-focal neurological deficits [80, 81]. In the situation with seizures in septic patients, PRES is often underdiagnosed [82]. The actual frequency of PRES among septic patients may be much higher compared with our current understanding of the place of PRES in the structure of noninfectious sepsis-associated brain injury. Favorable outcomes are typical for PRES; however, lethal outcome can develop [82]. The possibility of an unfavorable outcome in PRES makes its early verification and effective correction an extremely promising direction of treatment of noninfectious sepsis-associated brain injury.

39.5 Conclusions

Sepsis is an issue of great importance for both the global specialty of critical care and the subspecialty of neurocritical care. There are intimate links between critical care, neurocritical care, and sepsis. Primary brain injury leads to immunodepression, which, in turn, is a cause of sepsis. In other words, brain injury predisposes to sepsis. On the other hand, sepsis is a trigger of a plethora of mechanisms, which eventually leads to sepsis-associated brain injury. In other words, sepsis turns neurocritical care pathology into critical care disease.

Such understanding of relationships between brain injury, brain injury-associated immunodepression, sepsis, and sepsis-associated brain injury allows to create several important avenues for the management of neurocritical patients and septic critical care patients. Therapy, oriented to prophylaxis and effective correction of brain injury-associated immunodepression, may decrease the development of sepsis and improve outcomes in neurocritical care. Therapy, oriented to prophylaxis and effective correction of sepsis-associated brain injury, may decrease the development of brain damage and improve outcomes in critical care. Further research in this actual field is extremely warranted.

References

1. Noskova OA, Anganova E, Gvak G, Savilov ED. Epidemiological aspects of sepsis. J Microbiol Epidemiol Immunobiol. 2018;95:121–6.
2. Cohen J, Vincent JL, Adhikari NK, et al. Sepsis: a road- map for future research. Lancet Infect Dis. 2015;15:581–614.
3. Yealy DM, Huang DT, Delaney A, et al. Recognizing and managing sepsis: what needs to be done? BMC Med. 2015;13:98.
4. Fleischmann C, Scherag A, Adhikari NK, et al. Assessment of global incidence and mortality of hospital-treated sepsis—Current estimates and limitations. Am J Respir Crit Care Med. 2016;193:259–72.
5. Shankar-Hari M, Harrison DA, Rubenfeld GD, Rowan K. Epidemiology of sepsis and septic shock in critical care units: comparison between sepsis-2 and sepsis-3 populations using a national critical care database. Br J Anaesth. 2017;119:626–36.
6. Vincent JL, Sakr Y, Sprung CL, et al. Sepsis in European intensive care units: results of the SOAP study. Crit Care Med. 2006;34:344–53.
7. Kaukonen KM, Bailey M, Suzuki S, et al. Mortality related to severe sepsis and septic shock among critically ill patients in Australia and New Zealand. JAMA. 2014;311:1308–16.
8. Rolston JD, Han SJ, Lau CY, et al. Frequency and predictors of complications in neurological surgery: national trends from 2006 to 2011. J Neurosurg. 2014;120:736–45.
9. Burton BN, Hu JQ, Jafari A, et al. An updated assessment of morbidity and mortality following skull base surgical approaches. Clin Neurol Neurosurg. 2018;171:109–15.
10. Murthy SB, Moradiya Y, Shah J, et al. Nosocomial infections and outcomes after intracerebral hemorrhage: a population-based study. Neurocrit Care. 2016;25:178–84.
11. Lord AS, Langefeld CD, Sekar P, et al. Infection after intracerebral hemorrhage: risk factors and association with outcomes in the ethnic/racial variations of intracerebral hemorrhage study. Stroke. 2014;45:3535–42.
12. Hinduja A, Dibu J, Achi E, et al. Nosocomial infections in patients with spontaneous intracerebral hemorrhage. Am J Crit Care. 2015;24:227–31.
13. Berger B, Gumbinger C, Steiner T, Sykora M. Epidemiologic features, risk factors, and outcome of sepsis in stroke patients treated on a neurologic intensive care unit. J Crit Care. 2014;29:241–8.
14. Stösser S, Isakeit J, Bode FJ, et al. Sepsis in patients with large vessel occlusion stroke-clinical characteristics and outcome. Front Neurol. 2022;13:902809.
15. Dhar R, Diringer MN. The burden of the systemic inflammatory response predicts vasospasm and outcome after subarachnoid hemorrhage. Neurocrit Care. 2008;8:404–12.
16. Papadimitriou-Olivgeris M, Zotou A, Koutsileou K, et al. Risk factors for mortality after subarachnoid hemorrhage: a retrospective observational study. Rev Bras Anestesiol. 2019;69:448–54.
17. Mazeraud A, Robba C, Rebora P, et al. Acute distress respiratory syndrome after subarachnoid hemorrhage: incidence and impact on the outcome in a large multicenter, retrospective cohort. Neurocrit Care. 2020;34:1000–8.
18. Frontera JA, Fernandez A, Schmidt JM, et al. Impact of nosocomial infectious complications after subarachnoid hemorrhage. Neurosurgery. 2008;62:80–7.
19. Corral L, Javierre CF, Ventura JL, et al. Impact of non-neurological complications in severe traumatic brain injury outcome. Crit Care. 2012;16:R44.
20. Levy MM, Fink MP, Marshall JC, et al. SCCM/ESICM/ACCP/ATS/SIS international sepsis definitions conference. Crit Care Med. 2003;3:1250–6.
21. Bone RC, Balk RA, Cerra FB, et al. Definitions for sepsis and organ failure and guidelines for the use of innovative therapies in sepsis. The ACCP/SCCM Consensus Conference Committee. American College of Chest Physicians/Society of Critical Care Medicine. Chest. 1992;101:1644–55.
22. Gonçalves B, Kurtz P, Turon R, et al. Incidence and impact of sepsis on long-term outcomes after subarachnoid hemorrhage: a prospective observational study. Ann Intensive Care. 2019;9:94.
23. Connolly ES Jr, Rabinstein AA, Carhuapoma JR, et al. Guidelines for the management of aneurysmal subarachnoid hemorrhage: a guideline for healthcare professionals from the American Heart Association/American Stroke Association. Stroke. 2012;43:1711–37.
24. Angus DC, Seymour CW, Coopersmith CM, et al. A framework for the development and interpretation of different sepsis definitions and clinical criteria. Crit Care Med. 2016;44:e113–21.
25. Singer M, Deutschman CS, Seymour CW, et al. The third international consensus definitions for sepsis and septic shock (Sepsis-3). JAMA. 2016;315:801–10.
26. Centner FS, Schoettler JJ, Fairley AM, et al. Impact of different consensus definition criteria on sepsis diagnosis in a cohort of critically ill patients—insights from a new mathematical probabilistic approach to mortality-based validation of sepsis criteria. PLoS One. 2020;15:e0238548.
27. Henig O, Putler RK, Albin O, et al. The performance of sepsis-3 criteria to predict mortality among patients

with hematologic malignancy and post-transplant who have suspected infection. Open Forum Infect Dis. 2021;8:ofab529.
28. Wu F, Zhou X. The comparisons and limitations of sepsis 2.0 and sepsis 3.0. J Crit Care. 2018;47:350–1.
29. Yoon J, Kym D, Hur J, et al. Comparative usefulness of sepsis-3, burn sepsis, and conventional sepsis criteria in patients with major burns. Crit Care Med. 2018;46:e656–62.
30. Sprung CL, Schein RM, Balk RA. The new sepsis consensus definitions: the good, the bad and the ugly. Intensive Care Med. 2016;42:2024–6.
31. Centner FS, Oster ME, Dally FJ, et al. Comparative analyses of the impact of different criteria for sepsis diagnosis on outcome in patients with spontaneous subarachnoid hemorrhage. J Clin Med. 2022;11:3873.
32. Bogossian EG, Attanasio L, Creteur J, et al. The impact of extracerebral infection after subarachnoid hemorrhage: a single-center cohort study. World Neurosurg. 2020;144:e883–97.
33. Laban KG, Rinkel GJ, Vergouwen MD. Nosocomial infections after aneurysmal subarachnoid hemorrhage: time course and causative pathogens. Int J Stroke. 2015;10:763–6.
34. Dasenbrock HH, Rudy RF, Smith TR, et al. Hospital-acquired infections after aneurysmal subarachnoid hemorrhage: a nationwide analysis. World Neurosurg. 2016;88:459–74.
35. Sarrafzadeh A, Schlenk F, Meisel A, et al. Immunodepression after aneurysmal subarachnoid hemorrhage. Stroke. 2011;42:53–8.
36. Cardozo Junior LC, Silva RR. Sepsis in intensive care unit patients with traumatic brain injury: factors associated with higher mortality. Rev Bras Ter Intensiva. 2014;26:148–54.
37. Selassie AW, Fakhry SM, Ford DW. Population-based study of the risk of in-hospital death after traumatic brain injury: the role of sepsis. J Trauma. 2011;71:1226–34.
38. Divani AA, Hevesi M, Pulivarthi S, et al. Predictors of nosocomial pneumonia in intracerebral hemorrhage patients: a multi-center observational study. Neurocrit Care. 2015;22:234–42.
39. Meisel C, Schwab JM, Prass K, et al. Central nervous system injury-induced immune deficiency syndrome. Nat Rev Neurosci. 2005;6:775–86.
40. Dziedzic T, Slowik A, Szczudlik A. Nosocomial infections and immunity: lesson from brain-injured patients. Crit Care. 2004;8:266–70.
41. Deyo RA, Cherkin DC, Ciol MA. Adapting a clinical comorbidity index for use with ICD-9-CM administrative databases. J Clin Epidemiol. 1992;45:613–9.
42. Steinhagen V, Grossmann A, Benecke R, Walter U. Swallowing disturbance pattern relates to brain lesion location in acute stroke patients. Stroke. 2009;40:1903–6.
43. Harms H, Reimnitz P, Bohner G, et al. Influence of stroke localization on autonomic activation, immunodepression, and post-stroke infection. Cerebrovasc Dis. 2011;32:552–60.
44. Prass K, Meisel C, Hoflich C, et al. Stroke-induced immunodeficiency promotes spontaneous bacterial infections and is mediated by sympathetic activation reversal by poststroke T helper cell type 1-like immunostimulation. J Exp Med. 2003;198:725–36.
45. Morotti A, Marini S, Jessel MJ, et al. Lymphopenia, infectious complications, and outcome in spontaneous intracerebral hemorrhage. Neurocrit Care. 2017;26:160–6.
46. Marini S, Morotti A, Lena UK, et al. Men experience higher risk of pneumonia and death after intracerebral hemorrhage. Neurocrit Care. 2018;28:77–82.
47. Kammersgaard LP, Jørgensen HS, Reith J, et al. Early infection and prognosis after acute stroke: the Copenhagen stroke study. J Stroke Cerebrovasc Dis. 2001;10:217–21.
48. Aslanyan S, Weir CJ, Diener HC, et al. Pneumonia and urinary tract infection after acute ischaemic stroke: a tertiary analysis of the GAIN international trial. Eur J Neurol. 2004;11:49–53.
49. Kwon HM, Jeong SW, Lee SH, Yoon BW. The pneumonia score: a simple grading scale for prediction of pneumonia after acute stroke. Am J Infect Control. 2006;34:64–8.
50. Katzan IL, Cebul RD, Husak SH, et al. The effect of pneumonia on mortality among patients hospitalized for acute stroke. Neurology. 2003;60:620–5.
51. Klein SL. The effects of hormones on sex differences in infection: from genes to behavior. Neurosci Biobehav Rev. 2000;24:627–38.
52. Muenchhoff M, Goulder PJR. Sex differences in pediatric infectious diseases. J Infect Dis. 2014;209:S120–6.
53. Fish EN. The X-files in immunity: sex-based differences pre- dispose immune responses. Nat Rev Immunol. 2008;8:737–44.
54. Chamorro A, Urra X, Planas AM. Infection after acute ischemic stroke: a manifestation of brain-induced immunodepression. Stroke. 2007;38:1097–103.
55. Klehmet J, Harms H, Richter M, et al. Stroke-induced immunodepression and post-stroke infections: lessons from the preventive antibacterial therapy in stroke trial. Neuroscience. 2009;158:1184–93.
56. Berger JR, Houff S. Opportunistic infections and other risks with newer multiple sclerosis therapies. Ann Neurol. 2009;65:367–77.
57. Arvin AM, Wolinsky JS, Kappos L, et al. Varicella-zoster virus infections in patients treated with fingolimod: risk assessment and consensus recommendations for management. JAMA Neurol. 2015;72:31–9.
58. Gergely P. Drug-induced lymphopenia: focus on $CD4^+$ and $CD8^+$ cells. Drug Saf. 1999;21:91–100.
59. Salvana EMT, Salata RA. Infectious complications associated with monoclonal antibodies and related small molecules. Clin Microbiol Rev. 2009;22:274–90.
60. Kamel H, Iadecola C. Brain-immune interactions and ischemic stroke: clinical implications. Arch Neurol. 2012;69:576–81.

61. Schmutzhard E, Pfausler B. Neurologic complications of sepsis. Handb Clin Neurol. 2017;141:675–83.
62. Eidelman LA, Putterman D, Putterman C, Sprung CL. The spectrum of septic encephalopathy: definitions, etiologies, and mortalities. JAMA. 1996; 275:470–3.
63. Bolton CF, Young GB, Zochodne DW. The neurological complications of sepsis. Ann Neurol. 1993;33:94–100.
64. Hocker SE, Wijdicks EF. Neurologic complications of sepsis. Continuum (Minneap Minn). 2014;20: 598–613.
65. Ebersoldt M, Sharshar T, Annane D. Sepsis-associated delirium. Intensive Care Med. 2007;33:941–50.
66. Ely EW, Gautam S, Margolin R, et al. The impact of delirium in the intensive care unit on hospital length of stay. Intensive Care Med. 2001;27:1892–900.
67. Wilson JX, Young GB. Progress in clinical neurosciences: sepsis-associated encephalopathy: evolving concepts. Can J Neurol Sci. 2003;30:98–105.
68. Boehme AK, Ranawat P, Luna J, et al. Risk of acute stroke after hospitalization for sepsis: a case-crossover study. Stroke. 2017;48:574–80.
69. Neligan A, Rajakulendran S, Nortley R, Manji H. Extensive cerebral microhemorrhages caused by acute disseminated intravascular coagulation secondary to sepsis. JAMA Neurol. 2014;71:510–1.
70. Gusmao-Flores D, Salluh JI, Chalhub RÁ, Quarantini LC. The confusion assessment method for the intensive care unit (CAM-ICU) and intensive care delirium screening checklist (ICDSC) for the diagnosis of delirium: a systematic review and meta-analysis of clinical studies. Crit Care. 2012;16:R115.
71. Ali M, Cascella M. ICU delirium. Treasure Island: StatPearls Publishing; 2023.
72. Chung HY, Wickel J, Brunkhorst FM, Geis C. Sepsis-associated encephalopathy: from delirium to dementia? J Clin Med. 2020;9:703.
73. Westover MB, Shafi MM, Bianchi MT, et al. The probability of seizures during EEG monitoring in critically ill adults. Clin Neurophysiol. 2015;126:463–71.
74. Claassen J, Mayer SA, Kowalski RG, et al. Detection of electrographic seizures with continuous EEG monitoring in critically ill patients. Neurology. 2004;62:1743–8.
75. Alessandri F, Badenes R, Bilotta F. Seizures and sepsis: a narrative review. J Clin Med. 2021;10:1041.
76. Vezzani A, Moneta D, Richichi C, et al. Functional role of proinflammatory and anti-inflammatory cytokines in seizures. Adv Exp Med Biol. 2004;548:123–33.
77. Sewal RK, Modi M, Saikia UN, et al. Increase in seizure susceptibility in sepsis like condition explained by spiking cytokines and altered adhesion molecules level with impaired blood brain barrier integrity in experimental model of rats treated with lipopolysaccharides. Epilepsy Res. 2017;135:176–86.
78. Hinchey J, Chaves C, Appignani B, et al. A reversible posterior leukoencephalopathy syndrome. N Engl J Med. 1996;334:494–500.
79. Fugate JE, Rabinstein AA. Posterior reversible encephalopathy syndrome: clinical and radiological manifestations, pathophysiology, and outstanding questions. Lancet Neurol. 2015;14:914–25.
80. Bartynski WS. Posterior reversible encephalopathy syndrome, part 2: controversies surrounding pathophysiology of vasogenic edema. AJNR Am J Neuroradiol. 2008;29:1043–9.
81. Gofton TE, Young GB. Sepsis-associated encephalopathy. Nat Rev Neurol. 2012;8:557–66.
82. Orhun G, Sencer S, Tüzün E, et al. Posterior reversible encephalopathy in sepsis-associated encephalopathy: experience from a single center. Neurocrit Care. 2022;36:372–86.

40 Cerebral Resuscitation in Neurocritical Care

Prashant Kumar, Manisha Manohar, Kiranpreet Kaur, and Jyoti Sharma

40.1 Introduction

"**RESUSCITATION**" is derived from the Latin "Resuscitare," re: again + suscitare: to raise. Cerebral resuscitation includes the strategies that restore and protect cerebral function after the initial primary damage due to ischemic, hemorrhagic, traumatic, and nontraumatic injury. Neurologic deficits following cerebral injury result from the primary insult and secondary changes that occur during the resuscitative period. The clinicians have no dominion over the primary injury. Still, they can prevent secondary injury cascade by implementing evidence-based strategies to prevent and minimize secondary damage, revive neuronal function, hasten the recovery process, and improve the outcome of the patients. The goal of cerebral resuscitation is to provide an optimal macro- and micro-milieu to the stunned neuronal tissue by optimizing hemodynamics, glycemic control, metabolic status, and nutrition (Fig. 40.1).

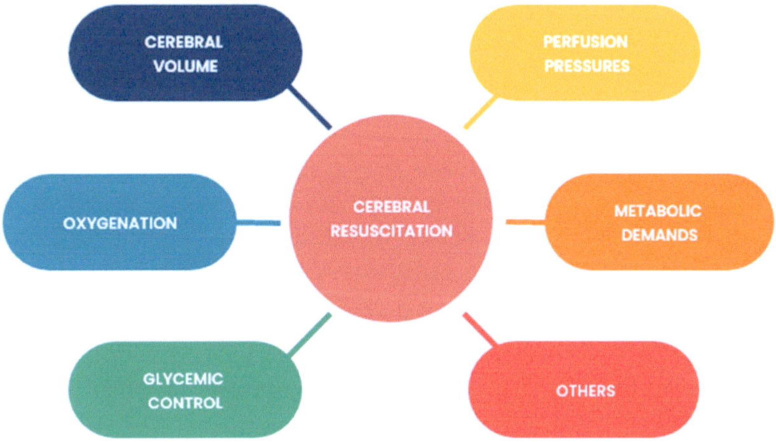

Fig. 40.1 Focus areas of cerebral resuscitation

P. Kumar (✉) · M. Manohar · K. Kaur
Department of Anaesthesiology and Critical Care, Pt BDS, PGIMS Rohtak, Rohtak, Haryana, India

J. Sharma
Department of Anaesthesiology and Critical Care, AIIMS, Bathinda, Punjab, India

H. Prabhakar et al. (eds.), *Principles and Practice of Neurocritical Care*,
https://doi.org/10.1007/978-981-99-8059-8_40

40.2 Optimizing Perfusion Pressures

The human brain has a high metabolic rate sustained by a high cerebral blood flow (CBF) of 50 mL/100 g/min. CBF is autoregulated and tightly coupled to local metabolism and electrophysiologic activity. The pressure gradient that drives cerebral blood flow depends on mean arterial pressure and intracranial pressure. The difference between systemic mean arterial pressure (MAP) and intracranial pressure (ICP) is cerebral perfusion pressure (CPP). MAP is considered a surrogate marker for CPP. It is autoregulated between 70 and 150 mmHg MAP in the normal healthy brain. However, above and below the autoregulatory limits, the CPP becomes passive.

The optimization of blood pressures in neurosurgical intensive care units is challenging as over, and under-correction can lead to unfavorable outcomes in stroke. High blood pressure can lead to cerebral edema, hemorrhagic conversions, and hematoma expansions. In contrast, low blood pressure reduces cerebral perfusion, especially in the ischemic penumbra, leading to worsening neurologic injury. The ideal blood pressure in ischemic and hemorrhagic stroke settings is still controversial.

40.2.1 Ischemic Stroke

The threshold for the treatment is generally higher in patients with acute ischemic stroke. American and European Stroke Association guidelines recommend cautiously lowering blood pressure only if it is greater than 220/120 mmHg [1] (Fig. 40.2). Patients with ischemic coronary disease, heart failure, aortic dissection, hypertensive encephalopathy, acute renal failure or eclampsia, and preeclampsia should also be maintained below 220/120 [2, 3]. A reasonable goal in the initial 24 h would be to avoid lowering blood pressure by 15–25% in the initial 24 h. Patients who are planning for thrombolytic therapy in acute ischemic stroke should have strict blood pressure control before and 24 h after the thrombolytic treatment as they are at high risk of developing intracranial hemorrhage. Blood pressures above 185/110 should be treated with intravenous antihypertensives. Frequent blood pressure monitoring is recommended in the first 24 h of thrombolysis to maintain blood pressure below 180/105 [2].

40.2.2 Hemorrhagic Stroke

Intracranial hemorrhage accounts for 10% of all strokes [4]. Hypertension, coagulopathy, head trauma, and congenital and acquired vascular lesions can lead to intracranial hemorrhage. Blood pressure higher than 160 mmHg is associated with a higher risk of aneurysmal rebleeding. AHA guidelines recommend maintaining systolic blood pressure below 160 mmHg [5] and ensuring mean arterial pressure above 90 mmHg to ensure cerebral perfusion in patients with aneurysmal bleeding

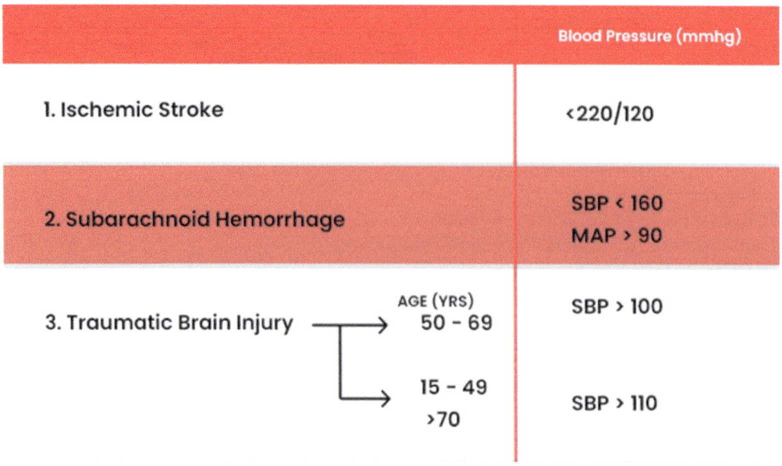

Fig. 40.2 Perfusion pressure targets

(Fig. 40.2). Cautious prescription of titratable antihypertensive agents should be done to balance the risk of stroke, hypertension-related rebleeding, and maintenance of cerebral perfusion. Antifibrinolytics can lower the risk of rebleeding. However, the finding of a recent trial suggests an association between aminocaproic acid and deep venous thrombosis [6]. Hence, caution is required in the administration of antifibrinolytics.

40.2.3 Traumatic Brain Injury

Systolic blood pressure is critical in the secondary injury cascade after severe traumatic brain injury. A mortality rate of 35% is reported in patients with SBP less than 85 mmHg, in contrast to 6% in patients with higher blood pressures [7]. If the cerebral autoregulation is not intact, cerebral perfusion becomes dependent on the systemic blood pressure; however, if it is intact, a fall in systolic blood pressure triggers autoregulatory vasodilation to maintain adequate cerebral perfusion, leading to increased cerebral blood volume and raised intracranial pressure. Guidelines recommend maintaining a systolic blood pressure of more than 100 mmHg for patients between 50 and 69 years of age and more than 110 mmHg for patients 15–49 or over 70 [8] (Fig. 40.2).

40.2.4 Sepsis and Septic Shock

Cerebral dysfunction is seen in sepsis and septic shock patients due to regional brain perfusion abnormalities in microcirculation. Fifty-three percent of the patients with sepsis develop septic encephalopathy [9], which is diffuse brain dysfunction, resulting from a systemic inflammatory response to infection. The outcome correlates with the management of sepsis. There are no specific treatments.

40.2.5 Promoting Macrocirculation

Early restoration of blood flow to the ischemic penumbra can prevent further damage and facilitate neuronal recovery. Thrombolysis should be initiated within one hour of the patient's arrival. Restoration of the microcirculation can be done using intravenous, intraarterial, or combined thrombolysis (intravenous + intraarterial thrombolysis). In patients with acute ischemic stroke, intravenous thrombolysis with recombinant tissue plasminogen activator is recommended within 4.5 h of onset after carefully excluding the contraindications for thrombolysis [10]. Intraarterial thrombolysis with recombinant prourokinase has shown higher rates of arterial recanalization but is also associated with a higher incidence of intracranial hemorrhage. A combination of intravenous and intraarterial thrombolysis techniques appears attractive but is yet to be established in clinical practice. Stent retrievers and aspiration catheters can help achieve intraarterial revascularization. The Merci retrieval system is an FDA-approved device that can retrieve clots. Mechanical thrombectomy using stent retrievers or aspiration catheters within 6 h of onset is recommended in addition to medical therapy if the patient meets the following criteria: acute occlusion of the internal carotid artery or M1 segment of a middle cerebral artery, modified Rankin score 0 or 1 before onset, Alberta stroke program early CT score >6 in CT, National Institute of Health Stroke Scale >6, and age >18. Apart from the failure to reperfuse, these therapies can lead to intracranial hemorrhage, ischemic reperfusion injury, and catheter-related complications.

Sonothrombolysis involves using ultrasonic exposure, which can cause reversible disaggregation of uncrosslinked fibrin fibers, microcavity formation in the shallow layers of thrombus, and increased transport of r TPA improving its uptake and penetration of TPA into clots and residual flow enhancement with vessel dilation. The lytic activity of intravenous tissue plasminogen activator can be safely augmented with transcranial Doppler (TCD) monitoring in human beings.

40.3 Optimizing Brain Volume

Cerebral edema is a pathologic brain swelling that develops in a focal or diffuse pattern after a primary brain insult. Cerebral edema can be cytotoxic, vasogenic, or interstitial. It results from an increase in one brain volume parenchymal compartment at the expense of another. Cytotoxic or intracellular edema results from fluid accumulation within the cells due to cellular injury from ischemia, hypoxia, or toxins. While cytotoxic edema involves gray and white matter, vasogenic edema is predominantly seen in white matter. Interstitial edema results from CSF migration into the periventricular white matter. Multiple pathophysiologic pathways are initiated after primary or secondary insult to the brain, leading to cerebral edema. As the intracranial pressure increases, brain tissue displacement can lead to cerebral herniation resulting in disability and death. Identifying and treating cerebral edema are a critical component of cerebral resuscitation.

The administration of hypertonic or hypotonic intravenous solutions leads to dramatic changes in the volume of the brain. Hyperosmolar agents partially reduce intracranial pressure by simple brain dehydration and reducing blood viscosity, leading to an improved microcirculatory flow of blood constituents and consequent constriction of pial arterioles resulting in decreased cerebral volume and intracranial pressures. Despite lowering the intracranial pressures, none of these agents has been shown to improve neurologic outcomes. Mannitol and hypertonic saline are the commonly used hyperosmolar agents. Hypertonic saline has a rapid onset of action and a prolonged effect on ICP reduction and can be advantageous for patients who do not respond to mannitol. Insufficient evidence is available to recommend the formal use of one agent over another. However, the patient-specific factors guide the initial agent choice. Acute kidney injury (AKI) is estimated at 6–12% of patients receiving mannitol [11, 12]. Renal function and electrolyte levels, especially sodium and chloride, should be monitored closely in patients receiving hyperosmolar therapy due to the risk of AKI. The osmolar gap appears to correlate best with mannitol concentration, and elevated mannitol concentration is best related to toxicity [13–16]. Hence, the osmolar gap is recommended over serum osmolarity to monitor the risk of acute kidney injury. An osmolar gap of 20 mOsm/kg is used in clinical practice to assess the risk of AKI, but adequate evidence to recommend a specific value is still unavailable. Hypertonic saline administration can lead to hypernatremia and hyperchloremia, which are linked to acute kidney injury and poor outcomes in critical care patients [17, 18]. Although a sodium range of 155–165 meq/L and serum chloride range of 110–115 meq/L are recommended to decrease the risk of acute renal injury, the clinician should evaluate the appropriate concentrations in individual patients keeping in mind the clinical context, renal function, acid-base status, and need for acute treatment of brain edema [19]. Guidelines recommend using symptom-based bolus dosing of hypertonic sodium solutions rather than sodium target target-based management of cerebral edema in SAH patients. Hyperosmolar therapy is recommended in SAH, acute ischemic stroke, intracranial hemorrhage, and hepatic encephalopathy (Fig. 40.3). However, in patients with meningitis, there is insufficient evidence to determine whether hyperosmolar agents reduce cerebral edema.

Aneurysmal SAH-associated acute symptomatic hydrocephalus should be managed by cerebrospinal fluid diversion. External ventricular drain is indicated in patients with obstructive hydrocephalus associated with intraventricular hemorrhage in the fourth or third ventricle. At the same time, lumbar drainage is preferred in patients communicating hydrocephalus without IVH and possibly supratentorial herniation. Permanent cerebrospinal fluid diversion with ventriculoperitoneal or ventricular atrial shunting is recommended in chronic symptomatic hydrocephalus.

Glucocorticoids are beneficial in patients with intracranial tumors. Steroids have been shown to restore altered vascular permeability in brain edema, reduce CSF production, and attenuate free radical production. However, their use in traumatic brain injury patients is no longer recommended for reducing intracranial pressure or improving neurologic outcomes. The CRASH trial in 2004 reported that

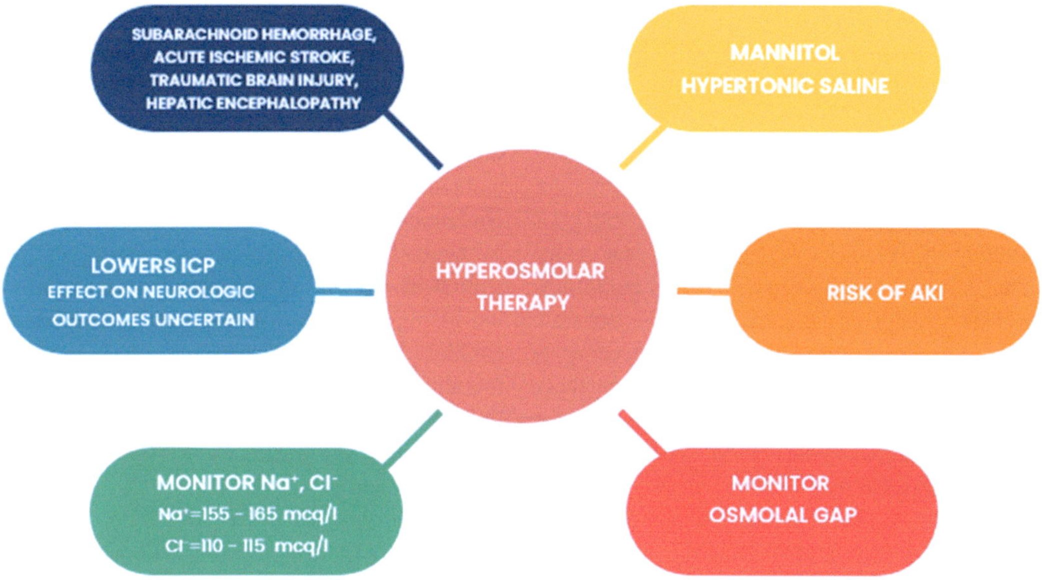

Fig. 40.3 Considerations while administering hyperosmolar therapy

the administration of methylprednisolone is associated with a 1.18 relative risk of death. The increase persisted even when the results were adjusted for extracranial injuries. The authors stated that the cause of death was not due to infection or gastrointestinal bleeding [20, 21]. Due to the potential for increased mortality and infectious complications, steroid use is not recommended to improve the neurologic outcome in patients with intracerebral hemorrhage. A two-week course of steroids is recommended in tubercular meningitis to reduce mortality in such patients. Dexamethasone 10 mg intravenously, 6-hourly, for 4 days, is strongly recommended before or with the first dose of antibiotic in patients with community-acquired bacterial meningitis to reduce the neurological sequelae in bacterial meningitis. However, clinicians should use patient-specific responses and factors to determine the duration of optimal steroid therapy.

40.3.1 Nonpharmacological Management

Nonpharmacological intervention decreases intracranial pressure through mechanical or structural changes. Elevation of the head end by 30 degrees, CSF diversion, and transient hyperventilation are effective for acute elevations of intracranial pressure. Still, there is insufficient evidence to prove that they are effective for treating any specific physiological change that produces brain swelling related to the brain. Bed rest is recommended to prevent increased intracranial pressure in aneurysmal SAH cases. Antiemetics and laxatives should be administered to avoid vomiting and constipation, which can lead to elevated intracranial pressure and cause rebleeding. Severe headaches due to dural irritation and increased ICP should be managed with analgesics before the obliteration of the aneurysm.

Surgical Decompression

A giant frontotemporoparietal decompressive craniectomy (DC) is recommended by Brain Trauma Foundation guidelines to relieve intracranial pressure in patients with traumatic brain injury. Although DC minimizes the ICU stay, recent guidelines do not recommend bifrontal decompressive craniectomy to enhance the patient outcome post-injury in severe traumatic brain trauma with diffuse injury and ICP values more than 20 mmHg, refractory to first-tier therapy.

40.4 Optimizing Glycemic Control

A critical component of cerebral resuscitation is preventing physiological imbalances induced by the cascade of events following an initial insult to the brain. Both hyperglycemia and hypoglycemia are deleterious. Hyperglycemia is associated with poor neurological outcomes in traumatic brain injury (TBI), aneurysmal subarachnoid hemorrhage (aSAH), intracranial hemorrhage (ICH), ischemic stroke, and anoxic brain injury. Hypoglycemia is also deleterious in neurocritical care since these patients depend on glucose as an energy source for the central nervous system. Pronounced neuroglycopenia symptoms may occur even with a moderate reduction in glucose levels. Impairment of glucose metabolism occurs in one-third of the patients with aneurysmal SAH who have no history of diabetes mellitus. The optimal glucose target for neurocritical patients is 110–180 mg/dL. Intensive glycemic control does not reduce mortality in neurocritical care patients. However, it poses a higher risk of hypoglycemia. Hyperglycemia over 200 mg/dL should be controlled with insulin.

40.4.1 Optimizing Oxygenation and Ventilation

Patients with acute brain injury experience respiratory failure due to loss of airway protective reflexes or decreased respiratory drive. Neurological injuries are not confined to the intracranial structures. The lung appears most vulnerable to damage following an acute brain injury [22, 23]. Brain injury induces systemic and pulmonary inflammation. Studies in brain-injured patients and animal models indicate massive intracranial production of proinflammatory cytokines. An impaired blood-brain barrier releases these cytokines into the systemic circulation, activating the inflammatory cascade [24, 25] immunosuppression and infection. Patients with severe brain injury and dysphagia have a higher risk of ventilator-associated pneumonia.

The extravasation of protein-rich fluid into the interstitial and alveolar space of the lungs after primary brain injury leads to neurogenic pulmonary edema. The diagnosis is based on respiratory distress, bilateral alveolar opacities, hypoxemia, and lack of evidence of left heart failure without other causes of ARDS. An abrupt increase in the intracranial pressure leads to sympathetic stimulation and massive release of catecholamines in the systemic circulation resulting in generalized vasoconstriction. The blood is shifted from systemic to pulmonary circulation, increasing hydrostatic pressure in the pulmonary capillaries. The increase in hydrostatic pressure in pulmonary vasculature leads to transudation of fluid and damage of the alveolar-capillary barrier, which results in leakage of protein-rich fluid into interstitial spaces and alveoli.

Acute lung injury (ALI)/ARDS is common in brain-injured patients [26, 27] with an incidence varying between 5 and 30%. Hypoxemia in the first few hours of brain injury is associated with a twofold mortality risk [28]. Hypoxemia leads to decreased cerebral oxygen delivery, which can cause intracranial hypertension due to hypoxemia-mediated vasodilation [29]. High-flow nasal cannula oxygen therapy may be considered in selected patients with acute brain injury who have hypoxemic respiratory failure refractory to conventional oxygen therapy. Both hypoxia and hyperoxia are associated with poor outcomes. European Society of Intensive Care Medicine recommends the optimal range of PaO_2 between 80 and 120 mmHg in acute brain injury patients on mechanical ventilation.

Invasive ventilation is used in acute brain injury to counter dysregulated breathing patterns and to maintain PaO_2 and $PaCO_2$ within the physiologic range. A combination of factors should guide the decision to intubate patients with acute brain injury (ABI). Endotracheal intubation should be considered in patients with ABI who have GCS <8, loss of protective airway reflexes, significantly elevated intracranial pressure, evidence of cerebral herniation, and non-neurological indications for intubation (Fig. 40.4).

Lung protective ventilator strategy leads to hypercapnia. Cerebral blood flow is linearly responsive to $PaCO_2$ between 20 and 80 mmHg. Hypercapnia can lead to cerebral hyperemia,

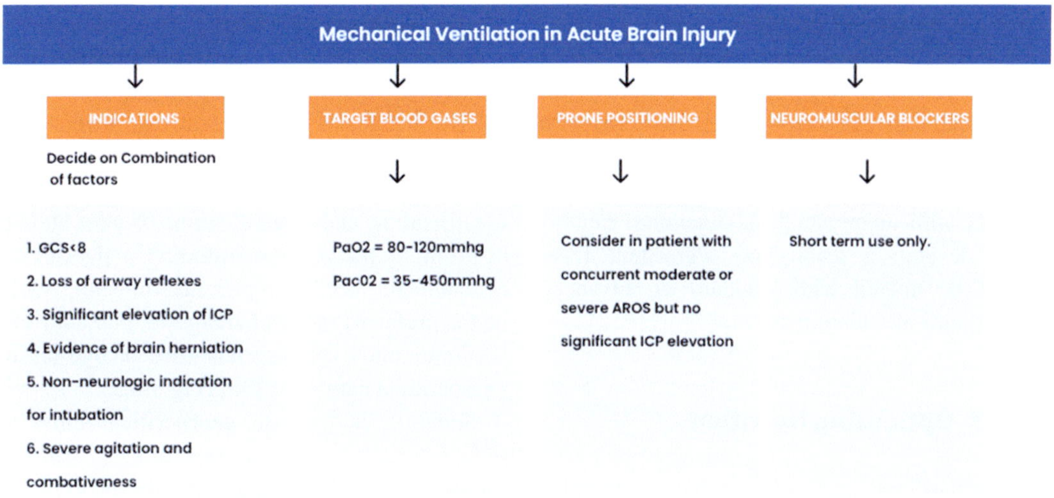

Fig. 40.4 Mechanical ventilation in acute brain injury

altering intracranial pressures, while low $PaCO_2$ can result in low cerebral blood flow. PEEP is a part of lung protective ventilation. In brain injury patients, PEEP may alter cerebral blood flow, reduce cerebral venous return, and increase ICP through complex mechanisms [30–32]. Consensus recommendations suggest that patients with ABI who do not have raised ICP should receive lung protective ventilation and PEEP like other mechanically ventilated patients. Traditionally, brain injury patients were treated with hyperventilation to keep intracranial pressures on the lower end. However, hypocapnia is deleterious in the setting of brain injury. Transient hyperventilation may be used to treat cerebral herniation. Prolonged prophylactic hyperventilation with the partial pressure of carbon dioxide of 25 mmHg is no longer recommended. The current recommendation is to maintain partial pressure of arterial CO_2 between 35 and 45 mmHg in patients with severe brain injury without cerebral herniation (Fig. 40.4).

Timely tracheotomy is an effective means of weaning sedation and ventilator liberation in patients who can breathe spontaneously but require an artificial airway. The optimal time for tracheostomy is still controversial. However, it should be considered in ABI patients who are persistently unconscious or when extubation trials have failed. Traumatic brain injury patients mostly require prolonged mechanical ventilation due to the risk of pulmonary aspiration or compromised respiratory drive and function. Even though early tracheostomy does not reduce mortality or rate of nosocomial pneumonia, it is recommended in traumatic brain injury patients to reduce mechanical ventilation days.

Resuscitative Hypothermia: Targeted temperature management is used in neurocritical care to minimize secondary neurologic injury and to improve outcomes. It encompasses therapeutic hypothermia, controlled normothermia, and treatment of fever. It is the current clinical standard in cerebral neuroprotection after cardiac arrest in patients in and out of hospital cardiac arrest. AHA 2020 recommends maintaining a constant temperature between 32 and 36 °C for at least 24 h after achieving the target temperature [33]. Hypothermia reduces cerebral metabolism and tissue edema, modifies inflammation, and reduces intracranial pressure. It is associated with the risk of immunosuppression, coagulopathy, cardiac arrhythmia, and death. Pediatric trials have failed to demonstrate the benefit of prophylactic hypothermia for traumatic brain injury. Insufficient evidence exists to support prophylactic hypothermia in traumatic brain injury patients.

40.4.2 Control of Fever

Regardless of the cause, fever in patients with acute brain injury is shown to be associated with adverse outcomes. It is an independent prognostic factor in SAH. Forty to seventy percent of the patients with aneurysmal subarachnoid hemorrhage develop a fever [34]. Persistent fever should be treated with standard or advanced temperature-modulating systems.

40.4.3 Optimizing Nutrition

The human body and nutrition have a complex interaction, especially in the setting of acute illness. Traumatic brain injury increases energy expenditure [35]. Comprehensive guidelines addressing all the unquestioned answers related to nutritional support, specifically in neurocritical illness, are still unavailable. Feeding should be started by at least the fifth day and, at the most, by the seventh day post-traumatic brain injury to reduce mortality. Transgastric jejunal feedings are recommended by the Brain Trauma Foundation to reduce the incidence of ventilator-associated pneumonia.

40.4.4 Analgosedation

All neurologic and neurosurgical patients should receive analgesics before sedatives. Severe pain induces tachycardia, hypertension, and desaturation, critically jeopardizing cerebral perfusion. Identification and quantification of pain should be promptly made before initiating analgesics. In mechanically ventilated patients, infusion should be the preferred mode of analgesia. Fentanyl and acetaminophen are recommended analgesics in neurocritical care units [36] (Fig. 40.5).

Sedation is used in neurocritical units to reduce cerebral metabolic rate, anxiety, ventilator asynchrony, ICP reduction, and seizure control. Depressed cerebral metabolism and reduced oxygen consumption are neuroprotective [37]. An objective sedation assessment should be done using the Richmond agitation sedation scale and Ramsay sedation scale. Unless contraindicated sedation vacation, every morning is the consensus of the experts (Fig. 40.5). Anesthetics and sedatives like barbiturates control intracranial pressures by suppressing metabolism, altering vascular tone, preventing coughing, and straining against the endotracheal tubes. They couple the regional blood flow to the metabolic demands and inhibit

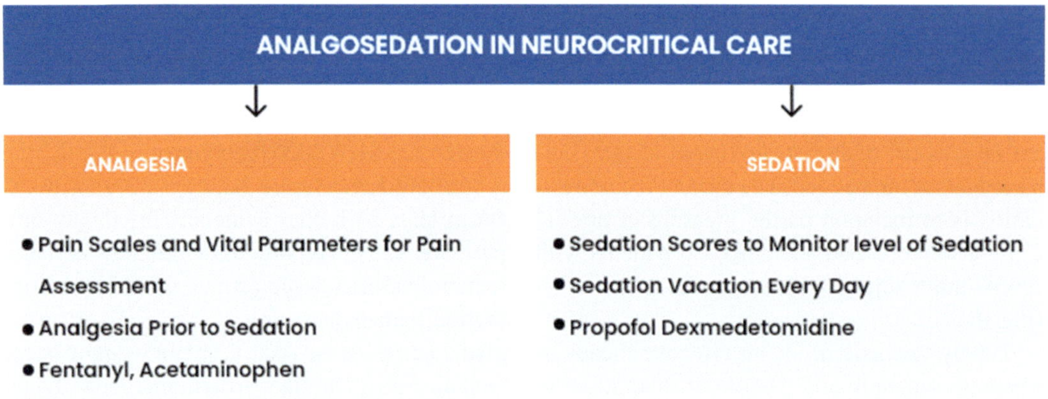

Fig. 40.5 Analgosedation in neurocritical care

oxygen radical-mediated lipid peroxidation. High-dose barbiturate administration is recommended to control elevated intracranial pressures refractory to standard medical and surgical interventions. Since decreased cardiac output and hypotension associated with these drugs can lead to hypoxia and decreased cerebral perfusion, diligent monitoring is required while using these medications. Propofol, although recommended for controlling ICP, does not have any effect on long-term mortality. Experts also recommend dexmedetomidine as the preferred sedative in neurocritical care units [36]. A deep level of sedation should be maintained in patients with refractory status epileptics, paroxysmal sympathetic activity, targeted temperature management, or refractory intracranial hypertension in the NCC set unit. The effectiveness of using volatile anesthetics for nontraditional sedation using special devices for rapid titration and faster wake-up needs to be explored in neurocritical care units.

40.4.5 Optimizing Hemoglobin

The presence of anemia is associated with poor outcomes in TBI, aSAH, ICH, and stroke. In the presence of anemia, compromised oxygen delivery to the brain, can exacerbate delayed cerebral ischemia. Studies report that blood transfusion can improve treatment outcomes and reduce mortality. Packed red blood cell transfusion is recommended in patients at risk of developing cerebral ischemia in aneurysmal SAH. A minimum hemoglobin level of 11 g/dL is recommended for patients with aSAH and those at high risk of vasospasm [34].

40.4.6 Electrolyte Abnormalities

The most common electrolyte imbalance seen in aneurysmal subarachnoid hemorrhage (aSAH) is hyponatremia. It is an independent risk factor associated with poor clinical outcomes in aSAH [38, 39]. Hyponatremia exacerbates cerebral edema, elevates intracranial pressure, and leads to seizures and further neurologic damage [40]. Irrespective of the etiology, conditions such as cerebral salt wasting, diuretic therapy, excessive fluid, and hyponatremia should be aggressively treated. AHA 2012 guidelines recommended using fludrocortisone acetate and hypertonic saline to prevent and correct hyponatremia [5].

40.4.7 Seizure Control

The incidence of seizures after aneurysmal SAH is reported to be 20%. Seizures are known to be the independent risk factor for poor clinical outcomes in patients with subarachnoid hemorrhage. Convulsions may worsen the outcome by precipitating a second bleed. While most guidelines recommend that seizures should always be treated with antiepileptic medications, prophylactic anticonvulsants are generally not recommended except in cases with a high risk of seizures. Patients with delayed seizures, Hunt Hess grades 4 and 5, cerebral infarction, and aneurysm in the middle cerebral artery are at increased risk of developing seizures and should receive prophylactic anticonvulsants [34].

Seizures occurring in the initial 7 days of traumatic brain injury are called early, while those manifesting after 7 days are called late seizures. Early post-traumatic seizures are seen in patients with GCS <10, immediate seizures, post-traumatic amnesia lasting longer than 30 min, linear or depressed skull fracture, penetrating head injury, subdural epidural, intracerebral hematoma, cortical contusion, age less than 65 years, and chronic alcoholism [41]. The risk of developing post-traumatic epilepsy is substantially higher than the risk of epilepsy in the general population. Prophylactic use of phenytoin or valproate is not recommended for preventing late post-traumatic seizures. Phenytoin, however, is recommended to decrease the incidence of early post-traumatic seizures if the benefits outweigh the risk of complications [8].

40.5 Conclusion

The goal of cerebral resuscitation strategies is to improve survival and minimize disability. Focus areas of cerebral resuscitation include blood pressure control, glycemic optimization, avoidance of high cerebral pressure, appropriate oxygen and carbon dioxide levels, optimal analgosedation, and timely surgical/radiological interventions if indicated. However, a single intervention addressing a single physiological variable is never enough to enhance the long and short outcomes. A comprehensive approach to cerebral resuscitation must be adopted to ensure improved outcomes. General principles of ICU care, such as adequate nutrition, physiotherapy, and adequate nutrition, are equally important.

References

1. European Stroke Organisation (ESO) Executive Committee; ESO Writing Committee. Guidelines for management of ischaemic stroke and transient ischaemic attack 2008. Cerebrovasc Dis. 2008;25(5):457–507.
2. Jauch EC, Saver JL, Adams HP Jr, Bruno A, Connors JJ, Demaerschalk BM, et al. Guidelines for the early management of patients with acute ischemic stroke: a guideline for healthcare professionals from the American Heart Association/American Stroke Association. Stroke. 2013;44(3):870–947.
3. Patarroyo SX, Anderson C. Blood pressure lowering in acute phase of stroke: latest evidence and clinical implications. Ther Adv Chronic Dis. 2012;3(4):163–71.
4. Loscalzo J, Fauci A, Kasper D, Hauser S, Longo D, Jameson J, editors. Harrison's principles of internal medicine, 21st ed. McGraw Hill; 2022.
5. Connolly ES Jr, Rabinstein AA, Carhuapoma JR, Derdeyn CP, Dion J, Higashida RT, et al.; American Heart Association Stroke Council; Council on Cardiovascular Radiology and Intervention; Council on Cardiovascular Nursing; Council on Cardiovascular Surgery and Anesthesia; Council on Clinical Cardiology. Guidelines for the management of aneurysmal subarachnoid hemorrhage: a guideline for healthcare professionals from the American Heart Association/American Stroke Association. Stroke. 2012;43(6):1711–1737.
6. Foreman PM, Chua M, Harrigan MR, Fisher WS 3rd, Tubbs RS, Shoja MM, et al. Antifibrinolytic therapy in aneurysmal subarachnoid hemorrhage increases the risk for deep venous thrombosis: a case-control study. Clin Neurol Neurosurg. 2015;139:66–9.
7. Klauber MR, Marshall LF, Luerssen TG, Frankowski R, Tabaddor K, Eisenberg HM. Determinants of head injury mortality: importance of the low risk patient. Neurosurgery. 1989;24(1):31–6.
8. Carney N, Totten AM, O'Reilly C, Ullman JS, Hawryluk GW, Bell MJ, Bratton SL, Chesnut R, Harris OA, Kissoon N, Rubiano AM, Shutter L, Tasker RC, Vavilala MS, Wilberger J, Wright DW, Ghajar J. Guidelines for the management of severe traumatic brain injury, fourth edition. Neurosurgery. 2017;80(1):6–15.
9. Sonneville R, de Montmollin E, Poujade J, Garrouste-Orgeas M, Souweine B, Darmon M, et al. Potentially modifiable factors contributing to sepsis-associated encephalopathy. Intensive Care Med. 2017;43(8):1075–84.
10. Miyamoto S, Ogasawara K, Kuroda S, Itabashi R, Toyoda K, Itoh Y, et al. Committee for Stroke Guideline 2021, the Japan Stroke Society. Japan Stroke Society guideline 2021 for the treatment of stroke. Int J Stroke. 2022;17(9):1039–1049.
11. Gondim Fde A, Aiyagari V, Shackleford A, Diringer MN. Osmolality not predictive of mannitol-induced acute renal insufficiency. J Neurosurg. 2005;103(3):444–7.
12. Lin SY, Tang SC, Tsai LK, Yeh SJ, Shen LJ, Wu FL, Jeng JS. Incidence and risk factors for acute kidney injury following mannitol infusion in patients with acute stroke: a retrospective cohort study. Medicine (Baltimore). 2015;94(47):e2032.
13. Dorman HR, Sondheimer JH, Cadnapaphornchai P. Mannitol-induced acute renal failure. Medicine (Baltimore). 1990;69(3):153–9.
14. García-Morales EJ, Cariappa R, Parvin CA, Scott MG, Diringer MN. Osmole gap in neurologic-neurosurgical intensive care unit: its normal value, calculation, and relationship with mannitol serum concentrations. Crit Care Med. 2004;32(4):986–91.
15. Fisher LA, Ko N, Miss J, Tung PP, Kopelnik A, Banki NM, Gardner D, Smith WS, Lawton MT, Zaroff JG. Hypernatremia predicts adverse cardiovascular and neurological outcomes after SAH. Neurocrit Care. 2006;5(3):180–5.
16. Stelfox HT, Ahmed SB, Zygun D, Khandwala F, Laupland K. Characterization of intensive care unit acquired hyponatremia and hypernatremia following cardiac surgery. Can J Anaesth. 2010;57(7):650–8.
17. Yunos NM, Bellomo R, Hegarty C, Story D, Ho L, Bailey M. Association between a chloride-liberal vs chloride-restrictive intravenous fluid administration strategy and kidney injury in critically ill adults. JAMA. 2012;308(15):1566–72.
18. Boland T, Henderson GV, Gibbons FK, Brouwers HB, Greenberg SM, Raffeld M, Kourkoulis CE, Rosand J, Christopher KB. Hypernatremia at hospital discharge and out of hospital mortality following primary intracerebral hemorrhage. Neurocrit Care. 2016;25(1):110–6.

19. Cook AM, Morgan Jones G, Hawryluk GWJ, Mailloux P, McLaughlin D, Papangelou A, Samuel S, Tokumaru S, Venkatasubramanian C, Zacko C, Zimmermann LL, Hirsch K, Shutter L. Guidelines for the acute treatment of cerebral edema in neurocritical care patients. Neurocrit Care. 2020;32(3):647–66. https://doi.org/10.1007/s12028-020-00959-7. PMID: 32227294; PMCID: PMC7272487.
20. Roberts I, Yates D, Sandercock P, Farrell B, Wasserberg J, Lomas G, et al. Effect of intravenous corticosteroids on death within 14 days in 10008 adults with clinically significant head injury (MRC CRASH trial): randomised placebo-controlled trial. Lancet. 2004;364(9442):1321–8.
21. Edwards P, Arango M, Balica L, Cottingham R, El-Sayed H, Farrell B, et al. Final results of MRC CRASH, a randomised placebo-controlled trial of intravenous corticosteroid in adults with head injury-outcomes at 6 months. Lancet. 2005;365(9475):1957–9. https://doi.org/10.1016/S0140-6736(05)66552-X. PMID: 15936423.
22. McDonald SJ, Sharkey JM, Sun M, Kaukas LM, Shultz SR, Turner RJ, Leonard AV, Brady RD, Corrigan F. Beyond the brain: peripheral interactions after traumatic brain injury. J Neurotrauma. 2020;37(5):770–81.
23. Mascia L. Acute lung injury in patients with severe brain injury: a double hit model. Neurocrit Care. 2009;11(3):417–26.
24. Ott L, McClain CJ, Gillespie M, Young B. Cytokines and metabolic dysfunction after severe head injury. J Neurotrauma. 1994;11(5):447–72.
25. Abraham E, Glauser MP, Butler T, Garbino J, Gelmont D, Laterre PF, Kudsk K, Bruining HA, Otto C, Tobin E, Zwingelstein C, Lesslauer W, Leighton A. p55 tumor necrosis factor receptor fusion protein in the treatment of patients with severe sepsis and septic shock. A randomized controlled multicenter trial. Ro 45-2081 Study Group. JAMA. 1997;277(19):1531–8.
26. Mrozek S, Constantin JM, Geeraerts T. Brain-lung crosstalk: implications for neurocritical care patients. World J Crit Care Med. 2015;4(3):163–78.
27. Mrozek S, Gobin J, Constantin JM, Fourcade O, Geeraerts T. Crosstalk between brain, lung and heart in critical care. Anaesth Crit Care Pain Med. 2020;39(4):519–30.
28. Rowat AM, Dennis MS, Wardlaw JM. Hypoxaemia in acute stroke is frequent and worsens outcome. Cerebrovasc Dis. 2006;21(3):166–72.
29. Gupta AK, Menon DK, Czosnyka M, Smielewski P, Jones JG. Thresholds for hypoxic cerebral vasodilation in volunteers. Anesth Analg. 1997;85(4):817–20.
30. Della Torre V, Badenes R, Corradi F, Racca F, Lavinio A, Matta B, Bilotta F, Robba C. Acute respiratory distress syndrome in traumatic brain injury: how do we manage it? J Thorac Dis. 2017;9(12):5368–81.
31. Blanch L, Fernández R, Benito S, Mancebo J, Net A. Effect of PEEP on the arterial minus end-tidal carbon dioxide gradient. Chest. 1987;92(3):451–4.
32. Doblar DD, Santiago TV, Kahn AU, Edelman NH. The effect of positive end-expiratory pressure ventilation (PEEP) on cerebral blood flow and cerebrospinal fluid pressure in goats. Anesthesiology. 1981;55(3):244–50.
33. Panchal AR, Bartos JA, Cabañas JG, Donnino MW, Drennan IR, Hirsch KG, Kudenchuk PJ, et al. 2020 American Heart Association guidelines for cardiopulmonary resuscitation and emergency cardiovascular care. Circulation. 2020;142(Suppl 2):S366–468.
34. Cho WS, Kim JE, Park SQ, Ko JK, Kim DW, Park JC, et al. Korean clinical practice guidelines for aneurysmal subarachnoid hemorrhage. J Korean Neurosurg Soc. 2018;61(2):127–66.
35. Clifton GL, Robertson CS, Choi SC. Assessment of nutritional requirements of head-injured patients. J Neurosurg. 1986;64(6):895–901.
36. Prabhakar H, Tripathy S, Gupta N, Singhal V, Mahajan C, Kapoor I, Wanchoo J, Kalaivani M. Consensus statement on analgo-sedation in neurocritical care and review of literature. Indian J Crit Care Med. 2021;25(2):126–33.
37. Roberts I, Sydenham E. Barbiturates for acute traumatic brain injury. Cochrane Database Syst Rev. 2012;12(12):CD000033.
38. Hasan D, Wijdicks EF, Vermeulen M. Hyponatremia is associated with cerebral ischemia in patients with aneurysmal subarachnoid hemorrhage. Ann Neurol. 1990;27(1):106–8.
39. Sayama T, Inamura T, Matsushima T, Inoha S, Inoue T, Fukui M. High incidence of hyponatremia in patients with ruptured anterior communicating artery aneurysms. Neurol Res. 2000;22(2):151–5.
40. Mount DB. The brain in hyponatremia: both culprit and victim. Semin Nephrol. 2009;29(3):196–215.
41. Torbic H, Forni AA, Anger KE, Degrado JR, Greenwood BC. Use of antiepileptics for seizure prophylaxis after traumatic brain injury. Am J Health Syst Pharm. 2013;70(9):759–66.

Coma in Neurocritical Care

41

Masao Nagayama

41.1 Introduction

Although acute and prolonged coma is a challenging condition, many of them are treatable, and also, many of them remain comatose with or without appropriate diagnostic work-up and treatment. In this chapter, the most important and often overlooked points and related issues in the differential diagnosis and management of comatose patients will be introduced from the standpoint of critical care neurology.

41.2 Consciousness Level and Content

The components of consciousness are separated into two groups: level of alertness (arousal, being awake) and content of thinking (awareness). Although many acute and chronic neurologic disorders affect both components, these two components are sometimes dissociated. For example, a patient can be awake but not aware (mental alteration or alteration of consciousness) with abnormal or odd behavior in patients with encephalitis, encephalopathy, and eye-open coma. Table 41.1 shows a differential diagnosis of mental alteration.

Table 41.1 Differential diagnosis of mental alteration

Category	Representative cause and pathophysiology
Acute encephalopathy crisis	Uremic, Hepatic, Hyper-ammonemic, Hypoglycemic, Hyperglycemic, Septic, Sepsis-related, Na↓, Na↑, Ca↑, Wernicke, Hypertensive, COVID-19, Porphyria, Thyroid crisis, Pituitary, Parathyroid, Adrenal, Carcinoid syndrome
Cerebrovascular diseases	Stroke with aphasia due to middle cerebral artery occlusion mainly of dominant hemisphere Subarachnoid hemorrhage due to anterior communicating artery aneurysm rupture
CNS infection	Encephalitis; Herpes Simplex, Limbic, Meningitis, Abscess, Whipple disease, COVID-19
Systemic infection	Pneumonia, Sepsis
Intoxication withdrawal side effect	Alcohol, Psychiatric, anti-Parkinson, Benzodiazepines, Narcotics, Opioids, Barbiturates, Digitalis anti-cholinergics, non-steroidal anti-inflammatory drugs, H_2 blockers, Antibiotics; Penicillin, Antihypertensives; Methyldopa, β-Blocker, Lidocaine, CO_2↓, O_2↑, Pneumonia, CO_2 narcosis
Functional	Epilepsy, especially non-convulsive status epileptics (NCSE)
Brain tumor	Brain tumor, especially at right hemisphere
Others	Prion diseases, Traumatic brain injury, Congestive heart failure, ICU syndrome, Heat stroke, Mental and psychiatric diseases
Mimics	Locked-in syndrome

M. Nagayama (✉)
Department of Neurology, International University of Health and Welfare Graduate School of Medicine, Narita, Japan
e-mail: nagay001@sj8.so-net.ne.jp

H. Prabhakar et al. (eds.), *Principles and Practice of Neurocritical Care*,
https://doi.org/10.1007/978-981-99-8059-8_41

41.3 Pathophysiological Basis of Disorders of Consciousness

Coma is often due to an extensive structural injury or physiologic dysfunction. Coma results from damage to structures such as the ascending reticular activating system (ARAS) or the reticular activating system in brainstem, thalamus, anterior cingulate cortex, and association cortex (precuneus and cuneus). So, a small unilateral lesion in the hemisphere cannot cause disorders of consciousness (DoC), and contrary, a very small brainstem lesion affecting ARAS can cause a comatose state. Thus, the pathophysiological basis of DoC consists of either or a mixture of (1) diffuse disturbance of the cerebral cortex usually of both sides, (2) disturbance of the ARAS located mainly in the dorsal upper pons and mesencephalon, (3) psychogenic, and (4) disturbance of general condition.

41.4 Causes of DoC at Emergency Department

DoC is often simplistically considered to be caused by neurological diseases. However, it is not true and final diagnosis of patients with DoC on arrival at the University of Virginia was reported to be neurologic (28%) and toxicologic (21%) followed by trauma (14%), psychiatric (14%), infectious (10%), endocrine/metabolic (5%), pulmonary (3%), oncologic (3%), cardiovascular (1%), gastrointestinal (1%), and renal (1%). So, the whole body including mental status must be fully evaluated by the emergency department [1].

41.5 Neurologic Complications of Critical Medical Illnesses

Critically ill non-neurological patients are very likely to be complicated by neurological diseases and conditions, especially including DoC. In 1993, Thomas P. Bleck, founder of the Neurocritical Care Society, reported that neurologic complications were observed in more than 12.3% of non-neurological patients admitted to the general medical intensive care unit (ICU) and cardiac/coronary care unit ($n = 217$) [2]. Details of the neurologic complications were as follows: metabolic encephalopathy (62 patients (28.6%)), seizure (61 (28.1%)), hypoxic/anoxic ischemic encephalopathy (51 (23.5%)), stroke (48 (22.1%)), and others (50 (23.0%)). In conjunction with our findings described in the invited review, which disclosed novel manifestations of non-convulsive status epilepticus (NCSE) and higher frequency of NCSE than convulsive status epilepticus [3], neurologic complications are estimated to be observed in more than 20% of critically ill non-neurological patients.

41.6 Diagnostic Step at Emergency Department

In many patients suspected of stroke, brain imaging with CT and MR would disclose the diagnosis rapidly. However, the same report from the University of Virginia disclosed the importance of medical interview and physical examination as follows: Contribution to the diagnosis was max in the history of present event (51%) followed by past medical history (43%), physical examination (41%), radiographs (16%), 12-lead electrocardiogram (7%), and various laboratory studies (chemistry panel [5%], complete blood count [1%], coagulation panel [0], and urinalysis [11%]) [1]. So, physicians and medical team need to decide on diagnostic steps flexibly titrating to each patient.

41.7 Determination of the Depth of the DoC

The most used coma scale is the Glasgow Coma Scale (GCS), which is well established and is the scale used most often for trauma patients and by emergency medical services personnel. It incorporates three unequally weighted responses: motor, verbal, and eye-opening, with a total score ranging from 3 to 15 [4]. To remedy a defect of the GCS such as inability to use in intubated patients, Professor Eelco F. M. Wijdicks at Mayo Clinic and Mayo Medical School created the Full Outline of Unresponsiveness (FOUR) score, which assesses four responses: eyelid opening and tracking, motor response, brainstem reflexes, and respiratory drive and regularity. This score has become widely used in the world, especially in those critically ill patients in the ICU. The usefulness of the FOUR score can be summarized as follows: (1) can be used in intubated patients, (2) capable of evaluating brain stem function, and (3) not only as the consciousness level scale but also as the neurocritical severity scale.

41.8 Non-convulsive Status Epilepticus (NCSE)

In 2012, the Neurocritical Care Society defined status epilepticus (SE) as 5 min or more of continuous clinical and/or electrographic seizure or recurrent seizure activity without recovery between seizures [5]. In 2015, the International League Against Epilepsy (ILAE) issued a new SE classification, including a detailed semiologic axis [6]. In this classification, NCSE was classified into "NCSE with coma" and "NCSE without coma." A separate manifestation of "NCSE in coma" has been increasingly identified since the advent of continuous EEG monitoring. Also, NCSE has rapidly expanded from classical features such as staring, repetitive blinking, chewing, swallowing, and automatism to include acute coma, prolonged apnea, dementia, higher brain dysfunction, and cardiac arrest, which were demonstrated mainly after the 2000s by us and other groups [3].

In adults, NCSE is not rare and frequently observed in acute critically ill neurological conditions such as stroke in 22%, metabolic abnormalities in 15%, hypoxia in 13%, systemic infections in 7%, anoxia in 5%, and trauma, drug overdose, and central nervous system (CNS) infection in 3% [7]. NCSE is also frequently observed in chronic neurological conditions such as low concentration of antiepileptics in 34%, remote symptomatic in 25%, alcohol misuse in 13%, and tumor in 7%. Furthermore, mortality of NCSE is high in both acute and chronic critically ill neurological conditions as much as 71% in anoxia, 53% in hypoxia, 33% in acute stroke, and 30% in metabolic abnormalities and tumors. We need to be aware that epileptic seizure can coexist with acute encephalopathy and that NCSE and convulsive seizure can coexist in a patient.

Regarding prolonged DoC, we studied six nontraumatic patients awakened from a coma of one month or more and with a total Glasgow Coma Scale score of seven or less [8]. Among them, two cases of NCSE were identified. One of these with symptomatic epilepsy was awakened after the start of phenytoin therapy, while the other, with viral encephalitis, was awakened after carbamazepine therapy. In case 1, the estimated duration of NCSE was 2 weeks, and in case 2, it was several months [8].

Although medical interview is more important than electroencephalogram (EEG) for the diagnosis of seizure, especially of NCSE, conventional and continuous EEG monitoring needs to be performed as soon as possible. Also, the most important clues to the bedside diagnosis of NCSE are spontaneous nystagmus and conjugate deviation of eyes in addition to classical clinical features such as staring and repetitive blinking, small amplitude myoclonus of the face and extremities, and neurological deficits of an unexplained, episodic, fluctuating, or recurrent nature. NCSE is very frequently observed in patients with acute and chronic phases of critically ill neurological conditions, and mortality is very high. However, although NCSE is potentially treatable, NCSE is very frequently overlooked in clinical practice. Not only in patients with acute coma but also in those with a variety of neurological manifestations including prolonged DoC, and especially in those without readily available cause of DoC, physicians need to consider NCSE in the differential diagnosis.

41.9 Diagnostic Bedside Tools and Devices in the Critically Ill Update

1. **Automated Electric Pupillometer**

   Classical manual pupillary examination is confounded by interobserver and intraobserver discrepancies and errors in detecting a reflex under certain conditions. The automated electric pupillometer is a computer-based infrared digital video device that can obtain objective measurements of pupillary size and reactivity (Fig. 41.1). This pupillometer has been already

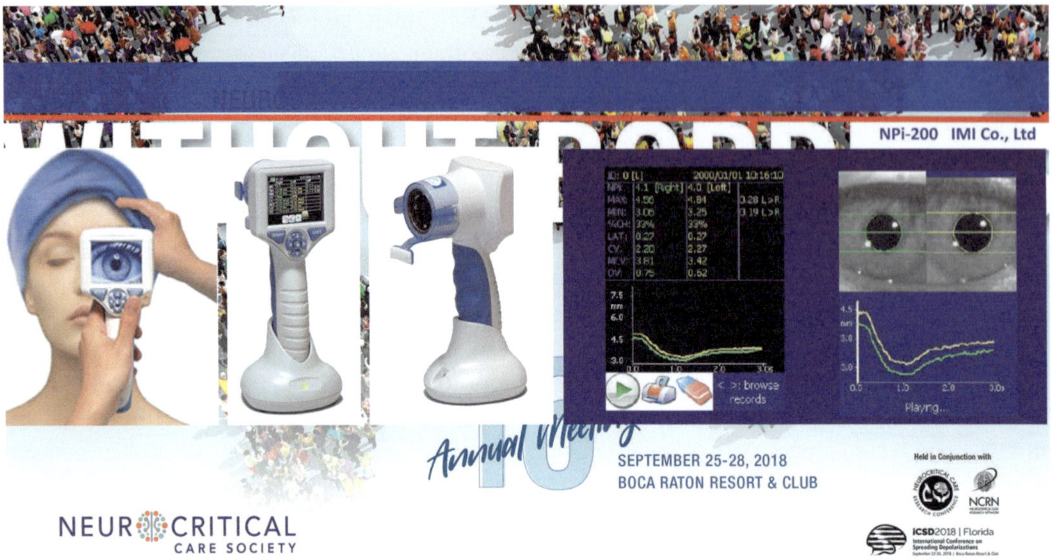

Fig. 41.1 Quantitative pupillometer

widely used in the world especially for neurologically critically ill.

2. **Capnometry and Tongue Protrusion**

   Although not a novel tool, the evaluation of tongue protrusion is important in the neurologically critically ill. Those severe patients with intracranial lesions such as stroke and neuromuscular diseases such as Guillain-Barré syndrome can lapse into alveolar hypoventilation, in other words acute (type II) respiratory failure with arterial $PaCO_2$ retention (Table 41.2) possibly with narcotic further worsening of the consciousness level. For the early detection of hypercapnia, bedside evaluation of tongue protrusion before comatose phase is very useful in addition to the arterial blood gases analysis, capnometry, and spirometry.

3. **Measurement of Optic Nerve Sheath Diameter (ONSD) by Transorbital Sonography**

   Clinical evaluation of manifestations including the Cushing phenomenon and ocular fundi examination is quite important for the diagnosis of the raised intracranial pressure (ICP). Although direct intracranial pressure monitoring is the gold standard, it is invasive and several noninvasive approaches have become available. Among them, transorbital sonography, which measures optic nerve sheath diameter (ONSD), can detect raised ICP well in traumatic brain injury and many other neurocritical conditions (Fig. 41.2). At the moment, it can be concluded that ONSD measurement by transorbital sonography is recommended and better than nothing for the early and noninvasive detection of raised ICP.

Table 41.2 Arterial blood gases of respiratory dysfunction

Arterial blood gases (ABGs)	PaO_2 ↓	$PaCO_2$ ↑
Diffusion impairment	○	×
Shunt	○	×
Ventilation perfusion ratio mismatch	○	×
Alveolar hypoventilation	○	○

Severe neurological diseases are often complicated by alveolar hypoventilation

4. **Novel Electrode and Headset for Rapid EEG**

   We created a novel electrode and headset, which enables rapid and continuous EEG monitoring from the emergency department to the neuro-ICU by (a) employment of an active amplifier and disposable gel electrodes for sustainable and stable usage, (b) a wireless device by using Bluetooth technology, and (c) an easy attachment of electrode contacts by employing the headset style (Figs. 41.3 and 41.4). This device was made

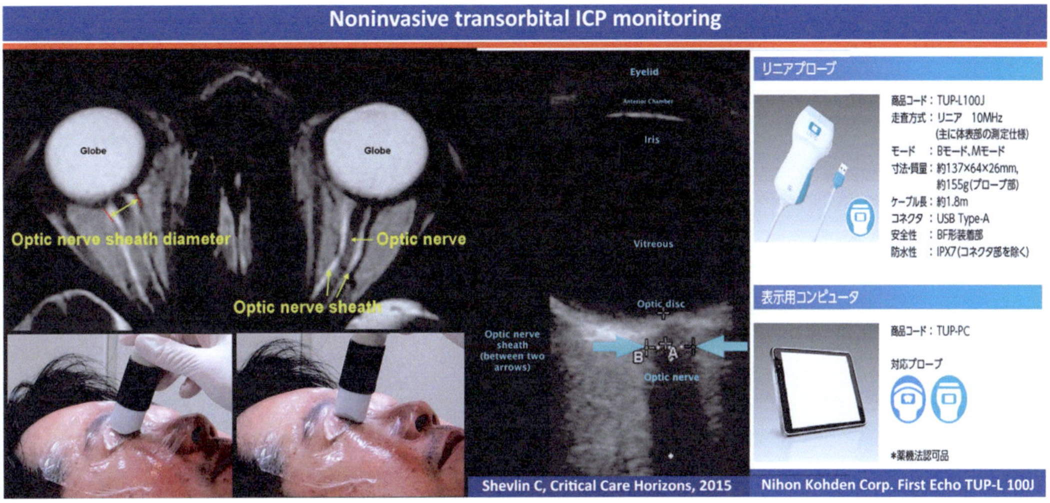

Fig. 41.2 Optic nerve sheath ultrasound for ICP monitoring

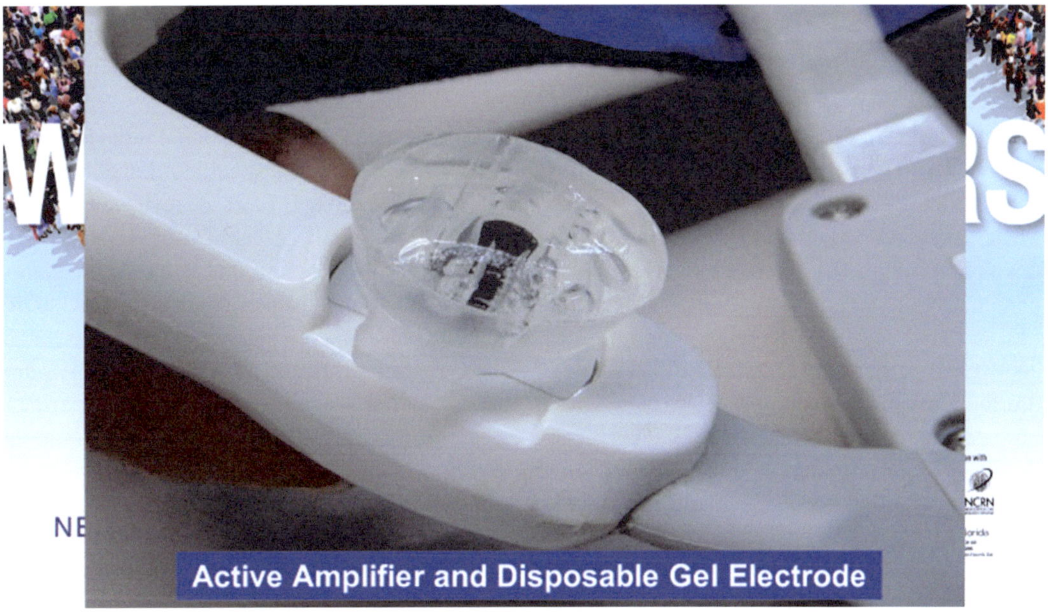

Fig. 41.3 Novel electrodes and headset

possible with novel industry-academia collaboration with Nihon Kohden Corporation and approved for practical use by the Ministry of Health, Labour and Welfare, Japan, at the year of 2016. Rapid EEG monitoring would improve the diagnosis of NCSE and might further expand the clinical spectrum of NCSE.

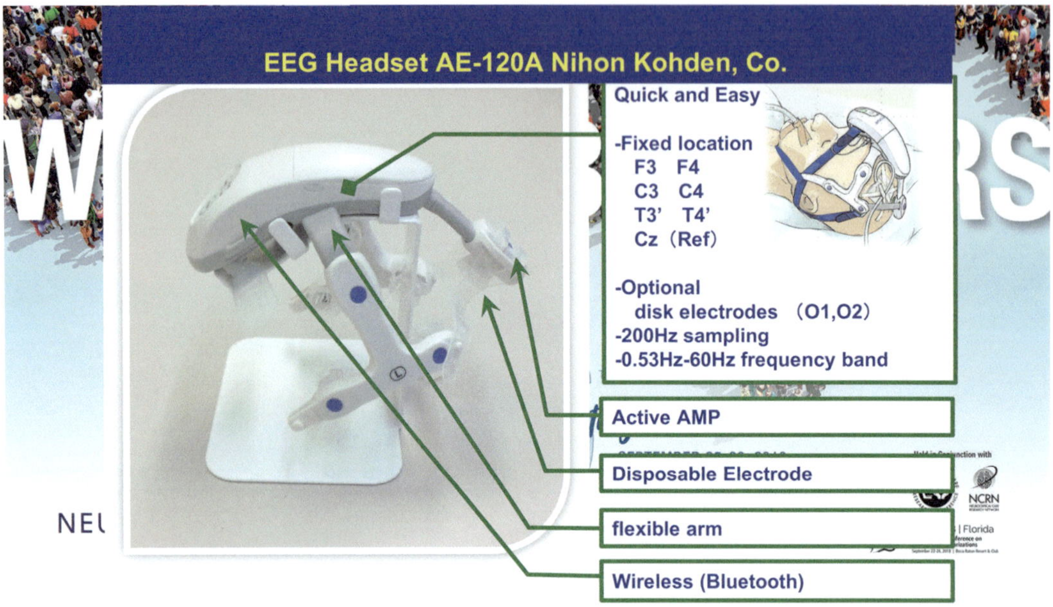

Fig. 41.4 Novel electrodes and headset

41.10 Therapeutic Interventions in Prolonged DoC

Management of patients with severe brain injuries and prolonged DoC raises challenging issues, particularly on therapeutic options. Thibaut et al. (2019) found several randomized controlled trials (RCTs) particularly focused on the effects of drugs or use of noninvasive brain stimulation; however, no definite results were obtained on any drugs or brain stimulation due to either small sample and/or heterogeneous results [9].

In 2018, the American Academy of Neurology, the American Congress of Rehabilitation Medicine, and the National Institute on Disability, Independent Living, and Rehabilitation Research jointly reported that clinicians should counsel families that for adults, minimally conscious state (MCS) (vs vegetative state [VS]/unresponsive wakefulness syndrome [UWS]) and traumatic (vs nontraumatic) etiology are associated with more favorable outcomes (level B) and clinicians should prescribe amantadine (100–200 mg bid) for adults with traumatic VS/UWS or MCS (4–16 weeks post-injury) to hasten functional recovery and reduce disability early in recovery (level B). Recent evidence indicates that the term chronic VS/UWS should replace permanent VS, with duration specified (Level B) [10].

In 2021, Edlow B.L. et al. reviewed the current status of recovery from DoC [11]. Points can be summarized as follows: A common pathophysiological mechanism underlying DoC is the withdrawal of excitatory synaptic activity across the cerebrum produced by deafferentation or disfacilitation of neocortical, thalamic, and striatal neurons. Recovery from coma involves various mechanisms, culminating in the restoration of excitatory neurotransmission across long-range corticocortical, thalamocortical, and thalamostriatal connections. Re-emergence of consciousness is associated with a shift in patterns of neuronal activity across the corticothalamic system that can be measured with EEG, PET, or resting-state functional MRI. Task-based functional MRI and EEG can reveal cognitive motor dissociation in up to 15–20% of patients who seem unresponsive on behavioral examination, and emerging evidence suggests that early detection of cognitive motor dissociation in the ICU predicts 1-year functional outcomes. Amantadine is the only therapy that has been associated with the acceleration of recovery of consciousness in an RCT of patients with subacute traumatic DoC, but multiple pharmacological and neuromodulatory therapies are now being tested. Emerging advances in diagnostic and prognostic techniques provide new opportunities to detect consciousness, monitor its recovery, elucidate its neuronal substrate, and identify the therapeutic potential of promoting the re-emergence of consciousness in a subset of patients with DoC.

41.11 Personal View on the Therapeutic Interventions for Refractory Prolonged DoC

Effective treatment of prolonged DoC especially of refractory cases needs to be done fundamentally by exploring novel medication or surgery including stimulation. It might be done most quickly by finding out deficient or excess humoral factors and systems such as extrapyramidal system, which may pave the way to novel pharmacotherapy including by existing agents.

For example, in my personal experiences, the improvement of consciousness level was obtained after weeks to months of administration of amantadine, bromocriptine, L-dopa, and so on in those comatose patients without medical history of Parkinson's disease. These experiences might be supported by the recent report published in the journal *Brain*, which disclosed presynaptic dopamine deficit in posttraumatic MCS [12]. Here, physicians must not rely on the past medical history of Parkinson's disease. There are so many patients with Parkinson's disease and related movement disorders and dementing illnesses or cognitive impairment without prior diagnosis and instead suffer from related complications such as paralytic ileus, aspiration pneumonia, vocal cord paralysis, central respiratory abnormality, dysautonomia, neuroleptic malignant syndrome, serotonin syndrome, frailty, and perioperative state in advance. Thus, neurological examination especially on muscle tonus, involuntary movements, and gathering information on cognitive function are critically important in those with DoC.

Table 41.3 summarizes my personal view on the therapeutic interventions for refractory and prolonged DoC.

Table 41.3 Personal view on the therapeutic interventions for refractory and prolonged DoC

Therapeutic interventions	Personal view
Antiepileptics	Levetiracetam, Carbamazepine, etc. Consider if non-convulsive status epilepticus (NCSE) is suspected clinically One patient fully recovered from coma of 1.5 year duration soon after starting antiepileptics Should not abuse antiepileptics in those not suspected of NCSE
Protirelin	In Japan, approved for subarachnoid hemorrhage, traumatic brain injury, spinocerebellar degeneration Although DoC improved dramatically in several patients, efficacy ratio is very low Rarely cause convulsive seizure
Amantadine	Consider in those suspected of dopamine deficiency from positive extrapyramidal signs Rarely cause convulsive seizure and aspiration
Bromocriptine	May consider in those suspected of dopamine deficiency from positive extrapyramidal signs Although DoC improved in several patients, efficacy ratio is very low
L-Dopa	Consider in those suspected of dopamine deficiency from positive extrapyramidal signs Although effective sometimes, efficacy ratio is low
Zolpidem	Although very effective case was reported in the literature and media, no experience personally Be cautious of possible aspiration due to further decrease of arousal
Steroid	Long-term administration for several months to one year is sometimes effective in encephalitis
Tapering/cessation of medications which can decrease arousal	Sedatives, Clonazepam, Neuroleptics, Muscle relaxants, Antiepileptics, if appropriate Many experiences of consciousness level improvement after cessation of sedatives and/or clonazepam

Table 41.3 (continued)

Therapeutic interventions	Personal view
Change of attending physician	To comprehensive work-up and treatment especially including NCSE
Intensive rehabilitation	Basically important in facilitating consciousness recovery

DoC disorders of consciousness

41.12 Curing Coma Campaign

Curing coma has become the worldwide topic of neurocritical care after the advent of the Curing Coma Campaign (CCC) by the Neurocritical Care Society and the National Institutes of Health (NIH) which was officially kicked off in 2019 and led by Professor J. Claude Hemphill III and Professor DaiWai M. Olson [13]. CCC is the platform to enable two interrelated goals: (a) focus the science of acute DoC on identifying and testing therapeutic interventions and (b) form an enduring community of medical providers, scientists, and advocates to test and implement these advances. The administrative structure consists of Steering Committees, Advisory Council, seven Modules, and seven Working Groups. The 10-year scientific roadmap consists of three domains: discovery science, clinical trial readiness, and curing coma treatments. Specific efforts of the CCC include two NIH Symposia and the World Coma Day on March 22 every year. All interested individuals and institutions can sign on as collaborators via the CCC website (https://www.curingcoma.org) to receive ongoing notifications and participate in CCC initiatives and studies.

The author is joining the CCC Common Data Elements Working Group (Chair; Professor Jose I. Suarez) representing Japan and also will chair the Annual Meeting of the Japan Coma Society in August 2024 in Tokyo. We know that curing coma is a truly grand challenge. The CCC represents a collaboration intended to leverage science and community. This work is challenging, but possible, and our patients and their families stand at the center (by Professor DaiWai M. Olson). Irrespective of nationality, specialty, subspecialty, and occupation, we need to collaborate together for the progress of Neurocritical Care and Critical Care Neurology including DoC.

References

1. Kanich W, Brady WJ, Huff JS, Perron AD, Holstege C, Lindbeck G, Carter CT. Altered mental status: evaluation and etiology in the ED. Am J Emerg Med. 2002;20(7):613–7.
2. Bleck TP, Smith MC, Pierre-Louis SJ, Jares JJ, Murray J, Hansen CA. Neurologic complications of critical medical illnesses. Crit Care Med. 1993;21(1):98–103.
3. Nagayama M, Yang S, Geocadin RG, et al. Novel clinical features of nonconvulsive status epilepticus. F1000Res. 2017;6:1690.
4. Wijdicks EFM, et al., editors. Mayo Clinic Critical and Neurocritical Care Board Review, Mayo Clinic Scientific Press (New York, 2019; online edn, Oxford Academic, 1 July 2019).
5. Brophy GM, Bell R, Claassen J, Alldredge B, Bleck TP, Glauser T, Laroche SM, Riviello JJ Jr, Shutter L, Sperling MR, Treiman DM, Vespa PM, Neurocritical Care Society Status Epilepticus Guideline Writing Committee. Guidelines for the evaluation and management of status epilepticus. Neurocrit Care. 2012;17:3–23.
6. Trinka E, Cock H, Hesdorffer D, Rossetti AO, Scheffer IE, Shinnar S, Shorvon S, Lowenstein DH. A definition and classification of status epilepticus—Report of the ILAE Task Force on Classification of Status Epilepticus. Epilepsia. 2015;56:1515–23.
7. Betjemann JP, Lowenstein DH. Status epilepticus in adults. Lancet Neurol. 2015;14(6):615–24.
8. Nagayama M, Matsushima K, Nagayama T, Shinohara Y. Persistent but reversible coma in encephalitis. Neurocrit Care. 2005;2:252–7.
9. Thibaut A, Schiff N, Giacino J, Laureys S, Gosseries O. Therapeutic interventions in patients with prolonged disorders of consciousness. Lancet Neurol. 2019;18(6):600–14.
10. Giacino JT, Katz DI, Schiff ND, Whyte J, Ashman EJ, Ashwal S, Barbano R, Hammond FM, Laureys S, Ling GSF, Nakase-Richardson R, Seel RT, Yablon S, Getchius TSD, Gronseth GS, Armstrong MJ. Practice guideline update recommendations summary: disorders of consciousness: report of the guideline development, dissemination, and implementation Subcommittee of the American Academy of Neurology; the American Congress of Rehabilitation Medicine; and the National Institute on Disability, Independent Living, and Rehabilitation Research. Neurology. 2018;91(10):450–60.
11. Edlow BL, Claassen J, Schiff ND, Greer DM. Recovery from disorders of consciousness: mechanisms, prognosis and emerging therapies. Nat Rev Neurol. 2021;17(3):135–56.
12. Fridman EA, Osborne JR, Mozley PD, Victor JD, Schiff ND. Presynaptic dopamine deficit in minimally conscious state patients following traumatic brain injury. Brain. 2019;142(7):1887–93.
13. Olson DM, Hemphill JC 3rd, Curing Coma Campaign and its Executive Committee. The Curing Coma Campaign: challenging the paradigm for disorders of consciousness. Neurocrit Care. 2021;35(Suppl 1):1–3.

42 Physiotherapeutic Management in Neurocritical Care

Rajeev Aggarwal, Vandana Dua,
and Harpreet S. Sachdev

42.1 Introduction

Neuro-critical care units (NCCUs) have emerged as a subspeciality of intensive care units (ICUs) in tertiary care hospitals. It is more challenging to manage critically ill neurological patients as compared to other critical patients. With the advent of scientific advancements in monitoring, diagnostics, and therapeutic interventions, the survival rate of critically ill neurological patients is steadily rising. Hand in hand, it has resulted in certain long-term health-related consequences in such patients ranging from cognitive, physical, to psychological impairments [1]. The success of interventions for critical illness depends not only on the diagnosis or availability of supportive care but also on individual vulnerability, considering the age, past clinical status, and genetic predisposition in addition to the present clinical status. Retrieving functional independence and quality of life (QoL) and societal reintegration of these patients post-discharge is perplexing for healthcare providers. The mounting need for rehabilitation of critically ill neurological patients requires an early intervention to improve the outcome.

Physiotherapeutic management in NCCU involves the implementation of a feasible, cost-effective, and individualized therapeutic program by a team of physiotherapists considering safety as a prime concern and thereby avoiding adverse effects. Physiotherapists deal with a unique set of impairments in critically ill neurological patients ranging from impaired sensorium, inability to communicate, sensory impairments, motor deficits, systemic manifestations, and secondary complications of neurological insult summarized in Table 42.1. Patients in NCCU are often sedated and paralyzed limiting their participation, and hence, initiation of self-activities and mobilization is frequently delayed leading to enormous multi-organ complications. Physiotherapy plays a vital role in the prevention and management of secondary complications and in maximizing functional activities to improve their survival and QoL.

R. Aggarwal (✉) · V. Dua · H. S. Sachdev
Department of Neurology, All India Institute of Medical Sciences, New Delhi, India

H. Prabhakar et al. (eds.), *Principles and Practice of Neurocritical Care*,
https://doi.org/10.1007/978-981-99-8059-8_42

Table 42.1 Concerns in critically ill neurological patients for consideration by physiotherapists

	Concerns
Respiratory	Impaired lung expansion/atelectasis
	Retention of tracheobronchial secretions
	Inability to maintain patent airways
	Ventilation-perfusion mismatch
	Difficult weaning from mechanical ventilation
Musculoskeletal	ICU acquired weakness
	Osteoporosis
	Muscle tightness, joint stiffness, contractures, deformities
	Muscular pains
	Muscle paresis/paralysis
	Impaired muscle tone: increased/decreased, dystonia
Altered state of consciousness	Delirium, coma, vegetative state, minimally conscious state, locked-in syndrome
Psychological functions	Anxiety, depression, apathy, posttraumatic stress
Sleep dysfunction	Insomnia, hypersomnolence
Cardiovascular	Deep vein thrombosis
Integumentary	Decubitus ulcers
Sensory	Hypoesthesia, hyperesthesia, paraesthesia, neuropathic pain
Cognitive	Attention, perception, executive functioning, verbal fluency, memory, visuospatial skills

42.2 Physiotherapy in Respiratory Impairments

Critically ill neurological patients often present with actual/impending type I or type II respiratory failure. Type I respiratory failure is characterized by hypoxemia with normocapnia, while type II respiratory failure is characterized by hypoxemia along with hypercapnia. Patients with traumatic brain injury with neurogenic pulmonary edema, associated lung injury, acute respiratory distress syndrome, aspiration pneumonitis, and varied degrees of atelectasis are commonly seen with type I respiratory failure in NCCU. Patients with neuro-muscular diseases such as Guillain-Barre syndrome, myasthenia gravis, myopathies, high spinal cord injury, and central respiratory depression in brain injury patients often present with type II respiratory failure.

Respiratory failure is the outcome of mismatch between load and efforts of respiratory system. Efforts of respiratory system are attributed to work done by respiratory muscles known as work of breathing. Work of breathing is broadly required to overcome the load, i.e., elasticity of lung tissues and airway resistance. Reduction in lung compliance and increase in airway resistance increase the load demanding higher work of breathing, while weakness in respiratory muscle strength reduces the efforts, hence leading to respiratory failure. Oxygen therapy and ventilatory support are instituted to manage hypoxemia and hypercapnia. Diligence in correction of blood gas level is warranted as both hypoxia and hyperoxia are detrimental. Hypoxia causes cerebral ischemia to produce functional deficits, whereas hyperoxia generates oxygen-free radicals and oxidative stress. It impairs cerebral autoregulation to cause damage to lungs and brain. Similarly, hypercapnia and hypocapnia have significant effects on cerebral blood flow that alters intracranial pressure. Hypercapnia leads to vasodilatation and increases the cerebral blood flow that, in turn, may increase the intracranial pressure, while hypocapnia leads to reduction in cerebral blood flow that leads to cerebral hypoxia [2].

Delineation of pathomechanics behind the clinical presentation, comprehensive understanding of oxygen cascade, and various threats at different levels of oxygen transport system foster clinical decision-making in the selection of appropriate chest physiotherapy technique.

42.2.1 Chest Physiotherapy

Chest physiotherapy (CPT) is a collection of therapeutic techniques deliberated to facilitate the clearance of airway secretions, re-expand the atelectatic areas, minimize ventilation-perfusion mismatch, reduce work of breathing, and enhance the respiratory muscles' strength and endurance. These techniques include therapeutic body positioning, postural drainage, percussion, vibration, directed coughing, huffing, respiratory muscles training, diaphragmatic breathing, thoracic expansion, and conditioning exercises. Various adjuncts such as humidification, mechanical vibrators, oscillators, nebulization, and positive airway pressure devices facilitate to achieve the desired goals. Chest physiotherapy techniques can be used as standalone or in combination.

42.2.2 Techniques of Chest Physiotherapy

Therapeutic Body Positioning

Positioning a patient to facilitate the physiologic functions and minimize the complications is termed as *therapeutic body positioning*. Human body composes two-third of water subjected to gravity. Gravity plays a crucial role in maintaining physiological functions of human body. In NCCU, patients are treated in recumbent or semi-recumbent position. Clinical parameters with therapeutic positioning and turning of the patient in NCCU should be reviewed periodically as physiologically advantageous position at one point of time becomes disadvantageous after sometime [3].

Regular turning of the body to promote lung expansion and improve oxygen transport 2 hourly should be done unless constrained due to hemodynamic and/or musculoskeletal instability. The frequency of turning can be altered as per the need and response of the patient. The patient can be positioned at varied degrees of rotations such as half-side lying, semi-prone, or in prone positions. Semi fowler (head end of bed raised between 30 and 45°), fowler (head end of bed raised between 45 and 60°), high fowler (head end of bed raised between 60 and 90°), and Trendelenburg (head end of bed lowered between 15 and 30°) positions are used to capitalize effect of gravity for conditioning of cardiopulmonary and musculoskeletal system. Trendelenburg positions are avoided in traumatic brain injury patients with raised intracranial pressure, unsecured airways with risk of aspirations, patients with Ryle's tubes, recent hemoptysis, uncontrolled hypertension, and distended abdomen. Fowler positions are avoided in hypotensive patients.

Postural drainage refers to positioning specific to each bronchopulmonary segment to facilitate gravity-assisted drainage of secretions. The affected segment is positioned in such a way that it remains higher than carina so that secretions are drained toward the main bronchus from where these can be cleared by coughing or suctioning. These positions can be modified as per the need of the patient and tolerance.

Percussion

Percussion is rhythmical striking of the thorax with a cupped hand directly over the lung segments to be drained. Clapping, cupping, and tapotement are the other terms used for percussion. During percussion, intermittently kinetic energy is applied to the chest wall to loosen the secretions in airways in patients with poor ventilatory muscle force who have impaired mucociliary clearance and viscous secretions. Percussion is done in both inspiratory and expiratory phases of the breathing.

Vibrations

Vibration is the application of a fine vibratory force over the lung segments to be drained during the expiratory phase of the breathing. The direction of vibratory force is inward and upward toward the central airways. Coarse vibratory movements are referred to as shaking. These are required in patients with weak cough reflex.

Percussion and vibrations should be avoided in patients with high intracranial pressure, unstable hemodynamic conditions, active hemoptysis, large pleural effusion, pulmonary embolism, pulmonary edema due to congestive heart failure, osteomyelitis of ribs, osteoporosis, unstable head and neck injury, flail chest, or surgical wound on chest.

42.2.3 Manual Hyperinflation

Manual hyperinflation is inflating the lungs with a larger tidal volume using a manual resuscitator bag. It provides slow deep inspiration and inspiratory hold followed by sudden and fast expiratory release to mimic a cough. It helps in the removal of stagnant secretions and the prevention of pulmonary atelectasis. Manual hyperinflation should be avoided in patients with undrained pneumothorax, hypotension, severe bronchospasm, unexplained hemoptysis intracranial hypertension, and high PEEP.

42.2.4 Active Cycle of Breathing Technique (ACBT)

ACBT is an active airway clearance technique employed in patients who have good ventilatory effort and poor mucociliary clearance. It involves three phases: breathing control, thoracic expansion exercises, and forced expiratory technique, repeated in a cyclic manner. Breathing control is relaxed tidal diaphragmatic breathing to relieve any anxiety or stress. Its importance is more pertinent in patients with bronchospasm. Thoracic expansion exercises constitute deep inhalation with relaxed exhalation at vital capacity with or without chest percussion/vibration/shaking. It is followed by huffing, which is a forced expiratory technique against open glottis performed to move the secretions from peripheral airways to central airways. During huffing, the air is exhaled forcefully using abdominal contractions after deep inspiration. Treatment is terminated when there is non-productive huff from a medium-sized inspiration through complete expiration and there is dry sound for two cycles in a row [4].

42.2.5 Autogenic Drainage (AD)

AD is a system of diaphragmatic breathing by varying expiratory flow to mobilize secretions from tracheobronchial tree; indicated in patients with chronic secretion retention. Good ventilatory efforts are a prerequisite for AD [5]. It consists of three phases.

Unsticking Phase: In this phase, the patient breaths at low lung volume (from tidal volume to expiratory reserve volume), i.e., an inspiration followed by a breath hold of 2–3 s to ensure equal filling of lung segments by collateral filling and then a deep exhalation into the expiratory reserve volume (ERV) range. By lowering mid-tidal volume below functional residual capacity, secretions from peripheral lung regions are mobilized by compression of peripheral alveolar ducts hence referred to as "unsticking." It continues until the mucus is loosened and starts to move into larger airways.

Collecting Phase: It consists of tidal breathing so that breathing is changed gradually from ERV into the inspiratory reserve volume (IRV) to mobilize secretions from the larger airways to central airways. The velocity of airflow is controlled so that the maximal expiratory flow is reached without collapsing the airways. This low to mid-lung volume continues until the sound of the mucus decreases, signaling its movement into central airways to be evacuated.

Evacuating Phase: It consists of deep inspiration into the IRV range. This middle to high lung volume breathing continues until the secretions are in the trachea and are ready to be expectorated. Control of airflow during this final phase is essential to avoid uncontrolled unproductive coughing, since it may result in the collapse of airways.

CPT can mobilize the tracheobronchial secretions and re-expand the lung segments, but it can transiently increase the ICP [6]. Many studies have found CPT techniques safe and effective in critically ill neurological patients [7, 8].

42.2.6 Positive Airway Pressure Techniques

Positive airway pressure techniques include application of positive pressure to the airways either in inspiration or in expiration. Expiratory positive airway pressure (EPAP) devices are used in patients who are prone to alveolar collapse like in obstructive airway disease. EPAP devices may be fixed orifice resistors or threshold resistors. A fixed orifice resistor is variable resistance device, whereas threshold resistors provide fixed and predictable resistance to the airways. EPAP device may offer vibratory movements during exhalation to mobilize the secretions from airways. Flutter®, Acapella®, Aerobika®, and VibraPEP® (Fig. 42.1) are commonly used oscillatory PEP devices in clinical practice.

42.2.7 Respiratory Muscle Training

Respiratory muscle strength and endurance are vital for optimal oxygen delivery. Ventilator-induced diaphragmatic dysfunction is found to occur in 80% of patients with IC acquired weakness (ICUAW) [9]. Prolonged controlled positive pressure ventilation deconditions the diaphragmatic muscle fibers. The ongoing sepsis and electrolyte imbalance further accelerate the

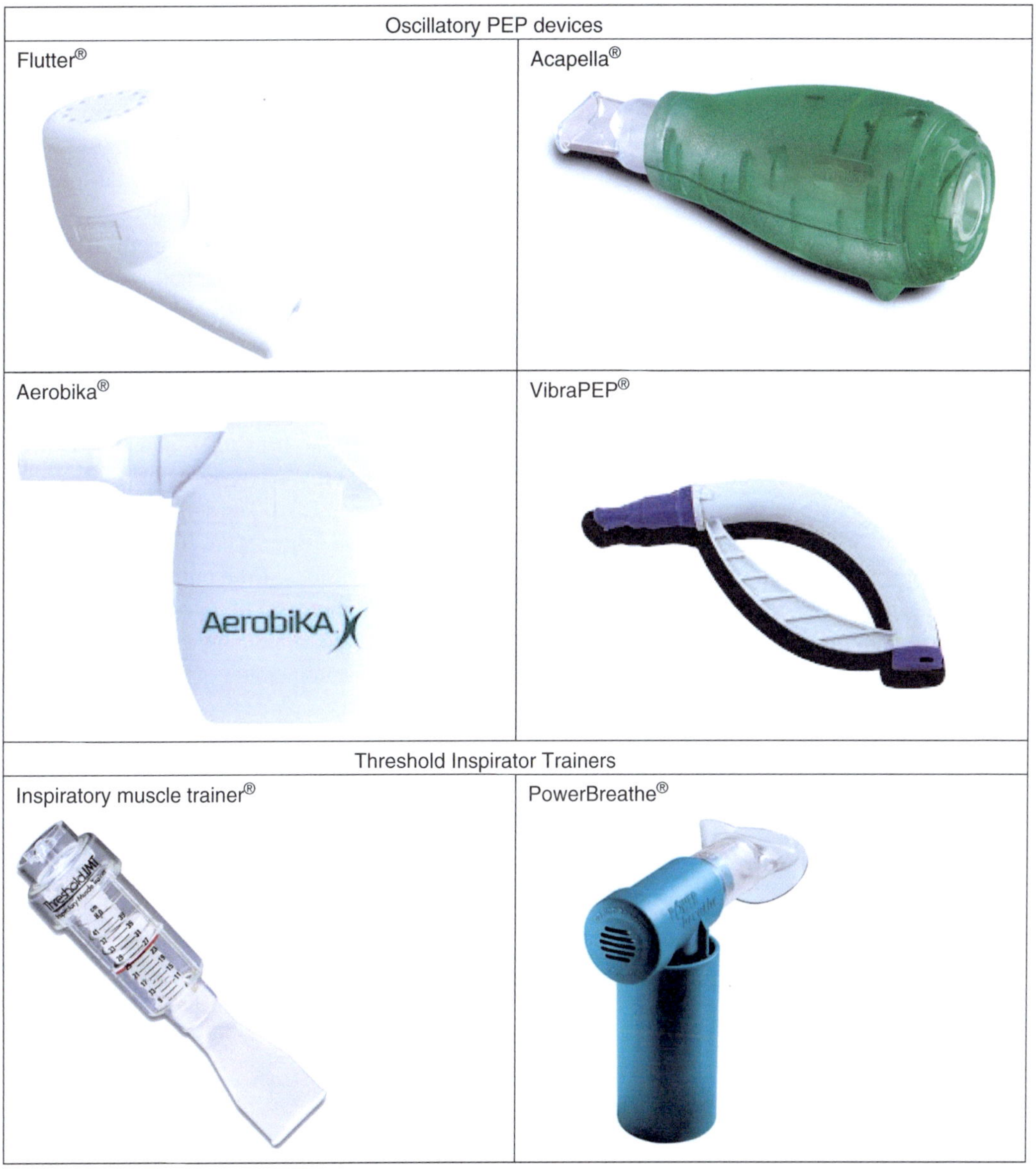

Fig. 42.1 Oscillatory positive expiratory pressure devices and threshold inspiratory pressure devices

diaphragmatic dysfunction. This, in addition to, atelectasis, fluid overload, neuromuscular dysfunction innate to various neurological conditions, results in difficult weaning of patients from ventilator. Therefore, respiratory, particularly inspiratory, muscle training has got attention of critical care practitioners in recent past. Muscle training works on principles of overload, specificity, and reversibility. Overload means a muscle is loaded with a higher load compared with its usual load to activate more motor units. The muscles respond to this overload by hypertrophy of muscle fibers and improved metabolic activities. The specificity principle pertains to training of a muscle in similar circumstances, posture, and range of movement where a muscle function is intended. For example, the performance of a cyclist can be improved by overloading the muscles in cycling but not by swimming. Reversibility refers to the reversal of training effect when a muscle is not used for a prolonged period.

Isocapnic hyperventilation and *inspiratory resistance training* are two methods for inspiratory muscle training. Isocapnic hyperventilation is a dynamic strengthening protocol to increase the endurance of the inspiratory muscles. A person is asked to breath at the highest rate that he can manage for 15–30 min. A rebreathing circuit is used with this technique to prevent hypocapnia. This technique has limited usage due to the usage of rebreathing bag [10].

Inspiratory resistance training is used for both strength and endurance training. It incorporates both isometrics and isotonic contractions. Devices used to train the inspiratory muscles are non-linear devices and threshold inspiratory muscle training devices. Non-linear devices are narrow tubes that provide resistance while inspiring and expiring through these tubes. At low flow, resistance is low, but with an increase in the flow of air, the resistance increases exponentially. Threshold inspiratory muscle training devices provide a fixed resistance irrespective of airflow.

Threshold loading (Fig. 42.2) is the most common mode of inspiratory muscle training (IMT). Initially, training is started at five sets of six breaths each at 50% of maximum inspiratory pressure (PIMax) once a day, and it is increased on daily basis in such a way that the patient can achieve only six breaths in single set [11]. IMT can also be given as interval training of seven sessions of 2-min duration each interspersed by 1 min of rest or continuous training of 30 min in one session or multiple sessions at lower intensity.

A systematic review on IMT in critically ill patients [12] that included 28 studies (1185 subjects) reported IMT is feasible and well-tolerated in critically ill patients and improves both inspiratory and expiratory muscle strength. IMT was started during early mechanical ventilation in eight studies, in difficult-to-wean patients in 14 studies, and after extubation in three studies, whereas three studies did not report exact timing. Strength-training regimens were employed by 13 studies, and endurance training regimens were employed by 11 studies, whereas four studies could not be classified. The study found that IMT was feasible, and there were few adverse events during IMT sessions. IMT improved PIMax (15 RCTs; mean increase of 6 cm H_2O, 95% CI 5–8 cm H_2O) and maximum expiratory pressure (four RCTs, mean increase of 9 cm H_2O, 95% CI 5–14 cm H_2O) compared to control. IMT resulted with a shorter duration of ventilation (nine trials, mean difference 4.1 days, 95% CI 0.8–7.4 days) and duration of weaning (eight trials, mean difference 2.3 days, 95% CI 0.7–4.0 days). Confidence in these pooled estimates was low due to methodological limitations including substantial statistical and methodological heterogeneity. Most studies of IMT in critically ill patients employed inspiratory threshold loading. The

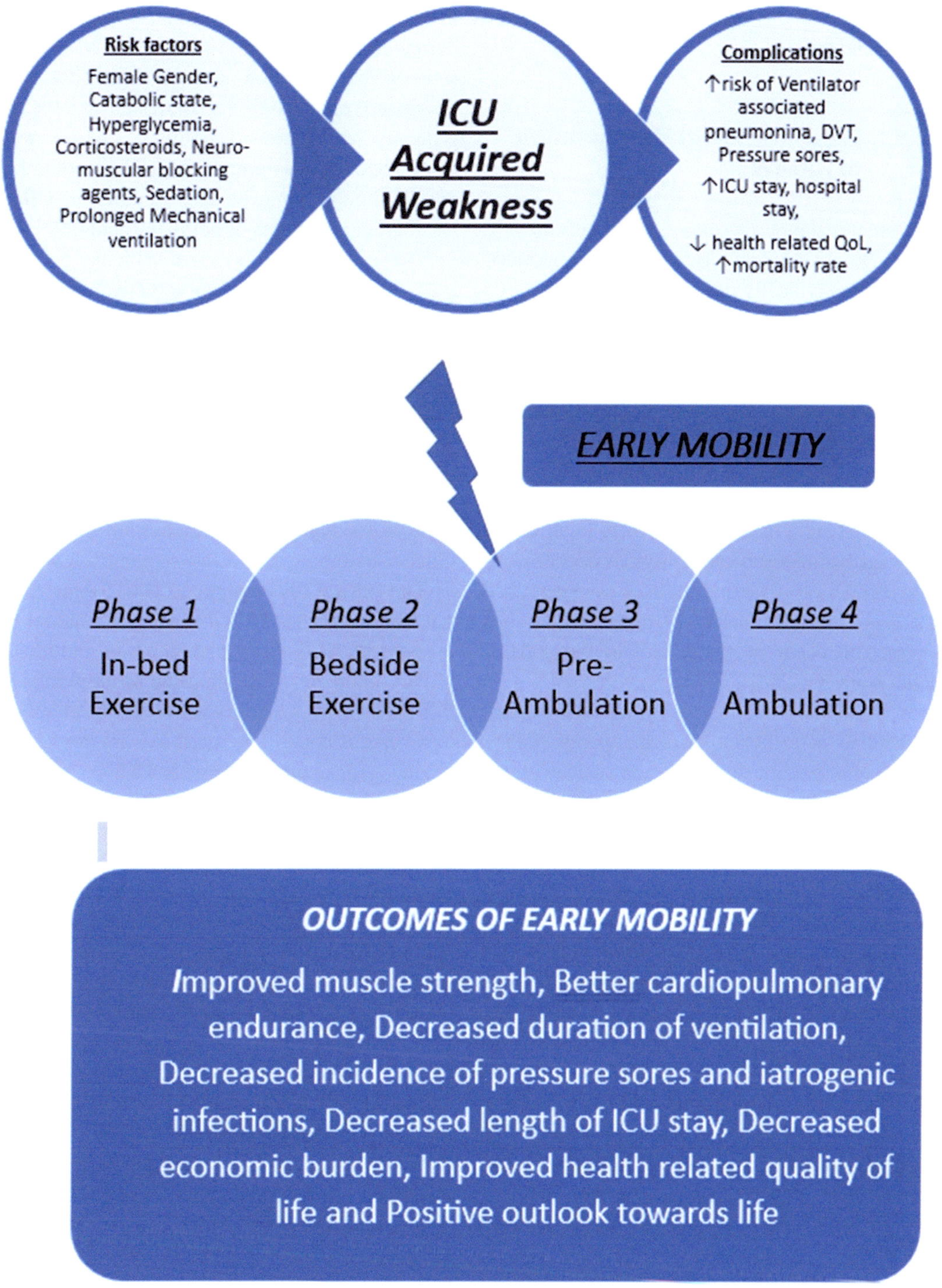

Fig. 42.2 Physiotherapeutic management of ICU Acquired Weakness through early mobility

impact of IMT on clinical outcomes requires future confirmation [12].

42.3 Prevention and Management of ICUAW

A symmetrical motor weakness ranging from mild paresis to quadriplegia typically sparing facial muscles in a critically ill patient, which cannot be attributed to any cause prior to admission to ICU, is considered ICU Acquired Weakness (ICUAW) [13]. ICUAW must be differentiated from disuse atrophy/deconditioning, which occurs as a result of prolonged inactivity. Respiratory muscles being the skeletal muscles are not spared and may prolong the duration of mechanical ventilation, and hence, the length of ICU stay, which, in turn, prolongs the bed rest and causes further deconditioning. This acts as a vicious circle of weakness, bed rest, and debility ultimately affecting the QoL. It is reported to occur in nearly half of the patients admitted in ICU [14].

ICUAW may manifest in myopathic pattern referred to as critical illness myopathy (CIM), neuropathic pattern referred to as critical illness polyneuropathy (CIP), or mixed pattern viz. critical illness poly-neuromyopathy (CIPM). Both clinical assessment and electrophysiological studies and/or biopsy are warranted for its diagnosis. Clinically, ICUAW is said to set in if muscle strength scores ≤48/60 on Medical Research Council (MRC)-Sum Score (MRC-SS) when assessed for shoulder abduction, elbow flexion, wrist extension, hip flexion, knee extension, and ankle dorsiflexion [13, 15]. CIP is characterized by acute, acquired length-dependent sensorimotor polyneuropathy due to axonal damage of the predominantly thick myelinated fibers and occasionally small fibers (sympathetic and C fibers) degeneration with distal muscles being affected more than proximal ones. Apart from muscle weakness and wasting, patients may present with symptoms related to temperature, pain, and sweat dysfunction. CIM, on the other hand, shows flaccid symmetrical paralysis with/without muscle atrophy, worse proximally than distally. Although the diagnosis can be made on clinical findings, electrodiagnostic tests give a definite diagnosis. CIP, on electromyography, reveals typical features suggestive of polyneuropathy with reduced compound muscle action potential (CMAP) and sensory nerve action potential (SNAP) with decreased motor unit recruitment, while CIM typically shows low amplitude CMAP with spared SNAP with normal motor unit recruitment pattern though it may be of short duration. CIPM shows mixed features of both CIM and CIP [16].

The sedated or comatose patients on prolonged mechanical ventilation, patients in sepsis with hyperglycemia, and patients on corticosteroids and/or neuromuscular blocking agents are reported to be at a higher risk of developing ICUAW [17]. Multi-faceted pathophysiological mechanisms underlying ICUAW are reported in the literature. Impaired protein synthesis, increased protein degradation, impaired excitability of skeletal muscle membranes, impaired glucose metabolism, etc., are to name a few [18].

The phrase "prevention is better than cure" goes apt with ICUAW as it can be prevented to an extent with meticulous planning and multidisciplinary approach since the time of admission to ICU. However, no intervention has been shown to reverse it completely once sets in. Prevention begins with avoiding the risk factors. Minimal use of corticosteroids and neuromuscular blocking agents and maintaining an optimum glycemic control and electrolyte balance have been shown to reduce morbidity and mortality in critically ill patients [19]. Maintaining optimum hydration and adequate calorie intake with appropriate protein proportion has been shown to maintain the muscle mass and improve muscle function. Minimizing sedation and giving daily sedation breaks have been shown to decrease the duration of mechanical ventilation and ICU dependency, thereby promoting early mobility [20].

Just like stagnant water favors the growth of microbes, bed rest leads to multi-organ dysfunction and predisposes the body to infection. Prolonged bed rest is known to affect lung volumes and capacities, cardiovascular endurance, musculoskeletal health and endurance, increased blood viscosity, impaired glucose metabolism, disrupted gastro-intestinal motility, depression, and impaired stress tolerance [21, 22]. Van Aerde et al. [23] in 2020 showed that muscle strength at ICU discharge is directly associated with mortality 5 years after discharge (hazard ratio 0.946, 95% CI: 0.928–0.968 per point increase in the MRC score). Hence, avoiding prolonged bed rest via early mobility is the mainstay of prevention.

Early mobility (EM), in literal terms, means adding *mobility* in a patient *early,* i.e., when he is still on mechanical ventilation (Fig. 42.2). EM has been shown to be safe and feasible and leads to less delirium, better cognition, improved functional recovery, early extubation, reduced length of ICU and hospital stay, and reduced mortality in critically ill patients [24–27]. In addition, EM in neurological patients helps in encashing the narrow window of neuroplasticity and neuronal reorganization to compensate for the insult to neurons [28]. EM of ventilated patients is safe and feasible with <2% reported adverse events, almost all of them being transient with no long-term consequences [29]. There is evidence of decreased muscle mass within the first 72 h of ICU admission so the timing of rehabilitation is an important variable to consider [30]. The mobility of critical patients is, however, frequently delayed due to multiple factors. There is no reported standard protocol for early mobility till date. It varies according to patient condition and willingness, ICU policies, sedation practices, outlook of ICU personnel toward it, staffing ratios, equipment safety and availability, funding policies, etc. Additionally, a neuro-critical care setup has its own unique challenges such as therapeutic flat head positioning to promote cerebral blood flow, cognitive impairment, altered sensorium, hemiplegia, visual deficit, altered cerebral autoregulation, ICP monitoring, external ventricular drainage, and lumbar drains.

Therefore, a multidisciplinary team including the physician, intensivist, physiotherapist, and nurse should take a decision regarding early mobility in neuro-critical care. Patient's willingness, level of alertness, present condition, past medical history, pre-ICU activity status, hemodynamic stability over the period of last 24 h, management of lines, tubes and equipment, and availability of staff should be considered while planning the protocol. Hemodynamic stability is considered if there is stable heart rate, rhythm, and blood pressure without any active titration of vasoactive drugs over the past 24 h. Acceptable respiratory reserve is determined by a respiratory rate of ≤30 with a minimal work of breathing, and if the patient is on mechanical ventilation, the oxygen saturation is ≥90% with $PaO_2/FiO_2 > 300$, PEEP <15 cm H_2O, and clear and secure airway with no change in oxygen requirements over past few hours. Neurological stability is considered if the patient is conscious, oriented, obeying com-

Table 42.2 Special considerations, contraindications, and termination criteria

Special considerations for mobilization in a neuro-critical care setup
1. It is recommended to initiate the bed mobility exercises within first 24 h of stroke; however, head of bed elevation should be attempted after initial 24 h of ischemic stroke [31]
2. Upright and out-of-bed activities initiated within 24–48 h of stroke onset have shown to reduce mortality and adverse events and improve functional capacity [32]
3. Hemorrhagic volume must be stabilized for at least 24 h before out-of-bed mobilization of a patient with hemorrhagic stroke [33]
4. Out-of-bed mobility can be initiated in patients after 24 h of recombinant tissue plasminogen activator administration or endovascular thrombectomy [33]
5. Early mobilization in patients with subarachnoid hemorrhage after clipping is safe and feasible. It is shown not to aggravate rather alleviate the cerebral vasospasm with mobility [34]
6. Mobilization with external ventricular drain is safe provided ICP < 20 mmHg, and the drain is clamped to avoid extra drainage [35]
7. Mobilization with femoral catheters is safe and feasible with no reported dislodgment or thrombotic/mechanical event once secured [36]
8. In neurosurgical patients where a bone flap is removed, protective helmets should be used while handling to avoid direct pressure on brain tissue
9. Early mobilization of spinal injury patients is recommended provided the spine is stabilized and orthostatic hypotension is taken care of
10. In case of elective spinal surgeries, bed exercises on the day of surgery itself and ambulation on first postoperative day are recommended for better functional outcomes [37]

(continued)

Table 42.2 (continued)

Contraindications and termination criteria to out-of-bed Mobility [38]	
Contraindications	Termination criteria
• Level of consciousness of patient –Richmond agitation sedation scale score: −4, −5, 3, and 4 • Recent myocardial ischemia and/or arrhythmias • Heart rate <40 and >130 beats/min • Mean arterial pressure <60 mmHg and >110 mmHg • Intracranial pressure >20 mmHg • Oxygen saturation <90% • Respiratory reserve (PaO_2/FiO_2) <200 • Parameters of ventilation –Fractional concentration of inspired oxygen >0.6 –Positive end-expiratory pressure > 10 cm H_2O –Partial pressure of arterial carbon dioxide >50 mmHg • Respiratory frequency >40 breath/min • Respiratory distress • Hemoglobin <7 g/dL • Platelet count <20,000 • High inotrope doses –Dopamine ≥10 mcg/kg/min –Noradrenaline/adrenaline ≥0.1 mcg/kg/min • Temperature > 38.5 °C or <36 °C • Spinal instability • Patients with active bleeding • Untreated deep venous thrombosis • Medically uncontrolled seizures • Ongoing renal replacement therapy • Ongoing intravenous sedation Relative contraindications: • Patient unwillingness • Emotional instability • Inadequate safety measures • Fatigue • Disturbance in monitoring • Intractable pain • Orthostatic hypotension • Intracranial pressure monitoring	• Oxygen desaturation <88% with supplemental oxygen during activity, unless otherwise specified by physician • Hypotension associated with dizziness, fainting, and/or diaphoresis • Tachycardia>130 bpm • Change in heart rhythm • Worsening of breathing pattern with an increase in accessory muscle use, paradoxical pattern, nasal flaring, or an appearance of facial distress • Extreme fatigue • Severe intolerable dyspnea with respiratory rate greater than baseline by >20/min • Significant chest pain • Excessive pallor or flushing of skin • Request of patient to stop

mands, Confusion Assessment Method for ICU (CAM-ICU) negative for delirium, ICP stable with no active titration of drugs/fluid over past 24 h, drains clamped if any, and spine is stabilized. Hemorrhagic volume is stabilized over 24 h in case of intracranial hemorrhage. In case of aneurysm, mobilization should be considered after appropriate medical/surgical intervention. The patient is not only assessed before attempting mobilization but also throughout the session. Special considerations to be considered while mobilizing a patient in neuro-critical care, and the contraindications and termination criteria for out-of-bed mobility are summarized in Table 42.2. There are a few tools available to objectively assess the patient's level of mobility in ICU. ICU Mobility Scale [39], Surgical Intensive Care Optimal Mobility Score [40], and Perme ICU Mobility Score [41] are a few validated ones, which can be utilized clinically both to assess the present level of mobility and to objectively assess the progression achieved through early mobility. National Guidelines for Prevention and Management of Stroke recommends that every stroke patient should be attended by a physiotherapist within 48 hours of admission [42].

Early mobility can be divided into four phases in succession to each other. *Phase 1* includes in-bed mobility and range of motion (ROM) exercises. The ROM exercises can be passive, active-assisted, active, or resisted in increasing proportion of patient participation. Bedsides sitting, sitting balance training and trunk mobility comprise *phase 2*. While *phase 3* implies out-of-bed activity including sit to stand, standing balance training, and pre-ambulation activities such as weight shifting, step marching, front/side stepping exercises, *phase 4* includes ambulation with/without assistance. The level of assistance, repetition of exercises, amount of resistance, duration of intervention, number of rest periods, and frequency of sessions are individualized throughout the protocol. The technological adjuncts such as tilt table, walking aids, arm/leg pedaling, cycle ergometer, and electrical stimulation are utilized wherever required (Table 42.3). Neuromuscular electrical stimulation (NMES) can be potentially considered an alternative to overcome barriers such as poor sensorium and lack of corporation with exercise, and a few studies have shown that it can be effectively utilized as a bridge till the patient is alert enough to participate in exercises [44]. Cognitive strategies such as mental imagery in addition to passive exercises have been

Table 42.3 Modalities used for early mobility

Modality	Advantages	Drawbacks	Dosage
Cycle ergometry	Exercises in debilitated population Used in bed-ridden patients No adverse effects Improves subjective feeling of well-being	Expensive Space requirements Time consuming in install-uninstall process	Once or twice daily 20- to 30-min session
Electrical muscle stimulation	Does not require volition Used in patients who cannot participate actively, maintains muscle mass (prevents disuse atrophy) Safe Can be started early	Minimal evidence regarding long-term functional benefits	Once daily 30-min session
Inspiratory muscle training	Prevents respiratory muscle atrophy Prevents pulmonary complications Early weaning from ventilator Decreases Length of stay in ICU	Not suitable for every patient [11]	15–20 min, twice daily
Tilt table	Improves respiratory and hemodynamic parameters Encourages weight bearing on joints	Space and personnel requirement	15–30 min daily
Standing hoists	Better alertness Physiological weight bearing on joints		15–20 min daily
Passive range of motion exercises (PROM)	Increases oxygen consumption in muscles [43] Safe; Maintains muscles and joint properties		15 min daily
Continuous passive motion (CPM) device	Maintains ROM, decreases loss of muscle proteins, improves circulation [43]		20–30 min daily

reported to be potentially beneficial in neurological patients with no active muscle control [45, 46]. Novel technological advancements such as whole body vibration, robotics such as LOKOMAT®, body weight supported treadmill training, and virtual reality have been utilized by researchers to combat ICUAW.

42.4 Prevention and Management of Deep Vein Thrombosis

Deep vein thrombosis and pulmonary embolism are common yet preventable cause of mortality in ICU patients. It is reported to occur in 2.9% of patients admitted to neuro-critical care [47] with its incidence as high as 1.7–34% in patients undergoing neurosurgery [48]. Immobility, intravenous catheters, coagulation disorders, dehydration, active cancer, and paralysis are some of the known risk factors in neurological ICU for developing thrombosis of deep veins in lower limbs [49]. Patient education, early mobility, leg elevation, and prophylactic anticoagulant cover can decrease the risk of the same. Intermittent pneumatic compression and/or use of compressive elastic stocking remains the mainstay of prevention in patients with contraindications to anticoagulants such as those with polytrauma, intracranial bleed, and thrombocytopenia, who received tissue plasminogen activator, etc. [50]. However, the sole use of graduated compressive stockings in the prevention of DVT is limited in high-risk patients [51] Almost 50% of the patients with DVT present with pain, edema, redness with tenderness, and warmth on examination. The clinical examination alone is unreliable to diagnose DVT. It is recommended to use D-dimer and Doppler ultrasound along with the coagulation profile to reach the diagnosis. Once diagnosed, the affected limb is immobilized with the initiation of anticoagulant cover. The mobilization of the limb must be initiated as soon as the therapeutic levels of anticoagulation are achieved, i.e., within 24–48 h of use of unfractionated heparin and 3–5 h of low molecular weight heparin [50] Early initiation of weight-bearing exercise can prevent post-thrombotic sequelae of severe pain, edema, and venous ulcers [52].

Table 42.4 Classification of states of altered consciousness

State of consciousness	Arousal	Awareness
Coma	–	–
Vegetative state (UWS)	+	–
Minimally conscious states (MCS)	+ (Fluctuating, not reliable but reproducible)	+ (Fluctuating, not reliable but reproducible)
Conscious	+ (May have complete/partial motor paralysis and language disorder)	+
Locked-in syndrome	+ (Preserved eye movements)	+

+ present, – absent, *UWS* unresponsive wakefulness syndrome [53]

42.5 Physiotherapy Management of Altered State of Consciousness

Altered state of consciousness is common and unique presentation in NCCU. Consciousness describes a combination of arousal and awareness components (Table 42.4).

Altered consciousness presents with fluctuating and variable levels of clinical signs and behaviors, of which many cannot be reproduced reliably and some are not perceived on bedside clinically. The presence of covert consciousness can be detected by measures such as functional magnetic resonance imaging (fMRI), positron-emission tomography (PET) scans, or electroencephalography (EEG), which have been used to augment clinical findings. Patients who are low-responsive or unresponsive to bedside stimuli could appear unresponsive but still be following commands indicating cognitive activity and hence categorized as cognitive motor dissociation (non-behavioral minimally conscious states) [53].

There are various physiotherapeutic techniques utilized to improve sensorium and hence responsiveness in patients presenting with altered sensorium in NCCU.

A ***multimodality sensory stimulation program*** (SSP) has shown significant improvements

Table 42.5 Multimodal Sensory Stimulation Program

Sensation type	Stimulation program
Touch	Family-directed social-tactile intervention Pressure devices
Taste (gustatory)	Familiar tastes
Smell (olfactory)	Familiar and daily olfaction objects
Proprioceptive	ROM exercises, transfers, and turning Early mobilization
Sight (visual)	Preferably outdoor, natural settings Green environment
Hearing (auditory)	Communication, preferably family delivered Use of music, as it engages emotion
Factors determining sensory stimulation	
Why?	It is noninvasive, simple to apply, inexpensive
What?	Should be simple, frequent, repetitive, autobiographical, emotional content Structured and meaningful stimuli: enrich environment
How?	Multiple sensory modalities Stimulate both input and output processing Moderate-to-high intensity (stimuli with sharp onset, strong energy)
Avoid?	Meaningless inputs (quality) Sensory deprivation (intensity) Habituation (response decrement by repeated stimulation)

in the levels of arousal, responsiveness, cognition, and sensorimotor behavior in patients with altered sensorium [54] SSP targets neuroplasticity promoting recovery and reducing long-term disability. It involves a safe, noninvasive, non-pharmacologic introduction of sensory stimulation addressing multiple sensations (Table 42.5).

Physiotherapists, in conjunction with the healthcare team and family members, design a personalized and specific sessions including necessary sensory stimuli and modality and determine threshold of exposure. Therapist varies the intensity and frequency of stimulus and also the number, duration, and frequency of each session. Each session includes use of simple, frequent, and repetitive sensory inputs with autobiographical and emotional content, and these are preferred over meaningless and repetitive sensory inputs, which could easily lead to habituation. Prolonged and unimodal SSP sessions should be avoided [55, 56]. ***Environmental enrichment*** is the manipulation of external environment of the patients targeting not only sensory stimulation but also increasing the environmental engagement. These structured and personalized sensory interactions replicate multimodal sensory inputs to the cortices as happens during activities of daily living (ADLs), preferred to unimodal sensory stimulation methods [54, 55].

Transcranial direct current stimulation (tDCS) is a relatively safe method of modulating the excitatory neurotransmission within the glutamate system. This has been used over the dorsolateral prefrontal cortex (DLPFC) as a noninvasive modulatory method, small amplitude direct currents over the scalp. Similarly, magnetic stimulation as ***transcranial magnetic stimulation (TMS) or repetitive TMS (rTMS)*** has shown both short-term and long-term effects on brain activity [57].

Right median nerve electrical stimulation (RMNS) is a simple, inexpensive, and noninvasive technique delivering electrical currents for coma arousal [58]. Right median nerve is selected for its disproportionately large sensory representation in the cortex and its association with the ascending reticular activating system (ARAS), neurotrophins, increasing the cerebral blood flow [59]. It influences the Glasgow Coma Scores irrespective of the cause, although other methods including bilateral MNS, electroacupuncture, transcutaneous peripheral nerve stimulation have been tried with mixed results.

Transcutaneous auricular vagal nerve stimulation (tVNS) is an emerging therapeutic modality used in improving the functional and cognitive recovery in impaired consciousness. Vagus nerve has extensive connections with nucleus tractus solitarius, which modulates the control of physiological states, body representation, and awareness. VNS targets the nor-epinephrine, GABA, and acetylcholine (Ach) in the nervous system and thus possesses the ability to modulate related cognitive systems [60] and neuroplasticity. Safety, feasibility, and efficacy of home-based VNS in patients after stroke have also been demonstrated in a small pilot study [61].

42.5.1 Brain-Computer Interface (BCI)

Behavioral assessment and neurological examination in patients with disorders of consciousness at bedside are difficult and unreliable due to inconsistent responsiveness, fluctuating alertness, lack of communication ability, and motor paralysis, which makes responding to stimuli difficult. Apart from being costly, it is human resource-dependent [62].

One such EEG-based system, brain-computer interface (BCI), has been used to detect covert-level consciousness and ability to follow commands in states of altered consciousness [63]. Research demonstrates its accuracy and sensitivity in ability to communicate with external world in patients who show no detectable command following behaviors but with clear evidence of command following brain activities (cognitive motor dissociation patients) [64]. BCI systems thus become an important tool to augment communication, through covert responses and training using BCI-controlled external environment.

42.6 Management of Spasticity, Muscle Tightness, and Contractures

Spasticity and hypertonicity are states of muscle overactivity, resistance, stiffness in response to movement, indicating abnormal neural mechanisms, and reduced threshold of spinal reflex mechanism. With time, this alters the mechanical properties of the muscle, non-neural reason for resistance to movement, atrophy, loss of sarcomeres and fibrosis, and accumulation of connective tissue and fat [65] Spasticity is a common feature following CNS insults such as stroke, brain injury, and spinal cord injury. Managing spasticity is crucial considering the high economic cost and social burden. It is seen that spasticity is more frequent (59–89%) and more severe (61.5% of patients had more than grade 3 spasticity on the Modified Ashworth scale) in patients with altered consciousness than in others with brain injury (25–42%) [65].

Spasticity varies depending on the type, location, and severity of the neural insult. Apart from leading to abnormal postures and movement, it also leads to pain, spasms, and skin ulcers [66]. In awake patients, it leads to loss of function, difficulty performing ADLs, and being socially active, and in unconscious states, it leads to weakness, improper positioning, abnormal postures, restricted mobility, difficulty transferring from bed, wheelchairs and toilet seats, and nursing care. It can be classified as focal (Fig. 42.3), segmental, or generalized. While planning treatment, the selection of methods not only depends on the grade of hypertonicity but also on factors such as behavioral and cognitive status, ability to communicate, sensory disturbance, motor ability, and affordability.

Abnormal posturing (Fig. 42.4) of the trunk and extremities is often observed after cerebral insults [67]. Such stereotypical pathological postures and movements typically occur in response to noxious stimuli or to internal or external envi-

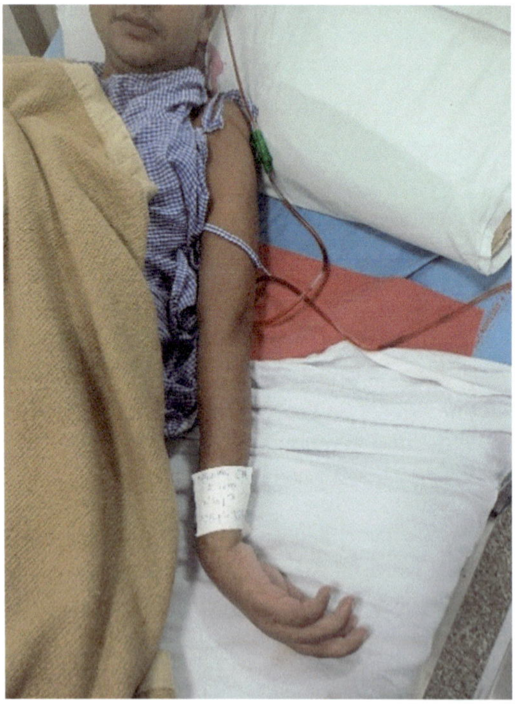

Fig. 42.3 Focal spasticity of upper extremity in a conscious patient

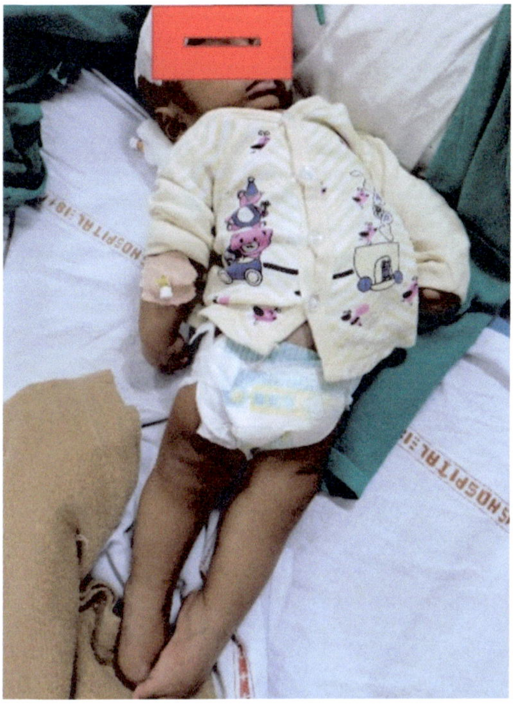

Fig. 42.4 Decerebrate posturing (opisthotonos), typical extension posturing

ronmental stimuli including fever, hypoxia, sensory irritation, metabolic factors, hypoglycemia, and meningeal irritation. These postures to some degree, point out to location of pathology as supratentorial and infratentorial, with their numerous causes.

Management of spasticity is a combination of pharmacological, non-pharmacological, and surgical interventions. Interventions can act locally on the muscle, termed "focal" or systemic acting through the central nervous system, termed "generalized" (Table 42.6). Management usually is directed at reversing the possible causes; in irreversible causes, supportive therapies are employed including a combination of pharmacological and non-pharmacological interventions. Physiotherapy interventions have a negative correlation with the degree of spasticity, i.e., the more frequent the session, the better outcomes of spasticity. Within the realm of existing non-pharmacological therapies for spasticity, noninvasive neuromodulation methods, namely tDCS and rTMS [68], have recently gained significance, but would need to gather more evidence on effectiveness.

Table 42.6 Management of spasticity

Focal measures	General measures
Stretching and flexibility exercises Serial casting and splinting Heat and cold therapeutic application Pressure garments Electrotherapy Robot-based therapies Botox injections Phenol injections Tendon/joint surgeries	Physical activity and seating devices Tilt tables and standing frames Positioning methods Relaxation methods Hydrotherapy and aquatic rehabilitation Noninvasive neuromodulation Medical management (oral drugs)

42.7 Conclusion

Early rehabilitation of neurological patients within the critical care unit is crucial especially with the steadily improving survival rates in the advent of technological advancements. At the same time, critically ill neurological patients present with unique challenges to physiotherapists such as altered state of consciousness, cognitive impairments, respiratory impairments, ICU-acquired weakness, hemiplegia, and altered cerebral autoregulation. It, therefore, requires expertise to individualize each physiotherapeutic session and hence encash the critical window period of recovery with utmost precision and care. The physiotherapeutic techniques and modalities are directed to prepone weaning from mechanical ventilation, improve sensorium, improve respiratory and peripheral muscle strength and endurance, manage muscle tone, and prevent tightness, contractures, deformities, venous thromboembolism, pressure sores, and other deleterious effects of bed rest and critical illness.

References

1. LaBuzetta JN, Rosand J, Vranceanu A-M. Review: post-intensive care syndrome: unique challenges in the neurointensive care unit. Neurocrit Care. 2019;31(3):534–45. https://doi.org/10.1007/s12028-019-00826-0.
2. Grüne F, Kazmaier S, Stolker RJ, Visser GH, Weyland A. Carbon dioxide induced changes in cerebral blood flow and flow velocity: role of cerebrovascular resistance and effective cerebral perfusion pressure. J

Cereb Blood Flow Metab. 2015;35(9):1470–7. https://doi.org/10.1038/jcbfm.2015.63. Epub 2015 Apr 15. PMID: 25873428; PMCID: PMC4640336.

3. Frownfelter DL, Dean E, editors. Principles and practice of cardiopulmonary physical therapy. 3rd ed. St. Louis: Mosby; 1996.
4. Pryor JA, Webber BA. Physiotherapy for respiratory and cardiac problems. 2nd ed. London: Churchill Livingstone; 1998.
5. Agostini P, Knowles N. Autogenic drainage: the technique, physiological basis and evidence. Physiotherapy. 2007;93(2):157–63. https://doi.org/10.1016/j.physio.2006.07.005.
6. Ferreira LL, Valenti VE, Vanderlei LC. Chest physiotherapy on intracranial pressure of critically ill patients admitted to the intensive care unit: a systematic review. Rev Bras Ter Intensiva. 2013;25(4):327–33. https://doi.org/10.5935/0103-507X.20130055. PMID: 24553515; PMCID: PMC4031870.
7. Harvey J, Hurst B. An evaluation of the effect of respiratory physiotherapy on intracranial pressure and cerebral perfusion pressure in ventilated, adult neurotrauma patients. Physiotherapy. 2016;102:e88. https://doi.org/10.1016/j.physio.2016.10.088.
8. Tomar GS, Singh GP, Bithal PK. To compare the effects of 2 different techniques of chest physiotherapy on intracranial pressure in traumatic brain injury patients: a randomized cross over study. J Neurosurg Anesthesiol. 2016;28:S18. https://doi.org/10.1097/ANA.0000000000000287.
9. Jung B, Moury PH, Mahul M, de Jong A, Galia F, Prades A, et al. Diaphragmatic dysfunction in patients with ICU-acquired weakness and its impact on extubation failure. Intensive Care Med. 2016;42:853–61.
10. McConnell A. Chapter 5. Methods of respiratory muscle training. In: Respiratory muscle training: theory and practice. Elsevier; 2013.
11. Bissett B, et al. Inspiratory muscle training for intensive care patients: a multidisciplinary practical guide for clinicians. Aust Crit Care. 2019;32(3):249–55.
12. Vorona S, Sabatini U, Al-Maqbali S, Bertoni M, Dres M, Bissett B, et al. Inspiratory muscle rehabilitation in critically ill adults. A systematic review and meta-analysis. Ann Am Thorac Soc. 2018;15(6):735–44. https://doi.org/10.1513/AnnalsATS.201712-961OC. PMID: 29584447; PMCID: PMC6137679.
13. Schefold JC, Wollersheim T, Grunow JJ, Luedi MM, Z'Graggen WJ, Weber-Carstens S. Muscular weakness and muscle wasting in the critically ill. J Cachexia Sarcopenia Muscle. 2020;11(6):1399–412. https://doi.org/10.1002/jcsm.12620. Epub 2020 Sep 7. PMID: 32893974; PMCID: PMC7749542.
14. Panahi A, Malekmohammad M, Soleymani F, Hashemian SM. The prevalence and outcome of intensive care unit acquired weakness (ICUAW). Tanaffos. 2020;19(3):250–5. PMID: 33815546; PMCID: PMC8008407
15. Fan E, Cheek F, Chlan L, Gosselink R, Hart N, Herridge MS, et al. An official American Thoracic Society clinical practice guideline: the diagnosis of intensive care unit-acquired weakness in adults. Am J Respir Crit Care Med. 2014;190:1437–46.
16. Zorowitz RD. ICU–acquired weakness: a rehabilitation perspective of diagnosis, treatment, and functional management. Chest. 2016;150(4):966–71, issn:0012-3692. https://doi.org/10.1016/j.chest.2016.06.006.
17. Hermans G, Van den Berghe G. Clinical review: intensive care unit acquired weakness. Crit Care. 2015;19:274. https://doi.org/10.1186/s13054-015-0993-7.
18. Kanova M, Kohout P. Molecular mechanisms underlying intensive care unit-acquired weakness and sarcopenia. Int J Mol Sci. 2022;23(15):8396. https://doi.org/10.3390/ijms23158396. PMID: 35955530; PMCID: PMC9368893.
19. Vanhorebeek I, Latronico N, Van den Berghe G. ICU-acquired weakness. Intensive Care Med. 2020;46(4):637–53. https://doi.org/10.1007/s00134-020-05944-4. Epub 2020 Feb 19. PMID: 32076765; PMCID: PMC7224132.
20. Kress JP, Pohlman AS, O'Connor MF, Hall JB. Daily interruption of sedative infusions in critically ill patients undergoing mechanical ventilation. N Engl J Med. 2000;342:1471–7.
21. Harper CM, Lyles YM. Physiology and complications of bed rest. J Am Geriatr Soc. 1988;36:1047–54.
22. Truong AD, Fan E, Brower RG, Needham DM. Bench-to-bedside review: mobilizing patients in the intensive care unit—from pathophysiology to clinical trials. Crit Care. 2009;13(4):216. https://doi.org/10.1186/cc7885. Epub 2009 Jul 13. PMID: 19664166; PMCID: PMC2750129.
23. Van Aerde N, Meersseman P, Debaveye Y, Wilmer A, Gunst J, Casaer MP, et al. Five-year impact of ICU-acquired neuromuscular complications: a prospective, observational study. Intensive Care Med. 2020;46:1184–93.
24. Schweickert WD, Pohlman MC, Pohlman AS, et al. Early physical and occupational therapy in mechanically ventilated, critically ill patients: a randomised controlled trial. Lancet. 2009;373:1874–82.
25. Tipping CJ, Harrold M, Holland A, et al. The effects of active mobilisation and rehabilitation in ICU on mortality and function: a systematic review. Intensive Care Med. 2017;43:171–83.
26. Zhang L, Hu W, Cai Z, et al. Early mobilization of critically ill patients in the intensive care unit: a systematic review and meta-analysis. PLoS One. 2019;14:e0223185.
27. Aggarwal R, Chauhan S, Behari M, Gupta C, Dua V. Effect of early mobility in mechanically ventilated patients with myasthenia crisis on duration of mechanical ventilation and length of intensive care unit stay. Physiother J Indian Assoc Physiother. 2020;14:74–9.
28. Murphy TH, Corbett D. Plasticity during stroke recovery: from synapse to behaviour. Nat Rev Neurosci. 2009;10:861–72.

29. Green M, Marzano V, Leditschke IA, Mitchell I, Bissett B. Mobilization of intensive care patients: a multidisciplinary practical guide for clinicians. J Multidiscip Healthc. 2016;9:247–56. https://doi.org/10.2147/JMDH.S99811. PMID: 27307746; PMCID: PMC4889100.
30. Anekwe DE, Biswas S, Bussières A, Spahija J. Early rehabilitation reduces the likelihood of developing intensive care unit-acquired weakness: a systematic review and meta-analysis. Physiotherapy. 2020;107:1–10. https://doi.org/10.1016/j.physio.2019.12.004. Epub 2019 Dec 19. PMID: 32135387.
31. Kumar MA, Romero FG, Dharaneeswaran K. Early mobilization in neurocritical care patients. Curr Opin Crit Care. 2020;26(2):147–54. https://doi.org/10.1097/MCC.0000000000000709. PMID: 32068582.
32. de Aquino Miranda JM, Mendes Borges V, Bazan R, José Luvizutto G, Shinosaki JSM. Early mobilization in acute stroke phase: a systematic review. Top Stroke Rehabil. 2023;30(2):157–68. https://doi.org/10.1080/10749357.2021.2008595. Epub ahead of print. PMID: 34927568.
33. Olkowski BF, Shah SO. Early mobilization in the neuro-ICU: how far can we go? Neurocrit Care. 2017;27(1):141–50.
34. Karic T, Roe C, Nordenmark T, et al. Effect of early mobilization and rehabilitation on complications in aneurysmal subarachnoid hemorrhage. J Neurosurg. 2017;126:518–26.
35. Moyer MT, Hinkle JL, Mendez JD. An integrative review: early mobilization of patients with external ventriculostomy drains in the neurological intensive care unit. J Neurosci Nurs. 2021;53(5):220–4. https://doi.org/10.1097/JNN.0000000000000609. PMID: 34369431.
36. Perme C, Nalty T, Winkelman C, Kenji Nawa R, Masud F. Safety and efficacy of mobility interventions in patients with femoral catheters in the ICU: a prospective observational study. Cardiopulm Phys Ther J. 2013;24(2):12–7. PMID: 23801900; PMCID: PMC3691704.
37. Burgess LC, Wainwright TW. What is the evidence for early mobilisation in elective spine surgery? A narrative review. Healthcare. 2019;7(3):92. https://doi.org/10.3390/healthcare703009.
38. Aggarwal R, Dua V. Physiotherapeutic management of critically ill neurological patients. In: Prabhakar H, Ali Z, editors. Textbook of neuroanesthesia and neurocritical care. Singapore: Springer; 2019. https://doi.org/10.1007/978-981-13-3390-3_19.
39. Hodgson C, Needham D, Haines K, Bailey M, Ward A, Harrold M, Young P, Zanni J, Buhr H, Higgins A, Presneill J. Feasibility and inter-rater reliability of the ICU mobility scale. Heart Lung. 2014;43(1):19–24.
40. Kasotakis G, Schmidt U, Perry D, Grosse-Sundrup M, Benjamin J, Ryan C, et al. The surgical intensive care unit optimal mobility score predicts mortality and length of stay. Crit Care Med. 2012;40(4):1122–8.
41. Perme C, Nawa RK, Winkelman C, Masud F. A tool to assess mobility status in critically ill patients: the Perme intensive care unit mobility score. Methodist Debakey Cardiovasc J. 2014;10(1):41–9.
42. https://mohfw.gov.in/sites/default/files/GuidelinesforPreventionandManagmentofStroke.pdf.
43. Newman ANL, Gravesande J, Rotella S, Wu SS, Topp-Nguyen N, Kho ME, Harris JE, Fox-Robichaud A, Solomon P. Physiotherapy in the neurotrauma intensive care unit: a scoping review. J Crit Care. 2018;48:390–406. https://doi.org/10.1016/j.jcrc.2018.09.037. Epub 2018 Oct 3. PMID: 30316038.
44. Zayed Y, Kheiri B, Barbarawi M, Chahine A, Rashdan L, Chintalapati S, Bachuwa G, Al-Sanouri I. Effects of neuromuscular electrical stimulation in critically ill patients: a systematic review and meta-analysis of randomised controlled trials. Aust Crit Care. 2019;50:280. https://doi.org/10.1016/j.aucc.2019.04.003.
45. McEwen SE, Huijbregts MP, Ryan JD, Polatajko HJ. Cognitive strategy use to enhance motor skill acquisition post-stroke: a critical review. Brain Inj. 2009;23(4):263–77.
46. Aikat R, Dua V. Mental imagery in spinal cord injury: a systematic review. J Spine. 2016;5:310. http://www.omicsgroup.org/journals/mentalimagery-in-spinal-cord-injury-a-systematicreview-2165-7939-1000310.php?aid=75087.
47. Browd SR, Ragel BT, Davis GE, Scott AM, Skalabrin EJ, Couldwell WT. Prophylaxis for deep venous thrombosis in neurosurgery: a review of the literature. Neurosurg Focus. 2004;17(4):E1. https://doi.org/10.3171/foc.2004.17.4.1. PMID: 15633987.
48. Li J, Ren X, Zhu X, Chen H, Lin Z, Huang M, Gu Z. Clinical predictive factors of lower extremity deep vein thrombosis in relative high-risk patients after neurosurgery: a retrospective study. Dis Markers. 2020;2020:5820749. https://doi.org/10.1155/2020/5820749. PMID: 32587639; PMCID: PMC7294362.
49. Sharma S. Deep vein thrombosis in neurocritical care. J Neuroanaesthesiol Crit Care. 2016;3(4):29.
50. Hillegass E, Puthoff M, Frese EM, Thigpen M, Sobush DC, Auten B, et al. Role of physical therapists in the management of individuals at risk for or diagnosed with venous thromboembolism: evidence-based clinical practice guideline. Phys Ther. 2016;96(2):143–66.
51. Dennis M, Sandercock PA, Reid J, Graham C, Murray G, Venables G, Rudd A, Bowler G. Effectiveness of thigh-length graduated compression stockings to reduce the risk of deep vein thrombosis after stroke (CLOTS trial 1): a multicentre, randomised controlled trial. Lancet. 2009;373(9679):1958–65.
52. Kahn SR, Shrier I, Kearon C. Physical activity in patients with deep venous thrombosis: a systematic review. Thromb Res. 2008;122(6):763–73.
53. Kondziella D, Bender A, Diserens K, van Erp W, Estraneo A, Formisano R, Laureys S, Naccache L, Ozturk S, Rohaut B, Sitt JD, Stender J, Tiainen M, Rossetti AO, Gosseries O, Chatelle C, EAN Panel

on Coma. Disorders of consciousness. European Academy of Neurology guideline on the diagnosis of coma and other disorders of consciousness. Eur J Neurol. 2020;27(5):741–56. https://doi.org/10.1111/ene.14151. Epub 2020 Feb 23. PMID: 32090418.
54. Abbate C, Trimarchi PD, Basile I, Mazzucchi A, Devalle G. Sensory stimulation for patients with disorders of consciousness: from stimulation to rehabilitation. Front Hum Neurosci. 2014;8:616. https://doi.org/10.3389/fnhum.2014.00616. PMID: 25157226; PMCID: PMC4127462.
55. Norwood MF, Lakhani A, Watling DP, Marsh CH, Zeeman H. Efficacy of multimodal sensory therapy in adult acquired brain injury: a systematic review. Neuropsychol Rev. 2023;33(4):693–713. https://doi.org/10.1007/s11065-022-09560-5. Epub ahead of print. PMID: 36056243.
56. Bondi CO, Klitsch KC, Leary JB, Kline AE. Environmental enrichment as a viable neurorehabilitation strategy for experimental traumatic brain injury. J Neurotrauma. 2014;31(10):873–88. https://doi.org/10.1089/neu.2014.3328. Epub 2014 Apr 17. PMID: 24555571; PMCID: PMC4012629.
57. Di Sarno L, Curatola A, Cammisa I, Capossela L, Eftimiadi G, Gatto A, Chiaretti A. Non-pharmacologic approaches to neurological stimulation in patients with severe brain injuries: a systematic review. Eur Rev Med Pharmacol Sci. 2022;26(18):6856–70. https://doi.org/10.26355/eurrev_202209_29789. PMID: 36196734.
58. Wang P, Cao W, Zhou H, et al. Efficacy of median nerve electrical stimulation on the recovery of patients with consciousness disorders: a systematic review and meta-analysis. J Int Med Res. 2022;50(12):3000605221134467. https://doi.org/10.1177/03000605221134467.
59. Wu X, Zhang C, Feng J, Mao Q, Gao G, Jiang J. Right median nerve electrical stimulation for acute traumatic coma (the Asia Coma Electrical Stimulation trial): study protocol for a randomised controlled trial. Trials. 2017;18(1):311. https://doi.org/10.1186/s13063-017-2045-x. PMID: 28693604; PMCID: PMC5504835.
60. Van Leusden JWR, Sellaro R, Colzato LS. Transcutaneous vagal nerve stimulation (VNS) a new neuromodulation tool in healthy humans? Front Psychol. 2015;6:102.
61. Kimberley TJ, Pierce D, et al. Vagus nerve stimulation paired with upper limb rehabilitation after chronic stroke: a blinded randomized pilot study. Stroke. 2018;49:2789–92.
62. Spataro R, Xu Y, Xu R, Mandalà G, Allison BZ, Ortner R, Heilinger A, La Bella V, Guger C. How brain-computer interface technology may improve the diagnosis of the disorders of consciousness: a comparative study. Front Neurosci. 2022;16:959339. https://doi.org/10.3389/fnins.2022.959339. PMID: 36033632; PMCID: PMC9404379.
63. Huang J, et al. Hybrid asynchronous brain–computer interface for yes/no communication in patients with disorders of consciousness. J Neural Eng. 2021;18:056001.
64. Pan J, Xie Q, Qin P, Chen Y, He Y, Huang H, Wang F, Ni X, Cichocki A, Yu R, Li Y. Prognosis for patients with cognitive motor dissociation identified by brain-computer interface. Brain. 2020;143(4):1177–89. https://doi.org/10.1093/brain/awaa026. Erratum in: Brain. 2020 Aug 1;143(8):e70. PMID: 32101603; PMCID: PMC7174053.
65. Thibaut FA, Chatelle C, Wannez S, Deltombe T, Stender J, Schnakers C, Laureys S, Gosseries O. Spasticity in disorders of consciousness: a behavioral study. Eur J Phys Rehabil Med. 2015;51(4):389–97. Epub 2014 Nov 6. PMID: 25375186.
66. Synnot A, Chau M, Pitt V, O'Connor D, Gruen RL, Wasiak J, Clavisi O, Pattuwage L, Phillips K. Interventions for managing skeletal muscle spasticity following traumatic brain injury. Cochrane Database Syst Rev. 2017;11:CD008929. https://doi.org/10.1002/14651858.CD008929.pub2. Accessed 10 March 2023.
67. Rauf W, et al. Effect of position on gross motor function and spasticity in spastic cerebral palsy children. J Pak Med Assoc. 2021;71(3):801. https://doi.org/10.47391/JPMA.1213.
68. Leo A, Naro A, Molonia F, Tomasello P, Saccà I, Bramanti A, Russo M, Bramanti P, Quartarone A, Calabrò RS. Spasticity management: the current state of transcranial neuromodulation. PM R. 2017;9(10):1020–9. https://doi.org/10.1016/j.pmrj.2017.03.014. Epub 2017 Apr 20. PMID: 28433830.

43 Palliative Care in Neurocritical Care

Sushma K. Gurav and Aditya Bang

Not to treat patients who are overmastered by their disease realizing that in such cases medicine is powerless—Hippocrates and Aristotle

43.1 Introduction

Neuro-critical care is the branch of medicine that deals with critical illness related to brain, spinal cord, and neuromuscular system [1]. It is often a sudden and catastrophic event for the family and the patient himself. With the ever-increasing sedentary lifestyle, use of recreational drugs, and dependence of human beings on technology, the incidence of neurological disorders requiring critical care has been on the rise for the last three decades [2, 3] The death rate in ICU is 20–35%. Public opinion surveys in the United States report that a majority of people would prefer to die at home. This might hold true even in India, but the rate of ICU use in the last month of life has increased, with 29.2% of decedents experiencing an ICU in the last months of life [4]. Teno et al. confirmed that persons aged 65 years and older in critical care in the last month of life have increased [5]. In these groups of patients, palliative care can be addressed to improve the quality of death. He found that in these group of patients either has multiorgan failure not responding to any treatment or patient are on life support which are not proportionate to prognosis. Continuation of this support will increase the burden on the family of the patient as the demise of the patient is imminent. Palliative care consultation has been reported to be requested in less than a quarter of patients [6].

Palliative care is a science that involves both the patient and patient family. The intent of palliative care is to optimize the quality of life where there is no definitive cure. This can be done by anticipation, preventative measures, and some therapeutic modalities to address the symptomatology of the patient. Thus, palliative care revolves around the alleviation of symptoms or symptom relief or any specific reversible aspects within that non-curable disease that the patient may have. Another important component of palliative care is ongoing good and careful communication with family members with the intent to set the goals of care encompassing the patient preferences and the values that will govern the care [7]. EOL is one of the components in this science of palliative care. It is for patients approaching death.

Recently, the World Health Assembly has suggested that palliative care is "an ethical responsibility of health systems" [8].

S. K. Gurav (✉) · A. Bang
Neurotrauma Unit, Ruby Hall Clinic, Pune, Maharashtra, India
e-mail: adityabang@cloud.com

H. Prabhakar et al. (eds.), *Principles and Practice of Neurocritical Care*,
https://doi.org/10.1007/978-981-99-8059-8_43

43.2 Palliative Care in Neuro-critical Care: Is There a Need?

Neuro-critical care deals with patients suffering from severe traumatic brain injury, ruptured aneurysms, malignant ischemic infarcts, intracerebral hemorrhage, and conditions that affect the CNS and neuromuscular systems. These patients are subjected to unclear prognostication, and their inability to participate in shared decision places considerable strain on the family members. Pottash et al. in their study on early (within 4 days of admission) vs late palliative care consultations (after 4 days of admission) for patients admitted in neuro-intensive care unit with devastating brain injuries showed that early palliative care consultations were associated with decreased length of stay in the hospital without any effect on the mortality rates [9]. Study revealed that an early palliative care consultation leads to early documentation of goals of care, and concretely, decision-making was easier, leading to reduced length of stay. Pottash et al. in their study put forth the importance and need of incorporating palliative care in patients getting admitted to neuro-intensive care units secondary to devastating brain injury.

In medical terms, neuro-critical illnesses are at the forefront of increasing disability-adjusted life years (DALY) all over the world [1]. Mortality and functional independence rates of adult patients suffering from the neurological disorders that require critical care are high (see Table 43.1).

43.2.1 Issues of Palliative Care in Neuro-intensive Care

Palliative care needs of neuro-ICU patients are considered different from patients in other ICUs [10, 11]. Prognostic uncertainty remains one of the most challenging issues in neuro-ICU. The most common reason for consultation of palliative care services was to discuss goals of care and treatment options with emphasis on prognosis. Issues related to symptom management appeared less common in neuro-ICU. The reason behind this was the neurologic catastrophe that led to loss of neurologic function rather than discomfort and pain.

43.2.2 Unique Issues for Palliative Care in Neuro-intensive Care Unit: [6] See Table 43.2

1. Devastated Condition/Catastrophic Presentation: Onset of neuro-critical illness is usually abrupt. Neuro-patients go from life to near death in seconds, which is specifically different from other speciality intensive care units. Patients may lose decision-making capacity without warning. The progress in neuro-critical care is slow and takes several months, leaving the patient in a severely disabled state [1].
2. Substantial Uncertainty: Despite substantial research into prognostic models in various neurological diseases, prognostic uncertainty remains

Table 43.1 Mortality and functional independence rates of adult patients suffering from neurological disorders

Condition	Incidence in the USA (annual)	Mortality rates (%) In hospital	Mortality rates (%) 30 days	Functional independence at 3 and 12 months
Traumatic brain injury	2,500,000	7.5%	21%	25–32%
Ischemic stroke	795,000	4.3–70%	16–23%	50%
Anoxic brain injury	424,000 out-of-hospital cardiac arrests	52–90%	25–40%	48–55%
Status epilepticus	200,000	14–50%	19–65%	42%
Intracerebral hemorrhage	63,000	30%	34–50%	12–39%
Subarachnoid hemorrhage	25,000	20–26%	45%	16–55%

Table 43.2 Characteristics of neuro-patients that changes the palliative care needs in neuro-critical care unit

Catastrophic presentation	Acutely neurologically devastation (go from life to near death in seconds)
Communication	Task to assess and manage without the ability to communicate Loss of sound mental health Patients lose the ability to decision-making without warning
Prognosis	Prognosis uncertain/complex
Quality of life	Severe disability that is incompatible

the most challenging issue in neuro-ICU states. The prognosis is more complex. Decision-making in neurology patients is further complicated by the unpredictable and extended course of many forms of neuro-critical illness.

3. Communication Difficulty: The clinician and family members have the challenge to assess and manage the needs without the ability to communicate.
4. Quality of Life: Brain injury has more profound effect on patients' quality of life. These patients are faced with severe disability, which is incompatible .

43.3 WHO Should Be Offered Palliative Care in Neuro-intensive Care

Patient needs to be screened by the prognostic scale for specific neurological disease along with other multiorgan dysfunctions, which are not responding to any treatment (see Fig. 43.1). This will help us to define futility in patient. The futility can be physiological [physiologically derange parameters/conditions that are not going to improve in spite of any therapeutic measures], quantitative [tremendous utilization of resources are not going to change the prognosis], qualitative [patient bed bound with neurological insult such as stroke will further compromise the quality of life], and lethal [no reversibility of disease like advanced cancer (space-occupying lesions) with metastasis]. Despite optimizing other physiological parameters, brain condition is not going to improve or the patient has chronic progressive degenerative neurological disease (Parkinson's disease, dementia, motor neuron disease, and metastatic cancer).

Neurological injury to a patient brings about a lot of anxiety and distress to both patient and their family members. Hence, the mere introduc-

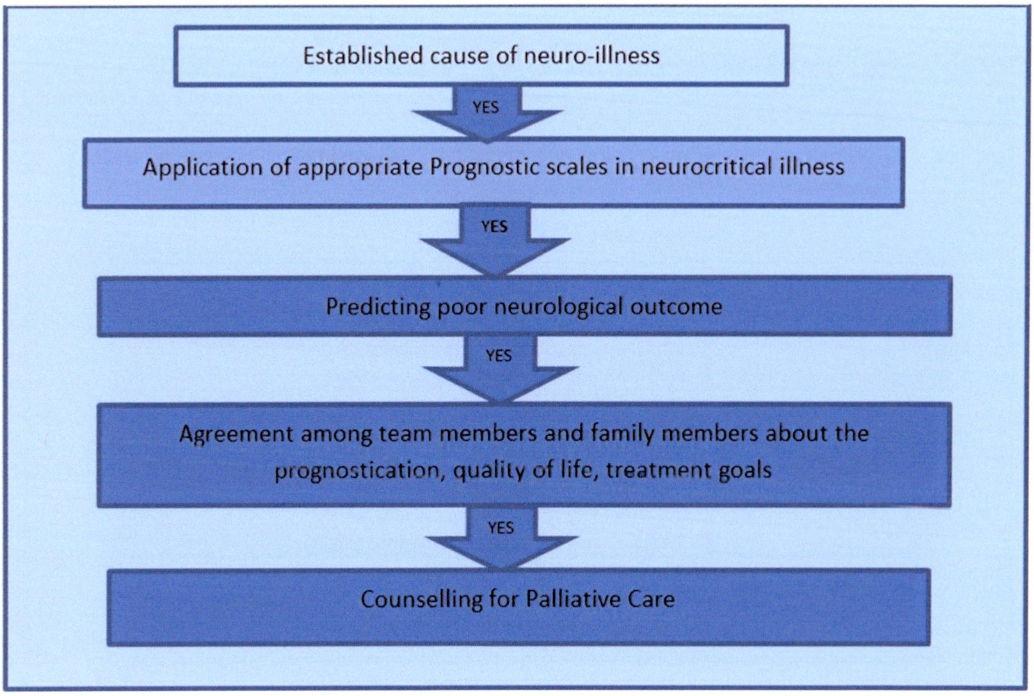

Fig. 43.1 Palliative care screening tools: predicting poor neurological outcome

tion of palliative care to a patient's care plan suffering from a neurological insult can bring about a lot of anxiety, depression, later posttraumatic stress disorder, and questions from the family members [1, 12]. Thus, it becomes imperative to know which kind of neurological injuries is associated with decreased and worse functional outcomes, so that an early attempt is made to introduce the concept of palliative care to the family members followed by incorporation of the same into the care plan of the respective patient. Injuries associated with poor functional outcomes [1, 13], which when encountered in neurocritical care should be considered for palliative care, are depicted in Table 43.3.

43.3.1 Advanced Directive [14, 15]

For the patients who are on advanced life support, it will be difficult to enquire about his consent to be on advanced life support.

In neuro-critical care with end-stage disease, one needs to have good communication with family members. Intensivist and palliative care specialists need to discuss with relatives the advanced directive made by the patient about his will to be on advanced life support.

As explained previously, neuro-patients have acute devastating stage; thus, it is difficult to discuss with the patient himself.

43.4 Palliative Care Plan: How to Communicate?

Initiation of palliative care in the setting of an acute serious neurological insult can be more challenging as the family has no idea about the nature of the insult and poor functional outcomes associated with it. Hence, the dictum used to discuss palliative care in cases of terminally ill cancer patients cannot be used for patients suffering from an acute serious neurological insult. The issues addressed in the neuro-ICU focus on the prognosis for a patient's functional recovery, patient values for living a life with neurological limitations, and medical options for prolonging life that involve long-term care [16]. Thus, combining method of "BREAKING BAD NEWS," i.e., discussing prognostication of neuro-illness and quality of life along with "DISCUSSING INITIATION OF PALLIATIVE CARE," needs to be adopted. GRIEV_ING is a tool used to ensure successful information transfer and empathic communication with the family members opting for palliative care

Table 43.3 Injuries associated with poor functional outcomes where palliative care must be initiated

Neurological insult	Features predictive of poor prognosis	Time frame of outcome measurement
Hemispheric ischemic stroke*	1. Coma with loss of pontomesencephalic brainstem reflexes 2. Midline shift of the pineal gland >4 mm within 48 h of onset 3. Age > 60 years	14 days–6 months
Cerebellar ischemic stroke	Coma after decompressive neurosurgery	3 months
Lobar intracerebral hemorrhage	1. Coma with extensor posturing and absent pontomesencephalic brainstem reflexes 2. Coma with midline septum pellucidum shift >6 mm within 48 h of onset	1–15 months
Deep basal ganglion intracerebral hemorrhage	1. Coma with hydrocephalus and bleed volume > 60 mL	1–3 months
Pontine hemorrhage	1. Coma with hyperthermia and tachycardia 2. Coma with hemorrhage extension into the midbrain or thalamus and acute hydrocephalus	3–12 months
Cerebellar hemorrhage	1. Absent oculocephalic reflexes with hydrocephalus 2. Absent corneal reflexes	3 months
Aneurysmal subarachnoid hemorrhage	1. Persistent deep coma or Hunt Hess grade 5 after attempts to lower ICP	12 months

[17]. Following are the steps to be followed while counseling relatives/patient for palliative care.

Step 1: **GATHER**: Assemble the family in a calm, closed, and considerate space. The counseling room should have bright light and adequate comfortable sitting arrangement (chairs/sofa). Try to gather as many family members possible so as to mitigate the risk of explaining the situation again and again.

Step 2: **RESOURCES**: If need be asked for additional help such as social workers, healthcare professional from speciality associated with the patients' care, an interpreter in case of a language barrier, or foreign national hospital representative.

Step 3: IDENTIFY: Upon entering the room with the family:

(a) Identify yourself
(b) Identify other members sitting along with you
(c) Ask how are family members related to the patient
(d) Identify the family's state of knowledge regarding the patient's clinical condition

Step 4: **EDUCATE**: In a concise manner, explain to the family the events that have transpired since the time the patient entered the hospital premises and the current clinical condition. Inform them about the severity of the injury.

Step 5: **VERIFY**: Confirm that relatives have understood the clinical condition and the severity of the illness by asking them about the same in a polite and empathetic manner, if possible in their own language. If needed, go back to the previous step and re-educate the family members.

Step 6: **SILENCE OR SPACE**: Stop talking. Allow the news to settle and give them time to process the information.

Step 7: **ENQUIRE**: After a brief interval, ask relatives if they have any questions. Note them down and answer them during the next step of discussing the prognosis and need for incorporating palliative care into the care plan of the patient.

Step 8: **DISCUSS PROGNOSIS AND NEED FOR PALLIATIVE CARE**: Discuss the patient's chance of recovery and the possible functional outcome post-injury while answering the queries asked by the patient's family during the INQUIRE phase of the discussion. Introduce the patient's family toward the need for incorporating palliative care in patients' care plan.

Step 9: **PATIENT AND FAMILY VALUES**: This involves anecdotes and stories about the patient and family and eliciting family member descriptions of who this patient was as a person prior to their injury.

Step 10: **UNDERSTANDING MEDICAL OPTIONS:** This involves the families' understanding of the patient's illness, available medical treatments, and the consequences of each treatment option.

Step 11: **IDENTIFYING CONFLICT**: It involves naming discord between the primary team and family and eliciting detailed views of families and providers in these situations, occasionally between the primary team and consulting teams.

43.5 Treatment Domains of Palliative Care in Neuro-ICU (See Fig. 43.2)

Palliative care prioritizes alleviating suffering and improving quality of life. The palliative care plan also focuses on prolonging life but with comfortness. Palliative care continues after curative options are no longer there. Thus, both survivors and dying patients are included. Palliative care skills are now been included in critical care competency programme [18].

Palliative care is patient and family-centered care that aims to optimize quality of life by addressing the physical, emotional, intellectual, and spiritual needs of the patient and family. Utilization of palliative care in the neuro-intensive care unit is less explored [19]. Palliative care is appropriate in the context of any serious illness, regardless of stage or prognosis. Palliative

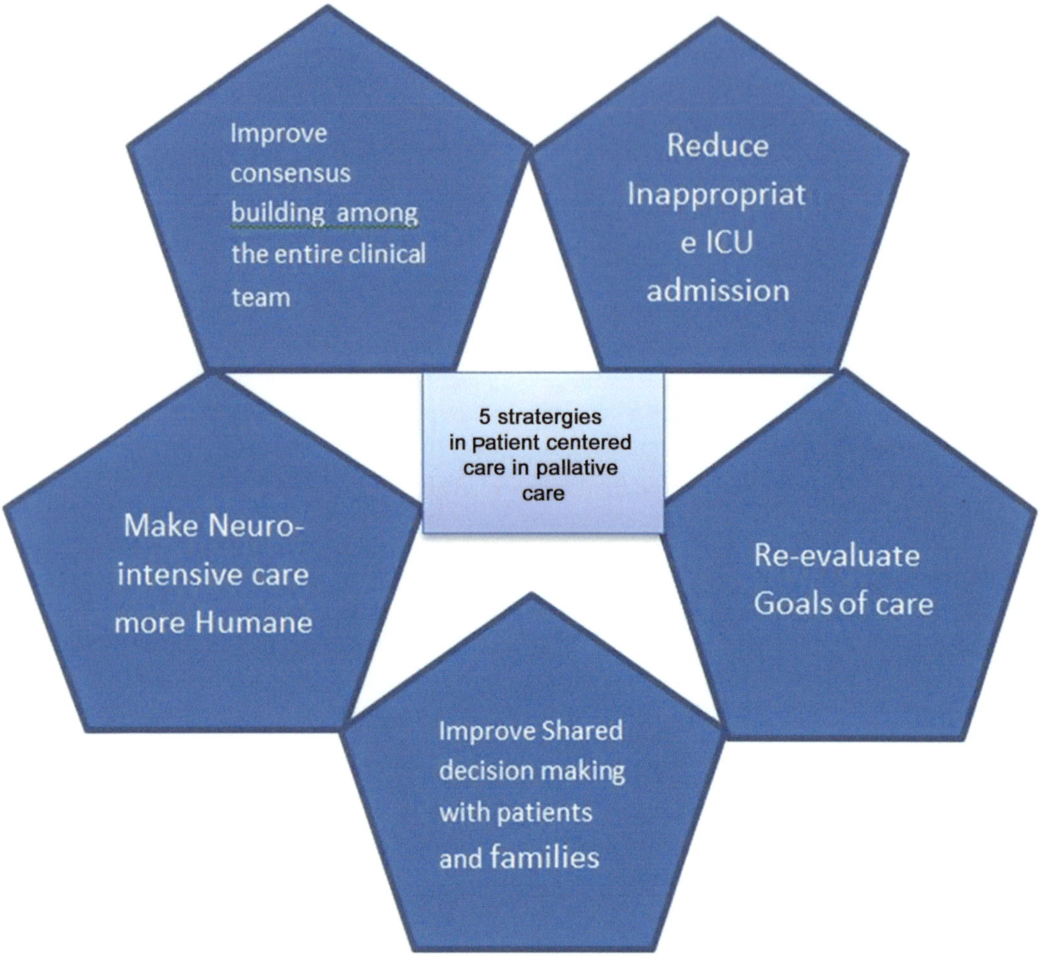

Fig. 43.2 Domains of palliative care

care is an interprofessional specialty, but also an approach for all clinicians caring for seriously ill patients who are expected to provide excellent "generalist"-level palliative care.

1. **Symptom Alleviation and Prevention of Discomfort and Delirium**

   Physical, psychological, and spiritual comfortness should be considered for patient opting for palliative care. Good pharmacological help can be taken to achieve comfortness. This can be achieved by:

   (a) Good pain control
   (b) Ensure adequate sleep and circadian rhythm
   (c) Delirium prevention
   (d) Liberal visit policy for family involvement
   (e) Environment modulation

   Periodic assessment should be part of daily monitoring and documentation of pain control.

2. Good Careful on Going Communication [20]

This is crucial intervention to build trust between family/patient and the healthcare team. Communication needs to be simple, clear, timely, and concise. A protocol must be developed for allotting dedicated time for communication. Staff need to trained specifically for communication with palliative care patient/family. Tools for alternative means of communication should be arranged in case requirement arises.

Daily discussion about patient's update needs to be carried out. Healthcare team needs to tackle the queries raised by the family members. Documentation of discussed issues need to be done to fulfill ethical obligations of autonomy, beneficence, and nonmaleficence. Opportunity for the participation of relatives in patient care should be discussed.

3. Psychological Support

   Detect and support the emotional and psychological needs of the families. Ensure availability of psychological support for patient and family members. We need to take care of comfort issues like overnight stay of relatives. Healthcare team needs to pick up postintensive care syndrome signs [21].

4. Spiritual Needs

   As curative pathway doors are closed, relatives might opt for spiritual options. Healthcare team needs to adjust as per the requirement and keep in mind the ethical/legal practice.

5. End-of-Life Care [22]

   As the neurological illness enters a phase of terminal illness, aggressive care may be harmful and expensive and may not go with patients/family members' wishes. Several interdisciplinary meetings with family need to be carried. This will help to build trust. Here, the healthcare team needs to open conversations about the transition to effective palliative care plan. Ethical decision-making involves the integration of four principles of bioethics: autonomy, beneficence, nonmaleficence, and justice.

   Conflicts are resolved through repeated meetings, conversations, and second opinions and referral to institutional end-of-life care committee.

43.6 Strategies to Help Ensure the Delivery of Appropriate and Optimal Patient-Centered Care for Patients at High Risk of Death or Severe Disability [23] (See Fig. 43.3)

1. **Reduce Inappropriate ICU Admissions**

   Palliative care specialist or intensivist need to interact with the patient and patient family members about the disease process and the various complications at various disease stages.

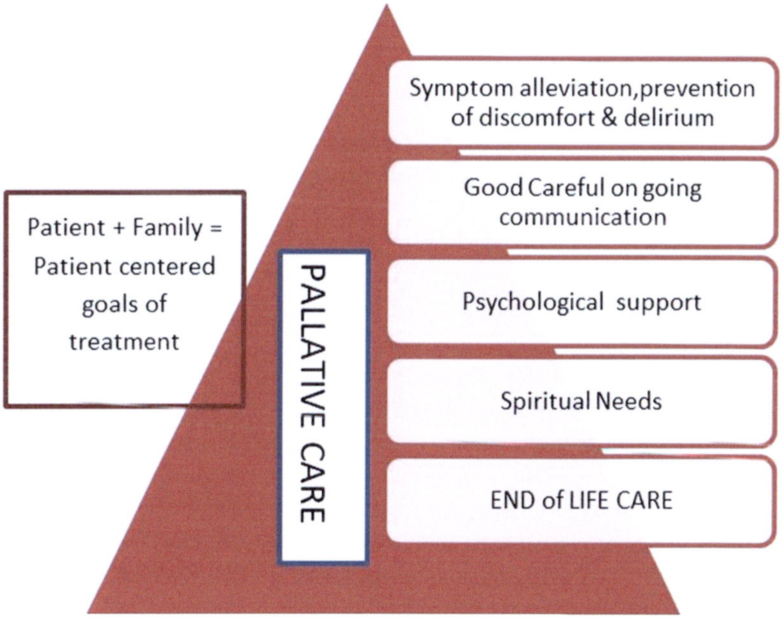

Fig. 43.3 Five strategies to help ensure the delivery of appropriate and optimal patient-centered care for patients at high risk of death or severe disability

Clinicians must discuss and help patients and families to understand in advance of acute serious illness or severe clinical deterioration. Further intensivist/clinician can guide them to decide in advance whether ICU admission is warranted in case if condition arises. The important challenges here is to ensure that advanced care planning realistically reflects ICU care scenarios or to simulate the acute deterioration scenario to the family members. For example, if bed-ridden stroke patient develops some infection, antibiotics can be delivered by home care personnel. The next challenge is the need for broad societal changes in expectations about end-of-life care.

2. **Reevaluate Goals of Care During the ICU Stay**

   Once the severity of disease is identified, the focus changes from cure to care. The treating doctor should regularly review and discuss with patients and families regarding appropriateness of continued therapy and the goals of therapy. Assessment should be done whether the patient is achieving milestones in treatment journey and patient is relieved of distressing symptoms and patients' comfortness is taken care of. With the tendency to accept the path of least resistance, these conversations are challenging and often ICU care is continued.

3. **Improve Shared Decision-Making with Patients and Families**

   Compassion and empathy are seen in the conversations with families of patients at the end-of-life care. Communication skills are an important step in palliative care science. With appropriate discussions with the families, the goals of treatment can be planned along. Healthcare team needs to give opportunity to relative for participation in patient care.

4. **Improve Consensus Building among the Entire Clinical Team**

   Palliative care team is a multidisciplinary team consisting of physician/intensivist/palliative care specialist/nurse/family members/oncologist. Different members of the clinical team may have different views on both prognosis and goals of care. The team members should communicate with each other and reach consensus about the prognosis of the illness of the patient and goal of treatment. To achieve this, the team should implement strategies that emphasize communication, respect for teamwork, recognizing burnout, and finally reaching consensus.

5. **Make Neuro-Intensive Care More Humane** [24]

   Instead of making stay in neuro-intensive care more stressful and painful, let us add a zone of comfortness to the patient and their family members stay in neuro-intensive care. The room should have proper natural light, if not at least should have bright light, curtains should have fresh color, blankets should be of different color than that of other patients, favorite food, small celebrations(birthday), and prevent noise and light pollution. Other areas of improvement are reduction in unnecessary testing and invasive monitoring. Open visiting hours allow friends and near and dear ones to spend quality time with patient. Least restrictive barriers for infection control is used in the patients' room. Using advance technologies, one can arrange Zoom meetings with distant friends. Allowing the patient to do his office work will keep him engage. Liberal visiting policies should be allowed for palliative care patient.

   The strategies to eliminate pain, incapacitation, and mental stress will require to implement safer and more effective analgesics and sedatives and the adoption of a more holistic agenda to make the ICU more humane.

43.6.1 Barriers of Palliative Care

Inpatient palliative care and hospice services have the advantage of significantly reducing the odds of rehospitalization, lowering the intensity of futile care provided, and improving the quality of death of terminally ill patients [25]. Despite these evidence-based advantages, the implementation of palliative care services is underutilized. The barriers recognized are categorized into three domains [26]

Barrier 1: Lack of awareness/education (related to patients, caregivers, and providers): The patient himself is unaware about his illness progress and thus unaware about palliative care services. Caregivers are emotionally stressed; thus, decision about this supportive care becomes difficult. The degree of difficulty increases if the patient is young and conscious. Provider himself might be uncertain about the importance of initiating a discussion of supportive services, more specifically palliative care.

Barrier 2: Lack of manpower/implementation (related to understaffed palliative care teams)

Barrier 3: Lack of policy (such as lack of guidelines for triggering referrals and consults): Multidisciplinary team might be in place, but lack of proper protocol in the institute or lack of awareness of trigger factors for the need of palliative care services leads to the non-usage of palliative care.

43.6.2 Precision Palliative Care Plan

As we are now practicing "precision medicine," let us also implement "precision palliative care." The primary devastating cause is different, and patient and family values and requirements are also different; thus, one size does not fit all [1]. Thus, palliative care should be individualized or planned as per patient and family requirements. Palliative care plan is depicted in Fig. 43.4.

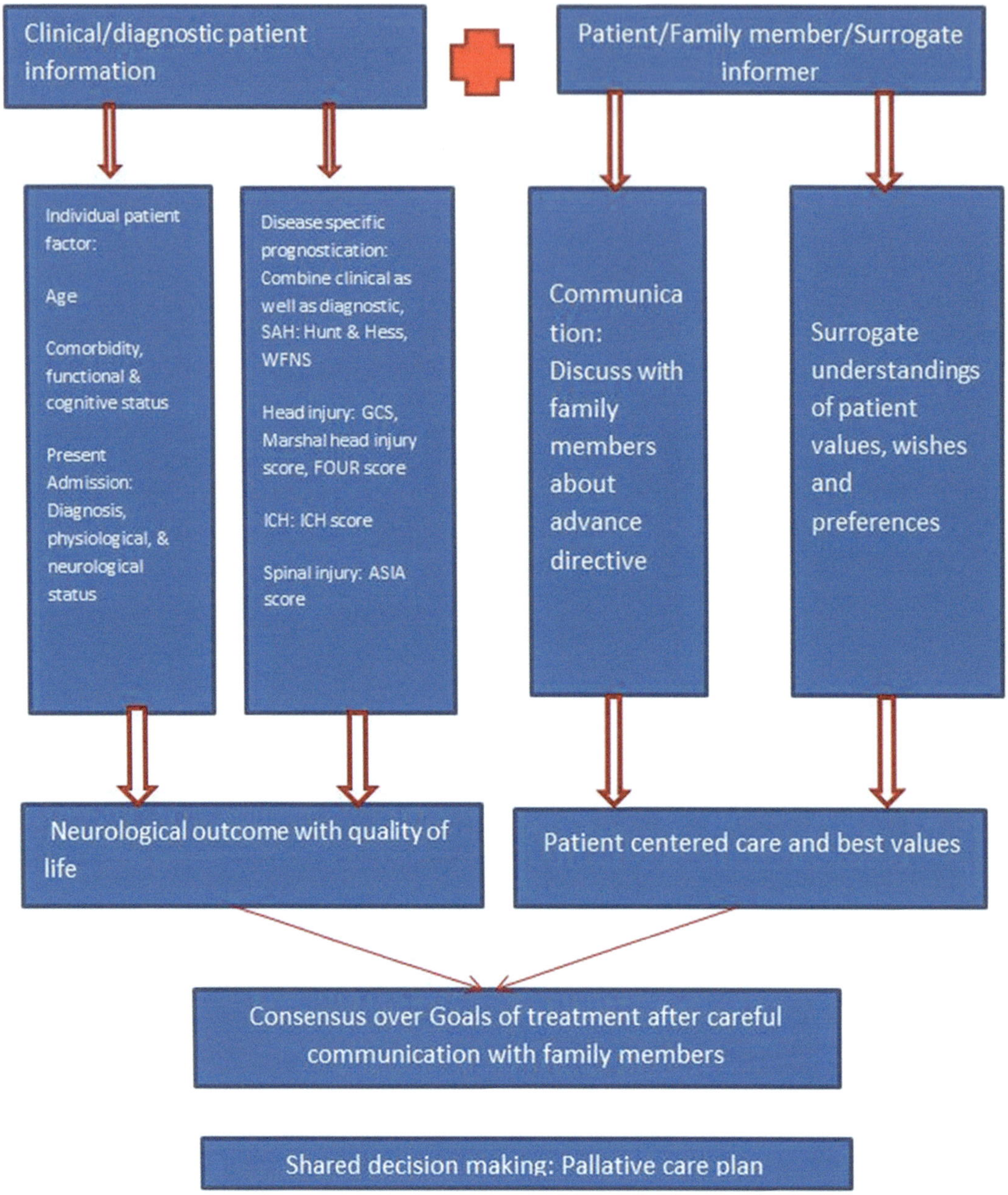

Fig. 43.4 Individualized palliative care protocol

43.7 Conclusion

The World Health Assembly has suggested that palliative care is "an ethical responsibility of health systems" and "integration of palliative care into public health care systems is essential for the achievement of the sustainable development goal on universal health coverage." Palliative care must respect principles of autonomy. Healthcare team needs to humanize critical care and thus improve the quality of palliative care, thus helping the patient to pass away from this world with a quality death. Let us hope that in the years to come palliative care finds its calling in the field of neuro-intensive care.

References

1. Frontera JA, Curtis JR, Nelson JE, Campbell M, Gabriel M, Hays RM, Mosenthal AC, Mulkerin C, Puntillo KA, Ray DE, Bassett R. Integrating palliative care into the care of neurocritically ill patients: a report from the IPAL-ICU (improving palliative care in the intensive care unit) project advisory board and the center to advance palliative care. Crit Care Med. 2015;43(9):1964.
2. Mehndiratta MM, Aggarwal V. Neurological disorders in India: past, present, and next steps. Lancet Glob Health. 2021;9(8):e1043–4.
3. Feigin VL, Vos T, Alahdab F, Amit AM, Bärnighausen TW, Beghi E, Beheshti M, Chavan PP, Criqui MH, Desai R, Dharmaratne SD. Burden of neurological disorders across the US from 1990-2017: a global burden of disease study. JAMA Neurol. 2021;78(2):165–76.
4. Gallup GH. Health, United States, 2010: with special feature on death and dying. National Center for Health Statistics. http://www.cdc.gov/nchs/data/hus/hus10.pdf.
5. Teno JM, Gozalo PL, Bynum JPW, Leland NE, Miller SC, Morden NE, et al. Change in end-of-life care for medicare beneficiaries site of death, place of care, and health care transitions in 2000, 2005, and 2009. JAMA. 2013;309(5):470–7.
6. Bar B, Creutzfeldt CJ, Rubin MA. Palliative care in the neuroICU: perceptions, practice patterns, and preferences of neurointensivists. Neurocrit Care. 2020;32(1):302.
7. McDonagh JR, Elliott TB, Engelberg RA, Treece PD, Shannon SE, Rubenfeld G, et al. Family satisfaction with family conference about end of life care in intensive care unit: increased speech is associated with increased satisfaction. Crit Care Med. 2004;32(7):1484–8.
8. World Health Organization. Implementing world health assembly resolution on palliative care. [online]. 2021. https://www.who.int/news/item/12-10-2021-Implementing-world-health-assembly-resolution-on-pallative-care. Accessed February 2023.
9. Pottash M, McCamey D, Groninger H, Aulisi EF, Chang JJ. Palliative care consultation and effect on length of stay in a tertiary-level neurological intensive care unit. Palliat Med Rep. 2020;1(1):161–5.
10. Morris M, Mroz EL, Popescu C, Baron-Lee J, Busl KM. Am J Hosp Palliat Med. 2021;38(11):1342–7.
11. Creutzfeldt CJ, Engelberg RA, Healey L, et al. Palliative care needs in the neuro-ICU. Crit Care Med. 2015;43:1677–84.
12. Azoulay E, Pochard F. Communication with family members of patients dying in intensive care unit. Curr Opin Crit Care. 2003;9(6):545–50.
13. Wijdicks EF, Rabinstein AA. Absolutely no hope? Some ambiguity of futility of care in devastating acute stroke. Crit Care Med. 2004;32(11):2332–42. [PubMed: 15640651].
14. del V Pérez M, Macchi J, Agranatti AF. Advance directives in the context of end-of-life palliative care. Curr Opin Support Palliat Care. 2013;7(4):406–10.
15. Sedini C, Biotto M, Crespi Bel'skij LM, Grandini REM, Cesar M. Advance care planning and advance directives: an overview of the main critical issues. Aging Clin Exp Res. 2022;34:325–30.
16. Tran LN, Back AL, Creutzfeldt CJ. Palliative care consultations in the neuro-ICU—a qualitative study. Neurocrit Care. 2016;25:266–72.
17. Hobgood C, Harward D, Newton K, Davis W. The educational intervention "GRIEV_ING" improves the death notification skills of residents. Acad Emerg Med. 2005;12(4):296–301.
18. European Society of Intensive Care Medicine. CoBaTrICE [online]. https://www.escim.org/education/cobatrice/. Accessed February 2023.
19. Forst DA. Palliative and supportive care in neuro-oncology. Continuum (Minneap Minn). 2020;26(6):1673–168.
20. Curtis JR, White DB. Practical guidance for evidence based ICU family conferences. Chest. 2008;134:835–43.
21. Jackson JC, Pandharipande PP, Girard TD, Brummel NE, Thompson JL, Hughes CG, et al. Depression post-traumatic stress disorder and functional disability in survivors of critical illness in the BRAIN-ICU study: a longitudinal cohort study. Lancet Respir Med. 2014;2(5):369–79.
22. Myatra SN, Salins N, Iyer S, Macaden SC, Divatia JV, Muckaden M, et al. End of life care policy: an integrated care plan for dying. Indian J Crit care Med. 2014;18:615–35.
23. Angus DC, Truo RD. Toward better ICU use at the end of life. JAMA. 2016;315(3):255–6.
24. Velasco Bueno JM, La Calle GH. Humanizing intensive care from theory to practice. Crit Care Nurs Clin North Am. 2020;32(2):135–47.
25. Brinkman-Stoppelenburg A, Witkamp FE, van Zuylen L, et al. Palliative care team consultation and quality of death and dying in a university hospital: a secondary analysis of a prospective study. PLoS One. 2018;13(8):e0201191.
26. Aldridge MD, Hasselaar J, Garralda E, et al. Education, implementation, and policy barriers to greater integration of palliative care: a literature review. Palliat Med. 2016;30(3):224–39.

44 Neurocritical Care Nursing

M. Anjali Devi

44.1 Introduction

The neuro-ICU cares for patients with all types of neurosurgical and neurological injuries, including stroke, brain haemorrhage, trauma and tumours. Comprehensive and continuous bedside care is focused on healing the patient in the ICU [1].

Nurses working in neuro-critical care units treat patients suffering from various neurological and neurosurgical disorders. Nurses give at most care and attention to neuro-critical care unit patients. Nurses working in ICUs should know how to treat neuro-patients and to operate and manage the monitors that are used in ICUs. Neuro-nurses need continuous monitoring and assessment while caring for neuro-critical care patients. Neuro-critical care depends on the whole healthcare team, especially neuro-nurses who work closely with dependent neuro-patients [2].

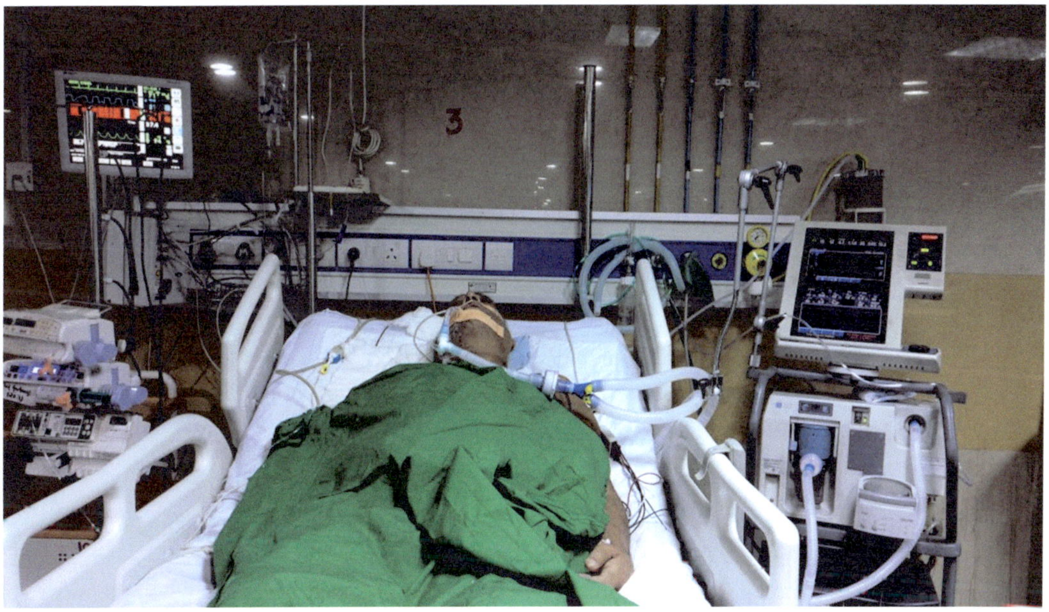

M. Anjali Devi (✉)
Neuro Sciences Centre, All India Institute of Medical Sciences, New Delhi, India

H. Prabhakar et al. (eds.), *Principles and Practice of Neurocritical Care*,
https://doi.org/10.1007/978-981-99-8059-8_44

44.2 Neuro-critical Care Nurse

A neuro-ICU nurse is a neuroscience nurse who works specifically in the intensive care unit (ICU). The responsibilities of a neuro-ICU nurse are to care for critically ill neurologically compromised patients. Due to the critical nature of these problems, the neuro-ICU nurse will experience a lot of death and dying as well. Neuro-patients are unique in that typically neuro-disease processes requiring intensive care monitoring typically happen very abruptly and suddenly, leaving patients and loved ones in a state of utter shock. Thus, the neuro-nurse must be clinically sound but also emotionally intelligent enough to support patients and family members actively experiencing trauma [3].

The essential skills for neuro-critical care nurses are communication, attitude and confidence, teamwork, critical thinking and creative problem-solving, professionalism, empathy, conflict resolution, adaptability, initiative and strong work ethic [2].

44.3 Features of Neuro-critical Care Nursing

- A focus on recognizing altered function in the brain and spinal cord and immediate intervention to prevent secondary injury improves outcomes and lowers hospitalization costs.
- A 24-bed state-of-the-art neurosurgical/neurological intensive care unit (ICU) directed by a neuro-intensivist along with neurosurgical and neurological attending and residents.
- An elite team of neuroscience nurses, respiratory technologists, EEG technologists and nurse managers provides minute-to-minute ICU care.
- Multimodality monitoring of the nervous system includes electroencephalography (EEG), evoked potentials (EPs), transcranial Doppler (TCD), intracranial pressure monitoring, single-photon emission computed tomography (SPECT) and positron-emission tomography (PET).
- Continuous EEG monitoring (cEEG) in the ICU detects silent seizures, which occur in 20% of comatose brain trauma patients and lead to worsening intracranial pressure [1].

44.4 Familiarity with Neuro-disease Processes and Diagnostics

Neuro-nursing is a pretty vast specialty; however, neuro-ICU nurse narrows it down quite a bit. There are many neuro-issues out there, but only a handful will land a patient in an intensive care unit. Below are some common patients of neuro-ICU nurses: stroke, head injury, brain tumours, hydrocephalus, spinal injuries, central nervous system infections, seizures and status epilepticus and more [3].

Neuro-critical care nurse needs to be familiar with common diagnostics. Those include CT, MRI, cerebral angiogram, transcranial Doppler, EEG and blood work [3].

44.5 Communication

Successful patient care in neuro-critical care units is based on effective communication between healthcare team members including neurologists, neurosurgeons, anaesthesiologists, nurses, physical therapists, occupational therapists, nutritionists and social workers. Constant communication between all team members is imperative to the recovery of the patients. Neuro-nurses play a pivotal role in communication between the neuro-critical care team [4].

The ability to communicate effectively is presumably the most important skill in a hospital. Neuro-nurses possess the ability to convey and receive information calmly and quickly, whether written or verbal, which can literally be a matter of life and death. Correctly documenting patient and treatment information is equally important, as these notes can be used as legal evidence if needed. Thorough handover to the next shift is important to avoid mistakes and to assure patient safety [4].

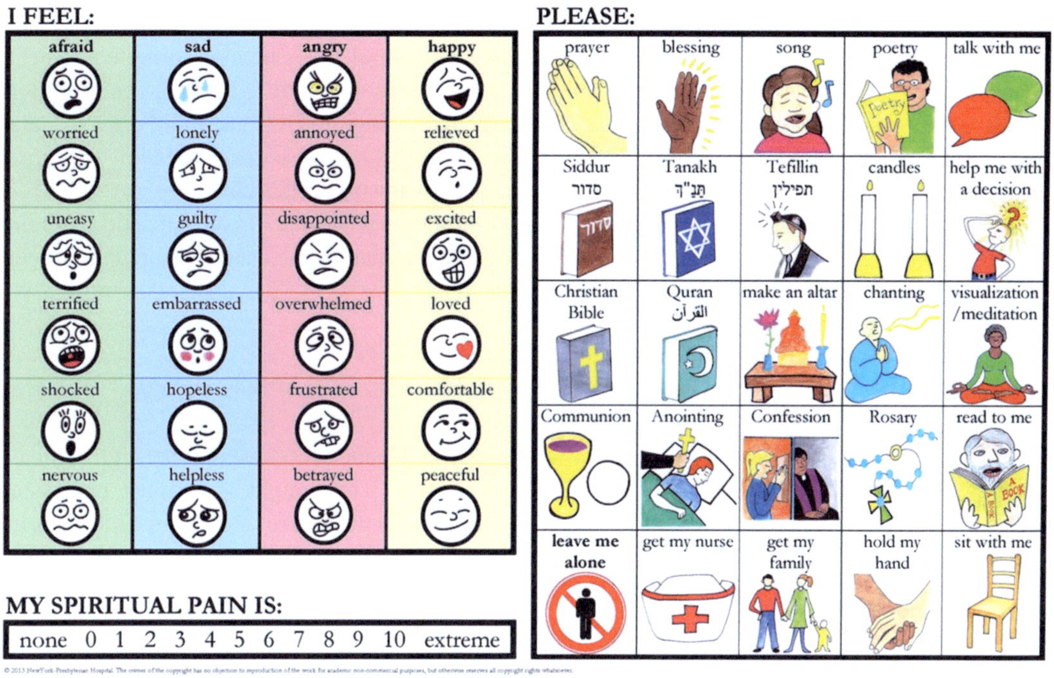

44.6 Teamwork, Confidence and Attitude

Neuro-nurses have enough self-confidence to alert the healthcare team when know about the patients' classic signs and symptoms of brain function deterioration. A quick neurological assessment and prompt actions are essential roles of neuro-nurses who have the courage and confidence to manage the neuro-critical care unit patients without fear of having doubts about patient assessment. Collaborate with other team members for better patient care [4].

In a neuro-critical care setting, confidence is not about thinking that you know everything, but about having faith in your abilities and training. Giving the impression of assuredness is important, especially in patient and/or family member's interactions. If neuro-nurse appears nervous when about to perform a basic procedure, the patient will be left feeling apprehensive. However, nurses portray themselves as calm and confident, and then, this will immediately put them at ease and make them more compliant [4].

A neuro-ICU is typically staffed by a diverse set of healthcare professionals. Constant communication between all team members is imperative to the recovery of the neuro-patients. For example, all staff members meet at least once a day to discuss their patients' progress and treatment plans [5].

44.7 Attention to Detail

It is vital to be aware of the finer details when working closely with drug doses and administrations. It can be easy to make a mistake, especially when nurses are on hectic shifts. Nurses are legally required to check serial numbers, batch numbers and expiry dates, and you need to be able to spot when something is amiss. Possessing attention to detail can also help you identify certain behavioural patterns or symptoms in patients that could potentially be a red flag. For example, if nurses overlook something important during an initial consultation, they could be scrutinised and even face legal action for professional negligence [4].

44.8 Decision-Making

Nurses too have the levels of responsibility, which means that in some instances, neuro-nurses may be expected to make certain calls based on their own opinion and analysis. On these occasions, it is critical to exercise solid decision-making skills, as the consequences could potentially have serious effects. The situation might also be time-sensitive, or it could be within a high-pressure environment, especially in critical care [4].

44.9 Focus and Dedication

Patients in the neurointensive care units (NICUs) are vulnerable due to their primary injury and in need of help with all their personal hygiene. When planning for nursing interventions, it is beneficial to be aware of the patient's intracranial adaptive capacity, i.e. intracranial compliance, to avoid the development of elevated ICP. All nursing interventions are performed with the aim of benefit for the patient, such as hygienic interventions, preventing pressure ulcers, surgery wound management and endotracheal suctioning when artificial ventilation is needed, among other things. However, nursing interventions might as well be stressful and can result in high ICP [4].

Therefore, it is the nurse's obligation to plan for the interventions so that a balance is achieved between the benefits for the patient's well-being and the risk of raised ICP, which might cause secondary insults. High ICP can be prevented by giving extra sedation before intervention and optimizing the patient's position with a raised head and stretched neck to avoid venous stasis. When ICP is >15 mmHg only, the most important interventions are to be performed, to minimize the probabilities of secondary insults.

Caring for patients with neurological illnesses requires close vigilance and the ability to closely monitor each patient's condition. Neuro-unit nursing responsibilities include continually assessing a patient's vital signs, his ability to speak and his reflexes and responses. They also rely on several types of monitoring equipment. Neuro-patients depend on brain oxygen monitoring, neuroimaging, EEG and monitoring of cerebral blood flow, intracranial pressure and brain tissue chemistry. This technology gives nurses a glimpse into what is going on in a patient's brain, even when that person cannot communicate with them [5].

44.10 Technical Proficiency

Neuro-ICU nurses frequently perform delicate procedures. They might also assist physicians with bedside procedures such as inserting a drain in the patient's skull to reduce pressure. Some neurointensive care units specialize in trauma in addition to neurological diseases [4].

Nurses working in trauma/neuro-ICU must understand not only how to treat and monitor neurological issues, but also how to evaluate patients with a devastating brain injury that could impact the rest of the body [5].

44.11 Compassion and Patience

Neurological disorders and brain injuries can affect everything from a person's ability to speak to his ability to walk and care for himself. In many cases, these patients cannot communicate with nurses and other caregivers. They may also suffer severe and devastating emotional and cognitive disabilities. The patient's family members must cope with the trauma of seeing their loved one incapacitated and not knowing if he will recover [5].

Neuro-ICU nurses must be sensitive to trauma, in educating the family members on the long-term implications of the patient's condition. Other important qualities of a neuro-ICU nurse include empathy, understanding and emotional intelligence. Neuro-unit nursing also requires the mental strength to work in an area of specialization that routinely deals with issues of death and dying [5].

44.12 Reporting/Handover

ICU patients are not always going to be stable and things change so incredibly quickly; sometimes, it is moment-to-moment… literally second-to-second. Occasionally, you are receiving a report in the midst of a soon-to-be code or urgent situation. Yes, shift change codes happen. You truly have to be ready to pivot any second. Verify orders and corresponding alarms. Check to make sure the bedside monitor has its alarms set to match the orders. During the report, check to make sure that the drips have enough volume in them for a few hours and are not going to run dry mid-med pass and also check when the tubing needs to be changed [4].

44.12.1 Assessment

Standardized neurologic assessments include the level of consciousness, spinal cord injury/function, sedation, pupillary response and dermatome level. Neurologically compromised patients will require very frequent neuro-assessments. This is because when something changes in the brain, it is evident in our bedside assessments, not vital sign changes. Neuro-nurses will focus more on their bedside neuro-checks to gauge if the patient is deteriorating. The signs are subtle [4].

As the oncoming nurse, you will be receiving all of this information and need to be aware of it throughout your shift. At the end of the day, you will provide it to the next shift. Once you obtain a report on all of your patients, get everything you need for an assessment and start to do an assessment from head to foot and specifically neurological assessment is vital. Analyse the patient's stability, drip titration, vital parameters, time-sensitive medication, arterial line levelled and zeroed, blood pressure, bedside monitor's accuracy, patient's tubing, etc. [4]

After completion of the assessment, check out the equipment, lines, drains, airway and monitoring and then give meds. Many ICU patients receive meds through a feeding tube, so it can take some additional time to crush these, mix them appropriately and flush them down, in addition to an IV push or IV piggyback medications. Of course, throughout this process, you have to watch their vitals and drips closely, to see if they are tolerating their medications. ICU patients can change in a matter of moments; therefore, it is the **ICU nurse's** responsibility to keep a vigilant eye on them. One must know their vital signs and assessment trends to know when they have deviated [4].

44.12.2 Codes

It is no surprise that codes happen more frequently in the neuro-ICU. Neuro-nurses quickly become acclimated to those adrenaline-filled scenarios when a patient starts to not look so hot that things are about to go down. Neuro-nurses become familiar with a code cart and the various roles within the code (chest compressions, meds, considerations, ACLS algorithms and the person running the code) and also know that some people will help with the code, while others have to continue to care for the rest of the unit who is not actively dying. These happen unexpectedly, so ICU nurses must always try to stay caught up on their tasks because you never know when you, or your co-worker, will be dealing with a coding patient.

ICU nurses have to be ready to receive any patients who may code out in nursing units or step-downs. (A patient who codes on a regular med Surg floor has to be emergently transferred to an ICU bed once they are ready to move.) Because of this, a bed in the ICU must be ready for this… and it is typically called "the code bed" because it is reserved for that unexpected patient.

44.12.3 Physicians Round

Physicians round once per day and many times the neuro-ICU physicians are housed within the unit for constantly changing needs. However, it is still up to the bedside nurse who is constantly monitoring the patient to update the physician as needs change. Interdisciplinary rounds occur daily and in many facilities. The attending physician, the nursing staff, therapy services (PT/OT/ST), chaplain, dietician, pharmacy, case management, social work and nursing leadership typically go through each patient and their needs. Physicians and their support staff round on their patients once a day. In addition to rounds, you update the physician whenever the patient declines or new needs arise.

44.12.4 Nursing Care

Provide continuous monitoring of respiratory functions, neurological functions, vital signs, fluid intake and output, bowel and bladder movements, nutritional status and skin integrity. Follow strict aseptic precautions while caring for the patients' lines. Carefully monitor the side effects of sedatives and narcotics. The nurse should give special focus to the patients who are under mechanical ventilation about monitoring the status of the patient, ventilator settings, prevention of complications and infections, oral hygiene, suctioning, position changes, eye care and ear care [3].

Prevent pressure ulcers by frequent position changes. Each neuro-nurse is responsible for his or her patient's entire care and communicates with other healthcare providers. All patients will have neurological problems hourly using the Glasgow Coma Scale. All critical care patients will have mouth care on every shift. The environment will be maintained in a safe condition by dry floors, proper placement of machineries and cleanliness freedom from any hazards [3].

In CCU/ICU at any time, life-threatening events may occur and require immediate response to save the life of the patients [3].

44.12.5 Documentation

As you can imagine, documentation for an ICU nurse is incredibly detailed. In addition to all that the neuro-nurse must document, every 15-min vitals (or even more frequently) and neurological assessments occur more often. Some patients change frequently, and these changes must be reflected in the documentation. Also, patients typically have many invasive lines and it is paramount to prevent infection. Therefore, meticulously document whatever is done to clean and prevent infection.

44.12.6 Furthering the Care Plan: Working Towards a Transfer

The ICU nurse's goal is transferring the patient out of the ICU. Progress them to a point in which they do not need constant monitoring. There is a lot to consider, all at once, in a very fast-paced, constantly changing environment. It is also important to get them out of the ICU as fast as possible because of something called ICU Delirium. Basically, when a patient is critically ill, in a different environment, receiving many different treatments, medications and interventions and hearing many different alarms, buzzes and sounds while being cared for by strangers, it is terrifying and people become delirious. People who seem totally fine neurologically can suffer from this, and it may impact individual's years later and result in long-term cognitive impairment. This is another reason why it is crucial to transfer patients out of the ICU as soon as it is medically appropriate.

44.12.7 Patient Flow

While transfer or discharges are a big focus for nurses, admissions are more of a focal point for the ICU nurse. An ICU admission is typically an unstable patient who needs the typical tasks completed like (good IV access, admission documentation and medication administration), a very solid baseline assessment, labs/diagnostics and so forth, but they also need to be stabilized FIRST! Stabilization is the key!

In addition to transfers when patients are ready, there is another piece to the puzzle. Sometimes, the ICU is full and there is no room to admit another patient. However, you get a call that there is a patient who needs to come who is incredibly unstable and must be in the ICU. Well, what happens is one patient must be transferred to another ICU with open beds or the nursing staff (or medical staff if it is a closed unit) must analyse which patient is most appropriate to transfer out to either step down or the floor to make room for this new patient. You may be in a situation in which you have to urgently give a report to another unit to get one patient out, only to get a much sicker patient back.

44.12.8 Dealing with Death

Patients die in all areas of the hospital, but it is a bit different for ICU nurses. It is more frequent than many other units, which can be ugly and traumatic. Patients die after long and brutal codes and are completely out of the blue. Dealing with trauma and death on a routine basis does take an emotional toll on an individual. Therefore, ICU nurses have capability to counsel the patient and their family members.

44.12.9 Finishing Up

After 12 h of assessing, monitoring, pivoting, stabilizing, tweaking, educating and documenting, it is time to give a report to the next shift. Documentation is important, but it is not more important than providing in-the-moment, time-sensitive care to the patient. Neuro-ICU work is challenging and exhausting, but when you are regularly dealing with urgent or emergent situations, it is hard to just turn that off after you clock out. Like a workout, it is helpful to have a post-work cool-down routine.

Neuro-nurses typically get off work earlier, and the sooner you can relax and calm down post-shift, the better you will sleep and the more mentally prepared you will be for your next shift.

44.13 Conclusion

Working as a neuro-ICU is extremely rewarding, but also extraordinarily challenging. Your normal day of work will be someone else's worst nightmare, and you are looked at to be the calm and confident nurse in control of the situation [6].

References

1. UCLA Health Neurotrauma and Neuro Critical Care. Introduction to the Neuro Intensive Care Unit. https://www.uclahealth.org/medical-services/neurosurgery/neurotrauma/neurocritical-care-program/neuro-icu-family-guide.
2. Bonsall L. Lippincott Nursing Centre. Ten essential skills for nurses. 2021. https://www.nursingcenter.com/ncblog/january-2021/essential-skills-for-nurse.
3. Kleber K. Neuro ICU nurse—what you need to know. Fresh RN. 2022. https://www.freshrn.com/neuro-icu-nurse-what-you-need-to-know/.
4. Perkins S. Characteristics of an effective nurse CHRON. 2022. https://work.chron.com/characteristics-effective-nurse-9429.html.
5. Phillpott S. 15 essential skills you need to become a nursecareer addict. https://www.careeraddict.com/nurse-skills.
6. Neurointensive care. Wikipedia, the free encyclopedia. https://en.wikipedia.org/wiki/Neurointensive_care.

Part VII

Case-Based Neurocritical Care

45 Traumatic Brain Injury and Neurocritical Care

Urvi Shukla and Savali Sultane

Case

A 23-year-old pillion rider without helmet fell off his bike when it hit the divider. He fell backwards with a laceration on occipital region of the head and bleeding from the wound. He had no other obvious injuries. He was brought to the ER by bystanders. On examination, there was ongoing bleeding from his occipital wound. He was found to be under the influence of alcohol and his GCS was 8/15. He was obtunded, responding to pain by flexion of hands and opening of eyes. His pupils were bilaterally equal and reacting. His wound was cleaned, bleeder identified and ligated. He was intubated with Cervical spine (C-spine) protection and a cervical collar was applied. A non-contrast CT(NCCT) scan of the brain and screening of spine were done which showed a large extradural hematoma over the right parietal region with 11 mm midline shift and screening of spine was normal. Relatives were anxious to know his prognosis and outcome.

U. Shukla (✉)
Symbiosis University Hospital and Research Center, Symbiosis International University, Pune, Maharashtra, India

S. Sultane
Symbiosis University Hospital and Research Center, Symbiosis International University, Pune, Maharashtra, India

Department of Neurology, Aditya Birla Memorial Hospital, Pune, India

45.1 Introduction

India has the highest incidence of head injuries in the world [1]. Majority of traumatic brain injuries(TBI) are linked to road traffic accidents (RTA). Every year, more than 1.5 lakh deaths are reported, with more than 5 lakh road accidents. It amounts to a death rate of 11.32 for every lakh population [2]. Road traffic accidents account for 44.5% total accidental deaths. Thirty one percent of the victims are in the age range of 30–45 years, 26% in the range of 18–30 years of age [3, 4]. The ratio of male: female is roughly 4:1, in contrast to high-income countries where male:female ratio is 1.4:1, and it is a more older population who fall victim to head injury. Most of the TBI in high-income countries are due to domestic falls in contrast to LMICs where injuries occur because of road traffic accidents [5]. A report published by NIMHANS say that unto 45% of deaths from road traffic accidents were among pedestrians and they seem to be increasing over the last decade [3]. They are more likely to be associated with lower Glasgow Coma score (GCS) on presentation and unfavorable long-term outcomes. Loss of economically productive lives impacts the national economy and also leaves behind families that struggle financially and psychologically.

Prevention of road traffic accidents and therefore head injuries will need road safety mechanisms and policies in place. Till then,

H. Prabhakar et al. (eds.), *Principles and Practice of Neurocritical Care*,
https://doi.org/10.1007/978-981-99-8059-8_45

Table 45.1 Criteria to classify severity of TBI [9]

Criteria	Mild	Moderate	Severe
Structural imaging	Normal	Normal/abnormal	Abnormal
Loss of consciousness	<30 min	30 min–24 h	> 24 h
Alteration in consciousness/mental state	Few seconds to 24 h	> 24 h	> 24 h
Post-traumatic amnesia	0–1 day	> 1 day to <7 days	> 7 days
GCS (best available score in 24 h)	13–15	9–12	3–8

evidence-based trauma care for victims of TBI will significantly impact early mortality and long-term outcomes. In this chapter, we look at ATLS principles [6] of managing a severe head injury and discuss evidence for the numerous interventions that follow.

45.2 Classification of TBI

- There are two broad types of TBI depending upon the mechanism of injury—Penetrating and Nonpenetrating type.
  - Penetrating TBI (open TBI) occurs when an object pierces the skull (e.g., a bullet, shrapnel, or a weapon like a hammer or a knife) and enters the brain tissue.

    Laceration of brain tissues primarily causes focal damage, intracranial hemorrhage, and secondary damage due to cerebral edema and ischemia. The type and severity of neurological damage are dependent on the size, speed, route, and strength of the external body penetrating the brain. Due to exposure of brain tissue to foreign body and the outside environment, the risk of infection is high in this form of TBI. The cognitive decline and residual deficit are related to the location of the injury and the amount of tissue lost [7].
  - Nonpenetrating TBI (closed head injury or blunt TBI) is caused by an external force strong enough to move the brain within the skull. Causes include falls, motor vehicle crashes, sports injuries, blast injury, or being struck by an object.

    The strong blunt and compression contact force disrupts normal functioning of the brain directly underneath the site of impact, thus causing immediate damage to brain vasculature and neuronal cells. Brain displacement due to vibrations generated during the impact can also lead to compression of brain tissues and reduction of cerebral blood flow. Both mechanisms can result in focal contusions or diffuse injury to other brain regions.
- TBI is also classified depending on clinical assessment, injury characteristics, and GCS as mild, moderate, and severe.
  - Mild TBI/concussion (GCS 13–15)—It comprises 70–80% of all cases. It occurs due to acceleration-deceleration or direct force to the brain that affects the structural integrity of neurons. Symptoms can be subtle and less often recognized. Majority of these individuals recover fully within the first year, but a few may develop persistent cognitive, emotional, behavioral, and physical impairments that may last up to 1 year [8].
  - Moderate to severe (Moderate GCS 9–12) (Severe GCS < 8)—These injuries more often require intensive medical care, and 40% of those hospitalized with nonfatal TBIs sustain long-term disability [9]. Table 45.1 describes the criteria of mild, moderate, and severe TBI.

45.3 Pathophysiology of TBI

45.3.1 Primary Traumatic Brain Damage

This type of TBI is the result of mechanical forces producing tissue deformation at the moment of injury. This occurs from direct damage to the blood vessels and neural tissue in a focal, multifocal, or a diffuse pattern of involvement. Focal injuries are hematomas, diffuse injuries are contusions, concussions, axonal or vascular injuries [10]. The injury initiates a complex cascade of events that results in complex cellular, inflammatory, neurochemical, and metabolic alterations [11]. There may be a second impact syndrome where an injured person gets another primary injury to the brain before he/she has recovered completely from the first episode. This usually happens in athletes following a concussion [10]. Contusional lesions can be a coup-contrecoup injury. The site of impact leads to coup, whereas contrecoup injuries happen on the contralateral side, usually the basi-frontal lobe and anterior temporal lobe due to contact with the bony prominences on base of the skull [11]. A subdural hematoma (collection of blood between dura and arachnoid mater) occurs due to bleeding from bridging veins, extradural hematoma (collection of blood between skull and dura mater) occurs due to rupture of middle meningeal artery. Traumatic subarachnoid hemorrhage occurs due to bleeding of small capillaries into the subarachnoid space. Diffuse lesions are seen more commonly in acceleration/deceleration or rotational injuries. Axonal injury results from any shearing, stretching, or twisting injuries to the neurons. These injuries are commonly seen at the junction of the gray and white matter. The axons are stretched, and the subsequent damage to the cytoskeleton may lead to axonal swelling, increased permeability, calcium influx, detachment, and axonal death. Diffuse vascular injury is almost always associated with diffuse axonal injury and there is widespread small arterial, venous, and capillary hemorrhages throughout the brain following trauma. Common sites are the frontal and temporal white matter and pontine tegmentum. They are seen with high-intensity dynamic force, especially rotation before impact.

45.3.2 Secondary Brain Damage

It occurs as a result of physiological response to the primary insult. It evolves over a period of hours to days and occurs due to chemical and vascular changes that will further brain destruction. It follows changes that occur in cerebral blood flow, both hypoperfusion and hyperperfusion, vascular dysautoregulation, cerebral metabolic changes, release of neuroexcitatory transmitters, and apoptotic cell death as a result [11]. As per the Monro-Kellie hypothesis, the cranium is a closed and nonexpansile bony cavity and the total intracranial volume (brain tissue, cerebrospinal fluid, and blood venous, and arterial) should always remain constant.

Any increase in one compartment will cause compensatory reduction in another to prevent intracranial hypertension. Cerebral perfusion pressure (CPP) = mean arterial pressure (MAP)–intracranial pressure (ICP). When the ICP increases, the CPP will drop and can lead to secondary cerebral ischemia and infarct [10]. This is an important consideration in the management of secondary brain damage and the entire focus of treatment lies in its prevention, early detection, and mitigation.

Cellular Metabolism and Cell Death

The first stage of cerebral injury after TBI is characterized by direct tissue damage and impaired regulation of cerebral blood flow (CBF) and metabolism. This "ischemia-like" pattern leads to accumulation of lactic acid due to anaerobic glycolysis, increased membrane permeability, and consecutive edema formation. Since the anaerobic metabolism is inadequate to maintain cellular energy states, the ATP-stores deplete and failure of energy-dependent membrane ion pumps occurs. The second stage of the pathophysiological cascade is characterized by terminal membrane depolarization along with excessive release of excitatory neurotransmitters (i.e., glutamate, aspartate), activation of *N*-methyl-d-aspartate, α-amino-3-hydroxy-5-methyl-4-isoxazole propionate, and voltage-dependent Ca^{2+}- and Na^{+}-channels. The consecutive Ca^{2+}- and Na^{+}-influx leads to self-digesting (catabolic) intracellular processes. Ca^{2+} activates lipid peroxidases, proteases, and phospholipases which in turn increase the intracellular concentration of free fatty acids and free radicals. Additionally, activation of caspases (ICE-like proteins), translocases, and endonucleases initiates progressive structural changes of biological membranes and the nucleosomal DNA (DNA fragmentation and inhibition of DNA repair). Together, these events lead to membrane degradation of vascular and cellular structures and ultimately necrotic or programmed cell death (apoptosis) (Fig. 45.1).

Cerebral Blood Flow

Acute head injury is associated with low cerebral blood flow states. There are multiple animal and human studies that have demonstrated this finding. Xenon-enhanced computed tomography (Xe-CT)of the brain done at various time intervals in severely head injured patients showed a global reduction in blood flow in the first 24–48 h following head injury [12–15]. Ultra early Xe-CT [15] performed in 30 comatose brain injured patients showed a 31.4% incidence of brain ischemia where cerebral blood flow was less than 18 mL/100 gm/min. CBF has a protective mechanism called autoregulation—whereby CBF remains constant despite changes in mean arterial pressure(MAP) and cerebral metabolism. The CBF remains constant across a MAP of 60–160 mmHg [12]. Changes in vascular tone in response to MAP is an important feature of autoregulation. When MAP increases, it increases vascular tone which reduces CBF and maintains ICP. This needs an intact blood–brain barrier (BBB). In TBI, when BBB is lost, autoregulation may be lost too and an increase in MAP can increase CBF leading to hyperemia [16] and vice versa. Most cerebral hypoperfusion was followed by hyperperfusion [16] after 24–48 h following

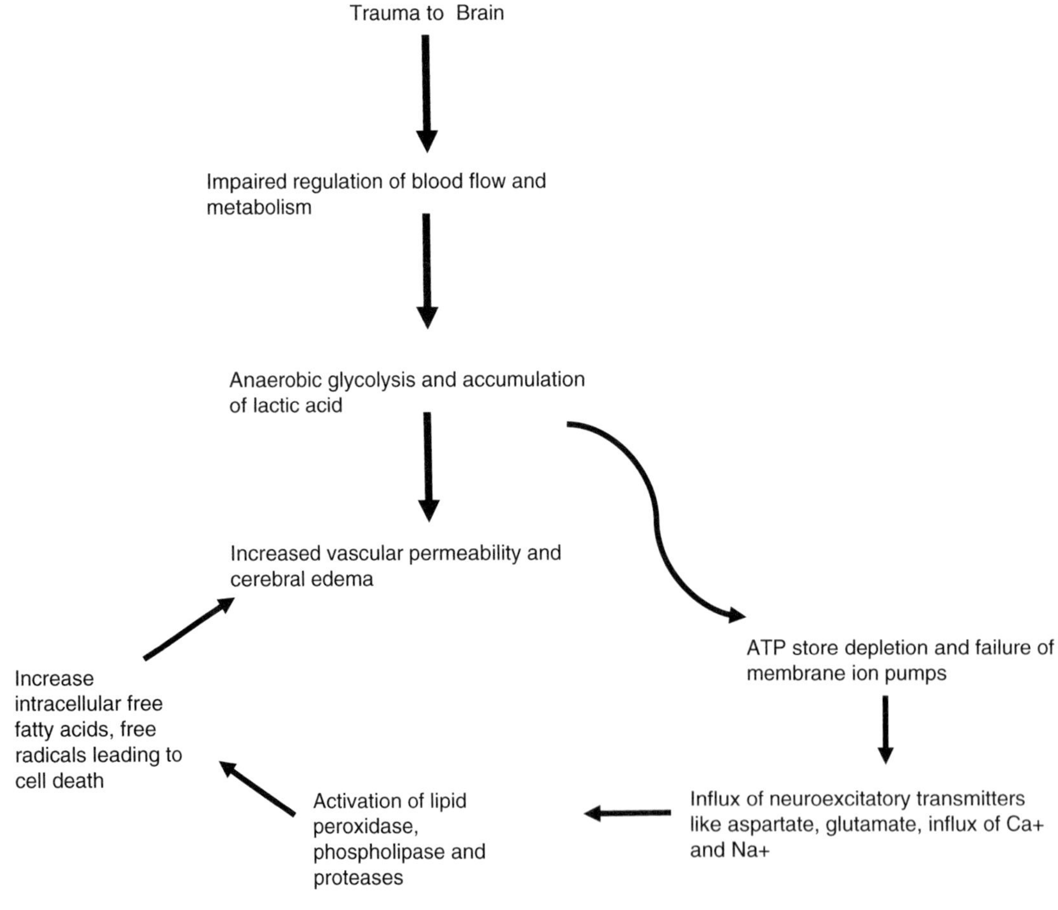

Fig. 45.1 Cascade of cellular metabolism and cell death (excerpt reused with permission from https://doi.org/10.1093/bja/aem131 [11])

brain trauma. In patients with diffuse TBI, the blood flow increased after the first 24 h leading to a hyperemic stage. Inoue et al. [15] studied CBF patterns in 20 head injured patients over 2–3 weeks post injury. They showed that patients whose CBF returned to normal within 2–3 weeks had a better outcome than those who had persistently abnormal/low CBF. This has been proved in other studies as well [13, 14]. It seems that coupling of blood flow to cerebral metabolism decides whether a patient develops ischemia or raised intracranial pressure (ICP). For instance, a patient with a low blood flow but normal or increased cerebral metabolism will experience ischemia and vice versa. Both situations will prove detrimental to neurological outcomes.

Cerebral Autoregulation and Carbon Dioxide (CO_2) Reactivity

Impaired autoregulation is a significant contributor to secondary brain damage. The temporal profile of autoregulation is unpredictable and variable. Currently, there are no validated and accurate methods of measuring autoregulatory changes leading to changes in cerebral blood flow [17]. Multiple methods are proposed to measure cerebral autoregulation, but their accuracy and clinical utility still remain unproven. Methods include spontaneous or induced changes in arterial blood pressure (ABP) as a surrogate for cerebral blood flow, transcranial Doppler (TCD)and its related indices, direct CBF measurements [15, 16], and cerebrovascular pressure reactivity (PRx). In a head injured patient with normal vascular reactivity, a rise in mean arterial blood pressure (MAP) causes cerebral vasoconstriction and vice versa. This response reduces ICP. In case of loss of autoregulation, rise in MAP would increase cerebral blood volume leading to a rise in ICP. This can be calculated as cerebrovascular pressure reactivity, i.e., the ability of the vessels to react to changes in intramural pressure [18]. PRx may be a helpful index in continuous monitoring of autoregulation. It is impaired during extremes of CPP [19]. CO_2 reactivity remains intact for the first 2–3 weeks after moderate to severe brain injuries in most patients [20]. Raised ICP, a low baseline CPP, hypotension, and hypoxia impair CO_2 reactivity in most patients. Impaired CO_2 reactivity significantly affected long-term outcomes.

Post-Traumatic Vasospasm

Post TBI vasospasm is known to be present in 45% patients with moderate—severe brain injury. TCD-related indices like velocities in middle cerebral artery or basilar artery, spasm index, Lindgaard ratio > 3 can ascertain presence of cerebral vasospasm. Incidence peaks at 2 days post injury and could continue till 14 days.

Risk factors for vasospasm include low baseline CPP, younger age, and low GCS score. Vasospasm occurs more commonly in anterior circulation and it was shown to resolve in 2.5 days [21, 22].

Cerebral Oxygenation

TBI induces a mismatch of oxygen delivery and consumption. This occurs due to various hemodynamic changes occurring at the time of injury and discussed above.

Increase in CPP, whether spontaneous or induced, is associated with increase in brain tissue oxygenation ($PbtO_2$) and reduced oxygen extraction fraction. The critically low level of $PbtO_2$ is 14 mmHg below which risk of cerebral ischemia increases. Manipulation of CPP can be considered as an effective strategy in preventing secondary hypoxic brain damage.

Edema

Cerebral edema after TBI increases intracranial volume and leads to raised ICP. This edema can be either vasogenic or cytotoxic. Vasogenic edema occurs with mechanical disruption or dysfunctional endothelial barrier. It causes net water and protein accumulation in extracellular space. Cytotoxic edema occurs due to dysfunctional ionic pumps and increase in net intracellular osmoles. Both types of edemas cause secondary ischemia due to raised ICP [23, 24], reduced CPP and CBF.

Inflammation and Cell Death

Mechanical injury to the brain causes release of inflammatory cytokines, prostaglandins, complement, and free radicals. These stimulate a cascade of events that lead to cell death (Fig. 45.1) [9], it also stimulates edema formation, reduced CPP, and secondary ischemia which results in a self-propagating vicious cycle.

45.4 Monitoring of Brain Trauma Patient

Monitoring a patient with moderate to severe head injury should include standard critical care monitoring plus specific for prevention or early diagnosis of secondary brain damage. It is clear from multiple studies that a simplistic approach of clinical neuromonitoring, CT scan, and ICP monitoring does not improve outcomes in TBI.

The concept of multimodal neuromonitoring was introduced in 1990 and integrated monitoring of cerebral blood flow, oxygenation, and metabolism evolved. Currently we are in the stage of multimodal monitoring and individualized neurophysiologic approach to the management of TBI.

45.4.1 Intracranial Pressure Monitoring

Measurement of ICP and MAP is used to derive CPP. It is integral to neurointensive care monitoring and helps guide therapy. Brain trauma foundation laid guidelines for the management of TBI recommend ICP monitoring in patients with risk of intracranial hypertension: GCS < 8, abnormal CT scan of the head (hematomas, contusions, effaced basal cisterns). In patients who have a normal initial CT scan, the following conditions indicate the need for ICP monitoring: age > 40 years, systolic blood pressure < 90 mmHg, bilateral or unilateral motor posturing [25].

There are two ways in which ICP can be measured, intraparenchymal microsensor and intraventricular catheter. Either method has its own advantages and further discussion is beyond the scope of this chapter. For more details on the type of ICP monitoring, refer here [26]. The critical threshold of ICP above which treatment should be initiated is debatable and treatment based on a singular threshold may not improve outcomes. Overall, ICP monitoring is based on evidence that untreated sustained intracranial hypertension is associated with poor outcome. Recent studies challenge the current rigid threshold of ICP > 20 mmHg for at least 15 min in 1 h as a trigger for treatment. However, extreme rises in ICP > 40 mmHg are associated with mortality [26]. A range of 20–25 mmHg is an acceptable trigger for treating intracranial hypertension used in conjunction with clinical and radiologic examination [27].

45.4.2 Brain Oxygen Tension ($PtiO_2$)

$PtiO_2$ is a measure of cerebral oxygenation. It is measured by intraparenchymal Clark-O_2 probe that may be inserted surgically in an uninjured area of the brain. It usually accompanies ICP monitoring, $PtiO_2$ < 15 mmHg indicates hypoxia. When used in severe TBI, it is strongly influenced by CPP [25]. Rise in CPP shows a rise in $PtiO_2$. In a study published by Marin-Caballos et al., CPP <60 mmHg was associated with hypoxia in half the samples tested. As CPP increased to 70 mmHg, this reduced to less than 10% [28]. Hypoxia can also occur in patients without any correlation to CPP. Factors like low arterial oxygen-carrying capacity, low hemoglobin levels, low fraction of inspired oxygen, impaired diffusion capacity, presence of arteriovenous shunt, and increased metabolic requirements may play a role. $PtiO_2$ reflects local oxygenation and is not synonymous with ischemia. There is no consensus on how to treat a low $PtiO_2$ and it is the severity, duration, and trend of $PtiO_2$ that determines outcomes rather than a single absolute value. Jugular venous oximetry and Near infra-red spectroscopy are alternative methods to measure oxygenation.

45.4.3 Transcranial Doppler (TCD)

It measures cerebral blood flow. Other methods like Kety-Schmidt and radioactive tracer techniques measure cerebral blood flow intermittently. Laser

Doppler flowmetry and thermal diffusion flowmetry are invasive continuous techniques for CBF measurement. Transcranial Doppler is a noninvasive, real-time method, conducted at the bedside and measures blood flow velocity (FV). It uses the Doppler principle to measure blood flow through the large cerebral vessels. It measures relative changes than actual blood flow. TCD is routinely used in intensive care and perioperatively. Middle cerebral artery FV > 120 cm/s–140 cm/s or a rise in FV > 50 cm/s above baseline is associated with established or evolving vasospasm. There is considerable interobserver variation and a very high incidence of false negatives. TCD values alone should not decide treatment decisions [29]. For detailed review on use of TCD, readers are referred elsewhere [30].

45.4.4 Cerebral Microdialysis (MD)

It monitors brain tissue biochemistry to give us information about cellular metabolism. The procedure consists of placing a mini electrode in the brain tissue that allows diffusion of molecules across a semipermeable dialysis membrane at its tip. It collects substances from the extracellular fluid in its microdialysate and allows an offline analysis [30]. Glucose, lactate, pyruvate, glycerol, and glutamate analyzers are now commercially available. It provides hourly sampling and levels of glucose, lactate, lactate-pyruvate ratio (LPR), and glutamate correlate with impending ischemia and reducing levels of $PtiO_2$ [31]. It is recommended that the catheter be placed as close to the at risk/vulnerable site as possible to allow for biochemical changes to be measured [32]. Most clinical experience of MD comes from monitoring of TBI and Subarachnoid hemorrhage patients [33]. A LPR more than 25 and glycerol levels more than 100 micromol/L are strongly associated with impending intracranial hypertension according to a recent study [34]. However, there are limitations to cerebral MD interpretation. Lactates may be a substrate and not necessarily indicate anaerobic metabolism [35], high glycerol levels may be present due to triglyceride breakdown systemically [33]. MD values, therefore, should be interpreted in correlation with clinical examination and outputs from other monitoring devices.

45.4.5 Continuous Electroencephalography (cEEG)

Up to 30% patients with acute brain injury develop nonconvulsive seizures (NCS) or nonconvulsive status epilepticus (NCSE). These can be detected only with cEEG, hence it is now a part of multimodal monitoring. Presence of seizures can affect cerebral metabolism and intracranial pressure [36]. cEEG can give real-time information about brain function, presence of new or worsening ischemia, seizures, increased intracranial pressure [37]. Its amelioration may change the outcomes of the patients. It is resource intensive, needs skilled personnel to interpret and its interpretation gets attenuated by anesthetic or sedative agents. EEG also helps to detect cortical spreading depolarizations(CSD). CSD are found in nearly half of patients with TBI and > 70% patients with subarachnoid hemorrhage [38]. They are characterized by sustained depolarizations of neurons and astrocytes, resulting in secondary injury. Detection of CSD requires placing the electrode strip directly on the brain surface, hence its use is limited. The physiological importance of detection of CSD is still unknown, but its control could be a therapeutic target [39]. Occurrence of CSD is associated with worse outcomes.

45.5 Principles of Management of Head Injured Patient

45.5.1 Management of Mild TBI (GCS 13–15)

Most of these patients will have sustained a concussion, which is a transient loss of neurological function. These patients may have loss of consciousness, amnesia, disorientation that may be difficult to elicit especially if under influence of drugs/alcohol. If the patient is talking, determine the history of the event, any past medical history, time of last meal, and mechanism of injury. The Canadian CT scan rules for mild TBI state that CT head should be done in all patients who have even one of the following features—loss of consciousness >5 min, amnesia >30 min, suspected or depressed fracture, penetrating TBI, any sign of basal skull fracture, vomiting > 2 episodes, anticoagulant use, age > 65 years, dangerous mechanism of injury, GCS <15 after 2 h [40].

45.5.2 Prehospital Care for Moderate to Severe Head Injury

Care of TBI patients should start at the site of injury. Rapid response from emergency medical teams, rapid resuscitation, prevention of secondary brain damage by preventing hypoxia and hypotension, and rapid referral to a neurosurgical center all play a vital role in the chain of survival and neurological outcome [41]. Prevention of hypoxia and hypotension is the single most important intervention as even a single episode of hypotension (systolic BP < 90 mmHg) is associated with doubling of mortality and poor outcomes. The Excellence in Prehospital Injury Care (EPIC) study [42] was started in 2014, with plans to enroll 25,000 patients. This study aims to test the hypothesis that implementation of prehospital TBI guidelines, as explained in Fig. 45.2, will reduce mortality and morbidity in moderate to severe head injured patients. These guidelines will focus on prevention and treatment of hypoxia, hypotension and hypocarbia.

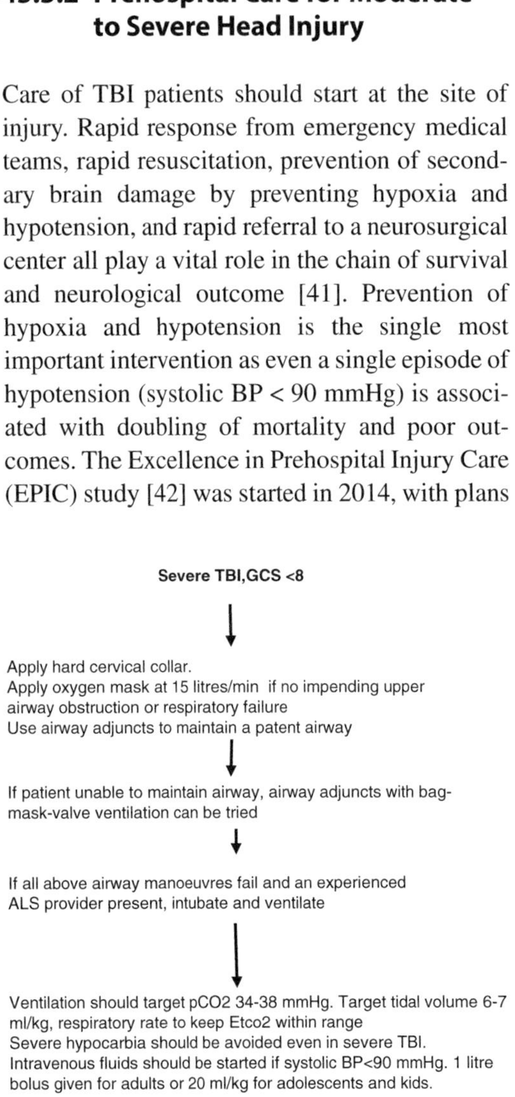

Fig. 45.2 Charts prehospital approach to a patient with severe TBI. (adapted from EPIC trial)

45.5.3 Hospital Care

Once a patient is in hospital, Glasgow coma scale (GCS) score, originally published by Teasdale and Jennett [43] is the most common tool for neurological clinical assessment along with pupillary reaction. There are limitations with GCS as it has poor interobserver variability, but other scores like simplified motor score or Full outline of Unresponsiveness score have not found widespread acceptance.

1. Airway and ventilatory therapies—Patients with severe TBI should have a definitive airway. However, intubation by inexperienced personnel at the site of injury has shown a fourfold increase in mortality. Basic airway maneuvers performed well in the prehospital setting may be significantly better [44, 45]. Patients with TBI have a 5–6% incidence of an unstable cervical spine (C-Spine) injury [27]. All attempts at intubation should have a manual in-line stabilization of the C-spine. Use of drug-assisted intubation allows for rapid control of airway and prevents rise in intracranial pressure. Drugs like propofol, thiopentone, etomidate, and ketamine can be used. They have different side effect profiles that may have to be considered depending on the clinical situation. Similarly use of succinylcholine or rocuronium for rapid sequence intubation is acceptable. Ventilation should target an arterial oxygen level (PaO_2) of 90 mmHg, lower PaO_2 may lead to hypoxia, and higher PaO_2 can cause hyperoxia-induced vasoconstriction. PEEP of 5–10cmH_2O is used to prevent atelectasis and does not hamper venous return [46]. $PaCO_2$ should be closely monitored and targeted to 34–38 mmHg. Hypocarbia ($PaCO_2$ < 25)

induces cerebral vasoconstriction even when instituted for a short duration.

2. Blood pressure and CPP—Use of vasopressors to treat hypotension and to augment CPP is common clinical practice. It helps to increase CPP to achieve the Brain Trauma Foundation (BTF) target of CPP between 50 and 70 mmHg [25]. However, there is no clear data on which vasopressor to use and evidence regarding the same is at best patchy. Noradrenaline has a more consistent effect on CPP, dopamine raises ICP [47]. Some studies have advocated use of phenylephrine as a single vasopressor agent. However, no significant difference in outcomes was found with either noradrenaline or phenylephrine [48]. The fourth edition of the BTF guidelines recommend: (a) Maintaining SBP at ≥100 mmHg for patients 50 to 69 years old or at ≥110 mmHg or above for patients 15 to 49 or over 70 years old to decrease mortality and improve outcomes (Level III); (b) The recommended target CPP value for survival and favorable outcomes is between 60 and 70 mmHg. Whether 60 or 70 mmHg is the minimum optimal CPP threshold is unclear and may depend upon the patient's autoregulatory status (Level IIB) (c) Avoiding aggressive attempts to maintain CPP above 70 mmHg with fluids and pressors may be considered because of risk of adult respiratory failure.
3. Management of intracranial hypertension—ICP monitoring is recommended by BTF and American College of Surgeons-Trauma Quality Improvement Program(ACS-TQIP) [49]. Raised ICP more than 20–25 mmHg is a trigger to treat. The Table 45.2 below explains the three tier approach to treat raised ICP.
4. Osmotherapy—Mannitol and hypertonic saline (HTS) have been used to treat raised ICP but controversy remains as to which agent is better. Mannitol increases CBF via volume expansion, reduces blood viscosity, and induces osmotic diuresis. Hypertonic saline also increases blood volume and offers better migration of water across the blood–brain barrier. In a study by Cottenceau, hypertonic saline and mannitol were equally effective in reducing ICP but HTS effect lasted longer and was significantly stronger [50].
5. Anticonvulsant therapy—Current BTS guidelines recommend the use of phenytoin (Level IIA) to prevent early post-traumatic seizures within 7 days. It does not provide any recommendation for use of levetiracetam. Clinical trials comparing levetiracetam and phenytoin have showed no significant difference in prevention of early post-traumatic seizures [51].
6. Temperature management—BTS guidelines say that early (within 2.5 h), short-term (up to 48 h) prophylactic hypothermia is not recommended to improve outcomes (Level IIB). Clinically, even mild hypothermia is associated with poor neurological outcomes and longer ICU stays. It increases inflammation and edema in injured brain tissue [52]. A Eurotherm trial was initiated to define the association of hypothermia and functional neurological outcomes. It was stopped prema-

Table 45.2 ACS-TQIP three tier approach to ICP treatment

Tier 1 GCS < 8, ICP > 22 mmHg
Intubate and ventilate Head end elevation to 30° Sedation and intermittent boluses of paralytic agents
$PaCO_2$ target 35–40 mmHg
External ventricular drain for intermittent CSF drainage Repeat neurological/radiological exam to assess progress of surgical mass lesion if any
Tier 2
Hyperosmolar therapy Mannitol 0.25–1 gm/kg OR hypertonic saline 3% 250 mL over 1/2 h Check serum sodium and osmolality frequently Maintain $PaCO_2$ 35–40 mmHg if there is no hypoxia Repeat CT and neurological exam as frequently as necessary
Tier 3
Decompressive Craniectomy if tier 1 and 2 (above) treatments fail
Barbiturate or Propofol coma if persistently raised ICP. Neuromuscular paralysis by continuous infusion
Hypothermia 34–36°C may be used as a rescue therapy if everything fails

turely as the treatment arm showed signs of harm [53].

7. Glycemic control—The surge of catecholamines post injury induces stress hyperglycemia. Anaerobic metabolism of glucose leading to accumulation of lactates and impaired autoregulation resulting from hyperglycemia all lead to poor outcomes.
8. Decompressive craniectomy—This is a surgical procedure where a large portion of the skull bone is removed to make space for increasing brain volume. Surgery for TBI patients is most commonly performed for extradural, subdural, intracranial hematomas that cause significant midline shift. Patients with a large hematoma who present to emergency comatose should be taken for surgery sooner rather than later. CT scan that shows evidence of high ICP like compression of basal cisterns, midline shift > 5 mm, effaced ventricles is an indication for surgical evacuation [54]. In patients who have a delayed progression of hematoma, surgery is indicated in order to reduce ICP and save lives. BTF recommends a large frontoparietotemporal craniectomy of 15 cm diameter rather than a smaller one (Level IIB) for reducing mortality and improving neurological outcomes [25]. A bifrontal craniectomy for diffuse injury (without mass lesion) is not recommended [55]. DECRA trial which enrolled 155 patients with severe and diffuse TBI found that early bifrontal craniectomy reduced ICP with minimal interventions and reduced length of stay in the ICU. However, the treatment arm had a higher risk for an unfavorable outcome. The RESCUE-ICP trial compared secondary craniectomy in 409 patients randomly assigned to the treatment arm. The craniectomy was associated with reduced mortality but a higher number of participants with poor neurological recovery [54].
9. Other considerations—Thromboprophylaxis, nutrition, prevention of bed sores are now part of standard critical care and severe TBI patients should be ensured the same. Nutrition should be started early or as soon as the patient is hemodynamically stable and rapidly progresses to full caloric intake usually within 7 days. Enteral feeding is still the preferred route. Postpyloric feeds may reduce the incidence of pneumonia. Thromboprophylaxis can be provided by compression stockings, sequential compression devices or both. Use of pharmacological agents may expand hematomas and fall as Level III evidence as per BTF guidelines [25]. There is uncertainty regarding the initiation, dose, drug, and duration of thromboprophylactic agents.

45.6 Outcomes

Patients with mild TBI (GCS—13–15)—Most recover over 1–2 weeks but a few may recover over many weeks. Approximately 40% patients develop persistent postconcussion syndrome—a patient experiences persistent headache, dizziness, irritability, difficulty to concentrate that lasts beyond 3 months [56].

These cases are managed symptomatically and might be considered for advanced imaging [57].

Patients with moderate TBI take a longer time to recover. Approximately 60% patients have good outcome, 25% will be left with moderate residual deficit, 0.9–8% will progress to death or persistent vegetative state, and remaining have a severe degree of disability [58, 59].

Patients with severe TBI have worse outcomes. Only 10% of patients have a positive outcome. About 65% of these patients do not survive and remaining are left with moderate to severe deficits or land in persistent vegetative states [60].

References

1. https://indianheadinjuryfoundation.org/traumatic-brain-injury/
2. Road Accidents in India 2018. Ministry of Road Transport and Highways, Government of India. http://morth.nic.in/showfile.asp?lid=835 .
3. Pruthi N, Ashok M, Kumar VS, Jhavar K, Sampath S, Devi BI. Magnitude of pedestrian head injuries & fatalities in Bangalore, South India: a retrospective study from an apex neurotrauma center. Indian J Med Res. 2012;136(6):1039–43.

4. National Crime Records Bureau Ministry of home affairs government of India, 2021. Accidental deaths and suicides in India 2021; pp. 7–322.
5. Massenburg BB, Veetil DK, Raykar NP, Agrawal A, Roy N, Gerdin M. A systematic review of quantitative research on traumatic brain injury in India. Neurol India. 2017;65:305–14.
6. Advanced Trauma Life Support. Student course Manual 10th edition. https://www.facs.org/quality-programs/trauma/education/advanced-trauma-life-support/
7. Ginsburg J, Huff JS. Closed head trauma. In: StatPearls. Treasure Island (FL): StatPearls Publishing; 2022;https://www.ncbi.nlm.nih.gov/books/NBK557861/.
8. Arciniegas DB, Anderson CA, Topkoff J, McAllister TW. Mild traumatic brain injury: a neuropsychiatric approach to diagnosis, evaluation, and treatment. Neuropsychiatr Dis Treat. 2005;1(4):311–27.
9. Brasure M, Lamberty GJ, Sayer NA, et al. Multidisciplinary Postacute rehabilitation for moderate to severe traumatic brain injury in adults. Rockville (MD): Agency for Healthcare Research and Quality (US); 2012. (comparative effectiveness reviews, no. 72.) executive summary. Executive Summary - Multidisciplinary Postacute Rehabilitation for Moderate to Severe Traumatic Brain Injury in Adults - NCBI Bookshelf
10. Georges A, Das JM. Traumatic brain injury. In: StatPearls. Treasure Island (FL): StatPearls Publishing; 2022;https://www.ncbi.nlm.nih.gov/books/NBK459300/.
11. Werner C, Engelhard K. Pathophysiology of traumatic brain injury, BJA. Br J Anaesth. 2007;99(1):4–9. https://doi.org/10.1093/bja/aem131.
12. Kinoshita K. Traumatic brain injury: pathophysiology for neurocritical care. J Intensive Care. 2016;4:29. https://doi.org/10.1186/s40560-016-0138-3.
13. Shaikh F, Waseem M. Head trauma. In: StatPearls. Treasure Island (FL): StatPearls Publishing; 2022.
14. Huffman JC, Brennan MM, Smith FA, Stern TA. Patients with neurologic conditions I. Seizure disorders (including nonepileptic seizures), cerebrovascular disease, and traumatic brain injury. In: Massachusetts General Hospital handbook of general hospital psychiatry; 2010. p. 237–53. https://doi.org/10.1016/b978-1-4377-1927-7.00019-4.
15. Inoue Y, Shiozaki T, Tasaki O, Hayakata T, Ikegawa H, Yoshiya K, Fujinaka T, Tanaka H, Shimazu T, Sugimoto H. Changes in cerebral blood flow from the acute to the chronic phase of severe head injury. J Neurotrauma. 2005;22(12):1411–8. https://doi.org/10.1089/neu.2005.22.1411.
16. Marion DW, Darby J, Yonas H. Acute regional cerebral blood flow changes caused by severe head injuries. J Neurosurg. 1991;74(3):407–14. https://doi.org/10.3171/jns.1991.74.3.0407.
17. Bouma GJ, Muizelaar JP, Choi SC, Newlon PG, Young HF. Cerebral circulation and metabolism after severe traumatic brain injury: the elusive role of ischemia. J Neurosurg. 1991;75(5):685–93. https://doi.org/10.3171/jns.1991.75.5.0685.
18. Kelly DF, Martin NA, Kordestani R, Counelis G, Hovda DA, Bergsneider M, McBride DQ, Shalmon E, Herman D, Becker DP. Cerebral blood flow as a predictor of outcome following traumatic brain injury. J Neurosurg. 1997;86(4):633–41. https://doi.org/10.3171/jns.1997.86.4.0633.
19. Steiner LA, Czosnyka M, Piechnik SK, Smielewski P, Chatfield D, Menon DK, Pickard JD. Continuous monitoring of cerebrovascular pressure reactivity allows determination of optimal cerebral perfusion pressure in patients with traumatic brain injury. Crit Care Med. 2002;30(4):733–8. https://doi.org/10.1097/00003246-200204000-00002.
20. Depreitere B, Citerio G, Smith M, Adelson PD, Aries MJ, Bleck TP, Bouzat P, Chesnut R, De Sloovere V, Diringer M, Dureanteau J, Ercole A, Hawryluk G, Hawthorne C, Helbok R, Klein SP, Neumann JO, Robba C, Steiner L, Stocchetti N, Taccone FS, Valadka A, Wolf S, Zeiler FA, Meyfroidt G. Cerebrovascular autoregulation monitoring in the Management of Adult Severe Traumatic Brain Injury: A Delphi consensus of clinicians. Neurocrit Care. 2021;34(3):731–8. https://doi.org/10.1007/s12028-020-01185-x.
21. Lee JH, Kelly DF, Oertel M, McArthur DL, Glenn TC, Vespa P, Boscardin WJ, Martin NA. Carbon dioxide reactivity, pressure autoregulation, and metabolic suppression reactivity after head injury: a transcranial Doppler study. J Neurosurg. 2001;95(2):222–32. https://doi.org/10.3171/jns.2001.95.2.0222.
22. Czosnyka M, Brady K, Reinhard M, Smielewski P, Steiner LA. Monitoring of cerebrovascular autoregulation: facts, myths, and missing links. Neurocrit Care. 2009;10(3):373–86. https://doi.org/10.1007/s12028-008-9175-7. Epub 2009 Jan 6
23. Oertel M, Boscardin WJ, Obrist WD, Glenn TC, McArthur DL, Gravori T, Lee JH, Martin NA. Posttraumatic vasospasm: the epidemiology, severity, and time course of an underestimated phenomenon: a prospective study performed in 299 patients. J Neurosurg. 2005;103(5):812–24. https://doi.org/10.3171/jns.2005.103.5.0812.
24. Johnston AJ, Steiner LA, Coles JP, Chatfield DA, Fryer TD, Smielewski P, Hutchinson PJ, O'Connell MT, Al-Rawi PG, Aigbirihio FI, Clark JC, Pickard JD, Gupta AK, Menon DK. Effect of cerebral perfusion pressure augmentation on regional oxygenation and metabolism after head injury. Crit Care Med. 2005;33(1):189–95; discussion 255–7. https://doi.org/10.1097/01.ccm.0000149837.09225.bd.
25. Brain Trauma Foundation, American Association of Neurological Surgeons, Congress of Neurological Surgeons, Joint Section on Neurotrauma and Critical Care, AANS/CNS, Bratton SL, Chestnut RM, Ghajar J, FF MCH, Harris OA, Hartl R, Manley GT, Nemecek A, Newell DW, Rosenthal G, Schouten J, Shutter L, Timmons SD, Ullman JS, Videtta W, Wilberger JE, Wright DW. Guidelines for the management of severe traumatic brain injury. VI. Indications for intracranial

pressure monitoring. J Neurotrauma. 2007;24(Suppl 1):S37–44. https://doi.org/10.1089/neu.2007.9990; Erratum in: J Neurotrauma. 2008 Mar;25(3):276-8. multiple author names added.
26. Unterberg AW, Stover J, Kress B, Kiening KL. Edema and brain trauma. Neuroscience. 2004;129(4):1021–9. https://doi.org/10.1016/j.neuroscience.2004.06.046.
27. Dash HH, Chavali S. Management of traumatic brain injury patients. Korean J Anesthesiol. 2018;71(1):12–21. https://doi.org/10.4097/kjae.2018.71.1.12.
28. Le Roux P. Intracranial pressure monitoring and management. In: Laskowitz D, Grant G, editors. Translational research in traumatic brain injury. Boca Raton (FL): CRC Press/Taylor and Francis Group; 2016. Chapter 15. https://www.ncbi.nlm.nih.gov/books/NBK326713/.
29. Kirkman MA, et al. Intracranial pressure monitoring, cerebral perfusion pressure estimation, and ICP/CPP-guided therapy: a standard of care or optional extra after brain injury? Br J Anaesth. 2014;112(1):35–46.
30. Marín-Caballos AJ, Murillo-Cabezas F, Cayuela-Domínguez A, Domínguez-Roldán JM, Rincón-Ferrari MD, Valencia-Anguita J, Flores-Cordero JM, Muñoz-Sánchez MA. Cerebral perfusion pressure and risk of brain hypoxia in severe head injury: a prospective observational study. Crit Care. 2005;9(6):R670–6. https://doi.org/10.1186/cc3822.
31. Kirkman MA, Smith M. Multimodal intracranial monitoring: implications for clinical practice. Anesthesiol Clin. 2012;30(2):269–87. https://doi.org/10.1016/j.anclin.2012.05.007.
32. Springborg JB, Frederiksen HJ, Eskesen V, Olsen NV. Trends in monitoring patients with aneurysmal subarachnoid haemorrhage. Br J Anaesth. 2005;94:259–70.
33. Kett-White R, Hutchinson PJ, Czosnyka M, et al. Effects of variation in cerebral haemodynamics during aneurysm surgery on brain tissue oxygen and metabolism. Acta Neurochir Suppl. 2002;81:327–9.
34. Bellander BM, Cantais E, Enblad P, et al. Consensus meeting on microdialysis in neurointensive care. Intensive Care Med. 2004;30:2166–9.
35. Hillered L, Vespa PM, Hovda DA. Translational neurochemical research in acute human brain injury: the current status and potential futur e for cerebral microdial- ysis. J Neurotrauma. 2005;22:3–41.
36. Belli A, Sen J, Petzold A, et al. Metabolic failure precedes intracranial pressure rises in traumatic brain injury: a microdialysis study. Acta Neurochir. 2008;150:461–9.
37. Friedman D, Claassen J, Hirsch LJ. Continuous electroencephalogram monitoring in the intensive care unit. Anesth Analg. 2009;109:506–23.
38. Gallagher CN, Carpenter KL, Grice P, et al. The human brain utilizes lactate via the tricarboxylic acid cycle: a 13C-labeled microdialysis and high-resolution nuclear magnetic resonance study. Brain. 2009;132:2839–49.
39. Dreier JP, Woitzik J, Fabricius M, et al. Delayed ischaemic neurological deficits after subarachnoid hemorrhage are associated with clusters of spreading depolarizations. Brain. 2006;129:3224–37.
40. Stiell IG, Wells GA, Vandemheen K, et al. The Canadian CT head rule for patients with minor head injury. Lancet. 2001;357(9266):1391–6.
41. Chesnut RM, Marshall LF, Klauber MR, Blunt BA, Baldwin N, Eisenberg HM, Jane JA, Marmarou A, Foulkes MA. The role of secondary brain injury in determining outcome from severe head injury. J Trauma. 1993;34(2):216–22. https://doi.org/10.1097/00005373-199302000-00006.
42. Spaite DW, Bobrow BJ, Stolz U, Sherrill D, Chikani V, Barnhart B, Sotelo M, Gaither JB, Viscusi C, Adelson PD, Denninghoff KR. Evaluation of the impact of implementing the emergency medical services traumatic brain injury guidelines in Arizona: the excellence in prehospital injury care (EPIC) study methodology. Acad Emerg Med. 2014;21(7):818–30. https://doi.org/10.1111/acem.12411.
43. Teasdale G, Jennett B. Assessment of coma and impaired consciousness. A practical scale. Lancet. 1974;2:81–4.
44. Davis DP. Prehospital intubation of brain-injured patients. Curr Opin Crit Care. 2008;14(2):142–8. https://doi.org/10.1097/MCC.0b013e3282f63c40.
45. Sobuwa S, Hartzenberg HB, Geduld H, Uys C. Outcomes following prehospital airway management in severe traumatic brain injury. S Afr Med J. 2013;103:644–6.
46. Caricato A, Conti G, Della Corte F, Mancino A, Santilli F, Sandroni C, et al. Effects of PEEP on the intracranial system of patients with head injury and subarachnoid hemorrhage: the role of respiratory system compliance. J Trauma. 2005;58:571–6.
47. Fontanilla L. Dopamine raises ICP. Crit Care. 2001;5:73300.
48. Toro C, Temkin N, Barber J, Manley G, Jain S, Ohnuma T, Komisarow J, Foreman B, Korley FK, Vavilala MS, Laskowitz DT, Mathew JP, Hernandez A, Sampson J, James ML, Goldstein BA, Markowitz AJ, Krishnamoorthy V, Investigators TRACK-TBI. Association of Vasopressor Choice with clinical and functional outcomes following moderate to severe traumatic brain injury: A TRACK-TBI study. Neurocrit Care. 2022;36(1):180–91. https://doi.org/10.1007/s12028-021-01280-7. Epub 2021 Aug 2
49. ACS TQIP: Best practices in the management of traumatic brain injury. https://doh.wa.gov/sites/default/files/legacy/Documents/2900//MgmtTBI.pdf
50. Cottenceau V, Masson F, Mahamid E, Petit L, Shik V, Sztark F, Zaaroor M, Soustiel JF. Comparison of effects of equiosmolar doses of mannitol and hypertonic saline on cerebral blood flow and metabolism in traumatic brain injury. J Neurotrauma. 2011;28(10):2003–12. https://doi.org/10.1089/neu.2011.1929.
51. Yang Y, Zheng F, Xu X, Wang X. Levetiracetam versus phenytoin for seizure prophylaxis following

traumatic brain injury: a systematic review and meta-analysis. CNS Drugs. 2016;30:677–88.
52. Sadaka F, Veremakis C. Therapeutic hypothermia for the management of intracranial hypertension in severe traumatic brain injury: a systematic review. Brain Inj. 2012;26:899–908.
53. Andrews PJ, Sinclair HL, Rodriguez A, Harris BA, Battison CG, Rhodes JK, et al. Hypothermia for intracranial hypertension after traumatic brain injury. N Engl J Med. 2015;373:2403–12.
54. Hutchinson PJ, Kolias AG, Timofeev IS, Corteen EA, Czosnyka M, Timothy J. Trial of decompressive craniectomy for traumatic intracranial hypertension. N Engl J Med. 2016;375:1119–30.
55. Cooper DJ, Rosenfeld JV, Murray L, Arabi YM, Davies AR, D'Urso P, et al. Decompressive craniectomy in diffuse traumatic brain injury. N Engl J Med. 2011;364:1493–502.
56. Ingebrigtsen T, Waterloo K, Marup-Jensen S, et al. Quantification of post-concussion symptoms 3 months after minor head injury in 100 consecutive patients. J Neurol. 1998;245:609–12.
57. Bazarian JJ, Zhong J, Blyth B, Zhu T, Kavcic V, Peterson D. Diffusion tensor imaging detects clinically important axonal damage after mild traumatic brain injury: a pilot study. J Neurotrauma. 2007;24:1447–59.
58. Fabbri A, Servadei F, Marchesini G, Stein SC, A. Vandelli early predictors of unfavorable outcome in subjects with moderate head injury in the emergency department. J Neurol Neurosurg Psychiatry. 2008;79:567–73.
59. Compagnone C, d'Avella D, Servadei F, Angileri FF, Brambilla G, Conti C, et al. Patients with moderate head injury: a prospective multicenter study of 315 patients. Neurosurgery. 2009;64:690–6.
60. Demetriades D, Kuncir E, Velmahos GC, Rhee P, Alo K, Chan LS. Outcome and prognostic factors in head injuries with an admission Glasgow coma scale score of 3. Arch Surg. 2004;139(10):1066–8. https://doi.org/10.1001/archsurg.139.10.1066).

46 Epilepsy and Neurocritical Care

Mariangela Panebianco

46.1 Introduction

A *seizure* is a paroxysmal alteration of neurologic function caused by the excessive, hypersynchronous discharge of neurons in the brain. It can cause changes in behavior, movements, feelings, and levels of consciousness. Most seizures last from 30 s to 2 min. A seizure that lasts longer than 5 min is a medical emergency [1]. Seizures are a considerable complication in critically ill patients and their incidence is significantly high in neurosciences care unit patients. *Epilepsy* is a disorder of the brain characterized by recurrent epileptic seizures [2].

A *neurological critical care unit* provides the optimal management of acutely ill patients with life-threatening neurologic and neurosurgical disease or with life-threatening neurologic manifestations of systemic disease [3]. Indeed, utilizing a multidisciplinary approach allows to manage the most challenging and highest acuity patients providing care for patients also with seizure disorders [4].

M. Panebianco (✉)
Department of Molecular and Clinical Pharmacology, Institute of Translational Medicine, University of Liverpool, Liverpool, UK
e-mail: m.panebianco@liverpool.ac.uk

46.2 Epileptic Seizures in Neurocritical Care Unit

A seizure can be a single event due to an acute cause: this is termed "*sporadic seizures.*" Diagnostic of sporadic seizure disorders with or without the disturbance of consciousness belong between the more difficult performances in the clinical practice [5, 6].

Most seizures in critical ill patients are nonconvulsive. *Nonconvulsive seizures* (NCS) are a highly heterogeneous clinical condition and broadly defined as a paroxysmal change in behavior and/or mental processes from baseline without convulsive activity [7, 8].

Many people with epilepsy report seizures which occur in close successions: these are called "*seizure clusters*" (SC) or "*acute repetitive seizures*" (ARS) [9, 10]. While no definition has been universally accepted, it is generally agreed that a seizure cluster represents closely grouped seizures over minutes to 2 days, representing an increase in seizure frequency compared with baseline [11]. These tightly grouped seizures represent an alarming clinical condition, and if not treated vigorously and efficiently, may lead to "*status epilepticus*" (SE), a very serious life-threatening condition [12]. Previously, SE was defined as a seizure with a duration equal to or greater than 30 min or a series of seizures in which the patient does not regain normal mental status between seizures. The Neurocritical Care

H. Prabhakar et al. (eds.), *Principles and Practice of Neurocritical Care*,
https://doi.org/10.1007/978-981-99-8059-8_46

Society guidelines from 2012 revised the definition of SE to a seizure with 5 min or more of continuous clinical and/or electrographic seizure activity or recurrent seizure activity without recovery between seizures [13]. Protracted seizure duration itself has the potential to result in maladaptive neuronal responses that can not only further increase seizure duration and worsen clinical outcomes but also lead to reduced responsiveness to pharmacotherapy. Seizure clusters and status epilepticus are neurologic emergencies.

Status epilepticus may be convulsive or nonconvulsive. *Generalized convulsive status epilepticus* (GCSE) consists of generalized tonic-clonic movements with impairment consciousness [14].

Nonconvulsive status epilepticus (NCSE) is defined as state of continuous or repetitive seizures for at least 30 min, with cognitive or behavioral changes, without a prominent motor component [15].

Refractory Status Epilepticus (RSE) is defined as persistent seizure activity after initiation of a first-line and 1 s-line antiseizure medications, while others suggest a duration of SE more than 60 min. RSE is usually managed in the Intensive Care Unit [16].

46.3 Recognizing Seizures in Neurocritical Care Unit

46.3.1 Clinical Presentation

Seizures can be difficult to recognize in critically ill patients. Prompt recognition of NCS or NCSE is crucial.

The following clinical presentations can indicate the ongoing NCS: (1) a prolonged reduction of alertness from an operative procedure or neurologic insult; (2) acute onset of impaired consciousness or fluctuating picture with episodes of normal mentation; (3) impaired mentation or consciousness with myoclonus of facial muscles or nystagmoid eye movements; (4) episodic blank staring, aphasia, automatisms (lip smacking, fumbling with fingers), perseverative activity; (5) aphasia without an acute structural lesion; (6) other acutely altered behavior without other obvious etiology [17].

A high degree of clinical suspicion is required to recognize these clinical presentations. Timely recognition is critical as NCSE is associated with a mortality rate of 33% [18]. The most common factors associated with missing seizures diagnosis are: (1) no prior history of epilepsy; (2) older age (mean 76.4 years); (3) Multimorbidities; (4) computed tomography (CT) brain showing cerebrovascular lesion; (5) seizure phenomenon (e.g., aphasia, lock of consciousness, paresis) and lack of tongue biting [19].

46.3.2 Continuous Electroencephalography Monitoring

The incidence of seizures in the neurological critical care unit ranges from 3.3–34.0%. When continuous electroencephalography monitoring (cEEG) is used, the incidence is highest [20]. cEEG monitoring is commonly used in critically ill patients in the neurological critical care unit and can identify NCS and NCSE [21]. The duration of cEEG monitoring is also an important aspect in diagnosing seizures in neurocritical care units [22].

The main indications for cEEG: (1) recent clinical seizure without return to baseline; (2) screening for nonconvulsive seizures (NCS) or nonconvulsive status (NCSE) in at-risk patients; (3) monitoring and treatment of known nonconvulsive seizures [23].

cEEG monitoring can be helpful in conditions lacking sufficient evidence to support the use of ASM for prophylactic use.

46.4 Seizure Prophylaxis in Neurocritical Care Unit

In various acute neurological insults including traumatic brain injury, epidural hemorrhage, subdural hemorrhage, aneurysmal subarachnoid hemorrhage, intracerebral hemorrhage, brain neoplasms, cerebral venous sinus thrombosis, posterior reversible encephalopathy syndrome, and meningitis are used ASMs for seizure prophylaxis [24].

Given the high incidence of seizures in *traumatic brain injury*, ASMs are frequently used as prophylactic therapy [25]. Post-traumatic seizures in traumatic brain injury are classified as early seizures (within 7 days of injury) with incidence rate between 4% and 25%, and late seizures (after 7 days of injury) with incidence rate between 49% and 42%. The most risk factors for seizure in patients with traumatic brain injury are: (1) Glasgow Coma Scale <10; (2) acute intracerebral or subdural hematoma; (3) penetrating brain injuries [26].

Incidence of seizures in patients with *neurosurgical intervention of craniotomy* varies greatly and depends upon the type of procedure performed and underlying pathology. Incidence rate of seizures in patients with postsupratentorial craniotomy is estimated to be 15–20%. There is limited evidence to support the prophylactic use of ASM in postneurosurgery patients [27].

Clinical seizures occur in about 1–7% of patients with *aneurysmal subarachnoid hemorrhage* and typically are manifestations of rebleeding of an unsecured aneurysm [28, 29]. Risk factors for seizures in aneurysmal subarachnoid hemorrhage are: (1) prior seizures; (2) intraparenchymal hemorrhage; (3) middle cerebral artery aneurysm; (4) rebleeding; (5) type of intervention (endovascular coiling associated with a lower risk of seizure compared to open craniotomy for clipping). According to Neurocritical Care Society guidelines (2011) and American Heart Association/American Stroke Association (AHA/ASA) guidelines (2012) for management of patients with aneurysmal subarachnoid hemorrhage, the prophylactic use of ASM can be considered for patients with known risk factors for delayed seizure disorder, such as prior seizure, intracerebral hematoma, intractable hypertension, infarction, or aneurysm at the middle cerebral artery [30].

Seizures are commonly reported in patients with *brain neoplasms* [31]. Risk factors for seizures in patients with brain neoplasm vary according to: (1) type of tumor (primary tumor > metastatic lesions); (2) grade of tumor (low-grade glioma > high-grade glioma); (3) specific tumor types (dysembryoplastic neuroepithelial tumors > meningiomas) [32]. ASMs are not recommended for routine prophylactic use in patients with newly diagnosed brain neoplasm, as they are not effective in preventing first seizures and have potential side effects. In patients with neurosurgical intervention for brain neoplasm, who never had seizures, discontinuation or taper of ASM after the first postoperative week is recommended. This is particularly suggested in medically stable patients or in those experiencing side effects [33].

The risk of seizures is highest within the first few days in patients with *intracerebral hemorrhage.* In fact, more than 50% of seizures occur in the first 24 h (early seizures). The incidence of early seizures in patients with intracerebral hemorrhage is reported to be 28–31% [34]. Late seizures are seen less frequently in patients with intracerebral hemorrhage and are believed to be due underlying gliotic scarring [35, 36]. As per the AHA/ASA guidelines for management of patients with intracerebral hemorrhage: (1) prophylactic use of ASM is not recommended; (2) clinical seizures should be treated with ASMs; (3) patients with a change in mental status who are found to have electrographic seizures on EEG should be treated with ASMs [37].

Ischemic stroke is the most common cause of seizure in elderly patients with an incidence rate from 4% to 23% [38]. A higher risk for seizure development exist in certain patients: hemorrhagic stroke or with hemorrhagic transformation are at higher risk of developing seizures (12.5%) as compared to ischemic stroke without hemorrhagic transformation (4.2%); cortical involvement in stroke patients predisposes them to higher seizure risk (9.8%) as compared to those with subcortical involvement (3.8%); patients with involvement of more than one lobe are higher risk (21.2%) as compared to those with single lobe involvement (5.2%) [39, 40]. As per the AHA guidelines for management of patients with acute ischemic stroke (2013) and malignant cerebral edema, the prophylactic use of ASM is not recommended in patients with ischemic stroke [41, 42].

Seizure prophylaxis in *vascular lesions, cavernous,* and *arteriovenous malformations* is controversial. In according with ASA guidelines, surgical or radiosurgical obliteration of arteriovenous malformation is generally considered effective in reducing seizure activity. Currently there are not enough studies available to formulate recommendations regarding type and duration of ASM prophylaxis after treatment [43].

Seizures occur in about 40% of patients with *cerebral venous thrombosis*. As per the AHA guidelines for management of patients with acute cerebral venous thrombosis in absence of seizure, routine use of ASM in patients with cerebral venous thrombosis is not recommended [44].

Febrile infection-related epilepsy syndrome (FIRES) is an intractable neurological disease characterized by an unexplained refractory status epilepticus triggered by febrile infection. The basic approach to the management of FIRES, like other forms of epilepsy, is based on the control of seizures, however seizures are extremely intractable and require intravenous administration of large doses of anticonvulsants [45].

In conclusion, guidelines for prophylactic use of ASMs in various neurological conditions encountered in the neurocritical care unit are generally derived from supporting evidence provided by various randomized controlled trials. For the majority of conditions, currently, there are not enough studies available to formulate recommendations regarding type and duration of ASM prophylaxis. In conditions without definite recommendations, the decision regarding prophylactic use of ASM is usually derived from physician's personal belief and local practice trends. However, under such circumstances, an ideal approach should be diagnosing seizure or epileptiform abnormalities rather than prophylaxis [46, 47].

46.5 Management of Seizures in Neurocritical Care Unit

An algorithm for the management of seizures in neurocritical care unit is provided in Fig. 46.1.

46.5.1 Seizures Prophylaxis

Patients with severe traumatic brain injury and aneurysmal subarachnoid hemorrhage seem to benefit with a short course of ASMs [24]. According to the latest brain trauma foundation (BTF) guidelines (2016), phenytoin (PHT) is recommended for prevention of early post-traumatic seizures and it should be used for the first 7 days after traumatic brain injury. Given its safety profile, levetiracetam (LEV) to the dosage 1000–2000 mg, could be a potential alternative to PHT for prophylaxis against early seizures postictus or postintracerebral hemorrhage [48, 49]. In addition, the use of lacosamide (LCM) 100–200 mg for seizure prophylaxis has favorable safety profiles [50]. See Table 46.1.

46.5.2 Treatment of Seizures

The treatment of seizures in neurocritical care unit must be individualized. It must depend on the type, frequency, severity, and duration of seizures, and whether episodes have been known to progress to prolonged seizures or seizure clusters or status epilepticus [51].

Benzodiazepines (BDZ) are consistently recommended as first-line treatment in SE, due to their rapid onset and efficacy in terminating seizures, followed by the emergent administration of an antiseizure medication (ASM). Various BDZ and ASM options are recommended and can be utilized in this setting, all with their own unique advantages and challenges. With time at a premium, agents should be selected that can be rapidly administered and have an advantageous pharmacokinetic profile in order to limit seizure duration and optimize outcomes [52].

Control of seizure clusters and SE in neurocritical care units generally follows the intrave-

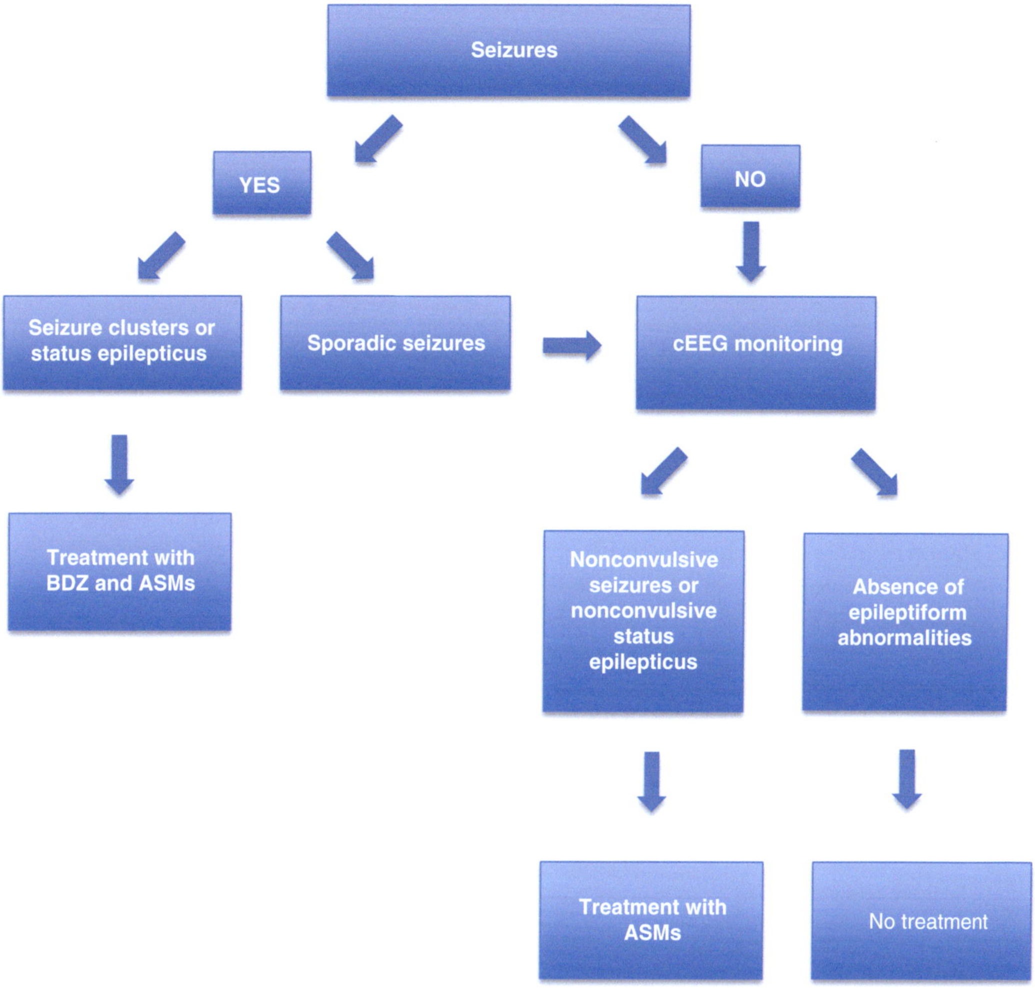

Fig. 46.1 Algorithm for management of seizures in neurocritical care unit

Table 46.1 Management of seizures in neurocritical care unit

Prophylaxis of seizures	**Antiseizures medications**	*Phenytoin*	*Levetiracetam*	*Lacosamide*
Treatment of seizures clusters or Status epilepticus	**Benzodiazepine** First-line treatment	*Lorazepam*	*Diazepam*	*Midazolam*
	Antiseizures medications Second-line treatment	*Valproate*	*Phenytoin*	*Levetiracetam*
		Brivaracetam	*Lacosamide*	*Perampanel*

nous administration of medications such as benzodiazepine (BDZ), and classical ASMs targeted at early resistant forms and longer-term coverage. In fact, first-line treatment involves the use of BDZ in the form of intravenous (IV) bolus of lorazepam 4–10 mg or midazolam 5–10 mg [53] or diazepam 5–10 mg [54]. Second-line treatment for seizure clusters involves some ASMs as IV valproate (VPA) 25–45 mg/Kg [55] or IV phenytoin (PHT) 20–30 mg/kg [56] or IV levetiracetam (LEV) 1000–2500 mg [57] or the newest drugs as IV brivaracetam (BRV) 50–400 mg [58, 59] or IV lacosamide (LCM) 400 mg [60] or perampanel (PER) administered per nasogastric tube (NGT) 4–12 mg [61]. See Table 46.1.

46.6 Conclusions

Seizures are well-described complications of acute brain injury and neurosurgery. Seizure prophylaxis with ASMs is common practice in neurocritical care units in patients with intracerebral tumors, traumatic brain injury, aneurysmal subarachnoid hemorrhage, craniotomy, ischemic stroke, and intracerebral hemorrhage [62]. The underlying risk for seizures varies significantly in all these disease states in neurocritical care unit [24].

In patients with injury to their brain, the use of cEEG monitoring in detecting early seizures would make sense rather than indiscriminately administering ASMs. Indeed, only observed seizures should be treated in such patients [17].

Treatment should depend on how severe the seizures are and how close they are to each other [63]. Seizure clusters and status epilepticus are frequent medical emergencies that require expedited treatment to avoid the ensuing high incidence of morbidity and mortality associated with prolonged seizures [13].

References

1. Stafstrom CE, Carmant L. Seizures and epilepsy: an overview for neuroscientists. Cold Spring Harb Perspect Med. 2015;5(6):a022426. https://doi.org/10.1101/cshperspect.a022426.
2. Panebianco M. Chapter 12: special considerations—epilepsy translational research. In: Prabhakar H, editor. Perioperative neuroscience: translational research. Elsevier, San Diego (USA): Academic Press; 2022. p. 179–88. https://doi.org/10.1016/C2020-0-02759-3.
3. Moheet AM, Livesay SL, Abdelhak T, Bleck TP, Human T, Karanjia N, Lamer-Rosen A, Medow J, Nyquist PA, Rosengart A, Smith W, Torbey MT, Chang CWJ. Standards for neurologic critical care units: a statement for healthcare professionals from the neurocritical care society. Neurocrit Care. 2018;29(2):145–60. https://doi.org/10.1007/s12028-018-0601-1;Erratum in: Neurocrit Care. 2019 May 22; PMID: 30251072.
4. Morris H, Hawkins A. Neuro critical care models improve outcomes in Epilepsy & Certified Stroke Centers. American Academy of Neurology; 2020.
5. Kollar B, Klobucnikova K, Fecikova A, Borovska J. Difficulties in diagnosis of solitary and sporadic epileptic seizures. Neuro Endocrinol Lett. 2010;31(6):814–7.
6. Varelas PN, Spanaki MV, Mirski MA. Seizures and the neurosurgical intensive care unit. Neurosurg Clin N Am. 2013;24(3):393–406. https://doi.org/10.1016/j.nec.2013.03.005.
7. Wang X, Yang F, Chen B, Jiang W. Non-convulsive seizures and non-convulsive status epilepticus in neuro-intensive care unit. Acta Neurol Scand. 2022;146(6):752–60. https://doi.org/10.1111/ane.13718.
8. Roodsari GS, Chari G, Mera B, Zehtabchi S. Can patients with non-convulsive seizure be identified in the emergency department? World J Emerg Med. 2017;8(3):190–4. https://doi.org/10.5847/wjem.j.1920-8642.2017.03.005.
9. Detyniecki K, O'Bryan J, Choezom T, et al. Prevalence and predictors of seizure clusters: a prospective observational study of adult patients with epilepsy. Epilepsy Behav. 2018;88:349–56.
10. Mesraoua B, Abou-Khalil B, Hosni Khodair R, Melikyan G, Al Hail H, Asadi-Pooya AA. Seizure clusters. J Drug Assess. 2021;10(1):86–90. https://doi.org/10.1080/21556660.2021.1962671.
11. Jafarpour S, Hirsch LJ, Gaínza-Lein M, et al. Seizure cluster: definition, prevalence, consequences, and management. Seizure. 2019;68:9–15.
12. Penovich PE, Buelow J, Steinberg K, et al. Burden of seizure clusters on patients with epilepsy and caregivers: survey of patient, caregiver, and clinician perspectives. Neurologist. 2017;22(6):207–14.
13. Wylie T, Sandhu DS, Murr N. Status Epilepticus. In: StatPearls. Treasure Island (FL): StatPearls Publishing; 2022;https://www.ncbi.nlm.nih.gov/books/NBK430686/.
14. Der-Nigoghossian C, Rubinos C, Alkhachroum A, Claassen J. Status epilepticus—time is brain and treatment considerations. Curr Opin Crit Care. 2019;25(6):638–46. https://doi.org/10.1097/MCC.0000000000000661.
15. Sutter R, Rüegg S, Kaplan PW. Epidemiology, diagnosis, and management of nonconvulsive status epilepticus: opening Pandora's box. Neurol Clin Pract. 2012;2(4):275–86. https://doi.org/10.1212/CPJ.0b013e318278be75.
16. Panebianco M, Marson A. Chapter 17: refractory status epilepticus. In: Prabhakar H, editor. Essential of Neuroanaesthesia. Elsevier, San Diego (USA): Academic Press; 2017. p. 309–14. 10.1016/B978-0-12-805299-0.00017-8.
17. Drislane FW. Presentation, evaluation, and treatment of nonconvulsive status epilepticus. Epilepsy Behav. 2000;1:301–14.
18. Young GB, Jordan KG, Doig GS. An assessment of nonconvulsive seizures in the intensive care unit using continuous EEG monitoring: an investigation of variables associated with mortality. Neurology. 1996;47:83–9.
19. Boesebeck F, Freermann S, Kellinghaus C, Evers S. Misdiagnosis of epileptic and non-epileptic seizures in a neurological intensive care unit. Acta Neurol Scand. 2010;122:189–95.

20. Abend NS, Dlugos DJ, Hahn CD, Hirsch LJ, Herman ST. Use of EEG monitoring and management of non-convulsive seizures in critically ill patients: a survey of neurologists. Neurocrit Care. 2010;12:382–9.
21. Newey CR, Sarwal A, Hantus S. Continuous electroencephalography (cEEG) changes precede clinical changes in a case of progressive cerebral edema. J Neurocrit Care. 2013;18:261–5.
22. Rubinos C, Alkhachroum A, Der-Nigoghossian C, Claassen J. Electroencephalogram monitoring in critical care. Semin Neurol. 2020;40(6):675–80. https://doi.org/10.1055/s-0040-1719073.
23. Herman ST, Abend NS, Bleck TP, Chapman KE, Drislane FW, Emerson RG, Gerard EE, Hahn CD, Husain AM, Kaplan PW, LaRoche SM, Nuwer MR, Quigg M, Riviello JJ, Schmitt SE, Simmons LA, Tsuchida TN, Hirsch LJ, Critical Care Continuous EEG Task Force of the American Clinical Neurophysiology Society. Consensus statement on continuous EEG in critically ill adults and children, part I: indications. J Clin Neurophysiol. 2015;32(2):87–95. https://doi.org/10.1097/WNP.0000000000000166.
24. Yerram S, Katyal N, Premkumar K, Nattanmai P, Newey CR. Seizure prophylaxis in the neuroscience intensive care unit. J Intensive Care. 2018;5(6):17. https://doi.org/10.1186/s40560-018-0288-6.
25. Yablon SA. Posttraumatic seizures. Arch Phys Med Rehabil. 1993;74:983–1001.
26. Frey LC. Epidemiology of posttraumatic epilepsy: a critical review. Epilepsia. 2003;44(s10):11–7. https://doi.org/10.1046/j.1528-1157.44.s10.4.x.
27. Pulman J, Greenhalgh J, Marson AG. Antiepileptic drugs as prophylaxis for post-craniotomy seizures. Cochrane Database Syst Rev. 2013;2:CD007286.
28. Molyneux AJ, Kerr RS, Yu LM, et al. International subarachnoid aneurysm trial (ISAT) of neurosurgical clipping versus endovascular coiling in 2143 patients with ruptured intracranial aneurysms: a randomized comparison of effects on survival, dependency, seizures, rebleeding, subgroups, and aneurysm occlusion. Lancet. 2005;366(809–17):15.
29. Claassen J, Peery S, Kreiter KT, et al. Predictors and clinical impact of epilepsy after subarachnoid hemorrhage. Neurology. 2003;60:208–14.
30. Connolly ES Jr, Rabinstein AA, Carhuapoma JR, Derdeyn CP, Dion J, Higashida RT, Hoh BL, Kirkness CJ, Naidech AM, Ogilvy CS, Patel AB, Thompson BG, Vespa P, American Heart Association Stroke Council; Council on Cardiovascular Radiology and Intervention; Council on Cardiovascular Nursing; Council on Cardiovascular Surgery and Anesthesia; Council on Clinical Cardiology. Guidelines for the management of aneurysmal subarachnoid hemorrhage: a guideline for healthcare professionals from the American Heart Association/American Stroke Association. Stroke. 2012;43:1711–137.
31. Glantz MJ, Cole BF, Forsyth PA, et al. Practice parameter: anticonvulsant prophylaxis in patients with newly diagnosed brain tumors. Report of the quality standards Subcommittee of the American Academy of neurology. Neurology. 2000;10:1886–93.
32. van Breemen MS, Wilms EB, Vecht CJ. Epilepsy in patients with brain tumours: epidemiology, mechanisms, and management. Lancet Neurol. 2007;5:421–30.
33. Komotar RJ, Raper DM, Starke RM, Iorgulescu JB, Gutin PH. Prophylactic antiepileptic drug therapy in patients undergoing supratentorial meningioma resection: a systematic analysis of efficacy. J Neurosurg. 2011;3:483–90.
34. Beghi E, D'Alessandro R, Beretta S, et al. Incidence and predictors of acute symptomatic seizures after stroke. Neurology. 2011;20:1785–93.
35. De Herdt V, Dumont F, Henon H, et al. Early seizures in intracerebral hemorrhage: incidence, associated factors, and outcome. Neurology. 2011;20(1794–800):40.
36. Lamy C, Domigo V, Semah F, et al. Early and late seizures after cryptogenic ischemic stroke in young adults. Neurology. 2003;3:400–4.
37. Morgenstern LB, Hemphill JC III, Anderson C, et al. Guidelines for the management of spontaneous intracerebral hemorrhage: a guideline for healthcare professionals from the American Heart Association/American Stroke Association. Stroke. 2010;9:2108–29.
38. Forsgren L, Bucht G, Eriksson S, Bergmark L. Incidence and clinical characterization of unprovoked seizures in adults: a prospective population based study. Epilepsia. 1996;3:224–9.
39. Gupta SR, Naheedy MH, Elias D, Rubino FA. Postinfarction seizures. A clinical study. Stroke. 1988;12(1477–81):50.
40. Lancman ME, Golimstok A, Norscini J, Granillo R. Risk factors for developing seizures after a stroke. Epilepsia. 1993;1:141–3.
41. Jauch EC, Saver JL, Adams HP Jr, Bruno A, Connors JJ, Demaerschalk BM, Khatri P, McMullan PW Jr, Qureshi AI, Rosenfield K, Scott PA, Summers DR, Wang DZ, Wintermark M, Yonas H, American Heart Association Stroke Council, Council on Cardiovascular Nursing, Council on Peripheral Vascular Disease, Council on Clinical Cardiology. Guidelines for the early management of patients with acute ischemic stroke: a guideline for healthcare professionals from the American Heart Association/American Stroke Association. Stroke. 2013;44(3):870–947.
42. Wijdicks EF, Sheth KN, Carter BS, Greer DM, Kasner SE, Kimberly WT, Schwab S, Smith EE, Tamargo RJ, Wintermark M, American Heart Association Stroke Council. Recommendations for the management of cerebral and cerebellar infarction with swelling: a statement for healthcare professionals from the American Heart Association/American Stroke Association. Stroke. 2014;45:1222–38.
43. Ogilvy CS, Stieg PE, Awad I, et al. AHA scientific statement: recommendations for the management of intracranial arteriovenous malformations: a state-

ment for healthcare professionals from a special writing group of the stroke council, American Stroke Association. Stroke. 2001;6:1458–71.
44. Ferro JM, Canhão P, Bousser MG, Stam J, Barinagarrementeria F, Investigators ISCVT. Early seizures in cerebral vein and dural sinus thrombosis: risk factors and role of antiepileptics. Stroke. 2008;39:1152–8.
45. Sakuma H, Horino A, Kuki I. Neurocritical care and target immunotherapy for febrile infection-related epilepsy syndrome. Biom J. 2020 Jun;43(3):205–10. https://doi.org/10.1016/j.bj.2020.03.009.
46. Kastrup O, Gerwig M, Frings M, Diener HC. Posterior reversible encephalopathy syndrome (PRES): electroencephalographic findings and eizure patterns. J Neurol. 2012;259:1383–9.
47. Rosman NP, Peterson DB, Kaye EM, Colton T. Seizures in bacterial meningitis: prevalence, patterns, pathogenesis, and prognosis. Pediatr Neurol. 1985;1:278–85.
48. Carney N, Totten AM, O'Reilly C, Ullman JS, Hawryluk GWJ, Bell MJ, Bratton SL, Chesnut R, Harris OA, Kissoon N, Rubiano AM, Shutter L, Tasker RC, Vavilala MS, Wilberger J, Wright DW, Ghajar J. Guidelines for the management of severe traumatic brain injury, fourth edition. Neurosurgery. 2017;80:6–15.
49. Fang T, Valdes E, Frontera JA. Levetiracetam for seizure prophylaxis in Neurocritical care: a systematic review and meta-analysis. Neurocrit Care. 2022 Feb;36(1):248–58. https://doi.org/10.1007/s12028-021-01296-z.
50. Luk ME, Tatum WO, Patel AV, Nau KM, Freeman WD. The safety of lacosamide for treatment of seizures and seizure prophylaxis in adult hospitalized patients. Neurohospitalist. 2012;2(3):77–81. https://doi.org/10.1177/1941874412446200.
51. Osman GM, Hocker SE. Status epilepticus in older adults: diagnostic and treatment considerations. Drugs Aging. 2023;40(2):91–103. https://doi.org/10.1007/s40266-022-00998-z.
52. Weant KA, Gregory H. Optimizing status epilepticus Management in the Emergency Department: It's about time. Adv Emerg Nurs J. 2023;45(1):11–22. https://doi.org/10.1097/TME.0000000000000440.
53. McKee HR, Abou-Khalil B. Outpatient pharmacotherapy and modes of administration for acute repetitive and prolonged seizures. CNS Drugs. 2015;29(1):55Y70. https://doi.org/10.1007/s40263-014-0219-6.
54. McMullan J, Sasson C, Pancioli A, Silbergleit R. Midazolam versus diazepam for the treatment of status epilepticus in children and young adults: a meta-analysis. Acad Emerg Med. 2010;17(6):575–82. https://doi.org/10.1111/j.1553-2712.2010.00751.x.
55. Gilad R, Izkovitz N, Dabby R, Rapoport A, Sadeh M, Weller B, et al. Treatment of status epilepticus and acute repetitive seizures with i.v. valproic acid vs phenytoin. Acta Neurol Scand. 2008;118(5):296–300. https://doi.org/10.1111/j.1600-0404.2008.01097.x.
56. Burman RJ, Ackermann S, Shapson-Coe A, Ndondo A, Buys H, Wilmshurst JM. A comparison of parenteral phenobarbital vs. parenteral phenytoin as second-line Management for Pediatric Convulsive Status Epilepticus in a resource-limited setting. Front Neurol. 2019;15(10):506. https://doi.org/10.3389/fneur.2019.00506.
57. Deshpande LS, Delorenzo RJ. Mechanisms of levetiracetam in the control of status epilepticus and epilepsy. Front Neurol. 2014;5:11. https://doi.org/10.3389/fneur.2014.00011.
58. Brigo F, Lattanzi S, Nardone R, Trinka E. Intravenous Brivaracetam in the treatment of status epilepticus: a systematic review. CNS Drugs. 2019;33(8):771–81. https://doi.org/10.1007/s40263-019-00652-0.
59. Lee K, Klein P, Dongre P, Choi EJ, Rhoney DH. Intravenous Brivaracetam in the Management of Acute Seizures in the hospital setting: a scoping review. J Intensive Care Med. 2022;37(9):1133–45. https://doi.org/10.1177/08850666211073598.
60. Höfler J, Trinka E. Lacosamide as a new treatment option in status epilepticus. Epilepsia. 2013;54(3):393–404. https://doi.org/10.1111/epi.12058.
61. Perez DQ, Espiritu AI, Jamora RDG. Perampanel in achieving status epilepticus cessation: a systematic review. Epilepsy Behav. 2022;128:108583. https://doi.org/10.1016/j.yebeh.2022.108583.
62. Rowe AS, Goodwin H, Brophy GM, Bushwitz J, Castle A, Deen D, Johnson D, Lesch C, Liang N, Potter E, Roels C, Samaan K, Rhoney DH, Neurocritical Care Society Pharmacy Section. Seizure prophylaxis in neurocritical care: a review of evidence-based support. Pharmacotherapy. 2014;34(4):396–409. https://doi.org/10.1002/phar.1374.
63. Gidal B, Klein P, Hirsch LJ. Seizure clusters, rescue treatments, seizure action plans: unmet needs and emerging formulations. Epilepsy Behav. 2020;112:107391.

Brain Tumors and Neurocritical Care

47

Liubov M. Tsentsiper, Anna O. Petrova,
Anatoly N. Kondratiev,
and Konstantin A. Samochernykh

47.1 Introduction

Brain tumors are ranked eighth among oncological diseases in adults over 40 years old [1, 2]. The perioperative period is largely determined by localization and size of the tumor, its histostructure, comorbid background, age. The development of postoperative complications is influenced by fact was it primary intervention or repeated and the experience of the neurosurgeon [2].

After an elective uncomplicated surgical intervention, the patient requires careful observation for 12–24 h. During this period, it is necessary to carry out monitoring of vital functions, neurological symptoms, laboratory data, maintenance of normovolemia, continuation of perioperative antibacterial therapy, resumption of preoperative medications: antihypertensive, antiarrhythmic, anticonvulsant, etc., if necessary, decongestant therapy with corticosteroids (CS) continues [3, 4].

The most frequent complications of the perioperative period in neuro-oncological patients are headache, nausea and vomiting, pneumocephaly seizures, water-electrolyte disorders, cerebral edema, hormonal insufficiency, disorders of carbohydrate metabolism, cerebrocardial syndrome, sympathetic, hyperactivity, dysphagia.

Patients with initial symptoms of pathological functioning of the central nervous system (CNS) (significant intracranial hypertension, dislocation syndrome, epileptic status, autonomic disorders), intraoperative complications (massive blood loss, hemodynamic reactions, changes in spontaneous and induced bioelectric activity of the brain during tumor removal, intraoperative brain swelling) before awakening from anesthesia need a detailed analysis of these changes. Most of these patients need the following therapeutic coma (TC) with opioid analgesics and alpha-2 adrenoagonists (clonidine or dexmedetomidine) until the stabilization of the condition (from 6 h to 72 h). This technique contributes to the formation of a sanogenetic dominant with the switching of brain functioning to a phylogenetically older level that implements the necessary protective reactions. The main objective of a TC is to create neurovegetative stability, a protective reaction in response to brain damage and the formation of an adequate level of its functioning, with preservation of compensatory, adaptive reactions and integrative activity necessary for sanogenesis [5, 6].

Pain syndrome (PS) ranks first among all complications. Headache is often one of the first symptoms of the brain tumor. In the postoperative period, pain stimuli come from the skin, periosteum, dura mater. The use of nonsteroidal anti-inflammatory drugs (acetaminophen, ibu-

L. M. Tsentsiper (✉) · A. O. Petrova ·
A. N. Kondratiev · K. A. Samochernykh
Almazov National Medical Research Centre,
St-Petersburg, Russia

H. Prabhakar et al. (eds.), *Principles and Practice of Neurocritical Care*,
https://doi.org/10.1007/978-981-99-8059-8_47

profen, ketorolac) for pain relief is usually sufficient, and only in extreme cases opioid analgesics are used. Intraoperative administration of dexmedetomidine allows not only to reduce opioids doses intraoperatively, but also to reduce the severity of the postoperative PS [7].

Perioperative nausea and vomiting are perhaps the second most common complications. The main causes are: increased ICP; cerebrospinal hyper—or hypotension; defeat of trigger zones, especially in patients with posterior fossa tumors; pneumocephaly; irritation of the stomach with blood and/or cerebrospinal fluid; exposure to medications. The appearance of nausea and vomiting together with the increase of headaches is one of the symptoms of increased ICP, which requires a thorough examination of the patient together with a neurosurgeon, neuroimaging examination [8]. Effective drugs for the prevention and relief of nausea and vomiting of central genesis are: ondansetron, metoclopramide hydrochloride, droperidol, dexamethasone [8].

Pneumocephaly is common in patients operated in a sitting position or on their side, if a significant amount of cerebrospinal fluid was released during the operation. Symptoms of pneumocephaly include: disturbances of consciousness like depression or psychomotor arousal; headache, nausea, vomiting; seizures; autonomic instability. In order to resolve pneumocephaly as soon as possible, the patient is given a horizontal position and humidified oxygen inhalation. In mechanically ventilated patients, increased FiO_2 up to 0.8–1.0 for 20–30 min every 2–3 h could be used. It is important to avoid hypovolemia. In case of intense pneumocephaly, surgical treatment is indicated [9].

47.2 Decongestant Therapy and Treatment of Intracranial Hypertension (ICH)

Basic rules in cases of cerebral edema and ICH are necessary:

- Ensuring adequate blood gas composition: PaO_2 more than 100 mmHg.
- $PaCO_2$—35–40 mmHg.
- Correct position of the head, not allowing flexion and overextension of the neck (without clamping the veins of the neck), elevated position of the head end 15–45°.
- Maintaining hemodynamics, it is possible to create a moderate hyperdynamic type of blood circulation.
- Maintaining normothermy.
- Monitoring of ICP (parenchymal or ventricular measurement).

ICH in neuro-oncological patients can be caused both by the mass effect of the tumor and by peritumorous edema. In some cases, if the tumor sprouts or compresses the sinuses and the veins of the brain, edema may be due to a violation of venous outflow. ICH also develops with impaired cerebrospinal fluid circulation, due to cerebrospinal fluid pathways occlusion by the tumor [10–14].

In 1945, Prados et al. [15] noted that spraying the brain with an extract, the adrenal glands protected it from the development of edema. Since that time, CS have been widely used in neurointensive therapy. They contribute to the restoration of normal BBB permeability, and reduce neuroinflammation [16, 17]. Besides it, CS have an antiemetic and analgesic effect, improve appetite and mood [3, 12].

In neuro-oncological patients, dexamethasone is currently the most common CS for the treatment of brain edema [3, 12]. It does not have mineralocorticoid activity; accordingly, it does not cause fluid and sodium retention, it has minimal psychotic side effects, a long half-life (34–54 h) and high efficacy [10–13]. If it is impossible to use dexamethasone, the use of other CS in equivalent doses is recommended. CS are not used as preventive therapy. Therapy begins in the presence of clinical and/or neuroimaging, signs of brain edema, and ICH [11, 12].

There are no standardized recommendations on the timing, dose, duration, and schedule of dose reduction of CS [12, 18]. Usually the initial dose is from 4 to 16 mg/day [11, 12] with the subsequent reduction to a sufficiently effective and gradual withdrawal after the tumor removal (a short course of 4–6 days does not require gradual withdrawal) [19, 20]. The frequency of administration of dexamethasone can vary from two to four times a day, depending on the duration of the clinical effect.

Various studies have shown the lack of benefits of previously recommended high doses (up to 100 mg of dexamethasone per day) in comparison with 8–16 mg/day [10–13, 20]. High doses of dexamethasone may cause more side effects (hyperglycemia, hypertension, psychosis, proximal myopathy, Cushing's disease, gastrointestinal ulcers, decreased immunity, impaired wound healing, suppression of adrenal function), but not necessarily lead to an improvement in clinical condition [11, 12, 19, 20]. In emergency situations, short-term (30–60 min) moderate hyperventilation (PaCO 2—30–35 mmHg) is used to reduce ICH. Prolonged hypocapnia can lead to brain ischemia due to vasospasm [3].

Loop and osmodiuretics (in particular Mannitol 30 mg/kg and hypertonic (3–5%) NaCl solutions) are used. Osmodiuretics can cause serious changes in plasma electrolytes level, and the so-called "rebound phenomenon" [3, 10, 11]. The absolute contraindication for mannitol therapy are: plasma hyperosmolarity of more than 320 mosm/L, plasma sodium level more than 150 mmol/L, severe renal and heart failure. In those cases, a hypertonic NaCl solution is safer. The phenomenon of "rebound" can be prevented by the administration of furosemide during or after mannitol infusion. The use of osmotic agents is advisable mainly in seriously ill patients in the pre—and intraoperative periods when it is necessary to avoid the use of steroids, for example, in patients with suspected lymphoma, until a tissue sample is obtained for histological evaluation [10].

For long-term edema control and in refractory cases, antiangiogenic agents are prescribed, such as bevacizumab (monoclonal antibody against VEGF) and cediranib (VEGF receptor tyrosine kinase inhibitor) [11].

The optimal method of treatment for ICH caused by disorders of venous outflow and hydrocephalus is surgical—total removal of the tumor or cytoreduction, or cerebrospinal fluid drainage [2, 3].

Seizures are one of the most common clinical symptoms in neuro-oncological patients [21]. In 25–60% of patients with brain tumors, epilepsy develops as the first symptom of the disease [22]. Patients with preoperative seizures have a significantly higher risk of developing postoperative seizures [21].

Antiepileptic drugs are prescribed to patients with brain tumors who have developed at least one seizure episode [22, 23]. The need in anticonvulsant therapy in the postoperative period depends on the EEG data. Usually in the absence of seizures for 4–6 months, anticonvulsants are gradually canceled [23].

However, in a significant number of patients, seizures persist after surgery [21]. Subtotal and total, in contrast to partial removal, provides more reliable control of seizures [22, 23]. Patients aged over 45 years old and patients with short anamnesis of seizures have the best postoperative prognosis [23]. Prevention of early postoperative seizures is usually carried out within 1–2 weeks [23].

When choosing anticonvulsants, one should follow the general recommendations for the treatment of epilepsy of nontumor etiology. Currently, the drugs of choice are levetiracetam and valproic acid (VPA) [23].

One of the most serious complications of seizures is the development of epileptic status (ES). The frequency of this complication during neurosurgical interventions reaches 5–20%, depending on the tumor localization [24].

Asymptomatic (nonconvulsive) epileptic syndrome, and especially, nonconvulsive epileptic status, may be the reason of neurological symptoms deterioration, up to the development of a comatose state. Nonconvulsive epileptic status accounts for 20% of all postoperative ES in neuro-oncological patients [24]. The therapy of nonconvulsive epileptic status does not differ from the therapy of convulsive ES. It is recommended to start therapy with intravenous administration of benzodiazepines: Lorazepam at a dose of 2–4 mg or diazepam—10–20 mg, or clonazepam—1–3 mg. Other drugs are VPA, phenobarbital (intravenous bolus dose of 10 mg/kg with at a maximum rate of 100 mg/min), levetiracetam 20–30 mg/kg or phenytoin 18 mg/kg or fosphenytoin. Phenytoin should be administered as a continuous infusion at a rate of 50 mg/min [25]. VPA is most often recommended to use intravenously in doses of 30–40 mg/kg of body weight for 10–20 min [24]. Initial serum levels decrease earlier than valproate is distributed in adipose tissue, therefore, a maintenance dose of 100–200 mg/h should be started after 30–60 min over the next 24 h. Alternatively, a maintenance dose of about 5 mg/kg every 6 h can be used. It is recommended to monitor the concentration of valproate in the blood serum [26].

Therapy of resistant ES is started with midazolam infusion (0.2 mg/kg IV bolus, and then 0.1–0.4 mg/kg/h) or propofol (2–3 mg/kg IV bolus, and then 1–2 mg/kg/h) or thiopental (3–5 mg/kg bolus, then further bolus administration of 1–2 mg/kg every 2–3 min until the cessation of seizures, then continued infusion 3–7 mg/kg/h). You can use Pentobarbital, VPA or Levetiracetam. Currently, due to the lack of comparative studies, there is no definitive clarity which of these drugs is more effective [25, 27, 28]. With refractory ES, the possibility of using anesthetics, that is, conducting a TC should be considered. The recommended anesthetics are propofol, midazolam or barbiturates, especially phenobarbital. Loading doses and infusion rates vary markedly in the literature, ranging from 0.5 to 20 mg/kg/h for barbiturates, 0.1–24 mg/kg/h for propofol and 0.02–1.8 mg/kg/h for midazolam [26].

The effectiveness of therapy is confirmed by EEG monitoring [28].

Cerebrocardial syndrome (CCS) is a special case of cerebrovisceral pathology and indicates an inextricable relationship between cerebral and systemic hemodynamics. The most frequent manifestations of CCS in patients with brain tumors are different types of tachyarrhythmias, arterial hypertension, cardialgia. The CCS is characterized by rapid dynamics, which does not always correspond the cerebral process. ECG changes are not specific and do not depend much on the localization of the process [29]. One of the manifestations of CCS is takotsubo cardiomyopathy (CMPT)—transient spherical expansion and akinesia of the upper and middle segments of the left ventricle in combination with hyperkinesia of its basal parts [30].

The possibilities of conservative treatment of CCS are extremely limited. They include the use of infusion therapy, including hyperosmolar solutions, change of ventilation parameters, CS to reduce the brain edema [3, 29–31].

Understanding the leading role of centrogenic vagosympathetic disorders in pathogenesis of CCS in brain tumors leads to the need to influence the central adreno—and opioid receptors located in the brainstem. There are no special methods of treating CCS [29].

From the onset of the disease and in the long-term, beta-blockers, alpha-2 adrenoagonists dexmedetomidine or clonidine (0.2–0.7 mcg/kg/h) may be useful [5, 6, 32]. CCS do not exclude the development of myocardial ischemia, rhythm, and conduction disturbances, as an aggravation of the concomitant coronary heart disease.

47.3 Intravascular Thrombosis and Thromboembolism

Patients with malignant brain tumors have the highest risk of venous thromboembolism (VTE) among all cancer patients, the rates reach 7.5–39%, depending on the use of thromboprophylaxis and the method of detection. In the postoperative period, the incidence of deep vein thrombosis (DVT) in meningiomas is 72% and 20% in metastatic tumors [11]. In the postoperative period, the incidence of deep vein thrombosis (DVT) in meningiomas is 72% and 20% in metastatic tumors, symptomatic VTE occurs in 18% of patients with primary CNS lymphoma [11].

Risk factors for the development of DVT and VTE include: the presence of paresis, age over 75 years, increased BMI, diabetes, blood group A or AB; a high degree of malignancy of the tumor and its size exceeding 5 cm, subtotal surgical resection compared with total resection, long-term CS therapy, pregnant women at the end of the second and third trimesters [11].

Pathological thrombosis is the result of both excessive release of coagulation activators and intraoperative release of tissue thromboplastin [11].

Biomarkers suitable for assessing the risk of VTE in patients with malignant gliomas are: platelet count, D-dimers, sP-selectin levels, factor VIII activity, prothrombin fragment 1 + 2, and white blood cell count [11]. Compression or duplex ultrasound in combination with clinical evaluation usually provides an accurate and noninvasive approach to the diagnosis of DVT [33].

Optimal methods of VTE prevention have not been definitively determined [34]. In oncologic patients, pharmacological thromboprophylaxis in the perioperative period is recommended and low-molecular weight heparins are used (LMH) [11, 35]. In neuro-oncological patients, this method remains controversial due to the high risk of intracranial hemorrhage [11, 35]. Gliomas, metastases from lung, and breast tumors have a relatively low frequency of spontaneous hemorrhage and should not be considered as a serious contraindication to anticoagulants [11, 35, 36]. Anticoagulants are often avoided in metastases of melanoma and renal cell carcinoma due to the high frequency of hemorrhage [37]. The use of unfractionated heparin (UFH) or LMH in combination with compression stockings proved to be more effective in preventing VTE compared to only with mechanical devices [38]. The timing of pharmacological prophylaxis may be crucial. In the postoperative period, prevention of VTE with LMH should be started within 24 h [39]. The beginning of prevention in 48 h after surgery is associated with an increased risk of thrombosis by 25% [40]. The most commonly used drugs are enoxaparin, dalteparin, enoxaparin, and nadroparin [41]. An alternative to anticoagulant therapy is to install a filter in vena cava inferior. However, filters have not shown reliable effectiveness in the prevention of VTE [13].

47.4 Antiulcer Gastroprotective Therapy (GPT)

Surgical stress, the development of sympathotonia, hypercatabolism, CS intake, impaired functions of the brain stem, coagulopathy, thrombocytopenia, and sepsis contribute to the violation of the gastrointestinal mucosa trophic [42]. The risk of gastrointestinal bleeding increases significantly when patients receive both CS and NSAIDs [43].

GPT should begin from the moment the patient enters the ICU. In the postoperative period, GPT includes the early enteral nutrition. Special therapy should be prescribed in the presence of risk factors, gastric ulcer, and duodenal ulcer in the anamnesis. It is possible to use H_2-histamine blockers. A contraindication to their appointment is violation of cardiac conduction, since H_2-receptor blockers have a negative inotropic and chronotropic effect. Recently, the advantage has been given to hydrogen pump inhibitors [42, 44].

The balance between the benefits and harms of preventing stress ulcers is still being studied. With a decrease in acidity in the stomach, the risk of nosocomial infections may increase [42, 44].

47.5 Vegetative Instability, Sympathetic Hyperactivity, and Hypercatabolism

These conditions quite often develop in patients with pituitary tumors, but they can be also observed in the complicated postoperative period in other tumor localizations. Vegetative instability is often one of the first manifestations of ICH, hemorrage, brain stem ischemia. With symptoms of sympathicotonia persisting for more than 72 h, one should diagnose paroxysmal sympathetic hyperactivity syndrome (PSHS) [45].

PSHS is caused by pathological activation of the sympathoadrenal and hypothalamic-pituitary-adrenal systems: arterial hypertension, tachycardia, tachypnea, hyperisothermia, increased activity of the sebaceous glands, hyperhidrosis, muscle hypertonus, trophic disorders—neurodystrophic syndrome, hypercatabolism. Laboratory examination reveals hyperglycemia, increased enzyme levels, hypernitrogenemia, hypoalbuminemia, hypernatremia, increased levels of catecholamines and cortisol [46, 47].

The basis of therapy and prevention of PSHS is compliance with general resuscitation principles (adequate hemodynamics, gas exchange, volemic status, nutritional support, electrolyte balance, normoglycemia, normothermy) [47, 48]. Medication includes: β-adrenoblockers (β-AB), bromocriptine, phenytoin, Gabapeptin, benzodiazepines, valproates, dantrolene [46–48]. In case of no effect, it is recommended to switch to continuous administration of opioids and propofol. The onset of TC with opioid analgesic and alpha-2adrenoagonist immediately after complicated surgery, also prevents the development of PSH [47].

Attention should be paid to the daily estimation of the volemic balance, consider the pathological loss of fluid and electrolytes. Thus, in patients with hyperhidrosis, fluid recovery is sometimes sufficient to increase the level of consciousness, reduce the number of paroxysms [48].

The last 10–15 years after the introduction of dexmedetomidine, alpha-2 adrenoagonists began to be successfully used for the treatment of PSH [47, 49, 50]. As mentioned earlier, a constant intravenous infusion of opioid and clonidine or dexmedetomidine in combination with a hypnotic (barbiturates or benzodiazepines, or propofol) seems to be the most pathophysiologically justified in severe PSH. The combined effect on the opioid and adrenergic antinociceptive systems of the brain, which are an integral part of the neuroregulatory systems of the brainstem, contributes to the functional integration of numerous compensation mechanisms, caudalization of brainstem functions, and reduction of pathological activity of telencephalic and diencephalic structures [5, 6]. With severe PSHS, persistent hyperthermia, a good effect provides sessions of therapeutic hypothermia [47, 51].

Neuroleptic drugs should be avoided due to the risk of developing a malignant neuroleptic syndrome [47].

47.6 Perioperative Period in Patients with Pituitary Tumors

Patients with pituitary tumor should be examined by endocrinologist before surgery in order to timely detect excessive hormonal activity or insufficiency. Possible humoral disorders that may affect the perioperative period are presented in Table 47.1.

Patients who have undergone pituitary surgery are at a higher risk of developing sleep apnea [52]. Noninvasive positive pressure ventilation is usually avoided due to the increased risk of bleeding from an operating wound, pneumocephaly, and liquorrhea [7, 52].

One of the serious postoperative complications is adrenal insufficiency (AI). Preoperative secondary AI is registered in 10–27% of patients with pituitary tumor, in 58% of cases with craniopharyngiomas [53]. Patients at high risk of developing AI include patients with macroadenomas, craniopharyngiomas, intraoperative liquorrhea [7]. Cortisol level monitoring is necessary from 1 postoperative day. Cortisol level should be evaluated in the blood (the sample is taken in the morning, on an empty stomach) or in the daily urine [7]. Stimulation tests in the early postoperative period are not recommended [54]. With initially preserved adrenal function, postoperative AI usually develops in the first 24–48 h in 4–9% of patients, and up to 18% may experience early transient AI [55]. The risk of developing postoperative AI is associated with the size of the tumor, its spread into surrounding structures, as well as the experience of the surgeon [56]. Restoration of adrenal function occurs within 14 days. With preoperative AI, restoration of function occurs in 15–20% of patients, and this is usually associated with a younger age, a smaller tumor size (<2 cm), hormone inactive tumors, normal blood pressure (BP) [55, 57].

After the corticotropinomas removal, the cortisol level should be checked every 6 h, and replacement therapy begins only after the cortisol level reaches subphysiological (cortisol <5 mcg/dL and/or the presence of AI symptoms). The faster cortisol reaches a subphysiological level, the more likely the patient would achieve ultimate surgical remission [19].

Patients who received oral forms of CS are transferred to parenteral forms of drugs for the entire perioperative period. In the evening before the operation, 100 mg of hydrocortisone is administered intravenously, and then 100 mg every 8 h. In the uncomplicated postoperative

Table 47.1 Humoral disorders that may affect the perioperative period in patients with pituitary tumors

The impact of the tumor	Clinical manifestations	Important features of the perioperative period
Compression of normal adenohypophysis tissue	Hypopituitarism	Overt or latent adrenal and/or thyroid insufficiency
Compression of the pituitary pedicle and posterior pituitary lobe	Diabetes insipidus	Hypovolemia, hypernatremia
Increased secretion of GH somatotropinomas	Acromegaly Splanchnomegaly Arterial hypertension DM, Insulin resistance Dyslipidemia	Difficulties of intubation, extubation High risk of cardiovascular complications Difficulties in correcting hyperglycemia
Increased secretion ACTH-Corticotropinomas	Arterial hypertension DM, insulin resistance Myopathies	High risk of cardiovascular complications. Difficulties in correcting hyperglycemia Difficulties of weaning from the ventilator.
Increased secretion TSH-thyrotropinomas	Tachycardia Thyrotoxicosis	High risk of cardiovascular complications

period, as a rule, 300–500 mg of hydrocortisone per day parenterally is sufficient. After stabilization of the patients state, the intravenous CS doses are quickly (in 3 days) reduced and transferred to oral CS [19, 56, 58].

Secondary hypothyroidism usually occurs in a mild form [19]. If the thyroid function is not impaired before surgery, the incidence of postoperative hypothyroidism is approximately 3% [55]. Only 7% of patients with preexisting secondary hypothyroidism demonstrate the restoration of thyroid function [56]. When if early postoperative thyroid dysfunction is suspected, both free thyroxine (FT4) and the index of free thyroxine and thyroid-stimulating hormone (TSH) are examined. In the immediate postoperative period, early hyponatremia may be an indicator of thyroid dysfunction [19]. The administration of CS at a stressful dose or therapy with dopamine agonists may inhibit the release of TSH from the pituitary gland [59].

Levothyroxine can be started with a low dose of 25–50 mcg/day and titrated in increments of 25 mcg to achieve a full replacement dose [19]. The effectiveness of thyroid hormone replacement therapy is evaluated after 6 weeks, then 3 months after surgery [19, 56, 58]. With the simultaneous development of AI and hypothyroidism, therapy begins with the replacement of AI [19, 58].

In the early postoperative period, water-electrolyte disorders are common, but often transient. The most common are central diabetes insipidus (DI), syndrome of inadequate secretion of antidiuretic hormone (SIADH), and, less frequently, cerebral salt wasting syndrome (CSWS), their comparative characteristics are presented in Table 47.2.

Postoperative DI develops in 10–30% of patients [60]. In most patients, DI is transient, persistent DI develops in less than 10% [61]. In some cases, three-phase DI develops: the first phase is the rapid occurrence of DI which lasts 4–5 days; the second —during 4–5 days, the volume of urine decreases and its osmolarity increases until the development of SIADH; the third is permanent polyuria [19, 62, 63]. Risk factors for persistent DI include younger age, male gender, preoperative DI, excess body weight, and previous operations in sellar region [60].

In the case of combined vasopressin and cortisol deficiency, DI symptoms may be masked, as cortisol deficiency disrupts free fluid clearance in the kidneys [19, 60].

Hypovolemia and hypernatremia are absent in patients with preserved consciousness and thirst. They need the desmopressin to eliminate the discomfort of frequent urination and the need for copious drinking. Hypovolemic plasma hyperosmolarity, hypernatremia could develop with disor-

Table 47.2 Differential diagnosis and therapy of CSWS, SIADH, DI

Indicators	CSWS	SIADH	DI
Dehydratation	Yes	No	Yes/no
Thirst	No	No	Yes
Diuresis	Is increased	Decreased	Increased
CVP	Is decreased	Increased or normal	Decreased or normal
The concentration of sodium in plasma	Decreased	Decreased	Normal or increased
Concentration of potassium in plasma	Increased or not changed	Decreased or not changed	Not changed
Hematocrit	Increased	Normal	Normal or increased
Plasma ADH	Is normal	Increased	Decreased
Urine osmolality	Is decreased or normal	Increased	Decreased
Urine-specific gravity	Normal	Increased	Decreased
Urine sodium concentration	Increased	Moderately increased or normal	Normal or decreased
Fluid infusion	Blood volume replenishment	Limited replenishment	Blood volume replenishment
NaCl 3%	Recommended	Not recommended	Not recommended
Mineralocorticoids	Recommended	Not recommended	Not recommended
Desmopressin	Not recommended	Not recommended	Recommended

ders of consciousness and thirst. In such situations, it is necessary to replenish the blood volume and conduct desmopressin therapy with daily revision and, if necessary, dose adjustment (taking into account the transient form of DI) [19, 60, 63].

SIADH is a transient syndrome. It is characterized by hypervolemic hyponatremia. For its correction, the fluid infusion should be limited to 800–1000 mL/day [19, 64, 65]. CSWS is also a transient syndrome, but it is more severe and lasts longer than SIADH. It is represented by polyuria and symptoms of hyponatremia and hypovolemia. Laboratory data show a decrease in sodium and plasma osmolality, urine density is normal or at the lower limit of normal, sodium in urine is increased [64–66].

Treatment consists in saline solutions infusion, a diet rich in sodium chloride. With severe hyponatremia (less than 125 mmol/L), an infusion of 3% NaCl solution is performed, CS with mineralocorticoid activity—fludrocortisone acetate (0.2–0.4 mg/day) or hydrocortisone is used to reduce natriuresis and diuresis. Correction of hyponatremia should be performed at a rate of no more than 0.5–1 mmol/L/h until the level of 125–130 mmol/L is reached. Exceeding this rate can lead to spontaneous myelinolysis [66, 67].

In the early postoperative period, all patients need a daily monitoring of diuresis, electrolyte levels, plasma, and urine osmolarity to assess the development of water-electrolyte disorders.

47.7 Violations of Thermoregulation

The main thermoregulation center is the hypothalamus. Thyroid and adrenal hormones are also involved in the regulation of heat exchange. Central hyperthermia can develop when the bottom of the third ventricle is affected by a tumor or in the structure of the PSH. Fever of central genesis is characterized by a slight difference between rectal and axillary temperatures (less than 0.5 °C)—isothermy. There is often no correlation between heart rate, respiratory rate, and hyperthermia. It is necessary to carry out a thorough differential diagnosis between central and infectious hyperthermia, especially since their combination is not uncommon. The drugs of choice are: clonidine (0.2–1.5 mcg/kg/h), NSAIDs, beta-AB of central action, dopaminergic drugs (bromocriptine, amantadine), benzodiazepines [68]. An important component of therapy is therapeutic hypothermia.

The causes of hypothermia can be both primary thermoregulation disorders with damage to the hypothalamus, and secondary adrenal insufficiency or hypothyroidism.

47.8 Perioperative Period in Patients with Posterior Fossa Tumors

The leading symptoms are: bulbar disorders (dysphagia, dysphonia, dysarthria), paresis of the facial and oculomotor nerves, hearing loss, cerebellar ataxia, and ICH [2, 3, 69, 70]. The main complications of the early postoperative period are: impaired consciousness, pathological brainstem reflexes; cranial nerve dysfunctions, subcortical and diencephalic symptoms; hemodynamic and respiratory disorders. These complications develop against the background of pneumocephaly, cerebral circulation disorders, both ischemic and hemorrhagic type, cerebrospinal fluid disorders (cerebrospinal hypotension with liquorrhea or hydrocephalus with occlusion of the cerebrospinal fluid pathways) [2, 3].

In the early postoperative period, the timing of extubation and need in tracheostomy are the main issues. An essential role in decision-making plays the assessment of independent breathing pattern and risk of dysphagia [3, 71]. The risk of postoperative dysphagia is significantly higher in patients who had bulbar disorders and large tumor sizes in the preoperative period, tumors closely related to the caudal nerves, and, of course, this risk is largely determined by the skill of the surgeon. Interventions on the structures of the posterior fossa are complicated by neurogenic dysphagia in 29–66% of cases [72]. Extubation against the background of swallowing disorders leads to the development of aspiration pneumonia, which increases the risk of death [72]. The risks associated with reintubation and complications caused by delayed extubation require precise decision either in favor of extubation or performing an early tracheostomy [73]. Indications for extubation are: positive dynamics in the level of consciousness (12–14 points on the GCS), restoration of protective reflexes of the respiratory tract, adequate spontaneous breathing, normalization of ICP, absence of gross pseudobulbar and bulbar disorders, absence of pulmonary causes for the development of hypoxemia and hypercapnia [74]. Indications for tracheostomy are: one or more unsuccessful attempts of extubation; level of consciousness ≤ 8 points on GCS; persistent bulbar symptoms; central respiratory disorders; predicted prolonged ventilation (more than 14 days) [74, 75].

Currently, there are no clear recommendations regarding the timing of extubation and tracheostomy. It is only determined the necessity to separate the respiratory tract and gastrointestinal tract as soon as possible. In all cases when the duration of recovery from a coma state, the need for lung ventilation, or the need for airway protection from aspiration exceeds 7–10 days, it is recommended to perform tracheostomy. Most researchers and clinicians are inclined to the benefits of early tracheostomy (on 2–4 days), which leads to a decrease in the duration of ventilation, reducing the risk of infectious complications, creates opportunities for rehabilitation of swallowing function, reduces the risk of complications from reintubation [74, 75].

The development of arterial hypertension, especially in combination with bradycardia (Cushing's reflex) [76] may indicate an increase of ICP, stem ischemia or hemorrhage. The drugs of choice for the treatment of hypertension are α-2 adrenoagonists and β-AB [3]. Arterial hypotension is also dangerous, and can lead to brain stem ischemia, perioperative stroke [77]. Maintaining blood pressure at the "upper level of operating values" can prevent the development of many postoperative complications [78, 79]. Therapy consists of carrying out adequate volemic support and, if necessary, the introduction of vasopressors and/or inotropic agents. The drug of choice is norepinephrine [4].

Adequate replacement of vital functions until the stabilization of brain stem symptoms (within 7–14 days) allows to prevent delayed damage to the brainstem. Patients with bulbar disorders need early rehabilitation aimed at restoring the respiratory pattern, swallowing, and motor functions [4].

Concluding the chapter on intensive care, it should be noted that despite the significant successes of modern neuro-oncology, anesthesiology, and intensive care, postoperative disability and mortality remain high. Careful monitoring and adequate therapy can help to avoid many complications or minimize them.

References

1. Ostrom QT, Patil N, Cioffi G, Waite K, Kruchko C, Barnholtz-Sloan JS. CBTRUS statistical report: primary brain and other central nervous system tumors diagnosed in the United States in 2013–2017. Neuro-Oncology. 2020;22(12 Suppl 2):iv1–iv96. https://doi.org/10.1093/neuonc/noaa200.
2. Batchelor T, Nishikawa R, Tarbell N, Weller M, editors. Oxford textbook of neuro-oncology. Oxford University Press; 2017. p. 272.
3. Gropper M, Eriksson L, Fleisher L, Jeanine Wiener-Kronish JW, Cohen N, Leslie K, editors. Miller's anesthesia. 9th ed. Elsevier; 2019. p. 3112.
4. Brambrink AM, Kirsch JR, editors. Essential of neurosurgical anaesthesia and critical care. 2nd ed. Springer; 2020. p. 671p.
5. Kondratyev AN. Usage of alpha-2 agonists and opioids in neuroanesthesia: twenty years of experience. Seminars in anesthesia, perioperative medicine and pain WB Saunders, 2004;23(3):192–195.
6. Kondratyev AN, Tsentsiper LM, Kondratyeva EA, Nazarov RV. Neurovegetative stabilization as a pathogenetic therapy for brain damage. Anesteziol Reanimatol. 2014;1:82–4.
7. Esfahani K, Dunn LK. Anesthetic management during transsphenoidal pituitary surgery. Curr Opin Anesthesiol. 2021;34(5):575–81. https://doi.org/10.1097/ACO.0000000000001035.
8. Uribe AA, Stoicea N, Echeverria-Villalobos M, Todeschini AB, Esparza Gutierrez A, Folea AR, Bergese SD. Postoperative nausea and vomiting after craniotomy: an evidence-based review of general considerations, risk factors, and management. J Neurosurg Anesthesiol. 2021;33(3):212–20. https://doi.org/10.1097/ANA.0000000000000667.
9. Bichsel O, Hauck A, Oertel M. Air travel with pneumocephalus: a systematic review. Acta Neurochir. 2022;164(9):2395–400. https://doi.org/10.1007/s00701-022-05297-5.
10. Roth P, Regli L, Tonder M, Weller M. Tumor-associated edema in brain cancer patients: pathogenesis and management. Expert Rev Anticancer Ther. 2013;13(11):1319–25. https://doi.org/10.1586/14737140.2013.852473.
11. Zoccarato M, Nardetto L, Basile AM, Giometto B, Zagonel V and Lombardi G. Seizures, Edema, Thrombosis, and hemorrhages: an update review on the medical management of gliomas. Front Oncol 2021, 11:617966. doi: https://doi.org/10.3389/fonc.2021.617966;
12. Ryan R, Sara Booth S, Price S. Corticosteroid-use in primary and secondary brain tumour patients: a review. J Neuro-Oncol. 2012;106:449–59. https://doi.org/10.1007/s11060-011-0713-3.
13. Wen PY, Schiff D, Kesari S, Drappatz J, Gigas DC, Doherty L. Medical management of patients with brain tumors. J Neuro-Oncol. 2006;80(3):313–32. https://doi.org/10.1007/s11060-006-9193-2.
14. Gogorian SF, Bersnev VP, Kim AV, Samochernykh KA, Malkhosian ZG. Brain tumors combined with hydrocephalus. Zh Vopr Neirokhir Im N N Burdenko. 2008;4:39–42.
15. Prados M, Strowger B, Feindel WH. Studies on cerebral edema: reaction of the brain to air exposure; pathologic changes. Arch Neurol Psychiatr. 1945;54:163–74.
16. Kotsarini C, Griffiths PD, Wilkinson ID, Hoggard N. A systematic review of the literature on the effects of dexamethasone on the brain from in vivo human-based studies: implications for physiological brain imaging of patients with intracranial tumors. Neurosurgery. 2010;67(6):1799–815. https://doi.org/10.1227/NEU.0b013e3181fa775b.
17. Förster C, Waschke J, Burek M, Leers J, Drenckhahn D. Glucocorticoid effects on mouse microvascular endothelial barrier permeability are brain specific. J Physiol. 2006;573(Pt 2):413–25. https://doi.org/10.1113/jphysiol.2006.10638585.
18. Schiff D, Lee EQ, Nayak L, Norden AD, Reardon DA, Wen PY. Medical management of brain tumors and the sequelae of treatment. Neuro-Oncology. 2015;17(4):488–504. https://doi.org/10.1093/neuonc/nou304.
19. Lavin N, editor. Manual of endocrinology and metabolism. 5th ed. Lippincott Williams & Wilkins; 2018. p. 986.
20. Jessurun CAC, Hulsbergen AFC, Cho LD, Aglio LS, Nandoe Tewarie RDS, Broekman MLD. Evidence-based dexamethasone dosing in malignant brain tumors: what do we really know? J Neuro-Oncol. 2019;144(2):249–64. https://doi.org/10.1007/s11060-019-03238-4.
21. Baumgarten P, Sarlak M, Baumgarten G, Gerhard MG, Seifert V, Strzelczyk A, Rosenow F, Freiman TM. Focused review on seizures caused by meningiomas. Epilepsy Behav. 2018;88:146–51. https://doi.org/10.1016/j.yebeh.2018.09.002.
22. Chen DY, Chen CC, Crawford JR, Wang SG. Tumor-related epilepsy: epidemiology, pathogenesis and management. J Neuro-Oncology. 2018;139(1):13–21. https://doi.org/10.1007/s11060-018-2862-0.
23. van der Meera PB, Taphoorna MJB, Koekkoek JAF. Management of epilepsy in brain tumor patients. Curr Opin Oncol. 2022;34(6):685–90. https://doi.org/10.1097/CCO.0000000000000876.
24. Al-Mefty O, Wrubel D, Haddad N. Postoperative nonconvulsive encephalopathic status: identification

of syndrome responsible for dekayed progressive deterioration of neurological status after skull base surgery. Neurosurgery. 2009;111(5):1062–8. https://doi.org/10.3171/2008.12.JNS08418.
25. Vossler DG, Bainbridge JL, Boggs JG, Novotny EJ, Loddenkemper T, Faught E, et al. Treatment of refractory convulsive status epilepticus: a comprehensive review by the American Epilepsy Society treatments committee. Epilepsy Curr. 2020;20(5):245–64. https://doi.org/10.1177/1535759720928269.
26. Heuser K, Olsen KB, Ulvin LB, Gjerstad L, Taubøll E. Modern treatment of status epilepticus in adults. In: Czuczwar SJ, editor. Epilepsy. Brisbane (AU): Exon Publications; 2022. p. 55–78. Chapter 5. https://www.ncbi.nlm.nih.gov/books/NBK580620/. https://doi.org/10.36255/exon-publications-epilepsy-status-epilepticus.
27. Rail S, Drislane FW. Treatment of refractory and super-refractory status epilepticus. Neurotherapeutics. 2018;15(3):697–712. https://doi.org/10.1007/s13311-018-0640-5.
28. Sculier C, Gaspard N. New onset refractory status epilepticus (NORSE). Seizure. 2019;68:72–8. https://doi.org/10.1016/j.seizure.2018.09.01.
29. Prasad Hrishi A, Ruby Lionel K, Prathapadas U. Head rules over the heart: cardiac manifestations of cerebral disorders. Indian J Crit Care Med. 2019;23(7):329–35.
30. Amin HZ, Amin LZ, Pradipta A. Takotsubo cardiomyopathy: a brief review. J Med Life. 2020;13(1):3–7. https://doi.org/10.25122/jml-2018-0067.
31. Madias JE. Takotsubo cardiomyopathy: current treatment. J Clin Med. 2021;10(15):3440. https://www.mdpi.com/2077-0383/10/15/3440. https://doi.org/10.3390/jcm10153440.
32. Tasbihgou SR, Barends CRM, Absalom AR. The role of dexmedetomidine in neurosurgery. Best Pract Res Clin Anaesthesiol. 2021;35(2):221–9. https://doi.org/10.1016/j.bpa.2020.10.002.
33. McRae SJ. Ginsberg JS (2006) update in the diagnosis of deep-vein thrombosis and pulmonary embolism. Curr Opin Anaesthesiol. 2006;19(1):44–51. https://doi.org/10.1097/01.aco.0000192772.79032.f2.
34. Epstein NE. A review of the risks and benefits of differing prophylaxis regimens for the treatment of deep venous thrombosis and pulmonary embolism in neurosurgery. Surg Neurol. 2005;64(4):295–301. https://doi.org/10.1016/j.surneu.2005.04.039.
35. Jo J, Donahue J, Sarai G, Petroni G, Schiff D. Management of venous thromboembolism in high-grade glioma: Does low molecular weight heparin increase intracranial bleeding risk? Neuro-Oncology. 2022;24(3):455–64. https://doi.org/10.1093/neuonc/noab198.
36. Iorio A, Agnelli G. Low-molecular-weight and unfractionated heparin for prevention of venous thromboembolism in neurosurgery: a meta-analysis. Arch Intern Med. 2000;160(15):2327–32. https://doi.org/10.1001/archinte.160.15.2327.
37. Alvarado G, Noor R, Bassett R, et al. Risk of intracranial hemorrhage with anticoagulation therapy in melanoma patients with brain metastases. Melanoma Res. 2012;22(4):310–5. https://doi.org/10.1097/CMR.0b013e328353efd8.
38. Agnelli G, Piovella F, Buoncristiani P, Severi P, Pini M, D'Angelo A, et al. Enoxaparin plus compression stockings compared with compression stockings alone in the prevention of venous thromboembolism after elective neurosurgery. N Engl J Med. 1998;339(2):80–5. https://doi.org/10.1056/NEJM199807093390204.
39. Pace A, Dirven L, Koekkoek JAF, Golla H, Fleming J, Rudà R, et al. European Association for Neuro-Oncology (EANO) guidelines for palliative care in adults with glioma. Lancet Oncol. 2017;18(6):e330–40. https://doi.org/10.1016/S1470-2045(17)30345-5.
40. Dickinson LD, Miller LD, Patel CP, Gupta SK. Enoxaparin increases the incidence of postoperative intracranial hemorrhage when initiated preoperatively for deep venous thrombosis prophylaxis in patients with brain tumors. Neurosurgery. 1998;43(5):1074–81. https://doi.org/10.1097/00006123-199811000-00039.
41. Bates SM, Ginsberg JM. Clinical practice. Treatment of deep vein thrombosis. New Engl J Med. 2004;351(3):268–77. https://doi.org/10.1056/NEJMcp031676.
42. Marik PE, Vasu T, Hirani A, Pachinburavan M. Stress ulcer prophylaxis in the new millennium: a systematic review and meta-analysis. Crit Care Med. 2010;38(11):2222–8. https://doi.org/10.1097/CCM.0b013e3181f17adf.
43. Nielsen GL, Sorensen HT, Mellemkjoer L, Blot WJ, McLaughlin JK, Tage-Jensen U, Olsen JH. Risk of hospitalization resulting from upper gastrointestinal bleeding among patients taking corticosteroids: a register-based cohort study. Am J Med. 2001;111(7):541–5. https://doi.org/10.1016/s0002-9343(01)00941-x.
44. Marker S, Krag M, Moller MH. What's new with stress ulcer prophylaxis in the ICU? Intensive Care Med. 2017;43(8):1132–4. https://doi.org/10.1007/s00134-017-4733-0.
45. Baguley IJ, Perkes IE, Fernandez-Ortega JF, Rabinstein AA, Dolce G, Hendricks HT. Paroxysmal sympathetic hyperactivity after acquired brain injury: consensus on conceptual definition, nomenclature, and diagnostic criteria. J Neurotrauma. 2014;31(17):1515–20. https://doi.org/10.1089/neu.2013.3301.
46. Thomas A, Greenwald BD. Paroxysmal sympathetic hyperactivity and clinical considerations for patients with acquired brain injuries: a narrative review. Am J Phys Med Rehabil. 2019;98(1):65–72. https://doi.org/10.1097/PHM.0000000000000990.
47. Tsentsiper LM, Terekhov IS, Shevelev OA, Petrova MV, Kondratiev AN. Paroxysmal sympathetic hyperactivity syndrome (review). General Reanimatol. 2022;18(4):55–67. https://doi.org/10.15360/1813-9779-2022-4-55-67.
48. Ding H, Liao L, Zheng X, Wang Q, Liu Z, Xu G, Tu JSY, Reeve J, Deane AM, Plummer MP. Pharmacological management of paroxys-

mal sympathetic hyperactivity: a scoping review. J Neurotrauma. 2021;38(16):2221–37. https://doi.org/10.1089/neu.2020.7597.
49. Abdelhakiem AK, Torres-Reveron A, Padilla JM. Effectiveness of pharmacological agents and validation of diagnostic scales for the management of paroxysmal sympathetic hyperactivity in Hispanics. Front Neurol. 2020;11:603011. https://www.frontiersin.org/articles/10.3389/fneur.2020.603011/full. https://doi.org/10.3389/fneur.2020.603011.
50. Bozorgi H, Zamani M, Motaghi E, Eslami M. Dexmedetomidine as an analgesic agent with neuroprotective properties: experimental and clinical aspects. J Pain Palliat Care Pharmacother. 2021;35(3):215–25. https://doi.org/10.1080/15360288.2021.1914280.
51. Liu X, Wen S, Zhao S, Yan F, Zhao S, Wu D, Ji X. Mild therapeutic hypothermia protects the brain from ischemia/reperfusion injury through upregulation of iASPP. Aging Dis. 2018;9(3):401–11. https://doi.org/10.14336/AD.2017.0703.
52. Rieley W, Askari A, Akagami R, Gooderham PA, Swart PA, Flexman AM. Immediate use of continuous positive airway pressure in patients with obstructive sleep apnea following transsphenoidal pituitary surgery: a case series. J Neurosurg Anesthesiol. 2020 Jan;32(1):36–40. https://doi.org/10.1097/ANA.0000000000000573.
53. Carosi G, Malchiodi E, Ferrante E, Sala E, Verrua E, Profka E, et al. Hypothalamic-pituitary axis in non-functioning pituitary adenomas: focus on the prevalence of isolated central hypoadrenalism. Neuroendocrinology. 2015;102(4):267–73. https://doi.org/10.1159/000430815.
54. Inder WJ, Hunt PJ. Glucocorticoid replacement in pituitary surgery: guidelines for perioperative assessment and management. J Clin Endocrinol Metab. 2002;87(6):2745–50. https://doi.org/10.1210/jcem.87.6.8547.
55. Fatemi N, Dusick JR, Mattozo C, McArthur DL, Cohan P, Boscardin J, et al. Pituitary hormonal loss and recovery after transsphenoidal adenoma removal. Neurosurgery. 2008;63(4):709–18. https://doi.org/10.1227/01.NEU.0000325725.77132.90.
56. Buttan A, Mamelak AN. Endocrine Outcomes After Pituitary Surgery. Neurosurg Clin N Am. 2019;30(4):491–8. https://doi.org/10.1016/j.nec.2019.05.009.
57. Munro V, Tugwell B, Doucette S, Clarke DB, Lacroix A, Imran SA. Recovery of adrenal function after chronic secondary adrenal insufficiency in patients with hypopituitarism. Clin Endocrinol. 2016;85(2):216–22. https://doi.org/10.1111/cen.13048.
58. Alexandraki KI, Grossman A. Management of Hypopituitarism. J Clin Med. 2019;8(12):2153. https://www.mdpi.com/2077-0383/8/12/2153. https://doi.org/10.3390/jcm8122153.
59. Haugen BR. Drugs that suppress TSH or cause central hypothyroidism. Best Pract Res Clin Endocrinol Metab. 2009;23(6):793–800. https://doi.org/10.1016/j.beem.2009.08.003.
60. Araujo-Castro M, Pascual-Corrales E, Martínez San Millan JS, Rebolleda G, Pian H, Ruz-Caracuel I, et al. Postoperative management of patients with pituitary tumors submitted to pituitary surgery. Experience of a Spanish pituitary tumor Center of Excellence. Endocrine. 2020;69(1):5–17. https://doi.org/10.1007/s12020-020-02247-y.
61. Adams JR, Blevins LS, Allen GS, Verity DK, Devin JK. Disorders of water metabolism following transsphenoidal pituitary surgery:a single institution's experience. Pituitary. 2006;9(2):93–9. https://doi.org/10.1007/s11102-006-9276-2.
62. Christ-Crain M, Gaisl O. Diabetes insipidus. Presse Med. 2021;50(4):104093. ;https://www.sciencedirect.com/science/article/pii/S0755498221000300?via%3Dihub. https://doi.org/10.1016/j.lpm.2021.104093.
63. Garrahy A, Moran C, Thompson CJ. Diagnosis and management of central diabetes insipidus in adults. Clin Endocrinol. 2019;90(1):23–30. https://doi.org/10.1111/cen.13866.
64. Sterns RH, Silver SH. Cerebral salt wasting *versus* SIADH: what difference? J Am Soc Nephrol. 2008;19(2):194–6. https://doi.org/10.1681/ASN.2007101118.
65. Cui H, He G, Yang S, Lv Y, Jiang Z, Gang X. Wang G Inappropriate Antidiuretic Hormone Secretion and Cerebral Salt-Wasting Syndromes in Neurological Patients. Front Neurosci. 2019;13:1170. https://doi.org/10.3389/fnins.2019.01170.
66. Oh H, Seo W. An integrative review of cerebral salt wasting syndrome. J Neurosci Nurs. 2020;52(6):289–94. https://doi.org/10.1097/JNN.0000000000000548.
67. Lindner G, Schwarz C, Haidinger M, Ravioli S. Hyponatremia in the emergency department. Am J Emerg Med. 2022;60:1–8. https://doi.org/10.1016/j.ajem.2022.07.023.
68. Holgersson J, Ceric A, Sethi N, Nielsen N, Jakobsen JC. Fever therapy in febrile adults: systematic review with meta-analyses and trial sequential analyses. BMJ. 2022;378:e069620. https://doi.org/10.1136/bmj-2021-069620.
69. Muthukumar N. Hydrocephalus Associated with Posterior Fossa Tumors: How to Manage Effectively? Neurol India. 2021;69(Supplement):S342–9. https://doi.org/10.4103/0028-3886.332260.
70. Kim AV, Samochernykh KA, Soltan PS, Don OA, Zaharchuk EV, Khachatryan WA. Features of brain tumors and their surgical treatment in children of the first 2 years of life. Grekov's Bull Surg. 2011;170(4):68–72.
71. Goethe EA, Gadgil N, Stormes K, Wassef A, LoPresti M, Lam S. Predicting dysphagia in children undergoing surgery for posterior fossa tumors Childs. Nerv

Syst. 2020;36(5):925–31. https://doi.org/10.1007/s00381-019-04468-7.
72. Wadhwa R, Toms J, Chittiboina P, Tawfik T, Glenn C, Caldito G, Guthikonda B, Nanda A. Dysphagia following posterior fossa surgery in adults. World Neurosurg. 2014;82(5):822–7. https://doi.org/10.1016/j.wneu.2013.01.035.
73. Cooper JD. Tracheal injuries complicating prolonged intubation and tracheostomy. Thorac Surg Clin. 2018;28(2):139–44. https://doi.org/10.1016/j.thorsurg.2018.01.001.
74. Robba C, Poole D, McNett M, Asehnoune K, Bösel J, Bruder N, et al. Mechanical ventilation in patients with acute brain injury: recommendations of the European Society of Intensive Care Medicine consensus. Intensive Care Med. 2020;46(12):2397–410. https://doi.org/10.1007/s00134-020-06283-0.
75. Enrichi C. Clinical criteria for tracheostomy Decannulation in subjects with acquired. Brain Inj. 2017;62(10):1255–63. https://doi.org/10.4187/respcare.05470.
76. Cushing H. Concerning a definite regulatory mechanism of the vasomotor Centre which controls blood pressure during cerebral compression. Bull Johns Hopkins Hosp. 1901;12:290–2.
77. Kamiya-Matsuoka C, Cachia D, Yust-Katz S, Rodriguez YA, Garciarena P, Rodarte EM, et al. Ischemic stroke in patients with gliomas at the University of Texas-M.D. Anderson cancer center. J Neuro-Oncol. 2015;125(1):143–8. https://doi.org/10.1007/s11060-015-1880-4.
78. Komlodi-Pasztor E, Gilbert MR, Armstrong TS. Diagnosis and management of stroke in adults with primary brain tumor. Curr Oncol Report. 2022;24(10):1251–9. https://doi.org/10.1007/s11912-022-01280-6.
79. Pires PW, Dams Ramos CM, Matin N, Dorrance AM. The effects of hypertension on the cerebral circulation. Am J Physiol Heart Circ Physiol. 2013;304(12):H1598–614. https://doi.org/10.1152/ajpheart.00490.2012.

Liubov M. Tsentsiper —MD, PhD, Anesthesiologist, Endocrinologist, Leading Researcher of the Research Laboratory for Neuroprotection and Neurometabolic Disorders of the Russian Neurosurgery Research Institute named after Prof. A.L. Polenov, Branch of the Almazov National Medical Research Centre, professor of the Chair of Anesthesiology and Intensive Care of the Institute of Medical Education of the Almazov National Medical Research Centre (St. Petersburg, Russian Federation);

Anna O. Petrova —PhD, Anesthesiologist, Almazov National Medical Research Centre (St. Petersburg, Russian Federation);

Anatoly N. Kondratiev —MD, PhD, D.Sci, Professor, Chief Specialist of the Ministry of Healthcare of the Russian Federation (Anesthesiology and Intensive Care in the North-West Federal District), Anesthesiologist, Head of the Research Laboratory for Neuroprotection and Neurometabolic Disorders of the Russian Neurosurgery Research Institute named after Prof. A.L. Polenov, Branch of the Almazov National Medical Research Centre (St. Petersburg);

Konstantin A. Samochernykh —MD, PhD, D.Sci, Professor of the Russian Academy of Sciences, neurosurgeon, Director of the Russian Neurosurgical Institute named after prof. A. L. Polenov, Branch of the Almazov National Medical Research Centre (St. Petersburg, Russian Federation)

Spinal Surgery and Neurocritical Care

48

Maresa Santi, Samuel Ern Hung Tsan, and Argyro Zoumprouli

48.1 Introduction

Spinal surgery is associated with a high rate of systemic complications. Systematic reviews have found that the overall rate of early complications from spinal surgery ranged from 5.2% to 16.4% [1, 2]. The rates of early systemic complications differed based on the type of surgery and the surgical approaches. Major systemic complications, defined as clinical events that led to long-lasting sequelae or required further intervention, including repeat surgery, are as high as 28% in cervical spinal surgery and 24.2% in thoracic or lumbar spinal surgeries (Table 48.1) [3, 4]. In addition, perioperative spinal cord injury after spinal surgery is a devastating complication with incidence of 0–3%. High-risk surgical procedures include spinal stabilisation following trauma/tumours and correction of scoliosis. Furthermore, the care of high-level acute spinal cord injuries requires physiological monitoring and stabilisation preoperatively; spinal decompression and/or fixation are common surgical approaches with post-operative challenges due to intraoperative factors and long-term physiological changes.

The high rate of significant complications in the early post-operative period for certain spinal surgeries warrants more specialised care and a higher standard of monitoring, often provided in the intensive care unit (ICU). Indications for admission to the ICU include but are not limited to major intraoperative bleeding, post-operative airway oedema, haemodynamic instability due to neurogenic shock, prolonged surgical procedures (more than 6–8 h) and any pre-existing or new organ failures. The specific indications for intensive care admission are usually determined locally in each institution, subject to local expertise and safety standards.

The higher level of care provided in the ICU aims to prevent post-operative complications or

Table 48.1 List of common major complications following spinal surgery

Cervical spinal surgery[a]	Thoracic or lumbar spinal surgery[b]
• Deep wound infection • Pulmonary embolism • Sepsis • Death • Aspiration pneumonia • Ischaemic stroke • Congestive heart failure • Epidural haematoma • Cardiac arrest • Airway oedema • Reintubation	• Deep wound infection • Myocardial infarction • Pulmonary embolism • Durotomy • New weakness • Sepsis • Splenic rupture • Death

[a] Adapted from Campbell et al. [4]
[b] Adapted from Campbell et al [3]

M. Santi (✉) · S. E. H. Tsan · A. Zoumprouli
St. George's University Hospitals NHS Foundation Trust, London, UK
e-mail: maresa@doctors.org.uk

H. Prabhakar et al. (eds.), *Principles and Practice of Neurocritical Care*,
https://doi.org/10.1007/978-981-99-8059-8_48

manage them promptly should they be present to ensure the best patient outcomes. This chapter will discuss specific major complications arising in patients who underwent spinal surgery and their prevention or management in the ICU.

48.2 Airway and Respiratory System

48.2.1 Airway Complications

Spinal surgeries are primarily performed in the prone position via the posterior approach. This position has been associated with airway oedema, leading to potential airway obstruction after extubation [5]. Airway oedema (e.g. swelling of the tongue, oropharynx, larynx and glottis) may result from decreased venous drainage from lingual, pharyngeal and laryngeal veins. The mechanisms for reduced venous drainage include increased intra-abdominal and intra-thoracic pressures in the prone position, the dependent position of the head relative to the heart and neck flexion. There is evidence that there is a risk of tongue swelling occurring after spinal surgery in the prone position. In a recent study, an increase in the modified Mallampati class was observed in 92% of patients undergoing spinal surgery in the prone position, with maximal airway change in the first hour post-operatively [6]. Airway deterioration is also seen in patients undergoing cervical spinal surgery via the anterior approach. In these patients, airway oedema secondary to venous stasis and neck surgical haematoma, whether alone or in combination, may lead to catastrophic airway obstruction and a difficult airway management scenario.

Signs and symptoms of increased work of breathing characterise the clinical signs of upper airway obstruction. The patient may complain of difficulty breathing and appears diaphoretic and distressed with an increased respiratory rate. There may be noisy breathing with snoring or stridor. Usage of accessory respiratory muscles will be prominent, along with nasal flaring, tracheal tug and intercostal recessions. If airway obstruction is severe, there may be a paradoxical breathing pattern, where during inspiration, the abdomen expands while the thorax contracts. This is caused by the maximal contraction of the diaphragm moving into the abdomen, generating negative pressure in the thorax; however, due to the obstruction of airflow, the negative intrathoracic pressure causes the chest wall to be drawn inwards. There may be no breath sounds in complete airway obstruction due to complete respiratory arrest. Pulse oximetry is an invaluable tool, but it is essential to remember there is a lag between clinical hypoxia and the reading obtained. Due to hypoxia, there will be sympathetic overdrive, leading to tachycardia and hypertension. There will also be mental status changes with agitation preceding coma as hypoxia worsens. Eventually, severe hypoxia will lead to cardiac arrest. Arterial blood gas analysis could be helpful and can reveal hypoxaemia (low PaO_2) and hypercarbia (high $PaCO_2$). However, a normal $PaCO_2$ level may present when the patient becomes increasingly tired, a sign of imminent respiratory arrest.

The management of airway obstruction is a clinical emergency. A call for help should immediately be put out, explicitly calling for senior airway experts and additional assistants. In severe cases of airway obstruction, the otorhinolaryngology surgeon should also be called. The patient should be administered oxygen via a non-rebreather mask as the first-line therapy. Nebulised 1:1000 adrenaline 1–5 mg and repeated as necessary may be administered, along with high-dose steroids such as dexamethasone (8 mg, IV). Where possible, reintubation of severe airway obstruction should be performed in the operating theatre (OT), with the otorhinolaryngology surgeon on standby for emergency front-of-neck access. However, if the patient is too unstable to be transported to the OT, airway management should be carried out in the ICU following difficult airway guidelines (Difficult Airway Society and American Society of Anaesthesiologists) [7, 8]. For patients who underwent cervical spinal surgery via the anterior approach, the presence of a neck haematoma must be ruled out. If present, the haematoma should be emergently evacuated by reopening the surgical incision.

48.2.2 Extubation Process

The extubation process of spinal surgery patients should be systematically managed to avoid extubation failure (reintubation within 48 h). Reintubation is associated with an increased mortality rate (independent predictor of inpatient mortality) [9]. Extubation failure can be divided into two leading causes: airway failure (inability of the patient to breathe without an artificial airway) or weaning failure (inability of the patient to breathe without ventilator assistance). A thorough assessment of the airway and general risk factors needs to be undertaken in post-spinal surgery patients before extubation.

Potential airway risk factors leading to airway failure after spinal surgery include airway oedema and airway injury sustained during anaesthesia and surgery, reduced pharyngeal tone seen in obesity and patients with obstructive sleep apnoea and residual neuromuscular blockade. Additionally, copious secretions and the absence of a strong cough before extubation, which could be present in patients with high spinal cord injury, are independent predictors of airway failure [10]. A cuff-leak test should be undertaken before extubation in patients with suspected subglottic oedema to minimise the risk of airway failure. Additionally, oedema of the upper airway structures can be evaluated via a flexible fibreoptic scope or video laryngoscope. Regular steroids for at least 24 h should be administered in suspected airway oedema. Extubation to non-invasive ventilation or high-flow nasal oxygenation (HFNO) should be considered to maintain airway patency. For patients with inadequate respiratory secretion clearance, therapies to loosen airway secretions should be instituted in addition to regular chest physiotherapy.

General risk factors for weaning failure in patients post-spinal surgery include haemodynamic instability, respiratory insufficiency, neurological deficits/impaired consciousness, neuromuscular pathology and acid-base imbalance. A Sequential Organ Failure Assessment (SOFA) score of ≥8 independently predicts weaning failure [10]. These general risk factors should be optimised before attempting extubation. To anticipate weaning failure, a spontaneous breathing trial (SBT) should be performed using either low settings pressure support ventilation or T-piece ventilation. There is also evidence that echocardiography, in combination with diaphragm and lung ultrasound, can improve the positive and negative predictive values of SBT [11]. For patients with cardiovascular or respiratory risk factors for weaning failure, extubation to non-invasive ventilation or HFNO can be considered.

48.3 Cardiovascular System

Spinal surgery is classically associated with significant blood loss. As a result, there may be a considerable transfusion of blood products perioperatively. Patients presenting to the ICU after spinal surgery may be haemodynamically unstable, have ongoing bleeding, or suffer possible blood transfusion complications.

Clinical signs of ongoing bleeding are signs of hypovolaemic shock. In the presence of hypovolaemic shock and ongoing bleeding, the immediate priority is volume replacement and control of the source of bleeding. The patient may need a reoperation. Point-of-care investigations such as blood gases or HemoCue are invaluable to guiding blood transfusion and fluid administration. A transfusion ratio of 1:1:1 consisting of plasma:platelets:red blood cells is beneficial in patients with major bleeding. This transfusion ratio is associated with improved haemostasis and reduced mortality rate without evidence of increased complications [12]. Tranexamic acid to aid coagulation should also be considered in such situations.

Patients who have received significant blood transfusion intraoperatively may present in the

ICU with hypothermia, acidosis and coagulopathy, known as the lethal triad. This would lead to a vicious cycle where further bleeding ensues due to impaired blood clotting, worsening the triad. Correction of these factors is therefore paramount to controlling bleeding. The use of thromboelastography can guide the precise correction of coagulopathy. Post-spinal surgery patients may also suffer complications of blood transfusion (acute haemolytic reaction, acute allergic reaction, transfusion-related acute lung injury and transfusion-associated circulatory overload). A multidisciplinary team management approach should be used for these patients.

48.4 Neurological System

Patients presenting to the ICU after spinal surgeries may suffer from neurological complications. In adult patients undergoing spinal deformity surgery, surgical procedure-related neurologic conditions are as high as 13.7%. The most common neurological complications included radiculopathy, motor deficits, sensory deficits and altered mental status [13].

One of the most devastating complications in this population of patients is the development of spinal epidural haematoma, which, if left untreated, can progress to spinal cord compression and paralysis. The incidence of epidural haematoma has been reported as 0.07–5.71%. The incidence differed based on the location of the surgery and the surgical approach, with thoracic spinal surgery and the posterior approach associated with the highest rate [14]. Given the catastrophic nature of neurological complications in patients post-spinal surgery, it is crucial to carry out comprehensive neurological monitoring in these patients, including motor and sensory functions. Early detection of neurological deficits will allow prompt management, including optimising physiological parameters, repeat radiological imaging and surgical reoperation. In the case of an epidural haematoma, earlier surgical evacuation of haematoma has been associated with reduced neurological deficits and improved clinical outcomes.

48.5 Pain

Spinal surgery is associated with significant post-operative pain. The incidence of moderate to severe pain (defined as pain scores ≥4 out of 10 on a numerical rating scale) post-spinal surgery over the first four post-operative days ranges from 19% to 65%, depending on the type of surgeries done [15]. Many patients undergoing spinal surgery have pre-existing chronic pain and may already be on multiple pain medications. The pain in these patients is usually a combination of nociceptive and neuropathic pain. Considering all these, managing post-operative pain following spinal surgery may be complex and challenging.

Effective pain management following spinal surgery requires accurate pain assessment using a standardised method at regular intervals. Pain should also be evaluated pre- and post-interventions to determine whether further treatment modifications are needed. A comprehensive pain assessment will include pain intensity, quality and objective pain medication quantification. Pain intensity is usually measured using validated tools such as the numerical rating scale or visual analogue scale. The Behavioural Pain Score or Critical Care Pain Observational Tool can be used for intubated and ventilated patients. These instruments use behavioural changes to pain to quantify the severity of pain. The McGill pain questionnaire can be used to assess pain quality. It is a comprehensive, multidimensional tool that evaluates neurophysiologic and psychological aspects. Five main measures of pain are evaluated: location, intensity, quality, pattern and alleviating and aggravating factors.

The management of post-operative pain in post-spinal surgery patients should utilise the principle of multimodal analgesia, which is superior to opioids alone. Examples of analgesic medications that can reduce opioid usage include non-steroidal anti-inflammatory agents, paracetamol, gabapentinoids, ketamine, local anaesthetic agents, alpha-2-agonists and amitriptyline. A summary of the different classes of pharmacological agents used to control post-operative pain is found in Table 48.2.

Table 48.2 Pharmacological agents for post-operative pain

Pharmacological class	Mechanism of action	Method of administration	Examples	Side effects
Opioid	Act on opioid receptors (MOP, DOP, KOP and NOP) to mimic effects of endogenous opioids	Oral Intravenous Intramuscular Transdermal Intrathecal Epidural	Morphine Fentanyl Oxycodone Tramadol Codeine	Respiratory depression Sedation Nausea and vomiting Urinary retention Constipation Dependence and addiction
NSAID	Inhibition of cyclo-oxygenase enzyme	Oral Intravenous Intramuscular Per rectal	Ibuprofen Diclofenac Ketorolac Celecoxib Parecoxib	Renal impairment Platelet dysfunction Gastric ulcer Bronchospasm
Paracetamol	Unclear. May have effect on cyclo-oxygenase enzyme inhibition and prevention of prostaglandin production	Oral Intravascular Per rectal		Liver toxicity
Ketamine	NMDA receptor antagonist	Oral Intravascular Intramuscular		Hallucinations Delirium Tachycardia Hypersalivation
Gabapentinoids	Calcium channel blocker. Stimulate descending inhibition, inhibit descending serotonergic facilitation and inflammatory mediators, influence affective component of pain	Oral	Gabapentin Pregabalin	Drowsiness Dizziness Ataxia
Local anaesthetic agents	Sodium channel blockers preventing transmission of pain impulses	Intravenous Local infiltration Intrathecal Epidural Peripheral nerve/fascial plane blocks	Lidocaine Bupivacaine Ropivacaine	Local anaesthetic systemic toxicity
Alpha-2-agonist	Acts on central alpha-2-adrenoceptor to inhibit pain transmission by activating inhibitory G-proteins	Oral Intravenous	Clonidine Dexmedetomidine	Sedation Bradycardia Hypotension

Abbreviations: *DOP* delta opioid receptor, *KOP* kappa opioid receptor, *MOP* mu opioid receptor, *NOP* nociceptin opioid receptor, *NSAID* non-steroidal anti-inflammatory drug

48.6 Venous Thromboembolism

Patients undergoing spinal surgery are at high risk of thromboembolic complications. Post-spinal surgery thromboembolic occurrences have been reported to be as high as 31%, leading to increased morbidity and mortality in this population [16]. Risk factors for developing thromboembolic events in these patients include cancer, advanced age, reduced preoperative or post-operative mobility, a complex or multi-level procedure and prolonged surgery.

Prevention of thromboembolic complications can be divided into mechanical and chemical prophylaxis. The external compression device is the most used mechanical thromboprophylaxis and often the safest. Examples of external compression devices include sequential compression devices, thrombo-embolus deterrent stockings and intermittent pneumatic compression devices. These devices effectively reduce the risk of thromboembolism by improving venous return from the lower limbs, thereby preventing venous stasis. Another form of mechanical thromboprophylaxis is the inferior vena cava (IVC) filter, an intravascular device designed to prevent the propagation of thromboembolus into the pulmonary circulation. Although it is beneficial in preventing pulmonary embolism, the IVC filter is invasive and may cause complications such as displacement, bleeding and infection. Finally, the safest mechanical thromboprophylaxis is for post-spinal surgery patients to start early ambulation. A multidisciplinary team approach is required to facilitate this.

Chemical prophylaxis is the administration of drugs to prevent thromboembolic phenomena. Common drugs include subcutaneous heparin and low-molecular-weight heparin (LMWH). Although there is strong evidence of their effectiveness, this should be balanced with the increased risk of bleeding. Currently, the optimal timing of initiating chemical thromboprophylaxis is still controversial. Based on clinical judgement, the National Institute for Health and Care Excellence (NICE) recommends starting chemical prophylaxis within the first 48 h post-operatively [17]. Therefore, a detailed risk-benefit analysis must be undertaken for each patient before initiating chemoprophylaxis.

48.7 Perioperative Management of Patients with Acute Traumatic Spinal Cord Injury

Acute traumatic spinal cord injuries (SCI) often affect young and fit people and can have devastating long-term consequences, including reduced functional independence as a result of permanent disability as well as financial and social implications. Patients with SCI require intensive medical care and continuous monitoring to prevent and respond to airway, respiratory, cardiovascular and neurological complications. We recommend using an integrated care pathway to systematically optimise the care of these patients (Fig. 48.1).

48.7.1 Spinal Immobilisation

C-spine injuries account for 55% of SCI. ATLS advocates immobilisation of the c-spine as a priority in conjunction with airway management. Spinal immobilisation involves using a number of devices and strategies to stabilise the spinal column after injury and thus prevent spinal cord injury [18]. Manual spinal protection should be commenced immediately.

If the neck is not in a neutral position, an attempt should be made to achieve alignment. A cervical spine positioned and maintained in neutral alignment should preserve the space within the spinal canal that normally surrounds the spinal cord, thus ameliorating injury. Deviations from neutral alignment can decrease the diameter of the spinal canal and the space available for the spinal cord [19]. If the patient is awake and cooperative, they should actively move their neck into alignment. If unconscious or unable to co-operate, this is done passively. If there is any pain, neurological deterioration, or resistance to movement, the procedure should be abandoned, and the neck splinted in the current position [20].

The spine board should be removed as soon as possible once the patient is on a firm trolley. Full immobilisation should be maintained, and manual protection should be reinstated if restraints must be removed for examination or procedures (e.g. intubation). Potential immobilisation complications include airway difficulties, increased intracranial pressure, increased risk of aspiration and skin ulceration.

Log rolling is the standard manoeuvre to allow examination of the back and transfer on and off backboards. Rigid transfer slides (e.g. Patslides, trauma mattress) are useful for transferring patients from one surface to another (e.g. CT scan, operating table).

Patients who are agitated or restless may be impossible to immobilise adequately. Forced

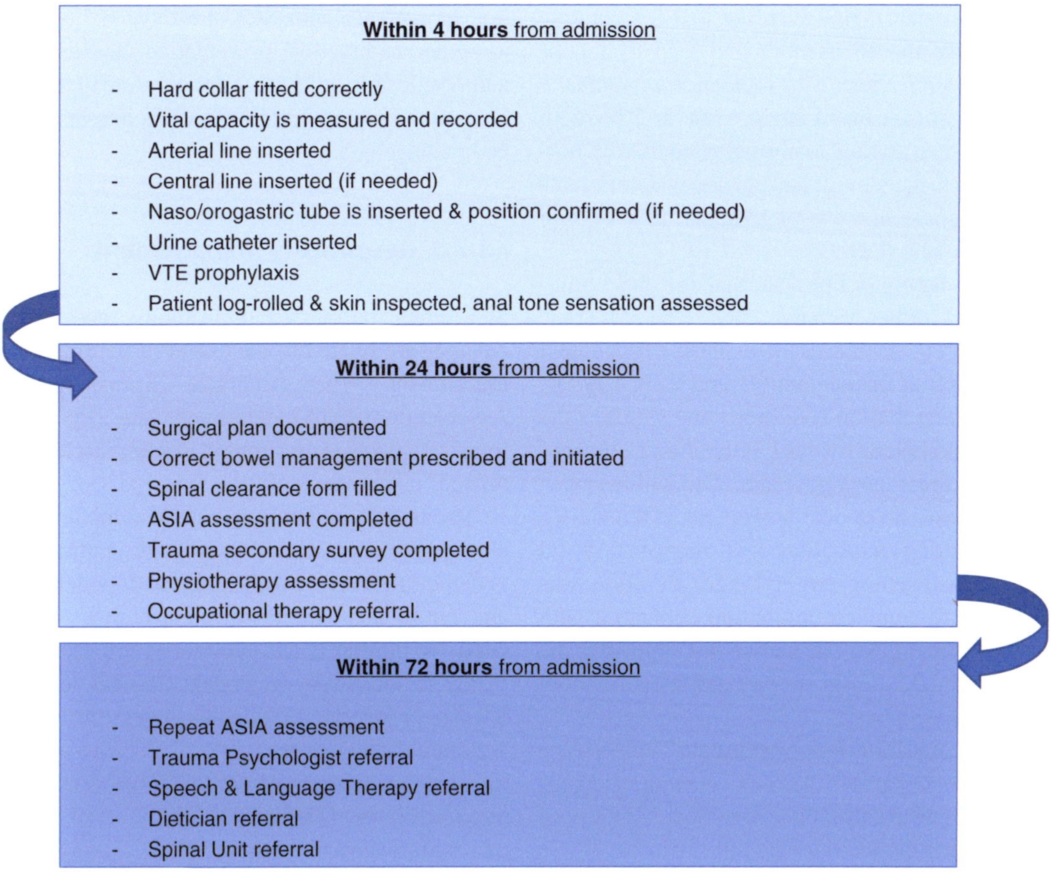

Fig. 48.1 The St. George's Hospital Integrated Care pathway for spinal cord injury patients. All patients with a spinal injury of T8 or above should be admitted to a neurocritical care unit

restraints or manual fixation of the head may risk further injury. Removing immobilisation devices and allowing the patient to move unhindered may be necessary. This should be a medical decision. Spinal immobilisation should continue until the spinal clearance is documented per existing guidelines.

48.7.2 Airway Management

C spine fractures can often cause soft tissue swelling, slowly compromising the airway. Therefore, the patient should be assessed for neck swelling; vital signs and arterial blood gases may be normal and should not be relied upon.

Tracheal intubation may be required for several reasons, including high-cord injury associated with respiratory failure and airway obstruction secondary to tissue swelling.

All airway manoeuvres will result in some degree of neck movement, and intubation has been ascribed to contribute to secondary injury. The most appropriate technique for tracheal intubation in patients with C-spine injury continues to be debated as no outcome studies exist [21].

Manual In-Line Stabilisation (MILS) should always be used when securing the airway. MILS aims to lessen C-spine movement during intubation by applying sufficient force to the head and neck to limit movement. The patient is supine with the head and the neck in a neutral position. Assistants either grasp the mastoid process with their fingertips and cradle the occiput in the palms of their hands (head-of-bed assistant) or cradle the mastoids and grasp the occiput (side-of-bed assistant). However, the MILS technique can reduce mouth opening and lead to a poor laryngoscopic view. The incidence of Grade 3 and 4 Cormack and Lehane view is 22% with MILS. When applied to normal patients with normal spines, the view at laryngoscopy deteriorates by one grade in 36% of patients, and by two grades in 10% [22].

Video laryngoscopes can manage these problems and prove valuable aids. The AirTraq® laryngoscope decreases the extension movement of C-spines at the occiput-C1 and C2-C4 levels, improves intubation conditions and shortens the time to complete tracheal intubation compared with a direct laryngoscope. The Glidescope® also decreased cervical movement in the C2-C5 levels during intubation and improved vocal cord visualisation, but a longer duration was required to complete intubation compared with other devices [23]. The person who intubates the patient should use the airway tool they are more confident with.

Clinical setting and practitioner's experience should be taken into account when considering the use of awake fibreoptic technique. The use of a technique by practitioners not skilled in its use carries risk. Failed awake intubations have been implicated in morbidity and mortality by the American Society of Anaesthesiologists. Awake fibreoptic intubation is not helpful in the management of the airway of an acute SCI. It requires special equipment and cannot be performed on uncooperative and unprepared patients; therefore, its use in the emergency setting is inappropriate.

Suxamethonium can be used up to 48 h post-injury. After this time, it can cause life-threatening hyperkalaemia [24]. In acute SCI, there is up-regulation of acetylcholine receptors (AChRs) spreading throughout the muscle membrane. The depolarisation of these AChRs that are spread throughout the muscle membrane by succinylcholine and its metabolites leads to potassium efflux from the muscle, resulting in hyperkalaemia.

During intubation, airway manipulation can lead to increased vagal activity causing bradycardia. In patients with SCI, pre-oxygenation and atropine are practical preventative measures. In addition to this, a MAP of 80–95 mmHg should be maintained (see cardiovascular complications and management).

48.7.3 Respiratory Management

SCI alters pulmonary physiology, and those changes are related to the extent of neurological impairment. The American Spinal Injury Association (ASIA) determines the degree of impairment based on strength in key muscles and sensory examinations [25].

The most common respiratory complications are respiratory failure, neurogenic pulmonary oedema (high cervical cord injuries), pneumonia and pulmonary embolism, contributing significantly to morbidity and mortality [26]. The incidence is increased on higher cervical lesions. Weakness of the diaphragm, chest wall and abdominal muscles lead to an ineffective cough, reduced secretion clearance, atelectasis and hypoventilation (Table 48.3). The level of injury can significantly affect lung volumes, and forced vital capacity (FVC) should be measured twice daily on non-intubated patients. The normal physiological range varies between men (70 mL/kg) and women (55 mL/kg).

SCI also leads to changes in lung and chest wall compliance, airflow limitation, bronchial hyper-responsiveness, secretion molecular composition and changes in ventilatory control. Signs of impending respiratory failure, such as increased respiratory rate, reducing FVC, rising $PaCO_2$ and falling PaO_2, are indications for intubation and mechanical ventilatory support. Invasive ventilation should be considered once the FVC falls below 15 mL/kg. Some patients have improved lung mechanics when lying flat due to an increase in FVC [27, 28].

For lesions above T11, prophylactic BIPAP of HFNO can be considered. Chest physiotherapy, including frequent suctioning and cough assist, should be initiated promptly to prevent atelectasis and pneumonia.

Table 48.3 Respiratory changes in spinal cord injury patients according to the level of injury

Injury level	Impaired respiratory muscles	Complications
Above C3	Near total ventilator muscle paralysis as a result of phrenic nerve disruption Denervation of intercostal, abdominal, sternocleidomastoid and trapezius muscles	Respiratory failure requiring immediate mechanical ventilation Unable to cough without assistance
C3-C5	Variable impairment of diaphragmatic strength and accessory muscles FVC is 20% of normal	Often develop respiratory failure requiring mechanical ventilation during the first few days–weeks Once accessory muscles strengthen, weaning from mechanical ventilation is possible Impaired cough
C6–8	Diaphragm and accessory muscles above the lesion are intact Exhalation occurs via passive recoil	Coughing is impaired and patients are therefore at increased risk of respiratory failure due to excess secretions.
Thoracic injuries	Intact diaphragm FVC 30–50% of normal	Impaired cough

48.7.4 Cardiovascular Complications and Management

Acute SCI to the cervical spinal cord is regularly accompanied by arrhythmias and haemodynamic abnormalities [29] and most frequently occur in the first 2 weeks after injury.

Neurogenic shock is a distributive shock resulting from sympathetic dysautonomia that follows a SCI. It manifests as hypotension, usually with bradycardia (especially injuries T6 and above) and poikilothermia, due to interruption of autonomic pathways in the spinal cord causing decreased vascular resistance. It is associated with cervical and high-thoracic SCI. Patients with traumatic SCI may also suffer from haemodynamic shock due to blood loss. A combination of careful fluid resuscitation, blood products and vasoconstrictors should be used in these cases.

Neurogenic shock differs from 'spinal shock'. The term 'spinal shock' applies to all phenomena surrounding physiologic or anatomic transection of the spinal cord that results in temporary loss or depression of all or most spinal reflex activity below the level of the injury.

Bradyarrhythmias, atrioventricular conduction block and hypotension are common following cervical lesions due to impaired sympathetic innervation in the setting of preserved parasympathetic function (vagus mediated). Stimulation of the bronchi by aggressive suctioning of secretions can also result in bradyarrhythmias or conduction block [30].

In the last decade, SCI management has focused on maintaining adequate spinal cord perfusion, thus minimising secondary injury. Mean arterial pressure (MAP) between 80 and 95 mmHg is believed to be important [31, 32]. This should be maintained for the first 7 days after acute SCI. Current guidelines are based on empirical data and expert opinion.

Increased vagal activity may cause bradycardia, often triggered by airway manipulation. In these cases, pre-oxygenation and atropine are helpful preventative measures. Severe bradycardia (especially SCI C1-C5) that does not respond to atropine may require external pacing and cardiology referral for temporary pacing.

Polytrauma patients often receive large amounts of intravenous fluids. Excess fluids can lead to further cord swelling, increasing secondary injury. The use of haemodynamic monitoring such as LiDCO® or Volume View® is recommended to guide fluid and vasopressor management. Urinary catheter insertion will allow an accurate measurement of fluid balance.

48.7.5 Autonomic Dysreflexia (AD)

AD is a life-threatening syndrome in high spinal cord lesions, normally above the T5 level [33]. It is unusual in the first month of SCI but usually appears within the first year. AD is an increase in systolic blood pressure by at least 20%, sometimes combined with bradycardia or cardiac dysrhythmia [34]. It can be accompanied by sweating in areas above the lesion, muscle spasms, paraesthesia in the neck and shoulders, headache, a feeling of fullness in the head and pallor followed by flushing of the face.

Symptoms resolve after the removal of the stimulus. Stimuli originate below the level of the lesion from the skin, abdominal (e.g. bowel impaction) or viscera, skeletal muscles or, most commonly, bladder distension (Fig. 48.2).

It manifests as the loss of coordinated autonomic responses to demands on heart rate and

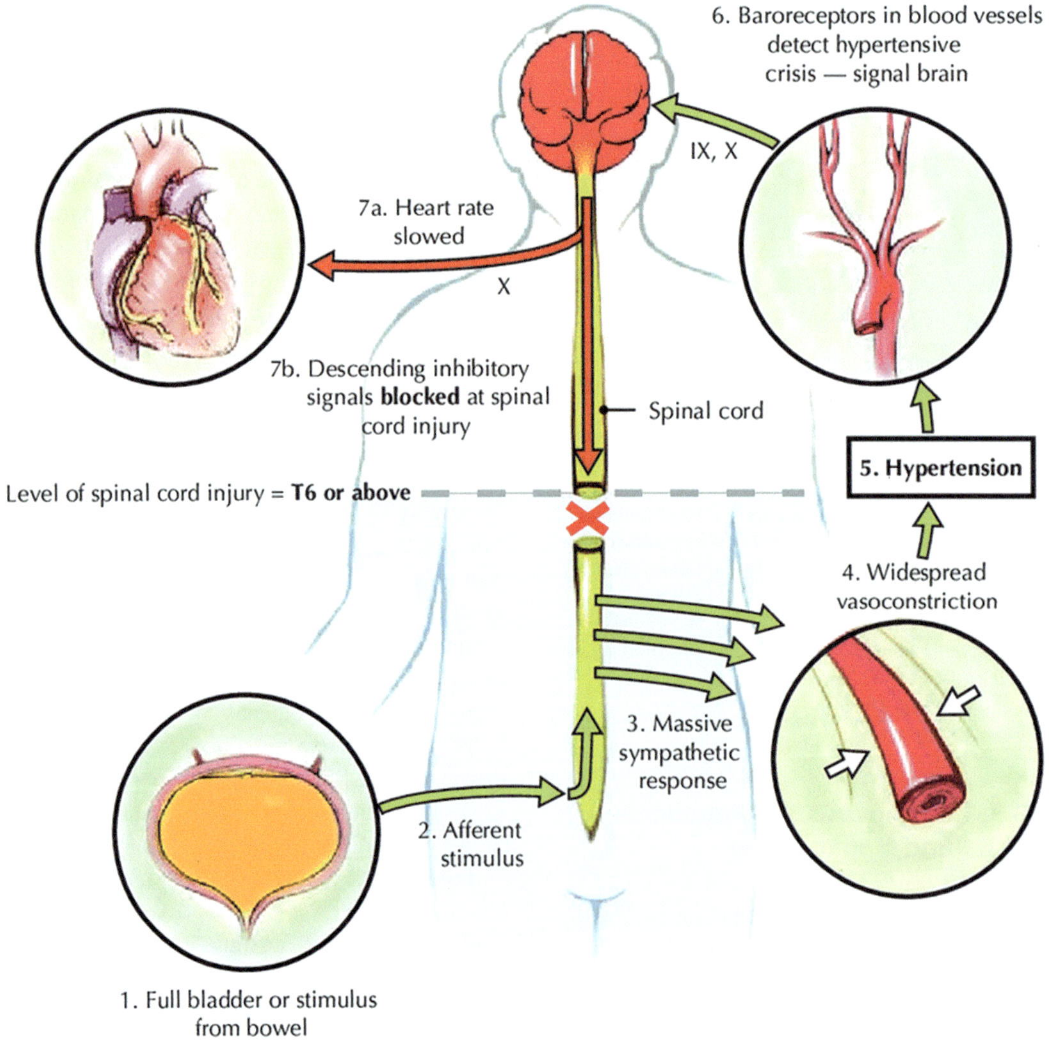

Fig. 48.2 Illustration of the pathophysiology of autonomic dysreflexia in spinal cord injury patients. The afferent stimulus, in this case a distended bladder, triggers a peripheral sympathetic response, which results in vasoconstriction and hypertension. Descending inhibitory signals, which normally counteract the rise in blood pressure, are blocked at the level of the spinal cord injury. The roman numerals (IX, X) refer to cranial nerves. (Source: Blackmer J. Rehabilitation medicine: 1. Autonomic dysreflexia. CMAJ. 2003 Oct 28;169(9):931–5)

vascular tone [35]. Uncontrolled sympathetic responses to noxious stimuli below the level of the injury lead to diffuse vasoconstriction and hypertension. A compensatory parasympathetic response produces bradycardia and vasodilation above the level of the lesion, but this is insufficient to reduce the elevated blood pressure. SCI lesions lower than T6 do not produce this complication because intact splanchnic innervation allows for compensatory dilatation of the splanchnic vascular bed.

The most important aspect of managing AD is preventing inciting stimuli (e.g. urological, gastrointestinal, musculoskeletal). Immediate measures should include sitting the patient upright to orthostatically lower blood pressure, removing tight-fitting clothes and searching for and correcting noxious inciting stimuli. Bladder distension and faecal impaction are the most common precipitants. Bladder catheterisation and evaluation for urinary tract infection should be undertaken; indwelling catheters should be checked for obstruction and a rectal examination should be performed. In addition, pharmacological management includes prompt blood pressure reduction with a rapid-onset/short-duration agent, depending on the severity of the attack and response to the above measures. Agents commonly used are intravenous administration of hydralazine (10 mg) or labetalol (10 mg). Oral agents include nifedipine (10 mg). Nitrates should be avoided in patients who may use sildenafil.

48.7.6 Thromboprophylaxis

Stasis and hypercoagulability are the two major factors contributing to the development of thrombosis in this patient population [36]. The incidence of deep vein thrombosis occurs in 50–100% of untreated patients in the first 12 weeks, with the first 2 weeks having the highest rate following acute injury. The 2016 Consortium for Spinal Cord Medicine guidelines and the Neurocritical Care Society suggest that all patients should receive pharmacological prophylaxis with subcutaneous LMWH unless there is a significant contraindication [37]. Full anticoagulation is not recommended in the acute phase due to bleeding risk. For patients in whom anticoagulation is contraindicated, mechanical methods should be used and an inferior vena cava filter can be considered. LMWH is safe within 24–48 h of surgical spine fixation [38].

48.7.7 Gastrointestinal Management

Bowel dysfunction is common after SCI and is increasingly recognised as a major physical and psychological difficulty for SCI patients [39]. The approach to bowel management should address faecal incontinence, constipation and functional mobility. The goal is a predictable and consistent regime to ensure bowel emptying and to avoid complications of bowel dysfunction (constipation, haemorrhoids, severe abdominal complications, superior mesenteric artery syndrome and AD). A typical routine includes regular laxatives to promote transit by keeping the stool soft. Suppositories should be started early to ensure effective colonic evacuation. Warm water should be given daily, followed by abdominal massage to stimulate the gastrocolic reflex to assist evacuation.

Paralytic ileus is expected, and the incidence of aspiration may be as high as 35%. A naso/orogastric tube should be inserted within 4 hours from admission. Feeding needs to be established slowly with the addition of prokinetics as needed.

Stress ulcer prophylaxis is mandatory for patients with acute SCI as they are at high risk of stress ulceration [40]. It is recommended for 4 weeks from admission.

48.7.8 Other Complications

Patients with high spinal cord injury have dysregulated temperature control due to disrupted autonomic pathways. Due to the lack of vasomotor control, they cannot sweat, which can lead to hyperthermia. Central hyperthermia responds poorly to antipyretics and can persist despite cooling wraps. There are case reports that central hyperthermia can be controlled by the administration of bromocriptine [41, 42] or baclofen [43, 44].

A pressure ulcer (PU) is an area of localised skin damage due to prolonged pressure alone or pressure in combination with shearing forces [45]. The loss of motor, sensory and autonomic control associated with a spinal cord injury (SCI) makes PUs the most common secondary medical complication associated with such an injury; up to 95% of adults with a SCI will develop at least one PU in their lifetime. PU can develop within hours, and the most common locations include the ischium, trochanter, sacrum and heel [46] (McKinley et al). Areas prone to PU formation should be examined daily. The application of emollients reduces friction over areas at risk. After spinal stabilisation, patients should log rolled every 2–3 h to minimise the risk for pressure sores. Early spinal fixation helps with the overall nursing of these patients.

48.7.9 Pain Management

Pain is a common consequence of a spinal cord injury (SCI) and has a major impact on quality of life through its impact on physical function, mood and participation in work, recreational and social activities. Several types of pain typically present following SCI, with central neuropathic pain being frequent and challenging to manage occurrence [47] (Siddall et al).

Surgical approaches usually relieve pain by reversing structural problems. Pharmacological options include pregabalin, anti-epileptic medication such as sodium valproate, anti-depressants, botulinum toxin injection, local anaesthetics and medical marijuana. Although opioids are sometimes regarded as relatively ineffective for the treatment of neuropathic pain, there is reasonably strong evidence to indicate the ability of opioids to produce a significant reduction in neuropathic SCI pain.

48.7.10 Steroids in SCI

The use of methylprednisolone after acute spinal cord injury has been under discussion for more than 20 years [48]. (Bresl. There is an ongoing debate about the efficacy and clinical impact of methylprednisolone in recovery from spinal cord injury, and studies show considerable variability in practice patterns among surgeons. Current guidelines do not recommend high doses of steroids [49] (Rouanet et al).

References

1. Kuo CC, Soliman MAR, Aguirre AO, et al. Risk factors of early complications after thoracic and lumbar spinal deformity surgery: a systematic review and meta-analysis. Eur Spine J. 2023;32(3):899–913. https://doi.org/10.1007/s00586-022-07486-3.
2. Nasser R, Yadla S, Maltenfort MG, et al. Complications in spinal surgery: a review. J Neurosurg Spine. 2010;13:144–57.
3. Campbell PG, Malone J, Yadla S, et al. Early complications related to approach in thoracic and lumbar spinal surgery: a single center prospective study. World Neurosurg. 2010;73:395–401.
4. Campbell PG, Yadla S, Malone J, et al. Early complications related to approach in cervical spinal surgery: single-center prospective study. World Neurosurg. 2010;74:363–8.
5. Membership of the Difficult Airway Society Extubation Guidelines Group, Popat M, Mitchell V, et al. Difficult airway society guidelines for the management of tracheal extubation. Anaesthesia. 2012;67:318–40.
6. Jain M, Lal J, Aggrawal D, Sharma J, Singh AK, Bansal T. A study to evaluate changes in modified Mallampati class in patients undergoing spinal surgery in prone position. Cureus. 2022;14:e25767. https://doi.org/10.7759/cureus.25767.
7. Apfelbaum JL, Hagberg CA, Connis RT, et al. 2022 American Society of Anesthesiologists practice guidelines for management of the difficult airway. Anesthesiology. 2022;136:31–81.
8. Higgs A, McGrath BA, Goddard C, et al. Guidelines for the management of tracheal intubation in critically ill adults. Br J Anaesth. 2018;120:323–52.
9. De la Garza RR, Passias PG, Schwab F, Bydon A, Lafage V, Sciubba DM. Incidence, risk factors, and mortality of reintubation in adult spinal deformity surgery. Clin Spine Surg. 2017;30:E896–900.
10. Jaber S, Quintard H, Cinotti R, et al. Risk factors and outcomes for airway failure versus non-airway failure in the intensive care unit: a multicenter observational study of 1514 extubation procedures. Crit Care. 2018;22:1–12.
11. De Jong A, Talmor D, Jaber S. How to optimize extubation? Intensive Care Med. 2023;49(3):337–40. https://doi.org/10.1007/s00134-022-06964-y.
12. Holcomb JB, Tilley BC, Baraniuk S, et al. Transfusion of plasma, platelets, and red blood cells in a 1: 1: 1 vs a 1: 1: 2 ratio and mortality in patients with severe

trauma: the PROPPR randomized clinical trial. JAMA. 2015;313:471–82.
13. Kim HJ, Iyer S, Zebala LP, et al. Perioperative neurologic complications in adult spinal deformity surgery: incidence and risk factors in 564 patients. Spinal. 2017;42:420–7.
14. Chen Q, Zhong X, Liu W, Wong C, He Q, Chen Y. Incidence of postoperative symptomatic spinal epidural hematoma requiring surgical evacuation: a systematic review and meta-analysis. Eur Spine J. 2022;31:3274–85. https://doi.org/10.1007/s00586-022-07421-6.
15. Sommer M, De Rijke JM, Van Kleef M, et al. The prevalence of postoperative pain in a sample of 1490 surgical inpatients. Eur J Anaesthesiol. 2008;25:267–74.
16. Mosenthal WP, Landy DC, Boyajian HH, et al. Thromboprophylaxis in spinal surgery. Spine. 2018;43:E474–E81.
17. NICE guideline. Venous thromboembolism in over 16s: reducing the risk of hospital-acquired deep vein thrombosis or pulmonary embolism 2018 [updated 13 Aug 2019]. https://www.nice.org.uk/guidance/ng89/chapter/recommendations#interventions-for-people-having-elective-spinal-surgery-or-cranial-surgery-or-people-with-spinal.
18. Kwan I, Bunn F, Roberts I. Spinal immobilisation for trauma patients. Cochrane Database Syst Rev. 2001;2001(2):CD002803. https://doi.org/10.1002/14651858.CD002803.
19. Swartz EE, Del Rossi G. Cervical spine alignment during on-field management of potential catastrophic spine injuries. Sports Health. 2009;1(3):247–52. https://doi.org/10.1177/1941738109334211.
20. Mills BM, Conrick KM, Anderson S, Bailes J, Boden BP, Conway D, Ellis J, Feld F, Grant M, Hainline B, Henry G, Herring SA, Hsu WK, Isakov A, Lindley TR, McNamara L, Mihalik JP, Neal TL, Putukian M, Rivara FP, Sills AK, Swartz EE, Vavilala MS, Courson R. Consensus recommendations on the prehospital Care of the Injured Athlete with a suspected catastrophic cervical spine injury. J Athl Train. 2020;55(6):563–72. https://doi.org/10.4085/1062-6050-0434.19.
21. Crosby ET. Airway management in adults after cervical spine trauma. Anesthesiology. 2006;104(6):1293–318. https://doi.org/10.1097/00000542-200606000-00026.
22. Adams JP, Bell D, McKinlay J. Neurocritical Care—a guide to practical management. Springer; 2010. https://doi.org/10.1007/978-1-84882-070-8.
23. Jung JY. Airway management of patients with traumatic brain injury/C-spine injury. Korean J Anesthesiol. 2015;68(3):213–9. https://doi.org/10.4097/kjac.2015.68.3.213.
24. Martyn JA, Richtsfeld M. Succinylcholine-induced hyperkalemia in acquired pathologic states: etiologic factors and molecular mechanisms. Anesthesiology. 2006;104(1):158–69. https://doi.org/10.1097/00000542-200601000-00022.
25. Kirshblum SC, Burns SP, Biering-Sorensen F, Donovan W, Graves DE, Jha A, Johansen M, Jones L, Krassioukov A, Mulcahey MJ, Schmidt-Read M, Waring W. International standards for neurological classification of spinal cord injury (revised 2011). J Spinal Cord Med. 2011;34(6):535–46. https://doi.org/10.1179/204577211X13207446293695.
26. Stevens RD, Bhardwaj A, Kirsch JR, Mirski MA. Critical care and perioperative management in traumatic spinal cord injury. J Neurosurg Anesthesiol. 2003;15(3):215–29. https://doi.org/10.1097/00008506-200307000-00009.
27. Estenne M, De Troyer A. Mechanism of the postural dependence of vital capacity in tetraplegic subjects. Am Rev Respir Dis. 1987;135(2):367–71. https://doi.org/10.1164/arrd.1987.135.2.367.
28. Baydur A, Adkins RH, Milic-Emili J. Lung mechanics in individuals with spinal cord injury: effects of injury level and posture. J Appl Physiol (1985). 2001;90(2):405–11. https://doi.org/10.1152/jappl.2001.90.2.405.
29. Lehmann KG, Lane JG, Piepmeier JM, Batsford WP. Cardiovascular abnormalities accompanying acute spinal cord injury in humans: incidence, time course and severity. J Am Coll Cardiol. 1987;10(1):46–52. https://doi.org/10.1016/s0735-1097(87)80158-4.
30. Atkinson PP, Atkinson JL. Spinal shock. Mayo Clin Proc. 1996;71(4):384–9. https://doi.org/10.4065/71.4.384.
31. Jia X, Kowalski RG, Sciubba DM, Geocadin RG. Critical care of traumatic spinal cord injury. J Intensive Care Med. 2013;28(1):12–23. https://doi.org/10.1177/0885066611403270.
32. Hadley MN, Walters BC, Grabb PA, Oyesiku NM, Przybylski GJ, Resnick DK, Ryken TC. Blood pressure management after acute spinal cord injury. Neurosurgery. 2002;50(3 Suppl):S58–62. https://doi.org/10.1097/00006123-200203001-00012.
33. Silver JR. Early autonomic dysreflexia. Spinal Cord. 2000;38(4):229–33. https://doi.org/10.1038/sj.sc.3100996.
34. Blackmer J. Rehabilitation medicine: 1. Autonomic dysreflexia. CMAJ. 2003;169(9):931–5.
35. Bycroft J, Shergill IS, Chung EA, Arya N, Shah PJ. Autonomic dysreflexia: a medical emergency. Postgrad Med J. 2005;81(954):232–5. https://doi.org/10.1136/pgmj.2004.024463. Erratum in: Postgrad Med J 2005 Oct;81(960):672. Choong, E A L [corrected to Chung, E A L]
36. Merli GJ, Crabbe S, Paluzzi RG, Fritz D. Etiology, incidence, and prevention of deep vein thrombosis in acute spinal cord injury. Arch Phys Med Rehabil. 1993;74(11):1199–205.
37. Nyquist P, Jichici D, Bautista C, Burns J, Chhangani S, DeFilippis M, Goldenberg FD, Kim K, Liu-DeRyke X, Mack W, Meyer K. Prophylaxis of venous thrombosis in Neurocritical care patients: an executive summary of evidence-based guidelines: a statement for healthcare professionals from the Neurocritical care society and Society of Critical Care Medicine. Crit Care Med. 2017;45(3):476–9. https://doi.org/10.1097/CCM.0000000000002247.

38. Kim DY, Kobayashi L, Chang D, Fortlage D, Coimbra R. Early pharmacological venous thromboembolism prophylaxis is safe after operative fixation of traumatic spine fractures. Spine (Phila Pa 1976). 2015;40(5):299–304. https://doi.org/10.1097/BRS.0000000000000754.
39. Lynch AC, Antony A, Dobbs BR, Frizelle FA. Bowel dysfunction following spinal cord injury. Spinal Cord. 2001;39(4):193–203. https://doi.org/10.1038/sj.sc.3101119.
40. Simons RK, Hoyt DB, Winchell RJ, Holbrook T, Eastman AB. A risk analysis of stress ulceration after trauma. J Trauma. 1995;39(2):289–93; discussion 293–4. https://doi.org/10.1097/00005373-199508000-00017.
41. Natteru P, George P, Bell R, Nattanmai P, Newey CR. Central hyperthermia treated with Bromocriptine. Case Rep Neurol Med. 2017;2017:1712083. https://doi.org/10.1155/2017/1712083.
42. Ge X, Luan X. Uncontrolled central hyperthermia by standard dose of bromocriptine: a case report. World J Clin Cases. 2020;8(23):6158–63. https://doi.org/10.12998/wjcc.v8.i23.6158.
43. Lee HC, Kim JM, Lim JK, Jo YS, Kim SK. Central hyperthermia treated with baclofen for patient with pontine hemorrhage. Ann Rehabil Med. 2014;38(2):269–72. https://doi.org/10.5535/arm.2014.38.2.269.
44. Huang YS, Hsiao MC, Lee M, Huang YC, Lee JD. Baclofen successfully abolished prolonged central hyperthermia in a patient with basilar artery occlusion. Acta Neurol Taiwanica. 2009;18(2):118–22.
45. Marin J, Nixon J, Gorecki C. A systematic review of risk factors for the development and recurrence of pressure ulcers in people with spinal cord injuries. Spinal Cord. 2013;51(7):522–7.
46. McKinley WO, Jackson AB, Cardenas DD, DeVivo MJ. Long-term medical complications after traumatic spinal cord injury: a regional model systems analysis. Arch Phys Med Rehabil. 1999;80(11):1402–10. https://doi.org/10.1016/s0003-9993(99)90251-4.
47. Siddall PJ, Middleton JW. Spinal cord injury-induced pain: mechanisms and treatments. Pain Manag. 2015;5(6):493–507. https://doi.org/10.2217/pmt.15.47.
48. Breslin K, Agrawal D. The use of methylprednisolone in acute spinal cord injury: a review of the evidence, controversies, and recommendations. Pediatr Emerg Care. 2012;28(11):1238–45.; quiz 1246-8. https://doi.org/10.1097/PEC.0b013e3182724434.
49. Rouanet C, Reges D, Rocha E, Gagliardi V, Silva GS. Traumatic spinal cord injury: current concepts and treatment update. Arq Neuropsiquiatr. 2017;75(6):387–93. https://doi.org/10.1590/0004-282X20170048.

Vascular Neurosurgery (Aneurysm) and Neurocritical Care

49

Deep Sengupta and Charu Mahajan

49.1 Introduction

Aneurysmal subarachnoid haemorrhage (aSAH) is an important health concern worldwide. Global incidence and prevalence of aSAH is ~6.1 per 100,000 person-years and eight million respectively [1, 2]. Women, especially of age > 55 years, have been reported to have a higher predilection for aSAH as compared to men [1, 3]. The significantly high morbidity and mortality (~13% in hospital and ~ 26% pre-hospital) associated with aSAH warrant improved treatment protocols in the management of such patients [4–6]. Key modifiable risk factors include history of smoking and hypertension [1]. Early brain injury associated with aSAH has multifactorial pathophysiological mechanisms which in turn drives the secondary complications and affects the overall outcome [7, 8]. Securing the ruptured aneurysm timely, prevention of rebleeding and multidisciplinary critical care management of the secondary complications like cerebral oedema, hydrocephalus, raised intracranial pressure (ICP), delayed cerebral ischaemia (DCI) is of utmost importance to improve the outcomes [9]. Literature confirms the adverse effects of aSAH on cognitive recovery, mood disorders and overall quality of life [7].

D. Sengupta
Department of Neuroanesthesiology and Critical Care, Max Superspeciality Hospital, Saket, New Delhi, India

C. Mahajan (✉)
Department of Neuroanaesthesiology and Critical Care, AIIMS, New Delhi, India

49.2 Diagnosis of aSAH

The classic clinical history of aSAH is a sudden onset headache reaching maximal intensity in a short time, often described as the 'worst imaginable' [10]. A sentinel headache preceding the aSAH is reported to occur in 10–43% of cases which represents minor leaks [11]. Patients may also present with neck pain, new focal neurological deficit, syncope or seizures. The Ottawa SAH rule, is reported to have 100% sensitivity but low specificity to identify high-risk patients [12]. According to Ottawa subarachnoid haemorrhage rule, presence of any of the following in an alert patient with severe headache—age ≥ 40 years, presence of neck pain or stiffness, loss of consciousness, onset during exertion, instantly peaking headache and limited neck flexion or examination alerts physician to evaluate patient for SAH [13].

Early diagnosis and prompt institution of therapy is essential and any delay in the identification of aSAH is catastrophic. A non-contrast head CT (NCCT) scan done within 6 h of symptom onset, has a high sensitivity (98.7%) and specificity (99.9%) [14]. CT angiography (CTA) and Lumbar puncture (LP) are recommended as addi-

H. Prabhakar et al. (eds.), *Principles and Practice of Neurocritical Care*,
https://doi.org/10.1007/978-981-99-8059-8_49

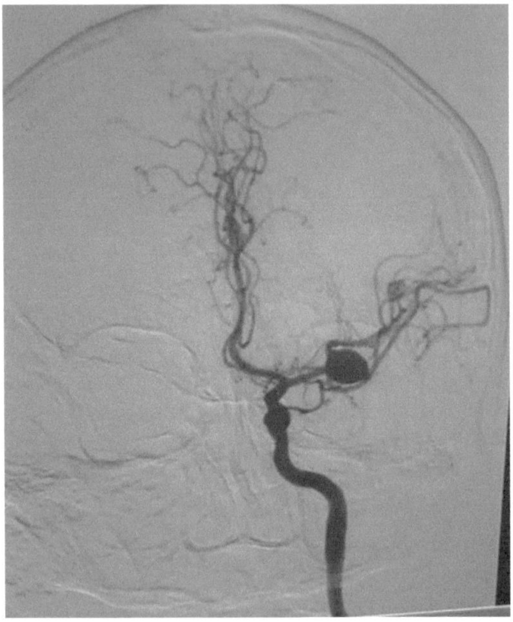

Fig. 49.1 DSA head showing 12 × 10 mm left MCA bifurcation aneurysm

tional diagnostic studies if NCCT head is inconclusive in a patient with high suspicion of SAH presenting with atypical symptoms [15]. Digital subtraction angiography (DSA) [Fig. 49.1] is considered the gold standard for evaluating aneurysmal anatomy and further aids in choosing the optimal treatment strategy [16]. Further studies are warranted to establish the diagnostic accuracy of established magnetic resonance imaging sequences in aSAH.

49.3 Outcome Prediction Based on Severity of aSAH Grading

Younger patients have more favourable outcomes (82% vs. 42%) compared to older patients (>65 years) as reported in Barrow Ruptured Aneurysm Trial (BRAT) [17]. Grading the severity of aSAH after initial stabilisation enables the physician to prognosticate and anticipate complications. Various scores like Hunt and Hess (HH), World Federation of Neurological Surgeons (WFNS), radiographic Fisher scale are commonly used in clinical practice. Composite grades like VASOGRADE, HAIR (HH grade, age, intraventricular haematoma, rebleed), SAHIT (Subarachnoid Haemorrhage International Trialists) consider important features to help in outcome prediction [18, 19].

The most commonly used HH score grades patients into 1–5 with grade 1: asymptomatic or mild headache, no neurological deficit, slight nuchal rigidity +; grade 2: moderate-severe headache, cranial nerve deficit +; grade 3: drowsy/confused, mild focal deficit+; grade 4: Stupor, hemiparesis, vegetative disturbances and grade 5: Comatose, moribund patients [20]. Presence of severe atherosclerosis, hypertension, diabetes, chronic pulmonary disease and severe vasospasm places the patient in next higher grade. World Federation of Neurological Surgeons (WFNS) considers patients' GCS and motor deficit to classify them into grades 1–5. High-grade SAH is clinically defined as grade 4 and 5 on either HH scale or WFNS scale.

49.4 Early Brain Injury

The aneurysm rupture heralds extravasation of blood into the subarachnoid space and it may also spill into ventricles and parenchyma. This causes rapid rise in ICP, decrease in cerebral blood flow (CBF) and compromised cerebral perfusion pressure (CPP) resulting in brain tissue hypoxia. This causes microcirculatory dysfunction, breakdown of blood–brain barrier, inflammation, cortical spreading depolarisation, impairment of autoregulation and global cerebral oedema. This period of early brain injury (EBI) (first 72 h) is believed to be harbinger of DCI and long-term poor outcome [21]. Higher grade of SAH scale scores are more likely to develop EBI and subsequent complications.

49.5 Stabilisation

It includes immediate care of airway, breathing by means of securing the airway if indicated and normalising the cardiovascular functions. These patients should be timely transferred to the hospital having facility of experienced surgeons, neuroendovascular interventionalists and neurointensive care services for an overall improved outcome.

49.6 ICU Concerns and Complications

Early major concerns like rebleeding, control of blood pressure and raised ICP require urgent intervention. Multiple complications like development of fever (infectious or non-infectious), dyselectrolytemia, DCI or vasospasm, venous thromboembolism, neurogenic stunned myocardium and neurogenic stunned myocardium can develop in patients as aftermath of aSAH [22, 23]. Early prevention, prompt diagnosis and treatment of these complications are the mainstays of critical care management in aSAH patients.

49.6.1 Rebleeding

One of the major early concerns is rebleeding which can be disabling and even fatal. Securing the ruptured aneurysm promptly is the most effective treatment to reduce the possibility of rebleeding [24, 25].

ULTRA (Ultra-Early Tranexamic Acid After Subarachnoid Haemorrhage) trial did not demonstrate any improvement in rate of rebleeding (10% in tranexamic group vs. 14% in control group) or functional outcomes (60% in Tranexamic group vs. 64% in control group) [26]. Antifibrinolytics are thus not routinely recommended to improve outcome, based on the current evidence [16, 27–29]. Other risk-factors for rebleeding are high blood pressure and patients receiving anticoagulation. Reversal of anticoagulation in any patient presenting with aSAH is advised based on the benefits demonstrated in other forms of intracranial haemorrhage [30, 31].

49.6.2 Blood Pressure Control

Blood pressure monitoring is recommended in all patients along with its control in those having severe hypertension at presentation (>180–200 mmHg). Short-acting medications are preferred to avoid severe hypotension. Hypotension (mean arterial pressure < 65 mmHg) must be avoided to prevent its deleterious effect on acutely injured brain [32, 33]. A systolic BP >160 mmHg was reported to be associated with a higher rate of rebleeding in a meta-analysis [34]. However, based on the current evidence, recent guidelines do not recommend any specific BP target [16]. This does not imply that blood pressure reduction is not helpful before aneurysm treatment but the evidence is not strong enough to recommend a specific reduction goal [27]. Increased blood pressure variability needs to be avoided as it is associated with worse outcomes. In cases where reduction of blood pressure is required, it is prudent to consider certain factors like BP at the time of presentation, cerebral oedema and renal impairment among others to help individualise the pressure targets. Future studies are required to comment conclusively on efficacy of therapeutic BP targets, usage of MAP as cut-off target or on minimisation of BP variability during BP reduction.

49.6.3 Hydrocephalus

Cerebrospinal fluid (CSF) flow is hindered due to obstruction caused by the blood products resulting in obstructive hydrocephalus (HCP). Subsequent adhesions at the arachnoid granulations result in reduced CSF absorption leading to the development of communicating HCP [35]. Incidence of hydrocephalus is reported to be between 15% and 87% in acute-stage post-aSAH [36].

CSF diversion procedures in the acute stage include insertion of either external ventricular drain (EVD) or lumbar drain. In the setting of acute neurological deterioration due to hydrocephalus, institution of a CSF diversion procedure has demonstrated improved neurological outcomes [37, 38]. Ventriculostomy-associated infection is a major concern in critical care management of such patients. Although various measures have been proposed to mitigate this hazard which include usage of antibiotic impregnated catheters, reduced frequency of sampling, bundled care and strict aseptic precautions while handling, no specific recommendation can be made for any intervention as there is not enough current evidence present in the literature [39, 40].

Chronic shunt-dependent hydrocephalus incidence has been reported in the literature to be 8.9% to 48% [36]. Risk factors for the development of shunt-dependent chronic hydrocephalus include high-grade aSAH, acute hydrocephalus, associated intraventricular haemorrhage, rebleeding, vasospasm and long duration of EVD requirement [41, 42]. Placement of a permanent shunt in patients with chronic hydrocephalus is shown to have better improved neurological outcomes.

49.6.4 Raised Intracranial Pressure

Acute aSAH causes activation of inflammatory cascade and breakdown of blood–brain barrier, resulting in cerebral oedema. Higher grades of aSAH are associated with more risk of oedema and intracranial hypertension. Conditions like development of HCP, cerebral infarct, hyponatraemia, increased intrathoracic pressure secondary to development of ARDS or neurogenic pulmonary oedema can lead to raised ICP. General principles like head up, administration of analgesics and osmotic diuretics are helpful. Either hypertonic saline or mannitol may be used for this purpose keeping a target of serum osmolality 320 mEq and serum sodium of 155 mEq as the upper threshold [43]. Specific management of underlying conditions is required to lower down ICP.

ICP monitoring is a reasonable option in critical care management, particularly in patients with high-grade SAH or acute hydrocephalus who are at risk of developing ICP [44]. This can be easily done via an EVD if it is in situ. Benefits conferred by ICP monitoring in patients without hydrocephalus is debatable. Baggiani et al. evaluated the variability in ICP monitoring practice across countries, treatment and effect on outcome in aSAH patients. The authors found high variability in ICP insertion practice across countries. In more severe patients, ICP monitoring was significantly associated with better 6-month neurological outcome [45].

49.6.5 Seizures

Incidence of seizures post-aSAH has been reported from as low as 2.3% to as high as 15.2% in various studies [46, 47]. Seizures can be categorised as onset (occurring at the time of haemorrhage), early (within a week of ictus) and late (after more than 7 days), with onset seizures having unfavourable prognosis and are predictive of poor long-term outcome [48]. American Clinical Neurophysiology Society defines seizures as 'epileptiform discharges averaging >2.5 Hz for ≥10 s (>25 discharges in 10 s) or any pattern with definite evolution and lasting ≥10 s' [49].

EEG monitoring can be considered in patients with high-risk characteristics for developing seizures [50]. Generalised tonic-clonic convulsions can precipitate rebleeding subjecting patient to high morbidity and mortality. Prophylactic administration of antiepileptic drugs can be considered in patients having risk factors like high-grade SAH, acute hydrocephalus, location of aneurysm in middle cerebral artery (MCA), cortical infarction and surgically clipped aneurysm [51]. At present, there is paucity of high-quality data supporting prophylactic administration of antiepileptic drugs post-aSAH [52]. In a recent meta-analysis, short-term (<3 days) administration of prophylactic antiepileptics is reported to have a favourable long-term outcome as compared to long-term (>3 days) administration, while the efficacy in preventing seizures was comparable in both the groups [46].

High suspicion for non-convulsive seizures is of vital importance as it may present with depressed level of consciousness or variable neurological examination, especially in the first 24–48 h. Treatment with newer generation antiepileptics is reasonable, while, usage of phenytoin has been reported to be associated with poorer cognitive outcomes [53]. In patients who present with seizures, administration of antiepileptics for less than 7 days is considered reasonable to reduce seizures-related complications in perioperative period [16].

49.6.6 Fever

Intracranial blood and breakdown products induce an inflammatory response manifesting as fever soon after ictus. This can exacerbate secondary brain injury by increase in cerebral metabolic rate, exacerbation of cerebral oedema and worsening of brain ischaemic injury. Fever is more commonly seen in poor-grade patients, those who have more bleed load and intraventricular haemorrhage [54, 55]. Control of fever has been observed to be associated with improved outcome [56]. Combination of non-pharmacological measures like cold sponging or cooling blankets, etc. along with administration of antipyretics is often utilised to control pyrexia. Infectious causes of fever should be sought and adequately treated. Institution of hypothermia as a neuroprotective therapy has not gained popularity because of lack of evidence.

49.6.7 Respiratory Complications

Altered sensorium, vomiting and aspiration can lead to pulmonary involvement and subsequent complications. Incidence of ARDS is ~3.6% within a week of ictus [57, 58]. An acute onset of pulmonary changes occurring after an aneurysm rupture is considered as neurogenic pulmonary oedema which is mainly caused by sympathetic hyperactivity secondary to release of catecholamines. The neurohaemodynamic theory postulates increase in systemic pressures leading to shift of blood from high-resistance systemic circulation to low-resistance pulmonary circulation, resulting in development of hydrostatic pulmonary oedema. The burst theory is based on acute increase in capillary pressure causing damage to alveolar-capillary membrane. The membrane becomes leaky resulting in development of protein-rich pulmonary oedema. The neurocardiac theory is based on direct injury to cardiomyocyte resulting in NPE. Other postulated mechanisms include release of inflammatory mediators that damage and alter the pulmonary capillaries permeability [59].

Clinical features include dyspnoea, tachypnoea, pink frothy secretions and hypoxia. The treatment focuses mainly on reduction of ICP to lessen the sympathetic hyperactivity. Rest of the management involves supportive treatment for pulmonary oedema. The need for mechanical ventilation >24 h requires implementation of standard ICU care bundle. Provision of bundled care which includes lung protective ventilation, moderate positive end-expiratory pressure application, institution of early enteral nutrition and adequate antibiotic therapy for pneumonia has shown to increase the ventilator-free days and reduces duration of ICU stay [60]. In cases of severe ARDS with refractory hypoxaemia, manoeuvres like alveolar recruitment and prone positioning may be implemented along with ICP monitoring [16].

49.6.8 Cardiac Complications

Acute left ventricular systolic dysfunction resulting from sympathetic surge, new ECG changes and increase in cardiac enzymes level is together referred to as neurogenic stunned myocardium (NSM) or neurogenic stress cardiomyopathy. This can result in complications such as arrhythmias, pulmonary oedema, wall motion abnormalities and heart failure. About 30% of the aSAH patients may experience NSM [61]. Common ECG changes observed are QT prolongation, ST-T wave changes, atrial fibrillation or flutter waves, sinus tachycardia and prominent U waves [62]. The ischaemic ECG changes do not follow a particular coronary vascular distribution and are associated with relatively low-troponin levels as compared to an acute coronary event. The wall motion abnormalities in NSM affect the left ventricle in global pattern. Takotsubo cardiomyopathy associated with apical ballooning is a type of a stress cardiomyopathy described in aSAH patients, that mimics acute coronary syndrome [63, 64]. NSM is generally considered to be reversible and coronary angiography is not routinely recommended for these new findings.

On admission, baseline 12-lead ECG and troponin levels should be sent, while echocardiography is prudent especially in patients with suspected myocardial dysfunction with data reporting an incidence of echocardiographic abnormalities in ~21% of patients [65]. Management remains supportive with administration of ionotropes for haemodynamic instability. The induction of hypertension as treatment for DCI can be a challenge in such patients and runs the risk of exacerbating cardiopulmonary dysfunction.

49.6.9 Intravascular Fluid and Electrolyte Abnormalities

Acute subarachnoid haemorrhage is associated with electrolyte abnormalities like hyponatraemia (20–40%), hypomagnesaemia (40%), hypokalaemia (25%) and hypernatraemia (20%) [66–69]. Hyponatraemia is secondary to hypothalamic injury which may lead to inappropriate secretion of antidiuretic hormone (SIADH) or cerebral salt wasting syndrome. Cerebral salt wasting is characterised by excessive renal sodium excretion due to increased atrial natriuretic factor [70]. Both these entities have similar laboratory parameters including hyponatraemia (<134 mEq/L), low-serum osmolality (<274 mosmol/kg), high urine sodium (>40 mEq/L) and high urine osmolality (>100 mosmol/kg), and are thus, difficult to distinguish. The major difference between them is that SIADH patients are usually euvolaemic to slightly hypervolaemic while cerebral salt wasting patients are hypovolaemic. The aSAH patients may be volume depleted in the acute stage. Associated natriuresis may also result in hypovolaemic state and is a risk factor for development of DCI and poor outcome. Close monitoring and early goal-directed fluid therapy within 24 h of ictus is shown to have been associated with decreased incidence of DCI and reduced length of ICU stay [71, 72]. There is no role of prophylactic or therapeutic hypervolaemia in management of DCI.

Administration of large-volume isotonic crystalloids and restriction of free-water intake should be applied to counteract potential hypovolaemia and to prevent inappropriate water retention. Hypertonic saline (3%) may be used to correct hyponatraemia [73, 74]. Treatment of symptomatic hyponatraemia in SIADH is hypertonic saline as volume restriction may lead to intravascular volume contraction and accentuate the vasospasm-related ischaemic injury SAH. Conivaptan is an arginine vasopressin receptor antagonist (V_{1A}/V_2) approved for the treatment of euvolaemic and hypervolaemic hyponatraemia [75]. Initial reports of its use in neurocritical care patients with hyponatraemia have yielded promising results [76]. Caution should be taken to avoid hypovolaemia with the use of conivaptan.

Fludrocortisone is effective in treating natriuresis but it does not reduce the incidence of DCI or affects outcome [77]. The recent guidelines state that mineralocorticoids use is reasonable to treat natriuresis and hyponatraemia (Class 2a) [16].

49.6.10 Cerebral Vasospasm and Delayed Cerebral Ischaemia

Cerebral vasospasm and DCI are a major cause of post-aSAH morbidity and mortality [25]. The incidence of DCI has been reported to be as high as 30%, most commonly between days 4 and 14 after aSAH. It is defined as the occurrence of focal neurological impairment (aphasia, hemiparesis) or a decrease of at least 2 points on the GCS, lasting for at least 1 h and is not apparent immediately after aneurysm obliteration, and cannot be attributed to other causes. New cerebral infarction has been defined as the presence of cerebral infarction on CT or magnetic resonance imaging scan of the brain within 6 weeks after aSAH not attributable to other causes [78–80]. Multiple pathophysiological mechanisms have been suggested for DCI which include EBI, microthrombosis, blood–brain barrier disruption, cortical spreading depolarisation and cerebral autoregulation failure among others [81]. Cerebral Vasospasm refers to the angiographic narrowing of the cerebral arteries leading to cerebral ischaemia that may result in impending cerebral infarction.

Repeated neurological examinations can be a good monitoring tool to identify the onset of any new neurological deficits attributable to cerebral ischaemia. This becomes unreliable in poor-grade patients who are comatose.

DSA is the gold standard for detection of narrowing of cerebral vessels and allows therapeutic instillation of intra-arterial vasodilators if vasospastic territory is identified. However, it is invasive and does not reveal the perfusion state of the cerebral tissue. Compared with DSA, CTA has been demonstrated to have a false-positive rate of 5% and diagnostic accuracy of 90% [82]. High specificity of CTA makes it a good tool for screening patients for vasospasm. CT Perfusion imaging aids in early detection of perfusion abnormalities, and both CTA and CTP can help guide the treatment decisions [83, 84].

Transcranial doppler (TCD) allows multiple, dynamic and non-invasive bedside assessment of vasospasm [85, 86]. Mean flow velocity (cm/sec), Lindegaard's ratio and Sviri ratio can be used to categorise vasospasm into mild, moderate and severe. Lindegaard's ratio is derived by dividing the mean flow velocities of the MCA by those of ipsilateral extracranial ICA and the Sviri ratio by dividing the mean flow velocities of basilar artery (BA) by those of extracranial vertebral artery (VA). For middle cerebral artery, vasospasm is deemed mild if mean flow velocity is 120–149 cm/s, moderate if it is 150–199 cm/s and severe if it is >200 cm/s with corresponding Lindegaard's ratio being 3–6 for mild to moderate vasospasm and > 6 for severe vasospasm. For basilar artery, a mean flow velocity of >70 cm/s is considered as mild to moderate vasospasm, and > 85 cm/s is severe vasospasm, while, a Sviri ratio of >2 is considered as mild, >2.5 is moderate and > 2.5 as severe vasospasm [87].

cEEG has been utilised in predicting DCI and the criterion includes decreasing alpha-to-delta power ratio, relative alpha power variability, epileptiform discharges, rhythmic and periodic ictal-interictal continuum patterns and isolated alpha suppression. Critical alpha power reduction of >40% for >5 h indicates an increased risk of poor functional outcome [88].

The cerebral ischaemia manifests as decrease in cerebral oxygenation when monitored by near infrared spectroscopy (NIRS), and brain tissue oxygenation ($PbtO_2$). However, utility of these monitors is limited by their focal assessment of brain milieu. Cerebral microdialysis allows detection of markers of anaerobic metabolism, excitotoxic metabolites and markers of cell membrane damage, depicting ongoing cerebral ischaemia. Bihemispheric cerebral microdialysis has been shown to have better predictive ability to detect DCI [89]. However, its high cost limits its wider applicability.

49.7 Prevention

Nimodipine administered at an oral dose of 60 mg four hourly is reported to be beneficial in improving functional outcome and reduction of cerebral infarction [90, 91]. In clinical practice, oral nimodipine should be started as soon as the diagnosis is confirmed. Intravenous nimodipine can be started at 15 mcg/kg/h for the first 2 h, if well-tolerated and no haemodynamic instability occurs, dose can be increased to 30 mcg/kg/h [92]. However, there is limited evidence to recommend the intravenous or intra-arterial administration of nimodipine [93]. The recent guidelines strongly recommend against administration of intravenous nicardipine for prevention of DCI [27].

Maintenance of euvolaemia, reduction of BP variability during the critical care period and prevention of secondary brain insults remains the mainstay for prevention of DCI. There is no role of prophylactic hypertensive therapy in aSAH patients at risk of DCI [16].

Drainage of CSF via an EVD or lumbar drain helps remove blood products which play an important role in development of DCI. A recent randomised controlled trial studied the effectiveness of early lumbar drain CSF drainage (within 72 h) in 144 aSAH patients after aneurysm treatment. Prophylactic insertion of lumbar drain decreased the incidence of secondary infarction and unfavourable 6-month outcome in aSAH patients [94].

49.8 Management

Current evidence lends credence to the fact that induced hypertension is a rational choice in managing patients with DCI [95, 96]. Induced hypertension is initiated by targeting a pressure of 20 mmHg above the baseline mean blood pressure or systolic blood pressure, with norepinephrine being the vasopressor of choice usually, and is titrated to a maximum of 220 mmHg systolic blood pressure in patients whom aneurysm has been definitively managed [97]. aSAH patients having symptomatic vasospasm should have systolic BP elevation and maintenance of euvolaemia to reduce the progression and severity of DCI [16].

Milrinone has emerged as a promising therapy for treating cerebral vasospasm owing to its selective inhibition of the low-Km cAMP-specific phosphodiesterase-3, which is associated with circulatory inotropic support and selective cerebral-vasodilatory effects [98, 99]. Intravenous milrinone is a reasonable option, but warrants future studies to more accurately define its role in the management of vasospasm [99, 100]. As per Montreal neurological hospital protocol, milrinone bolus 0.1–0.2 mg/kg IV was given followed by an infusion of 0.75 mcg/kg/min; infusion was titrated up to a maximum of 1.25 mcg/kg/min, while MAP was maintained >90 mmHg. If there was no recurrence of symptoms after 72 h, the infusion was tapered by 0.25 mcg/kg/min every 24–48 h until discontinuation [99]. Complications reported with IV milrinone therapy include new or worsening arrhythmia, hypokalaemia and pulmonary oedema [101]. In cases of refractory vasospasm, intra-arterial administration of milrinone has been reported with doses varying from 2 mg to 10 mg for each segment or 0.25 mg/min infusion until a satisfactory angiographic response is obtained [101, 102].

If neuro-worsening does not resolve, we need to proceed to endovascular rescue therapy. Intra-arterial administration of vasodilators is a reasonable modality to treat vasospasm effectively, but its overall benefit in preventing DCI and improving functional outcome requires further studies [103, 104]. The common agents used for this purpose include nimodipine and milrinone intermittent boluses through an intracranial microcatheter. Cerebral angioplasty is a reasonable option in refractory cerebral vasospasm, which is not amenable to pharmacological drugs. But it is associated with risk of cerebral vessel rupture and consequent high morbidity.

There is no evidence suggestive of improved outcomes in patients with aSAH with statins or magnesium sulphate and they are currently not recommended in routine management [106].

Promising measures which require robust future studies include neural ganglia blocks, administration of cisternal fibrinolytics to aid in clearance of subarachnoid blood and delivering medication intrathecally like (haptoglobin, deferoxamine, nimodipine, nicardipine, milrinone, nitric oxide) [16].

49.9 Other Neurocritical Care Concerns

49.9.1 Deep Vein Thrombosis

About 4%–24% of aSAH patients develop venous thromboembolism (VTE) making mechanical thromboprophylaxis, a part of standard neurocritical care. This is a safe approach prior to definitive treatment of ruptured aneurysm. Early pharmacological prophylaxis (<24 h after aneurysm occlusion) found no significant haemorrhagic complications as compared to late (>24 h) institution, in a case control study [106]. Based on this, AHA recommends (Class 1) that once the ruptured aneurysm is secured, mechanical or pharmacological venous thromboprophylaxis should be initiated to reduce the risk for VTE. However, optimal time of pharmacological prophylaxis and agent to be used remains inconclusive, and institutional protocol may be followed.

49.9.2 Anaemia

Anaemia can be deleterious for the injured brain and can accentuate ischaemic insult. Blood transfusion can increase cerebral oxygenation but optimal threshold remains inconclusive. Though theoretically a threshold of 9–10 gm/dl in patients with DCI should be preferable, the available literature fails to recommend using transfusion threshold higher than Hb > 7 g/dl in patients with aSAH [27]. Further studies are required to determine optimal haemoglobin thresholds and indication for transfusion in patients with aSAH.

49.9.3 Glucose Control

Hyperglycaemia and hypoglycaemia both induce secondary brain injury and need to be treated promptly. Increased glucose level is consistently associated with poor functional outcome. The optimal threshold for treatment has not been defined in guidelines but a limit of 180 mg/dl is considered reasonable in acute brain injury.

49.9.4 Nutritional Support

Enteral nutrition should be initiated as early as possible and established by 5–7 days. The principles of nutritional therapy remain the same as in other acutely brain injured patients. In the recovery stage, patients who are fit to be started on oral feeds should undergo a validated dysphagia screening protocol to help reduce aspiration and pneumonia [16].

49.9.5 Hypothalamic-Pituitary-Adrenal Axis Dysfunction

This may occur in acute stage and is difficult to differentiate from other causes of hypotension. A patient unresponsiveness to vasopressors (in absence of other apparent causes) might have underlying relative adrenal insufficiency. Hormonal testing may be difficult in critical care setting. A stress dose of steroid in selective patients (with refractory hypotension of unknown cause) might be reasonable to help recognise dysfunction, though high-dose steroids are clearly harmful. Hormonal replacement may be helpful in chronic state.

49.10 Post-aSAH Recovery—Cognitive Aspect

With the recent improvements in the understanding and management of aSAH, mortality has reduced over the last few decades. Though the recovery in terms of cognitive, functional, behavioural and overall quality of life, is deficient. Incidence of depression, anxiety, cognitive impairment and post-traumatic stress disorder is reported between 15% and 70% in literature [107, 108]. It is imperative that cognitive recovery should be a part of post-aSAH recovery using a multidisciplinary approach consisting of neuro-intensivists, rehabilitation specialists, physiotherapists, psychiatrists, occupational and speech therapist and cognitive screening should be done in all such patients [109].

49.11 Conclusion

Management of aSAH patients requires a complete understanding of interaction between the injured brain and all other organs. The basic principles of neurocritical care remain the same with several specific issues like early brain injury, vasospasm and DCI requiring our attention. The use of multimodal monitoring can be useful for management of these patients and can help guide the management strategies.

References

1. Etminan N, Chang HS, Hackenberg K, de Rooij NK, Vergouwen MDI, Rinkel GJE, Algra A. Worldwide incidence of aneurysmal subarachnoid hemorrhage according to region, time period, blood pressure, and smoking prevalence in the population: a systematic review and meta-analysis. JAMA Neurol. 2019;76:588–97. https://doi.org/10.1001/jamaneurol.2019.0006.
2. Tsao CW, Aday AW, Almarzooq ZI, Anderson CAM, Arora P, Avery CL, Baker-Smith CM, Beaton AZ, Boehme AK, Buxton AE, On behalf of the American Heart Association Council on Epidemiology and Prevention Statistics Committee and Stroke Statistics Subcommittee, et al. Heart disease and stroke statistics—2023 update: a report from the American Heart Association. Circulation. 2023;147:e93–e621. https://doi.org/10.1161/CIR.0000000000001123;[published correction appears in Circulation.2023;147:e622].
3. Fuentes AM, Stone McGuire L, Amin-Hanjani S. Sex differences in cerebral aneurysms and subarachnoid hemorrhage. Stroke. 2022;53:624–33. https://doi.org/10.1161/STROKEAHA.121.037147.
4. SVIN COVID-19 Global SAH Registry. Global impact of the COVID-19 pan- demic on subarachnoid haemorrhage hospitalisations, aneurysm treatment and in-hospital mortality: 1-year follow-up [published ahead of print July 28, 2022]. J Neurol Neurosurg Psychiatry. 2022;93(10):1028–38. https://doi.org/10.1136/jnnp-2022-329200. https://jnnp.bmj.com/content/93/10/1028.long.
5. Mackey J, Khoury JC, Alwell K, Moomaw CJ, Kissela BM, Flaherty ML, Adeoye O, Woo D, Ferioli S, De Los Rios La Rosa F, et al. Stable incidence but declining case-fatality rates of subarachnoid hemorrhage in a population. Neurology. 2016;87:2192–7. https://doi.org/10.1212/WNL.0000000000003353.
6. Mahlamäki K, Rautalin I, Korja M. Case fatality rates of subarachnoid hemorrhage are decreasing with substantial between-country variation: a systematic review of population-based studies between 1980 and 2020. Neuroepidemiology. 2022;56:402–12. https://doi.org/10.1159/000526983.
7. Chou SH. Subarachnoid hemorrhage. Continuum (Minneap Minn). 2021;27:1201–45. https://doi.org/10.1212/CON.0000000000001052.
8. Rass V, Helbok R. Early brain injury after poor-grade subarach- noid hemorrhage. Curr Neurol Neurosci Rep. 2019;19:78. https://doi.org/10.1007/s11910-019-0990-3.
9. Neifert SN, Chapman EK, Martini ML, Shuman WH, Schupper AJ, Oermann EK, Mocco J, Macdonald RL. Aneurysmal subarachnoidhem- orrhage: the last decade. Transl Stroke Res. 2021;12:428–46. https://doi.org/10.1007/s12975-020-00867-0.
10. Mark DG, Pines JM. The detection of nontraumatic subarachnoid hemorrhage: still a diagnostic challenge. Am J Emerg Med. 2006;24:859–63.
11. Matsuda S, Ikawa F, Hidaka T, Yamaguchi S, Inagawa T, Horie N, Kurisu K, Akiyama Y, Goto Y, Nakayama T, JIS Study Group, et al. Recent declining trend of incidence rate of subarachnoid hemorrhage in Shimane, Japan: the Japan Incidence of Subarachnoid Hemor- rhage (JIS) Study. Neurol Med Chir (Tokyo). 2022;62:458–64. https://doi.org/10.2176/jns-nmc.2022-0067.
12. Bellolio MF, Hess EP, Gilani WI, VanDyck TJ, Ostby SA, Schwarz JA, Lohse CM, Rabinstein AA. External validation of the Ottawa subarachnoid hemorrhage clinical decision rule in patients with acute headache. Am J Emerg Med. 2015;33:244–9. https://doi.org/10.1016/j.ajem.2014.11.049.
13. Perry JJ, Sivilotti MLA, Sutherland J, Hohl CM, Emond M, Calder LA, Vaillancourt C, Thirganasambandamoorthy V, Lesiuk H, Wells GA, et al. Vali- dation of the Ottawa subarachnoid hemorrhage rule in patients with acute headache. CMAJ. 2017;189:E1379–85. https://doi.org/10.1503/cmaj.170072.
14. Dubosh NM, Bellolio MF, Rabinstein AA, Edlow JA. Sensitivity of early brain computed tomography to exclude aneurysmal subarachnoid hemorrhage: a systematic review and meta-analysis. Stroke. 2016;47:750–5. https://doi.org/10.1161/STROKEAHA.115.011386.
15. Godwin SA, Cherkas DS, Panagos PD, Shih RD. Byyny R, wolf SJ; Ameri- can College of Emergency Physicians Clinical Policies Subcommittee (writ- ing committee) on acute headache. Clinical policy: critical issues in the evaluation and management of adult patients presenting to the emergency department with acute headache. Ann Emerg Med. 2019;74:e41–74. https://doi.org/10.1016/j.annemergmed.2019.07.009.
16. Hoh BL, Ko NU, Amin-Hanjani S, Hsiang-Yi Chou S, Cruz-Flores S, Dangayach NS, Derdeyn CP, Du R, Hänggi D, Hetts SW, Ifejika NL, Johnson R, Keigher KM, Leslie-Mazwi TM, Lucke-Wold B, Rabinstein AA, Robicsek SA, Stapleton CJ, Suarez JI, Tjoumakaris SI, Welch BG. 2023 guideline for the Management of Patients with aneurysmal subarachnoid hemorrhage: a guideline from the American Heart Association/American Stroke Association. Stroke. 2023;54(7):e314–70. https://doi.org/10.1161/STR.0000000000000436.
17. Catapano JS, Zeoli T, Frisoli FA, Burk-Hardt JK, Lawton MT. Long-term independence in older patients with aneurysmal subarachnoid hemorrhage in the Barrow ruptured aneurysm trial. World Neurosurg. 2021;147:e98–e104. https://doi.org/10.1016/j.wneu.2020.11.139.
18. Fang Y, Lu J, Zheng J, Wu H, Araujo C, Reis C, Lenahan C, Zhu S, Chen S, Zhang J. Comparison of aneurysmal subarachnoid hemorrhage grading scores in patients with aneurysm clipping and coiling. Sci Rep. 2020;10:9199. https://doi.org/10.1038/s41598-020-66160-0.
19. de Jong G, Aquarius R, Sanaan B, Bartels R, Grotenhuis JA, Henssen D, Boogaarts HD. Prediction

models in aneurysmal subarachnoid hemorrhage: forecasting clinical outcome with artificial intelligence. Neurosurgery. 2021;88:E427–34. https://doi.org/10.1093/neuros/nyaa581.
20. Mualem W, Durrani S, Ghaith AK, Bhandarkar AR, Wahood W, Tjoumakaris S, Jabbour P, Bydon M. Factors associated with increased inpatient charges following aneurysmal subarachnoid hemorrhage with vasospasm: a nationwide analysis. Clin Neurol Neurosurg. 2022;218:107259. https://doi.org/10.1016/j.clineuro.2022.107259.
21. Lauzier DC, Jayaraman K, Yuan JY, Diwan D, Vellimana AK, Osbun JW, Chatterjee AR, Athiraman U, Dhar R, Zipfel GJ. Early brain injury after subarachnoid hemorrhage: incidence and mechanisms. Stroke. 2023;54(5):1426–40. https://doi.org/10.1161/STROKEAHA.122.040072.
22. Roquilly A, Cinotti R, Jaber S, Vourc'h M, Pengam F, Mahe PJ, Lakhal K, Demeure Dit Latte D, Rondeau N, Loutrel O, et al. Implementation of an evidence-based extubation readiness bundle in 499 brain-injured patients. A before-after evaluation of a quality improvement project. Am J Respir Crit Care Med. 2013;188:958–66. https://doi.org/10.1164/rccm.201301-0116OC.
23. Wartenberg KE, Schmidt JM, Claassen J, Temes RE, Frontera JA, Ostapkovich N, Parra A, Connolly ES, Mayer SA. Impact of medical complications on out- come after subarachnoid hemorrhage. Crit Care Med. 2006;34:617–23s. https://doi.org/10.1097/01.ccm.0000201903.46435.35.
24. Vergouwen MD, Jong-Tjien-Fa AV, Algra A, Rinkel GJ. Time trends in causes of death after aneurysmal subarachnoid hemorrhage: a hospital-based study. Neurology. 2016;86:59–63. https://doi.org/10.1212/WNL.0000000000002239.
25. Kassell NF, Torner JC, Jane JA, Haley EC Jr, Adams HP. The international cooperative study on the timing of aneurysm surgery, part 2: surgical results. J Neurosurg. 1990;73:37–47. https://doi.org/10.3171/jns.1990.73.1.0037.
26. Post R, Germans MR, Tjerkstra MA, Vergouwen MDI, Jellema K, Koot RW, Kruyt ND, Willems PWA, Wolfs JFC, de Beer FC, et al. ULTRA Investigators. Ultra-early tranexamic acid after subarachnoid haemorrhage (ULTRA): a randomised controlled trial. Lancet. 2021;397:112–118. https://doi.org/10.1016/S0140-6736(20)32518-6.
27. Treggiari MM, Rabinstein AA, Busl KM, Caylor MM, Citerio G, Deem S, Diringer M, Fox E, Livesay S, Sheth KN, Suarez JI, Tjoumakaris S. Guidelines for the Neurocritical Care Management of Aneurysmal Subarachnoid Hemorrhage. Neurocrit Care. 2023;39(1):1–28. https://doi.org/10.1007/s12028-023-01713-5.
28. Shi M, Yang C, Chen ZH, Xiao LF, Zhao WY. Efficacy and safety of tranexamic acid in aneurysmal subarachnoid hemorrhage: a systematic review and meta-analysis of randomized controlled trials. Front Surg. 2021;8:790149. https://doi.org/10.3389/fsurg.2021.790149.
29. Baharoglu MI, Germans MR, Rinkel GJ, Algra A, Vermeulen M, van Gijn J, Roos YB. Antifibrinolytic therapy for aneurysmal subarachnoid haemorrhage. Cochrane Database Syst Rev. 2013;2013:Cd001245. https://doi.org/10.1002/14651858.CD001245.pub2.
30. Greenberg SM, Ziai WC. Cordonnier C, Dowlatshahi D, Francis B, Goldstein JN, Hemphill JC 3rd, Johnson R, Keigher KM, Mack WJ, et al; on behalf of the American Heart Association/American Stroke Association. 2022 guideline for the management of patients with spontaneous intracerebral hemorrhage: a guideline from the American Heart Association/American Stroke Association. Stroke. 2022;53:e282–361. https://doi.org/10.1161/STR.0000000000000407.
31. Kuramatsu JB, Gerner ST, Schellinger PD, Glahn J, Endres M, Sobesky J, Flechsenhar J, Neugebauer H, Juttler E, Grau A, et al. Anticoagulant re- versal, blood pressure levels, and anticoagulant resumption in patients with anticoagulation-related intracerebral hemorrhage. JAMA. 2015;313:824–36. https://doi.org/10.1001/jama.2015.0846.
32. Manley G, Knudson MM, Morabito D, Damron S, Erickson V, Pitts L. Hypotension, hypoxia, and head injury: frequency, duration, and consequences. Arch Surg. 2001;136(10):1118–23. https://doi.org/10.1001/archsurg.136.10.1118.
33. Ascanio LC, Enriquez-Marulanda A, Maragkos GA, Salem MM, Alturki AY, Ravindran K, Fehnel CR, Hanafy K, Ogilvy CS, Thomas AJ, et al. Effect of blood pressure variability during the acute period of subarachnoid hem- orrhage on functional outcomes. Neurosurgery. 2020;87:779–87. https://doi.org/10.1093/neuros/nyaa019.
34. Tang C, Zhang TS, Zhou LF. Risk factors for rebleeding of aneurysmal sub- arachnoid hemorrhage: a meta-analysis. PLoS One. 2014;9:e99536. https://doi.org/10.1371/journal.pone.0099536.
35. Douglas MR, Daniel M, Lagord C, et al. High CSF transforming growth factor beta levels after subarachnoid haemorrhage: association with chronic communicating hydrocephalus. J Neurol Neurosurg Psychiatry. 2009;80:545.
36. Xie Z, Hu X, Zan X, Lin S, Li H, You C. Predictors of shunt-dependent hydrocephalus after aneurysmal subarachnoid hemorrhage? A systematic review and meta-analysis. World Neurosurg. 2017;106:844–860.e6. https://doi.org/10.1016/j.wneu.2017.06.119.
37. Connolly ES Jr, Kader AA, Frazzini VI, Winfree CJ, Solomon RA. The safety of intraoperative lumbar subarachnoid drainage for acutely ruptured intracranial aneurysm: technical note. Surg Neurol. 1997;48:338–42. https://doi.org/10.1016/s0090-3019(96)00472-7.
38. Rajshekhar V, Harbaugh RE. Results of routine ventriculostomy with external ventricular drainage for acute hydrocephalus following sub- arachnoid haemorrhage. Acta Neurochir. 1992;115:8–14. https://doi.org/10.1007/BF01400584.
39. Olson DM, Zomorodi M, Britz GW, Zomorodi AR, Amato A, Graffagnino C. Continuous cerebral spi-

nal fluid drainage associated with complications in patients admitted with subarachnoid hemorrhage. J Neurosurg. 2013;119:974–80. https://doi.org/10.3171/2013.6.JNS122403.

40. Babu MA, Patel R, Marsh WR, Wijdicks EF. Strategies to decrease the risk of ventricular catheter infections: a review of the evidence. Neurocrit Care. 2012;16:194–202. https://doi.org/10.1007/s12028-011-9647-z.
41. O'Kelly CJ, Kulkarni AV, Austin PC, Urbach D, Wallace MC. Shunt- dependent hydrocephalus after aneurysmal subarachnoid hemorrhage: incidence, predictors, and revision rates: clinical article. J Neurosurg. 2009;111:1029–35. https://doi.org/10.3171/2008.9.JNS08881.
42. Hoh BL, Kleinhenz DT, Chi YY, Mocco J, Barker FG 2nd. Incidence of ven- tricular shunt placement for hydrocephalus with clipping versus coiling for ruptured and unruptured cerebral aneurysms in the Nationwide inpatient sample database: 2002 to 2007. World Neurosurg. 2011;76:548–54. https://doi.org/10.1016/j.wneu.2011.05.054.
43. Cook AM, Morgan Jones G, Hawryluk GWJ, Mailloux P, McLaughlin D, Papangelou A, Samuel S, Tokumaru S, Venkatasubramanian C, Zacko C, Zimmermann LL, Hirsch K, Shutter L. Guidelines for the acute treatment of cerebral edema in Neurocritical care patients. Neurocrit Care. 2020;32(3):647–66. https://doi.org/10.1007/s12028-020-00959-7.
44. Howard BM, Hu R, Barrow JW, Barrow DL. Comprehensive review of imaging of intracranial aneurysms and angiographically negative subarachnoid hemorrhage. Neurosurg Focus. 2019;47:E20. https://doi.org/10.3171/2019.9.FOCUS19653.
45. Baggiani M, Graziano F, Rebora P, Robba C, Guglielmi A, Galimberti S, Giussani C, Suarez JI, Helbok R, Citerio G. Intracranial pressure monitoring practice, treatment, and effect on outcome in aneurysmal subarachnoid hemorrhage. Neurocrit Care. 2023;38(3):741–51. https://doi.org/10.1007/s12028-022-01651-8.
46. Chen Y, Xia F, Cai C, Li H, Ma L, Hu X, You C. Duration and choices of prophylactic anticonvulsants in subarachnoid hemorrhage: a systematic review and meta-analysis. Neurosurg Rev. 2021;44:2459–67. https://doi.org/10.1007/s10143-020-01466-1.
47. Raper DM, Starke RM, Komotar RJ, Allan R, Connolly ES Jr. Seizures after aneurysmal subarachnoid hemorrhage: a systematic review of outcomes. World Neurosurg. 2013;79:682–90. https://doi.org/10.1016/j.wneu.2012.08.006.
48. Claassen J, Peery S, Kreiter KT, Hirsch LJ, Du EY, Connolly ES, Mayer SA. Predictors and clinical impact of epilepsy after subarachnoid hemorrhage. Neurology. 2003;60:208–14. https://doi.org/10.1212/01.wnl.0000038906.71394.de.
49. American Clinical Neurophysiology Society. ACNS standardized critical care EEG terminology 2021: reference chart. 2021. https://cdn-links.lww.com/permalink/jcnp/a/jcnp_2020_12_21_fong_00313_sdc099.pdf. Accessed 11 Apr 2021.
50. Rhoney DH, Tipps LB, Murry KR, Basham MC, Michael DB, Coplin WM. Anticonvulsant prophylaxis and timing of seizures after aneurysmal subarachnoid hemorrhage. Neurology. 2000;55:258–65. https://doi.org/10.1212/wnl.55.2.258.
51. Angriman F, Tirupakuzhi Vijayaraghavan BK, Dragoi L, Lopez Soto C, Chapman M, Scales DC. Antiepileptic drugs to prevent seizures after spontaneous intracerebral hemorrhage. Stroke. 2019;50:1095–9. https://doi.org/10.1161/STROKEAHA.118.024380.
52. Marigold R, Gunther A, Tiwari D, Kwan J. Antiepileptic drugs for the pri- mary and secondary prevention of seizures after subarachnoid haem- orrhage. Cochrane Database Syst Rev. 2013;2013:CD008710. https://doi.org/10.1002/14651858.CD008710.pub2.
53. Fiani B, Andraos C, Mabry I, Siddiqi J. A comparison of seizure prophy- laxis: phenytoin versus levetiracetam. Cureus. 2021;13:e14956. https://doi.org/10.7759/cureus.14956.
54. Commichau C, Scarmeas N, Mayer SA. Risk factors for fever in the neurologic intensive care unit. Neurology. 2003;60:837.
55. Fernandez A, Schmidt JM, Claassen J, et al. Fever after subarachnoid hemorrhage: risk factors and impact on outcome. Neurology. 2007;68:1013.
56. Badjatia N, Fernandez L, Schmidt JM, et al. Impact of induced normothermia on outcome after subarachnoid hemorrhage: a case- control study. Neurosurgery. 2010;66:696.
57. Dennis M, Sandercock P, Graham C, Forbes J, Smith J. CLOTS (Clots in legs or sTockings after stroke) trials collaboration. The Clots in legs or sTockings after stroke (CLOTS) 3 trial: a randomised controlled trial to determine whether or not intermittent pneumatic compression reduces the risk of post-stroke deep vein thrombosis and to estimate its cost-effectiveness. Health Technol Assess. 2015;19:1–90. https://doi.org/10.3310/hta19760.
58. Mazeraud A, Robba C, Rebora P, Iaquaniello C, Vargiolu A, Rass V, Bogossian EG, Helbok R, Taccone FS, Citerio G. Acute distress respiratory syndrome after subarachnoid hemorrhage: incidence and impact on the outcome in a large multicenter, retrospective cohort. Neurocrit Care. 2021;34:1000–8. https://doi.org/10.1007/s12028-020-01115-x.
59. Shrestha GS. Lung maladies following aneurysmal subarachnoid haemorrhage. J Neuroanaesthesiol Crit Care. 2017;4:S45–8.
60. Asehnoune K, Mrozek S, Perrigault PF, Seguin P, Dahyot-Fizelier C, Lasocki S, Pujol A, Martin M, Chabanne R, Muller L, BI-VILI Study Group, et al. A multi- faceted strategy to reduce ventilation-

associated mortality in brain-injured patients: the BI-VILI project: a nationwide quality improvement project. Intensive Care Med. 2017;43:957–70. https://doi.org/10.1007/s00134-017-4764-6.

61. Kopelnik A, Zaroff JG. Neurocardiogenic injury in neurovascular disorders. Crit Care Clin. 2006;22(4):733–52; abstract ix-x. https://doi.org/10.1016/j.ccc.2006.06.002.
62. Junttila E, Vaara M, Koskenkari J, et al. Repolarization abnormalities in patients with subarachnoid and intracerebral hemorrhage: predisposing factors and association with outcome. Anesth Analg. 2013;116:190.
63. Lee VH, Connolly HM, Fulgham JR, et al. Takotsubo cardiomyopathy in aneurysmal subarachnoid hemorrhage: an underappreciated ventricular dysfunction. J Neurosurg. 2006;105:264.
64. Hakeem A, Marks AD, Bhatti S, Chang SM. When the worst headache becomes the worst heartache! Stroke. 2007;38:3292.
65. Diringer MN, Bleck TP, Claude Hemphill J 3rd, et al. Critical care management of patients following aneurysmal subarachnoid hemorrhage: recommendations from the Neurocritical care Society's multidisciplinary consensus conference. Neurocrit Care. 2011;15:211.
66. McGirt MJ, Blessing R, Nimjee SM, et al. Correlation of serum brain natriuretic peptide with hyponatremia and delayed ischemic neurological deficits after subarachnoid hemorrhage. Neurosurgery. 2004;54(6):1369–73; discussion 1373–1374.
67. Qureshi AI, Suri MF, Sung GY, et al. Prognostic significance of hypernatremia and hyponatremia among patients with aneurysmal subarachnoid hemorrhage. Neurosurgery. 2002;50(4):749–55; discussion 755–756.
68. Fisher LA, Ko N, Miss J, et al. Hypernatremia predicts adverse cardiovascular and neurological outcomes after SAH. Neurocrit Care. 2006;5(3):180–5.
69. Wartenberg KE, Schmidt JM, Claassen J, et al. Impact of medical complications on outcome after subarachnoid hemorrhage. Crit Care Med. 2006;34(3):617–23; quiz 624.
70. Audibert G, Steinmann G, de Talancé N, et al. Endocrine response after severe subarachnoid hemorrhage related to sodium and blood volume regulation. Anesth Analg. 2009;108(6):1922–8.
71. Mutoh T, Kazumata K, Terasaka S, Taki Y, Suzuki A, Ishikawa T. Early intensive versus minimally invasive approach to postoperative hemodynamic management after subarachnoid hemorrhage. Stroke. 2014;45:1280–4. https://doi.org/10.1161/STROKEAHA.114.004739.
72. Kahn JM, Caldwell EC, Deem S, Newell DW, Heckbert SR, Rubenfeld GD. Acute lung injury in patients with subarachnoid hemorrhage: incidence, risk factors, and outcome. Crit Care Med. 2006;34:196–202. https://doi.org/10.1097/01.ccm.0000194540.44020.8e.
73. Woo MH, Kale-Pradhan PB. Fludrocortisone in the treatment of subarachnoid hemorrhage-induced hyponatremia. Ann Pharmacother. 1997;31(5):637–9.
74. Suarez JI, Qureshi AI, Parekh PD, et al. Administration of hypertonic (3%) sodium chloride/acetate in hyponatremic patients with symptomatic vasospasm following subarachnoid hemorrhage. J Neurosurg Anesthesiol. 1999;11(3):178–84.
75. Zeltser D, Rosansky S, van Rensburg H, Verbalis JG, Smith N. Assessment of the efficacy and safety of intravenous conivaptan in euvolemic and hypervolemic hyponatremia. Am J Nephrol. 2007;27(5):447–57.
76. Wright WL, Asbury WH, Gilmore JL, Samuels OB. Conivaptan for hyponatremia in the neurocritical care unit. Neurocrit Care. 2008;11(1):6–13.
77. Mistry AM, Mistry EA, Ganesh Kumar N, Froehler MT, Fusco MR, Chitale RV. Corticosteroids in the management of hyponatremia, hypovolemia, and vasospasm in subarachnoid hemorrhage: a meta-analysis. Cerebrovasc Dis. 2016;42:263–71. https://doi.org/10.1159/000446251.
78. Vergouwen MD, Vermeulen M, van Gijn J, Rinkel GJ, Wijdicks EF, Muizelaar JP, Mendelow AD, Juvela S, Yonas H, Terbrugge KG, et al. Definition of delayed cerebral ischemia after aneurysmal subarachnoid hemorrhage as an outcome event in clinical trials and observational studies: proposal of a multidisciplinary research group. Stroke. 2010;41:2391–5. https://doi.org/10.1161/STROKEAHA.110.589275.
79. Stienen MN, Visser-Meily JM, Schweizer TA, Hanggi D, Macdonald RL, Vergouwen MDI. Unruptured intracranial aneurysms and SAH CDE project investigators. Prioritization and timing of outcomes and endpoints after aneurysmal subarachnoid hemorrhage in clinical trials and observational studies: proposal of a multidisciplinary research group. Neurocrit Care. 2019;30(suppl 1):102–13. https://doi.org/10.1007/s12028-019-00737-0.
80. Suarez JI, Sheikh MK, Macdonald RL, Amin-Hanjani S, Brown RD Jr, de Oliveira Manoel AL, Derdeyn CP, Etminan N, Keller E, et al. Unruptured intracranial aneurysms and SAH CDE project investigators. Common data elements for unruptured intracranial aneurysms and subarachnoid hemorrhage clinical research: a National Institute for neurological disorders and stroke and National Library of medicine project. Neurocrit Care. 2019;30(suppl 1):4–19. https://doi.org/10.1007/s12028-019-00723-6.
81. Rowland MJ, Hadjipavlou G, Kelly M, Westbrook J, Pattinson KT. Delayed cerebral ischaemia after subarachnoid haemorrhage: looking beyond vasospasm. Br J Anaesth. 2012;109:315–29. https://doi.org/10.1093/bja/aes264.
82. Namyong J, Aurboonyawat T, Chankaew E, Chawalparit O, Tritrakarn S, Srirabheebhat P, Wongbhanuwich V, Songsaeng D, Boonma J. Computerized tomographic angiography for detec-

tion of cerebral vasospasm after ruptured intracranial aneurysm. J Med Assoc Thail. 2015;98:804–11.
83. Dankbaar JW, Rijsdijk M, vander Schaaf IC, Velthuis BK, Wermer MJ, Rinkel GJ. Relationship between vasospasm, cerebral perfusion, and delayed cerebral ischemia after aneurysmal subarachnoid hemorrhage. Neuroradiology. 2009;51:813–9. https://doi.org/10.1007/s00234-009-0575-y.
84. Maegawa T, Sasahara A, Ohbuchi H, Chernov M, Kasuya H. Cerebral vasospasm and hypoperfusion after traumatic brain injury: combined CT angiography and CT perfusion imaging study. Surg Neurol Int. 2021;12:361. https://doi.org/10.25259/SNI_859_2020.
85. Chen HY, Elmer J, Zafar SF, Ghanta M, Moura Junior V, Rosenthal ES, Gilmore EJ, Hirsch LJ, Zaveri HP, Sheth KN, et al. Combining transcranial Doppler and EEG data to predict delayed cerebral ischemia after subarachnoid hemorrhage. Neurology. 2022;98:e459–69. https://doi.org/10.1212/WNL.0000000000013126.
86. Kumar G, Shahripour RB, Harrigan MR. Vasospasm on transcranial Doppler is predictive of delayed cerebral ischemia in aneurysmal subarachnoid hemorrhage: a systematic review and meta-analysis. J Neurosurg. 2016;124:1257–64. https://doi.org/10.3171/2015.4.JNS15428.
87. Samagh N, Bhagat H, Jangra K. Monitoring cerebral vasospasm: how much can we rely on transcranial Doppler. J Anaesthesiol Clin Pharmacol. 2019;35(1):12–8. https://doi.org/10.4103/joacp.JOACP_192_17.
88. Gollwitzer S, Muller TM, Hopfengartner R, Rampp S, Merkel J, Hagge M, Jukic J, Lang J, Madzar D, Onugoren MD, et al. Quantitative EEG after subarachnoid hemorrhage predicts long-term functional outcome. J Clin Neurophysiol. 2019;36:25–31. https://doi.org/10.1097/WNP.0000000000000537.
89. Torne R, Culebras D, Sanchez-Etayo G, Garcia-Garcia S, Munoz G, Llull L, Amaro S, Heering C, Blasco J, Zavala E, et al. Double hemispheric micro- dialysis study in poor-grade SAH patients. Sci Rep. 2020;10:7466. https://doi.org/10.1038/s41598-020-64543-x.
90. Pickard JD, Murray GD, Illingworth R, et al. Effect of oral nimodipine on cerebral infarction and outcome after subarachnoid haemorrhage: British aneurysm nimodipine trial. BMJ. 1989;298:636–42.
91. Dorhout Mees SM, Rinkel GJ, Feigin VL, Algra A, van den Bergh WM, Vermeulen M, Van Gijn J. Calcium antagonists for aneurysmal subarachnoid haemorrhage. Cochrane Database Syst Rev. 2007;2007:CD000277. https://doi.org/10.1002/14651858.CD000277.pub3.
92. Das JM, Zito PM. Nimodipine. In: StatPearls [Internet]. Treasure Island (FL): StatPearls Publishing; 2023. https://www.ncbi.nlm.nih.gov/books/NBK534870/.
93. Geraldini F, De Cassai A, Diana P, Correale C, Boscolo A, Zampirollo S, Disarò L, Carere A, Cacco N, Navalesi P, et al. A comparison between enteral and intravenous nimodipine in subarachnoid hemorrhage: a systematic review and network meta-analysis. Neurocrit Care. 2022;36:1071–9. https://doi.org/10.1007/s12028-022-01493-4.
94. Wolf S, Mielke D, Barner C, Malinova V, Kerz T, Wostrack M, Czorlich P, Salih F, Engel DC, Ehlert A, Staykov D, Alturki AY, Sure U, Bardutzky J, HWS S, Schürer L, Beck J, Juratli TA, Fritsch M, Lemcke J, Pohrt A, Meyer B, Schwab S, Rohde V, Vajkoczy P, EARLYDRAIN Study Group. Effectiveness of lumbar cerebrospinal fluid drain among patients with aneurysmal subarachnoid hemorrhage: a randomized clinical trial. JAMA Neurol. 2023;80(8):833–42. https://doi.org/10.1001/jamaneurol.2023.1792. Erratum in: JAMA Neurol 2023 Aug 1;80(8):873.
95. Veldeman M, Weiss M, Albanna W et al. Incremental versus immediate induction of hypertension in the treatment of delayed cerebral ischemia after subarachnoid hemorrhage. Neurocrit Care. 2022;36:702–714. https://doi.org/10.1007/s12028-022-01466-7.
96. Francoeur CL, Mayer SA. Management of delayed cerebral ischemia after subarachnoid hemorrhage. Crit Care. 2016;20:1447–6. https://doi.org/10.1186/s13054-016-1447-6.
97. Haegens NM, Gathier CS, Horn J, Coert BA, Verbaan D, van den Bergh WM. Induced hypertension in preventing cerebral infarction in delayed cerebral ischemia after subarachnoid hemorrhage. Stroke. 2018;49(11):2630–6. https://doi.org/10.1161/STROKEAHA.118.022310.
98. Lannes M, Teitelbaum J, del Pilar CM, Cardoso M, Angle M. Milrinone and homeostasis to treat cerebral vasospasm associated with subarachnoid hemorrhage: the Montreal neurological hospital protocol. Neurocrit Care. 2012;16(3):354–62. https://doi.org/10.1007/s12028-012-9701-5.
99. Lakhal K, Hivert A, Alexandre PL, Fresco M, Robert-Edan V, Rodie-Talbere PA, Ambrosi X, Bourcier R, Rozec B, Cadiet J. Intravenous Milrinone for cerebral vasospasm in subarachnoid hemorrhage: the MILRISPASM controlled before-after study. Neurocrit Care. 2021;35(3):669–79. https://doi.org/10.1007/s12028-021-01331-z.
100. Bernier TD, Schontz MJ, Izzy S, Chung DY, Nelson SE, Leslie-Mazwi TM, Henderson GV, Dasenbrock H, Patel N, Aziz-Sultan MA, et al. Treatment of subarachnoid hemorrhage-associated delayed cerebral ischemia with milrinone: a review and proposal. J Neurosurg Anesthesiol. 2021;33:195–202. https://doi.org/10.1097/ANA.0000000000000755.
101. Abulhasan YB, Ortiz Jimenez J, Teitelbaum J, Simoneau G, Angle MR. Milrinone for refractory cerebral vasospasm with delayed cerebral ischemia. J Neurosurg. 2020;134(3):971–82. https://doi.org/10.3171/2020.1.JNS193107.
102. Duman E, Karakoç F, Pinar HU, Dogan R, Fırat A, Yıldırım E. Higher dose intra-arterial milrinone

and intra-arterial combined milrinone-nimodipine infusion as a rescue therapy for refractory cerebral vasospasm. Interv Neuroradiol. 2017;23(6):636–43. https://doi.org/10.1177/1591019917732288. Epub 2017 Sep 28
103. Jun P, Ko NU, English JD, Dowd CF, Halbach VV, Higashida RT, Lawton MT, Hetts SW. Endovascular treatment of medically refractory cerebral vasospasm following aneurysmal subarachnoid hemorrhage. AJNR Am J Neuroradiol. 2010;31:1911–6. https://doi.org/10.3174/ajnr.A2183.
104. Rabinstein AA, Friedman JA, Nichols DA, Pichelmann MA, McClelland RL, Manno EM, Atkinson JL, Wijdicks EF. Predictors of outcome after endovascular treatment of cerebral vasospasm. AJNR Am J Neuroradiol. 2004;25:1778–82.
105. Rabinstein AA. Vasospasm and statin therapy: yet another cautionary tale. Neurocrit Care. 2010;12:310–2. https://doi.org/10.1007/s12028-009-9267-z.
106. Manoel AL, Turkel-Parrella D, Germans M, Kouzmina E, Almendra Pda S, Marotta T, Spears J, Abrahamson S. Safety of early pharmacological thromboprophylaxis after subarachnoid hemorrhage. Can J Neurol Sci. 2014;41:554–61. https://doi.org/10.1017/cjn.2014.16.
107. Chun HY, Ford A, Kutlubaev MA, Almeida OP, Mead GE. Depression, anxiety, and suicide after stroke: a narrative review of the best available evidence. Stroke. 2022;53:1402–10. https://doi.org/10.1161/STROKEAHA.121.035499.
108. Nussbaum ES, Mikoff N, Paranjape GS. Cognitive deficits among patients surviving aneurysmal subarachnoid hemorrhage: a contemporary systematic review. Br J Neurosurg. 2021;35:384–401. https://doi.org/10.1080/02688697.2020.1859462.
109. Geraghty JR, Lara-Angulo MN, Spegar M, Reeh J, Testai FD. Severe cognitive impairment in aneurysmal subarachnoid hemorrhage: predictors and relationship to functional outcome. J Stroke Cerebrovasc Dis. 2020;29:105027. https://doi.org/10.1016/j.jstrokecerebrovasdis.2020.105027.

Vascular Neurosurgery - Cerebrovascular Malformations and Neurocritical Care

50

Cristiane Tavares, Ana Laura Lindner Latorre de Alcantara, Juan Carlos Ahumada Vizcaino, and Feres Eduardo Aparecido Chaddad Neto

50.1 Introduction

Cerebral vascular malformations refer to conditions related to abnormal vascular configurations in the brain. They can be congenital or acquired and are mainly classified as one of these below.

50.1.1 Cavernous Malformations

Cavernous malformations (CM), also called cavernous angiomas, are dilated, thin-walled dilated capillaries with a simple endothelial lining that does not contain smooth muscle or elastic fibers [1]. They account for approximately 5%–15% of all vascular abnormalities in the central nervous system and have a reported incidence of 0.15 to 0.56 per 100,000 in various populations [2].

Most CMs are asymptomatic and found incidentally on brain MRI [3, 4].

The most common locations in the brain are the rolandic and temporal subcortical areas and may present as hemorrhage, seizures, or progressive neurologic deficits. The risk of bleeding is expected to be from 0.25% to 1.1% per year, accordingly to several large series [5, 6].

Posterior fossa lesions are usually located in the pons and cerebellar hemispheres and account for approximately 10–23% of CMs [2]. Lesions in the brainstem usually have a worse natural history. They present as cranial neuropathies and long-tract signs leading to progressive neurologic decline due to the high volume of critical nuclei and fiber tracts in this area. The reported risk of bleeding is 2–3% per year, with recurrent rebleeding rates up to 17–21% [7].

Spinal cord CMs may be more common than traditionally thought and present as intramedullary lesions predominantly involving the cervical and thoracic regions [8, 9].

Diagnosis is based on neuroimaging (MRI) since they are often angiographically occult. Ideally, MRI should include gradient echo or susceptibility-weighted imaging to detect smaller CMs that may not be visible on conventional MRI sequences [1, 10, 11].

The management of patients with CMs depends on their risk of future bleeding or other neurologic sequelae. The routine care includes screening for asymptomatic AVMs "and" Heredi-

C. Tavares (✉)
Neuroanesthesiologist and Clinical Research Physician, Hospital das Clínicas of University of São Paulo School of Medicine (FMUSP), São Paulo, Brazil
e-mail: cristiane.tavares@hc.fm.usp.br

Ana Laura Lindner Latorre de Alcantara
Fernandes Figueira Institute, Rio de Janeiro, Brazil

J. C. A. Vizcaino
Feres Eduardo Aparecido Chaddad Neto
Department of Neurology and Neurosurgery, Federal University of Sao Paulo (UNIFESP), São Paulo, SP, Brazil

H. Prabhakar et al. (eds.), *Principles and Practice of Neurocritical Care*,
https://doi.org/10.1007/978-981-99-8059-8_50

tary hemorrhagic telangiectasia (HHT) or Moyamoya disease.

Asymptomatic cases are generally followed clinically, with annual neuroimaging [1].

Surgical resection may be indicated for accessible symptomatic lesions associated with progressive neurologic deficits, intractable epilepsy, or intracerebral hemorrhage (ICH). Accessible symptomatic cerebral and cerebellar lesions causing a progressive neurologic deficit, intractable epilepsy, and recurrent bleeding can also be surgically treated [1]. Stereotactic radiosurgery is an option for nonoperable lesions, but long-term safety is uncertain [12, 13].

In the clinical setting, patients with acute intracerebral hemorrhage (ICH) due to a CCM should be managed in the same way as those with ICH from other causes [1, 14].

Patients with a first seizure related to cerebral CCM should be managed with medical therapy using antiseizure medication. In contrast, prophylactic antiseizure medication treatment is not indicated for patients with asymptomatic or symptomatic CCMs who do not have seizures [15].

50.1.2 Developmental Venous Anomalies

Developmental venous anomalies (DVAs), previously known as venous angiomas, consist of a radially arranged configuration of medullary veins ("caput medusae") separated by normal brain parenchyma [16]. The lesions are usually solitary but can be multiple and occur with cavernous malformations. They are typically incidental findings on MRI, but cerebral angiography is considered the gold standard for its diagnosis. Most patients are followed without intervention since seizures or hemorrhages are infrequent [17].

They are reported in approximately 2% in autopsy series and are usually benign [18].

50.1.3 Capillary Telangiectasias

Capillary telangiectasias are small, dilated capillaries devoid of smooth muscle or elastic fibers. They are usually incidental findings on MRI, with an incidence of 0.7% and usually benign [19].

Their main locations are the pons, middle cerebellar peduncles, and dentate nuclei. Multiple lesions are common, not associated with morbidity, and intervention is usually unnecessary [20].

50.1.4 Arteriovenous Malformations (AVMs)

Traditionally thought to be congenital, their pathogenesis has yet to be entirely understood, since there are many well-documented reports of de novo brain AVM formation [21–23]. Growth, remodeling, or regression over time has also been observed in some patients [24, 25]. Genetic variation may influence brain AVM development and clinical course [26, 27].

50.1.5 Moyamoya Disease

A chronic progressive cerebrovascular disease is characterized by the progressive narrowing of large intracranial arteries and the development of prominent small-vessel collaterals [28].

50.1.6 Dural Arteriovenous Fistulas (DAVF)

DAVF are abnormal fistulous communications within the dural leaflets. The arterial component arises from any dural branches of the internal carotid artery, external carotid artery, vertebral carotid artery, or, more rarely, from pial branches

[29]. They usually occur near dural venous sinuses but can develop anywhere within the intracranial dura mater. The most common locations are the cavernous sinus, the cribriform plate, the transverse sigmoid sinus, and the tentorium [30]. They were recently reported to be acquired and not congenital lesions, presenting later in life compared to parenchymal AVMs [31]. The main difference between DAVF and cerebral AVM is the absence of parenchymal nidus and presence of dural arterial supply [32].

50.1.7 Carotid-Cavernous Fistulas (CCF)

An aberrant connection between branches of the carotid artery and the cavernous sinus leads to the shunting of blood from the high-pressure arterial system into the low-pressure venous circulation [33]. The first recorded patient presented proptosis, chemosis, and an ocular bruit [34]. Subsequent cases of CCFs have presented other physical examination findings, like pulsating exophthalmos. Understanding this disease's pathophysiology and treatment strategies, primarily via endovascular, have evolved [35].

This chapter focuses on AVMs and Moyamoya disease because they are more frequently operated and need special care in the perioperative period. We will present two clinical cases and describe how they were conducted in our service since evidence-based data regarding the best anesthetic and postoperative management are lacking.

50.2 Arteriovenous Malformations (AVMs)

50.2.1 Clinical Case

A 31-year-old woman presented with a history of minor depression and anxiety since 2008 that worsened in the last 6 months. She has never complained about headaches or any other symptoms. Neuropsychological assessment detected problems in working memory and arithmetical ability. Due to changes in the pattern of previous symptomatology, an MRI was performed and showed abnormal vessels in the right superior frontal gyrus, anterior to the prefrontal gyrus, with extension to the underlying white matter and intense paramagnetic contrast enhancement, with increased relative cerebral blood flow in the ASL sequence. Tractography revealed the nidus located anterior to the topography of the adjacent corticospinal tract without signs of involvement (Fig. 50.1). An AVM was suspected, and a digital subtraction angiography (DSA) was performed. It showed a right prefrontal AVM predominantly supplied by intermediate/posterior medial frontal branches of the right callosomarginal artery, the terminal branch of the anterior cerebral artery (Fig. 50.2). Also, it had some minor supply from branches of the right middle cerebral artery. Early venous drainage occurred from an ectatic and tortuous vein from the depth of the nidus toward the superior sagittal sinus.

We discussed this case with our multidisciplinary team and decided to operate it. Firstly, we performed a preoperative embolization with Squid focusing on the deepest and medial posterior parts (Fig. 50.3). As we know, it is easier for the neurosurgeon to deal with the superficial part of the AVM during surgery. Therefore, it is better to avoid embolizing the superficial parts of the AVM to avoid the flow deviation toward the most profound parts, which would increase the chances of bleeding and the complexity of the surgical resection.

A wide right frontoparietal craniotomy was performed. Bigger craniotomies are mandatory in order to expose the entire AVM and surrounding normal brain parenchyma.

We used an ICG video angiography to help assess the AVM feeders' surface anatomy, mainly the early draining vein.

After that, the first step of every AVM surgery consists of arachnoid dissection. Spending much time exposing the vasculature is essential to determine which vessels are going to the nidus and which are *en passage* vessels. Staying in the arachnoid plane can provide better control of the resection. It is better to avoid entering the nidus since there is a high probability of excessive bleeding on

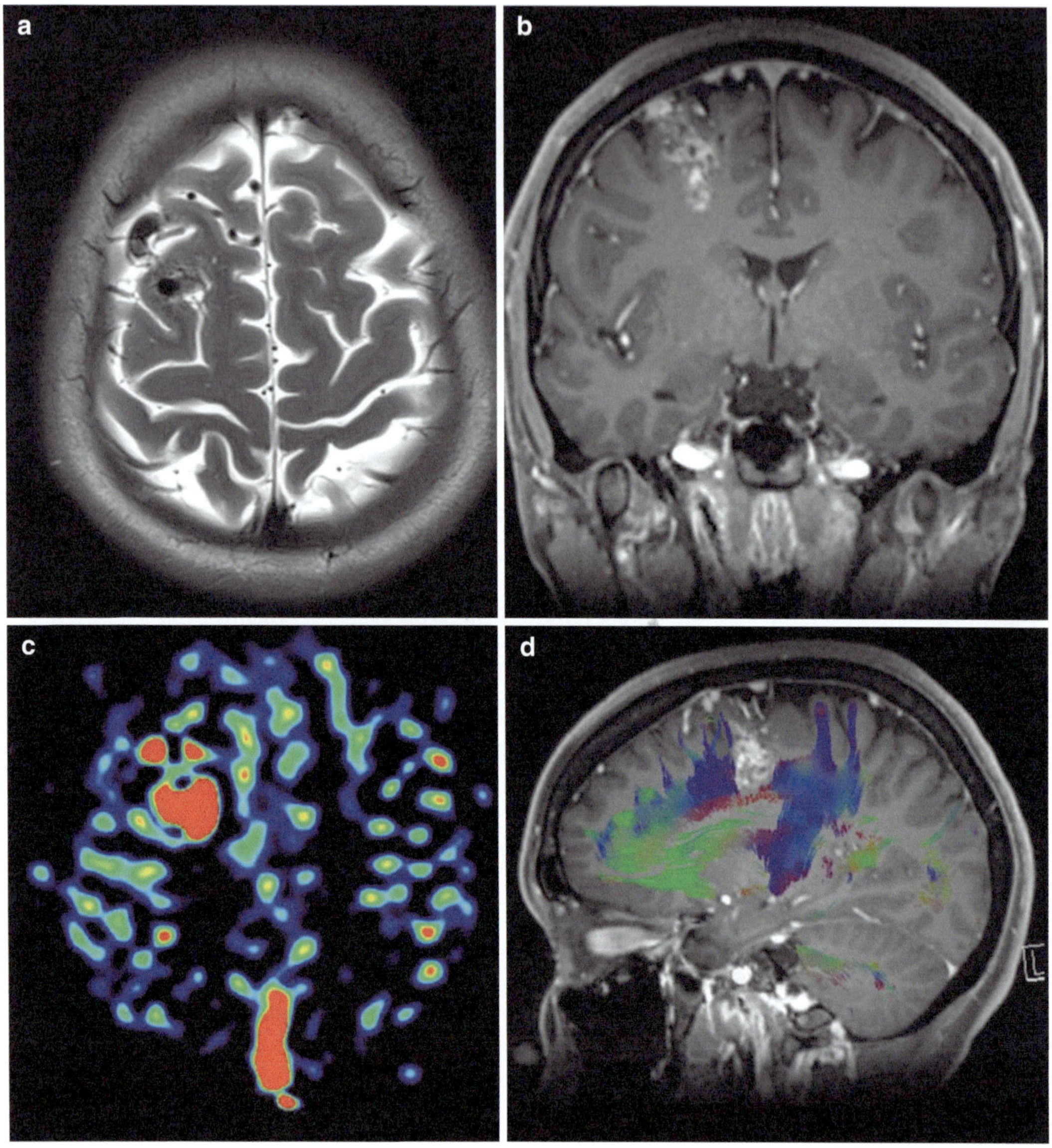

Fig. 50.1 MRI showed on T2-weighted image abnormal vessels in the right superior frontal gyrus, anterior to the prefrontal gyrus (**a**), with extension to the underlying white matter and intense paramagnetic contrast enhancement (**b**), with increased relative cerebral blood flow in the ASL sequence (**c**). Tractography (**d**) revealed the nidus located anterior to the topography of the adjacent corticospinal tract without signs of involvement

the surgical field, which can promote adhesion, and obscure the surrounding anatomical references, complicating the resection of the AVM.

The second step is the skeletonization of vessels, usually made circumferentially. In this stage, we identified, coagulated, and cut small branches going to the AVM nidus. After that, another ICG video angiography was performed to assess the disconnection status of the AVM.

The third step is parenchymal dissection. During this step, we visualized the embolic agent in the deepest and posterior parts. Deeper vessels, called "red devils," are challenging to coagulate and typically appear at the end of the resection. Once AVM was disconnected, another ICG video angiography confirmed the absence of flow into it.

The final step is coagulating and cutting the main draining vein (Fig. 50.4). A final ICG video

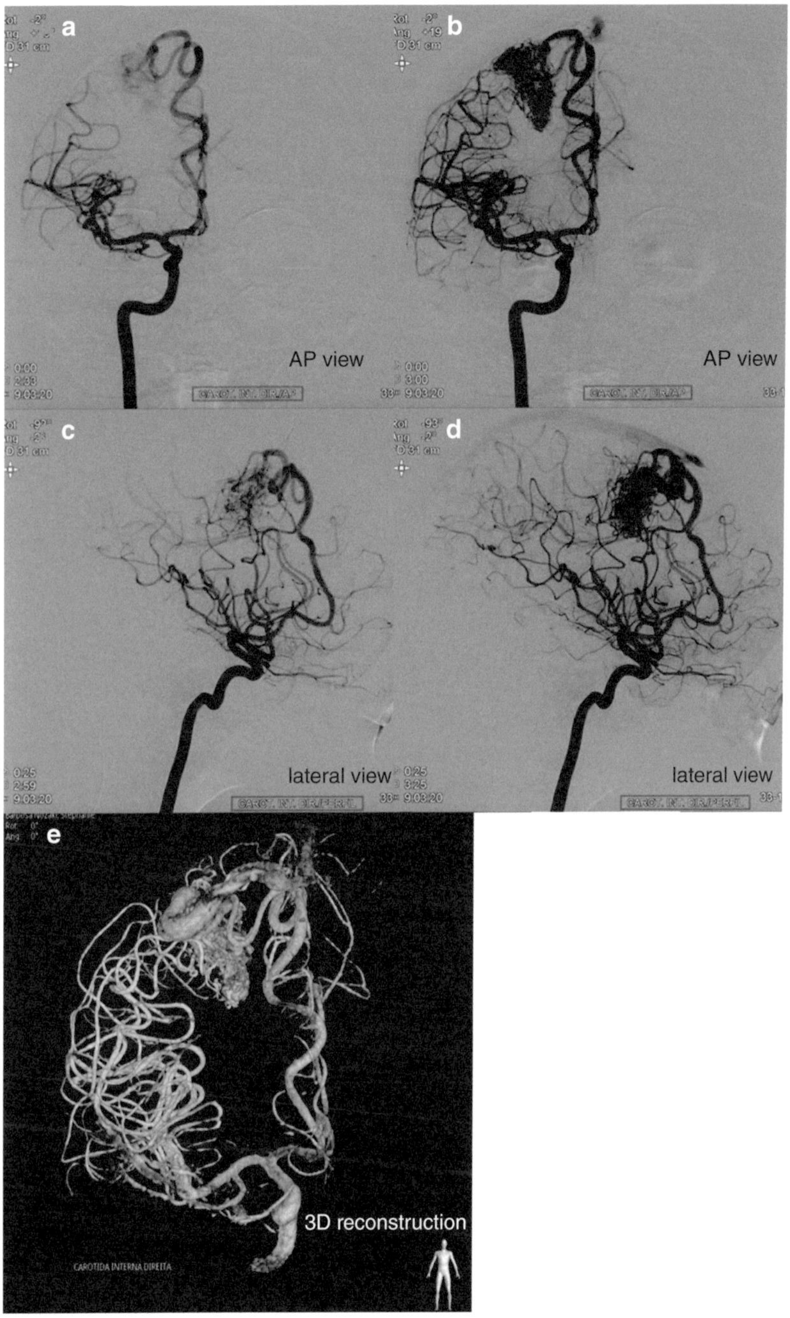

Fig. 50.2 Digital subtraction angiography (DSA) demonstrated an AVM on AP (**a** and **b**) and lateral (**c** and **d**), an AVM predominantly supplied by intermediate/posterior medial frontal branches of the right callosomarginal artery, terminal branch of the anterior cerebral artery. (**a**) AP view; (**b**) AP view; (**c**) lateral view; (**d**) lateral view; (**e**) 3D reconstruction

angiography assessed the surgical bed and surrounding vasculature. The closure was made in a typical manner.

The patient was extubated before going to the NeuroICU, where she stayed for 3 days. After three more days in the ward, she was discharged home with no postoperative deficits or complications.

Postoperative MRI and angiography confirmed a complete resection and cure of the AVM (Fig. 50.5).

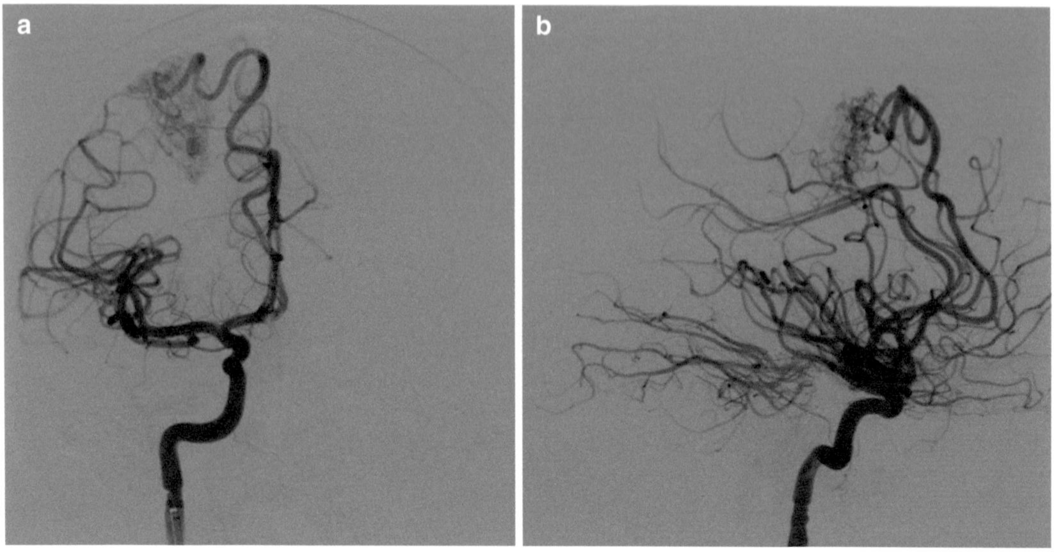

Fig. 50.3 Preoperative postembolization DSA showed reduced flow through the nidus. (**a** and **b**) AP view; lateral view; 3D reconstruction

50.2.2 Discussion

Arteriovenous malformations (AVMs) are the most dangerous of all cerebrovascular malformations, and their management usually is challenging for neurosurgeons, neuroanesthesiologists, neuro-interventionists, and neurocritical care specialists.

They are characterized by a direct arterial-venous connection without an intervening capillary network. There may be single or multiple vessels in the nidus, either on the arterial or the venous side. The high-flow arteriovenous communication potentiates the development of associated aneurysms and arterialization of the venous limb [36]. They are frequently surrounded by calcifications and ischemic or gliotic brain with abnormal autoregulation [24].

It is expected to be present in approximately 0.1% of the population, ten times less common than intracranial aneurysms [25]. About 90% are located in the supratentorial compartment and the remainder in the posterior fossa. They usually occur as single lesions, but as many as 9% are multiple [37]. They are generally diagnosed during childhood or between the ages of 30 and 50 [38, 39].

Clinical Manifestations

Many cases are incidental findings on brain imaging, either MRI or CT scan, performed for other reasons [22].

Other cases are symptomatic. The patient's age, as well as the size, location, and vascular features of the AVM, influence its clinical presentation [22, 25]:

Intraparenchymal, intraventricular, or subarachnoid hemorrhage are the most common clinical presentations (40–60%). Superficial AVM usually bleeds into the subarachnoid space, causing headaches [40].

Once diagnosed, the overall annual risk of hemorrhage is expected to be between 1% and 3% [41–44]. In the individual patient level meta-analysis, those with a previous hemorrhage are at higher risk of a second bleeding, around 4.5% per year [42]. AVMs with a deep brain location or exclusive deep venous drainage and associated aneurysms also have an increased risk of bleeding, reaching an annual risk of up to 30% [41, 43]. Pregnancy is not a risk factor, but it is controversial [45–47].

Other clinical features are seizure and epilepsy development, particularly in younger patients, with a nidus diameter > 3 cm, located

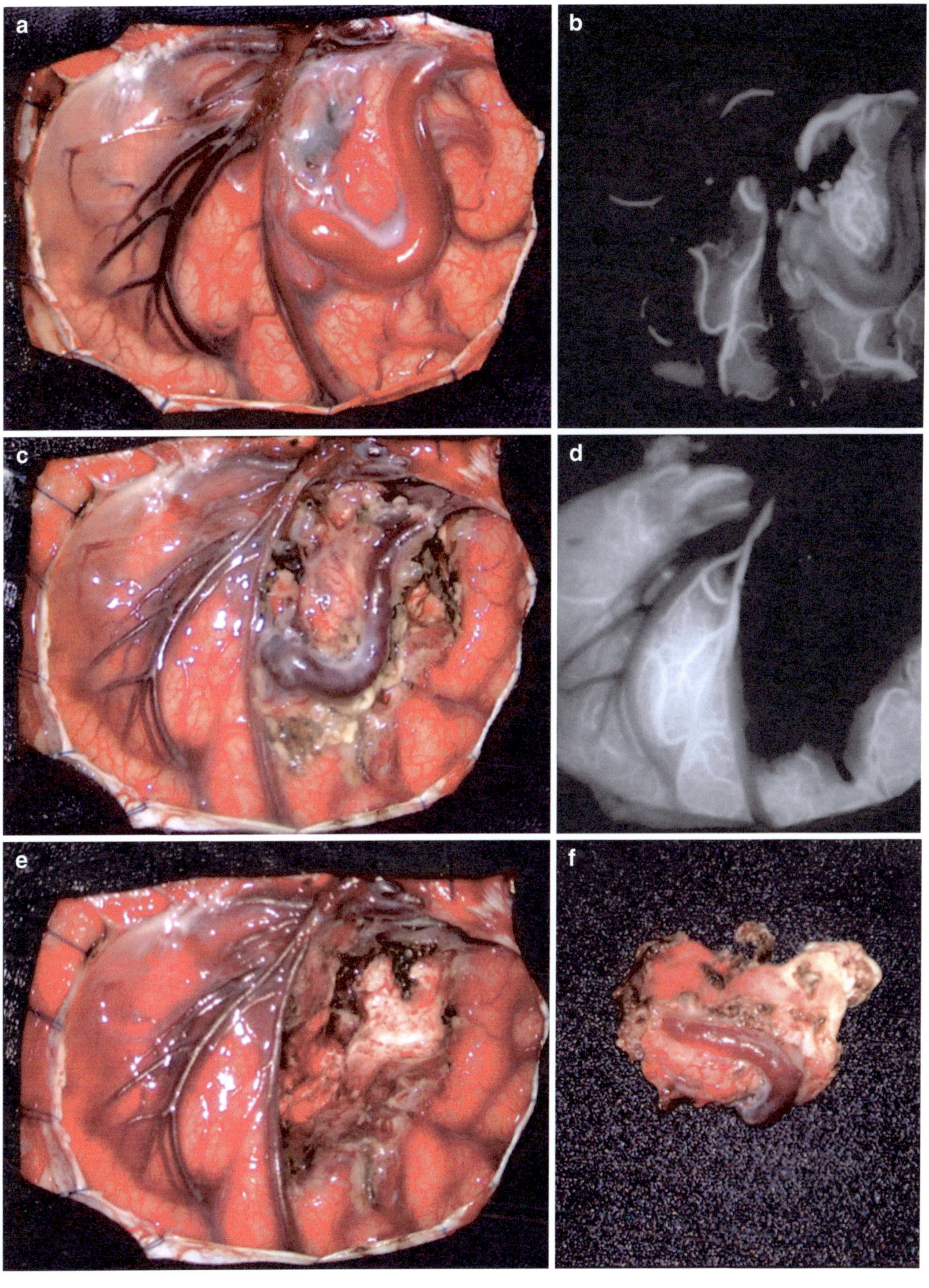

Fig. 50.4 AVM surgery. (**a**) Initial aspect of the AVM; (**b**) ICG video angiography showing arterial feeders, the superficial part of the nidus, and early draining vein; (**c**) aspect of the AVM after arachnoid and parenchymal dissection; (**d**) final ICG video angiography demonstrated an excluded AVM; (**e**) surgical bed after resection; (**f**) En bloc resection

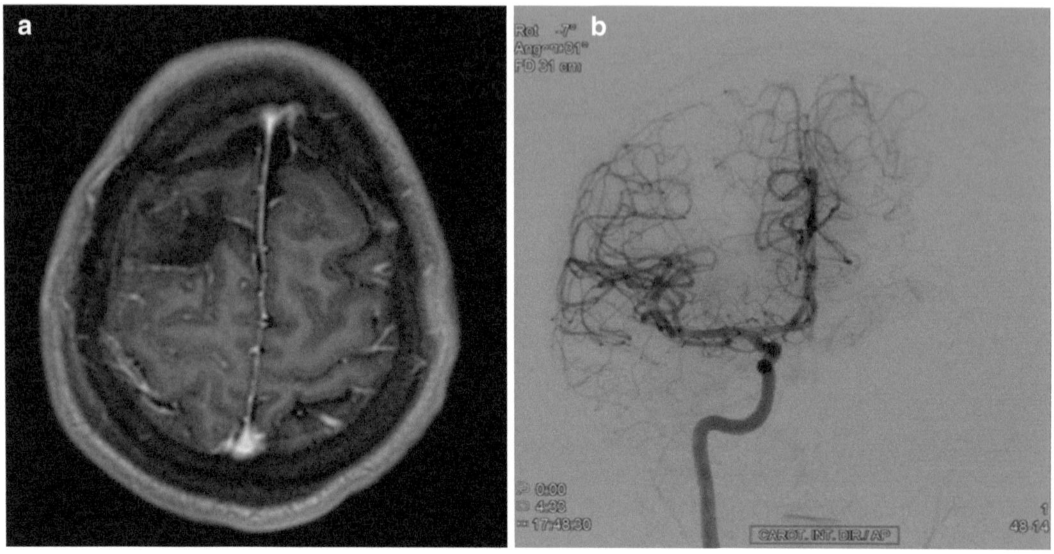

Fig. 50.5 Postoperative MRI (**a**) and angiography (**b**) demonstrated complete resection of AVM

on the temporal lobes, and with cortical involvement [48].

Patients with multiple, large, superficial-draining AVMs, located mainly in the cortex, are more likely to present with seizures. They are typically focal, simple, or complex with secondary generalization [48, 49].

More rarely, patients can develop a focal neurologic deficit due to hemorrhage, mass effect, disturbances of the cerebral blood flow autoregulation, or as a postictal effect of a seizure [25].

It is not indicated a routine screening of the general population or family members for brain AVMs [50, 51]. Brain AVMs are not hereditary, except for patients with hereditary hemorrhagic telangiectasia (Osler-Weber-Rendu syndrome). This diagnosis should be suspected in patients with spontaneous and recurrent epistaxis, multiple mucocutaneous telangiectasias at characteristic sites, gastrointestinal telangiectasia, pulmonary or hepatic arteriovenous malformation, or a first-degree relative with HHT [52].

Both computed tomography angiography (CTA) and magnetic resonance angiography (MRA) have good sensitivity and specificity (98 and 99%, respectively) to detect an underlying intracranial vascular malformation [53]. On the other hand, catheter contrast angiography (i.e., digital subtraction angiography [DSA]) is essential for treatment planning and posttreatment follow-up of brain AVMs since it provides crucial information such as the nidus configuration, its relationship to surrounding vessels, and localization of the draining or efferent portion and anatomical particularities like early draining vein without a visible nidus, venous outflow obstruction, and associated aneurysms that has not been detected using CTA or MRA [40]. However, there is a risk of immediate neurologic complications, mainly ischemic stroke, after performing angiography, but hopefully, this risk is low [54].

Treatment

The typical presentation of a brain AVM rupture is intracerebral hemorrhage (ICH), but concurrent intraventricular or subarachnoid hemorrhage may also be present, depending upon the AVM location [42]. Urgent surgery for ruptured AVMs is required in some cases, depending on the clinical status of the patient and the degree and location of the hemorrhage [40].

Antiseizure medications are indicated after the first seizure episode to prevent its recurrence but are not indicated prophylactically for those who have never had seizures [55].

Many factors should be considered when choosing between conservative medical management, microsurgical excision, radiosurgery, or

Table 50.1 Spetzler and Martin grading system [56]

Characteristic		Point (s) assigned
Size	Small (<3 cm)	1
	Medium (3–6 cm)	2
	Larger (>6 cm)	3
Eloquence area located	No	0
	Yes	1
Venous drainage	Superficial only	0
	Any deep	1

endovascular embolization. Several parameters are incorporated into the Spetzler-Martin grading scale [56] (Table 50.1).

The largest dimension of the nidus in centimeters on imaging determines AVM size. Eloquent brain areas include regions of the cortex devoted to sensorimotor, visual, and language functions and certain deeper structures: the internal capsules, basal ganglia, thalamus, hypothalamus, brain stem, cerebellar peduncles, and deep cerebellar nuclei [56, 57]. Deep venous drainage is considered present if any or all outflow occurs via deep veins such as internal cerebral veins, basal veins, and precentral cerebellar veins [40]. A higher Spetzler-Martin grading scale score correlates with an increased risk of surgical morbidity and neurologic deficits [58, 59].

Ruptured AVMs can be treated acutely or, preferably, four to six weeks after the hemorrhage. The anesthetic management of patients with acute bleeding is much more challenging because cerebral autoregulation is severely impaired soon after the intracranial hemorrhage. Moreover, absorption of the hematoma and resolution of any surrounding edema facilitates surgical access to the AVM [60].

Microsurgical excision has a higher rate of complete nidus obliteration and higher long-term durability compared to radiosurgery or endovascular embolization alone [40]. However, a more extended recovery period is needed. It may cause neurologic impairments related to the dissection of the normal adjacent brain parenchyma and neurovascular structures required to reach the AVM. Postoperative complications include arterial or venous infarction or hemorrhage from the resection cavity. Postoperative hemorrhage on the resection bed can occur despite documented complete resection of the lesion by angiography [61].

Some experts suggest that embolization can effectively adjunct surgery and radiosurgery [62]. Embolization before surgery can be performed to reduce blood loss and to occlude vessels that may be difficult to control during surgery [63]. However, this procedure is not risk-free; the embolic material can migrate and occlude vessels to healthy cerebral adjacent tissues. Also, post-procedural hemorrhage can occur due to venous occlusion from the embolic material [54, 64].

Anesthetic Management

Evaluation of associated aneurysms, signs of ischemia, or mass effect should be performed preoperatively.

It is essential to provide optimal brain relaxation for a better surgical field and euvolemia to maintain cerebral and systemic adequate perfusion.

In our service, besides the usual monitors (cardioscope, pulse oximeter, etCO2 and esophageal thermometer, urine output), we routinely get a central venous line and invasive arterial blood pressure catheter in order to obtain seriated arterial blood gases analysis, electrolytes, Hb, Ht, and lactate. In some cases, we also use processed EEG and cardiac output monitors, based on pulse wave analysis.

During the direct handling of the AVM, we maintain the MAP 20% below the patient's normal MAP. We avoid deliberate hypotension due to the increased risk of cerebral ischemia and venous thrombosis (outflow).

There are no conclusive studies on the benefits of the total intravenous anesthesia technique in these patients and the use of pharmacological or nonpharmacological cerebral protection maneuvers.

We prefer to use 1 CAM of sevoflurane instead propofol-based total intravenous anesthesia in most cases of AVM resections when intraoperative neurophysiological neuromonitoring is not being performed. It aims to help diminishing the amount of bleeding during the surgery. The neurophysiological reasoning for that could be that total intravenous anesthesia deviates blood from the normal brain to the AVM, and inhalation anesthesia could do the opposite. The same rationale applies for etCO2, that should be ideally kept in the higher normal range (40–45 mmHg) instead of the lower normal range (35–40 mmHg), with the advantage that it does not seem to interfere with the neuromonitoring.

Another important aspect during AVM manipulation is bleeding control since intense bleeding predisposes to malignant edema. Our transfusion trigger is Hb below 10 and we use the massive transfusion protocol when the AVM bleeds profusely.

We avoid using mannitol in order to have a better control of the volemic state of the patient, since it can induce osmotic diuresis. We use Plasmalyte and Ringer Lactate plus 5 mL of 20% NaCl to keep the solution isotonic or slightly hypertonic in relation to the plasma. In prolonged surgeries, we often use albumin.

In order to prevent intraoperative cerebral edema, we take special care avoiding seizures, that can occur spontaneously due to surgical manipulation depending on the AVM location. Therefore, we avoid superficial anesthesia.

We also use mild hypothermia, slight hypercapnia (within the normal range) and promptly correct acid-base and hydro electrolyte disturbances.

After total resection, blood pressure should be temporarily restored to normal levels or slightly above, to check the hemostasis of the surgical bed. Once the effectiveness of surgical hemostasis has been verified, blood pressure is reduced and maintained in this way in the postoperative period.

Ideally, the patients should be extubated in the OR and sent awake to the ICU, to have their neurological status easily assessed to promptly observe any neurologic deterioration or seizures. Dexmedetomidine can be used when a certain degree of sedation and analgesia is required.

Awake resection of AVMs can be performed in some specific cases, but its benefit is controversial [65].

Postoperative Care

Postoperative care in an intensive care unit is essential for better control of MAP, considering the altered cerebral autoregulation inside and outside the AVM resection bed.

Perilesional vessels are fragile and can predispose to complications such as rupture of small vessels, occlusive hyperemia, and the theoretical risk for Normal Perfusion Pressure Breakthrough Syndrome [66].

The phenomenon of breakthrough, also called hyperemia with normal perfusion pressure refers to a redistribution of blood flow after the resection of the AVM to areas that lived under a regime of chronic hypotension, with a different self-regulation curve. Therefore, even a normal perfusion pressure is supposed to cause hyperemia in these areas [67].

In occlusive hyperemia, cerebral edema occurs due to venous engorgement resulting from occlusion of the normal venous drainage of tissue adjacent to the AVM during surgery [68].

Induced hypotension demanding continuous intra-arterial monitoring to maintain systolic blood pressure < 120 mmHg during the postoperative period seems to be related to a lower incidence of hemorrhage in the postoperative period. An escalating drug regimen consisting of beta-blockers, sodium nitroprusside, oral nimodipine, and an angiotensin-converting enzyme inhibitor can be used in order to achieve this strict blood pressure control postoperatively [61].

50.3 Moyamoya Disease

50.3.1 Clinical Case

A 9-year-old boy presented to the emergency room with a sudden right hemiparesis, more evident on the upper extremities, and speech difficulty. There were no other associated symptoms. He reported previous events of transitory weakness on the right side, with complete recovery and without sequelae. He had no family history of vascular or neurological diseases. On admission, a neurological examination revealed a right-sided hemiparesis with mild dysarthria. Symptoms were suggestive of stroke, and an MRI was performed. T2-weighted image (T2WI) showed old infarcts in basal ganglia bilaterally and mild cortical atrophy in the left frontal lobe (Fig. 50.6a, b). Fluid-attenuated inversion recovery (FLAIR) sequence showed high-linear signals following a sulcal pattern on the left inferior frontal and precentral gyrus (Fig. 50.6c, d), with a contrast enhancement (Fig. 50.6e, f). This is called the "ivy sign." Three-dimensional time-of-flight MR angiography (3D TOF MRA) demonstrated reduced flow voids in the internal, middle, and anterior cerebral arteries coupled with prominent flow voids through the basal ganglia and thalamus, most evident on the left side (Fig. 50.7).

Suspicion of Moyamoya disease was high and a digital subtraction angiography was requested. Stenosis of the distal intracranial internal carotid artery, extending to the proximal anterior and middle arteries and extensive collateral network at the base of the brain along with the classic "puff of smoke" appearance was evident, predominantly on the left side (Fig. 50.8).

A diagnosis of Moyamoya disease was made, and surgical treatment was indicated to prevent future strokes by improving blood flow to the cerebral hemisphere. There is controversy about which type of revascularization is better for children. Indirect revascularization has a lower risk of complications, but the protective effect only appears months later. Direct revascularization offers an immediate increase in blood flow but is often technically challenging to perform because of the small size of both donor and recipient vessels.

In this case, we planned a combined direct and indirect revascularization. Although both sides were involved, the left side was chosen first because of the severity of stenosis and symptoms. Before initiating the surgery, the superficial temporal artery (STA) was mapped and marked using a doppler ultrasound probe. After the incision, STA was identified and dissected. Extremely care must be taken to protect STA. While we dissected the STA, we also elevated the temporal muscle, protecting the deep temporal fascia. We performed a frontotemporal craniotomy and opened the dura mater in a C-shape manner. At that time, we noticed ischemic changes in the arachnoid membrane (Fig. 50.9a). Therefore, we performed a comprehensive arachnoid dissection to expose the brain parenchyma and blood vessels (Fig. 50.9b). This arachnoid dissection enabled us to see better the cortical vasculature (Fig. 50.9c). Next step was to identify the best cortical (M4) branch of the middle cerebral artery as a recipient vessel for the direct bypass. After the preparation of STA (Fig. 50.9d), temporary clipping was placed in the recipient's vessel. A terminal-lateral anastomosis was performed with interrupted sutures (Fig. 50.9e). ICG confirmed bypass patency (Fig. 50.9f), and encephalomyoarteriosynangiosis was performed.

The procedure had no complications. MRA performed 3 months after surgery showed hypertrophied superficial temporal artery and profuse collateral vessel development on the left side (Fig. 50.10).

50.3.2 Discussion

Moyamoya is a rare arteriopathy characterized by progressive stenosis of the internal carotid arteries. The cause still needs to be better understood. There is a difference between Moyamoya disease and Moyamoya syndrome.

The Moyamoya disease (MMD) is an unusual, chronic, progressive, irreversible cerebrovascular disease characterized by progressive stenosis or occlusion, uni or bilateral, of the internal carotid arteries or their principal branches. As a result of this occlusion, a fragile vascular network is formed at the base of the brain that functions as a collateral pathway (the moyamoya vessels) [69]. In the angiographic image, the small collateral arteries appear as a "puff of smoke" [70–72].

Although it had already been described in 1957 by Takeuchi and Shimizu, it was only in 1969 that the term "moyamoya," which signifies something hazy, like a puff of cigarette smoke, began to be used [73].

The Moyamoya disease (MMD) seems to affect two age groups with different clinical presentations. The pediatric population (0–10 years) predominantly presents with ischemic strokes, and the adults (30–50 years) usually have the hemorrhagic form [74].

In the Moyamoya syndrome (congenital), this abnormal development may involve other systemic arteries, especially renal arteries [75].

This syndrome is more common in the Asian population than in the western hemisphere and

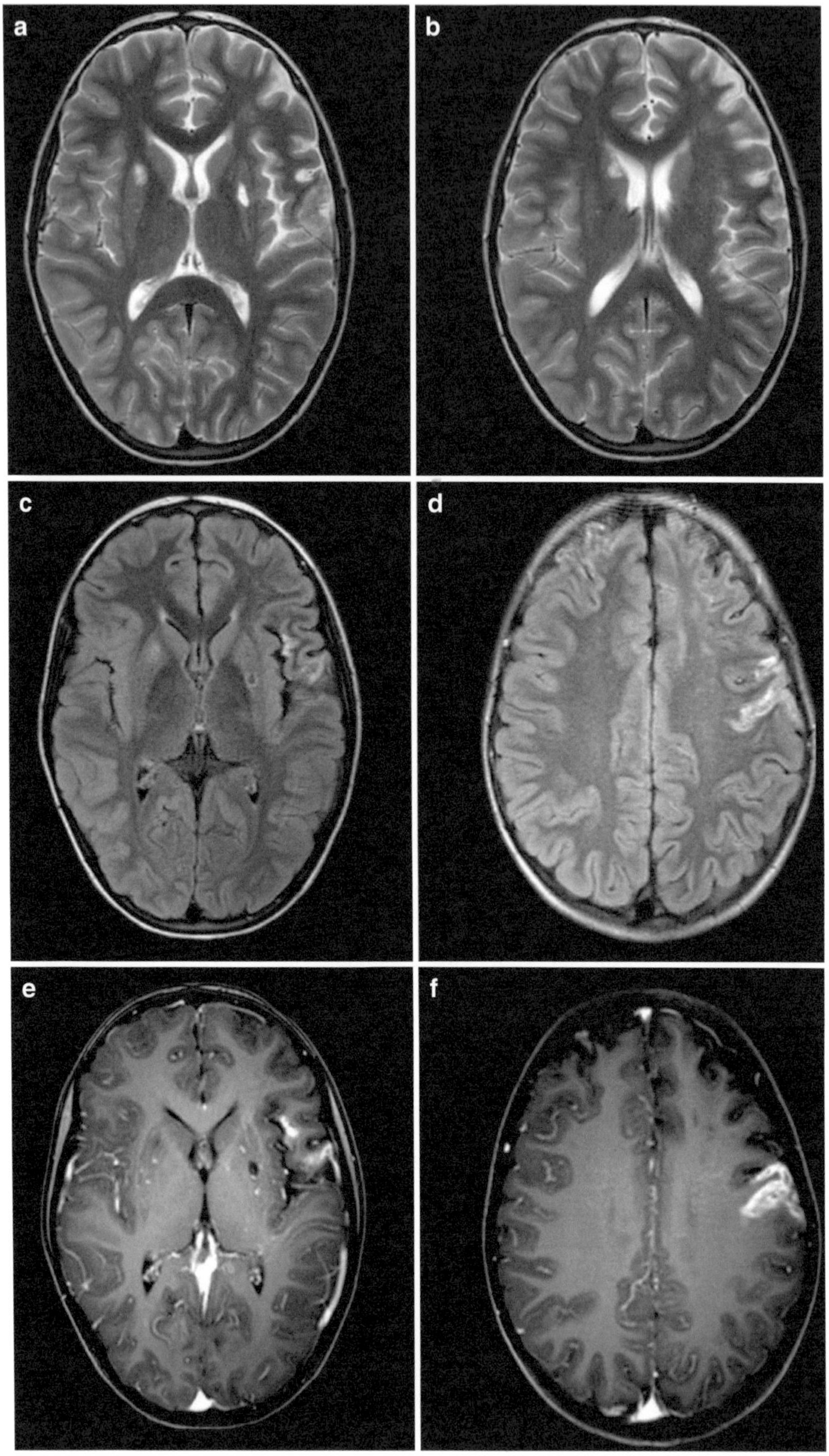

Fig. 50.6 MRI T2-weighted image revealed hyperintense signal lesions located in basal ganglia bilaterally and a mild cortical atrophy in the left frontal lobe (**a** and **b**); FLAIR sequence demonstrated linear high signals following a sulcal pattern on the left inferior frontal and precentral gyrus (**c**, **d**), with contrast enhancement (**e**, **f**)

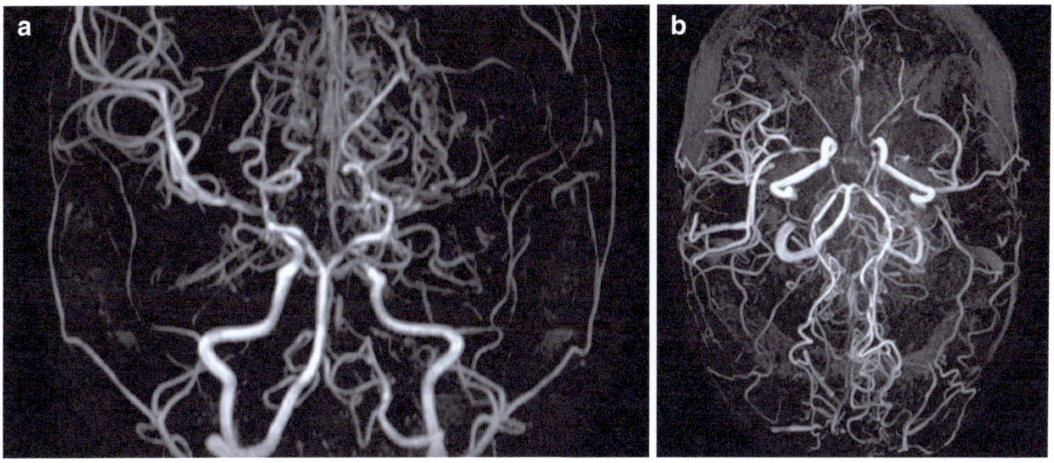

Fig. 50.7 Three-dimensional TOF MRA evidenced reduced flow voids in the internal, middle, and anterior cerebral arteries coupled with prominent flow voids through the basal ganglia and thalamus. (**a**) coronal view; (**b**) axial view

Europe. The reported incidence varies between 0.35 and 86 per 100,000 people [71].

Diagnosis is based on specific clinical signs and imaging methods such as conventional angiography and magnetic resonance imaging/angiography [71].

Clinical Manifestations

Stenosis of the internal carotid artery leads to symptoms related to decreased cerebral blood flow.

Signs and symptoms of ischemia prevail in the pediatric population, such as TIAs, headaches, ischemic strokes, seizures, and choreiform movements.

Hyperventilation can occur in everyday situations, for instance, when the child cries, exercises, coughs, or blow. They cause vasoconstriction of the normally dilated cerebral blood vessels, reducing cerebral blood flow and worsening ischemia [71].

In the adult population, intracranial hemorrhages are more common [71].

Treatment

Clinical treatment consists of antiplatelet drugs and calcium channel blockers that can control symptoms, reduce thrombotic phenomena, and maintain normal tension.

The surgical treatment improves cerebral perfusion distal to the lesion to prevent cerebral infarction. Direct and indirect cerebral revascularization techniques are used. The superficial temporal artery-to-middle cerebral artery bypass (STA-MCA) is more utilized in adults combined or not with pial synangiosis (more used in the pediatric population) [71, 74].

Anesthetic Management

Since cerebral autoregulation is affected in patients with MMD, the biggest challenge for the anesthesiologist is optimizing cerebral blood flow to reduce the risk of injury. On one side, arterial hypotension can cause graft thrombosis; on the other, hypertension can cause severe bleeding during surgery.

Therefore, the main challenge is to achieve strict control of arterial pressure. Moreover, it is crucial to maintain euvolemia, normothermia, adequate urine output [76], and normocapnia [77], avoiding both hypoperfusion and hyperperfusion [78].

Anticonvulsant medications and calcium channel blockers should be taken until the day of the surgery. Platelet antiaggregant should be suspended 7–10 days before surgery and reintroduced postoperatively. In this interval, patients should receive low-molecular-weight heparin.

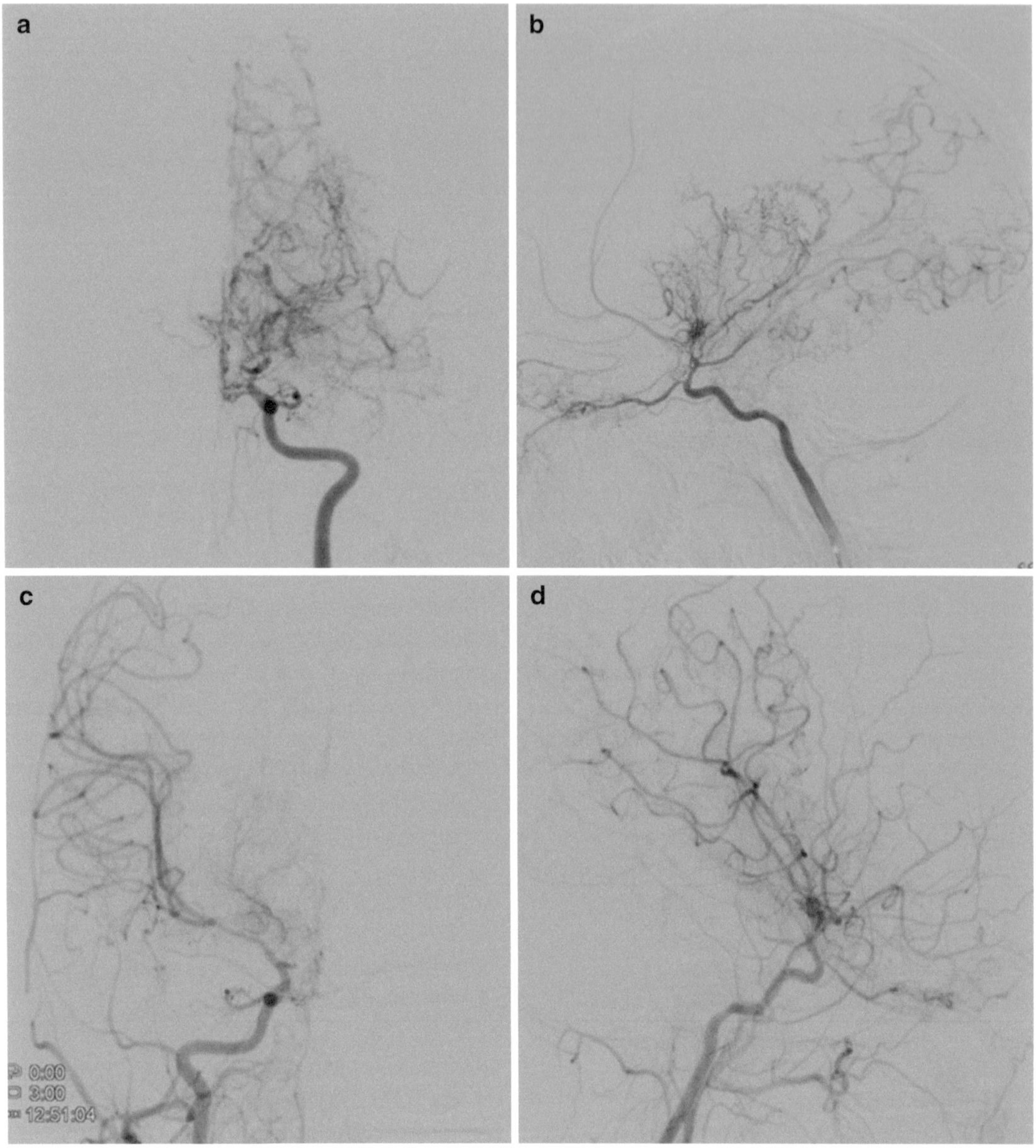

Fig. 50.8 Angiography demonstrated bilateral stenosis of the supraclinoid segment of internal carotid artery, with reduced blood flow through the anterior and middle arteries. Augmented collateral network at the basal ganglia giving the classic “puff of smoke” appearance; (**a**) left side; (**b**) left side; (**c**) right side; (**d**) right side

Preanesthetic medication should be used to prevent the child from crying and hyperventilating, which would cause cerebral vasoconstriction, decreased cerebral blood flow, and ischemia.

BP variations should be avoided during anesthetic induction and during anesthesia and awakening. Orotracheal intubation and extubation must be performed in a deep plane of anesthesia to prevent hypertensive peaks and ICP increase.

Hypercapnia can cause the stealing phenomenon. The Moyamoya-diseased vessels do not react to CO_2; therefore, hypercapnia can cause a cerebral blood flow deviation to normal brain areas, worsening the local ischemia of the perivascular regions. These areas have an altered cerebral blood flow autoregulation and are challenging because ischemia and hyperemia can occur more easily. Because of this, blood pres-

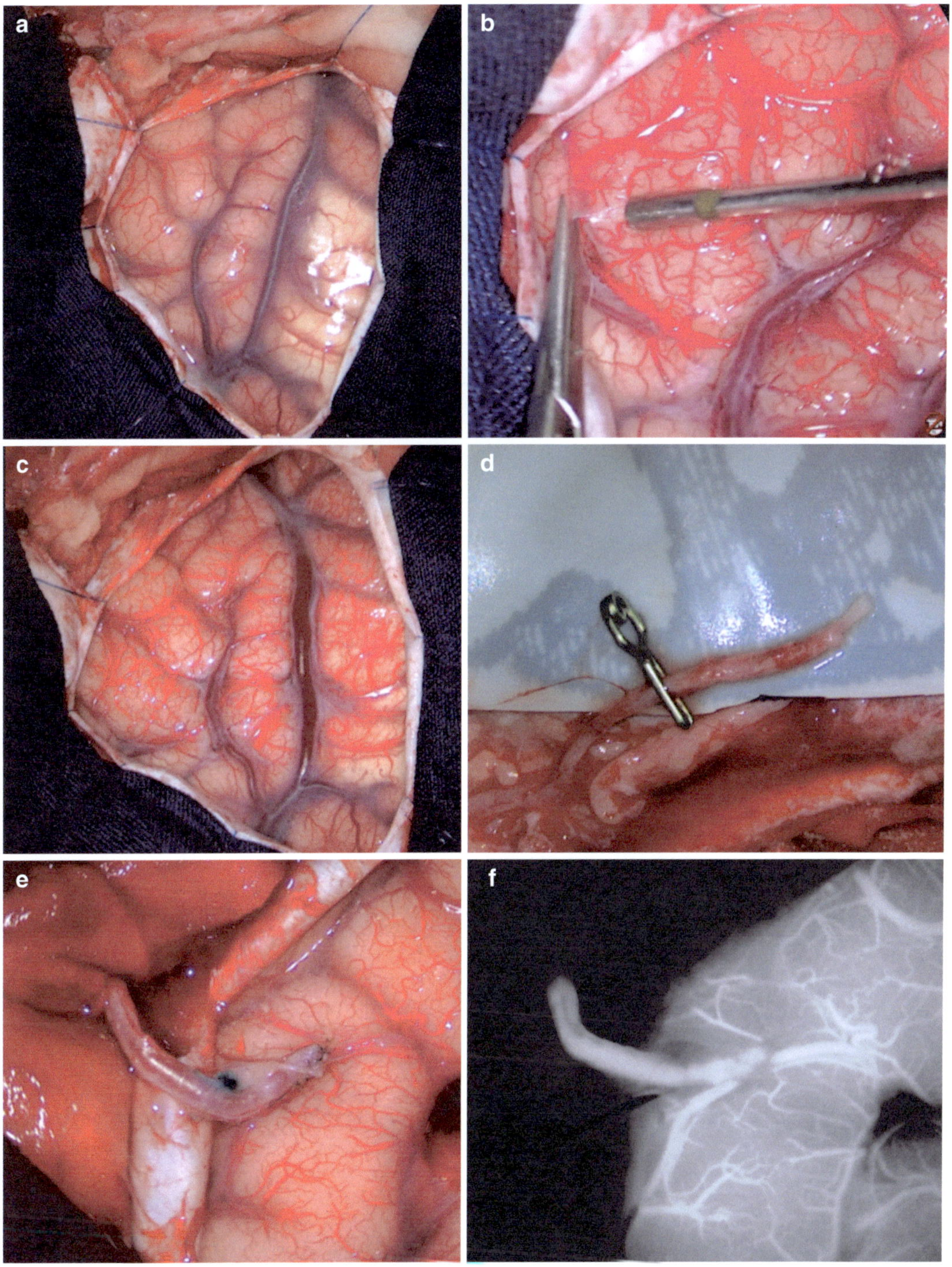

Fig. 50.9 Direct revascularization. (**a**) Initial aspect of the brain surface; (**b**) arachnoid dissection; (**c**) brain parenchyma after wide arachnoid dissection; (**d**) STA appearance after dissection and preparation; (**e**) final aspect after terminolateral anastomosis; (**f**) ICG videoangiography confirming bypass patency

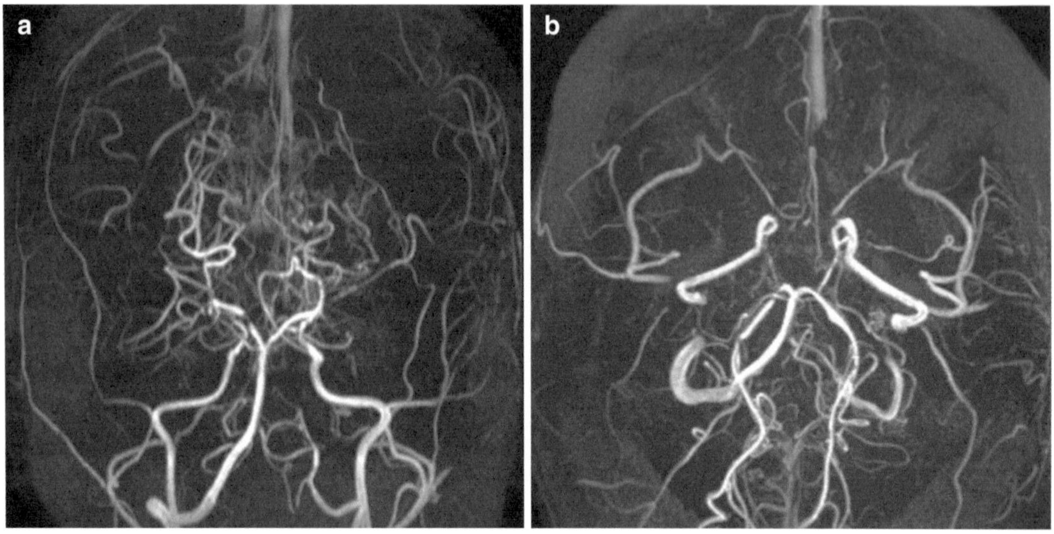

Fig. 50.10 Postoperative three-dimensional (3D) time-of-flight (TOF) magnetic resonance angiogram (MRA) showing collateral vessel development (**a** and **b**)

sure should be kept at normal or slightly higher levels. However, it is essential to avoid noradrenaline since it impairs microcirculation.

Mannitol should also be avoided, or at least used carefully, since it can cause osmotic diuresis and dehydration.

Polycythemia is undesirable as it causes increased viscosity and also impairs microcirculation. The hematocrit should be maintained between 30% and 42%. Mild hypothermia and thiopental boluses can be used aiming to burst suppression at critical moments of the bypass, although there is no robust evidence for this.

Neuromonitoring is advisable. EEG can be used to monitor ischemia and seizure intraoperatively and postoperatively [79]. Directly monitoring cerebral blood flow through Doppler flowmetry, micro-Doppler ultrasonography, and jugular bulb oxygen saturation measurements is not always available but may be helpful. Near-infrared spectroscopy (NIRS) can also be used [80].

Postoperative Care

The main complications in the postoperative period are TIA, infarction, subdural effusion, hyperperfusion syndrome (more common in adults), subdural hematoma, intracranial infection, and seizures [72, 76].

Essential issues are strict monitoring of blood pressure, hematocrit, urine output, and oxygen saturation to avoid neurologic complications. Optimizing analgesia and sedation levels is desirable in some cases, and preventing nausea and vomiting is mandatory [72, 76].

References

1. Akers A, Al-Shahi Salman R, Awad IA, Dahlem K, Flemming K, Hart B, Kim H, Jusue-Torres I, Kondziolka D, Lee C, Morrison L, Rigamonti D, Rebeiz T, Tournier-Lasserve E, Waggoner D, Whitehead K. Synopsis of guidelines for the clinical Management of Cerebral Cavernous Malformations: consensus recommendations based on systematic literature review by the Angioma Alliance scientific advisory board clinical experts panel. Neurosurgery. 2017;80(5):665–80. https://doi.org/10.1093/neuros/nyx091.
2. Goldstein HE, Solomon RA. Epidemiology of cavernous malformations. Handb Clin Neurol. 2017;143:241–7. https://doi.org/10.1016/B978-0-444-63640-9.00023-0.
3. Batra S, Lin D, Recinos PF, Zhang J, Rigamonti D. Cavernous malformations: natural history, diagnosis and treatment. Nat Rev Neurol. 2009;5(12):659–70. https://doi.org/10.1038/nrneurol.2009.177.
4. Flemming KD. Incidence, prevalence, and clinical presentation of cerebral cavernous malformations. Methods Mol Biol. 2020;2152:27–33. https://doi.org/10.1007/978-1-0716-0640-7_2.

5. Aiba T, Tanaka R, Koike T, Kameyama S, Takeda N, Komata T. Natural history of intracranial cavernous malformations. J Neurosurg. 1995;83(1):56–9. https://doi.org/10.3171/jns.1995.83.1.0056.
6. Robinson JR, Awad IA, Little JR. Natural history of the cavernous angioma. J Neurosurg. 1991;75(5):709–14. https://doi.org/10.3171/jns.1991.75.5.0709.
7. Fritschi JA, Reulen HJ, Spetzler RF, Zabramski JM. Cavernous malformations of the brain stem. A review of 139 cases. Acta Neurochir. 1994;130(1–4):35–46. https://doi.org/10.1007/BF01405501.
8. Badhiwala JH, Farrokhyar F, Alhazzani W, Yarascavitch B, Aref M, Algird A, Murty N, Kachur E, Cenic A, Reddy K, Almenawer SA. Surgical outcomes and natural history of intramedullary spinal cord cavernous malformations: a single-center series and meta-analysis of individual patient data: clinic article. J Neurosurg Spine. 2014;21(4):662–76. https://doi.org/10.3171/2014.6.SPINE13949.
9. Otten M, Mccormick P. Natural history of spinal cavernous malformations. Handb Clin Neurol. 2017;143:233–9. https://doi.org/10.1016/B978-0-444-63640-9.00022-9.
10. Liu C, Li W, Tong KA, Yeom KW, Kuzminski S. Susceptibility-weighted imaging and quantitative susceptibility mapping in the brain. J Magn Reson Imaging. 2015;42(1):23–41. https://doi.org/10.1002/jmri.24768.
11. Mokin M, Agazzi S, Dawson L, Primiani CT. Neuroimaging of cavernous malformations. Curr Pain Headache Rep. 2017;21(12):47. https://doi.org/10.1007/s11916-017-0649-1.
12. Mouchtouris N, Chalouhi N, Chitale A, Starke RM, Tjoumakaris SI, Rosenwasser RH, Jabbour PM. Management of cerebral cavernous malformations: from diagnosis to treatment. ScientificWorldJournal. 2015;2015:808314. https://doi.org/10.1155/2015/808314.
13. Kim BS, Kim KH, Lee MH, Lee JI. Stereotactic radiosurgery for brainstem cavernous malformations: an updated systematic review and meta-analysis. World Neurosurg. 2019;130:e648–59. https://doi.org/10.1016/j.wneu.2019.06.183.
14. Chohan MO, Marchiò S, Morrison LA, Sidman RL, Cavenee WK, Dejana E, Yonas H, Pasqualini R, Arap W. Emerging pharmacologic targets in cerebral cavernous malformation and potential strategies to Alter the natural history of a difficult disease: a review. JAMA Neurol. 2019;76(4):492–500. https://doi.org/10.1001/jamaneurol.2018.3634.
15. Rosenow F, Alonso-Vanegas MA, Baumgartner C, Blümcke I, Carreño M, Gizewski ER, Hamer HM, Knake S, Kahane P, Lüders HO, Mathern GW, Menzler K, Miller J, Otsuki T, Ozkara C, Pitkänen A, Roper SN, Sakamoto AC, Sure U, Walker MC, Steinhoff BJ, Surgical Task Force, Commission on Therapeutic Strategies of the ILAE. Cavernoma-related epilepsy: review and recommendations for management—report of the surgical task force of the ILAE commission on therapeutic strategies. Epilepsia. 2013;54(12):2025–35. https://doi.org/10.1111/epi.12402.
16. Mooney MA, Zabramski JM. Developmental venous anomalies. Handb Clin Neurol. 2017;143:279–82. https://doi.org/10.1016/B978-0-444-63640-9.00026-6.
17. Ruíz DS, Yilmaz H, Gailloud P. Cerebral developmental venous anomalies: current concepts. Ann Neurol. 2009;66(3):271–83. https://doi.org/10.1002/ana.21754.
18. McCormick WF. Pathology of vascular malformations of the brain. In: Wilson CB, Stein BM, editors. Intracranial arteriovenous malformations. Baltimore: Williams & Wilkins; 1984.
19. Al-Shahi R, Bhattacharya JJ, Currie DG, Papanastassiou V, Ritchie V, Roberts RC, Sellar RJ, Warlow CP. Scottish intracranial vascular malformation study collaborators. Prospective, population-based detection of intracranial vascular malformations in adults: the Scottish intracranial vascular malformation study (SIVMS). Stroke. 2003;34(5):1163–9. https://doi.org/10.1161/01.STR.0000069018.90456.C9.
20. Rigamonti D, Johnson PC, Spetzler RF, Hadley MN, Drayer BP. Cavernous malformations and capillary telangiectasia: a spectrum within a single pathological entity. Neurosurgery. 1991;28(1):60–4.
21. Pabaney AH, Rammo RA, Tahir RA, Seyfried D. Development of De novo arteriovenous malformation following ischemic stroke: case report and review of current literature. World Neurosurg. 2016;96:608.e5–608.e12. https://doi.org/10.1016/j.wneu.2016.09.062.
22. Flemming KD, Lanzino G. Management of unruptured intracranial aneurysms and cerebrovascular malformations. Continuum (Minneap Minn). 2017;23(1, Cerebrovascular Disease):181–210. https://doi.org/10.1212/CON.0000000000000418.
23. Dalton A, Dobson G, Prasad M, Mukerji N. De novo intracerebral arteriovenous malformations and a review of the theories of their formation. Br J Neurosurg. 2018;32(3):305–11. https://doi.org/10.1080/02688697.2018.1478060.
24. Moftakhar P, Hauptman JS, Malkasian D, Martin NA. Cerebral arteriovenous malformations. Part 1: cellular and molecular biology. Neurosurg Focus. 2009;26(5):E10. https://doi.org/10.3171/2009.2.FOCUS09316.
25. Mohr JP, Kejda-Scharler J, Pile-Spellman J. Diagnosis and treatment of arteriovenous malformations. Curr Neurol Neurosci Rep. 2013 Feb;13(2):324. https://doi.org/10.1007/s11910-012-0324-1.
26. Nikolaev SI, Vetiska S, Bonilla X, Boudreau E, Jauhiainen S, Rezai Jahromi B, Khyzha N, DiStefano PV, Suutarinen S, Kiehl TR, Mendes Pereira V, Herman AM, Krings T, Andrade-Barazarte H, Tung T, Valiante T, Zadeh G, Tymianski M, Rauramaa T, Ylä-Herttuala S, Wythe JD, Antonarakis SE, Frösen J, Fish JE, Radovanovic I. Somatic activating KRAS mutations in arteriovenous malformations of the brain. N Engl J Med. 2018;378(3):250–61. https://doi.org/10.1056/NEJMoa1709449.
27. Scimone C, Donato L, Marino S, Alafaci C, D'Angelo R, Sidoti A. Vis-à-Vis: a focus on genetic features

of cerebral cavernous malformations and brain arteriovenous malformations pathogenesis. Neurol Sci. 2019;40(2):243–51. https://doi.org/10.1007/s10072-018-3674-x.
28. Smith ER, Scott RM. Spontaneous occlusion of the circle of Willis in children: pediatric moyamoya summary with proposed evidence-based practice guidelines. A review. J Neurosurg Pediatr. 2012;9(4):353–60. https://doi.org/10.3171/2011.12.PEDS1172.
29. Martins C, Yasuda A, Campero A, Ulm AJ, Tanriover N, Rhoton A Jr. Microsurgical anatomy of the dural arteries. Neurosurgery. 2005;56(2 Suppl):211–51.; discussion 211-51. https://doi.org/10.1227/01.neu.0000144823.94402.3d.
30. Zipfel GJ, Shah MN, Refai D, Dacey RG Jr, Derdeyn CP. Cranial dural arteriovenous fistulas: modification of angiographic classification scales based on new natural history data. Neurosurg Focus. 2009;26(5):E14. https://doi.org/10.3171/2009.2.FOCUS0928.
31. Borden JA, Wu JK, Shucart WA. A proposed classification for spinal and cranial dural arteriovenous fistulous malformations and implications for treatment. J Neurosurg. 1995;82(2):166–79. https://doi.org/10.3171/jns.1995.82.2.0166.
32. Sinha PK, Neema PK, Rathod RC. Anesthesia and intracranial arteriovenous malformation. Neurol India. 2004;52(2):163–70.
33. Ellis JA, Goldstein H, Connolly ES Jr, Meyers PM. Carotid-cavernous fistulas. Neurosurg Focus. 2012;32(5):E9. https://doi.org/10.3171/2012.2.FOCUS1223.
34. Lang M, Habboub G, Mullin JP, Rasmussen PA. A brief history of carotid-cavernous fistula. J Neurosurg. 2017;126(6):1995–2001. https://doi.org/10.3171/2016.5.JNS152372.
35. De Stefano FA, Kaura S, Hankey PB, Dharia A, Heskett C, Peterson J, Ebersole K. A bibliometric analysis of the top 100 Most influential articles on carotid cavernous fistulas. World Neurosurg. 2022;167:44–54. https://doi.org/10.1016/j.wneu.2022.08.117.
36. Perata HJ, Tomsick TA, Tew JM Jr. Feeding artery pedicle aneurysms: association with parenchymal hemorrhage and arteriovenous malformation in the brain. J Neurosurg. 1994;80(4):631–4. https://doi.org/10.3171/jns.1994.80.4.0631.
37. Willinsky RA, Lasjaunias P, Terbrugge K, Burrows P. Multiple cerebral arteriovenous malformations (AVMs). Review of our experience from 203 patients with cerebral vascular lesions. Neuroradiology. 1990;32(3):207–10. https://doi.org/10.1007/BF00589113.
38. Al-Shahi R, Warlow C. A systematic review of the frequency and prognosis of arteriovenous malformations of the brain in adults. Brain. 2001;124(Pt 10):1900–26. https://doi.org/10.1093/brain/124.10.1900.
39. Friedlander RM. Clinical practice. Arteriovenous malformations of the brain. N Engl J Med. 2007;356(26):2704–12. https://doi.org/10.1056/NEJMcp067192.
40. Derdeyn CP, Zipfel GJ, Albuquerque FC, Cooke DL, Feldmann E, Sheehan JP, Torner JC, American Heart Association Stroke Council. Management of Brain Arteriovenous Malformations: a scientific statement for healthcare professionals from the American Heart Association/American Stroke Association. Stroke. 2017;48(8):e200–24. https://doi.org/10.1161/STR.0000000000000134.
41. Stapf C, Mast H, Sciacca RR, Choi JH, Khaw AV, Connolly ES, Pile-Spellman J, Mohr JP. Predictors of hemorrhage in patients with untreated brain arteriovenous malformation. Neurology. 2006;66(9):1350–5. https://doi.org/10.1212/01.wnl.0000210524.68507.87.
42. Gross BA, Du R. Natural history of cerebral arteriovenous malformations: a meta-analysis. J Neurosurg. 2013;118(2):437–43. https://doi.org/10.3171/2012.10.JNS121280.
43. Kim H, Al-Shahi Salman R, McCulloch CE, Stapf C, Young WL, Coinvestigators MARS. Untreated brain arteriovenous malformation: patient-level meta-analysis of hemorrhage predictors. Neurology. 2014;83(7):590–7. https://doi.org/10.1212/WNL.0000000000000688.
44. Mohr JP, Parides MK, Stapf C, Moquete E, Moy CS, Overbey JR, Al-Shahi Salman R, Vicaut E, Young WL, Houdart E, Cordonnier C, Stefani MA, Hartmann A, von Kummer R, Biondi A, Berkefeld J, Klijn CJ, Harkness K, Libman R, Barreau X, Moskowitz AJ, international ARUBA investigators. Medical management with or without interventional therapy for unruptured brain arteriovenous malformations (Aruba): a multicentre, non-blinded, randomised trial. Lancet. 2014;383(9917):614–21. https://doi.org/10.1016/S0140-6736(13)62302-8.
45. Horton JC, Chambers WA, Lyons SL, Adams RD, Kjellberg RN. Pregnancy and the risk of hemorrhage from cerebral arteriovenous malformations. Neurosurgery. 1990;27(6):867–71.; discussion 871-2. https://doi.org/10.1097/00006123-199012000-00002.
46. Liu XJ, Wang S, Zhao YL, Teo M, Guo P, Zhang D, Wang R, Cao Y, Ye X, Kang S, Zhao JZ. Risk of cerebral arteriovenous malformation rupture during pregnancy and puerperium. Neurology. 2014;82(20):1798–803. https://doi.org/10.1212/WNL.0000000000000436.
47. Porras JL, Yang W, Philadelphia E, Law J, Garzon-Muvdi T, Caplan JM, Colby GP, Coon AL, Tamargo RJ, Huang J. Hemorrhage risk of brain arteriovenous malformations during pregnancy and puerperium in a north American cohort. Stroke. 2017;48(6):1507–13. https://doi.org/10.1161/STROKEAHA.117.016828.
48. Al-Shahi SR. The outlook for adults with epileptic seizure(s) associated with cerebral cavernous malformations or arteriovenous malformations. Epilepsia. 2012;53(Suppl 4):34–42. https://doi.org/10.1111/j.1528-1167.2012.03611.x.
49. Garcin B, Houdart E, Porcher R, Manchon E, Saint-Maurice JP, Bresson D, Stapf C. Epileptic seizures at initial presentation in patients with brain arteriovenous malformation. Neurol-

ogy. 2012;78(9):626–31. https://doi.org/10.1212/WNL.0b013e3182494d40.
50. van Beijnum J, van der Worp HB, Schippers HM, van Nieuwenhuizen O, Kappelle LJ, Rinkel GJ, Berkelbach van der Sprenkel JW, Klijn CJ. Familial occurrence of brain arteriovenous malformations: a systematic review. J Neurol Neurosurg Psychiatry. 2007;78(11):1213–7. https://doi.org/10.1136/jnnp.2006.112227.
51. van Beijnum J, van der Worp HB, Algra A, Vandertop WP, van den Berg R, Brouwer PA, van der Sprenkel JW, Kappelle LJ, Rinkel GJ, Klijn CJ. Prevalence of brain arteriovenous malformations in first-degree relatives of patients with a brain arteriovenous malformation. Stroke. 2014;45(11):3231–5. https://doi.org/10.1161/STROKEAHA.114.005442.
52. Al-Samkari H, Eng W. A precision medicine approach to hereditary hemorrhagic telangiectasia and complex vascular anomalies. J Thromb Haemost. 2022;20(5):1077–88. https://doi.org/10.1111/jth.15715.
53. Josephson CB, White PM, Krishan A, Al-Shahi SR. Computed tomography angiography or magnetic resonance angiography for detection of intracranial vascular malformations in patients with intracerebral haemorrhage. Cochrane Database Syst Rev. 2014;2014(9):CD009372. https://doi.org/10.1002/14651858.CD009372.pub2.
54. Hartmann A, Pile-Spellman J, Stapf C, Sciacca RR, Faulstich A, Mohr JP, Schumacher HC, Mast H. Risk of endovascular treatment of brain arteriovenous malformations. Stroke. 2002;33(7):1816–20. https://doi.org/10.1161/01.str.0000020123.80940.b2.
55. Josephson CB, Leach JP, Duncan R, Roberts RC, Counsell CE, Al-Shahi Salman R. Scottish audit of intracranial vascular malformations (SAIVMs) steering committee and collaborators. Seizure risk from cavernous or arteriovenous malformations: prospective population-based study. Neurology. 2011;76(18):1548–54. https://doi.org/10.1212/WNL.0b013e3182190f37.
56. Spetzler RF, Martin NA. A proposed grading system for arteriovenous malformations. J Neurosurg. 1986;65(4):476–83. https://doi.org/10.3171/jns.1986.65.4.0476.
57. Ogilvy CS, Stieg PE, Awad I, Brown RD Jr, Kondziolka D, Rosenwasser R, Young WL, Hademenos G. Special writing Group of the Stroke Council, American Stroke Association. AHA scientific statement: recommendations for the management of intracranial arteriovenous malformations: a statement for healthcare professionals from a special writing group of the stroke council, American Stroke Association. Stroke. 2001;32(6):1458–71. https://doi.org/10.1161/01.str.32.6.1458.
58. Hamilton MG, Spetzler RF. The prospective application of a grading system for arteriovenous malformations. Neurosurgery. 1994;34(1):2–7.
59. Schaller C, Schramm J, Haun D. Significance of factors contributing to surgical complications and to late outcome after elective surgery of cerebral arteriovenous malformations. J Neurol Neurosurg Psychiatry. 1998;65(4):547–54. https://doi.org/10.1136/jnnp.65.4.547.
60. Barr JC, Ogilvy CS. Selection of treatment modalities or observation of arteriovenous malformations. Neurosurg Clin N Am. 2012;23(1):63–75. https://doi.org/10.1016/j.nec.2011.09.010.
61. Karbe AG, Vajkoczy P. Postoperative management and follow-up after resection of arteriovenous malformations. J Neurosurg Sci. 2018;62(4):484–9. https://doi.org/10.23736/S0390-5616.18.04417-X.
62. Krings T, Hans FJ, Geibprasert S, Terbrugge K. Partial "targeted" embolisation of brain arteriovenous malformations. Eur Radiol. 2010;20(11):2723–31. https://doi.org/10.1007/s00330-010-1834-3.
63. Brown RD Jr, Flemming KD, Meyer FB, Cloft HJ, Pollock BE, Link ML. Natural history, evaluation, and management of intracranial vascular malformations. Mayo Clin Proc. 2005;80(2):269–81. https://doi.org/10.4065/80.2.269.
64. Starke RM, Komotar RJ, Otten ML, Hahn DK, Fischer LE, Hwang BY, Garrett MC, Sciacca RR, Sisti MB, Solomon RA, Lavine SD, Connolly ES, Meyers PM. Adjuvant embolization with N-butyl cyanoacrylate in the treatment of cerebral arteriovenous malformations: outcomes, complications, and predictors of neurologic deficits. Stroke. 2009;40(8):2783–90. https://doi.org/10.1161/STROKEAHA.108.539775.
65. Richter KR, Turcotte EL, Hess RA, Patra DP, Rahme RJ, Tate MC, Bendok BR. Awake resection of an arteriovenous malformation. World Neurosurg. 2022;162:17. https://doi.org/10.1016/j.wneu.2021.06.146.
66. Chyatte D. Normal pressure perfusion breakthrough after resection of arteriovenous malformation. J Stroke Cerebrovasc Dis. 1997;6(3):130–6. https://doi.org/10.1016/s1052-3057(97)80229-7.
67. Spetzler RF, Wilson CB, Weinstein P, Mehdorn M, Townsend J, Telles D. Normal perfusion pressure breakthrough theory. Clin Neurosurg. 1978;25:651–72. https://doi.org/10.1093/neurosurgery/25.cn_suppl_1.651.
68. Al-Rodhan NR, Sundt TM Jr, Piepgras DG, Nichols DA, Rüfenacht D, Stevens LN. Occlusive hyperemia: a theory for the hemodynamic complications following resection of intracerebral arteriovenous malformations. J Neurosurg. 1993;78(2):167–75. https://doi.org/10.3171/jns.1993.78.2.0167.
69. Scott RM, Smith ER. Moyamoya disease and moyamoya syndrome. N Engl J Med. 2009;360(12):1226–37. https://doi.org/10.1056/NEJMra0804622.
70. Baaj AA, Agazzi S, Sayed ZA, Toledo M, Spetzler RF, van Loveren H. Surgical management of moyamoya disease: a review. Neurosurg Focus. 2009;26(4):E7. https://doi.org/10.3171/2009.01.FOCUS08293.
71. Ibrahimi DM, Tamargo RJ, Ahn ES. Moyamoya disease in children. Childs Nerv Syst. 2010;26(10):1297–308. https://doi.org/10.1007/s00381-010-1209-8.
72. Deng X, Ge P, Wang R, Zhang D, Zhao J, Zhang Y. Risk factors for postoperative ischemic complications in pediatric moyamoya disease. BMC Neurol.

2021;21(1):229. https://doi.org/10.1186/s12883-021-02283-9.
73. Suzuki J, Takaku A. Cerebrovascular "moyamoya" disease. Disease showing abnormal net-like vessels in base of brain. Arch Neurol. 1969;20(3):288–99. https://doi.org/10.1001/archneur.1969.00480090076012.
74. Sun J, Li ZY, Chen C, Ling C, Li H, Wang H. Postoperative neovascularization, cerebral hemodynamics, and clinical prognosis between combined and indirect bypass revascularization procedures in hemorrhagic moyamoya disease. Clin Neurol Neurosurg. 2021;208:106869. https://doi.org/10.1016/j.clineuro.2021.106869.
75. Ellison PH, Largent JA, Popp AJ. Moya-Moya disease associated with renal artery stenosis. Arch Neurol. 1981;38(7):467. https://doi.org/10.1001/archneur.1981.00510070101025.
76. Zhu B, He L. Transient ischemic attack after indirect revascularization surgery for pediatric patients with moyamoya disease: a retrospective study of intraoperative blood pressure. Anaesth Crit Care Pain Med. 2023;42(1):101168. https://doi.org/10.1016/j.accpm.2022.101168.
77. Kim EH, Park JB, Kang P, Ji SH, Jang YE, Lee JH, Kim JT, Kim HS. Response of internal carotid artery blood flow velocity to fluid challenge under general anesthesia in pediatric patients with moyamoya disease: a prospective observational study. Paediatr Anaesth. 2022;32(12):1330–8. https://doi.org/10.1111/pan.14558.
78. Song T, Liu X, Han R, Huang L, Zhang J, Xu H. Effects of end-tidal carbon dioxide levels in patients undergoing direct revascularization for Moyamoya disease and risk factors associated with postoperative complications. Medicine (Baltimore). 2021;100(7):e24527. https://doi.org/10.1097/MD.0000000000024527.
79. Huguenard AL, Guerriero RM, Tomko SR, Limbrick DD, Zipfel GJ, Guilliams KP, Strahle JM. Immediate postoperative electroencephalography monitoring in pediatric Moyamoya disease and syndrome. Pediatr Neurol. 2021;118:40–5. https://doi.org/10.1016/j.pediatrneurol.2021.02.004.
80. Lee JK, Williams M, Reyes M, Ahn ES. Cerebrovascular blood pressure autoregulation monitoring and postoperative transient ischemic attack in pediatric moyamoya vasculopathy. Paediatr Anaesth. 2018;28(2):94–102. https://doi.org/10.1111/pan.13293.

51 Ischemic Stroke Management in the ICU

Ali Alsarah, Lee A. Pfaff, Lilly Chau, Diana Greene-Chandos, and Michel T. Torbey

51.1 Introduction

Stroke is a significant public health concern and one of the leading causes of morbidity and mortality worldwide [1]. The management of acute stroke requires a multidisciplinary approach, and patients often require specialized care in the intensive care unit (ICU). ICU management of stroke patients is crucial for the prevention and management of complications such as cerebral edema, hemorrhagic transformation, and increased intracranial pressure (ICP). The optimal management of stroke patients in the ICU involves a careful balance between aggressive management of complications and minimizing the risk of further injury. This chapter will provide an overview of the current guidelines and best practices for the management of stroke patients in the ICU, including the recognition and treatment of complications and the use of advanced monitoring and treatment options.

A. Alsarah · L. A. Pfaff · L. Chau ·
D. Greene-Chandos · M. T. Torbey (✉)
Department of Neurology, University of New Mexico, Albuquerque, NM, USA
e-mail: dgreenechandos@salud.unm.edu; Lchau@salud.unm.edu; Mtorbey@salud.unm.edu

51.2 Brief Case History

Mrs. Smith is a 65-year-old female who was brought to the emergency department by ambulance after her daughter found her unresponsive on the floor of her bedroom. Mrs. Smith has a history of hypertension and diabetes mellitus and is a former smoker. On arrival, Mrs. Smith was found to have a left hemiparesis, a reduced level of consciousness, and a Glasgow Coma Scale score of 9. A non-contrast CT scan of the brain was normal, and her National Institutes of Health Stroke Scale (NIHSS) score was 20. She immediately received IV tissue plasminogen activator (tPA) in the emergency department. She also underwent a CT angiogram to assess for large vessel occlusion and was found to have a right MCA thrombus, for which she underwent endovascular mechanical thrombectomy with TICI 2 recanalization. Given the size and location of the infarct, the decision was made to admit Mrs. Smith to the intensive care unit (ICU) for close monitoring.

In the ICU, Mrs. Smith's condition worsened, and she developed cerebral edema and increased intracranial pressure (ICP). Despite receiving hypertonic saline therapy to manage her ICP, her neurological status continued to deteriorate. After careful consideration, the neurosurgical team decided to perform a hemicraniectomy. She underwent a successful hemicraniectomy, and her ICP returned to normal. Mrs. Smith remained

H. Prabhakar et al. (eds.), *Principles and Practice of Neurocritical Care*,
https://doi.org/10.1007/978-981-99-8059-8_51

in the ICU for several days under close observation and received appropriate medical management. Over time, Mrs. Smith's neurological status improved, and she was transferred to a rehabilitation facility for further recovery.

51.3 Neuro-Specific ICU Care

51.3.1 Neuro Checks

Stroke patients are often admitted to the neurocritical care unit for frequent neuro checks post rt-pa or thrombectomy. Current guidelines recommend repeat neuro checks and NIHSS every 15 min for 2 h, every 30 min for 6 h, then hourly for 16 h for patient. Clinically significant increase is usually defined as an increase in the NIHSS of > = 4. Acute imaging and bedside assessment is recommended to rule out a hemorrhagic transformation.

51.3.2 Seizure Prophylaxis

Seizures are uncommon in the setting of acute ischemic stroke, but can occur with both cortical and subcortical infarcts [2]. EEG changes in the form of periodic lateralized epileptiform discharges (PLEDs) are more common, but these are not associated with seizures or status epilepticus [3]. When seizures do occur, they can be classified as early (within 1 week) or late (>1 week). Patients with early seizures are at greater risk of developing late seizures [4, 5]. Primary prophylaxis for seizure prevention is not recommended. However, recurrent seizures in the case of post-stroke epilepsy should be treated with antiseizure medications [6, 7].

51.3.3 ICP Management

The pathophysiology of cerebral edema is generally thought to occur in two phases: cytotoxic edema followed by vasogenic edema. The initial ischemic insult causes disruption of cellular membrane homeostasis resulting in the influx of extracellular sodium and fluid into the cell (cytotoxic edema). Subsequent disruption of the blood-brain barrier results in protein and fluid accumulation in the extracellular space (vasogenic edema) [8]. General risk factors for malignant MCA strokes include young age, carotid artery occlusion with abnormal ipsilateral circle of Willis, early CT showing >50% MCA territory involvement, and history of heart failure or hypertension [9, 10]. Mounting evidence also suggests that cortical spreading depolarization contributes to the underlying pathophysiology [11].

Cerebral edema usually peaks at day 3–5 [12] and has the most clinical sequelae in hemispheric strokes due to large vessel occlusions, such as the ICA terminus or M1 branch of the MCA. Progressive edema can cause mass effect and increased ICP when compensatory mechanisms dictated by the Monroe-Kellie doctrine are exhausted and can result in life-threatening uncal and transtentorial herniation.

51.3.4 Medical Management

Medical management of increased ICP should proceed with a relatively tiered approach:

1. Elevate the head to 30° and ensure head is midline to optimize venous drainage.
2. Intubate (if not already previously done) and hyperventilate to goal $PaCO_2$ 30 mmHg to induce vasoconstriction. This should only be a transient measure as the resultant decrease in cerebral blood flow can cause further ischemia.
3. Osmotic therapy with mannitol or hypertonic saline. The choice between hypertonic saline and mannitol depends on the clinical scenario [13, 14]. Some small case series have shown hypertonic saline is more effective than mannitol in lowering ICP, but there is no randomized controlled trial comparing hypertonic saline and mannitol [15–17]. Osmotics should be dosed by intermittent boluses rather than continuous infusion to achieve a sodium goal. Serum sodium and serum osmolality, as well as osmolar gap in

the use of mannitol, should be monitored serially. Prophylactic osmotic therapy has not been shown to be effective in mitigating edema. In patients with hemispheric stroke and expected edema, it is reasonable to target normonatremia until clinical signs of elevated ICP develop [18].

4. Sedation with propofol and benzodiazepines to decrease cerebral metabolic rate.
5. Therapeutic hypothermia is a potential strategy. Prospective studies have shown hypothermia is effective in decreasing edema and lowering ICP, but may not prevent herniation [19–21]. If hypothermia is considered, a suggested target temperature is 33–36 °C for 24–72 h [18].
6. Corticosteroid therapy has not been shown to be effective for treating cerebral edema [22]. Likewise, barbiturate therapy has not been shown to be effective in decreasing ICP [23].

51.3.5 Surgical Management

Decompressive hemicraniectomy may be performed if edema progresses despite maximum medical management. In the case of slowly progressive edema, the need for and timing of decompression are varied. However, for large hemispheric strokes with rapidly progressive space-occupying cerebral edema, termed malignant MCA strokes, medical management has limited effect and acute surgical management is needed. In these cases, medical management is performed as a temporizing measure while the patient awaits surgery.

Multiple randomized controlled trials, DECIMAL, DESTINY, and HAMLET [24–26], as well as a pooled analysis of these trials [24], have shown that decompressive hemicraniectomy in malignant MCA stroke improves outcomes in patients aged 18–60 when decompression is performed within 48 h of stroke onset, with greater percentage of patients having modified Rankin Score of 4 or less. The efficacy of surgical decompression in patients age > 60 is less clear. In the DESTINY II trial, decompressive hemicraniectomy in patients >60 improved mortality but not morbidity in survivors [27]. In these patients, surgery may be a life-saving procedure with likely no improvement in functional outcome and families should be counseled appropriately.

51.4 Multimodal Monitoring

The utility of multimodal monitoring tools is unclear and routine monitoring is not recommended. Parenchymal ICP monitors may or may not be helpful in guiding clinical management. Some prospective studies have shown an association of high ICP with poor outcomes, whereas others show herniation and poor outcomes in normal ICP monitoring. These varying results may reflect the limitation of parenchymal ICP monitors, where local rather than global ICP is monitored [28–30]. Studies on cerebral microdialysis to monitor neurochemical levels (such as glutamate, glycerol, GABA, glycerol, lactate, pyruvate) and brain tissue oxygen monitoring have detected neurochemical states associated with ischemia (for example, increase in glutamate and decrease in tissue oxygen), but these studies have not shown utility for predicting poor outcomes [31–33].

Table 51.1 provides a detailed overview of the key elements of cerebral edema treatment for stroke patients.

Table 51.1 Management of Cerebral Edema in Stroke Patients

Treatment	Description	Dosage
Osmotic therapy	Hypertonic saline or mannitol can be used to reduce cerebral edema and intracranial pressure	Hypertonic saline: 3% sodium chloride solution administered at a rate of 50–150 mL/h. Mannitol: 0.25–1.0 g/kg administered intravenously over 20–30 min
Sedation	Sedation with medications such as propofol or dexmedetomidine may be used to reduce agitation and anxiety, which can contribute to increased intracranial pressure	Propofol: Initial infusion rate of 5–10 mcg/kg/min, titrated to effect Dexmedetomidine: Loading dose of 1 mcg/kg over 10 min, followed by a maintenance infusion rate of 0.2–0.7 mcg/kg/h
Hyperventilation	Hyperventilation can be used to rapidly reduce intracranial pressure by causing vasoconstriction and reducing cerebral blood flow However, it is important to monitor for potential ischemia due to decreased oxygen delivery to the brain.	Target PaCO2 of 30–35 mmHg
Steroids	Corticosteroids are not routinely recommended for cerebral edema in stroke patients, as they may worsen outcomes and increase the risk of infection	N/A
Decompressive Craniectomy	In severe cases of cerebral edema that do not respond to other treatments, decompressive craniectomy may be considered	N/A

51.5 General ICU Care

51.5.1 General ICU Management

Supplemental oxygen should be administered to maintain an SpO2 of 94%. Patients with decreased level of consciousness or bulbar dysfunction require evaluation for intubation to assist in maintaining optimal oxygenation [34]. There is no benefit of supplementing oxygen in patient to increase SpO2 beyond 94% [35–37]. Hyperbaric oxygen does not improve outcomes and should be reserved only for patients who have air embolism [38]. Patient should undergo monitoring for atrial fibrillation while admitted to the hospital [39]. Regular skin assessments with objective scaling such as Braden scale are recommended for all stroke patients. Skin breakdown can be prevented with frequent turns, low friction, dry surfaces, and good nutrition [40].

51.5.2 Airway Management

Respiratory failure in ischemic stroke can be caused by a combination of impaired consciousness with decreased respiratory drive and loss of bulbar reflexes with dysphagia. Dysphagia can also result in aspiration pneumonia and hypoxia. Endotracheal intubation is indicated for neurological decline, hypercarbic or hypoxemic respiratory failure due to any combination of neurological deterioration and/or pulmonary complications, and for surgery. Other criteria for intubation include GCS <10 or signs of increased intracranial pressure [41, 42].

Patients on mechanical ventilation should be maintained with normocapnia on control/assist control mode rather than support mode. Support mode ventilation is not preferred because sudden decrease in patient's respiratory drive can cause hypercapnia and resultant increase in intracranial pressure. However, prophylactic hypercapnia to prevent edema progression is not beneficial as vasoconstriction with persistently decreased cerebral blood flow can cause ischemia [43].

Persistent impairment in level of consciousness and dysphagia may cause difficulty with weaning ventilatory support for extubation and/or extubation failure. Successful extubation in the neurocritical care population is difficult to predict as standard respiratory weaning parameters, such as rapid shallow breathing index (RSBI), do not apply well to this population [44].

One small retrospective study found a trend towards successful extubation in patients with a GCS score ≥ 8 T [45].

The timing of safe extubation, if at all, is important as reintubation is associated with worsened outcome and increased mortality [46]. If patients cannot be safely extubated in a timely manner, generally by 14 days of intubation, tracheostomy is recommended. Multiple randomized controlled trials for early tracheostomy (4 days after intubation) have been performed. The SETPOINT trial showed early tracheostomy in neurocritical care patients, including ischemic stroke patients, was feasible and safe [47]. Subsequent to the SETPOINT2 efficacy study, which included only ischemic and hemorrhagic strokes, patients showed no difference in primary outcome, defined as modified Rankin Score of 4 or less at 6-month follow-up [48]. As such, clinical equipoise remains for timing of tracheostomy.

51.5.3 Blood Pressure Management

Hypertension is a well-established modifiable risk factor in stroke patients, and optimal management of blood pressure in the acute stroke is considered a cornerstone in the treatment [49]. When intravenous fibrinolytic therapy is indicated, before its administration blood pressure should be <185/110 mm Hg and < 180/105 mm Hg in the first 24 h after administration. If the patient is deemed to be a candidate for mechanical thrombectomy and intravenous thrombolytic therapy has not been given, BP should be ≤185/110 mm Hg before the procedure [6]. Post-procedural BP goal is typically determined by the revascularization grading, but if successful reperfusion is achieved, it may be reasonable to maintain BP <180/105 mm Hg. Blood pressure should be managed using intravenous agents like Labetalol or Nicardipine until the target is achieved.

In patients who don't receive either mechanical thrombectomy or intravenous thrombolytic therapy and BP is ≥220/120 mm Hg and there are no comorbid conditions requiring acute BP-lowering treatment, it is reasonable to initially lower BP by 15%. It might be a safe option to maintain the BP <220/120 mm Hg in the first 48–72 h in those patients to maximize salvaging the penumbra, but there are no established data to support the positive impact of this on the mortality or functional outcome. Following that stage and once the patient is stable neurologically, antihypertensive medication in patients who have a BP >140/90 mm Hg can be restarted.

51.5.4 Blood Glucose Management

Hyperglycemia is a common presentation in patients with acute ischemic stroke. It has been related to adverse clinical outcomes in several studies [50]. While intensive blood glucose control has not shown significant improvement compared to the standard glucose control [51], recent recommendations from the American Heart Association/American Stroke Association (AHA/ASA) suggest treating hyperglycemia to achieve a blood glucose level in the range of 140 to 180 mg/dL (7.8–10.0 mmol/L) and close monitoring to prevent hypoglycemia. Diabetes screening is recommended in all stroke patients with a Hemoglobin A1C [52].

51.5.5 Temperature Management

Fever can be seen in up to 60% in the acute setting in patients with ischemic stroke and has been identified as an independent factor that predicts poor outcome [53, 54]. Routine early administration of high-dose acetaminophen was not associated with improved functional outcome in patients with acute ischemic stroke [55]. It is recommended to maintain the state of normothermia (T < 99.6 °F; 37.6 °C) as the standard of care according to the (AHA/ASA) guidelines.

Temperatures of >99.6 °F should be addressed and managed aggressively including investigating any possible concurrent infections, treating the infections as well as symptomatically treating the fever with acetaminophen as standard first-line measure and physical cooling measures as a second line. Acetaminophen dose should not exceed 4 g per day and should be used with caution in patients with liver diseases or abnormal liver functions [56–58].

51.5.6 Ulcer Prophylaxis

There is currently no clear neurocritical care-specific evidence for ulcer prophylaxis. This is typically reserved for patient with prolonged intubation requiring blood pressure augmentation preventing good nutrition such as high levels of norepinephrine. PPIs have a higher risk of infection including C. Diff and pneumonias than H2 blockers such as famotidine. Utilization and choice of medication should be tailored to individual patient needs [59].

51.5.7 Urine Tract Infection (UTI) Prevention

Prevention of UTI is based around maintaining cleanliness with good nursing care. It is currently not recommended to insert a foley preemptively. This may be harmful and is associated with increased risk of infection and should be reserved for those patients with clear need for a foley such as a strict input and output, sacral/coccygeal pressure ulcer wound healing. Antibiotics should also not be used preemptively to prevent UTIs and serve to increase the risk of drug resistance [40].

51.5.8 Deep Venous Thrombosis (DVT) Prevention

DVT and PE are frequent complications of ischemic stroke as patients are at great risk due to their immobility. The incidence of DVT in stroke is approximately 3% and the incidence of PE among patients not receiving DVT prophylaxis is as high as 5.6% [42, 60]. In a large retrospective study of thirteen thousand patients with ischemic stroke, almost half of the patients who developed PE died during their hospital course [61]. Efforts should be made towards early mobilization to prevent DVT. DVT prophylaxis should begin as soon as possible with combination mechanical and chemical prophylaxis [62]. For mechanical prophylaxis, intermittent pneumatic compression should be used [63]. Compression stocking has not been shown to be effective in preventing DVT [64]. For chemical prophylaxis, lovenox is superior to unfractionated heparin and both have similar rate of hemorrhagic complications [65]. One advantage of unfractionated heparin is the antidote protamine sulfate, which becomes useful if there is hemorrhagic conversion. In the setting of hemorrhagic transformation, there are no clear guidelines for timing of initiation of systemic anticoagulation for PE. In the acute stroke period, an IVC filter can be placed until systemic heparin can be safely started.

51.5.9 Dysphagia

All stroke patients should have dysphagia screening at bedside which can be completed by nursing or speech language pathology before eating, drinking, or oral medications. Other modalities are available and can be used and are largely based on institutional standards and available equipment (i.e., video fluoroscopy). Oral hygiene protocols are reasonable as it may reduce the risk of aspiration pneumonia [66–69].

51.5.10 Nutrition

Nutrition should be started within 7 days of admission. If a patient does not pass swallow evaluation, a Nasogastric tube should be placed and G-tube should be considered in those patients who are not anticipated to be able to swallow within >2–3 weeks [70].

51.6 Stroke-Specific Complications

51.6.1 Suspected Intracranial Symptomatic Bleed

If an intracranial bleed is suspected after thrombolytics, the infusion should be stopped immediately. A CBC PT, aPTT, fibrinogen level, type, and cross match with STAT CT Head without contrast should be ordered. If CT scan showed hemorrhagic transformation, the patient should be treated with 10 units Cryoprecipitate over 10–30 min, repeat if fibrinogen <150; alternatively, tranexamic acid 1000 mg IV over 10 min or Epsilon-aminocaproic acid 4–5 g over 1 h then 1 g IV until bleeding is controlled if cryoprecipitate is not available or contraindicated. Neurosurgery should be consulted for any possible intervention and blood pressure should be managed per intraparenchymal hemorrhage protocols [40].

51.6.2 Angioedema from Rt-PA/TNK

Some patients may develop angioedema after treatment with thrombolytics. Consider intubation if more extensive than anterior tongue and lips. Patients with larynx, palate, floor of mouth, and oropharynx with progression within 30 min of infusion are at high risk and will likely need intubation. Awake fiberoptic or nasal-tracheal is preferred if intubation is required. Alteplase should be discontinued and ACE inhibitors should be held. You should administer methylprednisolone 125 mg IV, diphenhydramine 50 mg IV, ranitidine 50 mg, or famotidine 20 mg IV; if edema progressed despite treatment, 0.1% epinephrine, 0.3 mL subcutaneous, or 0.5 mL nebulizer [40].

51.7 Restarting Antithrombotic and Anticoagulation Poststroke

Restarting either anticoagulation or antiplatelet depends on size of stroke and extent of hemorrhagic transformation [71]. Patient with small petechial, non-confluent hemorrhages can start therapy without delay. Those with large territory hemorrhages should have a delay in starting treatment. There is currently no consensus on how long of a delay but usually no longer than 14 days from the bleed unless other complications exist. There has been no association with delayed anticoagulation with increased risk of stroke within the first 12 days [72]. The notable exception is in patient with hemorrhagic strokes from Central Venous Sinus Thrombosis (CVST) where anticoagulation remains the mainstay of treatment [73].

51.8 Cerebellar Strokes

Management of infratentorial strokes requires a slightly different approach. Due to the anatomical location as well as tight space in the posterior fossa, even mild edema in cerebellar strokes can lead to clinically significant mass effect with brainstem compression and obstructive hydrocephalus at the level of the fourth ventricle. Persistent edema progression and ICP elevation can lead to further infarction of the brainstem as well as brainstem herniation leading to death [74]. Clinically significant edema is particularly seen with occlusion of the PICA and SCA [75]. Cerebellar infarcts in younger patients are not uncommon due to vertebral artery dissection [76].

Early signs of clinical decline, such as decreased responsiveness with CT evidence of hydrocephalus (enlargement of the temporal horns), should prompt placement of an external ventricular drain (EVD) for CSF diversion. LP for CSF removal is generally contraindicated due to concern for downward herniation. Serial CT scans may be important to track progression of hydrocephalus, particularly if ICP is difficult to control [74]. Edema progression in cerebellar strokes may require suboccipital decompressive craniectomy.

Timing for surgical decompression is variable. After EVD placement, some neurosurgeons prefer to continue clinical monitoring while others proceed with suboccipital decompression before clinical deterioration to brainstem and/or tonsillar herniation [77–79]. As with supratentorial strokes, it may be difficult to predict which patients will require decompression. Case series have shown that patients may benefit from prophylactic decompression [80]. One retrospective study found that an infarct volume of 25-30 cc on restricted diffusion on MRI predicted deterioration and the need for decompression [81].

51.9 Conclusion

Stroke patients are admitted to ICU due to the risk of complications such as cerebral edema, hemorrhagic transformation, or increased ICP. ICU management can include close monitoring of vital signs, continuous neurological assessment, and specialized interventions such as mechanical ventilation, sedation, or neuromuscular blockade. Early recognition and treatment of stroke complications in the ICU can improve outcomes and reduce mortality rates. Therefore, prompt identification of stroke patients who require ICU care is crucial for optimizing acute stroke management.

References

1. Strilciuc S, et al. The economic burden of stroke: a systematic review of cost of illness studies. J Med Life. 2021;14(5):606–19.
2. Giroud M, et al. Early seizures after acute stroke: a study of 1,640 cases. Epilepsia. 1994;35(5):959–64.
3. Pohlmann-Eden B, et al. Periodic lateralized epileptiform discharges--a critical review. J Clin Neurophysiol. 1996;13(6):519–30.
4. Kilpatrick CJ, et al. Early seizures after acute stroke. Risk of late seizures. Arch Neurol. 1992;49(5):509–11.
5. So EL, et al. Population-based study of seizure disorders after cerebral infarction. Neurology. 1996;46(2):350–5.
6. Powers WJ, et al. Guidelines for the early Management of Patients with Acute Ischemic Stroke: 2019 update to the 2018 guidelines for the early Management of Acute Ischemic Stroke: A guideline for healthcare professionals from the American Heart Association/American Stroke Association. Stroke. 2019;50(12):e344–418.
7. Holtkamp M, et al. European stroke organisation guidelines for the management of post-stroke seizures and epilepsy. Eur Stroke J. 2017;2(2):103–15.
8. Astrup J, et al. Cortical evoked potential and extracellular K+ and H+ at critical levels of brain ischemia. Stroke. 1977;8(1):51–7.
9. Jaramillo A, et al. Predictors for malignant middle cerebral artery infarctions: a postmortem analysis. Neurology. 2006;66(6):815–20.
10. Kasner SE, et al. Predictors of fatal brain edema in massive hemispheric ischemic stroke. Stroke. 2001;32(9):2117–23.
11. Dohmen C, et al. Spreading depolarizations occur in human ischemic stroke with high incidence. Ann Neurol. 2008;63(6):720–8.
12. Huttner HB, Schwab S. Malignant middle cerebral artery infarction: clinical characteristics, treatment strategies, and future perspectives. Lancet Neurol. 2009;8(10):949–58.
13. Kempski O. Hypertonic saline and stroke. Crit Care Med. 2005;33(1):259–60.
14. Rabinstein AA. Treatment of cerebral edema. Neurologist. 2006;12(2):59–73.
15. Schwarz S, et al. Effects of hypertonic (10%) saline in patients with raised intracranial pressure after stroke. Stroke. 2002;33(1):136–40.
16. Vialet R, et al. Isovolume hypertonic solutes (sodium chloride or mannitol) in the treatment of refractory posttraumatic intracranial hypertension: 2 mL/kg 7.5% saline is more effective than 2 mL/kg 20% mannitol. Crit Care Med. 2003;31(6):1683–7.
17. Bardutzky J, Schwab S. Antiedema therapy in ischemic stroke. Stroke. 2007;38(11):3084–94.
18. Torbey MT, et al. Evidence-based guidelines for the Management of Large Hemispheric Infarction: A statement for health care professionals from the Neurocritical care society and the German Society for Neuro-Intensive Care and Emergency Medicine. Neurocrit Care. 2015;22(1):146–64.
19. Hong JM, et al. Therapeutic hypothermia after recanalization in patients with acute ischemic stroke. Stroke. 2014;45(1):134–40.
20. Schwab S, et al. Moderate hypothermia and brain temperature in patients with severe middle cerebral artery infarction. Acta Neurochir Suppl. 1998;71:131–4.
21. Steiner T, Ringleb P, Hacke W. Treatment options for large hemispheric stroke. Neurology. 2001;57(5 Suppl 2):S61–8.
22. Sandercock PA, Soane T. Corticosteroids for acute ischaemic stroke. Cochrane Database Syst Rev. 2011;2011(9):CD000064.
23. Schwab S, et al. Barbiturate coma in severe hemispheric stroke: useful or obsolete? Neurology. 1997;48(6):1608–13.
24. Vahedi K, et al. Early decompressive surgery in malignant infarction of the middle cerebral artery: a pooled analysis of three randomised controlled trials. Lancet Neurol. 2007;6(3):215–22.
25. Juttler E, et al. Decompressive surgery for the treatment of malignant infarction of the middle cerebral artery (DESTINY): a randomized, controlled trial. Stroke. 2007;38(9):2518–25.
26. Hofmeijer J, et al. Surgical decompression for space-occupying cerebral infarction (the Hemicraniectomy after middle cerebral artery infarction with life-threatening edema trial [HAMLET]): a multicentre, open, randomised trial. Lancet Neurol. 2009;8(4):326–33.
27. Jüttler E, et al. Hemicraniectomy in older patients with extensive middle-cerebral-artery stroke. N Engl J Med. 2014;370(12):1091–100.
28. Schwab S, et al. The value of intracranial pressure monitoring in acute hemispheric stroke. Neurology. 1996;47(2):393–8.

29. Frank JI. Large hemispheric infarction, deterioration, and intracranial pressure. Neurology. 1995;45(7):1286–90.
30. Poca MA, et al. Monitoring intracranial pressure in patients with malignant middle cerebral artery infarction: is it useful? J Neurosurg. 2010;112(3):648–57.
31. Berger C, Kiening K, Schwab S. Neurochemical monitoring of therapeutic effects in large human MCA infarction. Neurocrit Care. 2008;9(3):352–6.
32. Dohmen C, et al. Identification and clinical impact of impaired cerebrovascular autoregulation in patients with malignant middle cerebral artery infarction. Stroke. 2007;38(1):56–61.
33. Dohmen C, et al. Prediction of malignant course in MCA infarction by PET and microdialysis. Stroke. 2003;34(9):2152–8.
34. Powers WJ, Rabinstein AA, Ackerson T, Adeoye OM, Bambakidis NC, Becker K, Biller J, Brown M, Demaerschalk BM, Hoh B, Jauch EC, Kidwell CS, Leslie-Mazwi TM, Ovbiagele B, Scott PA, Sheth KN, Southerland AM, Summers DV, Tirschwell DL, American Heart Association Stroke Council. 2018 Guidelines for the early Management of Patients with Acute Ischemic Stroke: A guideline for healthcare professionals from the American Heart Association/American Stroke Association. Stroke. 2018;49(3):e46–99.
35. Christine Roffe TN, Sim J, Bishop J, Ives N, Ferdinand P, Gray R. Effect of routine low-dose oxygen supplementation on death and disability in adults with acute stroke: the stroke oxygen study randomized clinical trial. JAMA. 2017;318:1125–35.
36. Khalid Ali AW, Lally F, Sim J, Sills S, Pountain S, Nevatte T, Allen M, Roffe C, The stroke oxygen pilot study: a randomized controlled trial of the effects of routine oxygen supplementation early after acute stroke--effect on key outcomes at six months. PLoS One. 2013;8:e59274.
37. Rønning OM, Guldvog B. Should stroke victims routinely receive supplemental oxygen? A quasi-randomized controlled trial. Stroke. 1999;30:2033–7.
38. Bennett MH, Weibel S, Wasiak J, Schnabel A, French C, Kranke P. Hyperbaric oxygen therapy for acute ischaemic stroke. Cochrane Database Syst Rev. 2014;2014:CD004954.
39. Sposato LA, Cipriano LE, Saposnik G, Ruíz Vargas E, Riccio PM, Hachinski V. Diagnosis of atrial fibrillation after stroke and transient ischaemic attack: a systematic review and meta-analysis. Lancet Neurol. 2015;14:377–87.
40. Powers WJ, Rabinstein AA, Ackerson T, Adeoye OM, Bambakidis NC, Becker K, Biller J, Brown M, Demaerschalk BM, Hoh B, Jauch EC, Kidwell CS, Leslie-Mazwi TM, Ovbiagele B, Scott PA, Sheth KN, Southerland AM, Summers DV, Tirschwell DL. Guidelines for the Early Management of Patients With Acute Ischemic Stroke: 2019 Update to the 2018 guidelines for the early Management of Acute Ischemic Stroke: A guideline for healthcare professionals from the American Heart Association/American stroke. Stroke. 2019;50(12):e344–418.
41. Berrouschot J, et al. Mechanical ventilation in patients with hemispheric ischemic stroke. Crit Care Med. 2000;28(8):2956–61.
42. Wijdicks EF, Scott JP. Causes and outcome of mechanical ventilation in patients with hemispheric ischemic stroke. Mayo Clin Proc. 1997;72(3):210–3.
43. Christensen MS, et al. Cerebral apoplexy (stroke) treated with or without prolonged artificial hyperventilation. 1. Cerebral circulation, clinical course, and cause of death. Stroke. 1973;4(4):568–631.
44. Ko R, Ramos L, Chalela JA. Conventional weaning parameters do not predict extubation failure in neurocritical care patients. Neurocrit Care. 2009;10(3):269–73.
45. Wendell LC, et al. Predictors of extubation success in patients with middle cerebral artery acute ischemic stroke. Stroke Res Treat. 2011;2011:248789.
46. Esteban A, et al. Extubation outcome after spontaneous breathing trials with T-tube or pressure support ventilation. The Spanish lung failure collaborative group. Am J Respir Crit Care Med. 1997;156(2 Pt 1):459–65.
47. Bosel J, et al. Stroke-related early tracheostomy versus prolonged Orotracheal intubation in Neurocritical care trial (SETPOINT): a randomized pilot trial. Stroke. 2013;44(1):21–8.
48. Bösel J, et al. Effect of early vs standard approach to tracheostomy on functional outcome at 6 months among patients with severe stroke receiving mechanical ventilation: the SETPOINT2 randomized clinical trial. JAMA. 2022;327(19):1899–909.
49. Aiyagari V, Gorelick PB. Management of blood pressure for acute and recurrent stroke. Stroke. 2009;40(6):2251–6.
50. Desilles J-P, et al. Diabetes mellitus, admission glucose, and outcomes after stroke thrombolysis: a registry and systematic review. Stroke. 2013;44(7):1915–23.
51. Johnston KC, et al. Intensive vs standard treatment of hyperglycemia and functional outcome in patients with acute ischemic stroke: the SHINE randomized clinical trial. JAMA. 2019;322(4):326–35.
52. Nils Wahlgren NA, Eriksson N, Aichner F, Bluhmki E, Dávalos A, Erilä T, Ford GA, Grond M, Hacke W, Hennerici MG, Kaste M, Köhrmann M, Larrue V, Lees KR, Machnig T, et al. Multivariable analysis of outcome predictors and adjustment of main outcome results to baseline data profile in randomized controlled trials: safe implementation of thrombolysis in stroke-MOnitoring STudy (SITS-MOST). Stroke. 2008;39:3316–22.
53. Rincon F, et al. Brain injury as a risk factor for fever upon admission to the intensive care unit and association with in-hospital case fatality: a matched cohort study. J Intensive Care Med. 2015;30(2):107–14.
54. Azzimondi G, et al. Fever in acute stroke worsens prognosis. A prospective study. Stroke. 1995;26(11):2040–3.

55. den Hertog HM, et al. The paracetamol (acetaminophen) in stroke (PAIS) trial: a multicentre, randomised, placebo-controlled, phase III trial. Lancet Neurol. 2009;8(5):434–40.
56. Saxena M, Young P, Pilcher D, Bailey M, Harrison D, Bellomo R, Finfer S, Beasley R, Hyam J, Menon D, Rowan K, Myburgh J. Early temperature and mortality in critically ill patients with acute neurological diseases: trauma and stroke differ from infection. Intensive Care Med. 2015;41(5):823–32.
57. den Hertog HM, van der Worp HB, van Gemert HM, Algra A, Kappelle LJ, van Gijn J, Koudstaal PJ, Dippel DW. An early rise in body temperature is related to unfavorable outcome after stroke: data from the PAIS study. J Neurol. 2011;258:302–7.
58. Geurts M, Petersson J, Brizzi M, Olsson-Hau S, Luijckx GJ, Algra A, Dippel DW, Kappelle LJ, van der Worp HB. COOLIST (cooling for ischemic stroke trial): A multicenter, open, randomized, phase II, clinical trial. Stroke. 2017;48:219–21.
59. Barletta JF, Mangram AJ, Sucher JF, Zach V. Stress ulcer prophylaxis in neurocritical care. Neurocrit Care. 2018;29(3):344–57.
60. Douds GL, et al. Venous thromboembolism in the get with the guidelines-stroke acute ischemic stroke population: incidence and patterns of prophylaxis. J Stroke Cerebrovasc Dis. 2014;23(1):123–9.
61. Wijdicks EF, Scott JP. Pulmonary embolism associated with acute stroke. Mayo Clin Proc. 1997;72(4):297–300.
62. Heuschmann PU, et al. Predictors of in-hospital mortality and attributable risks of death after ischemic stroke: the German stroke registers study group. Arch Intern Med. 2004;164(16):1761–8.
63. Dennis M, et al. Effectiveness of intermittent pneumatic compression in reduction of risk of deep vein thrombosis in patients who have had a stroke (CLOTS 3): a multicentre randomised controlled trial. Lancet. 2013;382(9891):516–24.
64. Dennis M, et al. Effectiveness of thigh-length graduated compression stockings to reduce the risk of deep vein thrombosis after stroke (CLOTS trial 1): a multicentre, randomised controlled trial. Lancet. 2009;373(9679):1958–65.
65. Sherman DG, et al. The efficacy and safety of enoxaparin versus unfractionated heparin for the prevention of venous thromboembolism after acute ischaemic stroke (PREVAIL study): an open-label randomised comparison. Lancet. 2007;369(9570):1347–55.
66. Neha Rai KP, Bhatia R, Vibha D, Singh MB, Rai VK, Kumar A. Development and implementation of acute stroke care pathway in a tertiary care hospital in India: A cluster-randomized study. Neurol India. 2016;64 Suppl:s39–45.
67. Sandy Middleton PM, Ward J, Grimshaw JM, Dale S, D'Este C, Drury P, Griffiths R, Cheung NW, Quinn C, Evans M, Cadilhac D, Levi C, Q.T. Group. Implementation of evidence-based treatment protocols to manage fever, hyperglycaemia, and swallowing dysfunction in acute stroke (QASC): a cluster randomised controlled trial. Lancet. 2011;378(9804):1699–706.
68. Joundi RA, Martino R, Saposnik G, Giannakeas V, Fang J, Kapral MK. Predictors and outcomes of dysphagia screening after acute ischemic stroke. Stroke. 2017;48:900–6.
69. Sørensen RT, Rasmussen RS, Overgaard K, Lerche A, Johansen AM, Lindhardt T. Dysphagia screening and intensified oral hygiene reduce pneumonia after stroke. J Neurosci Nurs. 2013;45:139–1946.
70. Dennis M, Lewis S, Cranswick G, Forbes J, FOOD Trial Collaboration. FOOD: a multicentre randomised trial evaluating feeding policies in patients admitted to hospital with a recent stroke. Health Technol Assess. 2006;10:1–120.
71. Joon-Tae Kim S-HH, Park M-S, Chang J, Choi K-H, Cho K-H. Use of antithrombotics after hemorrhagic transformation in acute ischemic stroke. PLoS One. 2014;9(2):e89798.
72. Maurizio Paciaroni FB, Agnelli G, Tsivgoulis G, Yaghi S, Furie KL, Tadi P, Becattini C, Zedde M, Abdul-Rahim AH, Lees KR, Alberti A, Venti M, Acciarresi M, et al. Hemorrhagic transformation in patients with acute ischemic stroke and atrial fibrillation: time to initiation of Oral anticoagulant therapy and outcomes. J Am Heart Assoc. 2018;7:e010133.
73. Saposnik G, Barinagarrementeria F, Brown RD Jr, Bushnell CD, Cucchiara B, Cushman M, deVeber G, Ferro JM, Tsai FY. American Heart Association Stroke Council and the Council on epidemiology and prevention. Diagnosis and management of cerebral venous thrombosis: a statement for healthcare professionals from the American Heart Association/American Stroke Association. Stroke. 2011;42(4):1158–92.
74. Hornig CR, et al. Space-occupying cerebellar infarction. Clinical course and prognosis. Stroke. 1994;25(2):372–4.
75. Kase CS, et al. Cerebellar infarction. Clinical and anatomic observations in 66 cases. Stroke. 1993;24(1):76–83.
76. Malm J, et al. Clinical features and prognosis in young adults with infratentorial infarcts. Cerebrovasc Dis. 1999;9(5):282–9.
77. Khan M, et al. Massive cerebellar infarction: "conservative" management. Stroke. 1983;14(5):745–51.
78. Kudo H, et al. Controversy of surgical treatment for severe cerebellar infarction. J Stroke Cerebrovasc Dis. 2007;16(6):259–62.
79. Raco A, et al. Management of acute cerebellar infarction: one institution's experience. Neurosurgery. 2003;53(5):1061–5; discussion 1065–6
80. Wijdicks EF, et al. Recommendations for the management of cerebral and cerebellar infarction with swelling: a statement for healthcare professionals from the american heart association/american stroke association. Stroke. 2014;45(4):1222–38.
81. Tchopev Z, et al. Prediction of poor outcome in cerebellar infarction by diffusion MRI. Neurocrit Care. 2013;19(3):276–82.

Acute Hemorrhagic Stroke and Neurocritical Care

52

Murali T

52.1 Introduction

Intracerebral hemorrhage (ICH) is bleeding within the brain parenchymal tissue itself and it is a life-threatening type of stroke. Spontaneous intracerebral hemorrhage (ICH) is the second most common cause of stroke, forming 15–30% of all strokes and it is a deadly form of stroke. Blood vessels carry blood to and from the brain tissue; arteries or veins can rupture either from abnormally high blood pressure, abnormal development from birth, or degeneration due to age or due to injury.

Intracerebral hemorrhage (ICH) is one of the major medical emergencies that warrants immediate treatment, as it can lead to a high mortality of 40% within 1 month of the incidence and carries a very poor long-term outcome and neurological recovery [1]. Incidence of ICH is high in low and middle income countries as compared to high income countries [2]. Now-a-days, the incidence of intracerebral hemorrhage (ICH) is also increasing in India. Lack of awareness about the stroke in low and middle income countries leads to an increased mortality and morbidity. ICH is not a single entity and more than 80% of cases are due to small vessel disease, predominantly deep perforator arteriopathy, and cerebral amyloid angiopathy; rest resulting from vascular malformations.

Murali T. (✉)
KMCH Institute of Health Science and Research, Coimbatore, India

Primary intracerebral hemorrhage (ICH) is a term often applied to cases caused by cerebral small vessel disease. Hemorrhage in the internal capsule, basal ganglia, and brainstem accounts for two/third of the intracerebral hemorrhages; about 5–10% occurs in cerebellum [3]. The incidence of ICH also increases with increased use of anticoagulants, antiplatelets, and antithrombins, especially in the elderly age group.

52.2 Risk Factors

Risk factors belong to modifiable and non-modifiable groups. Modifiable risk factors include hypertension, cigarette smoking, excessive alcohol consumption, decreased low-density lipoprotein cholesterol, low triglycerides, and use of drugs including anticoagulants, antithrombotic agents, and sympathomimetics. Non-modifiable risk factors include old age, male sex, and Asian ethnicity (Table 52.1) [4, 5].

The most important risk factor which causes deep intracerebral hemorrhage (ICH) or lobar intracerebral hemorrhage (ICH) is hypertension [6]. Patients who currently continue to smoke and consume alcohol heavily [7] have an increased risk of intracerebral hemorrhage (ICH). There is also an increased risk of intracerebral hemorrhage (ICH) in patients with low total cholesterol and low-density lipoprotein cholesterol levels [8]. Now-a-days, there is an increased

H. Prabhakar et al. (eds.), *Principles and Practice of Neurocritical Care*,
https://doi.org/10.1007/978-981-99-8059-8_52

Table 52.1 Risk factors for intracerebral hemorrhage

Modifiable risk factors	Non-modifiable risk factors
1. Hypertension 2. Current smoking 3. Excessive alcohol consumption 4. Decreased low-density lipoprotein cholesterol and low-density triglycerides 5. Anticoagulants 6. Antiplatelets 7. Sympathomimetic agents—Cocaine, amphetamines, PPA, and ephedrine	1. Old age 2. Male sex 3. Asian ethnicity 4. Cerebral amyloid angiopathy 5. Cerebral microbleeds 6. Chronic kidney disease

incidence in patients on anticoagulants, especially in elderly population [9], and there is a two- to fivefold increase with the use of warfarin [10]. Use of warfarin accounts for 10% of all ICH incidences and other newer oral anticoagulants have also shown to increase the incidence of ICH, as their use has increased considerably in recent times. Increased use of antiplatelets now-a-days has also increased the risk of ICH, associated with expansion of hematoma in the early phase [11], along with increased mortality [12]. Dual antiplatelet therapy which is being used more commonly in patients with coronary artery disease and ischemic cerebrovascular accidents also leads onto an increased incidence of intracerebral hemorrhage.

Sympathomimetic drugs like cocaine, heroin, amphetamine, and ephedrine have also been shown to increase the incidence of ICH, especially in younger patients. High dose phenylpropanolamine is an independent risk factor for hemorrhagic stroke (ICH), especially in women [13]. Chronic kidney disease (CKD) which is common with small vessel disease, also increases the risk of ICH [14]; moreover, CKD is also associated with platelet dysfunction which may increase the risk of hemorrhagic stroke (ICH).

Other factors suggested to be related the risk:
Multiparity, poor work condition, long sleep duration

Many pathophysiological injuries have been postulated to cause ICH, but only a few are accepted and more common than the others.

52.2.1 Hypertensive Vascular Change

Long-standing hypertension causes degeneration of the media and smooth muscles of the blood vessels, leading to rupture and bleeding into the brain, ICH [15]. Fibroid necrosis giving rise to microaneurysm may be seen in some cases. Long-standing hypertension may also lead to lipohyalinosis which may produce ICH. Hypertensive ICH usually causes non-lobar ICH, common locations being internal capsule and basal ganglia.

52.2.2 Cerebral Amyloid Angiopathy (CAA)

Deposition of amyloid-β peptide occurs in capillaries, arterioles, and small- and medium-sized arteries of the cerebral cortex, leptomeninges, and cerebellum which is the hallmark of Cerebral Amyloid Angiopathy (CAA) [16]. CAA is more common with lobar ICH definitive diagnosis of CAA which requires pathologic demonstration of apple-green birefringence under polarized light microscopy of cortical vessels. One or more lobar ICH in non-hypertensive elderly patients should raise the suspicion of CAA. Susceptibility weighted MRI may show multiple deposits of hemosiderin in the cortex, immediately adjacent to white matter, which may be a reflection of ongoing micro bleeds. Rebleed may occur in 15% of cases, within 1 year, and 30–35% may show presence of CAA in autopsy [17].

52.2.3 Genetic

Genetic variations in the gene encoding apolipoprotein E epsilon 2 and 4 in chromosome 19 are seen in CAA [18]. Duplication of the APP locus on chromosome 21 is also found in families with familial early-onset Alzheimer disease and CAA. CAA-related ICHs occur mainly in the elderly subjects, while a rare familial syndrome may manifest in relatively younger patients [19].

52.2.4 Corticovenous Occlusion

Corticovenous occlusion is an important but rare cause of ICH. This usually occurs due to blockage of the venous drainage which raises the venous pressure leading to bleeding in the brain parenchyma.

When there is involvement of cortical veins, there will be lobar hemorrhagic infarcts, which will be difficult to diagnosis initially and needs a strong suspension to diagnose.

52.3 Causes of ICH

See Table 52.2.

Table 52.2 Causes of intracerebral hemorrhage

Most common causes	1. Hypertension 2. Cerebral amyloid angiopathy 3. Vascular malformations (arteriovenous fistula or malformations, cavernous angiomas) 4. Ruptured aneurysm 5. Hemorrhagic transformation of an ischemic stroke or neoplasm
Less common causes	1. Endocarditis with septic embolism and coagulopathy 2. Severe thrombocytopenia 3. Sympathomimetic drug abuse 4. Anticoagulant or antiplatelet therapy
Rare causes	1. Herpes simplex encephalitis 2. Cerebral vasculitis 3. Reversible cerebral vasoconstriction syndrome 4. Cerebrovenous occlusion 5. Moyamoya disease

52.4 Common Sites of ICH

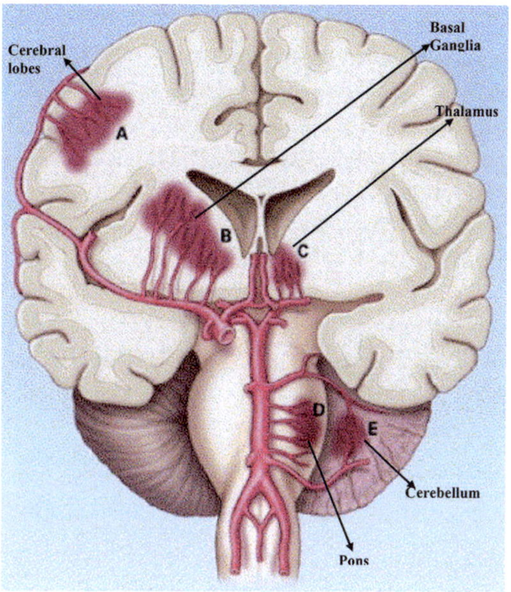

Common sites of intracerebral hemorrhage. (A) Cerebral lobes—originating from penetrating cortical branches of the anterior, middle, or posterior cerebral arteries. (B) Basal ganglia—originating from ascending lenticulostriate branches of the middle cerebral artery. (C) Thalamus—originating from ascending thalamogeniculate branches of the posterior cerebral artery. (D) Pons—originating from paramedian branches of the basilar artery. (E) Cerebellum—originating from penetrating branches of the posterior inferior, anterior inferior, or superior cerebellar arteries

Adapted from Qureshi A et al. N Engl J Med 2001; 344:1450–1460

52.5 Mechanisms for ICH-Related Brain Injury

Intracerebral hemorrhage (ICH) leads to both primary brain injury due to direct pressure of acutely expanding hematoma and through a secondary cellular and physiological pathway due to the hematoma and its metabolized blood products [20].

Direct Pressure Effects—Primary Injury: Includes local compression of the surrounding brain tissue adjacent to the hematoma and more widespread mechanical injury caused by increased intracranial pressure (ICP), hydrocephalus, or herniation. Early hematoma expansion, possibly due to mechanical shearing of surrounding vessels by the initial hematoma [21], which is more common and is considered to be a predictor of poor outcome [12].

Secondary Injury: It is due to physiological and cellular injury mechanisms triggered by ICH. Cerebral edema, inflammation, and biochemical toxicity of blood products such as hemoglobin, iron, and thrombin are the important mechanisms for secondary brain injury following ICH [20].

Several natural mechanisms and BP lowering agents help in reduction of hematoma expansion and prevent further injury to the brain (Fig. 52.1).

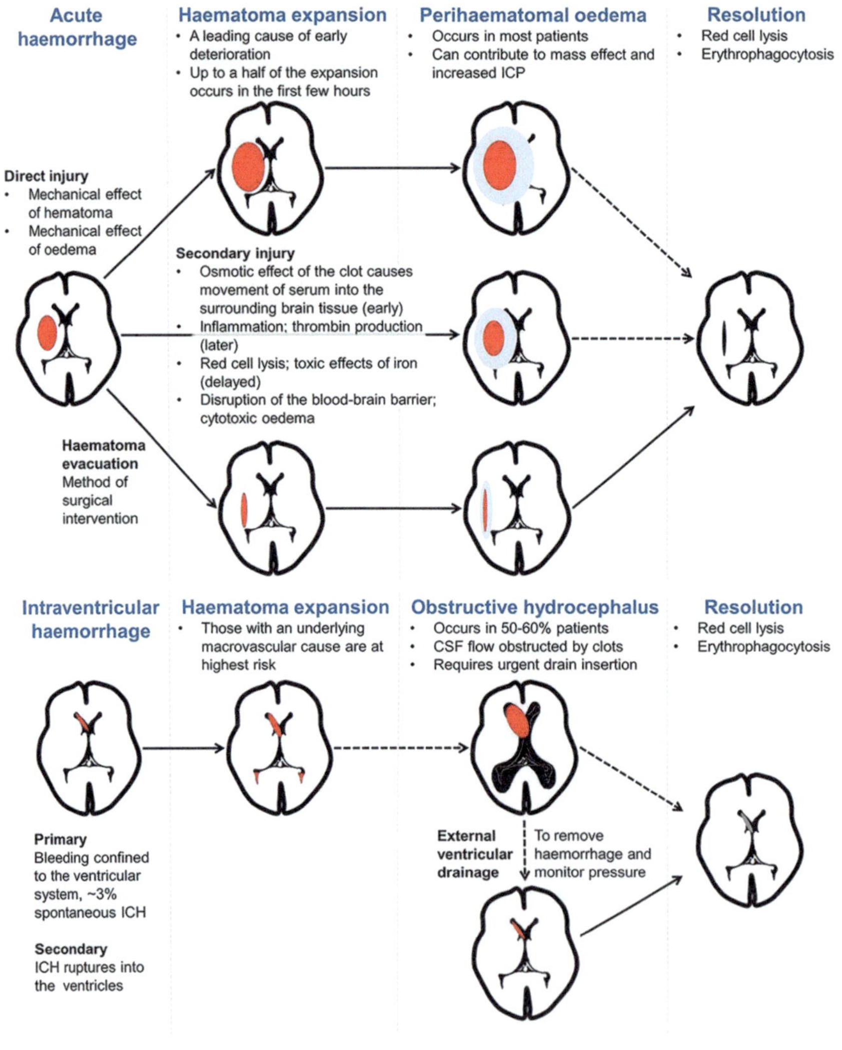

Fig. 52.1 Time course and mechanisms of secondary brain injury in intracerebral hemorrhage, including intraventricular hemorrhage [22]

Adapted from: McGurgan IJ, Ziai WC, Werring DJ, et al. Pract Neurol 2021;21:128–136

52.6 Diagnosis

52.6.1 History

History taking is very important in patients presenting with acute CNS symptoms which should focus on whether the problem is due to stroke, localization of the lesion, or likely mechanism of stroke.

Sudden onset of focal deficit may be seen, which may progress rapidly to even coma in a few hours [23]. As hypertension is an important risk factor for ICH, most patients will have a history of hypertension, treated or untreated. One must take into consideration a history of coronary artery disease, renal dysfunction, prior stroke, or retinal disease as all these are suggestive of preexisting hypertension. History of intake of drugs which increase the blood pressure should also be taken into consideration as well; also it is very important to rule out an intake of anticoagulants or antiplatelets which is one of the most important factors for causation or increase in the size of an intracerebral hemorrhage (ICH). Any history of seizures should raise an alert about vascular origin of intracerebral hemorrhage (ICH) and a history of previous intracerebral hemorrhage (ICH).

52.6.2 Symptoms and Signs Related to the Site of ICH

Putamen Hemorrhage: Presence of contralateral hemiparesis, hemisensory loss, or both due to involvement of the adjacent internal capsule may be seen in putamen hemorrhage. Smaller putamen hemorrhages may have pure motor hemiparesis, pure hemisensory sensory stroke, or ataxic hemiparesis which mimics lacunar infarcts; movement disorder like hemiballism may be seen sometimes. Larger putaminal hemorrhage results in cortical signs like aphasia, contralateral hemineglect, visual field disturbances, and ipsilateral gaze preferences. Massive putamen hematoma results in coma [24].

Caudate Hemorrhage: Bleeding into the caudate nucleus often extends into the ventricular system because of its proximity to the frontal horn, causing severe headache, nuchal rigidity, nausea, and vomiting. It may present with decreased verbal fluency or aphasia, but persistent language disturbance is uncommon. Hemiparesis is usually mild, seen in 30% cases of caudate nucleus hemorrhage and acute hydrocephalus, with coma and oculomotor palsies seen in severe cases of caudate hemorrhage. Prognosis is usually good in isolated caudate hemorrhage.

Thalamic Hemorrhage: Thalamic hemorrhage causes contralateral weakness and hemisensory loss to all modalities which occur rapidly; receptive aphasia or hemineglect may also be seen. Anterior and medial thalamic bleed causes amnesia or abulia with preserved motor and sensory function. Lateral thalamic hemorrhages rarely cause pure sensory stroke [25]. Thalamic bleed may dissect into midbrain and also extend into the ventricles rapidly progressing to cause coma. Few of the ocular signs peculiar to thalamic bleed are tonic, downward gaze deviation with upgaze palsy, horizontal gaze deviations to either the ipsilateral or contralateral side, midposition of unreactive pupils, and refractory nystagmus upon attempted upgaze. Thalamic bleed may cause a high mortality of 25–50% and severe refractory, contralateral thalamic pain syndrome may be seen in survivors.

Pontine Hemorrhage: Massive pontine hemorrhage is due to rupture of pontine perforating arteries that arise directly from the basilar artery. Ninety percent of the pontine bleed patients are hypertensives and 80% of patients progress rapidly into coma, accompanied by quadriplegia, stiffening of the limbs, extensor posturing, pinpoint reactive pupils, facial diplegia, absence of gag, and swallowing reflexes; they may also have loss of spontaneous, reflexic horizontal eye movements and loss of corneal reflexes. Rarely, patients may have symptoms of headache, deafness, numbness, or nausea, usually lasting for a few minutes, followed by coma. High fevers and respiratory abnormalities are frequently seen. It is very rare to see survivors from large pontine hemorrhage with coma.

Cerebellar Hemorrhage: It generally accounts for 10% of all intracerebral hemorrhages. Usually, patients have history of hypertension and they normally present with hypertension; few cerebellar bleeds may be due to AVM. The most common symptom is positional imbalances and inability to stand or walk independently. Vomiting, headache, neck pain, and stiffness are all common. Nystagmus, dysarthria, occasional ipsilateral peripheral facial and gaze palsy, and ipsilateral appendicular incoordination may often be seen on examination. Weakness of extremities is seen only when there is associated brain stem compression.

The level of consciousness may range from normal to coma. Hematomas greater than 3 cm in diameter are most often associated with decline in neurologic status and benefit from surgical decompression. When there is a hydrocephalus due to cerebellar hemorrhage, suboccipital craniotomy is preferred over external ventricular drainage to prevent upward herniation. Irrespective of size of bleed, it is very important to alert the neurosurgical team regarding cerebellar bleed [25].

52.7 Laboratory Investigations

Complete blood count and coagulation studies such as prothrombin time with INR and aPTT are important to determine the type of hemorrhage; they help to identify whether the spontaneous ICH is due to anticoagulant-related or coagulopathy-related causes, or due to thrombocytopenia <10,000. Anticoagulant-related hemorrhages are associated with increased hematoma volume and expansion and lead to increased morbidity and mortality [26]. Presence of anemia on admission is associated with poor outcome [27], and thrombocytopenia is associated with higher mortality for patients taking antiplatelets [28]. Patients taking warfarin, INR value on admission may predict the outcome; increased INR on admission has poor prognosis [29]. Elevation of troponin T on admission has a poor outcome [30]. Increased renal parameters on admission has also shown increased hospital and also1-year mortality [31]. Hyperglycemia on admission is also an important factor which increases mortality [32].

52.8 Investigations

1. Complete blood count including ESR
2. Renal function tests
3. Liver function tests
4. Blood glucose
5. CRP
6. PT/INR
7. aPTT
8. Troponin T
9. ECG
10. Urine toxicology—screening
11. Pregnancy test in child-bearing age females
12. Autoimmune panel in younger patients

52.9 Imaging (Table 52.3)

Brain imaging is essential to distinguish ICH from ischemic stroke and to determine ICH volume [33]. CT scan of the brain is the main modality for confirming presence of ICH. CT scan is widely available and has a high diagnostic accuracy for ICH. MRI brain with echo-planar gradient echo or Susceptibility-Weighted Sequences also can detect hyperacute ICH with

Table 52.3 Evolution of ICH signaling in the 1.5-Tesla MRI scanner [37]

ICH stage	Age of hematoma	T1	T2
Hyperacute	>24 h	**Isointense**	**Slightly hyperintense**
Acute	1–3 days	**Slightly hypointense**	**Hypointense**
Subacute early	>3 days	**Very hyperintense**	**Hypointense**
Subacute late	>7 days	**Very hyperintense**	**Very hyperintense**
Chronic center	>30 days	**Slightly isointense**	**Slightly hyperintense**
Chronic rim	>30 days	**Hypointense**	**Very hypointense**

Adapted from Allkemper et al.: Radiology 2004; 232:874–881

high accuracy [34], but availability and cost of MRI are limitations. Presence of heterogenous densities with hematoma, irregularities of the margins, or spot sign on CT angiogram are signs of ongoing bleed which indicate risk of hematoma expansion [35]. Repeating the CT angiogram is useful 48 h after the initial scan to evaluate for development of hematoma expansion [36], hydrocephalus, or perihematomal edema. CT angiogram may be needed in cases of suspected venous hemorrhage (Figs. 52.2, 52.3, and 52.4).

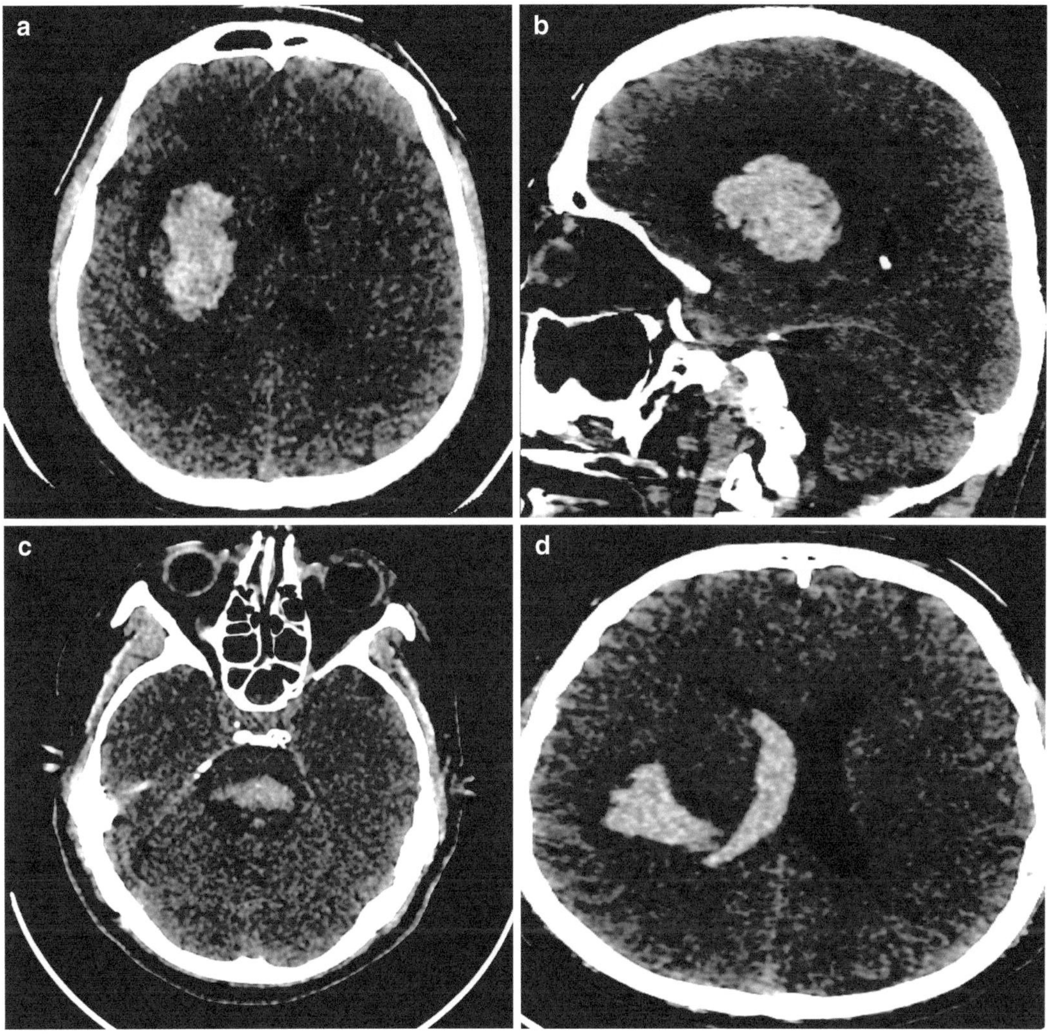

Fig. 52.2 CT scan CT scan (**a**) Axial section – showing gangliocapsular Bleed (**b**) Sagital section – showing gangliocapsular Bleed (**c**) Axial section – showing pontine Bleed (**d**) Axial section – showing gangliocapsular Bleed with intraventricalr extension

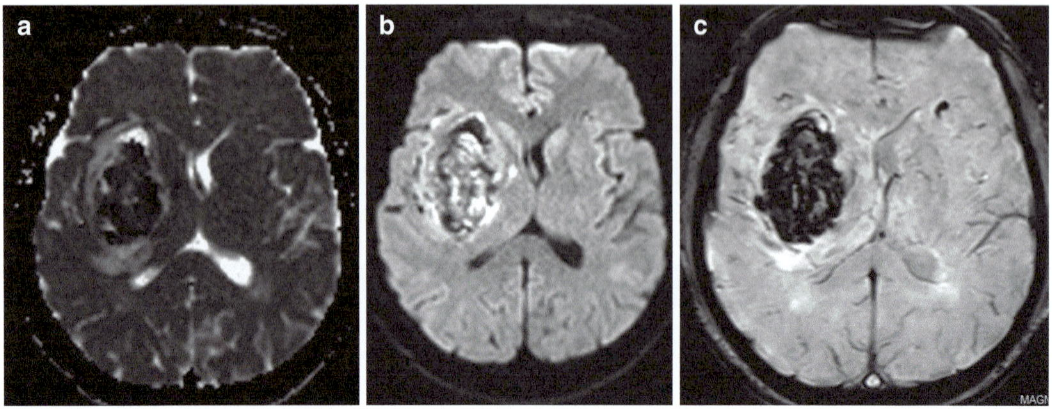

Fig. 52.3 MRI scan MRI scan (**a**) Apparent diffusion coefficient (ADC) image showing Gangliocapsular bleed (**b**) Diffusion weighted image (DWI) showing Gangliocapsular bleed (**c**) Susceptibility weighted image (SWI) showing Gangliocapsular bleed

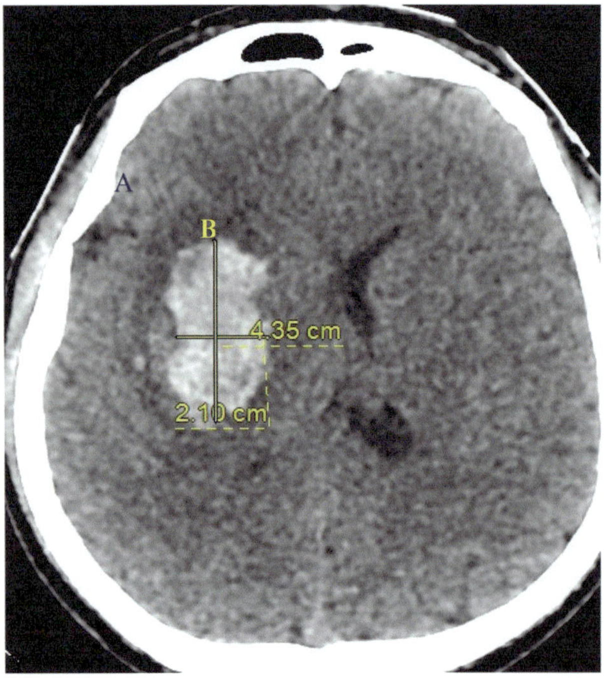

FIGURE 3 – VOLUME CALCULATION

ICH Volume = ABC/2

A = LARGEST DIAMETER OF HEMATOMA

B = DIAMETER PERPENDICULAR TO A

C = HEIGHT OF HEMATOMA - calculated by multiplying number of slices by the slice thickness

Fig. 52.4 ICH volume calculation
ICH Volume = $ABC/2$
A = Largest diameter of hematoma
B = Diameter perpendicular to A
C = Height of hematoma—calculated by multiplying number of slices by the slice thickness

52.10 Treatment

Intracerebral hemorrhage (ICH) is a neurological emergency. Presence of hematoma and vasogenic edema can lead to raised ICP as the brain is inside the fixed cranial vault. "Time is Brain" applies well to patients with ICH, as expanding hematoma increases the mortality of the patient. Rapid initiation of care, including intensive blood pressure management, reversal of anticoagulation, critical care management, and neurosurgical management, are all associated with improved mortality [38]. Patients with ICH need immediate admission to critical care unit or dedicated stroke unit. It has been shown that admission to dedicated stroke unit has reduced the mortality and improved functional outcome. It is important to have the full neurosurgical team inside the hospital which is treating stroke patients or else better to refer the patient to a higher center.

52.10.1 Initial Management

Airway, Breathing, and Circulation should always be in primary focus. Patients who are unable to protect airway (GCS <8) need intubation, and precautions should be taken to prevent sudden hemodynamic reflex changes during intubation, in order to minimize changes in intracranial pressure. It is better to sedate and paralyze the patients before intubation to protect the patient from developing severe intracranial hypertension which may again increase the hematoma size.

It is important to send all blood investigations and look for any abnormality in coagulation. Patients with low GCS presenting with seizures may have a large hematoma and hence an urgent neurosurgical intervention is warranted.

52.10.2 BP Management

Blood pressure management is very crucial in patients with spontaneous ICH, to prevent hematoma expansion and also to achieve good perfusion to the brain. In managing blood pressure, it is important to maintain continuous smooth and sustained control of blood pressure and to prevent large peaks and variabilities [39] as large fluctuations may lead to poor functional outcome. While lowering BP in acute severe hypertensive patients with ICH, it is important to start treatment within 2 h of ICH onset and the target should be reached within 1 h which reduces the risk of hematoma expansion and improves functional outcome [40]. Target blood pressure is SBP of 140 mmHg, and the goal of maintaining the BP should be in the range of 130–150 mmHg, which has shown to improve functional outcome [41]. It is important to make sure that blood pressure is not acutely lowered to <130 mmHg, which is very harmful and has poor prognosis [42] (Table 52.4).

Table 52.4 Drugs for Lowering BP [43]

Drugs	Intravenous bolus dose	Continuous infusion dose
Labetalol	5–20 mg every 15 min	2 mg/min
Nicardipine	NA	5–15 mg/min
Esmolol	250 mcg/kg loading dose	25–300 mcg/kg/min
Enalapril	1.25–5 mg every 6 h	NA
Hydralazine	5–20 mg every 30 min	1.5–5 mcg/kg/min
Nipride	NA	0.1–10 mcg/kg/min

52.10.3 Coagulopathy-Related ICH

In case of anticoagulation-related intracerebral hemorrhage (ICH), it is important to stop the anticoagulant immediately and attempts should be made to reverse it immediately [44]. In patients with VKA-associated spontaneous ICH and INR ≥2.0, 4-factor (4-F) prothrombin complex concentrate (PCC) is recommended in preference to fresh-frozen plasma (FFP) to achieve rapid correction of INR and limit HE [45]. Intravenous vitamin K should be directly administered after coagulopathy correction to prevent further hematoma expansion and later increase in INR in VKA-associated ICH [46]. In patients taking DOAC like dabigatran or factor Xa inhibitors-associated ICH, if taken orally within few hours, activated charcoal may be given to prevent absorption of remaining drug [47]. In dabigatran-associated ICH, idarucizumab is used to reverse the anticoagulant effect. When there is nonavailability of idarucizumab, 4 factor PCC can be given [48]. RRT can be tried to reduce the absorption of dabigatran. In patients with direct factor Xa inhibitor-associated spontaneous ICH, and exanet alfa is reasonable to reverse the anticoagulant effect of factor Xa inhibitors [49]. If it is not available, 4 factor PCC can be considered to improve hemostasis. In patient with unfractioned heparin-(UFH) associated ICH, intravenous protamine can be used for reversal. In case of LMWH, protamine is used which gives partial reversal of anticoagulation [50]. INR is repeated every 3–6 h until it gets normalized <1.4. Patients who are taking aspirin may be treated with platelet transfusion only when there is a planned neurosurgical intervention, to reduce postoperative bleeding and mortality [51]; when not planned for neurosurgical intervention, platelet transfusion is contraindicated and it increases mortality [52]. Use of tranaxemic acid for further bleeding control still remains controversial.

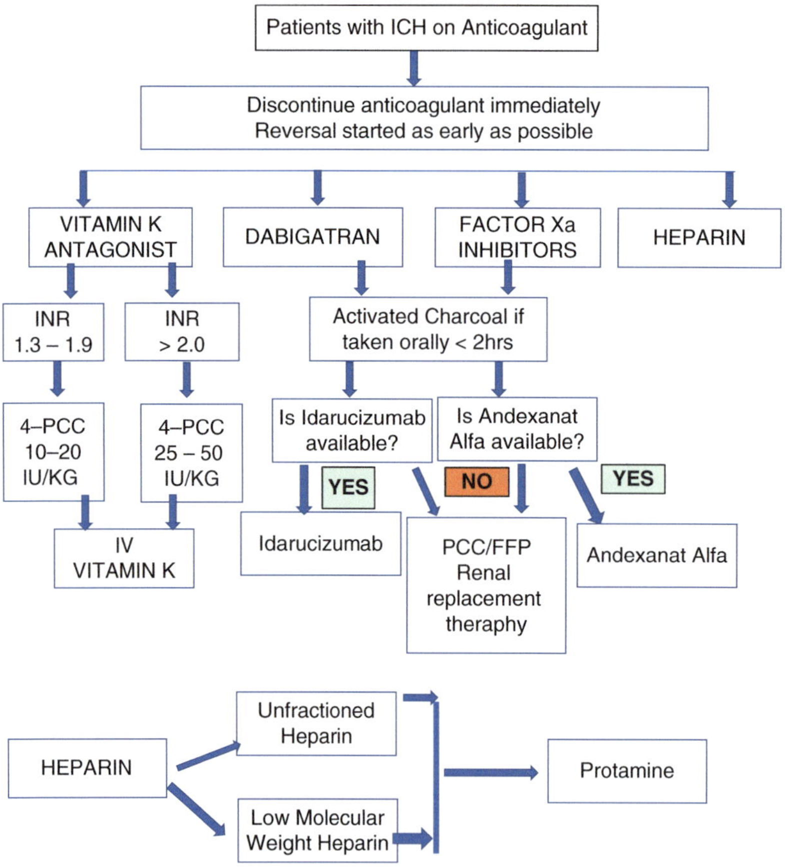

Adapted from: 2022 Guideline for the Management of Patients with Spontaneous Intracerebral Hemorrhage: A Guideline from the American Heart Association/ American Stroke Association

52.10.4 Seizure Management

New onset seizures are common with spontaneous intracerebral hemorrhage (ICH), which accounts for 2.8–28% within first 24 h of ICH [53]. So it is important to monitor the patients who have very low GCS on presentation, with continuous EEG for both clinical and electroencephalographic seizures. Prophylactic antiepileptic drugs do not help in preventing seizures. In patients with spontaneous ICH and clinical seizures, antiseizure drugs are recommended to improve functional outcomes and to prevent brain injury from prolonged recurrent seizures. In patients with spontaneous ICH, with impaired consciousness and confirmed electroencephalographic seizures, antiseizure drugs should be administered to reduce morbidity [54]. In patients with sudden loss of sensorium, one should have a suspicion of seizure, monitor EEG, and antiepileptics should be initiated.

52.10.5 Cerebral Edema and ICP

Cerebral edema may develop slowly within 48 h of onset of ICH; very rarely edema can develop after 2 weeks. ICP monitoring can help in managing the cerebral edema. Requirement of ICP monitoring in ICH doesn't have clear evidence. In ICH patients with a GCS of ≤8, ICP monitored treatment may be considered to reduce mortality and improve outcomes. In presence of hydrochepalus with IVH, placement of extraventricular drainage (EVD) can help in reducing the mortality [55]. Presence of EVD can also help in monitoring ICP and it is evident that ICP-targeted treatment has a reduced mortality. And it is clearly noted that elevated ICP in patients with ICH increases the mortality [56]. Hypertonic saline is the preferred agent and may be administered through a central venous catheter in a 50-mL bolus of 23% saline administered over 10 min or in 200-mL boluses of 3% saline. If hypertonic saline or central access is not readily available, mannitol may be administered in boluses of 0.25–1.0 g/kg to a target serum osmolality of 320 mOsm/L, although higher osmolalities may sometimes be accepted and may probably be safe. Hyperventilation to a $PaCO_2$ of 30–35 mmHg may also lower ICP, but the effect is transient, and this should be viewed as an emergent temporizing measure before more definitive therapy (e.g., surgery). Rebound increased ICP may occur when either mannitol or hyperventilation is withdrawn; so withdrawal should be done slowly. Prophylactic use of osmolar therapy doesn't show any benefit [57]. The goals for ICP and cerebral perfusion pressure (CPP) do not differ from those for traumatic brain injury, which suggests keeping an ICP <20 mmHg (in more recent guideline 22 mmHg) and a CPP >60 mmHg [58].

52.10.6 Surgical Management

There are only a few indications for surgical management of intracerebral hemorrhage (ICH), and when required, usually done late as early surgical management of ICH may lead to poor functional outcome.

Indication for Surgery [59]:

1. Superficial hemorrhage.
2. Clot volume between 20 and 80 mL
3. Worsening neurological status
4. Relatively young patients with poor GCS <5.
5. Hemorrhage causing midline shift/raised ICP
6. Cerebellar hematomas >3 cm or causing hydrocephalus or brain stem compression

Forty-five percent of patients with ICH may have associated intraventricular hemorrhage (IVH) [60] which has a poor prognosis. Patients with large IVH with significant hydrocephalus and a large hematoma with low GCS (<5) may require extra ventricular drain (EVD). For placement of EVD, minimally invasive surgery is preferred.

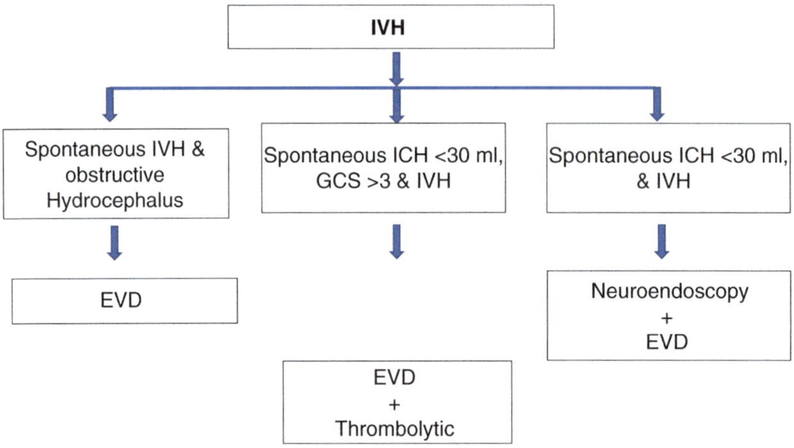

Adapted from: 2022 Guideline for the Management of Patients with Spontaneous Intracerebral Hemorrhage: A Guideline from the American Heart Association/ American Stroke Association

Open craniotomy for intracerebral hemorrhage (ICH) still remains controversial. In supratentorial ICH, open craniotomy and evacuation of hematoma are performed only as a lifesaving procedure in worsening patients [61]. In patients presenting with cerebellar ICH who are deteriorating or have brain stem compression, with ICH volume >15 mL, immediate surgical evacuation is preferred over medical management to reduce mortality [62].

52.10.7 General Management

Patients with intracerebral hemorrhage (ICH) is managed in a stroke unit or critical care setting having multidisciplinary team which has shown an improved outcome and reduced mortality [63]. Those patients who are stable initially may require monitoring in a stroke unit. Those patients who require transfer to higher center should be transferred after adequate airway protection and adequate oxygen support. Patients with large supratentorial ICH and patients with posterior infratentorial ICH should be treated in a setup where immediate neurosurgical consult is available [38].

Intubation is indicated for airway protection, to treat hypoxia and to maintain PaO_2 >60 mmHg. Hypoxia leads to cerebral damage which further worsens the ischemia, especially in the area surrounding ICH leading further to worst outcome. One should also make sure that $PaCO_2$ is within normal range (35–45 mmHg), as raise in $PaCO_2$ will increase the ICP and will lead to poor outcome. $PaCO_2$ <25 has been shown to cause cerebral vasoconstriction, leading to cerebral ischemia and worst outcome.

Patients with ICH require long-term ICU stay and are prone for infection. Infection control practices should be strictly followed like hand hygiene, VAP bundle in ventilated patients, CAUTI bundle, and CRBSI bundle in patients with central venous line according to the local protocol. Routine use of prophylactic antibiotics in the absence of infection is not recommended. Routine screening of infection is done on a regular basis depending on the local protocol [64]. Cardiac monitoring is done for at least 72 h to rule out new onset cardiac abnorality [65].

DVT prophylaxis is very important in these patients as most of them are bed-ridden. Mechanical DVT prophylaxis like pneumatic compression device is used as early as possible. Unfractioned heparin or low molecular weight heparin can be used after 48–96 h if there is no further contraindication to starting parenteral DVT prophylaxis [66]. In presence of DVT or pulmonary embolism, initially retrievable IVC filters can be used to prevent further embolization, and after 1–2 weeks if there are no contraindications, unfractionated heparin or low molecular heparin can be started [67].

It is important to maintain glucose levels between 140 and 180 mg/dL. Both hyperglycemia and hypogylcemia have poor prognosis. Very tight control of sugar has shown frequent hypoglycemic episodes leading to worst outcome, so it is not recommended [68]. Temperature management plays a crucial role in the management of ICH. It's very important that temperature is maintained within normal range avoiding hyperpyrexia. Hypothermia for neuroprotection has not shown any benefit in patients with ICH and hence it is not recommended [69].

52.11 Prognosis

Prognosis in case of intracerebral hemorrhage (ICH) predicts patients' survival and neurological recovery. If we are able to predict the prognosis early, it will be useful for the family members to decide early about the continuation or withdrawal of the support. Death may be due to catastrophic hematoma expansion, untreatable cerebral edema with herniation, or systemic complications such as pneumonia, or acute massive pulmonary embolism. Unfortunately, there is no clear recommendation or clear criteria to predict mortality. Clinical predictors of mortality include age, level of consciousness, size of the hematoma seen on CT scan, and location of the hematoma. ICH score is one such score which has reasonable prediction of mortality in patients with spontaneous intracerebral hemorrhage (ICH) (Table 52.5).

Table 52.5 ICH Score [70]

Component	Score
GCS	
3–4 5–12 13–15	2 1 0
ICH volume	
>30 mL <30 mL	1 0
Presence of IVH	
Yes No	1 0
Infratentorial origin	
Yes No	1 0
Age	
>80 years <80 years	1 0
Total score	**0–6**

ICH score predicts 30-day mortality with scores 1, 2, 3, 4, as 13%, 26%, 72%, and 97%, respectively

Families must be clearly told about the prognosis and survival of the patients with utmost care and comfort so that they can easily understand and take a decision to treat or withdraw.

52.12 Conclusion

Intracerebral hemorrhage (ICH) is a medical emergency which warrants immediate treatment. Patients usually present with sudden unresponsiveness and may also present with seizures. In history, presence of systemic hypertension is very important as it is the most common cause of ICH; also, it is important to know about the use of any anticoagulant drugs. CT brain is the preferred choice of imaging. Early airway protection, maintenance of oxygenation, and preventing hypercarbia and hyperpyrexia are essential. Equally important is effective management of cerebral edema and reducing ICP in reducing the mortality and improving functional outcome. Surgical option for ICH is present only in limited situations like young patients with poor GCS, large supratentorial hematoma >30 mL, superficial bleed, cerebellar hematoma >15 mL, and significant midline shift, as a life-saving procedure. ICH score is reasonable in prognostigating the patient and helps relatives to make a decision on continuing the treatment or withdrawing.

References

1. Feigin VL, Lawes CM, Bennett DA, et al. Worldwide stroke incidence and early case fatality reported in 56 population-based studies: a systematic review. Lancet Neurol. 2009;8:355–69.
2. Krishnamurthi RV, Ikeda T, Feigin VL. Global, regional and country-specific burden of ischaemic stroke, intracerebral haemorrhage and subarachnoid haemorrhage: a systematic analysis of the Global Burden of Disease Study 2017. Neuroepidemiology. 2020;54:171–9.
3. Rodrigues MA, Samarasekera N, Lerpiniere C, et al. The Edinburgh CT and genetic diagnostic criteria for lobar intra-cerebral haemorrhage associated with cerebral amyloid angiopathy: model development and diagnostic test accuracy study. Lancet Neurol. 2018;17:232–40.

4. Ariesen MJ, Claus SP, Rinkel GJ, Algra A. Risk factors for intracerebral hemorrhage in the general population: a systematic review. Stroke. 2003;34:2060–5.
5. Sturgeon JD, Folsom AR, Longstreth WT Jr, Shahar E, Rosamond WD, Cushman M. Risk factors for intracerebral hemorrhage in a pooled prospective study. Stroke. 2007;38:2718–25.
6. Martini SR, Flaherty ML, Brown WM, Haverbusch M, Comeau ME, Sauerbeck LR, et al. Risk factors for intracerebral hemorrhage differ according to hemorrhage location. Neurology. 2012;79:2275–82.
7. Grønbaek H, Johnsen SP, Jepsen P, Gislum M, Vilstrup H, TageJensen U, et al. Liver cirrhosis, other liver diseases, and risk of hospitalisation for intracerebral haemorrhage: a Danish population-based case-control study. BMC Gastroenterol. 2008;8:16.
8. Mustanoja S, Strbian D, Putaala J, Meretoja A, Curtze S, Haapaniemi E, et al. Association of prestroke statin use and lipid levels with outcome of intracerebral hemorrhage. Stroke. 2013;44:2330–2.
9. Flaherty ML, Kissela B, Woo D, Kleindorfer D, Alwell K, Sekar P, et al. The increasing incidence of anticoagulant-associated intracerebral hemorrhage. Neurology. 2007;68:116–21.
10. Flaherty ML, Tao H, Haverbusch M, Sekar P, Kleindorfer D, Kissela B, et al. Warfarin use leads to larger intracerebral hematomas. Neurology. 2008;71:1084–9.
11. Thompson BB, Béjot Y, Caso V, Castillo J, Christensen H, Flaherty ML, et al. Prior antiplatelet therapy and outcome following intracerebral hemorrhage: a systematic review. Neurology. 2010;75:1333–42.
12. Davis SM, Broderick J, Hennerici M, Brun NC, Diringer MN, Mayer SA, et al. Hematoma growth is a determinant of mortality and poor outcome after intracerebral hemorrhage. Neurology. 2006;66:1175–81.
13. Kernan WN, Viscoli CM, Brass LM, Broderick JP, Brott T, Feldmann E, et al. Phenylpropanolamine and the risk of hemorrhagic stroke. N Engl J Med. 2000;343:1826–32.
14. Ovbiagele B, Wing JJ, Menon RS, Burgess RE, Gibbons MC, Sobotka I, et al. Association of chronic kidney disease with cerebral microbleeds in patients with primary intracerebral hemorrhage. Stroke. 2013;44:2409–13.
15. Qureshi AI, Tuhrim S, Broderick JP, Batjer HH, Hondo H, Hanley DF. Spontaneous intracerebral hemorrhage. N Engl J Med. 2001;344:1450–60.
16. Rosand J, Hylek EM, O'Donnell HC, Greenberg SM. Warfarin-associated hemorrhage and cerebral amyloid angiopathy: a genetic and pathologic study. Neurology. 2000;55:947–51.
17. Boyle PA, Yu L, Wilson RS, Leurgans SE, Schneider JA, Bennett DA. Person-specific contribution of neuropathologies to cognitive loss in old age. Ann Neurol. 2018;83:74–83.
18. Phillips MC. Apolipoprotein E isoforms and lipoprotein metabolism. IUBMB Life. 2014;66:616–23.
19. Rost NS, Greenberg SM, Rosand J. The genetic architecture of intracerebral hemorrhage. Stroke. 2008;39:2166–73.
20. Wilkinson DA, Pandey AS, Thompson BG, Keep RF, Hua Y, Xi G. Injury mechanisms in acute intracerebral hemorrhage. Neuropharmacology. 2018;134(pt B):240–8.
21. Fisher CM. Pathological observations in hypertensive cerebral hemorrhage. J Neuropathol Exp Neurol. 1971;30:536–50.
22. McGurgan IJ, Ziai WC, Werring DJ, et al. Acute intracerebral haemorrhage: diagnosis and management. Pract Neurol. 2021;21:128136.
23. Kothari R, Hall K, Brott T, Broderick J. Early stroke recognition: developing an out-of-hospital NIH Stroke Scale. Acad Emerg Med. 1997;4:986–90.
24. Brott T, et al. Early hemorrhage growth in patients with intracerebral hemorrhage. Stroke. 1997;28:1.
25. Hemphill JC, et al. Guidelines for the management of spontaneous intracerebral hemorrhage. Stroke. 2015;46(7):2032–60.
26. Seiffge DJ, Goeldlin MB, Tatlisumak T, Lyrer P, Fischer U, Engelter ST, Werring DJ. Meta-analysis of haematoma volume, haematoma expansion and mortality in intracerebral haemorrhage associated with oral anticoagulant use. J Neurol. 2019;266:3126–35.
27. Roh DJ, Albers DJ, Magid-Bernstein J, Doyle K, Hod E, Eisenberger A, Murthy S, Witsch J, Park S, Agarwal S, et al. Low hemoglobin and hematoma expansion after intracerebral hemorrhage. Neurology. 2019;93:e372–80.
28. Mrochen A, Sprügel MI, Gerner ST, Sembill JA, Lang S, Lücking H, Kuramatsu JB, Huttner HB. Thrombocytopenia and clinical outcomes in intracerebral hemorrhage: a retrospective multicenter cohort study. Stroke. 2021;52:611–9.
29. Biffi A, Battey TW, Ayres AM, Cortellini L, Schwab K, Gilson AJ, Rost NS, Viswanathan A, Goldstein JN, Greenberg SM, et al. Warfarin-related intraventricular hemorrhage: imaging and outcome. Neurology. 2011;77:1840–6.
30. Sandhu R, Aronow WS, Rajdev A, Sukhija R, Amin H, D'aquila K, Sangha A. Relation of cardiac troponin I levels with in-hospital mortality in patients with ischemic stroke, intracerebral hemorrhage, and subarachnoid hemorrhage. Am J Cardiol. 2008;102:632–4.
31. Beuscher VD, Sprügel MI, Gerner ST, Sembill JA, Madzar D, Reindl C, Lücking H, Lang S, Hoelter P, Kuramatsu JB, et al. Chronic kidney disease and clinical outcomes in patients with intracerebral hemorrhage. J Stroke Cerebrovasc Dis. 2020;29:104802.
32. Guo X, Li H, Zhang Z, Li S, Zhang L, Zhang J, Han G. Hyperglycemia and mortality risk in patients with primary intracerebral hemorrhage: a meta-analysis. Mol Neurobiol. 2016;53:2269–75.
33. Kothari RU, Brott T, Broderick JP, Barsan WG, Sauerbeck LR, Zuccarello M, Khoury J. The ABCs of measuring intracerebral hemorrhage volumes. Stroke. 1996;27:1304–5.

34. Fiebach JB, Schellinger PD, Gass A, Kucinski T, Siebler M, Villringer A, Olkers P, Hirsch JG, Heiland S, Wilde P, et al. Kompetenznetzwerk Schlaganfall B5. Stroke magnetic resonance imaging is accurate in hyperacute intracerebral hemorrhage: a multicenter study on the validity of stroke imaging. Stroke. 2004;35:502–6.
35. Morotti A, Arba F, Boulouis G, Charidimou A. Noncontrast CT markers of intracerebral hemorrhage expansion and poor outcome: a meta-analysis. Neurology. 2020;95:632–43.
36. Van Asch CJ, Velthuis BK, Rinkel GJ, et al. Diagnostic yield and accuracy of CTangiography, MR angiography, and digital subtraction angiography for detection of macrovascular causes of intracerebral haemorrhage: prospective, multicentre cohort study. BMJ. 2015;351
37. Allkemper T, Tombach B, Schwindt W, Kugel H, Schilling M, Debus O, Mollmann F, Heindel W. Acute and subacute intracerebral hemorrhages: comparison of MR imaging at 1.5 and 3.0 T—initial experience. Radiology. 2004;232(3):874–81.
38. Parry-Jones AR, Sammut-Powell C, Paroutoglou K, et al. An intracerebral hemorrhage care bundle is associated with lower case fatality. Ann Neurol. 2019;86:495–503.
39. Moullaali TJ, Wang X, Martin RH, Shipes VB, Robinson TG, Chalmers J, Suarez JI, Qureshi AI, Palesch YY, Anderson CS. Blood pressure control and clinical outcomes in acute intracerebral haemorrhage: a preplanned pooled analysis of individual participant data. Lancet Neurol. 2019;18:857–64.
40. Li Q, Warren AD, Qureshi AI, Morotti A, Falcone GJ, Sheth KN, Shoamanesh A, Dowlatshahi D, Viswanathan A, Goldstein JN. Ultra-early blood pressure reduction attenuates hematoma growth and improves out- come in intracerebral hemorrhage. Ann Neurol. 2020;88:388–95.
41. Qureshi AI, Palesch YY, Barsan WG, Hanley DF, Hsu CY, Martin RL, Moy CS, Silbergleit R, Steiner T, Suarez JI, et al. ATACH-2 Trial Investigators and the Neurological Emergency Treatment Trials Network. Intensive blood- pressure lowering in patients with acute cerebral hemorrhage. N Engl J Med. 2016;375:1033–43.
42. Qureshi AI, Huang W, Lobanova I, Barsan WG, Hanley DF, Hsu CY, Lin CL, Silbergleit R, Steiner T, Suarez JI, et al. for ATACH-II Trial Investigators. Outcomes of intensive systolic blood pressure reduction in patients with intracerebral hemorrhage and excessively high initial systolic blood pressure: post hoc analysis of a randomized clinical trial. JAMA Neurol. 2020;77:1355–65.
43. Nyquist P. Management of acute intracranial and intraventricular hemorrhage. Crit Care Med. 2010;38:946–53.
44. Hanger HC, Geddes JA, Wilkinson TJ, Lee M, Baker AE. Warfarin-related intracerebral haemorrhage: better outcomes when reversal includes prothrombin complex concentrates. Intern Med J. 2013;43:308–16.
45. Steiner T, Poli S, Griebe M, Hüsing J, Hajda J, Freiberger A, Bendszus M, Bösel J, Christensen H, Dohmen C, et al. Fresh frozen plasma versus pro- thrombin complex concentrate in patients with intracranial haemorrhage related to vitamin K antagonists (INCH): a randomised trial. Lancet Neurol. 2016;15:566–73.
46. Dentali F, Ageno W, Crowther M. Treatment of coumarin-associated coagulopathy: a systematic review and proposed treatment algorithms. J Thromb Haemost. 2006;4:1853–63.
47. Ollier E, Hodin S, Lanoiselée J, Escal J, Accassat S, De Magalhaes E, Basset T, Bertoletti L, Mismetti P, Delavenne X. Effect of activated charcoal on rivaroxaban complex absorption. Clin Pharmacokinet. 2017;56:793–801.
48. Piran S, Khatib R, Schulman S, Majeed A, Holbrook A, Witt DM, Wiercioch W, Schünemann HJ, Nieuwlaat R. Management of direct factor Xa inhibitor-related major bleeding with prothrombin complex concentrate: a meta-analysis. Blood Adv. 2019;3:158.
49. Connolly SJ, Crowther M, Eikelboom JW, Gibson CM, Curnutte JT, Lawrence JH, Yue P, Bronson MD, Lu G, Conley PB, et al. ANNEXA-4 Investigators. Full study report of andexanet alfa for bleeding associated with factor Xa inhibitors. N Engl J Med. 2019;380:1326–35.
50. Schulman S, Bijsterveld NR. Anticoagulants and their reversal. Transfus Med Rev. 2007;21:37–48.
51. Li X, Sun Z, Zhao W, Zhang J, Chen J, Li Y, Ye Y, Zhao J, Yang X, Xiang Y, et al. Effect of acetylsalicylic acid usage and platelet transfusion on postoperative hemorrhage and activities of daily living in patients with acute intracerebral hemorrhage. J Neurosurg. 2013;118:94–103.
52. Baharoglu MI, Cordonnier C, Al-Shahi Salman R, de Gans K, Koopman MM, Brand A, Majoie CB, Beenen LF, Marquering HA, Vermeulen M, et al. PATCH Investigators. Platelet transfusion versus standard care after acute stroke due to spontaneous cerebral haemorrhage associated with anti- platelet therapy (PATCH): a randomised, open-label, phase 3 trial. Lancet. 2016;387:2605–13.
53. Claassen J, Jetté N, Chum F, Green R, Schmidt M, Choi H, Jirsch J, Frontera JA, Connolly ES, Emerson RG, et al. Electrographic seizures and periodic discharges after intracerebral hemorrhage. Neurology. 2007;69:1356–65.
54. Mehta A, Zusman BE, Shutter LA, Choxi R, Yassin A, Antony A, Thirumala PD. The prevalence and impact of status epilepticus secondary to intra- cerebral hemorrhage: results from the US Nationwide Inpatient Sample. Neurocrit Care. 2018;28:353–61.
55. Lovasik BP, McCracken DJ, McCracken CE, McDougal ME, Frerich JM, Samuels OB, Pradilla G. The effect of external ventricular drain use in intracerebral hemorrhage. World Neurosurg. 2016;94:309–18.
56. Godoy DA, Núñez-Patiño RA, Zorrilla-Vaca A, Ziai WC, Hemphill JC 3rd. Intracranial hypertension after

spontaneous intracerebral hemorrhage: a systematic review and meta-analysis of prevalence and mortality rate. Neurocrit Care. 2019;31:176–87.
57. Sun S, Li Y, Zhang H, Wang X, She L, Yan Z, Lu G. The effect of mannitol in the early stage of supratentorial hypertensive intracerebral hemorrhage: a systematic review and meta-analysis. World Neurosurg. 2019;124:386–96.
58. Hemphill JC, Lam A. Emergency neurological life support: intracerebral hemorrhage. Neurocrit Care. 2017;27:89–101.
59. Shahid Siddique M, et al. Surgical treatment of intracerebral haemorrhage. Br Med Bull. 2000;56(2):444–56.
60. Hallevi H, Albright KC, Aronowski J, Barreto AD, Martin-Schild S, Khaja AM, et al. Intraventricular hemorrhage: anatomic relationships and clinical implications. Neurology. 2008;70:848–52.
61. Li M, Mu F, Su D, Han Q, Guo Z, Chen T. Different surgical interventions for patients with spontaneous supratentorial intracranial hemorrhage: a network meta-analysis. Clin Neurol Neurosurg. 2020;188:105617.
62. Kuramatsu JB, Biffi A, Gerner ST, Sembill JA, Sprügel MI, Leasure A, Sansing L, Matouk C, Falcone GJ, Endres M, et al. Association of surgical hematoma evacuation vs conservative treatment with functional outcome in patients with cerebellar intracerebral hemorrhage. JAMA. 2019;322:1392–403.
63. Langhorne P, Fearon P, Ronning OM, Kaste M, Palomaki H, Vemmos K, Kalra L, Indredavik B, Blomstrand C, Rodgers H, et al. Stroke Unit Trialists' Collaboration. Stroke unit care benefits patients with intracerebral hemorrhage: systematic review and meta-analysis. Stroke. 2013;44:3044–9.
64. Lindner A, Kofler M, Rass V, Ianosi B, Gaasch M, Schiefecker AJ, Beer R, Loveys S, Rhomberg P, Pfausler B, et al. Early predictors for infectious complications in patients with spontaneous intracerebral hemorrhage and their impact on outcome. Front Neurol. 2019;10:817.
65. Alkhachroum AM, Miller B, Chami T, Tatsuoka C, Sila C. A troponin study on patients with ischemic stroke, intracerebral hemorrhage and subarachnoid hemorrhage: type II myocardial infarction is significantly associated with stroke severity, discharge disposition and mortality. J Clin Neurosci. 2019;64:83–8.
66. Boeer A, Voth E, Henze T, Prange HW. Early heparin therapy in patients with spontaneous intracerebral haemorrhage. J Neurol Neurosurg Psychiatry. 1991;54:466–7.
67. Muriel A, Jiménez D, Aujesky D, Bertoletti L, Decousus H, Laporte S, Mismetti P, Muñoz FJ, Yusen R, Monreal M, Investigators RIETE. Survival effects of inferior vena cava filter in patients with acute symptomatic venous thromboembolism and a significant bleeding risk. J Am Coll Cardiol. 2014;63:1675–83.
68. Oddo M, Schmidt JM, Carrera E, Badjatia N, Connolly ES, Presciutti M, Ostapkovich ND, Levine JM, Le Roux P, Mayer SA. Impact of tight glycemic control on cerebral glucose metabolism after severe brain injury: a microdialysis study. Crit Care Med. 2008;36:3233–8.
69. Taykov D, Schwab S, Dörfler A, Kollmar R. Hypothermia reduces perihemorrhagic edema after intracerebral hemorrhage: but does it influence functional outcome and mortality? Ther Hypothermia Temp Manag. 2011;1:105–6.
70. Hemphill JC, et al. The ICH Score. A simple, reliable grading scale for intracerebral hemorrhage. Stroke. 2001;32(4):891–7.

Myasthenia Gravis and Neurocritical Care

53

Birinder Singh Paul, Gunchan Paul, and Sidakbir Singh Paul

53.1 Introduction

Acquired myasthenia gravis (MG) is an autoimmune disorder directed against the neuromuscular junction (NMJ). The diagnosis of MG is based on the clinical history and examination demonstrating characteristic pattern of fluctuating, fatigable weakness in ocular, bulbar, respiratory, or limb muscles [1]. The presence of neuromuscular junction disorder needs to be confirmed by immunological and electrophysiological testing. MG is a rare disorder, but incidence is estimated to be 5 and 30 lacs cases per 1 million-person year [2, 3]. A bimodal peak is described with one peak around 30 year and another peak among 50 years [4, 5]. One should understand that as all patients might not have the classic clinical presentation, list of differential diagnosis for motor weakness and ocular weakness should be generated.

53.2 Pathogenesis

53.2.1 Autoantibodies

The autoimmune nature of MG was first proposed by Conti-Fine in 1960; subsequently many studies demonstrated the disruption of neuromuscular transmission across the NMJ by the binding of the autoantibodies to the acetylcholine receptors (AChR). Since then, a number of antibodies responsible for the pathological changes have been identified that are directed against either the acetylcholine receptors or postsynaptic neuromuscular junction proteins or signaling pathway [6, 7]. There are multiple mechanisms underlying the loss of functional integrity of AChRs or postsynaptic membrane that manifest as muscle weakness; (i) complement mediated lysis of the muscle endplate resulting in distortion and simplification of the postsynaptic muscle membrane, (ii) acceler-

B. S. Paul (✉)
Department of Neurology, Dayanand Medical College and Hospital, Ludhiana, Punjab, India

G. Paul
Department of Critical care, Dayanand Medical College and Hospital, Ludhiana, Punjab, India

S. S. Paul
Dayanand Medical College and Hospital, Ludhiana, Punjab, India

H. Prabhakar et al. (eds.), *Principles and Practice of Neurocritical Care*,
https://doi.org/10.1007/978-981-99-8059-8_53

ated internalization and degradation of AChRs by immunoglobulin (IgG), (iii) blockade of AChR by antibodies attached to the acetylcholine-binding sites, and (iv) loss of functional integrity of the NMJ due to inflammatory process [7].

53.2.2 Thymus Gland

Thymus plays an important role in the pathogenesis of MG manifesting as either hyperplasia or a thymoma in the majority of patients having AChRs antibodies-generalized MG. Hyperplasia is usually seen in 50% of postpubertal juvenile cases and early-onset adult cases. Thymic hyperplasia is usually not seen in anti-muscle-specific-tyrosine kinase (MuSK) antibody-positive MG and is less common in late onset or seronegative MG where thymus is either atrophic or absent. Thymoma is found in 10–20% with older individuals with MG; vice versa, myasthenic symptoms may be seen in 30%–50% of thymoma cases.

53.3 Fatigable Weakness—Physiology

Acetylcholine molecules released after a nerve action potential result in generation of end plate potential (EPP). The magnitude of EPP is always greater than the threshold required for the excitation threshold for depolarization and generation of action potential in the muscle fiber. The difference between the magnitude of EPP and the current required for firing of the muscle fiber potential is called *safety factor* of neuromuscular transmission. Under normal conditions, safety factor is several times larger than the threshold potential required for the generation of muscle fiber action potential. With repetitive (2–5 Hz) stimulation of the nerve, there is sequential decrease in the store of available acetylcholine molecules, and hence, decrease in the resultant magnitude of EPP, but there is no functional weakness noted since the safety factor is large.

In MG, the EPP is lessened because of loss of functional AChRs. Hence, physiological consequence is that EPP is significantly closer in magnitude to the threshold depolarization required for muscle fiber action potential generation. This reduction in safety factor is responsible for occurrence of fatigable muscle weakness on repetitive contractions as with sustained effort EPP falls below the threshold required for firing of the muscle fiber (Fig. 53.1). Baseline weakness may occur when the EPP amplitude is too small to generate muscle fiber action potential at rest when there is greater loss of functional integrity and postsynaptic receptor density [7].

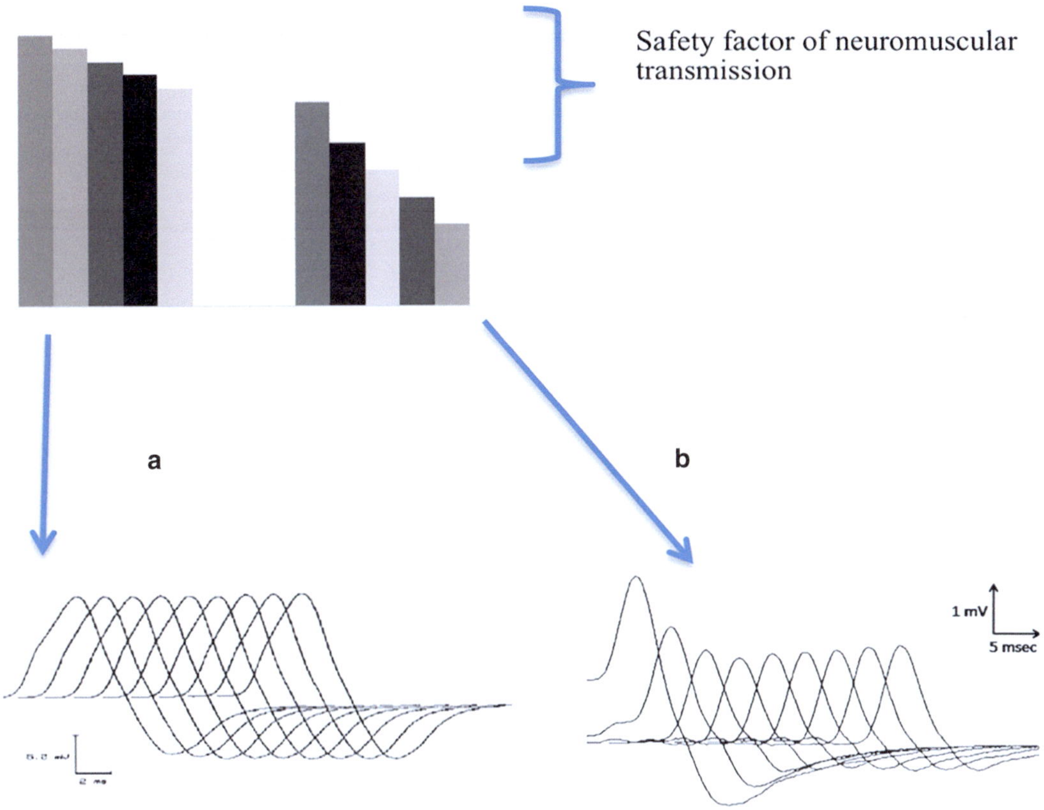

Fig. 53.1 (**a**) EPP amplitude is reduced in MG, narrowing of safety factor of NM transmission with repeated stimulation the EPP amplitude falls below the threshold for muscle fiber activation resulting in NM transmission failure. (**b**) When a critical number of EPP fails, s decremental response is seen on repetitive nerve stimulation studies

53.4 Clinical Characteristics

The clinical hallmark is the presence of distinctive pattern of muscle weakness, fluctuating in-group of muscles that is brought on by repetitive activity and improves with rest. This may be the reason for finding little or no weakness at the time of examination often masking the diagnosis.

Initial symptoms predominantly involve the ocular muscles in 85% of individuals as they report with asymmetrical ptosis, intermittent diplopia, or blurred vision with frequent change of eyeglasses. The remaining 15% MG patients may present with oropharyngeal weakness early in the disease course, including dysarthria, dysphagia, and chewing difficulty. This percentage may be higher up to 40%–50% in anti-muscle-specific-tyrosine kinase (MuSK) antibody-positive MG. Occasionally, the initial presentation is with respiratory muscle weakness without ocular or limb symptoms in 20%, while another 10% may have only diaphragmatic weakness with complaint of orthopnea as an early symptom. It is important to recognize these atypical presentations as early diagnosis changes the outcome, though motor neuron disease may always be in the differential diagnosis (Table 53.1).

On following the patients, majority (80%) of them with ocular muscle symptoms will subsequently develop generalized MG characterized by weakness of limb muscle predominantly proximal.

Examination and physical signs: The demonstration of physical signs of fluctuating or fixed weakness on examination or observing for pres-

Table 53.1 Differential diagnosis of myasthenia gravis

Diagnosis	Points of differentiation	Parameters
Botulism	Ptosis, ophthalmoplegia with blurred vision, facial weakness, poor pupillary reaction, and dry mouth	Neurophysiology suggests preganglionic neuromuscular junction disorder
Lambert-Eaton myasthenic syndrome	Relative sparing of ocular muscles, reduced or absent reflexes that may temporarily return, along with muscle strength following contraction (postexercise facilitation)	Anti-voltage-gated calcium channel antibody present, Incremental response at 30–50 Hz RNS
Inflammatory muscle disease (polymyositis)	Relative sparing of ocular and facial muscles, painful proximal> distal weakness	CPK >5 times EMG- myopathic pattern with spontaneous activity
Motor neuron disease	Presence of UMN + LMN signs (fasciculation, wasting, brisk reflexes)	NCV—low CMAP EMG—neurogenic pattern with fasciculations
Acute immune demyelinating polyneuropathy	Proximal weakness, no fluctuation, deep tendon reflexes absent, bilateral facial weakness	NCV—demyelination neuropathy with conduction block, CSF albumin-cytological dissociation
Thyroid ophthalmopathy	Proptosis, commonly medial rectus involvement	MRI demonstration of enlarged extraocular muscles with sparing of tendons
Congenital myasthenic syndrome	Onset in infancy or childhood, associated musculoskeletal abnormalities, no response to immunomodulation	AChR—antibodies absent Repetitive CMAP on RNST
Mitochondrial disorders	Gradual onset of symmetrical proximal weakness and ptosis, no diplopia despite ophthalmoplegia	EMG—myopathic RNS—no decremental response Muscle biopsy
CNS disorders causing cranial nerve dysfunction	Acute onset, impaired consciousness, pupillary involvement, corticospinal tract involvement	MRI brain

ence of fatigability in the muscles should prompt further investigations for a neuromuscular junction (NMJ) defect. Commonly noted physical signs include:

Ocular signs: The involvement of extraocular muscles and eyelid elevators to variable degrees with sparing of pupillary response is characteristic of neuromuscular junction disorder. Among the important signs, *Enhanced ptosis* sign is most commonly found during the course of disease. This is worsening of ptosis on the contralateral side by doing manual elevation of the more ptotic lid. In addition, the pattern of extraocular muscle weakness is typically asymmetrical and not isolated to the distribution of any individual III, IV, or VI nerve. As the pattern of weakness fluctuates and changes even during the course of a single examination, examination of extraocular movements should include a minimum 15–30 s of lateral and superior gaze holding. There are certain additional bedside maneuvers that may bring out occult signs of myasthenic weakness. Sustained upgaze for 60–180 s may bring out ptosis, while resting lid by closing the eyes for 30 s may improve ptosis demonstrating neuromuscular junctional weakness.

Involvement of facial muscles may produce a sagging appearance with loss of facial expression. Weakness of orbicularis oris may result in characteristic horizontal or snaling smiling while articulation abnormalities with labial or lingual consonant and vowel distortion because of facial and tongue weakness raise the possibility of MG. It is sometimes useful to ask MG patients with bulbar symptoms to count up to 50 and listen for the development of any nasal speech and labial or lingual dysarthria. Patient with dysphagia should be examined for presence of palatal weakness by observing the repetitive movement of soft palate on saying "AH" which will gradually reduce in amplitude. Chewing difficulty in MG is related to weakness of masseter and temporalis muscles, this pattern of weak jaw closure with relatively strong jaw opening is quite typical of MG. Having the patient clamp the jaws together while the examiner attempts to separate them by applying sustained downward pressure for period of 30 s checks the masseter and temporalis muscles.

Respiratory muscles: It is important to distinguish status of respiratory muscles from the functional status of lung. Simple observation is often quite revealing as respiratory muscle weakness presents with tachypnea and shallow breathing. Asking the subject to inspire forcefully and loudly through the nose (inspiratory sniff) gives indication of inspiratory muscle strength. However, expiratory muscle function can be checked by the ability to cough or clearing of throat. Outward protrusion of the abdomen against the examiner's hand is an indirect measure of diaphragmatic strength. Weak sniff, cough, tachypnea, and tachycardia are clinical signs of respiratory muscle weakness in MG. Given the fluctuating nature of disease, it is not uncommon for an MG patient to have intermittent symptomatic dyspnea on history with normal pulmonary function tests. Even in impending respiratory decompensation, it is to have normal arterial blood gas (ABG) measurement or it may show changes that are usually consistent with hyperventilation and may be falsely attributed to anxiety. It is important to mention here that by the time carbon dioxide retention occurs, the respiratory muscles have already begun to decompensate. The important clue to identify the failing respiratory muscles is to detect associated weakness of neck flexion also, which may be a useful sign if there is doubt about the respiratory decompensation and hence helps to initiate the optimal management of impending crisis. Sometimes neck flexors are weaker than extensors, resulting in "dropped head syndrome" seen as the presenting symptom.

Myasthenia Gravis with Anti-Muscle-Specific receptor tyrosine kinase antibodies (anti-MuSK-ab) may have atypical presentations characterized by prominent facial, bulbar, neck muscle involvement rather than ocular signs. Clinical presentations are similar to anti-AChR-positive disease, though respiratory crises are more frequent, with relative sparing of ocular muscles [8, 9]. Disease onset in anti-MuSK-positive MG tends to be more in males by third or fourth decade in addition to normal thymus histology seen in these patients.

53.5 Long-Term Outcome

Myasthenia gravis usually has fluctuating course lasting for months and rarely remission may be seen as permanent cure. Ocular MG is designated if symptoms are solely confined to the extraocular muscles for minimum duration of 2 years. On the other hand, in two-third of the patients with generalized MG, maximum disease severity is usually reached within 2 years of onset [10]. Myasthenia gravis has an active state lasting 5–7 years with frequent remission and replases. The active state is followed by inactive stage lasting approximately for 5–6 years with occasional disease exacerbation precipitated by intercurrent infections, exposure to drugs affecting neuromuscular transmission or pregnancy, and final state is burnt out.

MG is a fatal and severe disease, but advances in intensive care and immunotherapy have contributed to a very favorable prognosis in most patients.

53.6 Diagnostics

The MG starts with bedside clinical examination confirmed by electrophysiology and immunologic testing. Comparison of all three had been depicted in Table 53.2.

(a) ***Bedside:*** Ice pack test is the most commonly performed test at bedside for MG having sensitivity of 80–94%. It is done by placing an ice pack covered by towel over the eyelid for 2 to 5 minutes to look for improvement in lid ptosis (>2 mm). Fatiguing muscle before performing the test can increase the sensitivity of ice test. Ice test can also be performed

Table 53.2 Diagnostic tests based on distribution of myasthenic weakness

Distribution of weakness	Bedside test (sensitivity%)	Electro diagnostic test Muscle (sensitivity%)	Immunologic (sensitivity%)
Ocular	(i) Edrophonium (60–90%) (ii) Ice pack (89%)	SFEMG-facial (90%)	AChR-Ab (50%)
Oropharyngeal/ generalized	None	(i) RNS-limb/cranial (60%) (ii) SFEMG-limb/cranial (99%)	AChR-Ab (85%) MuSK-Ab (40–50%); if above is negative

for individuals with diplopia due to ocular weakness, as application of ice for 5–10 minutes may partially improve the degree of extraocular movement and diplopia in patients of MG [11, 12].

(b) ***Pharmacologic tests:*** Edrophonium test is the most commonly used pharmacological agent for diagnosing neuromuscular weakness. Edrophonium is acetylcholinesterase inhibitor that allows acetylcholine molecules to diffuse more widely throughout the synaptic cleft and interact with AChRs sequentially, increasing the amplitude and duration of EPP resulting in improvement of weakness in the involved muscles. Pharmacological properties such as rapid onset (30 seconds) and short duration of effect (5–10 minutes) make it an ideal agent.

    Method. Initially, 2 mg intravenous administration is done under cardiac monitoring followed by subsequent doses of 3 mg to 8 mg until a positive response is achieved or up to dose of 10 mg. The positive response is characterized by clinical improvement of the involved muscles. The sensitivity for this test is around 72–95%. In case edrophonium is not available, intramuscular neostigmine 1.5 mg dose challenge may also be used as an alternative. For neostigmine challenge, it is advisable to prime the patients with atropine (0.4 mg to 2 mg) to overcome the cholinergic side effects of AChEIs [13].

(c) ***Electrophysiological (EPS) tests:*** EPS is an important modality, which needs to be performed in all patients with suspicion of NMJ and to rule out other neurological disorders of the motor unit of the neuroaxis.

    Repetitive nerve stimulation test (RNST): This is most widely used EPS test of establishing the physiology of neuromuscular transmission. RNST at low frequency (2 Hz to 5 Hz) assesses the abnormalities at motor end plates by depleting the store of readily releasable acetylcholine on repetitive stimulation. A decremental response of more than 10% on repetitive stimulation at low frequency is characteristic of MG. The sensitivity of RNST is around 75% in generalized MG and 50% in purely ocular MG [13]. In order to increase the diagnostic yield, RNST should be performed in multiple muscles including facial, one proximal, and one distal muscle or clinically weaker muscle for elicitation of decremental response. The decremental response should be reproducible in at least two muscles before the test is considered positive. Technical factors, like temperature, inadequate mobilization of the tested muscle, strength of current, and AChEI drugs (if taken), need to be analyzed and controlled for accurate interpretation of the results.

    Single fiber EMG (SFEMG): It is considered to be the most sensitive test for neuromuscular disorders, though performed in specialized centers. It is selective recording of action potential from the individual muscle fibers. In those we record 2 to 4 muscle fiber action potential from a single motor unit at the same time using a specially constructed concentric needle. Physiologically, the time interval between onset of action potential in the two fibers is called *jitter*. Presence of normal or negative jitter during voluntary activation in a clinically weak muscle essentially excludes NMJ disorder. SFEMG has the highest specificity up to 99% when done in a clinically weak muscle, while sensitivity is around 85%. Normal SFEMG in weak muscles probably rules out MG [12, 14, 15].

(d) ***Immunologic tests:*** Acquired MG being an autoimmune disorder, antibodies against the AChR proteins are generally regarded as specific serological markers. Elevated AChR-binding antibodies in a patient with compatible clinical features and EPS findings confirm the diagnosis but normal antibody concentration does not exclude the diagnosis. Anti-AChR-binding antibodies are present in approximately 80% to 85% of patients with generalized MG, but only in 55% of those with purely ocular symptoms [12, 16].

A small proportion of patients who have generalized MG with anti-AChR-antibody-negative have been found to have anti-MuSK antibodies. Anti-MuSK antibodies are mostly of the non-compliment fixing IgG4 subclass that disrupt neuromuscular transmission by interfering with LRP4/MuSK interaction resulting in reduced AChR clustering at muscle end plate resulting in failure of NM transmission [17, 18].

Another specific antibody detected in MG is striated muscle antibody, which was the first autoantibody to be detected. Presence of striatal muscle antibodies is highly suggestive of thymoma that is seen in 75% to 80% of MG patients. However, this antibody may also be seen in non-thymomatous MG, particularly in older individuals.

Most recently, antibodies include that against LRP4, agrin and cortactin has been described in 10%–15% of seronegative generalized MG. Though the clinical features are less described but have similar response to treatment as in patients with anti-AChR antibody-positive MG [19].

(e) ***Ancillary testing:*** CT-chest should be performed in all patients with MG to exclude the presence of thymoma. CT chest is sensitive for identifying anterior mediastinum masses and anomalous occurrence of thymic tissue in the mediastinum.

Other autoimmune disorders can often coexist with MG particularly thyroid diseases, thus thyroid function tests as well as work up for other autoimmune serology should also be considered. It is important to treat the comorbid conditions along with myasthenic symptoms.

53.7 Treatment

The therapeutic goal in myasthenia gravis is to return the patient to normal functional status or minimal manifestation as rapidly as possible along with minimizing the side effects of symptomatic and immunosuppressive therapy. The treatment of MG must be individualized according to the age of onset, extent (ocular versus generalized), rate of progression, antibody status, childbearing potential, severity (mild to severe) of disease, and the presence or absence of concomitant diseases [20] (Box 53.1).

Before any pharmacological treatment of MG, the first step of management is patient education about the illness.

Box 53.1 Therapeutic Strategies

- For all patients of MG the treatment plan chosen must be tailored according to their disease severity, presence of comorbidities, and individualized therapeutic goals.
- The aim of immune-modulatory treatment is to achieve complete or near complete remission of myasthenic symptoms.
- Initial management in all cases of MG is to start cholinesterase inhibitors with optimization of dose for control of symptoms.
- Depending upon the type of MG, patient should be started on steroids followed by steroid sparing immune-modulatory therapy.
- MG patients with involvement of oropharyngeal or respiratory muscles should be treated with course of PE or IVIG along with initiation of steroids.
- Patients with mild or purely ocular MG may be initially treated with anticholinesterase inhibitors and non-improving patients should be started on low dose steroids.
- Early addition of steroid sparing drugs (AZA, MM, CYL) should be considered for patients with moderate or severe generalized disease.

- In addition steroid-sparing agent may be consider in even milder disease after failure of steroid tapering.
- In person with disease onset prior to age 50 years, thymectomy should be considered as a long-term option for immune modulation.
- Steroids can eventually be tapered to zero once the disease is controlled and also steroid-sparing agents should also be reduced very slowly to the minimum required maintenance dose.
- As patient response to therapy is variable in MG, a hierarchy of treatment choices is necessary if the first line drugs are ether ineffective of not tolerated (Fig. 53.2).
- Ranking order of immunosuppressive agents and there selection is dependent on number of factors, like desired course of improvement, burden of therapy, potential side effects, cost, patient preferences and physician experience.
- The non-steroid immunosuppressive agents are not typically effective until 1–14 months after initiating therapy.
- AZA, MM can also be given as initial monotherapy for mild disease or when steroids are contraindication.
- These immunosuppressive agents require frequent laboratory monitoring.
- In patients who's MG has been stable for 3–5 years, immunosuppressive dosage reduction can be considered.

53.7.1 Symptomatic (Nonimmune) Treatment

Cholinesterase inhibitors remain the cornerstone for symptomatic improvement, and among them, pyridostigmine bromide (mestinon) is the most commonly used agent. Dosage guidelines are depicted in Table 53.3. It is important to understand that treatment with cholinesterase inhibitors provide symptomatic treatment but does alter the disease progression. Muscarinic effects are the most common adverse events of cholinesterase inhibitors, which include cramps, diarrhea, seating, bradycardia, and bronchial and nasal secretions [21].

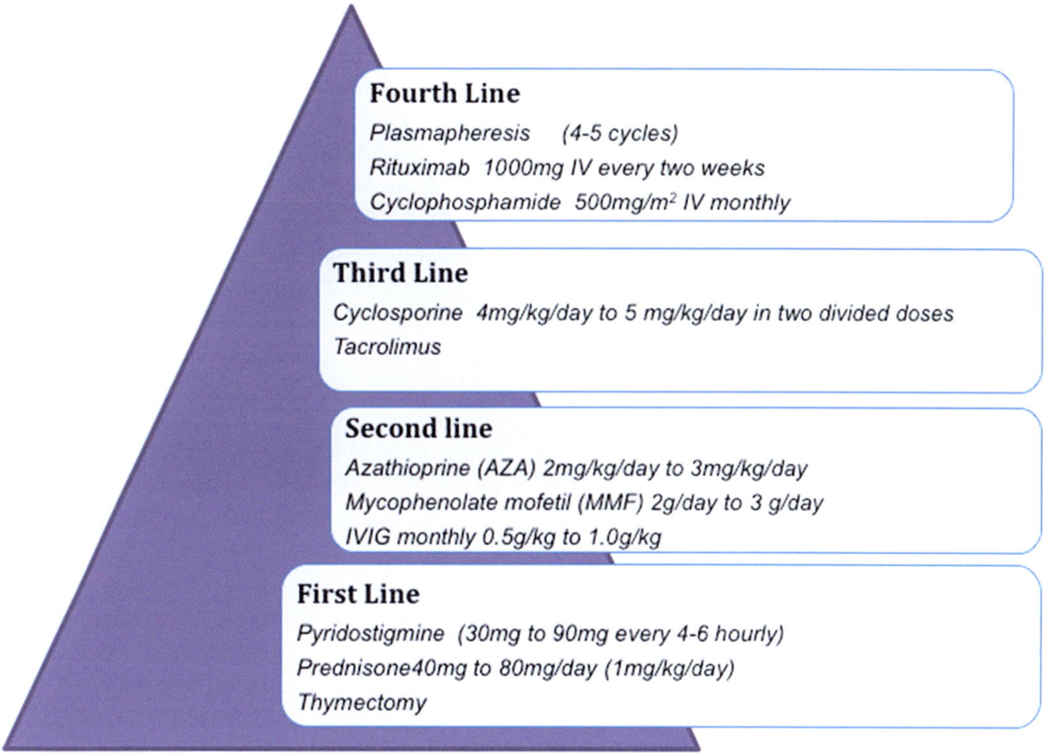

Fig. 53.2 Hierarchical therapeutic strategy for management of Myasthenia Gravis

Table 53.3 Anticholinesterase medication and drugs exacerbating myasthenia gravis

Anticholinesterase drugs				
Drug	Oral	Intramuscular	Intravenous	Pediatric oral
Pyridostigmine	30–60 mg 4–6 h	2.0 mg every 4–6 h	0.7 mg every 4–6 h	1.0 mg/kg to 7.0 mg/kg every 4–6 h
Neostigmine	15 mg every 4–6 h	1.5 mg every 4–6 h	0.5 mg every 4–6 h	0.3 mg/kg to 2.0 mg/kg in divided doses 3–4 times per day
Medications that may exacerbate Myasthenia Gravis				
Absolutely contraindicated	Affect neuromuscular transmission		Exacerbate weakness in some	
Curare D-Penicillamine Botulinum toxin Interferon alfa	Antibiotics Aminoglycosides (Gentamycin, amikacin, streptomycin) Macrolides (erthyromycin, azithromycin) Fluroquinolones (ciprofloxacin, levofloxacin, norfloxacin)	Quinine, quinidine Magnesium salt	Calcium channel blockers Beta-blockers	Iodinated contrast agents Lithium

53.8 Immune-Directed Therapy

The main goal of immune-directed therapy is to induce remission or near remission of myasthenic symptoms. Immune therapies are further divided into short-term (rapid onset) therapies and long-term therapies.

53.8.1 Short-Term Immune-Directed Therapies

Plasmapheresis (PE) is considered as the therapeutic modality for treatment of patients with MG in following clinical scenarios: (i) Myasthenic crisis, characterized by sudden worsening of bulbar or respiratory symptoms requiring need for ventilation, (ii) Prior to surgery or thymectomy to produce rapid improvement, (iii) in combination with high dose daily prednisone as a strategy to prevent steroid-induced worsening when rapid improvement is needed, and (iv) Serial PE may be the choice for refractory MG when other modalities of treatment fail [22].

PE is an extracorporeal blood purification procedure that temporarily reduces the level of circulating antibodies resulting in symptomatic improvement in few days. Usually, three to five cycles of exchange every alternate day are administered. This form of treatment is usually available at tertiary centers. Author had retrospectively analyzed the complication and outcome of PE in 35 patients of MG; 23 presented in crisis while 12 had progressive exacerbation of myasthenic symptoms in spite of optimal treatment. In all these patients, each session of therapeutic PE resulted in immediate improvement of clinical status and maximum improvement was observed after four exchanges (50 mL/kg of plasma removed per exchange). The complications noted in their study included citrate toxicity in 12 (6.8%), hypotension in 2 (1.14%), and catheter-related problems in 8 (4.6%). Infection was not observed in any and there was no mortality as a consequence of therapeutic PE. Hence, PE is a safe and efficacious mode of treatment option for management of MG with acceptance rate of 75% [23]. Although the general usefulness of PE lasts for brief duration and benefits begin to wear off after 3–4 weeks, combination with chronic immunosuppression is needed.

IV immunoglobulin (IVIG): IVIG is another form of short-term immune-directed treatment for MG. Multiple randomized trails have shown class I evidence for use of IVIG in MG exacerbations and literature suggests that it has comparable efficacy to PEin management of worsening myasthenic symptoms. IVIG results in rapid improvement in muscle strength, particularly in patients with moderate and severe MG with evolving oropharyngeal or respiratory symptoms. Hence, clinical indications of IVIG use are similar to those for PE. The induction of IVIG course is usually at a dose of 2 g/kg that is divided over 2–5 days with regular monitoring of renal and cardiac toxicity. Ease of administration makes it one of the most preferable agents of choice in certain clinical setting of MG [20]. In refractory cases of MG, maintenance dose of 0.5–1 g/kg may be used as monthly cycle for 4–6 months.

53.9 Long-Term Immune-Directed Therapies

Thymectomy: As it is known that thymus plays an important role in the pathogenesis of MG, therapeutic removal of gland is considered to have more marked and long-lasting beneficial effect on control of myasthenic symptoms. However, large randomized trails have expressed uncertainty over the observed improvement of myasthenic symptoms of thymectomy because the results were confounded by baseline differences between the surgical and nonsurgical groups. Still it is considered as an important immune-directed treatment modality [24].

The only absolute indication for thymectomy is the presence of thymoma observed in 10–20% of patients with MG. Surgical removal is recommended in thymoma with the understanding that thymectomy is not an emergency or urgent procedure, but it should be undertaken only after treatment of MG is optimized and myasthenic symptoms are well controlled with minimum dose of steroids (<30 mg/day).

Despite uncertainty of efficacy of thymectomy in nonthymomatus MG, most studies suggest that it should be a therapeutic option in AChR-antibody-positive adult patient who had generalized MG with disease onset before the age of 50 years [25]. Endoscopic surgery is a preferred approach for thymectomy, which is associated with low complication rate and shorter hospital stay. On the other hand, open thymectomy remains the preferred technique for invasive thymoma.

Corticosteroids: Oral steroids are the most widely and common form of immunomodulation in MG, though class I evidence is lacking. In a large series, prednisone induced complete remission of symptoms in 28%, marked improvement (minor symptoms, normal activities of daily living) in 53%, moderate improvement in 15%, and no improvement in only 5% patients of MG [26]. Prednisone is the preferred mode of immunosuppression in generalized or when cholinesterase inhibitors alone inadequately control ocular MG. It is generally recommended to start steroids at very low dose (10 mg/day) and then gradually build up the dose to approximately 1–1.5 mg/kg/day [27]. This slow escalation approach lessens the risk of transient worsening that is reported to occur in one-third to one-half of patients treated with high daily dose of prednisone in the beginning. Once, a remission in induced patients may be switched to alternate day regimen maintaining it for 1–2 months before initiating tapering along with addition of concurrent immunosuppressive agent. In ocular or mild MG, lower initial dose of prednisone (30–40 mg) may be effective in inducing remission. One should be vigilant for side effects noted in approximately two-third of the patients such as weight gain, impaired glucose tolerance, hypertension, osteoporosis, myopathy, cataract, and gastric ulcer. All patients should be placed on calcium (1000–1500 mg a day) and vitamin D (600–6000 units per week) supplementation to minimize bone loss along with regular monitoring of bone density performed every 6–12 months. Monitoring of serum electrolytes, glucose, weight, and blood pressure should be on a regular basis on patients taking steroid used for a long time.

Azathioprine (AZA): It is purine antimetabolite that interferes with T-cell and B-cell proliferation, and due to this property, it is another agent for immunosuppression in MG. Studies indicate that AZA is effective in 70%–90% of patients with MG. It plays an important role as a steroid-sparing agent, but can also be used for those having inadequate response to steroid and as a long-term immunomodulating agent in inducing remission [28]. AZA is initiated at 50 mg/day followed by gradual titration by 50 mg/week until a dose of 2–3 mg/kg/day is achieved, though its benefit may delay as long as 12 months. This drug is well tolerated by most, but 10%–15% of patients develop idiosyncratic reaction on administration of first dose. On the other hand, hepatotoxicity and leukopenia are important adverse effects for cumulative dose that should be watched for patients on AZA for a long time. White blood cell and liver enzymes should be monitored at least thrice monthly.

Myophenolate mofetil (MM): This molecule selectively blocks purine synthesis, thereby suppressing both T-cell and B-cell proliferation. MM is another stand-alone immune modulator as well as steroid sparing agent in the treatment of MG. Randomized studies have found MM to be 70%–80% effective as an oral drug in inducing remission in patients with MG. In these studies, onset of benefit was observed at a mean of 9–11 weeks [29–31]. The standard dose used was 1000 mg twice a day, but increasing up to 1500 mg twice a day in selected nonresponder patients was also found to be effective. In general side, effects of MM are mild and are most commonly diarrhea or abdominal pain. Long-term use is associated with myelosupression in a few of the patients.

Cyclosporine (CYL): It inhibits T-cell proliferation via disruption of calcineurin signaling which blocks synthesis of IL-2 and other protein essential to the function of CD4 T cells. CYL has been used as an immunomodulatory agent in whom MM/AZA is ether ineffective or not tolerated. The recommended initial dose of CYL is 6 mg/kg in two-divided dose with maintenance dosing of 3–4 mg/kg/day for remission of myasthenic symptoms [32–34]. The onset of effect may be seen within 1–2 months after starting the drug. Commonly noted side effects include hirsutism, tremor, gum hyperplasia, and anemia. The main limiting adverse reactions are hypertension and nephrotoxicity.

Cyclophosphamide: This alkylating agent is reserved for refractory cases of severe generalized MG. Studies recommend monthly IV pulses of cyclophosphamide (50 mg/m^2) for 3–4 months that results in improvement in weakness and also lowering the steroid dose [35, 36]. Reported side effects include myelosupression, cystitis, and increased risk of malignancy with increasing cumulative dose of cyclophosphamide.

Rituximab (RTX): It is one of the newer and evolving immune-directed treatment modalities for patients with generalized or refractory MG. Rituximab (RTX) is a chimeric human monoclonal antibody that selectively targets CD-20+ ß cells and leads to the depletion, making it as a first choice for therapeutic option in many autoimmune disorders. There have been multiple studies analyzing the efficacy and safety of RTX in generalized MG patients, though the dose and duration of treatment are variable among them. RTX was found to be more efficacious in patients with MuSK+Ab than with AChR+Ab and there was an inverse correlation between the disease duration and response rate. This difference may be due to selective depletion of cells producing IgG_4, which specifically produce MuSK antibodies. The generally accepted schedule for RTX dosage in majority of patients is four infusions of 375 mg/m^2 per dose [37–39]. Rituximab has an excellent safety profile, but opportunistic infections with bacteria or viral agents can occur in those receiving treatment for long time. One rare life-threatening infection that has been potentially linked to rituximab is progressive multifocal leucoencephalopathy (PML) [40].

53.10 Newer Agents for Management of Myasthenia Gravis

There are three newer agents that have been FDA-approved for MG. These complement and FcRn inhibitors open the doors for more target selective immunologic therapies in management of refractory or unresponsive MG. In addition, they offer advantages over conventional immunosuppressive treatment in terms of faster onset of action and favorable side effect profile. However, cost effectiveness of the new treatments is always a limiting factor for these newer drugs.

Eculizumab: It is the first complement inhibitor that has been approved by the FDA for the management of anti-AChR-positive generalized MG. Clinical improvement appears within 2 weeks following the first infusion, becomes maximal at 3 months for most patients, and remains stable for at least 3 years [41].

Ravulizumab: This newer agent is an engineered form of eculizumab with improved pharmacokinetics resulting in a long half-life that permits a maintenance-dosing interval of 1 infusion every 8 weeks. FDA recently approved its usage in adult anti-AChR-positive generalized MG [42].

Efgartigimod: This is the first FcRn inhibitor that has been approved by the FDA for the treatment of anti-AChR-positive generalized MG. Efgartigimod is an option for patients with MG who have an exacerbation or whose MG remains poorly controlled. Patients with MG were treated with cycles of four weekly efgartigimod infusions. It is administered as infusion; clinical improvement is apparent at 1 week, becomes maximal at 4–5 weeks, and then gradually declines in the following 4 weeks [43].

53.11 Special Therapeutic Situations: *Myasthenic Crisis*

Myasthenic crisis is clinically defined as weakness involving respiratory or oropharyngeal muscles severe enough to necessitate intubation and mechanical ventilation for ventilator support. The risk of exacerbation is generally highest within the first 3 years of symptom onset; such patients should always be managed in intensive care setting with close and frequent monitoring. Indication for mechanical ventilator support includes increasing tachypnea, forced vital capacity less than 1 L, and negative inspiratory force <20 cm of H_2O hypoxemia or hypercapnia. Use of noninvasive mechanical ventilation with bilevel-positive pressure ventilation may circumvent the need for intubation in selected myasthenic patients in whom Pco_2 is less than 50 mmHg. This noninvasive ventilation may reduce pulmonary complications and hospital stay. The second most important factor in treatment of myasthenic crisis is identification of the precipitating factor which may be infections, surgical procedure, thymectomy, rapid tapering of immune modulators, steroids-induced worsening, or use of drugs that increase myasthenic weakness [44–46]. Identifying and controlling the precipitating factors is equally important in management of MG.

Short-term immune directive treatments are favored for myasthenic crisis. Four to six plasma exchanges are the preferred treatment as it has rapid onset of action as required during crisis. As similar efficacy of IVIG has been reported, it can also be considered in situation where PE is not feasible [47]. Since effects of PE or IVIG are short term, long-acting immune-directed treatment should be added to have more prolonged therapeutic effect. Weaning trail should only be given once there is improvement in respiratory muscle strength with vital capacity >15 mL/kg in presence of anticholinesterase inhibitors. It is clinically helpful to look for improvement in strength of corresponding surrogate muscles such as neck flexors that mirror respiratory and bulbar muscle strength.

Important condition that needs to be considered in patients with features of acute worsening of symptoms is cholinergic crisis, though rare. Cholinergic crisis is related to excessive dosing of cholinesterase inhibitors. Signs of cholinergic hyperactivity include excessive salivation, increased bronchial secretion, muscle fasciculation, and abdominal cramps. The optimal management for such situations is to discontinue the use of cholinesterase inhibitors following intubation. The other condition that needs to be individualized is Myasthenia gravis in pregnancy, which needs a multidisciplinary approach as depicted in Box 53.2.

Box 53.2 Myasthenia Gravis in Pregnancy

Myasthenia in pregnant female may be the first manifestation of disease as noted by worsening of occult previously unrecognized symptoms occurring in the first trimester or a known patient with myasthenia gravis may becomes pregnant. The course of MG is unpredictable in pregnancy as worsening occurs in the first trimester of pregnancy. Steroids, PE and IVIG use is safe during pregnancy and are the agent of choice for treatment of MG exacerbation in a pregnant female. Cholinesterase inhibitors may induce uterine contractions hence use of higher dose needs caution. In general, immunosuppressant medications have potential teratogenicity so their use should preferable be avoided and discontinued 4–6 months prior to conceiving. Regional anesthesia is preferred for delivery or cesarean section. Magnesium sulfate should not be used for management of pre-eclampsia because of its adverse effect on neuromuscular junction.

53.12 Conclusion

Myasthenia is being the commonest among the neuromuscular disorders with good prognosis. Many newer diagnostic modalities are available with improved diagnostic accuracy, especially for patients who are seronegative for anti-AChR and anti-MuSK antibodies. Currently, many treatment options exist for MG, and with appropriately selected short- and long-term immunosuppression, most of the patients with MG are able to achieve favorable outcomes. However, many unresolved issues remain, including when and how to discontinue immunosuppressant therapy to avoid a relapse, role of thymectomy in late-onset, seronegative, and pediatric MG need to be explored. The development of new therapies for MG is truly exciting with the aim to induce long-term remission or cure.

References

1. Grob D, Arsura EL, Brunner NG, Namba T. The course of myasthenia gravis and therapies affecting outcome. Ann N Y Acad Sci. 1987;505:472–99.
2. McGrogan A, Sneddon S, de Vries CS. The incidence of myasthenia gravis: a systematic literature review. Neuroepidemiology. 2010;34(3):171–83.
3. Carr AS, Cardwell CR, McCarron PO, McConville J. A systematic review of population based epidemiological studies in myasthenia gravis. BMC Neurol. 2010;10:46.
4. Heldal AT, Owe JF, Gilhus NE, Romi F. Seropositive myasthenia gravis: a nationwide epidemiologic study. Neurology. 2009;73(2):150–1.
5. Andersen JB, Engeland A, Owe JF, Gilhus NE. Myasthenia gravis requiring pyridostigmine treatment in a national population cohort. Eur J Neurol. 2010;17(12):1445–50.
6. Grob D, Brunner N, Namba T, Pagala M. Lifetime course of myasthenia gravis. Muscle Nerve. 2008;37(2):141–9.
7. Gilhus NE. Myasthenia gravis. N Engl J Med. 2016;375(26):2570–81.
8. Pasnoor M, Wolfe GI, Nations S, et al. Clinical findings in MuSK-antibody positive myasthenia gravis: a U.S. experience. Muscle Nerve. 2010;41(3):370–4.
9. Guptill JT, Sanders DB, Evoli A. Anti-MuSK antibody myasthenia gravis: clinical findings and response to treatment in two large cohorts. Muscle Nerve. 2011;44(1):36–40.
10. Peeler CE, De Lott LB, Nagia L, et al. Clinical utility of acetylcholine receptor antibody testing in ocular myasthenia gravis. JAMA Neurol. 2015;72(10):1170–4.
11. Giannoccaro MP, Paolucci M, Zenesini C, et al. Comparison of ice pack test and single-fiber EMG diagnostic accuracy in patients referred for myasthenic ptosis. Neurology. 2020;95(13):e1800–6.
12. Benatar M. A systematic review of diagnostic studies in myasthenia gravis. Neuromuscul Disord. 2006;16(7):459–67.
13. Meriggioli MN. Diagnostic tests for neuromuscular junction disorders. In: Meriggioli MN, Howard JF, Harper CM, editors. Neuromuscular junction disorders: diagnosis and treatment. Marcel Dekker; 2003. p. 59–99.
14. Sanders DB, Arimura K, Cui L, et al. Guidelines for single fiber EMG. Clin Neurophysiol. 2019;130(8):1417–39.
15. Sarrigiannis PG, Kennett RP, Read S, Farrugia ME. Single-fiber EMG with a concentric needle electrode: validation in myasthenia gravis. Muscle Nerve. 2006;33:61–5.
16. Meriggioli MN, Sanders DB. Advances in the diagnosis of neuromuscular junction disorders. Am J Phys Med Rehabil. 2005;84(8):627–38.
17. Bokoliya SC, Kumar VP, Nashi S, et al. Anti-AChR, MuSK, and LRP4 antibodies coexistence: a rare and distinct subtype of myasthenia gravis from Indian subcontinent. Clin Chim Acta. 2018;486:34–5.
18. Shelly S, Paul P, Bi H, et al. Improving accuracy of myasthenia gravis autoantibody testing by reflex algorithm. Neurology. 2020;95(22):e3002–11.
19. Rivner MH, Quarles BM, Pan JX, et al. Clinical features of LRP4/agrin-antibody-positive myasthenia gravis: a multicenter study. Muscle Nerve. 2020;62(3):333–43.
20. Sanders DB, Wolfe GI, Benatar M, et al. International consensus guidance for management of myasthenia gravis: executive summary. Neurology. 2016;87(4):419–25.
21. Angelini C, Martignago S, Bisciglia M. New treatments for myasthenia: a focus on antisense oligonucleotides. Drug Des Devel Ther. 2013;7:13–7.
22. Gamez J, Salvado M, Carmona F, et al. Intravenous immunoglobulin to prevent myasthenic crisis after thymectomy and other procedures can be omitted in patients with well-controlled myasthenia gravis. Ther Adv Neurol Disord. 2019;12:1756286419864497.
23. Kumar R, Birinder SP, Gupta S, Singh G, Kaur A. Therapeutic plasma exchange in the treatment of myasthenia gravis. Indian J Crit Care Med. 2015;19(1):9–13.
24. Wolfe GI, Kaminski HJ, Aban IB, et al. Randomized trial of thymectomy in myasthenia gravis. N Engl J Med. 2016;375(6):511–22.
25. Brenna G, Antozzi C, Montomoli C, et al. A propensity score analysis for comparison of T-3b and VATET in myasthenia gravis. Neurology. 2017;89(2):189–95.
26. Muscle Study Group. A trial of mycophenolate mofetil with prednisone as initial immunotherapy in myasthenia gravis. Neurology. 2008;71(6):394–9.
27. Morren J, Li Y. Maintenance immunosuppression in myasthenia gravis, an update. J Neurol Sci. 2020;410:116648.
28. Palace J, Newsom-Davis J, Lecky B. A randomized double-blind trial of prednisolone alone or with azathioprine in myasthenia gravis. Myasthenia Gravis Study Group. Neurology. 1998;50(6):1778–83.
29. Hehir MK, Burns TM, Alpers J, et al. Mycophenolate mofetil in AChR-antibody-positive myasthenia gravis: outcomes in 102 patients. Muscle Nerve. 2010;41(5):593–8.
30. Sanders DB, Hart IK, Mantegazza R, et al. An international, phase III, randomized trial of mycophenolate mofetil in myasthenia gravis. Neurology. 2008;71(6):400–6.
31. Hobson-Webb LD, Hehir M, Crum B, et al. Can mycophenolate mofetil be tapered safely in myasthenia gravis? A retrospective, multicenter analysis. Muscle Nerve. 2015;52(2):211–5.
32. Rozsa C, Lovas G, Fornadi L, et al. Safety of long-term combined immunosuppressive treatment in myasthenia gravis—analysis of adverse effects of 163 patients. Eur J Neurol. 2006;13(9):947–52.
33. Farmakidis C, Dimachkie MM, Pasnoor M, Barohn RJ. Immunosuppressive and immunomodulatory

therapies for neuromuscular diseases. Part II: new and novel agents. Muscle Nerve. 2020;61(1):17–25.
34. Tindall RS, Phillips JT, Rollins JA, et al. A clinical therapeutic trial of cyclosporine in myasthenia gravis. Ann N Y Acad Sci. 1993;681:539–51.
35. Buzzard KA, Meyer NJ, Hardy TA, et al. Induction intravenous cyclophosphamide followed by maintenance oral immunosuppression in refractory myasthenia gravis. Muscle Nerve. 2015;52(2):204–10.
36. Cutter G, Xin H, Aban I, et al. Cross-sectional analysis of the myasthenia gravis patient registry: disability and treatment. Muscle Nerve. 2019;60(6):707–15.
37. Tandan R, Hehir MK 2nd, Waheed W, Howard DB. Rituximab treatment of myasthenia gravis: a systematic review. Muscle Nerve. 2017;56(2):185–96.
38. Nowak RJ, Coffey CS, Goldstein JM, et al. Phase 2 trial of rituximab in acetylcholine receptor antibody–positive generalized myasthenia gravis: the BeatMG study. Neurology. 2021;98(4):e376–89.
39. Brauner S, Eriksson-Dufva A, Hietala MA, et al. Comparison between rituximab treatment for new-onset generalized myasthenia gravis and refractory generalized myasthenia gravis. JAMA Neurol. 2020;77(8):974–81.
40. Doughty CT, Suh J, David WS, et al. Retrospective analysis of safety and outcomes of rituximab for myasthenia gravis in patients ≥65 years old. Muscle Nerve. 2021;64(6):651–6.
41. Trice JA, Touchette DR, Nikitin D, et al. Eculizumab and efgartigamod for the treatment of myasthenia gravis: effectiveness and value; final report. Institute for Clinical and Economic Review; 2021.
42. Vu T, Meisel A, Mantegazze R, et al. Terminal complement inhibitor ravulizumab in generalized myasthenia gravis. NEJM Evid. 2022;1(5)
43. Howard JF Jr, Bril V, Vu T, et al. Safety, efficacy, and tolerability of efgartigimod in patients with generalised myasthenia gravis (ADAPT): a multicentre, randomised, placebo-controlled, phase 3 trial. Lancet Neurol. 2021;20(7):526–36.
44. Jones SC, Sorbello A, Boucher RM. Fluoroquinolone-associated myasthenia gravis exacerbation: evaluation of postmarketing reports from the US FDA adverse event reporting system and a literature review. Drug Saf. 2011;34(10):839–47.
45. Sheikh S, Alvi U, Soliven B, Rezania K. Drugs that induce or cause deterioration of myasthenia gravis: an update. J Clin Med. 2021;10(7):1537.
46. Dubey D, David WS, Reynolds KL, et al. Severe neurological toxicity of immune checkpoint inhibitors: growing spectrum. Ann Neurol. 2020;87(5):659–69.
47. Utsugisawa K, Nagane Y, Akaishi T, et al. Early fast-acting treatment strategy against generalized myasthenia gravis. Muscle Nerve. 2017;55(6):794–801.

Guillain-Barré Syndrome and Neurocritical Care

54

Gentle Sunder Shrestha and Ankit Rimal

Case Vignette

A 21-year-old male was admitted to the hospital with acute onset of weakness in bilateral lower limbs since the last 2 days. A day back, he was able to ride his two-wheeler to college in the morning, but required assistance to get up on the level ground at the end of the day. This was associated with numbness and tingling sensation in his lower limbs. The next day, he had blurring of vision in the morning along with an unease while swallowing food and felt he had a lump in his throat. His parents noticed a change in the quality of his voice as well.

There was no history of fever, rash, headache, or vomiting. No history was suggestive of exposure to toxins. There was no history of a preceding respiratory or gastrointestinal illness.

He was previously well with no chronic disease, no previous hospital admissions, and no history of surgeries in the past. He was not under any regular medications. He did not have a positive family history for any other chronic disease. He was a full-time student and did not smoke or consume alcohol.

On examination, the patient was conscious and oriented to time, place, and person. He had a resting tachycardia of 130/min, blood pressure of 110/80 mm Hg, respiratory rate of 24/min, was afebrile with SpO_2 of 92% in ambient air. Higher mental functions were intact. In motor system examination, the patient had a power of 4/5 in the bilateral hip and knee joints in all muscle groups and a power of 3/5 in the bilateral shoulder, elbow joints, and small muscles of hands. Bilateral lateral recti were found to be weak. Deep tendon reflexes were absent in bilateral knee and ankle and in biceps, triceps, and supinator. Plantar reflex was down-going bilaterally. There was no sensory deficit and no bowel and bladder involvement. He displayed significant dysmetria on finger-to-nose test.

Other investigations at admission were as follows: hemoglobin 11.6 g/dL, total leukocyte count 9800/μL, platelet count 120,000/μL, liver function tests within normal limits, and renal function tests within normal limits. MRI brain and spine were normal. Antiganglioside antibody test could not be performed due to unavailability at the treating center. CSF studies were not performed since the onset was barely 2 days before presentation.

A clinical diagnosis of the Miller Fisher Syndrome variant of Guillain-Barré Syndrome was made and the patient was started with Intravenous Immune Globulin following admission to the ICU for supportive care and monitoring. The patient developed respiratory distress with a respiratory rate of 40/min and an inability

G. S. Shrestha (✉)
Department of Critical Care Medicine, Tribhuvan University Teaching Hospital, Kathmandu, Nepal

A. Rimal
Intensivist, Pokhara Academy of Health Sciences, Pokhara, Nepal

H. Prabhakar et al. (eds.), *Principles and Practice of Neurocritical Care*,
https://doi.org/10.1007/978-981-99-8059-8_54

to clear secretions the next day. He was placed under mechanical ventilation. Over the next few days, the patient gradually improved and was extubated on the fifth day. He did not suffer from any infective or other complications and was discharged from the ICU on the seventh day.

54.1 Introduction

Guillain-Barré syndrome (GBS) is an immune-mediated polyradiculoneuropathy and it is the most common cause of acute flaccid paralysis worldwide [1]. It is considered one of the serious neurological emergencies, with about 25% of patients developing respiratory insufficiency [2, 3]. An estimated 100,000 new cases of GBS are diagnosed globally each year [4].

Although described by Octave Landry initially in 1859 in a series of 10 patients, the eponymous disease was much widely recognized following the publication by Guillain, Barré, and Strohl in 1916 [5, 6]. The seminal paper by the three authors described in detail the condition of two French soldiers. They had a similar clinical picture involving motor difficulties, areflexia, muscle tenderness, preservation of cutaneous reflexes, paresthesias with impairment of objective sensations, alteration in nerve conduction and an increase in albumin in the absence of cells in the cerebrospinal fluid (CSF), commonly referred to as albumin-cytologic dissociation [6]. Their paper included longitudinal clinical observations of the progressive areflexic paralysis in great detail and these features are still the cornerstones in the diagnosis of GBS.

54.2 Pathogenesis

There is considerable evidence to justify an autoimmune cause of GBS. The syndrome is usually preceded by an infection or an immune provocation [7]. *Campylobacter jejuni* is the commonest organism identified to be associated with the subsequent development of GBS [8, 9]. Other organisms include, but are not limited to, Cytomegalovirus, Epstein-Barr virus, Varicella-Zoster virus, *Mycoplasma pneumoniae,* and Hepatitis E [10–12]. In the majority of cases, a subsequent aberrant autoimmune response attributable to molecular mimicry between nerve antigens and the microbial agent is central to the development of this syndrome [13]. This response generates autoantibodies that target gangliosides at nerve membranes, particularly in the peripheral nerves and the spinal roots. This leads to either nerve damage or a functional blockade of neural conduction [14]. Furthermore, autoantibody profiling has assisted confirmation of this typical clinical and electrophysiological relationship unique to GBS [15].

Importantly, more than 99% of all individuals who develop an infection with *C. jejuni*, and in all likelihood other organisms, do not develop immune response leading to the development of GBS [16]. This explains why GBS is a sporadic disease, although outbreaks of GBS following infection with *C. jejuni* have been reported [17]. Prevalence of GBS is also dependent on endemic infections leading to a transient rise in outbreaks. An example of this phenomenon is the surge followed by decline of cases of GBS following the Zika virus outbreak in French Polynesia [18]. Additionally, environmental and genetic factors that predispose an individual to develop GBS are not well elucidated [19].

Guillain-Barré syndrome was known to be a single disease entity causing demyelination leading to secondary axonal damage. On the basis of the site of target antigen, GBS was subsequently classified broadly into acute inflammatory demyelinating polyradiculoneuropathy (AIDP) and acute axonal motor neuropathy (AMAN) [20, 21]. AIDP is characterized by infiltrates of inflammatory T cells and macrophages leading to the stripping myelin [22]. Schwann cells suffer injury due to antibodies and membrane attack complexes. In contrast, AMAN is primarily an antibody-mediated condition [21]. Features include deposition of IgG and activated complement proteins on the nodal and internodal axolemma. Macrophages invade the periaxonal space between axon and myelin leading to axonal injury. Antibodies are known to interfere with nerve regeneration in AMAN. Antecedent infection with *C. jejuni* shows frequent association with AMAN [23]. Other axonal forms with sensory involvement have been described. These include acute motor and sensory axonal neuropathy (AMSAN).

Table 54.1 Variants of GBS, frequency, clinical features, and IgG autoantibodies detected [65, 92]

Variant	Frequency (% of GBS cases)	Clinical features	IgG autoantibodies
Classic sensorimotor GBS	30–85	Classic clinical features	None
Pure motor	5–70	Motor weakness with no sensory signs	GM1, GD1a
Paraparetic	5–10	Paresis limited to the legs	GM1, GD1a
Pharyngeal-cervical-brachial	<5	Weakness of pharyngeal, cervical, and brachial muscles without weakness of lower limbs	GT1a > GQ1b ≫ GD1a
Bilateral facial palsy with paresthesias	<5	Reduced reflexes seen	None
Pure sensory	<1	Acute or subacute sensory neuropathy without other deficits	None
Miller Fisher syndrome	5–25	Incomplete forms with isolated ataxia or ophthalmoplegia can be seen	GQ1b, GT1a
Bickerstaff brainstem encephalitis	<5	Ophthalmoplegia, ataxia, areflexia, pyramidal tract signs, and impaired consciousness	GQ1b, GT1a

The pathophysiology of axonal subtypes of GBS has recently been discovered to be characterized by reversible conduction failure [24]. Both AMAN and AMSAN share a common immunological profile, besides axonal degeneration. The electrophysiological features in these subtypes represent a continuum in the axonal GBS spectrum [25]. Subtypes and variants of GBS and the associated autoantibodies against glycolipids are listed in Table 54.1.

54.3 Clinical Symptoms

The classic clinical features of GBS are described as rapidly progressive, symmetrical weakness of the limbs along with hyporeflexia or areflexia [26–28]. At the bedside, however, the presentation of GBS is highly variable. There are considerable differences in terms of sensory symptoms, weakness, pain, ataxia, and autonomic dysfunction. Occurrence, distribution, and extent of cranial nerve deficits and course of the disease can be variable [26].

Swallowing difficulties, bilateral facial weakness, and extraocular motor dysfunction are seen in half of the patients [26]. The majority experience pain, including paresthesias, meningism, backache, and muscle pain. At times, these symptoms herald the onset of muscle weakness of GBS [27, 29]. About a fourth of patients develop respiratory insufficiency mandating requirement of mechanical ventilation [28]. The occurrence of autonomic dysfunction varies abundantly, is mainly related to the cardiovascular system, and is observed in about two-thirds of patients [29, 30].

The course of GBS typically follows an initial phase of progression, followed by a plateau phase and a recovery phase. GBS is known to be a monophasic disease with the majority of patients reaching a nadir of severity at the end of 4 weeks [28]. It is during the progressive phase that 20–30% of patients develop respiratory failure with need for mechanical ventilation [28]. The plateau phase lasts for months, while the recovery phase lasts from months to years, with variable degrees of disability.

54.4 Diagnosis

The typical patient with GBS develops rapidly progressive bilateral limb weakness with reduced or absent reflexes. Facial or bulbar palsy along with ophthalmoplegia and ataxia are common in some variants. However, the presentation is considerably heterogeneous. Some patients present with only localized weakness such as the pharyngeal–cervical–brachial variant. At times, despite sharing similar serological biomarkers, presentations can contrast immensely [15]. Disorders closely associated and usually considered variants of GBS include Miller Fisher syndrome (MFS) and Bickerstaff brainstem encephalitis [31, 32]. It is essential that the clinician acknowledges the different clinical patterns recognized under the broad spectrum of the diagnosis of GBS. Such an understanding allows for early diagnosis and prompt initiation of treatment [33]. Clinical, laboratory, and electrodiagnostic criteria aid in making the diagnosis.

54.4.1 Diagnostic Criteria

In the background of suspected association between GBS and the swine flu vaccination campaign of 1976–1977, the US National Institute of Neurological Disorders and Stroke (NINDS) developed case definitions for GBS. The diagnostic criteria and the modification were published in 1981 and 1990, respectively [26, 34]. These criteria, although developed for research purposes, are still widely used. The primary goal of the NINDS was to develop diagnostic criteria with high specificity, and hence, it was not designed to capture all cases in clinical practice. Additionally, the NINDS criteria are not strict in that predefined clinical features are grouped as 'supporting the diagnosis' or 'casting doubt on the diagnosis'. They do not clarify on the decision rules for inclusion or exclusion of individual patients.

Later during another vaccination campaign, a different group gave new case definitions. The Brighton Collaboration published case definitions for GBS in 2011 while evaluating for a possible association between the vaccination for H1N1 swine flu and GBS, during the campaign of 2009–2010 [35]. The Brighton criteria have the advantage of defining cases explicitly with classification of GBS in four levels of diagnostic certainty depending on patient characteristics and availability of data. The NINDS and Brighton criteria are given in Tables 54.2 and 54.3, respectively.

Table 54.2 Diagnostic criteria for Guillain–Barré syndrome developed by the National Institute of Neurological Disorders and Stroke (NINDS) and subsequently modified in a review paper [26, 33]. Criteria are not applicable to some specific variants of GBS

Features needed for diagnosis of Guillain-Barré syndrome in clinical practice
• Progressive weakness in legs and arms (sometimes initially only in legs)
Areflexia (or decreased tendon reflexes) in weak limbs
Additional symptoms
• Progressive phase lasts days to 4 weeks (often 2 weeks)
• Relative symmetry
• Mild sensory symptoms or signs (not present in acute motor axonal neuropathy)
• Cranial nerve involvement, especially bilateral weakness of facial muscles
• Autonomic dysfunction
• Pain
Features that should raise doubt about the diagnosis of Guillain-Barré syndrome
• CSF: Increased number of mononuclear cells or polymorphonuclear cells (>50 cells/μL)
• Severe pulmonary dysfunction with little or no limb weakness at onset
• Severe sensory signs with little or no weakness at onset
• Bladder or bowel dysfunction at onset
• Fever at onset
• Sharp spinal cord sensory level
• Marked, persistent asymmetry of weakness
• Persistent bladder or bowel dysfunction
• Slow progression of weakness and without respiratory involvement (consider subacute inflammatory demyelinating polyneuropathy or acute onset chronic inflammatory demyelinating polyneuropathy)
Nerve conduction studies
• Can be helpful in clinical practice, but are generally not required to diagnose Guillain-Barré syndrome
• Needed to meet all Brighton criteria for Guillain-Barré syndrome
• Essential for classification of Guillain-Barré syndrome in acute inflammatory demyelinating polyneuropathy or acute motor axonal neuropathy
• Acute inflammatory demyelinating polyneuropathy: Features of demyelination (decreased motor nerve conduction velocity, prolonged distal motor latency, increased F-wave latency, conduction blocks, and temporal dispersion) [93]
• Acute motor axonal neuropathy: No features of demyelination (one demyelinating feature in one nerve, if distal CMAP amplitude is less than 10% LLN, can be found; distal CMAP amplitude less than 80% LLN in at least two nerves [93]. Transient motor nerve conduction block might be present [94]

Table 54.3 Brighton Collaboration Diagnostic Criteria for Guillain-Barré syndrome [35]

Level 1	Level 2	Level 3
Bilateral flaccid paralysis of the limbs *AND*	Bilateral flaccid paralysis of the limbs *AND*	Bilateral flaccid paralysis of the limbs *AND*
Decreased or absent tendon reflexes in weak limbs *AND*	Decreased or absent tendon reflexes in weak limbs *AND*	Decreased or absent tendon reflexes in weak limbs *AND*
Monophasic illness pattern and interval between onset AND nadir of weakness between 12 h and 28 days with subsequent clinical plateau *AND*	Monophasic illness pattern and interval between onset and nadir of weakness between 12 h and 28 days with subsequent clinical plateau *AND*	Monophasic illness pattern, interval between onset and nadir of weakness between 12 h and 28 days, with subsequent clinical plateau *AND*
Electrophysiological findings consistent with Guillian-Barré syndrome (GBS) *AND*	CSF total white cell count <50 cells/μL (with or without CSF protein elevation above laboratory normal value) *OR*	Absence of an identified alternative diagnosis for weakness
Cerebrospinal fluid (CSF) protein level above laboratory normal value AND CSF total white cell count <50 cells/μL) *AND*	If CSF not collected or results not available, electrophysiologic studies consistent with GBS *AND*	
Absence of an identified alternative diagnosis for weakness	Absence of an identified alternative diagnosis for weakness	

These diagnostic criteria are not applicable to all variants of GBS; separate diagnostic criteria are found in the referred publication

Table 54.4 Differential diagnosis of GBS [92]

CNS	
• Inflammation or infection of the brainstem: sarcoidosis, Sjögren syndrome, neuromyelitis optica • Inflammation or infection of the spinal cord: sarcoidosis, Sjögren syndrome, or acute transverse myelitis • Malignancy: leptomeningeal metastases or neurolymphomatosis	• Compression of brainstem or spinal cord • Brainstem stroke • Vitamin deficiency: Wernicke encephalopathy (B1 deficiency, subacute combined degeneration of the spinal cord, B12 deficiency)
Anterior horn cells	
• Acute flaccid myelitis: polio, enterovirus, West Nile virus, Japanese encephalitis virus, or rabies virus	
Nerve roots	
• Compression • Leptomeningeal malignancy • Infection: lyme disease, cytomegalovirus, HIV, Epstein-Barr virus, or varicella zoster virus	
Peripheral nerves	

Table 54.4 (continued)

CNS	
• CIDP • Metabolic or electrolyte disorders: hypoglycemia, hypothyroidism, porphyria, or copper deficiency • Vitamin deficiency: B1 (Beriberi), B12, or E • Toxins: drugs, alcohol, vitamin B6, lead, thallium, arsenic, organophosphate, ethylene glycol, methanol	• Critical illness polyneuropathy • Neuralgic amyotrophy • Vasculitis • Infection: diphtheria, HIV
Neuromuscular junction	
• Myasthenia gravis • Lambert–Eaton myasthenic syndrome	• Neurotoxins: botulism, tetanus, tick paralysis, or snakebite envenomation • Organophosphate intoxication
Muscles	
• Metabolic or electrolyte disorders: hypokalemia, thyrotoxic hypokalemic periodic paralysis, hypomagnesaemia, or hypophosphatemia • Inflammatory myositis • Acute rhabdomyolysis	• Drug-induced toxic myopathy: colchicine, chloroquine, emetine, or statins • Mitochondrial disease
Other	
• Conversion or functional disorder	

54.4.2 Differential Diagnosis

The differential diagnosis of GBS is broad and depends on the clinical features of the patient. These are mentioned in Table 54.4.

54.5 Treatment

The treatment of GBS involves meticulous supportive care and immunotherapy [3, 36].

54.5.1 ICU Admission

Reasons to admit patients to the ICU include worsening respiratory distress with clinical evidence of impending respiratory failure, diminished cough and severe swallowing impairment, and severe autonomic cardiovascular dysfunction [37]. Clinical evidence of impending respiratory failure is defined by breathlessness at rest or during talking, use of accessory respiratory muscles, and inability to count to 15 in a single breath. Additionally, even in absence of these features, artificial mechanical ventilation may still be required in patients meeting at least one major or two minor criteria. Major criteria include hypercarbia (arterial $PaCO_2$ >48 mmHg), hypoxemia when breathing ambient air (arterial PaO_2 <56 mmHg), and a vital capacity less than 15 mL/kg of body weight and minor criteria include inefficient cough, atelectasis, and dysfunctional swallowing [38].

Respiratory insufficiency is the commonest indication for admission in these patients to the neurocritical care unit. The Erasmus GBS Respiratory Insufficiency Score (EGRIS) is used at hospital admission, to help determine the likelihood a patient will require mechanical ventilation within 1 week of assessment [39].

Risk factor for the requirement of prolonged mechanical ventilation is an inability to lift arms from the bed at 1 week following intubation and an axonal subtype or unexcitable nerves in electrophysiological studies [40]. These patients are considered for early tracheostomy.

54.5.2 General Supportive Care

Medical complications are responsible for deaths in GBS in 5% of patients, even in developed countries [36]. These complications include sepsis, pulmonary emboli, and unexplained cardiac arrest, most probably associated with dysautonomia. Early recognition of these complications is an integral part of the management, particularly in the ICU [27].

All patients with GBS should be admitted to the hospital for a few days. Patients with mild disease, with features limited to mild limb weakness and distal paresthesias, may not require treatment, but still should be observed for 2 weeks to assure that there is no further progression [41]. Another issue that needs to be addressed is thromboprophylaxis. Patients with GBS are predominantly admitted to the ICU for respiratory assistance. They are bed-bound in the acute phase and need thromboprophylaxis with subcutaneous heparin [36]. Constipation and urinary retention are commonly encountered. They are addressed with the use of laxatives and bladder catheterization, respectively [2].

Pain is common and is present in almost two thirds of patients. It can be severe and may persist for several months. The pain can be muscular, arthralgic, radicular, or even meningitic and has been described to precede weakness in almost a third of patients [29]. Early recognition and treatment with opioids, carbamazepine, and gabapentin may be effective but not glucocorticoids [42]. Patients are in early need of physiotherapy, rehabilitation, and psychosocial support [33].

54.5.3 Immunotherapy

Numerous studies over the past five decades have indicated immunotherapy with either plasmapheresis or intravenous immune globulin (IVIG) to be effective as a disease-modifying treatment in GBS [1, 43, 44]. In some cases, however, the eventual functional outcome may not be influenced by immunotherapy [45].

Plasmapheresis

In 1982, Osterman performed plasmapheresis in eight adult patients with the Guillain-Barré syndrome [46]. Although no apparent differences in clinical and neurophysiologic parameters were observed between those whose conditions improved and those whose conditions did not, only half of the patients improved. The Guillain-Barré Syndrome Study Group in 1985 published findings of their randomized trial comparing plasmapheresis versus conventional care among 245 patients severely ill with acute GBS [47]. Plasmapheresis was shown to be most effective when initiated within the first 2 weeks after disease onset among patients unable to walk. Functional improvement among those treated with plasmapheresis was earlier when compared against those assigned placebo (19 versus 40 days). Additionally, the median time to walking was 53 and 85 days, respectively, for patients unaided in the plasmapheresis and control groups.

Plasma exchange is known to nonspecifically remove antibodies and complement. When compared to standard supportive therapy alone, plasma exchange is associated with lesser nerve damage and hastened clinical improvement [47]. The standard empirical regimen involves five exchanges over a period of 2 weeks targeting a total exchange of five plasma volumes. Each exchange usually involves 2–3 L of plasma according to bodyweight. A French trial showed that patients who could walk with or without aid but could not run benefited from two exchanges of 1.5 plasma volumes [48]. In the same study, more severely affected patients were observed to require at least four exchanges for an improvement.

Plasma volume for adults is estimated with the following formula [49]:

$$\text{Estimated plasma volume}(\text{in L}) = 0.07 \times \text{weight}(\text{kg}) \times (1 - \text{hematocrit})$$

Venous access is achieved either with two large-bore intravenous lines or a single central line with a dual-lumen catheter. Hemodialysis catheters may be better suited since they have larger lumens. Use of peripheral veins eliminates issues related with central venous catheters, but is associated with slower blood flow and longer procedure times. These eventually render peripheral veins inefficient and create discomfort for the patient. Fluid loading prior to conducting plasma exchange reduces the incidence of hypotension during the procedure.

Intravenous Immune Globulin

Buoyed by its beneficial effects in chronic inflammatory demyelinating polyneuropathy [50, 51] and other autoimmune conditions [52, 53], Kleyweg et al. first used high dose IVIG in the treatment of GBS [54]. Although IVIG was observed to be beneficial in only one among the eight patients treated with IVIG, this study garnered a lot of interest.

The Dutch Guillain-Barré Study Group, in 1992, conducted a randomized trial comparing IVIG and plasma exchange in GBS [55]. Patients with GBS for less than 2 weeks duration and who were unable to walk were randomly assigned to two groups. The first group received five plasma exchanges (each of 200–250 mL/kg of body weight) and the second received five doses of a preparation of IVIG (0.4 g per/kg/day). The primary outcome measure was an improvement by at least one grade on a seven-point scale of motor function at 4 weeks. The median time to improvement by one grade was 41 days with plasma exchange and 27 days with immune globulin therapy ($P = 0.05$). Furthermore, the IVIG group had significantly fewer complications along with less need for mechanical ventilation.

Immune globulin is thought to act by neutralizing pathogenic antibodies and inhibiting autoantibody-mediated complement activation. This is thought to prevent and/or reduce nerve injury aiding in faster clinical improvement, when compared to no therapy [56, 57]. The standard treatment regimen consists of a total dose of 2 g per kilogram of body weight of immune globulin over a period of 5 days [55, 58]. With the pharmacokinetics of immune globulin unalike among patients, patients with a smaller rise in serum IgG following administration of IVIG are likely to have an inferior outcome [59]. Moreover, not all patients who receive IVIG benefit from treatment. This was true in one study among those with the mild form of the disease who were able to walk independently at enrolment [45].

Immune globulin may be administered for 2 days (1 g/kg per day). Any additional benefit from this accelerated administration is not known. The regimen of IVIG given over a total of 5 days seems more preferred since it might cause fewer adverse effects. Interestingly, children who receive a faster IVIG regimen have been reported to have more frequent treatment-related fluctuations (TRFs) [60]. IVIG is considered to be as effective as plasma exchange for treatment of GBS by the American Academy of Neurology guideline on IVIG for treatment of neuromuscular disorders [61].

Adverse effects of IVIG include headache, backache, nausea, vomiting, hypotension, rash, acute kidney injury, and transfusion reactions [62]. Rarely, patients may develop hyperviscosity leading to myocardial infarction or stroke [62].

Indications for Immunotherapy

Based on the available evidence, treatment with immunotherapy for nonambulatory adult patients with GBS is beneficial when initiated within 2 weeks, but uncertain after 4 weeks of symptom onset [1, 3]. Furthermore, treatment of ambulatory adult patients can be initiated if they are within 4 weeks of neuropathic symptom onset and not yet recovering. The severity of symptoms and duration of disease may serve as a rough guide to start immunotherapy.

- Severity of symptoms: All patients unable to walk a distance of 10 m independently should receive immunotherapy [43, 44]. Despite an absence of definitive evidence, patients with rapidly progressive weakness (loss of grip or antigravity arm strength over 24 h) and/or respiratory, bulbar, or autonomic involvement should be started on immunotherapy [48, 60, 63].
- Duration since onset of symptoms: Immunotherapy improves outcome when initiated within 2 weeks of symptom onset. Benefit is questionable after 4 weeks of symptom onset [43, 44].

Although most patients with MFS variant of GBS recover completely within 6 months without treatment [64], immunotherapy is reserved for those with severe respiratory and bulbar involvement [63, 65]. Immunotherapy is used in patients with Bickerstaff brainstem encephalitis in view of the severity of symptoms, despite no evidence of efficacy [66, 67]. An electrophysiological examination is not a requisite to initiate immunotherapy [2].

Selection of Modality

Early studies comparing plasma exchange and IVIG showed that plasma exchange was more likely among the two to be discontinued, even though both carried a similar risk of adverse events [68]. Overall, IVIG has substituted plasma exchange in many medical centers as the treatment of choice in GBS because of its greater availability and convenience in administration [2].

No trials have compared IVIG with placebo. Large trials have compared IVIG with plasma exchange with the two showing similar efficacy [55, 58, 69]. The choice between the use of plasma exchange and IVIG depends on the local availability of a modality and on patient preference, risk factors, and contraindications [48, 60, 63, 67]. Based on the clinical trials providing evidence on the use of plasma exchange and IVIG, they should be started within 4 weeks and within 2 weeks, respectively [43, 44]. The efficacy of IVIG within 2 weeks has favored its use beyond 2 weeks as well.

Most of the studies done in evaluation of both plasma exchange and IVIG were conducted in Europe and North America where the common variant is AIDP. Whether differences would arise had studies been conducted in areas where AMAN is the common variant is unknown. Future studies may be designed to look into the efficacy of immunotherapy according to the variant of GBS.

Apart from plasma exchange and IVIG, no procedures or drugs have been shown to be as efficacious in treating GBS. Due to the anti-inflammatory effects, corticosteroids were assumed to be beneficial in slowing disease progression in GBS. However, eight randomized controlled trials evaluating efficacy of corticosteroids for GBS showed no significant benefit [70]. Moreover, treatment with oral corticosteroids led to a negative effect on the outcome [71]. Even add-on treatment with intravenous methylprednisolone in IVIG treated patients has not been found to be beneficial [72].

Approximately 40% of patients treated with either modality do not improve within the first 4 weeks after initiation of therapy [63, 73]. It is essential that all patients who worsen following therapy be reevaluated clinically to ascertain the accuracy of the diagnosis.

For patients who do not improve following initial treatment, additional immunomodulatory treatment may be considered if severe symptoms persist. Retreatment with immunotherapy, although controversial, may have been contemplated in the past due to paucity of alternative options. One randomized placebo-controlled trial and another observational trial have both demonstrated a lack of benefit of a second dose of IVIG among patients with a poor prognosis defined by the EGOS [74, 75]. In fact, the second dose of IVIG entailed a risk of serious adverse events [74]. Switching from IVIG to plasma exchange may reduce the effectiveness of the initial IVIG therapy. For patients treated with plasma exchange initially, retreating with plasma exchange may be an option theoretically but has not been studied so far.

Eculizumab is a humanized monoclonal antibody. It specifically binds to complement component 5, potently inhibiting complement activation, and is believed to improve outcomes [76]. Following a randomized phase 2 trial [76], Eculizumab is being evaluated in a phase 3, prospective, multicenter, placebo-controlled, double blind, randomized study to investigate its efficacy and safety in participants with severe GBS, within 2 weeks from onset of weakness due to GBS [77].

54.5.4 Treatment-Related Fluctuations

Treatment-related fluctuations are deterioration following initial improvement in patients who have received either plasma exchange or IVIG [43, 78]. These are seen in almost 10% of cases and are common within the first 8 weeks of treatment [79]. These relapses are characteristically not as severe as the initial progressive phase of GBS before initiation of treatment. Patients who experience TRFs are thought to have a prolonged immune response. This results in continued nerve damage or functional blockade and needs an extended duration of treatment as compared to standard care.

Among patients who have progression of disease beyond 4 weeks, it becomes important to question whether the patient still has GBS or the patient has an acute-onset chronic inflammatory demyelinating polyneuropathy (CIDP). About 5% of patients initially diagnosed with GBS were eventually determined to have acute-onset CIDP, in one prospective study series [78]. The distinction between GBS with TRFs and acute-onset CIDP can be problematic, but some clinical patterns may be more indicative of CIDP rather than GBS. These include a deterioration beyond 8 weeks from onset of weakness, occurrence of 3 or more deteriorations, preservation of unaided ambulation, and absence of cranial nerve involvement [78].

Differentiating these two entities is significant since GBS with TRFs might improve following retreatment, while those diagnosed with acute-onset CIDP will require chronic maintenance treatment in the form of IVIG or corticosteroids [33].

54.5.5 Low Cost Alternatives for Treatment

An important factor to consider in our part of the world, especially in low-middle income countries (LMICs), is that most patients spend for medical treatment out of their pockets. Neither plasma exchange nor IVIG therapy is inexpensive. Alternatives to these therapies have been explored. Among them, small volume plasma exchange (SVPE) has been described as an economical and relatively safe alternative to conventional plasma exchange. SVPE was first described in literature in 1990 [80]. Islam et al. evaluated the feasibility and safety of SVPE for Guillain-Barré syndrome in their phase II study in Bangladesh and found it to be a valid alternative to conventional plasma exchange and IVIG [81]. The same technique has been used successfully in the treatment of Myasthenic crisis, an entity similar to GBS in its autoimmune nature [82]. Other low-cost techniques are modifications of conventional plasma exchange including centrifugal therapeutic plasma exchange and use of a variety of replacement fluids other than human albumin for the exchanged plasma [83]. Replacement fluids used in various studies include fresh frozen plasma, normal saline, and a combination of the two [83]. Efficacy of SVPE in treatment of SVPE is yet to be established in larger clinical trials.

54.6 Outcome

The majority of patients with GBS, including tetraplegics at nadir and those on mechanical ventilation for an extended period of time, show considerable recovery [84, 85]. Four in every five patients with GBS recover to be able to ambulate independently at 6 months following onset of disease [85]. Outcome in GBS is measured in terms of the probability of a patient to regain the ability to walk using the modified Erasmus GBS outcome score (mEGOS) prognostic tool (Table 54.5) [86]. Patient characteristics established to be related to poor prognostic outcome in GBS include age ≥40 years, a preceding diarrhea in the past 4 weeks, and severe disability at nadir.

Table 54.5 Modified Erasmus GBS Outcome Score (mEGOS) [86]

Prognostic factors	Categories	Score
Age at onset (years)	≤40	0
	41–60	1
	>60	2
Preceding diarrhea	Absent	0
	Present	1
MRC sum score[a] at day 7 of hospital	60–51	0
Admission	50–41	3
	40–31	6
	30–0	9
mEGOS 0–12		
0–6 = low risk (>90%)		
7–9 = intermediate risk (70–85%)		
9–12 = high risk (40–70%)		

Prognostic model based on a Dutch cohort predicting the ability to walk independently at 6 months [86]
[a]MRC sum score: sum of Medical Research Council scale scores for muscle strength of bilateral shoulder abduction, elbow flexion, wrist extension, hip flexion, knee extension, and ankle dorsiflexion

Table 54.6 The Erasmus GBS Respiratory Insufficiency Score (EGRIS) [39]

Measure	Categories	Score
Days between onset of weakness and hospital admission	>7 days	0
	4–7 days	1
	≤3 days	2
Facial and/or bulbar weakness at hospital admission	Absent	0
	Present	1
MRC sum score at hospital admission	60–51	0
	50–41	1
	40–31	2
	30–21	3
	≤20	4
EGRIS	NA	0–7

An EGRIS of 0–2 indicates a low risk of mechanical intervention (4%), 3–4 indicates an intermediate risk of mechanical intervention (24%), and ≥5 indicates a high risk of mechanical intervention (65%) [39]

Death still occurs in 3–10% of cases of GBS [87–89]. Patients die in the acute progressive stage, most commonly due to ventilatory insufficiency, pulmonary complications, and from autonomic dysfunction including dysrhythmias [33]. Death can occur following discharge from the neurocritical care unit to the neurology ward [89]. A prolonged monitoring of these patients is thus justified. Respiratory failure is linked to rate of disease progression, severity of limb weakness, and low vital capacity [39].

The risk of respiratory failure can be predicted for individual patients using the EGRIS (Table 54.6).

On the long run, patients with GBS can suffer from numerous residual problems. These include incomplete recovery of motor and sensory systems, pain, fatigue, and psychological distress [90]. Prior to discharge of the patient, possible long-term effects of GBS should be considered and addressed [36, 91].

References

1. Shahrizaila N, Lehmann HC, Kuwabara S. Guillain-Barré syndrome. Lancet (London, England). 2021;397(10280):1214–28.
2. Yuki N, Hartung H-P. Guillain-Barré syndrome. N Engl J Med. 2012;366(24):2294–304.

3. van den Berg B, Walgaard C, Drenthen J, Fokke C, Jacobs BC, van Doorn PA. Guillain-Barré syndrome: pathogenesis, diagnosis, treatment and prognosis. Nat Rev Neurol. 2014;10(8):469–82.
4. Sejvar JJ, Baughman AL, Wise M, Morgan OW. Population incidence of Guillain-Barré syndrome: a systematic review and meta-analysis. Neuroepidemiology. 2011;36(2):123–33.
5. Landry O. Note sur la paralysie ascendante aigue. Gaz Hebd Med Paris. 1859;472:486.
6. Guillain G, Barré JA, Strohl A. Radiculoneuritis syndrome with hyperalbuminosis of cerebrospinal fluid without cellular reaction. Notes on clinical features and graphs of tendon reflexes. 1916. Ann Med Interne (Paris). 1999;150(1):24–32.
7. Hughes RAC, Cornblath DR. Guillain-Barré syndrome. Lancet (London, England). 2005;366 (9497):1653–66.
8. Poropatich KO, Walker CLF, Black RE. Quantifying the association between campylobacter infection and Guillain-Barré syndrome: a systematic review. J Health Popul Nutr. 2010;28(6):545–52.
9. Willison HJ, Goodyear CS. Glycolipid antigens and autoantibodies in autoimmune neuropathies. Trends Immunol. 2013;34(9):453–9.
10. Jacobs BC, Rothbarth PH, van der Meché FG, Herbrink P, Schmitz PI, de Klerk MA, et al. The spectrum of antecedent infections in Guillain-Barré syndrome: a case-control study. Neurology. 1998;51(4):1110–5.
11. Hadden RD, Karch H, Hartung HP, Zielasek J, Weissbrich B, Schubert J, et al. Preceding infections, immune factors, and outcome in Guillain-Barré syndrome. Neurology. 2001;56(6):758–65.
12. Geurtsvankessel CH, Islam Z, Mohammad QD, Jacobs BC, Endtz HP, Osterhaus ADME. Hepatitis E and Guillain-Barre syndrome. Clin Infect Dis. 2013;57:1369–70.
13. Sheikh KA, Ho TW, Nachamkin I, Li CY, Cornblath DR, Asbury AK, et al. Molecular mimicry in Guillain-Barré syndrome. Ann N Y Acad Sci. 1998;845:307–21.
14. Yuki N, Susuki K, Koga M, Nishimoto Y, Odaka M, Hirata K, et al. Carbohydrate mimicry between human ganglioside GM1 and Campylobacter jejuni lipooligosaccharide causes Guillain-Barre syndrome. Proc Natl Acad Sci USA. 2004;101(31):11404–9.
15. Caudie C, Vial C, Bancel J, Petiot P, Antoine JC, Gonnaud PM. Antiganglioside autoantibody profiles in Guillain-Barré syndrome. Ann Biol Clin (Paris). 2002;60(5):589–97.
16. Huizinga R, van den Berg B, van Rijs W, Tio-Gillen AP, Fokkink WJR, Bakker-Jonges LE, et al. Innate immunity to Campylobacter jejuni in Guillain-Barré syndrome. Ann Neurol. 2015;78(3):343–54.
17. Jackson BR, Zegarra JA, López-Gatell H, Sejvar J, Arzate F, Waterman S, et al. Binational outbreak of Guillain-Barré syndrome associated with Campylobacter jejuni infection, Mexico and USA, 2011. Epidemiol Infect. 2014;142(5):1089–99.
18. Leonhard SE, Bresani-Salvi CC, Lyra Batista JD, Cunha S, Jacobs BC, Brito Ferreira ML, et al. Guillain-Barré syndrome related to Zika virus infection: a systematic review and meta-analysis of the clinical and electrophysiological phenotype. PLoS Negl Trop Dis. 2020;14(4):e0008264.
19. Blum S, McCombe PA. Genetics of Guillain-Barré syndrome (GBS) and chronic inflammatory demyelinating polyradiculoneuropathy (CIDP): current knowledge and future directions. J Peripher Nerv Syst. 2014;19(2):88–103.
20. Feasby TE, Gilbert JJ, Brown WF, Bolton CF, Hahn AF, Koopman WF, et al. An acute axonal form of Guillain-Barré polyneuropathy. Brain. 1986;109(Pt 6):1115–26.
21. McKhann GM, Cornblath DR, Ho T, Li CY, Bai AY, Wu HS, et al. Clinical and electrophysiological aspects of acute paralytic disease of children and young adults in northern China. Lancet (London, England). 1991;338(8767):593–7.
22. Wanschitz J, Maier H, Lassmann H, Budka H, Berger T. Distinct time pattern of complement activation and cytotoxic T cell response in Guillain-Barré syndrome. Brain. 2003;126(Pt 9):2034–42.
23. Kuwabara S, Yuki N. Axonal Guillain-Barré syndrome: concepts and controversies. Lancet Neurol. 2013;12(12):1180–8.
24. Uncini A, Manzoli C, Notturno F, Capasso M. Pitfalls in electrodiagnosis of Guillain-Barré syndrome subtypes. J Neurol Neurosurg Psychiatry. 2010;81(10):1157–63.
25. Capasso M, Notturno F, Manzoli C, Uncini A. Involvement of sensory fibres in axonal subtypes of Guillain-Barre syndrome. J Neurol Neurosurg Psychiatry. 2011;82(6):664–70.
26. Asbury AK, Cornblath DR. Assessment of current diagnostic criteria for Guillain-Barré syndrome. Ann Neurol. 1990;27(Suppl):S21–4.
27. van Doorn PA, Ruts L, Jacobs BC. Clinical features, pathogenesis, and treatment of Guillain-Barré syndrome. Lancet Neurol. 2008;7(10):939–50.
28. Fokke C, van den Berg B, Drenthen J, Walgaard C, van Doorn PA, Jacobs BC. Diagnosis of Guillain-Barré syndrome and validation of Brighton criteria. Brain. 2014;137(Pt 1):33–43.
29. Ruts L, Drenthen J, Jongen JLM, Hop WCJ, Visser GH, Jacobs BC, et al. Pain in Guillain-Barre syndrome: a long-term follow-up study. Neurology. 2010;75(16):1439–47.
30. Samadi M, Kazemi B, Golzari Oskoui S, Barzegar M. Assessment of autonomic dysfunction in childhood guillain-barré syndrome. J Cardiovasc Thorac Res. 2013;5(3):81–5.
31. Teener JW. Miller Fisher's syndrome. Semin Neurol. 2012;32(5):512–6.
32. Horton E, Krishnamoorthy S, Reynolds L. Bickerstaff's encephalitis. BMJ Case Rep. 2014;2014:bcr2014205336.

33. Willison HJ, Jacobs BC, van Doorn PA. Guillain-Barré syndrome. Lancet (London, England). 2016;388(10045):717–27.
34. Asbury AK. Diagnostic considerations in Guillain-Barré syndrome. Ann Neurol. 1981;9(Suppl):1–5.
35. Sejvar JJ, Kohl KS, Gidudu J, Amato A, Bakshi N, Baxter R, et al. Guillain-Barré syndrome and Fisher syndrome: case definitions and guidelines for collection, analysis, and presentation of immunization safety data. Vaccine. 2011;29(3):599–612.
36. Hughes RAC, Wijdicks EFM, Benson E, Cornblath DR, Hahn AF, Meythaler JM, et al. Supportive care for patients with Guillain-Barré syndrome. Arch Neurol. 2005;62(8):1194–8.
37. Mehta S. Neuromuscular disease causing acute respiratory failure. Respir Care. 2006;51(9):1013–6.
38. Burakgazi AZ, Höke A. Respiratory muscle weakness in peripheral neuropathies. J Peripher Nerv Syst. 2010;15(4):307–13.
39. Walgaard C, Lingsma HF, Ruts L, Drenthen J, van Koningsveld R, Garssen MJP, et al. Prediction of respiratory insufficiency in Guillain-Barré syndrome. Ann Neurol. 2010;67(6):781–7.
40. Walgaard C, Lingsma HF, van Doorn PA, van der Jagt M, Steyerberg EW, Jacobs BC. Tracheostomy or not: prediction of prolonged mechanical ventilation in Guillain-Barré syndrome. Neurocrit Care. 2017;26(1):6–13.
41. Ropper AH. The Guillain-Barré syndrome. N Engl J Med. 1992;326(17):1130–6.
42. Ruts L, van Koningsveld R, Jacobs BC, van Doorn PA. Determination of pain and response to methylprednisolone in Guillain-Barré syndrome. J Neurol. 2007;254(10):1318–22.
43. Hughes RAC, Swan AV, van Doorn PA. Intravenous immunoglobulin for Guillain-Barré syndrome. Cochrane Database Syst Rev. 2014;2014(9):CD002063.
44. Chevret S, Hughes RA, Annane D. Plasma exchange for Guillain-Barré syndrome. Cochrane Database Syst Rev. 2017;2(2):CD001798.
45. Verboon C, Harbo T, Cornblath DR, Hughes RAC, van Doorn PA, Lunn MP, et al. Intravenous immunoglobulin treatment for mild Guillain-Barré syndrome: an international observational study. J Neurol Neurosurg Psychiatry. 2021;92(10):1080–8.
46. Osterman PO, Fagius J, Säfwenberg J, Danersund A, Wallin BG, Nordesjö LO. Treatment of the Guillain-Barré syndrome by plasmapheresis. Arch Neurol. 1982;39(3):148–54.
47. The Guillain-Barré Syndrome Study Group. Plasmapheresis and acute Guillain-Barré syndrome. Neurology. 1985;35(8):1096–104.
48. The French Cooperative Group on Plasma Exchange in Guillain-Barré Syndrome. Appropriate number of plasma exchanges in Guillain-Barré syndrome. Ann Neurol. 1997;41(3):298–306.
49. Kaplan AA. A simple and accurate method for prescribing plasma exchange. ASAIO Trans. 1990;36(3):M597–9.
50. van der Meché FG, Vermeulen M, Busch HF. Chronic inflammatory demyelinating polyneuropathy. Conduction failure before and during immunoglobulin or plasma therapy. Brain. 1989;112(Pt 6):1563–71.
51. Vermeulen M, van der Meché FG, Speelman JD, Weber A, Busch HF. Plasma and gamma-globulin infusion in chronic inflammatory polyneuropathy. J Neurol Sci. 1985;70(3):317–26.
52. Sultan Y, Kazatchkine MD, Maisonneuve P, Nydegger UE. Anti-idiotypic suppression of autoantibodies to factor VIII (antihaemophilic factor) by high-dose intravenous gammaglobulin. Lancet (London, England). 1984;2(8406):765–8.
53. Arsura EL, Bick A, Brunner NG, Namba T, Grob D. High-dose intravenous immunoglobulin in the management of myasthenia gravis. Arch Intern Med. 1986;146(7):1365–8.
54. Kleyweg RP, van der Meché FG, Meulstee J. Treatment of Guillain-Barré syndrome with high-dose gammaglobulin. Neurology. 1988;38(10):1639–41.
55. van der Meché FG, Schmitz PI. A randomized trial comparing intravenous immune globulin and plasma exchange in Guillain-Barré syndrome. Dutch Guillain-Barré Study Group. N Engl J Med. 1992;326(17):1123–9.
56. Jacobs BC, O'Hanlon GM, Bullens RWM, Veitch J, Plomp JJ, Willison HJ. Immunoglobulins inhibit pathophysiological effects of anti-GQ1b-positive sera at motor nerve terminals through inhibition of antibody binding. Brain. 2003;126(Pt 10):2220–34.
57. Zhang G, Lopez PHH, Li CY, Mehta NR, Griffin JW, Schnaar RL, et al. Anti-ganglioside antibody-mediated neuronal cytotoxicity and its protection by intravenous immunoglobulin: implications for immune neuropathies. Brain. 2004;127(Pt 5):1085–100.
58. Plasma Exchange/Sandoglobulin Guillain-Barré Syndrome Trial Group. Randomised trial of plasma exchange, intravenous immunoglobulin, and combined treatments in Guillain-Barré syndrome. Lancet (London, England). 1997;349(9047):225–30.
59. Kuitwaard K, de Gelder J, Tio-Gillen AP, Hop WCJ, van Gelder T, van Toorenenbergen AW, et al. Pharmacokinetics of intravenous immunoglobulin and outcome in Guillain-Barré syndrome. Ann Neurol. 2009;66(5):597–603.
60. Korinthenberg R, Schessl J, Kirschner J, Mönting JS. Intravenously administered immunoglobulin in the treatment of childhood Guillain-Barré syndrome: a randomized trial. Pediatrics. 2005;116(1):8–14.
61. Patwa HS, Chaudhry V, Katzberg H, Rae-Grant AD, So YT. Evidence-based guideline: intravenous immunoglobulin in the treatment of neuromuscular disorders: report of the therapeutics and technology assessment subcommittee of the american academy of neurology. Neurology. 2012;78(13):1009–15.
62. Wiles CM, Brown P, Chapel H, Guerrini R, Hughes RAC, Martin TD, et al. Intravenous immunoglobulin in neurological disease: a specialist review. J Neurol Neu-

rosurg Psychiatry [Internet]. 2002;72(4):440 LP–448. http://jnnp.bmj.com/content/72/4/440.abstract
63. Verboon C, van Doorn PA, Jacobs BC. Treatment dilemmas in Guillain-Barré syndrome. J Neurol Neurosurg Psychiatry. 2017;88(4):346–52.
64. Overell JR, Hsieh ST, Odaka M, Yuki N, Willison HJ. Treatment for Fisher syndrome, Bickerstaff's brainstem encephalitis and related disorders. Cochrane Database Syst Rev. 2007;2007(1):CD004761.
65. Sekiguchi Y, Mori M, Misawa S, Sawai S, Yuki N, Beppu M, et al. How often and when Fisher syndrome is overlapped by Guillain-Barré syndrome or Bickerstaff brainstem encephalitis? Eur J Neurol. 2016;23(6):1058–63.
66. Odaka M, Yuki N, Yamada M, Koga M, Takemi T, Hirata K, et al. Bickerstaff's brainstem encephalitis: clinical features of 62 cases and a subgroup associated with Guillain-Barré syndrome. Brain. 2003;126(Pt 10):2279–90.
67. Verboon C, Doets AY, Galassi G, Davidson A, Waheed W, Péréon Y, et al. Current treatment practice of Guillain-Barré syndrome. Neurology. 2019;93(1):e59–76.
68. Raphaël JC, Chevret S, Hughes RAC, Annane D. Plasma exchange for Guillain-Barré syndrome. Cochrane Database Syst Rev. 2012;(7):CD001798.
69. Bril V, Ilse WK, Pearce R, Dhanani A, Sutton D, Kong K. Pilot trial of immunoglobulin versus plasma exchange in patients with Guillain-Barré syndrome. Neurology. 1996;46(1):100–3.
70. Hughes RA, Brassington R, Gunn AA, van Doorn PA. Corticosteroids for Guillain-Barré syndrome. Cochrane Database Syst Rev. 2016;10(10):CD001446.
71. Hughes RA, Newsom-Davis JM, Perkin GD, Pierce JM. Controlled trial prednisolone in acute polyneuropathy. Lancet (London, England). 1978;2(8093):750–3.
72. van Koningsveld R, Schmitz PIM, Meché FGA, Visser LH, Meulstee J, van Doorn PA. Effect of methylprednisolone when added to standard treatment with intravenous immunoglobulin for Guillain-Barré syndrome: randomised trial. Lancet (London, England). 2004;363(9404):192–6.
73. Hughes RAC, Swan AV, Raphaël J-C, Annane D, van Koningsveld R, van Doorn PA. Immunotherapy for Guillain-Barré syndrome: a systematic review. Brain. 2007;130(Pt 9):2245–57.
74. Walgaard C, Jacobs BC, Lingsma HF, Steyerberg EW, van den Berg B, Doets AY, et al. Second intravenous immunoglobulin dose in patients with Guillain-Barré syndrome with poor prognosis (SID-GBS): a double-blind, randomised, placebo-controlled trial. Lancet Neurol. 2021;20(4):275–83.
75. Verboon C, van den Berg B, Cornblath DR, Venema E, Gorson KC, Lunn MP, et al. Original research: second IVIg course in Guillain-Barré syndrome with poor prognosis: the non-randomised ISID study. J Neurol Neurosurg Psychiatry. 2020;91(2):113–21.
76. Misawa S, Kuwabara S, Sato Y, Yamaguchi N, Nagashima K, Katayama K, et al. Safety and efficacy of eculizumab in Guillain-Barré syndrome: a multicentre, double-blind, randomised phase 2 trial. Lancet Neurol. 2018;17(6):519–29.
77. A study to evaluate the efficacy and safety of eculizumab in guillain-barré syndrome—Full text view [Internet]. https://clinicaltrials.gov/ct2/show/NCT04752566
78. Ruts L, Drenthen J, Jacobs BC, van Doorn PA. Distinguishing acute-onset CIDP from fluctuating Guillain-Barre syndrome: a prospective study. Neurology. 2010;74(21):1680–6.
79. Kleyweg RP, van der Meché FG. Treatment related fluctuations in Guillain-Barré syndrome after high-dose immunoglobulins or plasma-exchange. J Neurol Neurosurg Psychiatry. 1991;54(11):957–60.
80. Tharakan J, Jayaprakash PA, Iyer VP. Small volume plasma exchange in Guillain-Barre syndrome: experience in 25 patients. J Assoc Physicians India. 1990;38(8):550–3.
81. Islam B, Islam Z, Rahman S, Endtz HP, Vos MC, van der Jagt M, et al. Small volume plasma exchange for Guillain-Barré syndrome in resource-limited settings: a phase II safety and feasibility study. BMJ Open. 2018;8(8):e022862.
82. Rimal A, Shrestha GS, Pradhan B, Acharya SP. Small volume plasma exchange as an alternative to conventional plasma exchange and intravenous immunoglobulin for myasthenic crisis: a case report. J Adv Intern Med [Internet]. 2023;11(2 SE-Case Reports):52–4. https://www.nepjol.info/index.php/JAIM/article/view/52407
83. Nepal G, Shrestha GS, Shing YK, Yadav JK, Coghlan MA, Ojha R. Low-cost alternatives for the management of Guillain-Barré syndrome in low- and middle-income countries. World Med Heal Policy [Internet]. 2021;13(4):749–57. https://onlinelibrary.wiley.com/doi/abs/10.1002/wmh3.474
84. van den Berg B, Storm EF, Garssen MJP, Blomkwist-Markens PH, Jacobs BC. Clinical outcome of Guillain-Barré syndrome after prolonged mechanical ventilation. J Neurol Neurosurg Psychiatry. 2018;89(9):949–54.
85. Doets AY, Verboon C, van den Berg B, Harbo T, Cornblath DR, Willison HJ, et al. Regional variation of Guillain-Barré syndrome. Brain. 2018;141(10):2866–77.
86. Walgaard C, Lingsma HF, Ruts L, van Doorn PA, Steyerberg EW, Jacobs BC. Early recognition of poor prognosis in Guillain-Barre syndrome. Neurology. 2011;76(11):968–75.
87. Islam Z, Jacobs BC, van Belkum A, Mohammad QD, Islam MB, Herbrink P, et al. Axonal variant of Guillain-Barre syndrome associated with Campylobacter infection in Bangladesh. Neurology. 2010;74(7):581–7.
88. Netto AB, Taly AB, Kulkarni GB, Rao UGS, Rao S. Mortality in mechanically ventilated patients of Guillain Barré Syndrome. Ann Indian Acad Neurol. 2011;14(4):262–6.
89. van den Berg B, Bunschoten C, van Doorn PA, Jacobs BC. Mortality in Guillain-Barre syndrome. Neurology. 2013;80(18):1650–4.
90. Forsberg A, Press R, Holmqvist LW. Residual disability 10 years after falling ill in Guillain-Barré syn-

drome: a prospective follow-up study. J Neurol Sci. 2012;317(1–2):74–9.
91. Davidson I, Wilson C, Walton T, Brissenden S. Physiotherapy and Guillain-Barré syndrome: results of a national survey. Physiotherapy. 2009;95(3):157–63.
92. Leonhard SE, Mandarakas MR, Gondim FAA, Bateman K, Ferreira MLB, Cornblath DR, et al. Diagnosis and management of Guillain-Barré syndrome in ten steps. Nat Rev Neurol. 2019;15(11):671–83.
93. Meulstee J, van der Meché FG. Electrodiagnostic criteria for polyneuropathy and demyelination: application in 135 patients with Guillain-Barré syndrome. Dutch Guillain-Barré Study Group. J Neurol Neurosurg Psychiatry. 1995;59(5):482–6.
94. Uncini A, Kuwabara S. Electrodiagnostic criteria for Guillain-Barrè syndrome: a critical revision and the need for an update. Clin Neurophysiol Off J Int Fed Clin Neurophysiol. 2012;123(8):1487–95.

Movement Disorders in Neurocritical Care

55

Kaustubh Aurangabadkar

55.1 Introduction

Mostly movement disorders have insidious onset and gradual progression. Due to complexity and distinctiveness, movement disorders are tough to diagnose properly. Rarely, neurologist is called to assess evolving movement disorder or to opine on acute complication of existing diseases. Any movement disorder emergency is defined as a situation evolving over hours to days in which failure to diagnose and treat promptly can lead to a significant morbidity and rarely mortality [1–3]. In this article we shall discuss diagnosis and management of some common movement disorders that require intensive care unit (ICU) management. Most of these emergencies are so rare that they lack large randomized double-blind placebo controlled trial-based guidelines.

55.2 Approach

A thorough history is the key. Some important questions regarding the time course (hours or days), evolution (Improving or static or deteriorating), triggering and ameliorating factors, voluntary suppressibility, and persistence of movements in sleep should be asked. Nothing can substitute the drug details, especially review of past and present medications. A recent change in the drug regimen in those who are already taking medications should be noted. Ask for change in the settings of deep brain stimulation device in those who have undergone surgery. Exposure to chemicals/toxins, use of illicit drugs, and family history of any similar illness also should be asked. Recent febrile illness like gastroenteritis or urinary tract infection and use of certain antibiotics like Imipenem or Linezolid, to name a few, can worsen the preexisting movement disorder.

Patient should be thoroughly observed and examined to define the phenomenology of the abnormal movement. Sometimes different types of movement abnormality can be seen concurrently. Coexisting abnormalities in mentation and vital parameters like pulse rate, blood pressure, and temperature should be recorded. Signs of chronic kidney or liver disease should be looked for in all patients. Syndromic approach based on recognizing the type of involuntary movement is usually most helpful.

55.3 Classification

Table 55.1 gives a practical classification based on the predominant phenomenology.

K. Aurangabadkar (✉)
Diamond Superspeciality Hospital, Kolhapur, India

H. Prabhakar et al. (eds.), *Principles and Practice of Neurocritical Care*,
https://doi.org/10.1007/978-981-99-8059-8_55

Table 55.1 Classification of movement disorder with examples

Type of movement disorder	Clinical features	Examples
Hypokinetic	Rigidity, bradykinesia, stiffness	Acute parkinsonism Parkinsonism hyperpyrexia Neuroleptic malignant syndrome
Hyperkinetic	Tremor, Chorea-hemiballism Myoclonus Tics Dyskinesia	Serotonin syndrome Acute parkinsonian dyskinesia Autoimmune encephalitis
Dystonic	Dystonia	Acute dystonic reaction Status dystonicus

55.4 Hypokinetic Movement Disorders

55.4.1 Acute Parkinsonism

Rarely, parkinsonian features evolve over hours to days requiring admission to ICU. It is typically seen after administration of dopa depleting agents [4]. Sometimes infections and toxins are the culprits [5, 6]. A review of drug list and appropriate imaging studies to rule out structural pathology are important.

Table 55.2 elicits various causes of acute parkinsonism.

Patient presents with acute/subacute onset parkinsonian features like bradykinesia, rigidity, and tremors. Toxic parkinsonism is often accompanied by signs of encephalopathy. Treatment is often aimed at removing the toxic cause. Stopping the offending drug is necessary. Sometimes antibiotics and antiviral drugs are used. Symptomatic treatment can be given with Dopaminergic drugs like levodopa carbidopa and anticholinergics in a selected patient.

Table 55.2 Various causes of acute parkinsonism

Drugs	Anti-arrhythmic— Amiodarone Chemotherapeutic— Cyclosporin Dopa antagonists— Neuroleptics Antiemetics Anticonvulsants— Valproic acid Lamotrigine Carbamazepine Lithium Tricyclic antidepressants Melatonin
Structural	Subdural hematoma Brain tumor Ischemic stroke
Poisoning	Carbon monoxide [8] Carbon disulphide Methanol
Autoimmune	Antiphospholipid antibody syndrome Systemic lupus erythematous
Infections	Epstein Barr virus Cytomegalovirus Japanese B Encephalitis [7] Human immunodeficiency virus
Systemic disease	Chronic liver diseases

55.4.2 Neuroleptic Malignant Syndrome (NMS)

This potentially lethal iatrogenic disorder was first described in 1960 [9]. It results from exposure to dopamine receptor blocking drugs. Most of the cases are caused by neuroleptics (both typical and atypical) [10–13]. Meoclopromide, Lithium, Promethazine, Droperidol, and Tetrabenazine [14–18] are some other culprits in a few patients. Reported risk factors include abrupt dose increase, concurrent use of lithium or Selective serotonin reuptake inhibitors (SSRIs), and prior NMS episode. Though the incidence is low(0.2%), NMS has high mortality(5–20%) [19]. A high index of clinical suspicion is necessary. Young and middle-aged men and postpartum women appear to be at increased risk. Pathophysiologic mechanism is secondary to abrupt changes in central dopamine transmission [20] (Table 55.3).

Table 55.3 DSM—V criteria for NEUROLEPTIC MALIGNANT SYNDROME

Exposure to dopamine antagonist or dopamine agonist withdrawal within past 72 h
Hyperthermia >100.4 on at-least 2 occasions
Rigidity
Altered mental status
Serum CK elevation 4 × upper limit of Normal
Hypermetabolism (heart rate increased 25% from baseline, respiratory rate increased 50% from baseline)
Sympathetic system lability: • Blood pressure systolic increase by >25 mmHg from baseline, diastolic BP >50 mmHg from baseline, or both >25% from baseline. • Diaphoresis • Urinary incontinence
Not attributable to any other cause.

Pathophysiologic mechanism is secondary to abrupt changes in central dopamine transmission [20].

NMS is a clinical diagnosis. It presents with fever, mental status changes, autonomic dysfunction (Labile blood pressure, Tachycardia), and rigidity. Tremor and dystonia are also seen. Myoclonus is uncommon. Key laboratory abnormalities include leucocytosis and raised creatine kinase. Serum iron level is often low. NMS usually increases in severity in 2–3 days and lasts for up to 2 weeks. Renal failure can result from rhabdomyolysis. Other complications include aspiration pneumonia and deep vein thrombosis. Death results from pneumonia, renal failure, or pulmonary embolism [20].

Key steps in treatment involve withdrawal of causative agent and treatment with dopaminergic agent. Intravenous fluids and antipyretic are used. If required, cooling blankets also must be used for hyperpyrexia [21]. Bromocriptine (2.5 mg twice a day upto a total dose of 45 mg/day) is the preferred drug. Dantrolene(1 mg/kg/day for 8 days and orally for next 7 days) reduces muscle rigidity and minimizes rhabdomyolysis [22]. It is a nonspecific muscle relaxant, sometimes used in addition to dopaminergic agents. It has class III evidence as a treatment for NMS. Levodopa/carbidopa and ropinirole are also effective. Anticholinergics are generally avoided as they may impair heat dissipation in febrile patients. Benzodiazepines may be used for agitation and rigidity. Electroconvulsive therapy is useful in refractory cases [22]. Treatment depends on the half life of the offending agent and should be continued for 1–2 weeks. If required, neuroleptic should be added after 2 weeks.

55.4.3 Parkinsonism Hyperpyrexia Syndrome (PHS)

This mimics neuroloeptic malignant syndrome, except that it occurs in patients with preexisting parkinsonism [3] Abrupt changes in first-line antiparkinsonian medications and discontinuation of amantidine or tolcapone are the usual precipitating factors [39, 40]. Rapid changes in the medication, especially after deep brain stimulation surgery, is another important scenario [38]. Time of onset of the symptoms after change in dopaminergic therapy ranges from 18 h to 7 days. Initial features are severe rigidity, dysautonomia, and tremors. Within 3–4 days, most of the patients develop altered mentation and are febrile. Creatine kinase and white blood cells are usually not as elevated as in NMS. Treatment involves supportive measures and reinstitution of dopaminergic therapy. High dose of intravenous methyprednisolone can also be effective [41]. Overall recovery is better than NMS. Despite treatment, permanent worsening has been reported [42].

55.4.4 Lethal Catatonia (LC)

This may be considered as a variant of NMS with high mortality, up to 50%. This is usually induced by neuroleptics. Other causes include cerebrovascular disorders involving the anterior cingulate gyri or temporal lobes, normal pressure hydrocephalus, head trauma, subacute sclerosing panencephalitis in early stages, viral encephalitis, bacterial meningitis, etc. [23]. Onset is usually rapid. Prominent features include fever and significant psycho motor disturbances. Rigidity, mutism, negativity, and posturing are present. It can progress to stupor, exhaustion, and coma. It needs to be excluded from other disorders like herpes simplex encephalitis and autoimmune encephalitis. In a suspected case CSF studies, MRI and evaluation for autoimmune encephalitis should be carried out [24].

Treatment includes removal of offending agent and supportive care. High dose of intravenous benzodiazepine is used. Sometimes electroconvulsive therapy (ECT) is considered in refractory cases.

55.4.5 Malignant Hyperthermia (MH)

This uncommon life threatening disorder is caused by exposure to certain volatile anesthetic agents and neuromuscular blocking agents like succinylcholine. Hyperthermia, rigidity, metabolic acidosis, and rhabdomyolysis are key features. MH is frequently inherited as an autosomal dominant pattern of which the most significant locus is the rynodione receptor gene. Caffeine contracture test is positive. Treatment includes discontinuation of anesthesia, cooling, and dantrolene [25].

Key points:- NMS, MH, LC and Serotonin Syndrome (to be discussed later) are the four frequently diagnosed hypermetabolic syndromes. They manifest with hyperthermia, muscular rigidity, and autonomic dysfunction. They are usually drug-induced and have high mortality. Prompt recognition is necessary. These groups of disorders require the discontinuation of the offending drug and management of complications like rhabdomyolysis, hyperthermia, and autonomic dysfunction.

55.5 Dystonic Movement Disorders

Dystonia refers to involuntary sustained muscle contractions that produce abnormal postures and twisting movements.

55.5.1 Status Dystonicus (SD)

It is a state of unremitting severe dystonia. It is defined as increasingly frequent and severe episodes of generalized dystonia requiring urgent hospitalization [5]. Tonic spasm characterized by sustained muscle contractions and postures is the common form. Phasic form is characterized by repetitive and rapid dystonic movements and is more common in secondary dystonias and in female patients. SD is common in patients between ages 5 and 16 years. It can occur in primary as well as secondary forms of dystonia. It is usually precipitated by infection, trauma, surgery, or abrupt failure of deep brain stimulation hardware. Use of dopamine receptor blockers like pimozide and haloperidol is known triggers. Initiation of chelation therapy with penicillamine or zinc sulphate in the treatment of Wilson disease has also been implicated [26]. Mortality is upto 10%.

First-line treatment involves specific anti-dystonia drugs like anticholinergic (trihexyphenidyl), dopamine blocker(haloperidol, tetrabenazine), baclofen, or clonidine. Status dystonicus in Wilson disease responds well to gabapentin [27]. However, first-line drugs are effective only in 10% patients. Second-line treatment usually requires sedation with midazolam accompanied by intubation and ventilation.

Usual response to oral anti-dystonia drugs is poor. Deep brain stimulation of bilateral globus pallidus interna [28] and intrathecal baclofen pump (ITB) has been found to be effective in refractory cases. They should be considered early, once infections are excluded.

55.5.2 Drug-Induced Acute Dystonic Reactions

Drug reactions are by far the most common cause of acute focal dystonia. It usually occurs within 24 h of drug exposure [29]. Usually, it manifests as orofacial dystonia. Sometimes, back arching, neck extension, and even life threatening laryngospasm are seen. They are common with high potency antipsychotics (typical ≫ newer atypical drugs) [30]. Acute dystonic reactions are more common in young men [31], whereas tardive dyskinesia and drug-induced parkinsonism are more common in the elderly [30]. SSRIs, tricyclic antidepressants, have also been reported to provoke acute dystonia.

Management

Acute dystonic reactions usually respond well to injectable diphenhydramine(25–50 mg). Anticholinergic drugs are also used for management as well as prevention. Because the possibility of reoccurence is high, a short course of an oral anticholinergic is necessary for 4–7 days.

55.6 Hyperkinetic Movement Disorders

55.6.1 Hemiballism-Hemichorea

Hemiballism refers to unilateral large amplitude, flailing movements caused by involvement of proximal muscle group [32]. These are rarely suppressible and they disappear in sleep. It represents an extreme end of the spectrum of chorea. Chorea is an involuntary, purposeless irregular movement that flows into one another in random fashion. Stroke and nonketotic hyperglycemia [33] are some of the common causes. Rarely, it is observed with CNS infections like cryptococcal granuloma and toxoplasmosis. Systemic lupus erythematosus (SLE) often with anticardiolipin antibodies, drugs like levodopa, ibuprofen, and oral contraceptives, is another rare cause [33].

MRI shows areas of infarction in the contralateral subthalamic nucleus in 50% cases. Sometimes, other parts of basal ganglia or contralateral cortex are also involved. Diabetic striatopathy describes classical changes of T1 hyperintensities involving putamen and/or caudate. CT scan in such cases shows uniform, slight hyperdense attenuation of putamen and/or caudate. Diffuse and uniform involvement of basal ganglia differentiates it from other etiologies like stroke.

Treatment is usually directed towards the cause. Tetrabenazene is the preferred symptomatic drug.(12.5 mg twice a day, titrate upto 250 mg/day if required). Sometimes, drugs like haloperidol and clonazepam are useful. Treatment is usually given for 3 months [33].

55.6.2 NMDA Receptor Encephalitis (Autoimmune Orobuccolingual Dyskinesia)

This syndrome was first described in 2005. Though usually progressive, it can present as an emergency with a prominent movement disorder. It is common in children and adults below the age of 50. Typical history involves prodromal illness followed by agitation, confusion, psychosis, poverty of speech, and seizures. Orobuccolingual dyskinesia is a prominent feature. Later, chorea and opisthotonus also occur. The presence of CSF NMDA receptor antibodies is diagnostic [34].

Early in the course, MRI and CSF studies are normal. Later, MRI shows typical mild to transient FLAIR or T2 hyperintensities involving hippocampi, cerebellum, or cortex. A thorough search of malignancy by imaging studies is necessary. Sixty percent of patients have ovarian teratoma [35]. Testicular teratoma is common in men. Neurologic syndrome improves with surgical treatment of malignancy. Even in absence of malignancy immunotherapy with corticosteroids, intravenous immunoglobulins and plasmapharesis are considered first-line treatments. Patients who do not have teratomas usually need aggressive second-line immunotherapy, such as rituximab and cyclophosphamide. Twenty five percent patients without teratoma relapse after months to years. Hence, periodic monitoring and addition of mycophenolate mofetil or azathioprine are preferred for at least 1 year. After the recovery from encephalitis, periodic screening for teratomas at least for 2 years is recommended [20].

There are certain important issues in consideration of management of these patients. In many patients who initially present with psychiatric manifestations and hence are on neuroleptic medications, the dyskinesias are often misinterpreted as tardive dyskinesia. NMS is also considered in these patients in view of fever and exposure to neuroleptic drugs. A strong clinical suspicion is necessary in young patients for correct and timely management.

55.6.3 Motor Fluctuations and Dyskinesia in Parkinson Disease

Motor fluctuations are common in patients of PD. They are seen in 40% patients by 4–6 years. Generally not dangerous, motor fluctuations are one of the common reasons for which patients seek emergency treatment. During off periods, patients become bradykinetic and rigid. These patients are often depressed and they can have tachycardia and labile blood pressure.

A careful evaluation to see recent drug changes is necessary. Exposure to dopamine depleting agents should also be asked. Subdural hematoma should be suspected in a patient who has falls. Concurrent urinary tract infection, pneumonia, and metabolic derangements like hyponatremia should be considered [3].

Sometimes levodopa-induced dyskinesia(LID) can be severe. They can lead to rhabdomyolysis and dehydration. Generalized LID may be complicated by involvement of respiratory muscles. Treatment should include lowering doses of levodopa. Benzodiazepine is used to treat anxiety. Neuroleptics are to be avoided. Long-term treatment of dyskinesia may involve addition of amantidine or deep brain stimulation [50].

55.6.4 Psychosis in Parkinson Disease (PD)

It is commonly encountered in patients with PD and dementia, occurring in 45–64% of patients [51]. Visual hallucinations are common. Paranoid delusions constitute a greater problem. PD psychosis may be precipitated by metabolic derangements, infections, and change in drug therapy.

Treatment includes thorough workup for metabolic or infectious disorders. Nonessential psychoactive medications should be discontinued. The daily dose of levodopa may need to be lowered. Antipsychotics like clozapine and quetiapne are used [52]. Agranulocytosis is associated with clozapine use. Complete blood counts should be frequently checked if clozapine is used.

55.6.5 Tic Status

Tics are brief paroxysmal movements or vocalizations, sometimes accompanied by premonitory urge. They may be stereotyped and may be voluntarily suppressed for a short period of time. Tic status is an increase in the frequency and severity of tics; enough to disrupt social, vocational, or daily activities. Self-injurious tics, coprolalia, copropraxia, or violent neck tics causing cervical myelopathy are tic emergencies. Change in medications, intercurrent illness, and worsened comorbid psychiatric illness are usual precipitating factors [20]. Several drugs like methylpheidate, pemoline, levodopa, phenytoin, carbamazepine, sertaline, and fluoxetine can worsen the tics.

First-line treatment includes benzodiazepines. Pimozide is the treatment of choice in acute disabling tics. Lowest possible dose is preferred. Tetrabenazine, a dopamine depleting agent, is second-line treatment. Dopamine receptor blockers like haloperidol are third-line agents. They are avoided as they can cause tardive syndromes. Rarely, botulinum toxin injection to accessible site can be used as a useful adjunct for tic treatment [37]. In refractory cases, trial of DBS to centromedian thalamic nucleus is useful.

55.6.6 Myoclonus

Myoclonus is a sudden brief, shock-like movement. It may be positive(caused by sudden muscle contraction) or negative (caused by sudden loss of muscle tone), usually not suppressible by the patient.

55.6.7 Serotonin Syndrome (SS)

This was first described in 1960 [43]. This is an iatrogenic condition which is caused by drugs either alone or in combination that enhances serotonin transmission. The greatest risk appears to be the combination of SSRI antidepressants with MAO inhibitors [44]. Many drugs can potentially be responsible for SS like MAO inhibitors, SSRIs, tricyclic antidepressants, lithium, buspirone, opiates, triptans, and fentanyl [45], to name a few. Diagnosis is clinical and should be suspected in any patient with a history of exposure to relevant medication. Examination shows confusion, restlessness, elevated mood, dysautonomia, myoclonus, generalized rigidity, hyperreflexia, and spontaneous or inducible clonus [46]. Compared to NMS, hyperreflexia, myoclonus, and dysautonomic features like mydriasis, sialorrhea, and hyperactive bowel sounds are more common in SS. White cell count and creatine kinase are raised. Some patients can have hyponatremia and hypocalcemia. If a patient is exhibiting signs of DIC, serotonin secreting tumors should be suspected [25].

Treatment involves removal of the offending agent and supportive measures like iv fluids antipyretics, antihypertensives, cardiac monitoring, and benzodiazepines for myoclonic jerks.

If needed, cyprohetadine can be used as an initial dose of 12 mg(oral or via nasogastric tube), followed by a maintenance dose of 8 mg four times a day once the patient is stabilized [47]. Occasionally, electroconvulsive therapy is used for the refractory SS [48].

Post-Hypoxic Myoclonus

Cerebral hypoxia can cause acute myoclonic status epilepticus as well as chronic post-hypoxic myoclonus [49].

Acute myoclonus manifests within 12–24 h after return of spontaneous circulation in a comatose patient and is usually an indicative of poor prognosis. EEG monitoring is of importance in such patients. Some benefits have been reported with valproic acid, levetiracetam, and benzodiazepine use.

Chronic post-hypoxic myoclonus (Lance Adams syndrome) is a late complication following recovery from anoxic brain injury. Clinical picture involves action and stimulus-sensitive myoclonus in awake patient. Cognitive functions may be preserved.

Valproic acid, Levetiracetam, piracetam, benzodiazepines, and fluoxetine have been tried in such patients.

Myoclonus in Other Conditions

Often, positive and negative myoclonus are seen in ICU patients, in the setting of encephalopathy. It can be generalized or multifocal. The common associations include renal failure, hepatic failure, sepsis, and hypercapnia.

General anesthetics(etomidate, enflurane), opioids, SSRIs, gabapentin, and pregabalin antibiotics like quinolones are some medications which characteristically provoke myoclonus. EEG is usually done to rule out seizures. Therapy is directed towards underlying cause and removing the offending agent. Sometimes oral clonazepam is used. Sodium oxybate can be used for both cortical and subcortical myoclonus.

55.7 Airway Emergencies

55.7.1 Laryngeal Adductor Dystonia

It occurs in both primary and secondary dystonia and rarely after exposure to neuroleptics. In acute situation, immediate endotracheal intubation is performed. It sometimes requires immediate tracheostomy or cricothyroidotomy as endotracheal intaubation is not easy in such situation [20].

55.7.2 Laryngeal Abductor Paralysis in Multiple System Atrophy

Multiple system atrophy is a progressive illness. Laryngeal paralysis usually occurs in advanced stage. Neurogenic atrophy of the posterior cricoarytenoid muscle, which is the abductor of the vocal cords, is caused by the neuronal loss in the nucleus ambiguss. Patients often have sleep apnoea and nocturnal stridor leading to fatal airway obstruction [36]. Fiberoptic laryngoscopy helps to decide the severity. Low-grade paralysis is managed by continuous positive airway ventilation at night. High-grade paralysis warrants tracheostomy [1].

55.8 Conclusion

Movement disorder emergencies are rare, and if not diagnosed quickly, they can be fatal. A detailed history including the drug prescription is very important. A syndromic approach based on the phenomenology is the key. Rapid clinical recognition in the ICU often results in effective treatment. Treating physician should be aware of drug interactions, as in most of the emergencies, drugs are the culprit. This article has discussed the rapidly evolving situations requiring emergency intervention. Several discussed disorders are so rare that treatment guidelines are not based on randomized, double blind, placebo-controlled trials.

References

1. Poston KL, Frucht SJ. Movement disorder emergencies. J Neurol. 2008;255(Suppl 4):2–13.
2. Frucht SJ. Movement disorder emergencies. Curr Neurol Neurosci Rep. 2005;5:284–93.
3. Robottom BJ, Shulman LM. Drug-induced movement disorders: emergencies and management. Neurol Clin. 2012;30:309–20.
4. Robottom BJ, Weiner WJ. Movement disorders emergencies part 1: hypokinetic movement disorders. Arch Neurol. 2011;68:567–72.
5. Fernandez HH, Friedman JH. Acute parkinsonism. In: Frucht SJ, Fahn S, editors. Movement disorder emergencies: diagnosis and treatment. Totowa: Humana Press; 2005. p. 9–28.
6. Howard RS, Lees AJ. Encephalitis lethargica: a report of four recent cases. Brain. 1987;110:19–33.
7. Pradhan S, Pandey N, Sbashank S, et al. Parkinsonism due to predominant involvement of substantianigra in Japanese encephalitis. Neurology. 1999;53:1781–6.
8. Choi IS. Parkinsonism after carbon monoxide poisoning. Eur Neurol. 2002;48:30–3.
9. Delay J, Pichot P, Lemperiere T. Un neuroleptique majeur non phenothiazine et non reserpinique l'haloperidal dans le traitement des psychoses. Ann Med Psychol. 1960;118:145–52. [in French].
10. Shalev A, Munitz H. The neuroleptic malignant syndrome: agent and host interaction. Acta Psychiatr Scand. 1986;50:18–25.
11. Caroff SN, Mann SC. Neuroleptic malignant syndrome. Psychopharmacol Bull. 1988;24:25–9.
12. Shalev A, Hermesh H, Munitz H. Mortality from neuroleptic malignant syndrome. J Clin Psychiatry. 1989;50:18–25.
13. Hasan S, Buckley P. Novel antipsychotics and the neuroleptic malignant syndrome: a review and critique. Am J Psychiatry. 1998;115:1113–6.
14. Caroff SN, Mann SC, Campbell EC. Neuroleptic malignant syndrome. Adverse Drug React Bull. 2001;209:799–802.
15. Khan FY, Qusad MJ. Neuroleptic malignant syndrome. Neuroscience. 2006;11(2):104–6.
16. Petzinger GM, Bressman SB. A case of tetrabenazine-induced neuroleptic malignant syndrome after prolonged treatment. Mov Disord. 1997;12(2):246–8.
17. Washington C, Haines KA, Tam CW. Amoxipine-induced neuroleptic malignant syndrome. DICP. 1989;23(9):713.
18. Gill J, Singh H, Nugent K. Acute lithium intoxication and neuroleptic malignant syndrome. Pharmacotherapy. 2003;23(6):811–5.
19. Shalev A, Munitz H. The neuroleptic malignant syndrome: agent and host interaction. Acta Psychiatr Scand. 1986;73:337–47.
20. Chang FCF, Frucht SJ. ICU Intensive Care Unit Movement Disorder Emergencies In: Non-movement disorders. Eds: Hall DA, Barton BR. Wiley Blackwell; 2017, pp 150–60.
21. Davis JM, Caroff SN, Mann SC. Treatment of neuroleptic malignant syndrome. Psychiatr Ann. 2000;30:325–31.
22. Caroff SN, Mann SC, Keck PE Jr. Specific treatment of the neuroleptic malignant syndrome. Biol Psychiatry. 1998;44:378–81.
23. Fricchione G, Bush G, Fozdar M, et al. Recognition and treatment of the catatonic syndrome. J Intensive Care Med. 1997;12:135–47.
24. Fricchione G, Mann SC, Caroff SN. Catatonia, lethal catatonia, and neuroleptic malignant syndrome. Psychiatr Ann. 2000;3:347–55.
25. Alekseeva N, Geller F. Urgent and emergent psychiatric disorders. Neurol Clin. 2012;30:321–44.
26. Svetel M, Stemic N, Pejovic S, Kostic VS. Penicillamine-induced lethal status dystonicus in a patient with Wilson's disease. Mov Disord. 2001;16:568–9.
27. Paliwal VK, Gupta PK, Pradhan S. Gabapentin as a rescue drug in D-penicillamine-induced status dystonicus in patients with Wilson disease. Neurol India. 2010;58:761–3.
28. Apetauerova D, Schirmer CM, Shils JL, Zani J, Arie JE. Successful bilateral deep brain stimulation of the globuspallidusinternus for persistent status dystonicus and generalized chorea. J Neurosurg. 2010;113:634–8.
29. Tousi B. Movement disorder emergencies in the elderly: recognizing and treating an often iatrogenic problem. Cleveland Clin J Med. 2008;75(6):449–57.
30. Pierre JM. Extrapyramidal symptoms with atypical antipsychotics: incidence. Prevention and management. Drug Sat. 2005;28(3):191–208.
31. van Harten PN, Hock HW, Kahn RS. Acute dystonia induced by drug treatment. BMJ. 1999;319:623–6.
32. Dewey RB, Jankovic J. Hemiballism-hemichorea. Arch Neurol. 1989;46:862–7.
33. Lee B, Hwang S, Chang G. Hemiballismus-hemichorea in older diabetic women: a clini-

cal syndrome with MRI correlation. Neurology. 1999;52:646–8.
34. Dalmau J, Lancaster E, Martinez-Hernandez E, Rosendeld MR, Balice Gordon R. Clinical experience and laborator investigation in patients with anti—NMDAR encephalitis. Lancet Neurol. 2011;10(1):63–7.
35. Kleinig TJ, Thompson PD, Matar W, Duggins A, Kimber TE, Morris JG, et al. The distinctive movement disorder ofovarian teratoma-associated encephalitis. Mov Disord. 2008;23(9):1256–61.
36. Isono S, Shiba K, Yamaguchi M, et al. Pathogenesis of laryngeal narrowing in patients with multiple system atrophy. J Physiol. 2001;536:237–49.
37. Jankovic J. Botulinum toxin in the treatment of dystonic tics. Mov Disord. 1994;9:347–9.
38. SA Factor et al parkinsonism-hyperpyrexia syndrome in a Parkinson disease patient while actively treated with deep brain stimulation. Mov Disorders. 2007;22(1):148–53.
39. Ito T, Shibata K, et al. Neuroleptic malignant syndrome following withdrawal of amantidine in a patient with influenza encephalopathy. Eur J Pediatr. 2001;160(6):401.
40. Iwuagwu CU, RIley D, et al. Neuroleptic malignant like syndrome in an elderly patient caused by abrupt withdrawal of tolcapone, a catechol-O-methyl transferase inhibitor. Am J Med. 2000;108(6):517–8.
41. Sato Y, Asoh T, et al. Efficacy of methylprednisolone pulse therapy on neuroleptic malignant syndrome in Parkinson disease. J Neurol Neurosurg Psychiatry. 2003;74:574–6.
42. Factor SA, Weiner MJ. Movement disorder emergencies: adults and children. American Academy of Neurology, 61 st Annual Meeting. Seattle, WA, April 25–May 2, 2009.
43. Oates JA, Sjoerdsma A. Neurologic effects of tryptophan in patients receiving a monoamine oxidase inhibitor. Neurology. 1960;10:1076–8.
44. Mason PJ, Morris VA, et al. Serotonin syndrome. Presentation of 2 cases and review of the literature. Medicine. 2000;79:201–9.
45. Kirschner R, Donovan JW. Serotonin syndrome precipitated by fentanyl during procedural sedation. J Emerg Med. 2010;38(4):477–80.
46. Radomski JW, Dursun SM, et al. An exploratory approach to the serotonin syndrome: an update on clinical phenomenology and revised diagnostic criteria. Med Hypotheses. 2000;55(3):218–24.
47. Hall M, Buckley N. Serotonin syndrome. Aust Prescr. 2003;26:62–23.
48. Okamoto N, Sakamoto K, et al. Electroconvulsive therapy as a potentially effective treatment for severe serotonin syndrome: two case reports. J Clin Psychopharmacol. 2010;30(3):191–208.
49. English WA, Giffin NJ, et al. Myoclonus after cardiac arrest: pitfalls in the diagnosis and prognosis. Anaesthesia. 2009;64(8):908–11.
50. Pahwa R, Factor SA, et al. Practice parameter: treatment of parkinson disease motor fluctuations and dyskinesia(an evidence based review): report of the Quality Standards Subcommittee of the American Academy of Neurology. Neurology. 2006;66:983–95.
51. Robottom BJ, Weiner WJ. Parkinsons disease dementia. Curr Psychiatr Rev. 2009;5(3):218–25.
52. Miyasaki JM, Shannon K, et al. Practice parameter: evaluation and treatment of depression, psychosis and dementia in Parkinson disease(an evidence based review). Neurology. 2006;66:996–1002.

Meningitis/Encephalitis and Neurocritical Care

56

Srinivas Samavedam

56.1 Introduction

Meningitis and Encephalitis are clinical syndromes commonly encountered in Neuro Critical Care Units (NCCUs), with significant morbidity and mortality. The aetiological causes are varied and include infectious and non-infectious entities. Diagnostic approach involves a combination of clinical, biochemical, radiological, and serological parameters. The availability of molecular diagnostic tools has contributed to the identification of several new organisms as the causative agents of infection of the Central Nervous System (CNS), than was possible in the past. Long-term neurological and cognitive sequelae are known to occur following CNS infections. It is therefore imperative to follow a structured approach for an appropriate and timely diagnosis and prompt effective treatment of these disorders.

Meningitis involves inflammation of the meninges and shows varied features or changes in the Cerebro Spinal Fluid (CSF). Meningitis could be acute (<5 days symptom duration), subacute (6–30 days symptom duration), or chronic (>30 days symptom duration). The anatomical location of the infection and the virulence of the infecting organism determine the clinical manifestations and severity of meningitis. Immunocompromised states and the presence of interventricular shunts will also play a role in the aetio-pathogenesis of meningitis.

Encephalitis, on the other hand, is caused by infection and resultant inflammation of the brain parenchyma. The major criterion to diagnose encephalitis is [1] Altered mental status >24 h with no alternate explanation. This has to be corroborated by several minor criteria which include

(i) Documented fever >38 °C in the 72 h prior to presentation
(ii) Un-explained seizures
(iii) New-onset Focal Neurological Deficit (FND)
(iv) CSF Leucocytosis (>5 WBC/cu.mm)
(v) New or Acute abnormalities on Neuro-Imaging consistent with encephalitis
(vi) Electro Encephalo - Graphic (EEG) abnormalities not correlating with other aetiologies and consistent with encephalitis.

Presence of two of these minor criteria is essential to make a diagnosis of encephalitis among patients who satisfy the major criteria. It is also likely that some of these criteria might manifest without evidence of CNS inflammation. Such a situation may be described as an "Encephalopathy". This review will discuss the common forms of both conditions. The salient differences between two disorders and overlapping Meningo-Encephalitis are shown in Table 56.1.

S. Samavedam (✉)
Ramdev Rao Hospital, Hyderabad, India

H. Prabhakar et al. (eds.), *Principles and Practice of Neurocritical Care*,
https://doi.org/10.1007/978-981-99-8059-8_56

Table 56.1 Salient features and differences between Meningitis, Meningo-Encephalitis, and Encephalitis

	Meningitis	Meningo-encephalitis	Encephalitis
Fever/Leucocytosis	Common	Common	Common
Signs of meningeal irritation	Consistent	Variable	Rare
Altered mental status	Rare	Variable	Consistent
Seizures	Less common		Common
Focal neurological findings	Seen in 50% Usually late		Hallmark feature Early
Typical pathogens	*S. pneumoniae* *H. influenzae* *N. meningitidis*	Herpes Simplex Varicella Zoster Listeria	Herpes Simplex Varicella Zoster Enteroviruses

56.2 Community Acquired Acute Bacterial Meningitis (CA-ABM)

The incidence of CA-ABM seems to be decreasing across the world consequent to the availability of vaccines for children. However, CA-ABM still contributes to significant number of adults getting admitted to NCCUs in developing countries. *Streptococcus pneumoniae, Neisseria meningitidis,* and *Hemophilus influenzae* still remain the aetiological agents for this condition [2]. Immunocompromised individuals and the elderly are more susceptible to infections with *Listeria monocytogenes* [2]. Aetiological agents responsible for CA-ABM among different age groups are listed in Table 56.2.

Table 56.2 Age-related aetiological agents for acute bacterial meningitis

Age category	Organism
Infants upto 4–6 weeks age	Streptococcus agalactiae *Escherichia coli* Enterobacteriacae *Listeria monocytogenes*
Children >6 weeks old and adults upto 50 years of age	*Streptococcus pneumoniae* *Neisseria meningitidis* *Hemophilus influenzae*
Adults over 50 years of age	*Streptococcus pneumoniae* *Neisseria meningitidis* *Hemophilus influenzae* *Listeria monocytogenes*
Immunocompromised host	*Streptococcus pneumoniae* *Neisseria meningitidis* *Hemophilus influenzae* *Listeria monocytogenes*

The portal of entry for the common aetiological agents seems to be upper respiratory tract. Breach of the mucosal barrier and consequent invasion of the blood stream sets the platform for breach of the Blood Brain Barrier (BBB). This step triggers the inflammatory response, which is perpetuated by the relatively low immunity in the CNS. The infection then causes a rise in the Intra Cranial Pressure (ICP), by multiple mechanisms including extra-cellular oedema, increased CSF volume, cytotoxic intra-cellular oedema, and hyperemia. Local and systemic complications can occur which contribute to the morbidity and mortality.

Clinical Features: The clinical symptoms of CA-ABM are dominated by fever, headache, and impaired mental status. Neck stiffness is also a fairly consistent manifestation. However, all four symptoms occur in 30–40% of patients [2]. Nausea, vomiting, photophobia, and hypersensitivity to sound are likely to be manifestations of CNS irritation and raised ICP. The well-described Kerning's and Brudzinski's signs lack sensitivity. The presence of a petechial rash usually suggests meningococcal infection and portends the possibility of Sepsis and Septic shock. The manifestations of ABM among the elderly are atypical and make the diagnosis difficult. New-onset seizures and FND can also be manifest in a smaller percentage of patients. The differential diagnosis of ABM includes viral encephalitis, cerebral mass lesions, and subarachnoid haemorrhage.

Initial Approach: Lumbar Puncture (LP) and CSF analysis are the cornerstones for the diagnosis of ABM [3]. Cloudy CSF with a high opening spinal pressure (>300 cm H_2O) manifests very early in the course. Leucocytosis in the CSF with polymorphonuclear pleocytosis, low CSF/serum Glucose ratio (<0.4), and elevated proteins (>100 mg/dL) occur within a few hours of the onset. While some authorities recommend a computerized tomography (CT) of the brain when raised ICP is suspected, the imaging modality is a poor predictor of cerebral herniation in ABM [4]. The decision to perform an LP with or without a CT should not delay the administration of appropriate antibiotics. However, a CT scan should aways precede an LP when a space occupying lesion (SOL) is more likely and if symptoms have been present for more than 4 days. Delayed LP may also have to be considered among patients with known bleeding abnormalities and among those on anticoagulants. It is advisable to perform the LP once the International Normalized Ratio (INR) has been corrected to <1.6 and /or the platelet count has been corrected to >30,000/cu.mm. The salient features of the CSF in various infective conditions are shown in Table 56.3.

Empiric Antibiotic Therapy: The choice of empirical antibiotic agent should be guided by the probable organisms, bactericidal properties, and ability to penetrate the BBB. The drugs of choice for the management of CA-ABM still remain third-generation cephalosporins (Cefotaxime or Ceftriaxone +/− Ampicillin). Ampicillin may have to be added if infection with Listeria is suspected (Elderly, diabetic, immunocompromised, and neonates). Vancomycin is recommended if local epidemiological data suggest high prevalence of resistant pneumococci [3]. Patients who have allergy to penicillin and cephalosporins should receive either monotherapy with meropenem or a combination therapy with moxifloxacin and either vancomycin or linezolid [3]. In such patients, trimethoprim-sulfamethoxazole can be considered to cover listeria [4]. The second step in the management is to tailor and modify the empirical combination based on the microbiology. The recommended doses of the antibiotics are listed in Table 56.4.

Role of Corticosteroids: The role of adjuvant corticosteroids in the management of CA-ABM is controversial. Decreased mortality and improved long-term outcome have been shown among adults with pneumococcal meningitis [5]. Similarly, sequelae with *H. influenzae* meningitis have been shown to be lower with the concomitant use of steroids [6]. Neutral effect has been reported for meningococcal meningitis. These effects, however, have been restricted to cohorts from the developed world. It is also clear that the use of steroids among patients with listeria infection is associated with inferior outcomes [7]. The corticosteroid that has been most studied is dexamethasone and has been administered in the dose of 0.5 mg/kg, upto a maximum of 10 mg, four times daily. This dose should accompany the first dose of antibiotic, but should not be delayed longer than 6 h after the first dose of antibiotic. The duration of corticosteroid treatment ranges between 2 and 4 days.

An algorithm showing the comprehensive management plan for CA-ABM is shown in Fig. 56.1.

Table 56.3 The salient features of the CSF in various infective conditions

Parameter	Normal	Bacterial	Viral	Tubercular	Fungal
Opening pressure	6–20 cm H_2O	20–50 cm H_2O	6–30 cm H_2O	20–40 cm H_2O	20–100 cm H_2O
Colour	Clear	Cloudy	Clear	Cloudy/yellow	Cloudy
Cells	<5/mm^3	Very high >1000/mm^3	Mild increase 10–1000/mm^3	Mild increase 10–1000/mm^3	Normal to high <1000/mm^3
Differential	Lymphocytic	Neutrophilic	Lymphocytic	Lymphocytic	Lymphocytic
CSF/blood glucose ratio	>0.5	<0.4	>0.5	<0.3	>0.5
Proteins	<0.45 g/L	>1 g/L	0.5–1 g/L	1–5 g/L	0.5–5 g/L

Table 56.4 Recommended doses of antibiotics for acute bacterial meningitis

Antibiotic	Adult dose	Dose in children	Total daily doses
Ceftriaxone	2 g q 12h	100 mg/kg	2
Cefotaxime	3 g q 6h	225–300 mg/kg	4–6
Penicillin G	3 g q 6h	300 mg/kg	4–6
Ampicillin	3 g q 6h	300 mg/kg	4–6
Meropenem	2 g q 8h	120 mg/kg	3
Vancomycin	1 g q 8h	60 mg/kg	2–3
Linezolid	600 mg q 12h	10 mg/kg	2
Moxifloxacin	400 mg q 24h	6–8 mg/kg	1

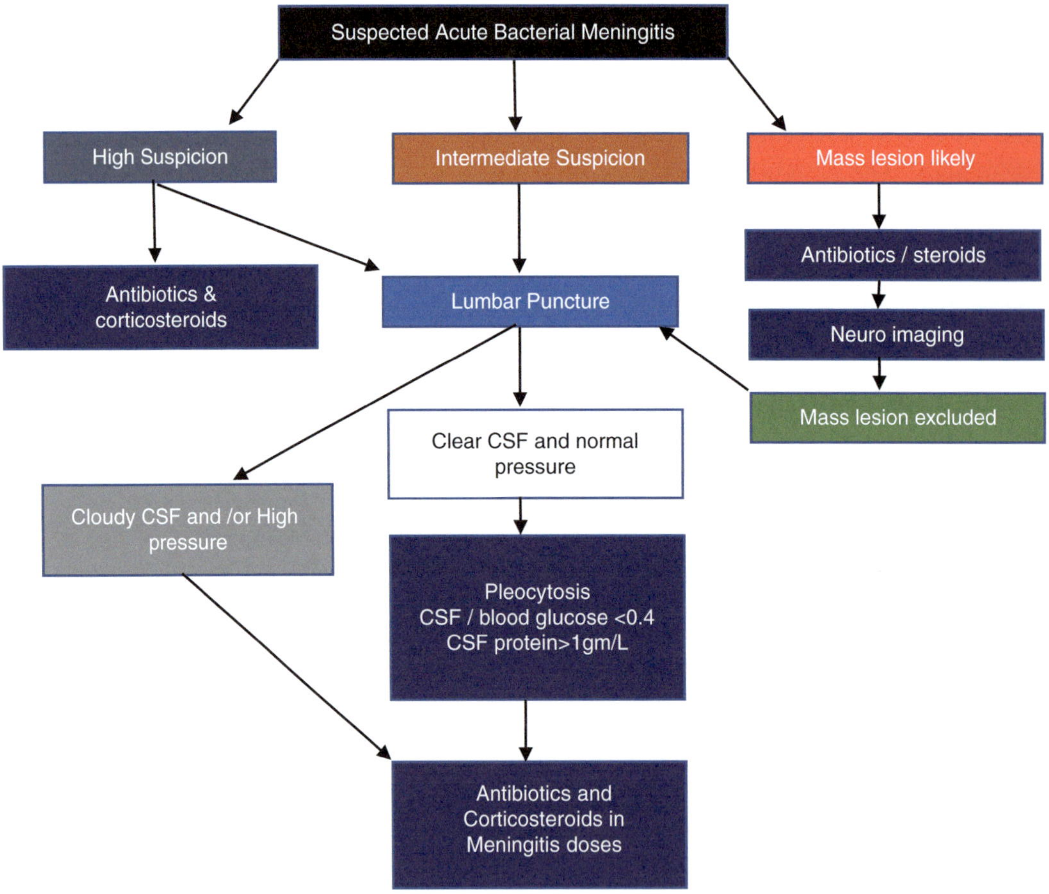

Fig. 56.1 Comprehensive management plan for Community-Acquired Acute Bacterial Meningitis (*CSF* Cerebro Spinal Fluid)

56.3 Health Care-Associated Meningitis and Ventriculitis (HA-MV)

This group of disorders includes infections that occur after LP, CSF drain/shunt placement, and after neurosurgical procedures where there has been a dural breach. The incidence of these infection ranges varies between 4% (post LP) and 10% (Drains and Shunts). The organisms causing HA-MV vary according to the temporal occurrence of the infection. Direct invasion can occur during surgical procedures, while shunts are likely to be infected through the peritoneal route.

Organisms that frequent the health care environment-*Staphylococcus aureus* and *S. epidermidis*, *E. coli*, *Klebsiella*, *Pseudomonas*, and *Acinetobacter*—are the most commonly isolated among patients with HA-MV. Rarely, infections with *Candida* may be encountered.

The clinical presentation of HA-MV could vary from acute and severe forms to mild and chronic variants depending on the virulence of the infecting organism. The presentations are also atypical, with isolated ventriculitis and shunt blockade being encountered frequently. Fever, headache, and altered mental status are less consistently encountered in this form of meningitis.

Evaluation of HA-MV proceeds along lines similar to those adopted for CA-ABM. Biomarker (Procalcitonin, C-Reactive Protein) elevation is not as consistent in HA-MV as in other infective conditions. The diagnostic value of CSF cell count, glucose, and protein diminishes in the context of shunt-related ventriculitis and is confounded by intra-cranial haemorrhage and neurosurgical interventions. In addition, it is important to remember that bone flap and sub-galeal infections could cause CSF leucocytosis in the absence of meningitis. Culture of the CSF is probably the most reliable method of diagnosing HA-MV. Anaerobic cultures are needed for the slow growing organisms that often cause HA-MV. More recently, the availability of Polymerase Chain Reaction- (PCR) based assays has added new tools in the workup of patients with HA-MV. Different categories of HA-MV may be identified based on the clinical and CSF parameters. These categories are listed in Table 56.5. The White Cell Count threshold for the diagnosis of CSF-Shunt-related ventriculitis is very low (<10/μL) owing to the minimal inflammation which is invoked by indolent organisms.

Treatment of HA-MV: One of the main challenges in managing HA-MV is the difficulty in achieving high concentrations of antibiotics in the CSF. Both intravenous and intraventricular antibiotics may have to be considered. Empirical therapy is quite often driven by local epidemiological data. However, a combination of fourth generation cephalosporins (Ceftazidime 2 gm q 8h or Cefepime 2 g q 8h) and vancomycin (as an infusion 60 mg/kg/day after a loading dose of 15 mg/kg) is quite effective in most instances. For patients with penicillin allergy, a combination of aztreonam (2 g q 6h) and vancomycin may be tried. Specific targeted antimicrobial therapy is enumerated in Table 56.6.

Lack of response to intravenous antibiotics should trigger an attempt to administer intrathecal or intraventricular antibiotics. The BBB is by-passed by this approach. This strategy has to be followed especially when the minimum inhibitory concentration (MIC) of cephalosporins exceeds 0.5 μg/mL, meropenem exceeds 0.25 μg/

Table 56.5 Categories of healthcare-associated meningitis and ventriculitis

Category	Description
Contamination	Isolated positive CSF culture or Gram stain. No symptoms and signs
Colonization	Multiple positive CSF cultures or Gram stain. No signs and symptoms
Possible ventriculitis	Progressive rise in cell index or progressive decrease in CSF/blood glucose ratio or an extreme value for CSF WBC count (>1000/μL) or CSF/blood glucose ratio (<0.2), with attributable symptoms or signs, but Negative Gram stain and cultures
Probable ventriculitis	CSF WBC count or CSF/blood glucose ratio more abnormal than expected, and stable with Attributable symptoms or signs and Positive Gram stain and cultures
Definitive ventriculitis	Progressive rise in cell index or progressive decrease in CSF/blood glucose ratio or Extreme value for CSF WBC count (>1000/μL) or CSF/blood glucose ratio (<0.2), With attributable symptoms or signs and A positive Gram stain and cultures

Table 56.6 Targeted Intravenous antimicrobial therapy for hospital-acquired meningitis and ventriculitis

Organism	First choice	Second choice
Pseudomonas	Ceftazidime 2 g q 8h or Cefepime 2 g q 8h	Meropenem 2 g q 8 h
E. coli	Ceftriaxone 2 g q 12h	Meropenem 2 g q 8 h
Enterobacter spp.	Cefepime 2 g q 8h	Meropenem 2 g q 8 h
Methicillin-sensitive Staphylococcus aureus and epidermidis	Oxacillin 2 g q 4h	
Methicillin-resistant Staphylococcus aureus	Vancomycin 60 mg/kg in 2–3 divided doses after a loading dose of 15 mg/kg + Rifampicin 300 mg q 12h if catheter cannot be removed	Linezolid 600 mg q 12h

Table 56.7 Recommended intraventricular/intrathecal doses of antibiotics

Antibiotic	Recommended dose
Gentamicin	4–8 mg
Tobramycin	5–20 mg
Amikacin	5–30 mg
Colistimethate sodium	125,000 IU
Daptomycin	2–5 mg

mL, and that of Vancomycin exceeds 1 μg/mL. Volume of CSF equal to the volume of drug diluent and flush should be aspirated and discarded prior to drug administration to avoid rise in ICP. The recommended intraventricular doses of antibiotics are shown in Table 56.7. Therapeutic drug monitoring may be used to assess drug levels in the CSF where available.

Explanting the infected device or shunt followed by replacing it through a second surgery has the best results. Prophylactic use of first- or second-generation cephalosporins with vancomycin may reduce the incidence of HA-MV, but the evidence in favour is not very robust. Catheters impregnated with either minocycline or clindamycin combined with rifampicin may be associated with a lesser incidence of HA-VM [8].

56.4 Acute Aseptic Meningitis (AAM)

This syndrome, first described by Wallgren in 1925, represents a combination of CSF pleocytosis and absence of a gram stain or culture proven infection, with parameningeal foci and systemic illnesses being excluded. The aetiology of AAM includes both infectious and non-infectious causes with viral infections being the most dominant. The list of aetiologies of AAM is shown in Table 56.8. Certain salient findings in the CSF help to differentiate viral from bacterial origin of AAM. A CSF glucose value of less than 34 mg/dL, a CSF/Blood glucose ratio <0.23, CSF protein concentration >220 mg/dL, and a cell count >2000/cu.mm argue in favour of a bacterial aetiology. Elevated CSF lactate values are also in favour of bacterial infections.

Table 56.8 Aetiological agents responsible for acute aseptic meningitis

Infectious etiology	Non-infectious aetiology
Viruses Enteroviruses Arboviruses Herpes viruses Mumps virus Lymphocytic Choriomeningitis virus HIV Influenza Measles	Intracranial tumours/ cysts
Bacteria Rickettsia Ehrlichia Brucella Nocardia Spirochetes Leptospira	**Drugs** NSAIDs Antimicrobials Azathioprine
Parasites Taenia Toxocara Strongyloides Angiostrongylus	**Systemic diseases** Systemic lupus Eryhthematosus Behcet's disease Sarcoidosis
Protozoa Naegleria	Post-procedure

While the general approach to meningitis and encephalitis has been alluded to in the preceding sections, certain specific types need to be discussed. These include (in order of relevance to developing countries) tubercular meningitis (TBM), Herpes Simplex Encephalitis (HSE), Cryptococcal Meningitis (CM), and Japanese B Encephalitis (JBE).

56.5 Tubercular Meningitis (TBM)

The CNS is the second most common site for extra-thoracic tuberculosis. Meningitis and tuberculoma are the most common manifestations. Immunocompromise increases the risk of developing TBM. Certain manifestations like cranial nerve palsies, hydrocephalus, brain abscess, and hyponatremia are more common with TBM than with other forms of CA-ABM. The CNS is usually seeded through the blood stream, with the lungs being the first portal of entry in 95% of cases. Majority of manifestations of TBM are due to a few pathophysiological mechanisms. Formation of a thick exudate around the base of the brain, development of oedema in the adjacent brain, CSF blockade resulting in hydrocephalus, and vasculitis with cerebral infarction are the major interlinked mechanisms.

The clinical manifestations of TBM are varied and are quite often atypical [9]. The extent of pathophysiological mechanisms described above determines the spectrum of manifestations. The clinical onset is gradual (over 1–3 weeks) which makes an early diagnosis difficult. A three-stage course was initially described as follows:

- The first stage characterized by irritability, anorexia, weight loss, fever, and personality changes
- The second stage characterized by neck stiffness, cranial nerve palsies, vomitings, seizures, and FNDs
- The third stage characterized by coma or stupor.

This classical three-stage temporal pattern is less commonly encountered in current practice. Difficulty in detecting the organism makes the diagnosis more difficult. Elevation of Erythrocyte Sedimentation Rate (ESR) which is seen in close to 80% of patients, however, is non-specific. The CSF is usually clear, but may show a clot on standing. The cell count usually does not exceed 1000/cu.mm, with lymphocyte predominance appearing early. The CSF protein concentration ranges between 100 and 500 mg/dL, with sudden elevation indicating an obstruction. The CSF glucose values tend to remain in low-normal range initially and tend to decrease as the disease advances. Measurement of CSF Adenosine De-Aminase (ADA) levels is commonly used to diagnose TBM, but the specificity varies from 60% to 90% [10]. Demonstration of the Acid Fast Bacilli (AFB) in the CSF can confirm the diagnosis. A negative test should, however, not be used to exclude TBM. Molecular diagnostic tools like PCR have high specificity, but sensitivity ranges between 50% and 85% [10].

Neuro-imaging plays a significant role in the assessment of patients with TBM. Hydrocephalus is the most common abnormality detected (80%–100% of patients), but the most sensitive feature is basal enhancement on a non-contrast-enhanced CT of the head. Presence of high density within the basal cisterns is the most specific neuroradiological feature of TBM. Neuro-imaging may also be needed to monitor the appearance and the progress of tuberculomas.

Treatment: Morbidity and mortality secondary to TBM have remained high despite the availability of effective Anti-Tubercular Therapy (ATT). Susceptible infection is usually treated with four drugs – Isoniazid (INH), Rifampicin (RMP), Pyrazinamide (PZA), and Ethambutol (ETM). Among these, INH and PZA penetrate the CSF well even in the absence of meningeal inflammation. The conventional dose of RMP (10–15 mg/kg/day) is considered ineffective and a dose of 20–30 mg/kg/day is now recommended [11]. An initial 3–4 drug regimen containing PZA is very effective and a total length of treatment of 9–12 months is currently advocated.

Management of inflammation is of critical importance in the management of TBM [12].

Corticosteroid therapy has long been prescribed for patients with TBM. Corticosteroids are postulated to reduce cerebral oedema and inflammation and for quicker radiographic resolution and lower mortality among non-HIV infected patients. They should always be initiated with ATT. The duration of therapy is usually 3–6 weeks and tapered gradually.

56.6 Herpes Simplex Encephalitis (HSE)

Infection with Herpes Simplex Virus (HSV) is a leading cause of meningoencephalitis. The reported incidence of HSE accounts for 15% of all cases of encephalitis. Nearly 22% of all deaths due to encephalitis are attributed to HSE [13]. Aseptic meningitis seems to be associated more often with HSV-2 infection in comparison to HSV-1 infection.

The initial cutaneous infection is associated with encephalitis in 30% of instances with the balance occurring due to reactivation. The ability of the virus to remain latent in the trigeminal ganglion and its propensity for a retrograde spread via the olfactory and trigeminal nerves explain the predilection of the temporal lobe to HSE.

Clinical Features: The spectrum of CNS involvement of HSV infection is wide. This includes encephalitis, meningitis, myelitis, radiculopathy, and acute retinal necrosis. The salient features of HSE are listed in Table 56.9.

The salient CSF and diagnostic features of HSE are listed in Table 56.10. Meningitis seems to occur more often in younger individuals with few comorbidities. A well-recognized form of recurrent meningitis—Mollaret's meningitis—is also attributed to HSV-2 infection

Treatment: Encephalitis caused by HSV is one of the few treatable causes of viral encephalitis. Therefore, it is recommended that Acyclovir be started for all patients with encephalitis. The standard dose of Acyclovir is 10 mg/kg intravenously, every 8 h for 3–4 weeks. The role of corticosteroids in the management of HSE is not established. The strategy to be followed for HSV meningitis is less clear.

Table 56.9 Clinical features of herpes simplex and varicella zoster encephalitis

Manifestation	Herpes simplex virus	Varicella zoster virus
Fever	80%	45–90%
Altered Sensorium	70%	70–80%
Headache	60%	80%
Seizures	50%	10–20%
Focal Neurological Deficit	40%	10–50%
Nausea/Vomiting	40%	30%
Coma	30%	Unknown
Rash	0%	30%

Table 56.10 Diagnostic features of Herpes Simplex and Varicella Zoster infections

Diagnostic feature	Herpes Simplex Virus	Varicella Zoster Virus
CSF WCC/cu.mm	70 (5–500)	150 (0–1200)
CSF Lymphocytosis	80%	80%
CSF Protein	50–200 mg/dL	20–500 mg/dL
Abnormal CT scan	50%	75%
Abnormal MRI	95%	65%
Abnormal EEG	45%	90%

56.7 Cryptococcal Meningitis (CM)

The genus Cryptococcus was first identified in 1894 and includes more than 30 species. Among them, *Cryptococcus neoformans* and *Cryptococcus gattii* [14] are known to cause infections in humans. *C.neoformans* accounts for more than 85% of the infections among human hosts. However, *C.gattii* is likely to cause more infections among immune-competent hosts. The most important predisposing factors for CM are hematologic malignancies, corticosteroid therapy, solid organ transplant, and sarcoidosis. The incidence of CM among Bone Marrow Transplant [15] recipients is low probably due to the routine use of azole prophylaxis among this cohort. The most well-described virulence factor of *C. neoformans* is its capsule, which helps it to evade phagocytosis. In addition, the capsule also triggers hypocomplementemia and inhibits T-Cell activation. The antigen-presenting capacity of monocytes is also down-regulated by the capsule. Other factors like prevention of oxidative stress by a laccase enzyme, thermotolerance, and enzymes that facilitate transcellular migration also contribute to the virulence of *C. neoformans*. The organism also has the ability to survive nutrient starvation in the brain.

Clinical Features: CM usually presents with fever, headache, altered mental status, cranial nerve palsies, and coma [14]. The onset of disease usually takes 2 weeks among HIV + patients in whom disseminated disease is more likely. HIV − patients are likely to be symptomatic earlier. Ocular involvement is quite often encountered among patients with CM.

Diagnosis: The CSF is the most informative source for investigating a patient with suspected CM. The protein and white cell counts are elevated especially among HIV − patients. Low levels of glucose and lymphocytic predominance are seen in both HIV + and HIV − patients [15]. The commonly recommended India Ink preparation is a rapid tool which is highly operator-dependent. The sensitivity of the test is higher among HIV + patients. The organism can be detected in cultures in 3–7 days. The most sensitive test for the diagnosis of CM is the detection of cryptococcal capsular polysaccharide antigen in both serum and CSF using latex agglutination. There are no radiologic findings which are pathognomonic of CM. MRI, which is more sensitive than CT, can show lesions in the basal ganglia and midbrain. In addition, hydrocephalus, non-enhancing nodules, pseudocysts, masses, gyral enhancement, and lacunar/cortical infarcts are also part of the radiological spectrum of CM.

Treatment: Untreated CM has a high mortality rate. Host factors and fungal burden determine the rate of progression. The treatment is usually stratified according to three risk groups:

- HIV-infected individuals
- Organ transplant recipients and
- Non-HIV-infected and Non-Organ transplant recipient hosts

The treatment is usually administered in three steps—induction, consolidation, and maintenance [16]. The mainstay of treatment is Amphotericin B in combination with Flucytosine. This combination has been shown to be associated with better survival, lower nephrotoxicity, and shorter length of hospital stay. Liposomal Amphotericin B (L-AmB) is recommended for those with renal dysfunction or are recipients of organ transplant. The treatment regimen for various categories is shown in Table 56.11.

Table 56.11 Treatment regimens for various categories of Cryptococcal Meningitis

Phase	Regimen	Duration	Alternatives
Induction HIV-related disease Transplant-related Non-HIV, Non-Transplant	Amphotericin B Deoxycholate 0.7 mg/kg/day + flucytosine 100 mg/kg/day orally Liposomal Amphotericin B 3–4 mg/kg/day + flucytosine Amphotericin B deoxycholate or Liposomal Amhotericin B Liposomal Amphotericin B 3–4 mg/kg/day + flucytosine Amphotericin B deoxycholate (0.7–1.0 mg/kg/day) + flucytosine (100 mg/kg/day) Liposomal amphotericin B (3–4 mg/kg/day)	2 weeks 2 weeks 6 weeks if Flucytosine is not tolerated 2 weeks Atleast 4 weeks 4 weeks	Amphotericin B deoxycholate + fluconazole Fluconazole + flucytosine Fluconazole Itraconazole Liposomal amphotericin B 6 mg/kg/day for 4–6 weeks
Consolidation HIV-related disease Transplant-related Non-HIV, Non-transplant-related	Fluconazole (400 mg/day) Fluconazole (400–800 mg/day) Fluconazole (400–800 mg/day)	8 weeks 8 weeks 8 weeks	
Maintenance HIV-related disease Transplant-related Non-HIV, Non-transplant-related	Fluconazole (200 mg/day) Fluconazole (200–400 mg/day) Fluconazole (200 mg/day)	Atleast 1 year 6–12 months 6–12 months	Itraconazole (400 mg/day) Amphotericin B deoxycholate (1 mg/kg/week)

Table 56.12 Comparison of encephalitis and meningitis

Comparison	Meningitis	Encephalitis
Definition	Inflammation of meninges	Inflammation of brain parenchyma
Causative Agents	Bacteria, Viruses and Fungi	Mostly Viruses
Incubation period	Hours to days	3–5 days
Symptoms	Fever, headache, neck pain	Headache, seizures, altered sensorium
Risk groups	Elderly, immunocompromised, steroid users Invasive Neurosurgical procedures	Extremes of age
CSF findings	Low sugar, pleocytosis, elevated protein	Normal Sugar Raised protein
Vaccine availability	*Streptococcus pneumoniae* *Hemophilus influenzae*	Japanese B Encephalitis

56.8 Japanese B Encephalitis (JE)

Japanese B Encephalitis is probably the most common cause of vaccine preventable encephalitis in South East Asia [17]. The causative agent isolated in 1935 is a small single stranded RNA virus belonging to the Flavivirus genus, the same as Dengue. Among the five different genotypes of the JE virus known, genotype I is the most commonly identified variant in the post-vaccination database [18].

The main vector for JE is the Culex mosquito, with swine as the major amplifier hosts and Humans as "dead-end" hosts. The disease becomes manifest only in 1 in 25 human infections. Involvement of the CNS occurs in 1:200 infections and causes a mortality rate of 30% [19].

The disease should be suspected among all patients presenting with an acute encephalitis syndrome. Seizures and extra-pyramidal manifestations occur in the acute phase, sometimes associated with meningitis and flaccid paralysis [20, 21]. Radiologic abnormalities are non-specific and are seen in the thalamus, basal ganglia, and midbrain. The CSF manifestations are similar to those seen in other forms of encephalitis. The diagnostic criteria for JE are as follows:

1. Presence of JE IgM in CSF
2. Detection of JE Virus antigen, virus itself, or its genome in body fluids
3. Four-fold rise in JE IgG during convalescent phase

Treatment: There is no specific antiviral treatment for JE. Supportive treatment for seizure control, cerebral oedema management, and hypoglycemia are the cornerstones of treatment [22].

From the preceding discussion, it is obvious that there is a significant overlap in the manifestations of meningitis and encephalitis. However, there are subtle differences between the two disorders. These differentiating features are listed in Table 56.12.

56.9 Conclusion

Meningitis and encephalitis are associated with significant morbidity and mortality. Bacteria and viruses are the predominant cause of meningitis and encephalitis. CSF analysis and serology play a major role in diagnosis. Immunocompromised state alters the clinical course of both the diseases. A structured approach helps in treating a significant number of these infections.

References

1. Venkatesan A, Tunkel AR, Bloch KC, Lauring AS, Sejvar J, Bitnun A, International Encephalitis Consortium, et al. Case definitions, diagnostic algorithms, and priorities in encephalitis: consensus statement of the international encephalitis consortium. Clin Infect Dis. 2013;57:1114–28.
2. van de Beek D, de Gans J, Spanjaard L, Weisfelt M, Reitsma JB, Vermeulen M. Clinical features and prog-

nostic factors in adults with bacterial meningitis. N Engl J Med. 2004;351(18):1849–59.
3. van de Beek D, Cabellos C, Dzupova O, et al. ESCMID guideline: diagnosis and treatment of acute bacterial meningitis. Clin Microbiol Infect. 2016;22(Suppl 3):S37–62.
4. Murray K, Walker C, Herrington E, Lewis JA, McCormick J, Beasley DW, et al. Persistent infection with West Nile virus years after initial infection. J Infect Dis. 2010;201(1):2–4.
5. Huhn GD, Austin C, Langkop C, Kelly K, Lucht R, Lampman R, et al. The emergence of West Nile virus during a large outbreak in Illinois in 2002. Am J Trop Med Hyg. 2005;72(6):768–76.
6. Ferguson DD, Gershman K, LeBailly A, Petersen LR. Characteristics of the rash associated with West Nile virus fever. Clin Infect Dis. 2005;41(8):1204–7.
7. Chowers MY, Lang R, Nassar F, Ben-David D, Giladi M, Rubinshtein E, et al. Clinical characteristics of the West Nile fever outbreak, Israel, 2000. Emerg Infect Dis. 2001;7(4):675–8.
8. Salazar L, Hasbun R. Cranial imaging before lumbar puncture in adults with community-acquired meningitis: clinical utility and adherence to the Infectious Diseases Society of America guidelines. Clin Infect Dis. 2017;64(12):1657–62.
9. Yaramis A, Gurkan F, Elevli M, et al. Central nervous system tuberculosis in children: a review of 254 cases. Pediatrics. 1998;102:e49.
10. Xu HB, Jiang RH, Li L, Sha W, Xiao HP. Diagnostic value of adenosine deaminase in cerebrospinal fluid for tuberculous meningitis: a meta-analysis. Int J Tuberc Lung Dis. 2010;14:1382–7.
11. Donald PR, Schoeman JF, Vanzyl LE, et al. Intensive short-course chemotherapy in the management of tuberculous meningitis. Int J Tuberc Lung Dis. 1998;2:704–11.
12. Wilkinson RJ, Rohlwink U, Misra UK, et al. Tuberculous meningitis. Nat Rev Neurol. 2017;13:581–98.
13. Bradshaw MJ, Venkatesan A. Herpes simplex virus-1 encephalitis in adults: pathophysiology, diagnosis, and management. Neurotherapeutics. 2016;13:493–508. https://doi.org/10.1007/s13311-016-0433-7.
14. Perfect JR. Cryptococcosis (Cryptococcus neoformans and Cryptococcus gattii). In: Bennett JE, Dolin R, Blaser MJ, editors. Mandell, Douglas, and Bennett's principles and practice of infectious diseases. 8th ed. Philadelphia: Elsevier; 2015. p. 2934–48.
15. Jarvis JN, Bicanic T, Loyse A, Namarika D, Jackson A, Nussbaum JC, et al. Determinants of mortality in a combined cohort of 501 patients with HIV-associated Cryptococcal meningitis: implications for improving outcomes. Clin Infect Dis. 2014;58(5):736–45.
16. Perfect JR, Dismukes WE, Dromer F, Goldman DL, Graybill JR, Hamill RJ, et al. Clinical practice guidelines for the management of cryptococcal disease: 2010 update by the infectious diseases society of America. Clin Infect Dis. 2010;50(3):291–322.
17. Japanese encephalitis vaccines: WHO position paper—February 2015. Wkly Epidemiol Rec. 2015;90:69–87.
18. Schuh AJ, Ward MJ, Brown AJL, Barrett ADT. Phylogeography of Japanese encephalitis virus: genotype is associated with climate. PLoS Negl Trop Dis. 2013;7:e2411. https://doi.org/10.1371/journal.pntd.0002411.
19. Solomon T. Flavivirus encephalitis. N Engl J Med. 2004;351:370–8. https://doi.org/10.1056/NEJMra030476.
20. Solomon T, Dung NM, Kneen R, Thao LTT, Gainsborough M, Nisalak A, et al. Seizures and raised intracranial pressure in Vietnamese patients with Japanese encephalitis. Brain J Neurol. 2002;125:1084–93.
21. Solomon T, Thao TT, Lewthwaite P, Ooi MH, Kneen R, Dung NM, et al. A cohort study to assess the new WHO Japanese encephalitis surveillance standards. Bull World Health Organ. 2008;86:178–86.
22. Rao PN. Japanese encephalitis. Indian Pediatr. 2001;38:1252–64.

Part VIII

Special Considerations in Neurocritical Care

57 Pediatric Patients and Neurocritical Care

Ritesh Lamsal and Navindra R. Bista

57.1 Introduction

Pediatric neurocritical care (PNCC) is a diverse specialty that deals with critically ill children with neurological diseases. Pediatric neurocritical illnesses constitute a substantial disease burden accounting for nearly 20–30% of all pediatric critical care admissions [1–3]. Children with neurologic injuries have a higher rate of critical care admission and mortality compared with non-neurologic illnesses [1]. Neurologic injury is the proximate cause of death in a large fraction of PNCC admissions [4–6].

Traumatic brain injury, seizure disorders, tumors, and central nervous system (CNS) infections are the most common diagnoses in pediatric neurocritical care. Many systemic illnesses also lead to life-threatening neurologic complications in children that require PNCC admission [7]. With the steady rise in the numbers of pediatric neurosurgery and neurointervention, post-surgical patients also comprise a large share of admissions.

Neurological illnesses manifest differently in children compared with adults and require different treatment approaches. There is also a significant practice difference among physicians managing children with neurologic injuries. Part of this problem is because of the vast heterogeneity in the types of neurological problems that afflict children. Equally important is the lack of evidence-based knowledge in pediatric neurocritical care as most of the accumulated evidence is largely empirical and extrapolation of related research in adults.

57.2 PNCC Subspecialty

In adults, neurocritical care is an established specialty with wide-ranging practitioners. These include general intensivists, neurointensivists, neurologists, neurosurgeons, critical care nurses, and other supporting specialists. Dedicated adult neurocritical care units are common in contemporary clinical practice. It has also been found that neurointensivist-led dedicated neurocritical care units improve clinical outcomes [8, 9]. However, the development of PNCC units is still in its early stages. The majority of PNCC services function as consultative services [10].

Several difficulties limit the development of dedicated PNCC units. The patient population in PNCC is more diverse and requires a larger multidisciplinary collaboration and more specialist referrals than in adults [11]. The management of neonates, infants, and larger children demands very different skill sets. Also, the volume of children admitted to PNCC may not be sufficient in

R. Lamsal (✉) · N. R. Bista
Department of Anaesthesiology, Tribhuvan University Teaching Hospital, Institute of Medicine, Kathmandu, Nepal
e-mail: ritesh.lamsal@mmc.tu.edu.np

H. Prabhakar et al. (eds.), *Principles and Practice of Neurocritical Care*,
https://doi.org/10.1007/978-981-99-8059-8_57

many centers to develop a separate unit and justify the added utilization of resources. Dedicated pediatric neurocritical care units are found in only some large tertiary-level institutions. In most cases, children are managed in general pediatric intensive care units (PICUs) or mixed adult-pediatric neuro ICUs. In resource-limited settings, there may be no distinction and all critically ill patients may be managed in the same ICU. Additionally, there is no consensus on the training required for specialized pediatric neuro-intensivists and the organizational structure of a pediatric neuro ICU.

57.3 Physiological Considerations in Children

There are considerable differences in the physiology of the central nervous system in adults and children pertinent to the management of critically ill children. As brain maturation is incomplete at birth, neurophysiology develops rapidly in the first few years of life, corresponding with the anatomic, functional, and organizational development of the brain. Global cerebral blood flow as a fraction of cardiac output peaks around 2 years of age and stabilizes to adult values by 7–8 years of life [12]. Human brain glucose demand also peaks during early childhood [13]. Cerebral blood flow represents nearly half of the cardiac output between the ages of 1 and 3 years, which highlights the vulnerability of this population to neurological injury, even with transient hemodynamic alterations in the ICU.

Full-term infants have intact cerebral autoregulation and carbon dioxide reactivity. However, cerebral autoregulation is in a very narrow range in preterm newborns and children with neurocritical illnesses [14]. The autoregulation thresholds are variable in different disease conditions [15–18]. The CBF velocity may be entirely passive in preterm neonates up to 33 weeks of gestation [19]. Tight control of blood pressure is important in preterm infants and those with neurological illnesses, as they are extremely vulnerable to the effects of hypoperfusion, reperfusion, and hyperemia.

There are also important pathophysiological considerations in children with open fontanels and cranial sutures. Open fontanels and sutures and a less rigid skull may permit a greater expansion of mass lesions before neurological signs are apparent. Thus, expanding intracranial lesions, such as an intracranial hematoma or an abscess, may manifest late in small children with severe consequences as a result of the delayed diagnosis.

57.4 General Approach to Pediatric Neurocritical Care

Even though the broad principles of airway management, ventilation strategies, fluid and hemodynamic management, antimicrobial use, and nutrition appear similar across various disciplines of critical care, considerable differences exist in pediatric neurocritical care. As the brain and spinal cord are extremely vulnerable to the effects of hypoxia, ischemia, and systemic medications, children admitted to PNCC require rigorous monitoring and prompt treatment of physiological perturbations. Multimodal neuromonitoring is helpful to detect acute changes in physiological parameters. Any delay in therapeutic intervention can lead to serious complications in these children. Recent advances in neuromonitoring and neuroimaging have helped to individualize management strategies in PNCC.

57.5 Multimodal Neuromonitoring

Multimodal neuromonitoring is the concomitant use of several neuro-monitors to detect real-time physiologic changes that are clinically important. These monitors can be invasive or noninvasive and have distinct benefits and limitations. Several types of neuromonitoring are available in PNCC, such as intracranial pressure (ICP) monitoring, monitoring of electrophysiological parameters, brain tissue oxygenation, cerebral microdialysis, jugular venous oximetry, near-infrared spectroscopy, transcranial Doppler (TCD), and other imaging modalities (Table 57.1). Although

Table 57.1 Common neuro-monitors in pediatric neurocritical care

Neuromonitoring	Common monitors
Cerebral oxygenation	Invasive • Jugular bulb oximetry • Brain tissue oxygen tension Noninvasive • Near-infrared spectroscope
Cerebral blood flow	Noninvasive • Neuroimaging • Transcranial Doppler
Intracranial pressure	Invasive • Ventricular catheter • Microtransducer device (parenchymal/subdural) Noninvasive • Optic nerve sheath diameter • Transcranial Doppler • Neuroimaging
Cerebral electrical activity	Noninvasive • Electroencephalography (EEG) • Evoked potentials • Derived EEG indices
Cerebral metabolism	Invasive • Cerebral microdialysis
Cerebral autoregulation	Invasive • Brain tissue oxygen monitor • Intracranial pressure monitor Noninvasive • Transcranial Doppler • Near-infrared spectroscope

widely utilized in adult neurocritical care, there is a general lack of consensus and clinical evidence for adopting neuromonitoring-guided treatment decisions in children. ICP monitoring and EEG are routinely employed in most pediatric neurocritical care units [20]. Monitors for other organ systems like pulse oximetry, blood pressure, electrocardiogram, arterial gases, temperature, cardiac output, and point-of-care ultrasonography are common in all critical care units.

Continuous electroencephalogram (cEEG) is useful in PNCC as there may be no clear association between electrographic seizures and clinical features in children. Important uses of cEEG in PNCC are for the detection of nonconvulsive seizure (NCS) and nonconvulsive status epilepticus (NCSE). The incidence of NCSE in PNCC is high and is associated with poor outcomes [21, 22].

ICP monitoring is frequently used in pediatric neurocritical care. Invasive ICP monitoring is considered the gold standard; noninvasive estimation of ICP using transcranial Doppler, optic nerve sheath diameter, and quantitative pupillometry are also useful tools in children. Even though guideline-based recommendations for the use of ICP monitoring in children are only available for managing traumatic brain injury, ICP monitoring can be used in other conditions that cause intracranial hypertension, like intracranial bleeding, CNS infections, and post-cardiac arrest hypoxic states. ICP data can provide early warning of clinical deterioration and neuro-prognostication of critically ill children [23]. Despite promising data, ICP monitoring is less commonly performed in children than in adults, even though children are at a higher risk of developing raised ICP [24]. Some important reasons include resource limitations, concerns of infection, hemorrhage, malposition, and malfunction, and a lack of strong evidence that ICP-targeted management approach leads to better clinical outcomes in children [25].

Transcranial Doppler has broad-ranging applications in pediatric neurocritical care. It can predict ICP in children when placing an ICP catheter is contraindicated or not possible because of resource constraints [26]. TCD helps diagnose and monitor the progression of cerebral vasospasm. Vasospasm is common in conditions like ruptured aneurysms and arteriovenous malformations, resection of brain tumors, and TBI. It can also be used to assess cerebral autoregulation. Valid TCD-based methods of testing both dynamic and static autoregulation exist [27]. There are several other uses of TCD described in critical care, including monitoring hemodynamic changes after stroke and diagnosis of brain death [28].

57.6 Important Pediatric Neurocritical Care Conditions

57.6.1 Traumatic Brain Injury

Primary traumatic brain injury is broadly divided into extra-parenchymal (epidural hematoma, subdural hematoma, subarachnoid hemorrhage, intraventricular hemorrhage), intraparenchymal (contusion, diffuse axonal injury), and vascular (dissection, carotid-cavernous fistula, pseudoaneurysm). TBI is an important cause of pediatric neurocritical care admission. Clinical presentation of traumatic brain injury may be distinct from adults and depends on the nature and site of brain injury, concurrent multisystem injury, the child's developmental stage, and difficulties associated with neurologic examination in children. TBI is a leading cause of mortality and physical disability in children [29, 30]. Many children who survive the initial injury have other long-term consequences, such as cognitive deficits, psychosocial problems, memory and learning problems, motor deficits, and neurodegenerative diseases [31–33].

Children with severe TBI require a period of mechanical ventilation and ICU management. Evidence-based treatment is often complicated as many experimental drugs have failed to demonstrate neuroprotective efficacy. Similarly, acute, subacute, and chronic CNS biomarkers have failed to add meaningful diagnostic, therapeutic, or prognostic insight in children [34].

Patients with severe TBI are at risk of developing intracranial hypertension, and ICP monitoring is useful to guide treatment decisions. Even though there is no robust evidence, children with severe TBI who have ICP monitoring may have a small survival benefit over those without ICP monitoring [35, 36]. The accepted threshold to start treatment for intracranial hypertension in children is 20 mmHg. Cerebral perfusion pressure (CPP) is maintained between 40 and 50 mmHg [37]. However, it may be prudent to maintain the CPP at the lower end of this spectrum in infants and at the higher end of the targeted CPP range in adolescents. Sedatives and analgesics are required for the general management of all children with severe TBI. A bolus of 3% hypertonic saline should be used to lower acute intracranial hypertension in children. Hypertonic saline may be better than mannitol to reduce ICP in children [38]. A continuous infusion or a higher concentration of saline may be needed in children with refractory rise of ICP. Like in adults, prophylactic antiseizure medications are indicated to control early (<7 days) post-traumatic seizures [39]. Steroids and prophylactic hypothermia should not be used to improve outcomes in children with severe TBI. The Guidelines for the Management of Pediatric Severe Traumatic Brain Injury are the most comprehensive set of guidelines to manage children who suffer a severe TBI [40].

57.6.2 Stroke

Stroke is a leading cause of mortality and morbidity in children. Long-term neurologic deficits are present in over 60% of children who survive stroke [41]. There is a high incidence of stroke in neonates and infants, accounting for nearly half of all pediatric strokes [42]. Stroke incidence then gradually declines and remains low in older children.

The etiopathogenesis and management of pediatric stroke differ from adults. In particular, the risk factors for stroke are markedly different, as atherosclerotic disease is not common in children. Similarly, the clinical presentation is highly variable depending on the age of the patient and whether the stroke is ischemic or hemorrhagic, and further, arterial, or venous. Hemorrhagic strokes are more common in children than adults [43]. Most children with arterial stroke have arteriopathy, congenital or acquired cardiac disorders, or some form of underlying infection [44]. Other risk factors include chronic systemic disorders and prothrombotic states. The diagnosis is often delayed in children, hindering the timely initiation of treatment for stroke.

Evidence-based treatment guidelines for pediatric stroke are lacking. Treatment depends on the specific stroke subtype and the underlying pathophysiology. Unlike in adults, thrombolysis for acute ischemic stroke is not universally accepted as the standard of care, mainly because of deficient outcome data after thrombolysis and the high rate of stroke mimics in children [45]. In experienced centers, tissue plasminogen activator (tPA) can be administered to selected children who can be treated within 3–4.5 h of stroke onset. The overall experience with intra-arterial thrombolysis and mechanical thrombectomy in pediatric stroke is even more limited. As only a small number of children with ischemic stroke are eligible for reperfusion strategies, neurocritical care management is mainly focused on the optimal delivery of other supportive measures to reduce secondary neurologic injury.

Fluid and electrolyte disturbances are common in all children with stroke and need careful consideration, especially in those with reduced oral intake. Maintenance isotonic fluids are usually required to prevent dehydration and ensure hemodynamic stability. Enteral feeding should be started as soon as possible depending on the patient's neurological condition. In neurocritical care practice, feeding is only started after a swallowing test. Seizure is one of the commonest presentations of pediatric stroke and needs to be aggressively controlled. Intracranial hypertension, fever, hemodynamic disturbances, and hypoglycemia should be treated. Patients with malignant cerebral edema after a large-vessel stroke or a significant hemorrhagic transformation may need decompressive craniectomy to lower the ICP [46].

57.6.3 Status Epilepticus

Status epilepticus is a life-threatening medical emergency in children defined as 5 min or more of continuous clinical or electrographic seizure or recurrent seizure without recovery to baseline [47]. Status epilepticus may develop because of underlying epilepsy or in response to an acute illness, such as a CNS infection, hypoxia, dyselectrolytemia, metabolic disorder, traumatic brain injury, or stroke [48].

The diagnosis of convulsive status epilepticus is clinical and treatment is time-tiered. The goal is to promptly terminate clinical and electrographic seizure activity. Treatment should begin with supportive care, which may include airway and breathing support, circulatory support, fever control, and correction of hypoglycemia and metabolic derangements. Supportive care should be provided concurrently with emergent pharmacologic control of seizures. Delay in the administration of anti-seizure drugs strongly correlates with prolonged status epilepticus and a lower response to anticonvulsants [49, 50]. The emergent anti-seizure drug is a rapid-acting benzodiazepine, such as lorazepam, diazepam, or midazolam. Emergent therapy is followed by urgent therapy with a long-acting non-benzodiazepine anti-seizure drug such as levetiracetam, phenytoin, or valproate [51, 52]. Urgent therapy with a second drug is required as short-acting benzodiazepines will achieve seizure control in only half the patients with an established status epilepticus [52]. The emergent medication may be repeated in 5–10 min depending on clinical response.

Refractory status epilepticus (>30 min) may occur in up to 40% of children with status epilepticus [53]. Patients with refractory status epilepticus will require endotracheal intubation and a continuous infusion of anti-seizure medication [54]. Propofol infusion is commonly used in adults with refractory status epilepticus; however, safety concerns limit its use in children. Midazolam infusion is common in PNCC. Additional diagnostic testing, such as brain imaging, cerebrospinal fluid analysis, arterial gases, toxicology profiling, and liver function tests, may be performed. Continuous electroencephalogram is useful for monitoring response to treatment and escalation or de-escalation of therapy. In refractory status, other antiseizure medications like lacosamide, topiramate, ketamine, and a ketogenic diet may also be useful.

57.6.4 Central Nervous System Infections

CNS infections are another important cause of morbidity and mortality in pediatric neurocritical care. The case fatality rate of acute CNS infections in children can be as high as 30% in resource-poor environments [55]. In children, CNS infections have distinct geographic, etiologic, and seasonal differences. There are also important differences in the burden of CNS infections in high and low-income countries. Easy access to antimicrobials and vaccination has reduced the burden of community-acquired CNS infections in resource-rich countries; whereas, it remains a significant problem in other countries [49, 56]. CNS infections are the commonest cause of status epilepticus in resource-poor environments [57]. There are also some infections common in certain endemic regions, like cerebral malaria and tuberculous meningitis, or in certain populations like fungal infections in immunocompromised children. Many children admitted to neurocritical care also have significant comorbid illnesses that increase their susceptibility to CNS infections.

Acute Bacterial Meningitis

The common pathogens responsible for bacterial meningitis in children differ by age group (Table 57.2). *Neisseria meningitides*, *Haemophilus influenzae*, and *Streptococcus pneumoniae* are the most common pathogens causing meningitis in children [58, 59]. In neonates and small infants, Group B *Streptococcus* and *Escherichia coli* are common causes. Nearly 50% of children with bacterial meningitis develop neurologic or systemic complications and require ICU care [59]. Children admitted to neurocritical care have a multitude of neurologic findings, such as irritability, lethargy, altered mental status, seizures, increased ICP, and depressed consciousness. There may be other major systemic manifestations like coagulopathy, septic shock, and acute respiratory distress syndrome.

Table 57.2 Common age-wise cause of bacterial meningitis[a]

Age-group	Bacteria
Neonates	Group B Streptococcus *Escherichia coli* *Enterococcus* *Listeria monocytogenes*
Infants <3 months	Group B Streptococcus *Escherichia coli* *Gram negative bacilli*
Young children	*Streptococcus pneumoniae* *Neisseria meningitides*
Adolescents	*Neisseria meningitides* *Streptococcus pneumoniae* *Haemophilus influenzae*

[a]There may be significant geographic differences in causative organisms

The major goals of treating bacterial meningitis in PNCC include antimicrobial therapy, supportive measures, and infective source control. Prompt parenteral antibiotic therapy is the cornerstone of treatment. This should be initiated immediately after blood and CSF samples are obtained. The initial antibiotic regimen depends on the suspected bacteria (based on the age of the child and geographic location) and local antibiotic sensitivity patterns. Vancomycin along with a third-generation cephalosporin is commonly used for empirical therapy in neurocritical care settings. Supportive measures like respiratory support, hemodynamic support with fluids and vasopressors, treatment of metabolic disturbances, and seizure control may be required in the ICU. In some cases, an intracranial device, such as an external ventricular drain, can be the source of infection and needs to be removed urgently. Surgical treatment may also be required to drain a brain or an ear abscess, or to treat meningitis-related complications like subdural empyema and hydrocephalus.

Aseptic Meningitis and Encephalitis

All nonbacterial meningitis, including those cases with no known cause, are classified as aseptic meningitis. Viral infections are the most common cause of aseptic meningitis in PNCC [60]. The causative organisms for viral meningitis differ in various age groups and different geographic locations. The clinical manifestations are similar to features of bacterial meningitis, but are usually less severe. Viral meningitis can progress to encephalitis, which commonly presents as seizures and focal neurologic signs. Enteroviruses are the most common cause of viral meningitis in children [61]. Multisystem involvement is common in meningitis/encephalitis caused by herpesviruses like herpes simplex virus, Epstein-Barr virus, and cytomegalovirus [62, 63]. Arthropod or insect-borne arbovirus encephalitis is common in some geographic locations [64].

In most cases of viral meningitis/encephalitis, treatment in PNCC is largely supportive, comprising intravascular volume support, analgesics, antiseizure drugs, and multisystem support for disseminated disease. Acyclovir is indicated in children of all age groups with suspected or proven herpes simplex virus encephalitis [65]. Antivirals are also recommended to treat influenza infections [66]. For other types of viral meningitis/encephalitis, specific antivirals either do not exist or have no strong evidence of benefit in children. Steroids, immunoglobulins, plasmapheresis, and other immunomodulators have a limited role in the treatment of viral encephalitis in children.

57.7 Conclusion

The diversity of pediatric illnesses requiring neurocritical care admission is vast. The increasing complexity of care requires a multidisciplinary approach for optimal treatment. It is vital to minimize secondary neurologic illnesses in PNCC by a prompt diagnosis, multimodal neuromonitoring, targeted therapy, lowering of intracranial hypertension, and multi-organ support. Improved understanding of various neurocritical care conditions, including advances in monitoring, neuroimaging, laboratory support, and therapeutics, has steadily improved clinical outcomes in PNCC. The way forward in pediatric neurocritical care is to foster the culture of clinical research, expand the quality of basic and translational research, focus on improving the quality of care, and increase collaboration between and within institutions.

References

1. Moreau JF, Fink EL, Hartman ME, Angus DC, Bell MJ, Linde-Zwirble WT, et al. Hospitalizations of children with neurologic disorders in the United States. Pediatr Crit Care Med. 2013;14(8):801–10. https://doi.org/10.1097/PCC.0b013e31828aa71f.
2. Fink EL, Kochanek PM, Tasker RC, Beca J, Bell MJ, Clark RS, et al. International survey of critically ill children with acute neurologic insults: the prevalence of acute critical neurological disease in children: a global epidemiological assessment study. Pediatr Crit Care Med. 2017;18(4):330–42. https://doi.org/10.1097/pcc.0000000000001093.
3. Chang N, Rasmussen L. Exploring trends in neuromonitoring use in a general pediatric ICU: the need for standardized guidance. Children (Basel). 2022;9(7) https://doi.org/10.3390/children9070934.
4. Au AK, Carcillo JA, Clark RS, Bell MJ. Brain injuries and neurological system failure are the most common proximate causes of death in children admitted to a pediatric intensive care unit. Pediatr Crit Care Med. 2011;12(5):566–71. https://doi.org/10.1097/PCC.0b013e3181fe3420.
5. Ruttimann UE, Pollack MM. Variability in duration of stay in pediatric intensive care units: a multiinstitutional study. J Pediatr. 1996;128(1):35–44. https://doi.org/10.1016/s0022-3476(96)70425-0.
6. Arias Y, Taylor DS, Marcin JP. Association between evening admissions and higher mortality rates in the pediatric intensive care unit. Pediatrics. 2004;113(6):e530–4. https://doi.org/10.1542/peds.113.6.e530.
7. Wainwright MS, Hansen G, Piantino J. Pediatric neurocritical care in the 21st century: from empiricism to evidence. Curr Opin Crit Care. 2016;22(2):106–12. https://doi.org/10.1097/mcc.0000000000000288.
8. Kramer AH, Zygun DA. Do neurocritical care units save lives? Measuring the impact of specialized ICUs. Neurocrit Care. 2011;14(3):329–33. https://doi.org/10.1007/s12028-011-9530-y.
9. Samuels O, Webb A, Culler S, Martin K, Barrow D. Impact of a dedicated neurocritical care team in treating patients with aneurysmal subarachnoid hemorrhage. Neurocrit Care. 2011;14(3):334–40. https://doi.org/10.1007/s12028-011-9505-z.
10. LaRovere KL, Murphy SA, Horak R, Vittner P, Kapur K, Proctor M, et al. Pediatric neurocritical care: evolution of a new clinical service in PICUs across the United States. Pediatr Crit Care Med. 2018;19(11):1039–45. https://doi.org/10.1097/pcc.0000000000001708.
11. Bell MJ, Carpenter J, Au AK, Keating RF, Myseros JS, Yaun A, et al. Development of a pediatric neurocritical care service. Neurocrit Care. 2009;10(1):4–10. https://doi.org/10.1007/s12028-008-9061-3.
12. Wintermark M, Lepori D, Cotting J, Roulet E, van Melle G, Meuli R, et al. Brain perfusion in children: evolution with age assessed by quantitative perfusion computed tomography. Pediatrics. 2004;113(6):1642–52. https://doi.org/10.1542/peds.113.6.1642.
13. Kuzawa CW, Chugani HT, Grossman LI, Lipovich L, Muzik O, Hof PR, et al. Metabolic costs and evolutionary implications of human brain development. Proc Natl Acad Sci USA. 2014;111(36):13010–5. https://doi.org/10.1073/pnas.1323099111.
14. Rhee CJ, da Costa CS, Austin T, Brady KM, Czosnyka M, Lee JK. Neonatal cerebrovascular autoregulation. Pediatr Res. 2018;84(5):602–10. https://doi.org/10.1038/s41390-018-0141-6.
15. Brady KM, Mytar JO, Lee JK, Cameron DE, Vricella LA, Thompson WR, et al. Monitoring cerebral blood flow pressure autoregulation in pediatric patients during cardiac surgery. Stroke. 2010;41(9):1957–62. https://doi.org/10.1161/strokeaha.109.575167.
16. Zipfel J, Hockel KL, Gerbig I, Heimberg E, Schuhmann MU, Neunhoeffer F. Impaired autoregulation following resuscitation correlates with

outcome in pediatric patients: a pilot study. Acta Neurochir Suppl. 2021;131:97–101. https://doi.org/10.1007/978-3-030-59436-7_21.
17. Lee JK, Williams M, Jennings JM, Jamrogowicz JL, Larson AC, Jordan LC, et al. Cerebrovascular autoregulation in pediatric moyamoya disease. Paediatr Anaesth. 2013;23(6):547–56. https://doi.org/10.1111/pan.12140.
18. Kooi EMW, Richter AE. Cerebral autoregulation in sick infants: current insights. Clin Perinatol. 2020;47(3):449–67. https://doi.org/10.1016/j.clp.2020.05.003.
19. Rhee CJ, Fraser CD 3rd, Kibler K, Easley RB, Andropoulos DB, Czosnyka M, et al. The ontogeny of cerebrovascular pressure autoregulation in premature infants. J Perinatol. 2014;34(12):926–31. https://doi.org/10.1038/jp.2014.122.
20. Kirschen MP, LaRovere K, Balakrishnan B, Erklauer J, Francoeur C, Ganesan SL, et al. A survey of neuromonitoring practices in North American pediatric intensive care units. Pediatr Neurol. 2022;126:125–30. https://doi.org/10.1016/j.pediatrneurol.2021.11.002.
21. Alehan FK, Morton LD, Pellock JM. Utility of electroencephalography in the pediatric emergency department. J Child Neurol. 2001;16(7):484–7. https://doi.org/10.1177/088307380101600704.
22. Topjian AA, Gutierrez-Colina AM, Sanchez SM, Berg RA, Friess SH, Dlugos DJ, et al. Electrographic status epilepticus is associated with mortality and worse short-term outcome in critically ill children. Crit Care Med. 2013;41(1):215–23. https://doi.org/10.1097/CCM.0b013e3182668035.
23. Güiza F, Depreitere B, Piper I, Citerio G, Jorens PG, Maas A, et al. Early detection of increased intracranial pressure episodes in traumatic brain injury: external validation in an adult and in a pediatric cohort. Crit Care Med. 2017;45(3):e316–e20. https://doi.org/10.1097/ccm.0000000000002080.
24. Keenan HT, Nocera M, Bratton SL. Frequency of intracranial pressure monitoring in infants and young toddlers with traumatic brain injury. Pediatr Crit Care Med. 2005;6(5):537–41. https://doi.org/10.1097/01.pcc.0000164638.44600.67.
25. Bennett TD, DeWitt PE, Greene TH, Srivastava R, Riva-Cambrin J, Nance ML, et al. Functional outcome after intracranial pressure monitoring for children with severe traumatic brain injury. JAMA Pediatr. 2017;171(10):965–71. https://doi.org/10.1001/jamapediatrics.2017.2127.
26. Melo JR, Di Rocco F, Blanot S, Cuttaree H, Sainte-Rose C, Oliveira-Filho J, et al. Transcranial Doppler can predict intracranial hypertension in children with severe traumatic brain injuries. Childs Nerv Syst. 2011;27(6):979–84. https://doi.org/10.1007/s00381-010-1367-8.
27. Panerai RB. Transcranial Doppler for evaluation of cerebral autoregulation. Clin Auton Res. 2009;19(4):197–211. https://doi.org/10.1007/s10286-009-0011-8.
28. LaRovere KL, O'Brien NF. Transcranial Doppler sonography in pediatric neurocritical care: a review of clinical applications and case illustrations in the pediatric intensive care unit. J Ultrasound Med. 2015;34(12):2121–32. https://doi.org/10.7863/ultra.15.02016.
29. Cheng P, Li R, Schwebel DC, Zhu M, Hu G. Traumatic brain injury mortality among U.S. children and adolescents ages 0-19 years, 1999-2017. J Saf Res. 2020;72:93–100. https://doi.org/10.1016/j.jsr.2019.12.013.
30. Dewan MC, Mummareddy N, Wellons JC 3rd, Bonfield CM. Epidemiology of global pediatric traumatic brain injury: qualitative review. World Neurosurg. 2016;91:497–509.e1. https://doi.org/10.1016/j.wneu.2016.03.045.
31. DeKosky ST, Asken BM. Injury cascades in TBI-related neurodegeneration. Brain Inj. 2017;31(9):1177–82. https://doi.org/10.1080/02699052.2017.1312528.
32. Johnson VE, Stewart JE, Begbie FD, Trojanowski JQ, Smith DH, Stewart W. Inflammation and white matter degeneration persist for years after a single traumatic brain injury. Brain. 2013;136(Pt 1):28–42. https://doi.org/10.1093/brain/aws322.
33. Herrero Babiloni A, Baril AA, Charlebois-Plante C, Jodoin M, Sanchez E, De Baets L, et al. The putative role of neuroinflammation in the interaction between traumatic brain injuries, sleep, pain and other neuropsychiatric outcomes: a state-of-the-art review. J Clin Med. 2023;12(5):1793. https://doi.org/10.3390/jcm12051793.
34. Wang KK, Yang Z, Zhu T, Shi Y, Rubenstein R, Tyndall JA, et al. An update on diagnostic and prognostic biomarkers for traumatic brain injury. Expert Rev Mol Diagn. 2018;18(2):165–80. https://doi.org/10.1080/14737159.2018.1428089.
35. Alkhoury F, Kyriakides TC. Intracranial pressure monitoring in children with severe traumatic brain injury: national trauma data bank-based review of outcomes. JAMA Surg. 2014;149(6):544–8. https://doi.org/10.1001/jamasurg.2013.4329.
36. Alali AS, Gomez D, Sathya C, Burd RS, Mainprize TG, Moulton R, et al. Intracranial pressure monitoring among children with severe traumatic brain injury. J Neurosurg Pediatr. 2015;16(5):523–32. https://doi.org/10.3171/2015.3.Peds14507.
37. Miller Ferguson N, Shein SL, Kochanek PM, Luther J, Wisniewski SR, Clark RS, et al. Intracranial hypertension and cerebral hypoperfusion in children with severe traumatic brain injury: thresholds and burden in accidental and abusive insults. Pediatr Crit Care Med. 2016;17(5):444–50. https://doi.org/10.1097/pcc.0000000000000709.
38. Shein SL, Ferguson NM, Kochanek PM, Bayir H, Clark RS, Fink EL, et al. Effectiveness of pharmacological therapies for intracranial hypertension in children with severe traumatic brain injury—results from an automated data collection system time-synched to drug administration. Pediatr Crit Care

Med. 2016;17(3):236–45. https://doi.org/10.1097/pcc.0000000000000610.

39. Liesemer K, Bratton SL, Zebrack CM, Brockmeyer D, Statler KD. Early post-traumatic seizures in moderate to severe pediatric traumatic brain injury: rates, risk factors, and clinical features. J Neurotrauma. 2011;28(5):755–62. https://doi.org/10.1089/neu.2010.1518.
40. Kochanek PM, Tasker RC, Carney N, Totten AM, Adelson PD, Selden NR, et al. Guidelines for the management of pediatric severe traumatic brain injury, third edition: update of the brain trauma foundation guidelines, executive summary. Neurosurgery. 2019;84(6):1169–78. https://doi.org/10.1093/neuros/nyz051.
41. Ganesan V, Hogan A, Shack N, Gordon A, Isaacs E, Kirkham FJ. Outcome after ischaemic stroke in childhood. Dev Med Child Neurol. 2000;42(7):455–61. https://doi.org/10.1017/s0012162200000852.
42. deVeber GA, Kirton A, Booth FA, Yager JY, Wirrell EC, Wood E, et al. Epidemiology and outcomes of arterial ischemic stroke in children: the Canadian Pediatric Ischemic Stroke Registry. Pediatr Neurol. 2017;69:58–70. https://doi.org/10.1016/j.pediatrneurol.2017.01.016.
43. Sporns PB, Fullerton HJ, Lee S, Kim H, Lo WD, Mackay MT, et al. Childhood stroke. Nat Rev Dis Primers. 2022;8(1):12. https://doi.org/10.1038/s41572-022-00337-x.
44. Mallick AA, Ganesan V, Kirkham FJ, Fallon P, Hedderly T, McShane T, et al. Childhood arterial ischaemic stroke incidence, presenting features, and risk factors: a prospective population-based study. Lancet Neurol. 2014;13(1):35–43. https://doi.org/10.1016/s1474-4422(13)70290-4.
45. Elbers J, Wainwright MS, Amlie-Lefond C. The pediatric stroke code: early management of the child with stroke. J Pediatr. 2015;167(1):19–24.e1–4. https://doi.org/10.1016/j.jpeds.2015.03.051.
46. Beez T, Munoz-Bendix C, Steiger HJ, Beseoglu K. Decompressive craniectomy for acute ischemic stroke. Crit Care. 2019;23(1):209. https://doi.org/10.1186/s13054-019-2490-x.
47. Brophy GM, Bell R, Claassen J, Alldredge B, Bleck TP, Glauser T, et al. Guidelines for the evaluation and management of status epilepticus. Neurocrit Care. 2012;17(1):3–23. https://doi.org/10.1007/s12028-012-9695-z.
48. Barcia Aguilar C, Sánchez Fernández I, Loddenkemper T. Status epilepticus-work-up and management in children. Semin Neurol. 2020;40(6):661–74. https://doi.org/10.1055/s-0040-1719076.
49. Chin RF, Neville BG, Peckham C, Wade A, Bedford H, Scott RC. Treatment of community-onset, childhood convulsive status epilepticus: a prospective, population-based study. Lancet Neurol. 2008;7(8):696–703. https://doi.org/10.1016/s1474-4422(08)70141-8.
50. Eriksson K, Metsäranta P, Huhtala H, Auvinen A, Kuusela AL, Koivikko M. Treatment delay and the risk of prolonged status epilepticus. Neurology. 2005;65(8):1316–8. https://doi.org/10.1212/01.wnl.0000180959.31355.92.
51. Chamberlain JM, Okada P, Holsti M, Mahajan P, Brown KM, Vance C, et al. Lorazepam vs diazepam for pediatric status epilepticus: a randomized clinical trial. JAMA. 2014;311(16):1652–60. https://doi.org/10.1001/jama.2014.2625.
52. Lewena S, Pennington V, Acworth J, Thornton S, Ngo P, McIntyre S, et al. Emergency management of pediatric convulsive status epilepticus: a multicenter study of 542 patients. Pediatr Emerg Care. 2009;25(2):83–7. https://doi.org/10.1097/PEC.0b013e318196ea6e.
53. Lewena S, Young S. When benzodiazepines fail: how effective is second line therapy for status epilepticus in children? Emerg Med Australas. 2006;18(1):45–50. https://doi.org/10.1111/j.1742-6723.2006.00807.x.
54. Abend NS, Dlugos DJ. Treatment of refractory status epilepticus: literature review and a proposed protocol. Pediatr Neurol. 2008;38(6):377–90. https://doi.org/10.1016/j.pediatrneurol.2008.01.001.
55. Expanding poliomyelitis and measles surveillance networks to establish surveillance for acute meningitis and encephalitis syndromes—Bangladesh, China, and India, 2006–2008. MMWR Morb Mortal Wkly Rep. 2012;61(49):1008–11.
56. O'Horo JC, Sampathkumar P. Infections in neurocritical care. Neurocrit Care. 2017;27(3):458–67. https://doi.org/10.1007/s12028-017-0420-9.
57. Singhi P. Central nervous system infections in children: an ongoing challenge! Indian J Pediatr. 2019;86(1):49–51. https://doi.org/10.1007/s12098-018-2745-6.
58. Okike IO, Ribeiro S, Ramsay ME, Heath PT, Sharland M, Ladhani SN. Trends in bacterial, mycobacterial, and fungal meningitis in England and Wales 2004-11: an observational study. Lancet Infect Dis. 2014;14(4):301–7. https://doi.org/10.1016/s1473-3099(13)70332-3.
59. Husain E, Chawla R, Dobson S, Dele DH. Epidemiology and outcome of bacterial meningitis in Canadian children: 1998-1999. Clin Invest Med. 2006;29(3):131–5.
60. Tapiainen T, Prevots R, Izurieta HS, Abramson J, Bilynsky R, Bonhoeffer J, et al. Aseptic meningitis: case definition and guidelines for collection, analysis and presentation of immunization safety data. Vaccine. 2007;25(31):5793–802. https://doi.org/10.1016/j.vaccine.2007.04.058.
61. McBride M, Williman J, Best E, Walls T, Sadarangani M, Grant CC, et al. The epidemiology of aseptic meningitis in New Zealand children from 1991 to 2020. J Paediatr Child Health. 2022;58(11):1980–9. https://doi.org/10.1111/jpc.16131.
62. Hudson JA, Broad J, Martin NG, Sadarangani M, Galal U, Kelly DF, et al. Outcomes beyond hospital discharge in infants and children with viral meningitis: a systematic review. Rev Med Virol. 2020;30(2):e2083. https://doi.org/10.1002/rmv.2083.

63. Nigrovic LE, Fine AM, Monuteaux MC, Shah SS, Neuman MI. Trends in the management of viral meningitis at United States children's hospitals. Pediatrics. 2013;131(4):670–6. https://doi.org/10.1542/peds.2012-3077.
64. Logan SA, MacMahon E. Viral meningitis. BMJ. 2008;336(7634):36–40. https://doi.org/10.1136/bmj.39409.673657.AE.
65. Sanders JE, Garcia SE. Pediatric herpes simplex virus infections: an evidence-based approach to treatment. Pediatr Emerg Med Pract. 2014;11(1):1–19; quiz.
66. Costa BKD, Sato DK. Viral encephalitis: a practical review on diagnostic approach and treatment. J Pediatr. 2020;96(Suppl 1):12–9. https://doi.org/10.1016/j.jped.2019.07.006.

58 Geriatric Neurocritical Care

Swagata Tripathy

58.1 Introduction

One of the most significant concerns of the twenty-first century is providing care for the aging population. An important component of medical care delivery for the elderly is the provision of critical care services. A combination of age, function, and social definitions is essential to define the aged population accurately. The global population demographics have transformed with economic development. Death rates have declined, and birth rates have steadily increased over the last 200 years. Termed as 'baby boom,' this has resulted in an imbalance, as a result of which, the global senior population will surpass the global youth population by 2050 for the first time in history [1].

The World Health Organization (WHO) reports that in 2019, the average life expectancy for people worldwide was 73.4 years. Nevertheless, the average life expectancy in emerging nations is only about 50 years [2]. Most wealthy countries use 65 as the threshold for defining old age, although this definition is only sometimes applicable in poorer nations. Although aging is a biological chronologic fact, it is also influenced by cultural and social constructs. In affluent countries such as the United States, chronologic age plays a fundamental role. However, in emerging nations, the shift in social roles greatly influences how the elderly are defined. People who can no longer contribute to their designated social position may be considered old.

58.2 Frailty in Geriatrics

As the population ages, the concept of frailty has gained importance [3]. Frailty is defined as a lifetime accumulation of deterioration in diverse physiological systems [4]. Due to the accumulation of the slow cumulative degradation, it is a state of susceptibility resulting from poor resolution of homeostasis following a stressor event. As this cumulative deterioration depletes homoeostatic reserves, exaggerated changes in health status are eventually brought on by modest stressor events. Research demonstrates the link between frailty and unfavorable health outcomes. Frailty is prevalent, especially in older people with severe chronic illnesses such as chronic obstructive lung disease and heart failure. While there is not yet any agreement on the optimal way to test and diagnose frailty, specific frailty markers, including premorbid slow gait speed, offer a promising and workable alternative. Eliciting a history suggestive of frailty in hospitals and ICUs may offer the chance to direct appropriate patient counselling and proactive preventative measures

S. Tripathy (✉)
AIIMS Bhubaneswar, Bhubaneswar, India

H. Prabhakar et al. (eds.), *Principles and Practice of Neurocritical Care*,
https://doi.org/10.1007/978-981-99-8059-8_58

when considering medical interventions. Identifying frailty may also aid in locating coexisting conditions that could affect or contribute to frailty and aid in their management [5].

Frailty and aging are not the same, although older people are likelier to be weak. It is estimated that 25% of people over 65 and over 50% of people over 85 are frail [6]. Properly selecting elderly patients for therapies would be greatly aided by effective methods to identify frailty and gauge its severity in routine clinical practice. This could additionally serve as the foundation for a change in the care of frail elderly patients from condition-specific care to more appropriate goal-directed care [4].

58.3 Frailty and Critical Care

Critically ill patients' baseline condition in terms of functional status and chronic health status has an important influence on patient outcomes. To better understand how frailty affects ICU outcomes, a metanalysis of 3030 patients—927 fragile and 2103 fit patients—was conducted. Frailty was linked to higher hospital and long-term mortality (RR 1.71; 95% CI 1.43, 2.05; *p* 0.00001 and RR 1.53; 95% CI 1.40, 1.68; *p* 0.00001), respectively. Frailty was prevalent at 30% (95% CI: 29–32%). Compared to fit patients, frail patients had a lower likelihood of being sent home (RR 0.59; 95% CI 0.49, 0.71; *p* 0.00001) [7].

Time Limited Trial (TLT) has been proposed as an approach to frail and elderly patients' ICU care and management since predicting their response to aggressive interventions is often difficult. A screening checklist and mnemonic, "F-R-A-I-L," has been suggested to stimulate TLT conversation while considering ICU admission: **F**unctional impairment, **R**ecurrent hospital stays, **A**dvanced chronic diseases or cancer, **I**rreversible organ failure, and a **L**engthy hospital stay are all examples of impairments. The symptoms of frailty syndrome, expected restricted recovery potential, and poor response to continuing therapy or other underlying conditions are all represented by these problems, which are associated with a worse clinical outcome. Conceptually, given the hazy incremental clinical value of ICU admission, patients who satisfy any one of these criteria are more likely to gain from an early TLT discussion [8].

58.4 Neurocritical Care and Geriatric Outcomes

58.4.1 Frailty and Traumatic Brain Injury

Recent estimates place the number of traumatic brain injuries (TBI) in senior patients at 155,000 per year, with over 12,000 deaths as a result. Its incidence has more than doubled in the last 18 years and is highest for people 83–90 [9]. In an elderly patient, brain damage can occur through simple head rotation or deceleration without needing an external force. Subdural hematomas, acute or chronic, are the most typical symptom following TBI in older people. Beyond the age of 50, subdural hematomas are more frequent than extradural hematomas. In individuals with TBI, contusions develop roughly at the same rate and expand considerably in about one-third of cases. Older adults are more likely to develop intracerebral hematomas, probably connected to the reduced blood vessel flexibility brought on by atherosclerosis [10].

A direct correlation has been noted between mortality at 6 months and post-fall hospital readmission of elderly individuals. Anticoagulation medications have less impact on death, suggesting that fragility is a more reliable indicator of readmission and mortality. In a recent study, about 40% of TBI patients experienced low-energy (LE) transfer events, confirming the rising percentage of elderly trauma patients in advanced trauma centres. The LE cohort was generally older (>65 years), female, and with greater comorbidity and anticoagulants than high-energy transfer accidents. More research is required to assess the relationship between energy transfer and the severity of TBI in the elderly [11]. When studying the effect of frailty and early postinjury measures on the long-term outcome after mild traumatic brain injury in elderly patients from 3 Dutch advanced trauma care centres, it was seen that the frail elderly had worse long-term outcomes. Early complaints were stronger predictors of unfavourable outcomes [12].

Multiple anticoagulant or antithrombotic drug usage, or polypharmacy, has been linked to more extensive, evolving, or progressing extracranial lesions and delayed intracranial hemorrhage. However, the effect on functional or clinical consequences is unclear. Frail patients are more likely to need hospitalization, are more vulnerable to adverse events, and may experience long-lasting posttraumatic deficits that reduce their quality of life. Furthermore, due to their age and pre-injury health status, the senior population has a higher likelihood of a negative result after TBI [13].

58.4.2 Decompressive Craniectomy

According to the updated guidelines, Decompressive Craniectomy (DC) after TBI or massive middle cerebral artery strokes is not considered in elderly patients due to robust evidence of the poor resultant quality of life, even if mortality reduces. However, the effect on reduced ICP and the resultant decrease in ICU length of stay is unclear [14]. The morbidity, poor outcome scores, and dismal quality of life in elderly patients in these scenarios have yielded recommendations against considering DC in older patients.

Acute subdural hematoma (SDH) surgical therapy is still up for dispute, particularly in senior patients. In order to determine the impact of craniotomy size in terms of clinical and radiological outcome, a retrospective study comparing two surgical approaches—standard (SC, craniotomy size >8 cm) and limited (LC, craniotomy size 8 cm), in 64 individuals (>75 years age) with aSDH as the only lesion showed that the SC group's mortality was considerably greater (68.4% vs. 31.6%; $p = 0.045$), indicating that for effective evacuation of an aSDH in the elderly, a modest craniotomy is enough to produce the same radiological and clinical results [15].

58.4.3 Mechanical Thrombectomy

Analysis of pooled patient level data from more than 12,000 patients with proximal anterior large vessel ischemic stroke across five randomized trials by the HERMES collaborators demonstrated that mechanical thrombectomy benefited patients across age [16].

Although superior to medical therapy alone, post-thrombectomy complications rise with age. Data suggest that the elderly have worse outcomes after endovasculat therapy(EVT), achieve less successful reperfusion, are at higher risk for hemorrhagic transformation, and are less likely to benefit from EVT [17].

Careful selection of patient population among elderly is done with special focus on premorbid quality of life, preexisting white matter disease (preexisting cognitive deficit and poor collateral circulation), size of the ischemic core, and pre-strike disability (neurologic or not). Proper planning for procedure with a low threshold for vessel imaging and direct carotid puncture in cases with difficult anatomy (higher rates of vessel tortuosity) has been suggested to optimize reperfusion at least risk to elderly patients [18, 19].

58.4.4 Post-neurocritical Care Morbidity and Mortality

With increasing age, the capacity of the human body to respond to and compensate for physiologic stress and insults of surgery and anesthesia get blunted. Dearth of good quality data on morbidity and mortality rates in the elderly patients undergoing elective neurosurgical procedures makes prognostication and decision-making tricky. Although over the last 25 years the mortality rates in this population have decreased (possibly attributed to improved anesthesis and surgical technology and skills), postoperative length of stay in the hospital and associated morbidities among elderly are much higher than their younger counterparts [20]. The tumor volume, local postoperative problems, and preexisting comorbidities like diabetes and hypertension all impact the postoperative outcomes. Intensive monitoring techniques like transcranial Doppler ultrasonography and ICP are helpful in this age group for early detection of intracranial complications after surgery because the warning signs and symptoms may be subtle [21]. Age-related dementia and changes in respiratory physiology expose the older postoperative patient to greater respiratory complications. Postoperative atelectasis is frequently caused by anesthetics, analgesics, discomfort, decreased mucociliary clearance, and fluid changes. The risk of postoperative aspiration may be increased by decreased cough, pharyngeal reflex, and related cranial nerve palsies, particularly in posterior fossa and cervical spine surgery. The neuro-ICU must implement strict analgesia, chest physical therapy, and toileting procedures to prevent aspiration. After surgery and anesthesia, geriatric people are more likely to experience postoperative delirium and probable cognitive deterioration due to a variety of causes. Anesthetic medications that cause age-associated anticholinergic deficit to worsen and other elements including a urinary tract infection, hypoxia, hypercarbia, hyperthermia, fluid changes, and electrolyte imbalance may all be contributing causes [22].

58.4.5 Immunosuppression in ICU

According to experimental research, age may enhance a person's susceptibility to ventilator-induced lung injury. Presenting signs and symptoms, like delirium and cognitive impairment, may result in increased mortality due to delays in diagnosis and treatment. According to numerous studies, age is independently related to mortality in patients needing mechanical ventilation and ARDS. Age was also linked to death, ICU length of stay, and longer duration of mechanical ventilation. After ARDS, long-term effects are more common and severe in older people. Patients older than 70 have a decreased capacity to maintain spontaneous respiration after extubation due to the inability to clear secretions and a higher prevalence of nosocomial pneumonia [23, 24].

Sepsis occurs more frequently as people age. Subtle clinical manifestations, hospitalization, use of invasive equipment, many drugs, decreased renal function, and poor nutritional status are further concerns. Sepsis is a leading source of morbidity and mortality in the older population, with about 60% of septic patients over 65 [25]. Fewer classic clinical signs of sepsis, like tachycardia, fever, and peripheral vasodilation, are present in older patients. Patients more frequently present with heart failure, arrhythmias, arterial hypertension, and impaired mental status, making early diagnosis difficult. They have reduced cardiac compliance, which makes managing fluid therapy more challenging because renal perfusion is more heart flow-dependent.

58.5 Conclusion

Because of the high hospitalization rate and institutionalization among the elderly, they account for a sizable share of the total healthcare spending. Increases in healthcare costs are proportional to the rising age of the population. With a 40–80% prevalence, multimorbidity is common among older people. It is expensive to treat, linked to a notable rise in mortality, and has a considerable impact on mental health, quality of life, and overall health outcomes. Elderly patients admitted to neuro critical care units (NICUs) are increasing as life expectance rises: high mortality and the drastically reduced physical function and general health of ICU survivors are significant.

References

1. Oliveira K, Maerz LL. Epidemiology of critical illness in the elderly. Principles of geriatric critical care. Cambridge University Press; 2018. p. 1–10. https://doi.org/10.1017/9781316676325.002.
2. https://www.who.int/data/gho/data/themes/mortality-and-global-health-estimates/ghe-life-expectancy-and-healthy-life-expectancy; n.d.
3. McDermid RC, Stelfox HT, Bagshaw SM. Frailty in the critically ill: a novel concept. Crit Care. 2011;15:301.
4. Clegg A, Young J, Iliffe S, Rikkert MO, Rockwood K. Frailty in older adults. Lancet. 2013;381, Elsevier B.V.:752–62. https://doi.org/10.1016/S0140-6736(12)62167-9.

5. Lee L, Fcfp C, Heckman G, Molnar FJ. Clinical review frailty identifying elderly patients at high risk of poor outcomes. Can Fam Physician. 2015;61(3):227–31. PMID: 25767167; PMCID: PMC4369632.
6. Hoover M, Rotermann M, Sanmartin C, Bernier J. Validation of an index to estimate the prevalence of frailty among community-dwelling seniors. Health Rep. 2013;24:10–7.
7. Muscedere J, Waters B, Varambally A, Bagshaw SM, Boyd JG, Maslove D, et al. The impact of frailty on intensive care unit outcomes: a systematic review and meta-analysis. Intensive Care Med. 2017;43:1105–22. https://doi.org/10.1007/s00134-017-4867-0.
8. Cheung EHL, Cheung JCH, Yip YY. Raising awareness for time-limited trial discussion upon ICU triage and admission. Intensive Care Med. 2022;48:240–1. https://doi.org/10.1007/s00134-021-06590-0.
9. Wilberger J, Geriatric neurotrauma. Geriatric trauma and critical care. 2nd ed. Springer International Publishing; 2017. p. 273–83. https://doi.org/10.1007/978-3-319-48687-1_26.
10. Mushkudiani NA, Engel DC, Steyerberg EW, Butcher I, Lu J, Marmarou A, et al. Prognostic value of demographic characteristics in traumatic brain injury: results from the IMPACT study. J Neurotrauma. 2007;24:259–69. https://doi.org/10.1089/neu.2006.0028.
11. Lecky FE, Otesile O, Marincowitz C, Majdan M, Nieboer D, Lingsma HF, et al. The burden of traumatic brain injury from low-energy falls among patients from 18 countries in the CENTER-TBI registry: a comparative cohort study. PLoS Med. 2021;18:18. https://doi.org/10.1371/journal.pmed.1003761.
12. Abdulle AE, De Koning ME, Van Der Horn HJ, Scheenen ME, Roks G, Hageman G, et al. Early predictors for long-term functional outcome after mild traumatic brain injury in frail elderly patients. J Head Trauma Rehabil. 2018;33:E9–67. https://doi.org/10.1097/HTR.0000000000000368.
13. Baggiani M, Guglielmi A, Citerio G. Acute traumatic brain injury in frail patients: the next pandemic. Curr Opin Crit Care. 2022;28:166–75. https://doi.org/10.1097/MCC.0000000000000915.
14. Hawryluk GWJ, Rubiano AM, Totten AM, O'Reilly C, Ullman JS, Bratton SL, et al. Guidelines for managing severe traumatic brain injury: 2020 update of the decompressive craniectomy recommendations. Neurosurgery. 2020;87:427–34. https://doi.org/10.1093/neuros/nyaa278.
15. Pinggera D, Bauer M, Unterhofer M, Thomé C, Unterhofer C. Craniotomy size for traumatic acute subdural hematomas in elderly patients—same procedure for every age? Neurosurg Rev. 2022;45:459–65. https://doi.org/10.1007/s10143-021-01548-8.
16. Goyal M, Menon BK, Van Zwam WH, Dippel DWJ, Mitchell PJ, Demchuk AM, et al. Endovascular thrombectomy after large-vessel ischaemic stroke: a meta-analysis of individual patient data from five randomised trials. Lancet. 2016;387:1723–31.
17. Chen H, Jindal G, Miller TR, Gandhi D, Chaturvedi S. Stroke thrombectomy in the elderly: efficacy, safety, and special considerations. Stroke Vasc Intervent Neurol. 2023;0:e000634. https://doi.org/10.1161/SVIN.122.000634.
18. Goda T, Oyama N, Kitano T, Iwamoto T, Yamashita S, Takai H, et al. Prestroke conditions of acute ischemic stroke patients are associated with functional outcome after mechanical thrombectomy. J Stroke Cerebrovasc Dis. 2020;29:104540.
19. Kurisu K, Sakurai J, Wada H, Takebayashi S, Kobayashi T, Takizawa K. Effects of clinical outcomes by modification of patient selection protocol based on premorbid independence for mechanical thrombectomy in older adult patients. Brain Circ. 2022;8:24.
20. Chibbaro S, Di Rocco F, Makiese O, Mirone G, Marsella M, Lukaszewicz AC, et al. Neurosurgery and elderly: analysis through the years. Neurosurg Rev. 2011;34:229–34.
21. Dodds C, Kumar C, Veering B. Oxford textbook of anaesthesia for the elderly patient. Oxford University Press; 2014.
22. Tripathy S. Geriatric neuroanesthesia. Essentials of neuroanesthesia. Elsevier; 2017. p. 653–9. https://doi.org/10.1016/B978-0-12-805299-0.00038-5.
23. Esteban A, Anzueto A, Frutos F, Alía I, Brochard L, Stewart TE, et al. Characteristics and outcomes in adult patients receiving mechanical ventilation a 28-day international study, vol. 287; 2002. p. 345.
24. Bellani G, Laffey JG, Pham T, Fan E, Brochard L, Esteban A, et al. Epidemiology, patterns of care, and mortality for patients with acute respiratory distress syndrome in intensive care units in 50 countries. JAMA. 2016;315:788–800. https://doi.org/10.1001/jama.2016.0291.
25. Angus DC, Linde-Zwirble WT, Lidicker J, Clermont G, Carcillo J, Pinsky MR. Epidemiology of severe sepsis in the United States: analysis of incidence, outcome, and associated costs of care, vol. 29; 2001. p. 1303.

Pregnant Patients and Neurocritical Care

59

Barkha Bindu

59.1 Introduction

Neurological emergencies in pregnant patients are a complicated and challenging situation for physicians owing to the physiological changes of pregnancy and the risks involved to both mother and fetus. While emergency surgeries in pregnancy are performed regardless of gestational age, elective surgeries are usually performed in second trimester. First trimester is avoided for elective surgeries due to ongoing organogenesis while third trimester is avoided due to the size of gravid uterus. Although neurological emergencies in pregnancy are rare, they can significantly increase morbidity and mortality. Management of these conditions prioritizes maternal outcome while minimizing fetal harm. Exclusion of pregnant patients in clinical trials is a major reason for lack of clinical data to guide management of pregnant neurocritical patients. Both diagnosis and management of neurological conditions in pregnancy are difficult and must take into consideration the risks involved to the fetus as well. This chapter will discuss various neurological conditions that can present during pregnancy and their management.

B. Bindu (✉)
Neuroanesthesiology and Neurocritical Care, Paras Hospital, Gurugram, India

59.2 Special Concerns in Pregnancy

Pregnancy involves numerous physiological changes in various systems. Profound hormonal, metabolic, and enzymatic changes take place during pregnancy. Table 59.1 enumerates various system-wise physiological changes seen in pregnancy which together predispose pregnant patients to some dreaded neurological complications.

Increased plasma volume, cardiac output and decreased systemic vascular resistance (SVR), and a hyperdynamic circulation in pregnancy result in increased perfusion to various organs. Cerebral circulation undergoes multiple structural and functional adaptations to maintain a constant cerebral blood flow (CBF) and prevent rise in intracranial pressure (ICP) despite a hyperdynamic circulation [1]. Failure of these autoregulatory adjustments leads to development of preeclampsia [2]. Posterior reversible encephalopathy syndrome (PRES) related to preeclampsia/eclampsia develops due to endothelial dysfunction leading to compromised cerebral autoregulation [3]. This leads to increased blood-brain-barrier (BBB) permeability and subsequent vasogenic edema, microbleeds, and inflammation.

Increased volume of distribution due to plasma volume expansion and increased renal clearance reduce the effect of drug boluses and lower serum concentrations of drugs during steady state. Drug

H. Prabhakar et al. (eds.), *Principles and Practice of Neurocritical Care*,
https://doi.org/10.1007/978-981-99-8059-8_59

Table 59.1 Physiological changes of pregnancy

System	Physiological Changes
Central nervous system	• Widened autoregulatory range of cerebral circulation • BBB permeability maintained • Neuronal hyperexcitability, decreased GABA levels, increased susceptibility to seizures • Congested epidural venous plexus causing compression of subarachnoid space and reduced CSF volume, reduced intracranial compliance, increased risk of intracranial hypertension • Increased sensitivity to epidural anesthetic agents
Cardiovascular system	• 40–50% increase in plasma volume and cardiac output • Compensatory decrease in SVR by 35–40% to maintain blood pressure • Decrease in MAP by 10–15 mmHg • Reflex increase in heart rate by 10–20 bpm • Physiological anemia • Hyperdynamic circulation • Aortocaval compression due to gravid uterus and increased intra-abdominal pressure from 20 weeks gestation • Hypercoagulable state
Renal system	• Increased sympathetic and renin-angiotensinogen tone • Increased renal blood flow and GFR • Hypervolemic hyponatremia
Respiratory system	• Hyperventilation • Respiratory alkalosis with a pH of 7.40–7.47 • Lowering of $PaCO_2$ to 28 mmHg • Decreased RLV, FRC • Increased susceptibility to hypoxemia • Difficult intubation, edematous, and vascular upper respiratory tract mucosa
Hepatobiliary system	• Reduced plasma protein concentration after second trimester • Variable effects on hepatic enzymes
Gastrointestinal system	• Reduced esophageal sphincter tone, increased gastric reflux • Delayed gastric emptying • Prone to aspiration

BBB Blood brain barrier, *GABA* Gamma-amino butyric acid, *CSF* Cerebrospinal fluid, *SVR* Systemic vascular resistance, *MAP* Mean arterial pressure, *GFR* Glomerular filtration rate, *RLV* Residual lung volume, *FRC* Functional residual capacity

binding capacity decreases by 20–30% by end of gestation due to reduced plasma protein concentrations [4]. As a result, highly protein bound drugs (like phenytoin, midazolam, valproic acid) are expected to have higher serum concentrations, whereas renally cleared drugs (like levetiracetam, heparin, opioids, aminoglycosides) are likely to have lower serum concentrations. Drugs metabolized predominantly by the liver (such as barbiturates) need tough concentrations monitoring as their levels can be variably affected [4, 5].

High concentrations of aromatized sex steroids in pregnancy confer a protective effect against rupture of cerebral aneurysms in pregnancy [6]. Apoptosis of vascular smooth muscles, disruption of elastic lamina, and breakdown of collagen and elastin contribute to aneurysm formation and rupture. Risk of rupture in pregnancy is, however, similar to that in general population [6]. Increased stroke volume, cardiac output, and plasma volume along with higher mean arterial pressure (MAP) in last trimester may contribute to the higher rate of aneurysmal rupture seen towards end of pregnancy. Hypertensive disorders of pregnancy may also play a contributory role. Labor-related increased blood pressure may also have an effect on rate of aneurysmal rupture.

Ability of various drugs to cross placental barrier is also an important factor to be considered. Drugs that cross placenta can reach dangerously high levels in fetus. Table 59.2 gives a brief overview of drugs used in pregnant neurocritical patients.

Table 59.2 Summary of medications used in pregnant neurocritical patients

Pharmacological agent	Safety considerations	Placental transfer	Fetal effects
1. Thrombolytic Agents			
Alteplase	Close monitoring for uterine bleeding needed	No	
Reteplase	Risk of increased bleeding. Close monitoring for uterine bleeding needed	No	
Tenecteplase	Close monitoring for uterine bleeding needed	No	
2. Antiplatelets			
Acetylsalicylic acid (ASA)	Expressed in breast milk. FDA Pregnancy category B.	Yes	Gastroschisis. No fetal malformations at low doses (60–100 mg). May increase risk of neonatal ICH.
Clopidogrel	Limited use in pregnancy advised. Black box warning regarding diminished platelet effect in patients with 2 loss-of-function alleles in CYP2C19 gene. Increased intra and postpartum bleeding. FDA pregnancy category B.	Unknown	
Cangrelor	FDA pregnancy category C.	Unknown	
Ticagrelor	Black box warning for bleeding risk. Can exacerbate bradyarrhythmias. FDA pregnancy category C.	Unknown	
3. Anticoagulants			
Enoxaparin	Black box warning for spinal/ epidural hematoma	No	
Heparin (UF)	Benzyl alcohol preservative contraindicated	No	Teratogenicity, increased fetal bleeding
Apixaban	Black box warning for spinal/ epidural hematoma	Yes	May increase risk of spontaneous abortions.
Rivaroxaban	Black box warning for spinal/ epidural hematoma	Yes	May increase risk of spontaneous abortions.
Warfarin	Black box warning for fatal bleeding	Yes	Craniofacial malformations
4. Anticoagulant Reversal Agents			
PCC, FFP, Vitamin K, Protamine sulphate	FDA pregnancy category C		
Andexanet alfa	Black box warning for arterial/ venous thrombotic events, cardiac arrest, sudden death, FDA category N (not yet classified). No data in pregnancy/lactation.	Unknown	
5. Antiepileptic Drugs			
Levetiracetam		Yes	No specific malformations
Phenytoin	Black box warning for cardiovascular risk	Yes	Cleft lip/palate, club foot
Valproic acid	Black box warning for fetal risk, hepatotoxicity, Pancreatitis, use in mitochondrial disease	Yes	Cleft lip/palate, club foot, hypospadias. Dose-dependent increase in risk of major malformations.

(continued)

Table 59.2 (continued)

Pharmacological agent	Safety considerations	Placental transfer	Fetal effects
Phenobarbital		Yes	Cleft lip/palate. Dose-dependent increase in risk of major malformations.
Lamotrigine	Black box warning for serious skin rashes	Yes	
6. Antihypertensives			
Amlodipine		Yes	
Clevidipine	Pregnancy class C drug. Rapid onset and elimination. Can cause tachyarrhythmias	Unknown	
Nicardipine	Rapid onset, 4–6 h duration of action. Pregnancy category C. Can cause tachyarrhythmias	Limited transfer	
Nifedipine	Can cause prematurity, perinatal asphyxia, IUGR. Pregnancy category C	Yes	
Nimodipine			Teratogenic
ACEI/ARB	Black box warning for fetal toxicity. Contraindicated in pregnancy.	Yes	CNS, CVS, urogenital malformations. Miscarriage, still birth.
Esmolol		Yes	
Labetalol	Pregnancy category C	Yes	Fetal bradycardia
Clonidine	Black box warning regarding usage as epidural agent	Yes	
Hydralazine	Pregnancy category C. Can increase ICP	Yes	
Sodium nitroprusside	Black box warning for hypotension and cyanide toxicity. Can increase ICP. Considered last resort. Pregnancy category C	Yes	
7. Immunomodulatory Agents			
Azathioprine	Black box warning for malignancy	Yes	
Tacrolimus	Black box warning for serious infections and malignancy. Higher risk of preeclampsia	Yes	Preterm birth, low birth weight
Intravenous Immunoglobulin	Black box warning for thrombosis, renal dysfunction, renal failure	Transfer is higher in later pregnancy.	
8. Sedatives/Analgesics/NMB			
Propofol	Short half-life. Myocardial depression. Risk of propofol infusion syndrome		Not teratogenic
Fentanyl	Less hemodynamic instability		Neonatal respiratory depression, withdrawal syndrome. Not teratogenic
Morphine	Histamine release, hypotension		Neonatal respiratory depression, withdrawal syndrome. Not teratogenic
Remifentanil	Less hemodynamic instability		Not teratogenic
Vecuronium	Contraindicated in renal or liver failure	Yes	Nil

Table 59.2 (continued)

Pharmacological agent	Safety considerations	Placental transfer	Fetal effects
Cisatracurium		Yes	Nil
Lorazepam	Lacks active metabolites, less residual effect. Long half-life.		Unclear teratogenic effects. Neonatal respiratory depression, floppy baby syndrome.
Midazolam	Active metabolites. Tolerance. Prolonged sedation.		Unclear teratogenic effects. Neonatal respiratory depression, floppy baby syndrome.
Dexmedetomidine	No respiratory depression		
Barbiturates	Immunosuppression	Yes	Spinal cord malformations, fetal hemorrhages, neonatal abstinence syndrome
Ketamine	Dose-dependent increase in uterine contractions. Reduced clearance in pregnancy	Yes	Increased risk of Hirschcprung disease, Treacher Collins syndrome, Waardenburg Shah syndrome, DiGeorge syndrome, CHARGE syndrome, neuroblastoma, melanoma. Lower APGAR scores. Neonatal respiratory depression.
9. Miscellaneous Drugs			
Mannitol	Can reduce amniotic fluid, cause electrolyte abnormalities, hypovolemia	Yes	
Hypertonic saline	May be more physiological		Known abortifacient (intrauterine instillation)
Pyridostigmine		Yes	
Acetylcholinesterase inhibitors	Can induce uterine contractions		
Steroids			Small risk of cleft palate
Rituximab	Transient decline in B-cell counts.		

Continuous fetal monitoring must be initiated as early as possible during maternal neurological emergency. For previable pregnancies, fetal heart monitoring (FHR) must be done before and after surgical procedure. For viable pregnancies, continuous FHR monitoring may be needed. As soon as preterm delivery becomes a possibility, corticosteroids should be administered. They help in lung maturity and maximum benefit is seen 2–7 days after administration [7]. Left lateral tilt must be given after 20 weeks of gestation to prevent compression of inferior vena cava by gravid uterus.

59.3 Imaging Modalities

Ionizing radiation exposure can lead to fetal demise (0–2 weeks gestation), fetal malformations, developmental delay and intellectual disability (2–8 weeks gestation), and increased risk of cancer. Occupational limit for fetal radiation is 5 mGy. Radiation exposure less than 50 mGy has negligible risk for the fetus [8].

X-ray of structures away from the uterus causes very low radiation exposure of the fetus. Use of abdominal shield can further reduce this exposure. Anteroposterior abdominal X-rays can cause upto 9 mGy of radiation exposure. Although X-rays are safe in pregnancy, it is advisable to minimize exposure by reducing number of views. Posteroanterior views carry one-tenth radiation exposure.

Non-contrast CT of head carries fetal radiation exposure of 0.001–0.01 mGy which is well below prescribed limits [9]. CT of lumbar spine carries radiation exposure of 2–20 mGy. CT scan of abdomen and pelvis can cause upto 50 mGy of exposure. Use of abdominal shield is sometimes questioned since radiation scatter to other body parts is majorly through internal tissue transfer. Also, newer CT machines have gating mechanism to reduce radiation exposure of abdomen which might be interrupted by the use of abdominal shield [10]. Further, weight of abdominal shield on the gravid uterus can cause IVC compression or increase intra-abdominal pressure and ICP.

Digital Subtraction Angiography (DSA) carries highest risk of radiation exposure to the fetus and is best avoided. Radiation dose higher than 1000 mGy may be seen in flow diversion or embolization procedures [11]. Dose can be reduced by using radial or carotid access.

MRI is the preferred imaging modality for diagnosis in pregnant patients because of nil exposure to ionizing radiation. Non-contrast MRI at 3 Tesla or less is safe in pregnancy. Earlier concerns over increased specific absorption rate of energy by fetus in 3 T MRI compared to 1.5 T MRI in first trimester have now been allayed [8, 9].

Ultrasonography is considered safe in pregnancy. There can be a rise in tissue temperature due to absorption of sound wave energy from ultrasonography. Association between high intensity ultrasonography and fetal risks like low birth weight, dyslexia, or rise in fetal tissue temperature of upto 2 °C has led to limitation of average intensity of transducers. Thermal effects of ultrasonography depend on exposure and dwell times. Risk of temperature elevation is least with B-mode and maximum with color and spectral Doppler. Ultrasonography machines are calibrated to reduce thermal effects in obstetric patients [12].

59.4 Contrast

59.4.1 Iodinated Agents

Modern low osmolality contrast agents are classified as pregnancy category B. Although they are absorbed by fetus and can cross blood-brain-barrier (BBB), mutagenic effects have not been reported so far.

59.4.2 Gadolinium-Based Contrast Agents

Gadolinium in repeated and high doses is teratogenic in animals. Free gadolinium is toxic and is therefore always administered with a chelating agent. In humans, gadolinium crosses placenta and has long half-life and unknown effects on fetus [13]. The fetus excretes gadolinium into amniotic fluid from where it is reingested and reabsorbed. The longer it persists in amniotic fluid, the more likely it is to become unbound from the chelating agent and increasing the risk of nephrogenic systemic fibrosis. Gadolinium-based contrast agents should therefore only be used when benefits outweigh risks [9].

59.5 Neurological Conditions in Pregnancy

Headache is the most common neurological symptom in pregnancy. A change in nature of headache or any new onset headache must prompt evaluation for neurological causes like worsening of migraine headache, preeclampsia, cerebral venous sinus thrombosis, or aneurysmal subarachnoid hemorrhage.

59.5.1 Cerebrovascular Disorders (CVD)

Risk of CVD is higher in intra- and postpartum period [14]. Pregnancy-related changes like increase in total body water, increased cardiac output, stroke volume and heart rate, venous stasis due to IVC compression by gravid uterus, decreased systemic vascular resistance, and pregnancy-induced hypercoagulable state predispose pregnant women to cerebrovascular disorders [15]. Acute ischemic stroke (AIS) is the most common CVD seen in pregnancy, followed by intracerebral hemorrhage (ICH), cerebral venous sinus thrombosis (CVT), and aneurysmal subarachnoid hemorrhage (aSAH) [16]. A noncontrast MRI is the imaging modality of choice.

Ischemic strokes in pregnancy account for 15% of maternal mortality. Risk of ischemic stroke is highest in last trimester of pregnancy and immediate postpartum [17] and remains high upto 12 weeks after pregnancy [18]. Age more than 35 years, autoimmune conditions like catastrophic antiphospholipid syndrome, immune thrombocytopenic purpura, and thrombotic microangiopathies of pregnancy increase the risk of AIS in pregnancy [19]. Cesarean delivery compared to vaginal delivery is also associated with increased chances of stroke [20, 21]. Pregnancy and postpartum-related cardiomyopathy can also manifest as embolic ischemic stroke.

Hemorrhagic strokes can occur due to hypertensive disorders of pregnancy, CVT, aneurysm rupture, or due to arteriovenous malformations (AVM) [22]. Upto 14%–55% of hemorrhagic strokes in pregnancy are attributed to hypertensive disorders of pregnancy [23]. In-hospital maternal mortality rate in hemorrhagic stroke is upto 20% [24]. Risk of AVM rupture in pregnancy is high, although data are conflicting.

CVT refers to presence of thrombosis in dural venous sinus. Incidence of CVT in pregnant women is around 0.012% [25]. Risk of venous thrombotic event is 4–5 times higher during pregnancy and 20 times higher in postpartum period [26]. Headache, seizures, visual symptoms, and focal neurological deficits are common presenting symptoms. Infection, increased maternal age, hypertension, dehydrated state, cesarean section, and hyperhomocysteinemia increase the risk of CVT [27].

Prevalence of aSAH is lower in pregnancy than in nonpregnant women. Most cases of aSAH in pregnancy occur in the last trimester followed by second and first trimesters, respectively. Aneurysmal rupture can also occur in puerperium and upto 2 weeks postpartum [28]. Risk factors include advanced age, tobacco use, and hypertension. Aneurysms are predominantly seen in anterior circulation. Clinical presentation is similar to that in general population.

Management

Principles of management of CVD are broadly the same as in nonpregnant patients. Treatment is focused on protecting the salvageable brain, preventing seizures, optimizing blood pressure and glucose levels, and preventing intracranial hypertension.

In ischemic stroke, further damage to brain must be avoided and reperfusion must be facilitated. Thrombolytic therapy, intravenous or intra-arterial, is the cornerstone of management of AIS in nonpregnant patients. Concerns regarding life-threatening hemorrhage in the mother and potential harm to fetus have resulted in pregnancy being considered a relative contraindication for thrombolytic therapy. However, thrombolytic medications do not cross placenta and their ability to cause fetal hemorrhage or teratogenicity is unknown. Potential for increased uterine bleeding during pregnancy does exist and it can be life-threatening in the first 48 h postpartum. The AHA/ASA 2018 AIS guidelines support consideration of intravenous (IV) tPA administration in pregnancy when the anticipated benefits of treating moderate or severe stroke outweigh the anticipated increased risk of uterine bleeding [29]. In pregnant patients who have not received thrombolysis or oral anticoagulants, aspirin is administered within 48 h of stroke onset [29]. Mechanical thrombectomy (MT) is the standard of care for anterior large vessel occlusions. However, most trials in this context excluded pregnant patients. Canadian Best Practice Consensus Statement on Acute Stroke Management in Pregnancy (2018) recommends not considering pregnancy a contraindication to angiography [30]. Angiography and MT should be performed without delay in pregnant patients with disabling stroke. Fetal radiation exposure during this procedure is reported to be minimal. Malignant cerebral edema due to AIS may need emergency decompressive craniectomy surgery.

Management of hemorrhagic stroke in pregnant patients is similar to that in general population. Control of blood pressure and reversal of coagulopathy are the mainstays of treatment along with management of mass effect. Continuous infusions of IV antihypertensives are preferred. Labetalol infusion is used as first line and esmolol and nicardipine infusions as second-line options. Clevidipine is now considered a first-line antihypertensive infusion in stroke in nonpregnant population [31]. Due to lack of data with clevidipine use in pregnancy, it is considered only in rare instances like flow limiting stenosis where maternal benefits outweigh fetal risks [12]. Reversal of coagulopathy may require prothrombin complex concentrates, fresh frozen plasma, vitamin K, etc. Hemorrhagic stroke due to AVM or aneurysmal rupture is managed with embolization or clipping. Assisted second-stage delivery or cesarean delivery might be required in these patients to minimize Valsalva-associated rise in intracranial pressure.

The mainstay of treatment in CVT is anticoagulant therapy with IV heparin (Pregnancy Category C) or low molecular weight heparin (LMWH) (Pregnancy Category B). Unfractionated heparin (UFH) has shorter half-life compared to LMWH. Both UFH and LMWH do not cross placenta and are considered safe in pregnancy. Warfarin, on the other hand, crosses placenta (pregnancy category D) and is avoided in pregnancy. Anticoagulation is warranted even if there is evidence of venous hemorrhage on imaging, as the hemorrhage size is expected to increase unless the clot burden is decreased. UFH may be transitioned to LMWH during pregnancy and postpartum period. Patients on LMWH are transitioned to UFH at 36 weeks of gestation to prevent intrapartum hemorrhage and allow for regional anesthesia. Anticoagulation with LMWH is continued until at least 6 weeks after delivery [27]. CVT is often associated with significant cerebral edema due to venous/arterial infarct or obstructive hydrocephalus due to intraventricular hemorrhage. Life-saving surgery in the form of decompressive craniectomy may be required [32]. Available data on use of direct oral anticoagulants during pregnancy do not support their use [33]. Underlying hypercoagulable disorders such as antiphospholipid antibody syndrome, factor V Leiden deficiency, prothrombin (factor II) gene mutation, antithrombin III deficiency, and protein S and C deficiencies must be looked for.

Management of aSAH focuses on control of blood pressure and securing the aneurysm. Aneurysm must be secured early. Use of stent or flow diverter for endovascular therapy needs antiplatelet therapy. Hence, endovascular therapy may be a less favorable approach in pregnancy. Calcium channel blockers (nimodipine) must be avoided, unless necessary [34]. Diuretics and antihypertensives can cause reduced placental perfusion. Hence, use of temporary clips instead of global hypotension is advised. At gestational age less than 24 weeks, attempts are made towards securing the aneurysm and aiming for a term delivery [35]. At gestational age more than 34 weeks, cesarean delivery may be planned [16]. At 24–34 weeks gestation, need for delivery must be decided on a case to case basis. Permissive hypertension to reduce the risk of vasospasm which is often achieved by using vasopressors can cause placental insufficiency and result in placental abruption, premature rupture of membranes and intrauterine growth restriction, etc. [36] Data to suggest a target blood pressure in pregnant patients with vasospasm are inadequate at present. A blood pressure of 150–180 mmHg during peak vasospasm is generally maintained. Endovascular treatment of vasospasm may reduce the need to maintain prolonged hypertension.

59.5.2 Hypertensive Disorders of Pregnancy

Hypertensive disorders of pregnancy account for 16% of maternal mortality [37]. Preeclampsia is defined as new-onset hypertension with either proteinuria or end-organ dysfunction. It affects 2%–8% of pregnancies [38]. Eclampsia is a severe variant of preeclampsia and is associated with new-onset seizure, with no other cause of seizure. Neurological sequelae of preeclampsia and eclampsia include seizures, ischemic stroke, intracerebral hemorrhage, and HELPP syndrome (hemolysis, elevated liver enzymes, low platelet count). HELPP syndrome can lead to disseminated intravascular coagulopathy and hemorrhage.

Blood Pressure Management

Due to limited data to guide blood pressure goals in neurological pregnant patients, general goals of pregnancy are followed. Blood pressure must be reduced to less than 160/110 mmHg [38]. Fall in blood pressure to less than 140/90 mmHg must be avoided to maintain uteroplacental blood flow. Continuous fetal monitoring is important. Until recently, IV hydralazine or labetalol were considered agents of choice for hypertensive disorders of pregnancy. Since hydralazine was shown to have higher number of side effects including lower birth weight [39], antihypertensives of choice currently are IV labetalol (20–40 mg every 15 min, maximum 300 mg), oral nifedipine (10–20 mg every 30 min, maximum 180 mg), methyldopa [40], while IV hydralazine (5–10 mg, maximum 20 mg), clonidine, and thiazide diuretics are considered second line.

Management of Eclampsia

Maternal injury and hypoxia must be prevented. Supplemental oxygen, left lateral tilt, and intravenous fluids must be administered. Fetal bradycardia might be noticed after seizure, which usually resolves within 10 min. Persistent fetal bradycardia lasting more than 15 min or persistent late decelerations might mandate expeditious delivery [41].

Intravenous magnesium sulphate (loading with 4–6 g diluted in 100 mL administered over 15–20 min followed by continuous infusion at 2 g/h till 24 h after delivery) is used in patients with eclampsia [42]. Intramuscular route (10 g loading dose given as 5 g dose in upper outer quadrant of each buttock, followed by 5 g IM injection every 4 h until 24 h after delivery) is used in patients without intravenous access [42]. The therapeutic range of serum magnesium level at which eclamptic seizures are prevented is 4–8 mEq/L. [38] Signs of magnesium toxicity begin at serum levels of 7–10 mEq/L with loss of deep tendon reflexes. Life-threatening side effects like respiratory paralysis occur at 10–13 mEq/L, altered cardiac conduction at >15 mEq/L, and cardiac arrest at >25 mEq/L. Calcium gluconate (1 g IV) can be administered to counteract magnesium toxicity. Magnesium is renally excreted and must be used cautiously in patients with renal failure. Delivery of fetus is the definitive treatment of preeclampsia and eclampsia. Recommended timing of delivery is between 34 and 37 weeks of gestation. Vaginal delivery is the preferred method.

59.5.3 Intracranial Neoplasms, Cerebral Edema, Intracranial Hypertension

Pregnancy is associated with several physiological changes like hormonal changes, fluid retention, and plasma volume expansion. These changes can cause tumor expansion and associated symptoms during pregnancy. Often, preexisting intracranial tumors present for the first time during pregnancy. Some tumors show accelerated growth in pregnancy. For example, meningiomas express estrogen and progesterone receptors, acoustic tumors express estrogen receptors [43], and pituitary adenomas might undergo lactotroph hyperplasia due to estrogen. Intravascular volume in pregnancy expands by upto 50% with maximum increase at 32 weeks of gestation. This volume expansion can increase tumor edema and enlarge vascular tumors.

Intracranial neoplasms present with symptoms similar to those in nonpregnant individuals including headache, nausea, vomiting, seizures, visual changes, etc. New onset headache or seizures, worsening of nausea, and vomiting in later stages of pregnancy must raise suspicion of an etiology other than that due to hormonal changes of pregnancy. Diagnosis can be made based on imaging.

Intracranial hypertension (IHT) during pregnancy can develop due to intracranial neoplasms, trauma, infection, preeclampsia, or vascular events. There is inadequate data regarding normal physiological range of intracranial pressure (ICP) in pregnancy. Noninvasive methods of ICP measurement like transcranial doppler, pupillometry, optic nerve sheath diameter, etc. are still in investigational stages. Indications for invasive ICP monitoring are similar to those in general population.

Management

First line therapy for IHT includes general measures to like elevation of head end of bed by 30° and neutral position of head. Physiological neuroprotection includes a set of measures that aim to maintain physiological homeostasis (Table 59.3) [44]. Intubation and mechanical ventilation, when indicated, are started with controlled mode, tidal volume 6–8 mL/kg, respiratory rate set to achieve a $PaCO_2$ of 30–32 mmHg, FiO_2 and PEEP set to achieve a PaO_2 >80 mmHg and SaO_2 >92%, plateau pressure <24 cmH_2O, and driving pressure <13 cmH_2O [45]. Hyperventilation, a commonly instituted temporizing measure in intracranial hypertension, can reduce placental oxygen transfer. Therefore, PaCO2 goal during hyperventilation in pregnancy is 26–28 mmHg and must be used as briefly as possible [46]. MAP must be adjusted to maintain cerebral perfusion pressure between 50 and 60 mmHg. Vasopressor of choice in pregnancy is phenylephrine since it does not alter uterine tone or fetal acid-base status [47]. Animal studies have shown norepinephrine to cause increased uterine tone, placental hypoperfusion, and fetal bradycardia [48]. Sedation and analgesia, when needed, are achieved using short acting agents. Fetal toxicity and respiratory depressive effects of various sedatives must be considered. Hyperosmolar agents can cause fetal dehydration and electrolyte abnormalities and are therefore avoided in pregnant patients. Hypertonic saline is a known abortifacient in first trimester. Anticonvulsants for seizure prophylaxis and steroids for tumor edema are used. Among steroids, both dexamethasone (pregnancy category C) and prednisone (pregnancy category D) can cross placenta.

Owing to the limitations associated with medical management modalities, surgical management may come earlier in the treatment algorithm for IHT in pregnant patients. Surgical excision of intracranial neoplasm is deferred until after delivery, if possible [49]. High grade tumors and severity of symptoms decide the need for surgery. Benefits of operating must be weighed against the risks involved in preterm delivery.

None of the second line therapies for IHT have been evaluated in pregnancy. High dose barbiturates are not a safe option (Table 59.2). Indomethacin, used as a rescue measure in refractory IHT in general population, is tocolytic and can cause oligohydramnios, jaundice, premature closure of arteriovenous ductus, necrotizing enterocolitis, and intraventricular hemorrhage in fetus [50]. Therapeutic hypothermia for IHT has not been studied in pregnancy.

Timing and mode of delivery are patient-specific to a large extent. In case of preterm labor, tocolytics (oxytocin receptor antagonists, beta agonists, calcium channel blockers) can be used, but their safety profile is unknown. Beyond 34 weeks gestation, it is generally advisable to proceed with cesarean delivery at the time of neurosurgery. Presence of IHT might warrant emergency cesarean section. Oxytocin and its

Table 59.3 Physiological neuroprotection

Parameter	Target
Central temperature	• <37.5 °C
Intravascular volume	• Avoid hypovolemia
Ventilation	• Arterial oxygen saturation >92%, PaO_2 >80 mmHg • $PaCO_2$ 30–32 mmHg
Sodium	• Avoid hyponatremia • Serum sodium level 135–145 mEq/L
Osmolality	• Avoid hypoosmolality
Hemoglobin	• Avoid hemoglobin <7 g/dL
Glycemia	• Serum glucose level 110–150 mg/dL

analogues have a good safety margin. However, owing to their potential to cause vasodilation, hypotension, and increased ICP, lowest possible dose at slow infusion rates must be used [51].

59.5.4 Seizures

Seizures in pregnancy are more commonly epileptic than eclamptic. Other causes include intracranial hemorrhage, trauma, infection, reversible cerebral vasoconstriction syndrome, posterior reversible encephalopathy syndrome, etc. Among pregnant patients with known seizure disorder, 14–32% reported an increase in seizure frequency during pregnancy [52, 53]. Change in serum antiepileptic drug levels due to plasma volume expansion and hormonal effects predisposes these patients to breakthrough seizures. Seizures increase lactic acid level, thereby decreasing uteroplacental blood flow, increasing cardiac output and intra-abdominal pressure, and causing shunting of blood flow to the brain and muscles away from the uterus. Treatment of seizures is therefore essential to avoid harm to the mother and fetus. MRI and EEG help in diagnostic workup.

Management

Airway, breathing, and circulation must be stabilized. Causes such as infection, electrolyte disturbances, and hypoglycemia should be treated. Hypotension and hypoxemia must be prevented. Fetal bradycardia might follow maternal seizures. If persisting more than 15 min, delivery needs to be expedited [41]. Left lateral tilt is given to prevent compression of inferior vena cava by the gravid uterus [41].

Lorazepam (0.1 mg/kg or 4 mg total intravenous, repeated every 5 min till cessation of seizure) or diazepam (5–10 mg intravenous boluses) may be used for controlling seizures [37]. Subsequently, levetiracetam 60 mg/kg may be administered over 15 min [42]. Phenytoin and valproic acid are avoided in pregnancy due to their teratogenicity. If seizure is not controlled, intubation and midazolam infusion may be needed [46].

Daily usage of antiepileptic drug (AED) in first trimester places the fetus at risk of major congenital malformations. Table 59.2 gives details of effects of AEDs in pregnancy. No significant change in rate of major congenital malformations was noted on increasing or adding AEDs in second or third trimesters [54]. Valproic acid, phenobarbital, and phenytoin are associated with increased congenital malformations, while levetiracetam is not [55]. AED levels in plasma might have to be checked as volume expansion and increased metabolism of pregnancy might lead to subtherapeutic levels of AEDs.

59.5.5 Postpartum Angiopathy

Postpartum angiopathy is a type of reversible cerebral vasoconstriction syndrome (RCVS). It can present as ischemic stroke, cortical SAH, intraparenchymal hemorrhage, or cerebral edema. Presenting features include sudden, severe headache with diffuse cerebral vasospasm, seizures, or focal neurological deficits [56, 57]. It is usually fully reversible with spontaneous resolution of vasospasm and symptoms within 12 weeks.

Supportive treatment with analgesics, maintenance of systolic blood pressure of 90–180 mmHg, and avoidance of vasoconstrictive medications are the cornerstones of management. Maintenance of a minimum systolic blood pressure of 90 mmHg is recommended to reduce the risk of ischemic stroke [58].

59.5.6 Posterior Reversible Encephalopathy Syndrome (PRES)

PRES, also known as reversible posterior leukoencephalopathy syndrome, occurs due to cerebral autoregulation dysfunction and endothelial malfunction. In pregnancy, it is usually a manifestation of eclampsia. A rapid change in blood pressure can cause BBB breakdown leading to extravasation of fluid and edema, which is usually reversible. Nonhypertensive causes like immunosuppressive and antineoplastic medications or renal disorders also can cause PRES.

While in nonpregnant state PRES is associated with SBP of 180–220 mmHg, in pregnant patients, SBP of 140 mmHg also may cause PRES, especially if there is a rapid change in blood pressure [59]. Headache, visual symptoms, and seizures are the usual presenting symptoms. Bilateral, asymmetrical occipital edema is commonly seen. Edema in watershed territories, bilateral cerebellar hemispheres, and pons may also occur.

Treatment focuses on blood pressure and seizure control. Blood pressure may have to be reduced by 10–25% of baseline while monitoring for signs of hypoperfusion. In most cases, PRES is fully reversible.

59.5.7 Ventriculoperitoneal Shunt Malfunction

Reportedly, upto 50% of VP shunts malfunction during pregnancy [60]. As pregnancy progresses, intra-abdominal pressure rises and can lead to disruption of peritoneal catheter flow. This can cause rise in ICP manifesting as nausea, vomiting, headache, lethargy, confusion, etc. Diagnosis is made based on brain imaging.

Management

Shunt revision might be needed if shunt malfunction occurs. First and second trimesters are suitable for shunt revision since the gravid uterus does not obstruct at this stage. In third trimester, a ventriculoatrial shunt or third ventriculostomy may have to be performed to avoid preterm labor and trauma to uterus [61]. In patients with functional shunt, vaginal delivery can be attempted. Vaginal delivery with shortened second stage or operative vaginal delivery may be needed to prevent ICP rise. In patients with malfunctioning shunt, cesarean delivery is recommended [61]. Prophylactic antibiotics must be administered to prevent shunt infection in patients undergoing surgical delivery.

59.5.8 Myasthenia Gravis (MG)

One-third patients with MG in pregnancy improve, one-third worsen, and one-third experience myasthenic crisis. Such crisis is more common in first trimester. Oral pyridostigmine is the first line agent used in pregnancy [62]. Acetylcholinesterase inhibitors can induce uterine contractions and are avoided. Plasma exchange and IV immunoglobulin (IVIg) can be used in myasthenic crisis [63]. Adjunct steroids and rituximab may be used in patients at risk of recurrent exacerbations, if benefits outweigh risks. Pain management using epidural anesthesia is preferred over local anesthetics and narcotics.

MG patients who develop preeclampsia are a difficult subset. Use of beta blockers and calcium channel blockers for control of BP in these patients can precipitate myasthenic crisis. Methyldopa and hydralazine are the first choice agents. Magnesium which is the treatment of choice for seizure prophylaxis in preeclampsia is contraindicated in MG [64]. Other AEDs like levetiracetam, valproic acid, and diazepam have been used. Phenytoin is used in refractory cases.

Vaginal delivery is the preferred method of delivery in these patients. Fatigue can develop in second stage of labor. Intramuscular neostigmine 1.5 mg or 0.5 mg IV (equivalent to 60 mg pyridostigmine) can assist through second stage of labor. Cesarean section, though performed, can precipitate myasthenic crisis. Use of epidural anesthesia and vacuum delivery has been shown to reduce maternal fatigue [65]. Transient myasthenia gravis called "floppy baby" may occur in the newborn and may present as respiratory weakness for upto a month after delivery [66].

59.5.9 Cardiac Arrest and Hypoxic Brain Injury

Cardiac arrest occurs in 1 in 30,000 pregnancies. Given the increased susceptibility of pregnant patients to hypoxia, early control of airway is recommended. Gravid uterus must be displaced to the left during resuscitation. Defibrillation and other medications are used similar to that in general population. Timely decision to deliver the fetus within 5 min of loss of circulation, especially when more than

24 weeks gestation, is needed when resuscitation efforts are failing. Such prompt decision making not only improves fetal chances of survival, but also improves maternal viability by improving cardiac output [67].

If return of spontaneous circulation is achieved, patient must be placed in left lateral decubitus position. While hypothermia to support neurological recovery in post-cardiac arrest patients is the standard of care in general population, there is a lack of data in pregnant patients [68]. Expert consensus recommends ultra-mild hypothermia (36 °C) for post-cardiac arrest care in pregnant patients [69]. Decreased fetal heart rate and variability might occur due to hypothermia, mandating the need for continuous fetal heart rate monitoring.

Brain death in pregnancy, although uncommon, can occur. Care of the fetus takes priority in such instances. If the fetus is of more than 28–32 weeks gestation, then cesarean section is performed [70]. But, if the fetus is less than 28 weeks gestation age, then the mother would require "somatic" support to improve chances of fetal viability. Literature has reports of brain dead maternal patients being cared for till fetus was over 25 weeks of gestation [71, 72]. Fetal survival in such cases depends on gestational age and maternal complications like hemodynamic instability, hypothermia, diabetes insipidus, etc. [73] Mother should be placed in left lateral decubitus position, MAP of atleast 65 mmHg must be maintained along with PaCO2 of 30–35 mmHg, normoxia, and euvolemia, and nutritional needs as per pregnancy demands must be met. There is a lack of clarity over optimum gestational age and timing of delivery in these patients. Ethical aspects of managing these cases also need to be looked into.

59.6 Recent Developments in Neurocritical Pregnant Patients

59.6.1 Ketamine

Ketamine is emerging as a treatment option for refractory status epilepticus (RSE) in pregnant patients as well. There is growing evidence of potential toxicity due to in-utero exposure to ketamine. Ketamine causes disruption of a NOTCH signaling pathway in neural crest development resulting in increased risk of several congenital malformations (Table 59.2) [74]. Despite the potential fetal toxicity, use of ketamine for RSE may be justified given the significant morbidity and mortality risks to both mother and fetus due to status epilepticus [75].

Ketamine can be used for postoperative pain relief after cesarean section. There are case reports of usage of ketamine for management of pain due to sickle cell crisis in pregnant patients that was refractory to high dose opioids [76].

59.6.2 Immunomodulators and Immunosuppressants

Autoimmune conditions like immune thrombocytopenic purpura and antiphospholipid syndrome can occur in pregnant patients [19]. IVIg mitigates inflammation without causing immunosuppression and can be used for treatment in these conditions. IVIg is also emerging as a treat option in status epilepticus [77].

Azathioprine and tacrolimus are used in post-transplant patients. Table 59.2 gives details of these drugs relevant to pregnancy.

59.7 Conclusion

Neurological emergencies in pregnancy are rare, but can be devastating. Special consideration must be given to early resuscitation, optimal diagnostic techniques, treatment options, and ethical concerns. Management goals broadly remain the same as in nonpregnant patients. However, both maternal and fetal factors must be taken into consideration while managing these patients. This chapter has provided a review of various neurological conditions in pregnancy including rare situations like brain death in pregnancy. However, there are several gaps in knowledge about management of these conditions in pregnancy highlighting the need for further research.

References

1. Cipolla MJ. The adaptation of the cerebral circulation to pregnancy: mechanisms and consequences. J Cereb Blood Flow Metab. 2013;33:465–78.
2. Janzarik WG, Jacob J, Katagis E, Markfeld-Erol F, Sommerlade L, Wuttke M, et al. Preeclampsia postpartum: impairment of cerebral autoregulation and reversible cerebral hyperperfusion. Pregnancy Hypertens. 2019;17:121–6.
3. Jones-Muhammad M, Warrington JP. Cerebral blood flow regulation in pregnancy, hypertension, and hypertensive disorders of pregnancy. Brain Sci. 2019;9:224.
4. Ansari J, Carvalho B, Shafer SL, Flood P. Pharmacokinetics and pharmacodynamics of drugs commonly used in pregnancy and parturition. Anesth Analg. 2016;122:786–804.
5. Pariente G, Leibson T, Carls A, Adams-Webber T, Ito S, Koren G. Pregnancy-associated changes in pharmacokinetics: a systematic review. PLoS Med. 2016;13:e1002160.
6. Desai M, Wali AR, Birk HS, Santiago-Dieppa DR, Khalessi AA. Role of pregnancy and female sex steroids on aneurysm formation, growth, and rupture: a systematic review of the literature. Neurosurg Focus. 2019;47:E8.
7. Roberts D, Dalziel S. Antenatal corticosteroids for accelerating fetal lung maturation for women at risk of preterm birth. Cochrane Database Syst Rev. 2006;3:CD004454.
8. ACR–SPR practice parameter for imaging pregnant or potentially pregnant adolescents and women with ionizing radiation. 2018. https://www.acr.org/Clinical-Resources/Radiology-Safety/Radiation-Safety.
9. Committee Opinion No. 723: guidelines for diagnostic imaging during pregnancy and lactation. Obstet Gynecol. 2017;130:e210–6. Erratum in: Obstet Gynecol. 2018; 132:786.
10. Ryckx N, Sans-Mercea M, Schmidt S, Poletti P-A, Verdun FR. The use of out-of-plane high Z patient shielding for fetal dose reduction in computed tomography: literature review and comparison with Monte-Carlo calculations of an alternative optimisation technique. Phys Med. 2018;48:156–61.
11. Colby GP, Lin L-M, Nundkumar N, Jiang B, Huang J, Tamargo RJ, et al. Radiation dose analysis of large and giant internal carotid artery aneurysm treatment with the pipeline embolization device versus traditional coiling techniques. J Neurointerv Surg. 2015;7:380–4.
12. Malaiyandi D, James E, Peglar L, Karim N, Henkel N, Guilliams K. Neurocritical care of the pregnant patient. Curr Treat Options Neurol. 2021;23:22.
13. Kanal E, Barkovich AJ, Bell C, Borgstede JP, Bradley WG Jr, Froelich JW, et al. ACR guidance document for safe MR practices: 2007. Am J Roentgenol. 2007;188:1447–74.
14. James AH, Bushnell CD, Jamison MG, Myers ER. Incidence and risk factors for stroke in pregnancy and the puerperium. Obstet Gynecol. 2005;106:509–16.
15. Grear KE, Bushnell CD. Stroke and pregnancy: clinical presentation, evaluation, treatment, and epidemiology. Clin Obstet Gynecol. 2013;56:350–9.
16. Robba C, Bacigaluppi S, Bragazzi NL, Bilotta F, Sekhon MS, Bertuetti R, et al. Aneurysmal subarachnoid hemorrhage in pregnancy-case series, review, and pooled data analysis. World Neurosurg. 2016;88:383–98.
17. Ban L, Sprigg N, Sultan AA, Nelson-Piercy C, Bath PM, Ludvigsson JF, et al. Incidence of first stroke in pregnant and nonpregnant women of childbearing age: a population-based cohort study from England. J Am Heart Assoc. 2017;6:e004601.
18. Kamel H, Navi BB, Sriram N, Hovsepian DA, Devereux RB, Elkind MSV. Risk of thrombotic event after the 6-week postpartum period. N Engl J Med. 2014;370:1307–15.
19. Silver RM. Catastrophic antiphospholipid syndrome and pregnancy. Semin Perinatol. 2018;42:26–32.
20. Moatti Z, Gupta M, Yadava R, Thamban S. A review of stroke and pregnancy: incidence, management and prevention. Eur J Obstet Gynecol Reprod Biol. 2014;181:20–7.
21. Feske SK. Stroke in pregnancy. Semin Neurol. 2007;27:442–52.
22. Marder CP, Narla V, Fink JR, Fink KRT. Subarachnoid hemorrhage: beyond aneurysms. Am J Roentgenol. 2014;202:25–37.
23. McDermott M, Miller EC, Rundek T, Hurn PD, Bushnell CD. Preeclampsia: association with posterior reversible encephalopathy syndrome and stroke. Stroke. 2018;49:524–30.
24. Ascanio LC, Maragkos GA, Young BC, Boone MD, Kasper EM. Spontaneous intracranial hemorrhage in pregnancy: a systematic review of the literature. Neurocrit Care. 2019;30:5–15.
25. Coutinho JM, Zuurbier SM, Aramideh M, Stam J. The incidence of cerebral venous thrombosis: a cross-sectional study. Stroke. 2012;2012(43):3375–7.
26. Heit JA, Kobbervig CE, James AH, Petterson TM, Bailey KR, Melton LJ 3rd. Trends in the incidence of venous thromboembolism during pregnancy or postpartum: a 30-year population-based study. Ann Intern Med. 2005;143:697–706.
27. Saposnik G, Barinagarrementeria F, Brown RD, Bushnell CD, Cucchiara B, Cushman M, et al. Diagnosis and management of cerebral venous thrombosis. A statement for healthcare professionals from the American Heart Association/American Stroke Association. Stroke. 2011;42:1158–92.
28. Bateman BT, Olbrecht VA, Berman MF, Minehart RD, Schwamm LH, Leffert LR. Peripartum subarachnoid hemorrhage: nationwide data and institutional experience. Anesthesiology. 2012;116:324–33.

29. Powers WJ, Rabinstein AA, Ackerson T, Adeoye OM, Bambakidis NC, Becker K, et al. 2018 guidelines for the early management of patients with acute ischemic stroke: a guideline for healthcare professionals from the American Heart Association/American Stroke Association. Stroke. 2018;49:e46–110.
30. Ladhani NNN, Swartz RH, Foley N, Nerenberg K, Smith EE, Gubitz G, et al. Canadian stroke best practice consensus statement: acute stroke management during pregnancy. Int J Stroke. 2018;13:743–58.
31. Watson K, Broscious R, Devabhakthuni S, Noel ZR. Focused update on pharmacologic management of hypertensive emergencies. Curr Hypertens Rep. 2018;20:56–73.
32. Ebke M, Jurgens KU, Tomandl B, Merten U, Kastrup A. Surgical treatment of space occupying edema and hemorrhage due to cerebral venous thrombosis during pregnancy. Neurocrit Care. 2011;15:166–9.
33. Ferro JM, Coutinho JM, Dentali F, Kobayashi A, Alasheev A, Canhão P, et al. Safety and efficacy of dabigatran etexilate vs dose-adjusted warfarin in patients with cerebral venous thrombosis: a randomized clinical trial. JAMA Neurol. 2019;76:1457–65.
34. Tranquilli AL, Giannubilo SR. Use and safety of calcium channel blockers in obstetrics. Curr Med Chem. 2009;16:3330–40.
35. Selo-Ojeme DO, Marshman LAG, Ikomi A, Ojutiku D, Aspoas RA, Chawda SJ, et al. Aneurysmal subarachnoid haemorrhage in pregnancy. Eur J Obstet Gynecol Reprod Biol. 2004;116:131–43.
36. Minzter BH, Johnson RF, Paschall RL, Ramasubramanian R, Ayers GD, Downing JW. The diverse effects of vasopressors on the fetoplacental circulation of the dual perfused human placenta. Anesth Analg. 2010;110:857–62.
37. Pollock W, Rose L, Dennis CL. Pregnant and postpartum admissions to the intensive care unit: a systematic review. Intensive Care Med. 2010;36:1465–74.
38. ACOG practice bulletin No. 202: gestational hypertension and preeclampsia. Obstet Gynecol. 2019;133:1.
39. Antza C, Doundoulakis I, Akrivos E, Dimou C, Stabouli S, Haidich A, et al. Hydralazine in pregnancy: a systematic review and meta-analysis. J Hypertens. 2019;37:e40.
40. Duley L, Henderson-Smart DJ, Meher S. Drugs for rapid treatment of very high blood pressure during pregnancy. Cochrane Database Syst Rev. 2006;3:CD001449.
41. Sibai BM. Diagnosis, prevention, and management of eclampsia. Obstet Gynecol. 2005;105:402–10.
42. Sheth SS, Sheth KN. Treatment of neurocritical care emergencies in pregnancy. Curr Treat Options Neurol. 2012;14:197–210.
43. Ostrom QT, Gittleman H, Truitt G, Boscia A, Kruchko C, Barnholtz-Sloan JS, et al. CBTRUS statistical report: primary brain and other central nervous system tumors diagnosed in the United States in 2011–2015. Neuro-Oncology. 2018;20:iv1–86.
44. Godoy DA, Robba C, Paiva WS, Rabinstein AA. Acute intracranial hypertension during pregnancy: special considerations and management adjustments. Neurocrit Care. 2022;36:302–16.
45. Pacheco LD, Saade GR, Hankins GDV. Mechanical ventilation during pregnancy: sedation, analgesia, and paralysis. Clin Obstet Gynecol. 2014;57:844–50.
46. Frontera JA, Ahmed W. Neurocritical care complications of pregnancy and puerperum. J Crit Care. 2014;29:1069–81.
47. Nag DS, Samaddar DP, Chatterjee A, Kumar H, Dembla A. Vasopressors in obstetric anesthesia: a current perspective. World J Clin Cases. 2015;3:58–64.
48. Stevens AD, Lumbers ER. Effects of intravenous infusions of noradrenaline into the pregnant ewe on uterine blood flow, fetal renal function, and lung liquid flow. Can J Physiol Pharmacol. 1995;73:202–8.
49. Stevenson CB, Thompson RC. The clinical management of intracranial neoplasms in pregnancy. Clin Obstet Gynecol. 2005;48:24–37.
50. Abou-Ghannam G, Usta IM, Nassar AH. Indomethacin in pregnancy: applications and safety. Am J Perinatol. 2012;29:175–86.
51. Unterrainer AF, Steiner H, Kundt MJ. Caesarean section and brain tumour resection. Br J Anaesth. 2011;107:111–2.
52. Harden CL, Hopp J, Ting TY, Pennell PB, French JA, Hauser WA, et al. Practice parameter update: management issues for women with epilepsy—focus on pregnancy (an evidence-based review): obstetrical complications and change in seizure frequency: report of the quality standards subcommittee and therapeutics and technology assessment subcommittee of the American Academy of neurology and American Epilepsy Society. Neurology. 2009;73:126–32.
53. Thomas SV, Syam U, Devi JS. Predictors of seizures during pregnancy in women with epilepsy. Epilepsia. 2012;53:e85–8.
54. Asranna A, Jose M, Philip RM, Sarma PS, Thomas SV. Do anti-epileptic drug modifications after first trimester of pregnancy influence fetal malformation or cognitive outcome? Epilepsy Res. 2018;146:121–5.
55. Veroniki AA, Cogo E, Rios P, Straus SE, Finkelstein Y, Kealey R, et al. Comparative safety of anti-epileptic drugs during pregnancy: a systematic review and network meta-analysis of congenital malformations and prenatal outcomes. BMC Med. 2017;15:95.
56. Singhal AB, Bernstein RA. Postpartum angiopathy and other cerebral vasoconstriction syndromes. Neurocrit Care. 2005;3:91–7.
57. Fugate JE, Ameriso SF, Ortiz G, Schottlaender LV, Wijdicks EFM, Flemming KD, et al. Variable presentations of postpartum angiopathy. Stroke. 2012;43:670–6.
58. Rosenbloom MH, Singhal AB. CT angiography and diffusion-perfusion MR imaging in a patient with ipsilateral reversible cerebral vasoconstriction after carotid endarterectomy. Am J Neuroradiol. 2007;28:920–2.

59. Macri E, Chandos DG. Neurological emergencies during pregnancy. Neurol Clin. 2021;39:649–70.
60. Maheut-Lourmie're J, Si CT. Hydrocephalus during pregnancy with or without neurosurgical history in childhood. Practical advice for management. Neurochirurgie. 2000;46:117–21.
61. Ng J, Kitchen N. Neurosurgery and pregnancy. J Neurol Neurosurg Psychiatry. 2008;79:745–52.
62. Bansal R, Goyal MK, Modi M. Management of myasthenia gravis during pregnancy. Indian J Pharmacol. 2018;50:302–8.
63. Gamez J, Salvado M, Casellas M, Manrique S, Castillo F. Intravenous immunoglobulin as monotherapy for myasthenia gravis during pregnancy. J Neurol Sci. 2017;383:118–22.
64. Hamel J, Ciafaloni E. An update: myasthenia gravis and pregnancy. Neurol Clin. 2018;36:355–65.
65. Tsurane K, Tanabe S, Miyasaka N, Matsuda M, Takahara M, Ida T, et al. Management of labor and delivery in myasthenia gravis: a new protocol. J Obstet Gynaecol Res. 2019;45:974–80.
66. Cialfaloni E, Massey JM. The management of myasthenia gravis in pregnancy. Semin Neurol. 2004;24:95–100.
67. Zelop CM, Einav S, Mhyre JM, Martin S. Cardiac arrest during pregnancy: ongoing clinical conundrum. Am J Obstet Gynecol. 2018;219:52–61.
68. Kikuchi J, Deering S. Cardiac arrest in pregnancy. Semin Perinatol. 2018;42:33–8.
69. Jeejeebhoy FM, Zelop CM, Lipman S, Carvalho B, Joglar J, Mhyre JM, et al. Cardiac arrest in pregnancy: a scientific statement from the American Heart Association. Circulation. 2015;132:1747–73.
70. Lewis A, Varelas P, Greer D. Pregnancy and brain death: lack of guidance in US Hospital policies. Am J Perinatol. 2016;33:1382–7.
71. Pikto-Pietkiewicz I, Okniński A, Wójtowicz R, Wójtowicz M. The management of a thirteen weeks pregnant woman rendered brain-dead following a ruptured aneurysm. J Crit Care Med (Targu Mures). 2019;5:111–4.
72. Staff L, Nash M. Brain death during pregnancy and prolonged corporeal support of the body: a critical discussion. Women Birth. 2017;30:354–60.
73. Esmaeilzadeh M, Dictus C, Kayvanpour E, Sedaghat-Hamedani F, Eichbaum M, Hofer S, et al. One life ends, another begins: management of a brain-dead pregnant mother—a systematic review. BMC Med. 2010;8:74.
74. Shi Y, Li J, Chen C, Xia Y, Li Y, Zhang P, et al. Ketamine modulates Zic5 expression via the Notch signaling pathway in neural crest induction. Front Mol Neurosci. 2018;11:9.
75. Talahma M, Sabharwal V, Bukovskaya Y, Khan F. Ketamine infusion used to successfully control refractory status epilepticus in a pregnant patient. Case Rep Neurol Med. 2018;2018:3041279.
76. Gimovsky AC, Fritton K, Viscusi E, Roman A. Evaluating the use of ketamine for pain control with sickle cell crisis in pregnancy: a report of 2 cases. A A Pract. 2018;10:20–2.
77. Zeiler FA, Matuszczak M, Teitelbaum J, Kazina CJ, Gillman LM. Intravenous immunoglobulins for refractory status epilepticus, part I: a scoping systematic review of the adult literature. Seizure. 2017;45:172–80.

Part IX

Ethics in Neurocritical Care

60 Ethical Issues in Neurocritical Care

Jaya Wanchoo

60.1 Introduction

A sense of ethical responsibility has always accompanied the profession of medicine. The Charaka Shapath is considered to be one of the oldest guiding principles for the medical professionals [1]. It lays emphasis on "complete trust between a physician and his patient, doing no harm to the patient and working for his best interests in every possible way." All these are relevant even today. The Hippocratic Oath is an oath of ethics derived from the Greek medical texts. It is a charter of ethical principles that physicians over the ages have sworn to uphold in the practice of their profession. The original oath is known to date back to the late third century AD. It provides moral guidelines and a code of conduct to doctors for their acceptable and dignified professional conduct.

The role of the World Medical Association (WMA) is to ensure the highest possible standard of ethical practice of the medical profession [2]. Since its establishment in 1947, the WMA has adopted a comprehensive range of declarations and resolutions to guide the medical practitioner. At the heart of the WMA's body of policies, three core documents are presented: the Declaration of Geneva: The Physician's Pledge, the Declaration of Helsinki, and the International Code of Medical Ethics. These outline the ethical principles and professional duties of the medical profession, including the physician's responsibilities toward patients, students, and society and towards other healthcare professionals. The Constitution of India also grants right to life as a fundamental right (Article 21). The Supreme Court has elaborated that the right to life includes proper diagnosis, proper medicine, and proper attendance.

Modern medicine has made enough technological progress to keep patients alive while supporting multi-organ failure. One of the greatest challenges clinicians face in the intensive care unit is to decide if and when it is appropriate to initiate 'end-of-life' care with the withdrawal of active measures in patients following severe brain damage.

60.2 Principles of Ethics

The four fundamental principles of ethics include Beneficence, nonmaleficence, autonomy and distributive justice [3, 4]. The basis of all ethical principles include avoiding harm to the patient, providing maximum benefit and respecting his/her wishes and preferences.

1. **Beneficence**

    The principle of beneficence is the obligation of physician to act for the benefit of the patient, to protect and defend their rights, pre-

J. Wanchoo (✉)
Medanta The Medicity, Gurugram, Haryana, India

H. Prabhakar et al. (eds.), *Principles and Practice of Neurocritical Care*,
https://doi.org/10.1007/978-981-99-8059-8_60

vent harm, remove conditions that will cause harm, help persons with disabilities, and rescue persons in danger. Healthcare providers have a duty to be of benefit to the patient, as well as to take positive steps to prevent and remove harm from the patient. The benefit may be at a physiologic, biomedical, or personal level. This principle is at the very heart of healthcare implying that a suffering supplicant (the patient) can enter into a relationship with one whom society has licensed as competent to provide medical care, trusting that the physician's chief objective is to help.

2. **Nonmaleficence**

   Nonmaleficence is the obligation of a physician not to harm the patient. This principle supports several moral rules—do not kill, do not cause pain or suffering, do not incapacitate, do not cause offense, and do not deprive others of the goods of life. The practical application of nonmaleficence is for the physician to weigh the benefits against burdens of all interventions and treatment and to choose the best course of action for the patient. This is particularly important and pertinent in difficult end-of-life care decisions on withholding or withdrawing life-sustaining treatment, medically administered nutrition and hydration, and in pain and other symptom control. A physician's obligation and intention to relieve the suffering of a patient by the use of appropriate drugs including opioids override the foreseen but unintended harmful effects or outcome (doctrine of double effect). The principle of nonmaleficence requires that we do not intentionally create harm or injury to the patient, either through acts of commission or omission. Medical mistakes may occur; however, this principle articulates a fundamental commitment on the part of healthcare professionals to protect their patients from harm [5, 6].

3. **Autonomy**

   Immanuel Kant (1724–1804) and John Stuart Mill (1806–1873) have interpreted and accepted autonomy as an ethical principle [7]. According to them, all persons have intrinsic and unconditional worth, and should have the power to make rational decisions and moral choices. This ethical principle was affirmed in a court decision by Justice Cardozo in 1914 with the dictum, "Every human being of adult years and sound mind has a right to determine what shall be done with his own body." The principle of autonomy cannot extend to persons who lack the capacity or competence to take independent decisions, examples being infants, children, and incompetence due to developmental, mental, or physical disorder. Competency is a legal term and all adults are legally competent unless a court of law has determined otherwise. On the other hand, capacity is a functional determination that the patients physician makes and can vary over time as the medical condition changes. A rigid distinction between incapacity to make healthcare decisions (assessed by health professionals) and incompetence (determined by court of law) is not always possible as a clinician's determination of a patient's lack of decision-making capacity based on physical or mental disorder has the same practical consequences as a legal determination of incompetence [8–10].

   For a patient to have capacity for a particular decision, he or she must be able to comprehend the information presented, compare the alternatives and their consequences, question information rationally, and communicate their decision in a meaningful way.

   Respecting the principle of autonomy obliges the physician to disclose medical information and treatment options available for a particular disease and supports the principles of informed consent, truth telling, and confidentiality.

60.2.1 Informed Consent

The requirements of an informed consent for a medical or surgical procedure, or for research, are that the patient or subject:

- Must be competent to understand and decide
- Receives a full disclosure

- Comprehends the disclosure
- Acts voluntarily
- Consents to the proposed action

An informed consent should include the following:

- Patient diagnosis
- Intervention proposed
- Benefits, risks, and burdens
- Consequences of withholding it
- Alternatives and their consequences

60.2.2 Truth Telling

Truth telling is a vital component in a physician-patient relationship; without this component, the physician loses the trust of the patient. A patient not only has the right to know of his/her diagnosis and prognosis, but also has the option to forgo this disclosure.

60.2.3 Confidentiality

Physicians are expected not to disclose confidential information given by a patient to another party without the patient's authorization. An exception may be considered when necessary information is shared from the primary physician to consultants and other healthcare teams. In the present-day modern hospitals with the use of electronic medical records, there can be an erosion of confidentiality. However, individual physicians must exercise discipline in not discussing patient specifics with their family members or in social gatherings and social media. There are some exceptions to patient confidentiality-reporting of medico-legal cases like road traffic accidents, gunshot wounds, sexually transmitted diseases, situations that may cause major harm to another, e.g., epidemics of infectious diseases, partner notification in HIV disease, and relative notification of certain genetic risks [11].

60.2.4 Distributive Justice

Distributive justice refers to the fair, equitable, and appropriate distribution of healthcare resources. There are different principles of distributive justice. These are distribution to each person (1) an equal share, (2) according to need, (3) according to effort, (4) according to contribution, (5) according to merit, and (6) according to free-market exchanges. Each principle is not exclusive, and can be combined in application. It is easy to see the difficulty in choosing, balancing, and refining these principles to form a coherent and workable solution to distribute medical. Despite all the ethics and rules laid down in theory, it is not always easy for the physician to follow them in practice. It may not be easy to prognosticate a patient, to quantify his term disabilities or predict the outcome [12, 13].

60.3 Dilemmas in Ethical Practice

Despite theoretical guidelines for ethical practice, there are several situations which pose a challenge for the physicians and it may become difficult to choose the correct path for an individual. The common examples are as follows:

1. Surrogate decision-making and role of a living will
2. Accurate prognostication
3. Declaring medical futility
4. Conflicts in organ donation

60.3.1 Role of Advance Directives and Surrogate Decision-Maker

Most of the patients in the neurocritical care unit have impaired capacity to make decisions regarding their line of treatment or even withdrawal of treatment. In these cases, the clinicians have to depend on the decisions based on advance directives (such as a living will), decisions taken by the family, or the decisions of a surrogate, assuming they are in the best interest of the patient. The neurointensivist has a very large and vital role to play in this shared decision-making process.

Has the living will be failed?

> *In pursuit of the dream that patients' exercise of autonomy could extend beyond their span of competence, living wills have passed from controversy to conventional wisdom, to widely promoted policy. But the policy has not produced results, and should be abandoned* [14].

Legally, a written directive would provide the most concrete evidence of the patient's decisions. The AMA's Council on Ethical and Judicial Affairs proclaims: "Physicians should encourage their patients to document their treatment preferences or to appoint a healthcare proxy with whom they can discuss their values regarding healthcare and treatment" [15].

The various reasons why a living will does not seem to work are that it may be signed years before it is used, the nature of illness, and the treatment modalities cannot be predicted beforehand. The proxy may not understand the wishes of the dying person.

The current status in India is that passive euthanasia was legalised in 2018 for people with a living will. This document required the counter signature of a first class judicial magistrate, and a judge serving in the lower rungs of Indian courts. The challenges faced were access to such a judge due to overburdened courts and lack of awareness among the judicial magistrates. It also required a three-tier check by the internal medical board at the hospital, district collector and a final physical verification of the patient by a judicial magistrate. To make matters simpler, the court has now done away with these processes. The living will can be attested by public notaries or a gazetted senior government officer. The three-tier check was also simplified. This does raise concerns of it being misused by some people. The people in support of these changes think that this was needed for dignified death by following the wishes of an individual when he was competent enough to put them forward [16].

The bioethical hierarchy of three decision-making standards is endorsed widely by both medicine and the law [17].

First and foremost, the explicit wishes of the patients or a living will are to be followed. Living wills typically apply only in the setting of terminal illness, permanent unconsciousness, or other end-stage conditions. A living will may not take effect in the common scenario of a patient facing serious illness with a high probability of death or disability. Written documents are generally given more weight than verbal statements, unless it is witnessed and documented by a physician.

If the patient's wishes are unknown, the next highest standard is based on the principle of substituted judgment, in which a surrogate decision has to be made based on an understanding of the patient's values and preferences. The typical hierarchy of surrogates is a spouse, followed by grown children, and then additional family members [18].

In some instances, when there is no appropriate surrogate, a court-appointed surrogate, often referred to as a legal guardian, may be necessary.

If clinicians are convinced that surrogates are not well-enough informed to do so, then the patients' best interests should guide surrogates' decision-making [19, 20]. If no information about the patient's values and preferences is available, decisions should be made according to the best interest standard. The best interest standard involves looking at risks and benefits of a treatment and making decisions according to how a reasonable person would be expected to balance it.

Despite laws and rules being laid down, decision-making is not without its problems.

Advance directives are usually not documented for most of the patients, and if so, they have their strengths and weaknesses. The family may have disagreements on the line of treatment or the interpretation of the living will if found. Surrogates are not always able to accurately predict patients' preferences, may overestimate the patients desire for life support and serving as a surrogate decision-maker can be a substantial emotional burden for a family member [21, 22].

The preferred approach is to discuss overall goals of care first. Common goals of care include prioritizing comfort over length of life, survival at any cost regardless of disability, or survival only if disability is minimized. Once the goals of care have been established, the treating team can help the family understand the patient's current condition and whether the various treatment options will be able to achieve the goals of care. If families seem unable to reach a consensus or are struggling with the emotional burden of the decision process, a specific treatment recommendation can be provided. The most important intervention on which surrogate decision-making rests is effective family meetings where mutual sharing of information and expertise—medical knowledge from the physician and knowledge pertaining to patients' values and priorities from family—will lead to optimum medical treatments and care most in accordance with patient preferences [23, 24].

60.3.2 Prognostication

Kondziella et al. argued that premature end-of-life care should be avoided. If a meaningful physical and cognitive recovery is very likely to occur, a strong case can be made for this decision. Making and effectively communicating an accurate neurological prognosis is an ethical duty as well as a medical responsibility. This is never easy due to the lack of adequate data base or good quality studies, which are usually observational. It becomes difficult to predict the outcome, more so in acute settings. Good communication and daily counselling with the patients' family is the key to building trust and good prognostication.

A systematic way to improve accuracy of prognosis is to rely on clinical factors like patient's age, general health, co-morbidities, and their level of frailty. Reversible factors such as sedatives, muscle relaxants, electrolyte disturbances, fever, sepsis, anaemia, seizures, and multi-organ failure may complicate or delay this decision-making [25–27].

60.3.3 Medical Futility

The biggest challenge is—How does one define medical futility? It may be defined in qualitative and quantitative terms. Qualitative futility would mean that the patient benefit from the proposed treatment is extremely low in terms of quality and length of life. Quantitative futility on the other hand means that therapy should not be performed because available data show that it will not improve the patient's medical condition, the dynamic variable being advance in medical science which makes futility a moving target. It is important for this reason that the healthcare team shares the progress with the family on a daily basis so that everyone understands the evolution of what is happening and the risks taken for the patient. Determining patient benefit requires discussing with patients families their values and goals as well as the burdens and benefits of further treatment. The disadvantage of futile treatment is both for the family, in terms of moral distress and the medical systems, in terms of using the scarce resources and denying them to someone who may benefit from them [28–31].

Recently revised Australian Medical Association (AMA) position statement on end-of-life care and advance care planning states that -in end-of-life care, medically futile treatment can be considered to be treatment that gives no, or an extremely small, chance of meaningful prolongation of survival and, at best, can only briefly delay the inevitable death of the patient [32].

60.3.4 Conflicts in Organ Donation

The neurocritical care physicians have an ethical and legal duty to offer organ donation to families of dying patients. The conflicts arise in two situations:

1. When a family member believes that a physician has more interest in the patient's organs than in the patient's welfare. These apparent conflicts between the duty to care for the dying patient and to offer organ donation can be minimized if critical care physicians and nurses adopt the attitude of "dual advocacy" in which

they simultaneously promote excellent end-of-life care and organ donation. The dual advocacy approach is founded on the belief that "given the opportunity, most people will choose to help others" which is the basis of a successful voluntary organ donation program.

2. Presumed Vs explicit consent-The near-universal acceptance of cadaveric organ donation has been based on the provision of explicit consent by the donor while alive, in the form of a formal signature to pledge his organs upon his death. In the event of untimely death of a potential donor with no explicit consent for organ donation, most countries accept 'consent' to donation being provided by his closest relatives (presumed consent). A presumption of consent is considered ethically sound and morally justified in organ retrieval for transplantation, provided information on the opt-out process is readily available in easily comprehensible formats, and families are given a say in the final decision. The next-of-kin have a considerable influence on the organ procurement process in both presumed and explicit consents [33–36]. Organ donation remains an important medical and social goal that should be supported fully because of the obvious good it provides to the recipients and the associated benefit to the donor family.

ICU clinicians should be competent in end-of-life care, including the use of sedatives, analgesics, and nonpharmacologic approaches to ease the suffering of the dying process. They should know when to withhold or withdraw treatment, improve communication skills with the family. In case the patient is an organ donor, this care extends even after the death of the patient. Comprehensive guidelines for improving end-of-life care should be in place in all neuro intensive care units [37].

60.3.5 Ethical Decision-Making Model

All over the world, people have tried to create do-not-resuscitate models, making end-of-life care simpler and more compassionate [38]. As advance directives are not very specific, being a surrogate decision-maker can pose its own challenges. Determining the appropriate course to take when faced with an ethical dilemma can be a challenge [39, 40]. The American counseling Association (ACA) Ethics Committee has developed a guide to ethical decision-making [41, 42]. The intent of this document is to offer professional counsellors a framework for sound ethical decision-making and involves the following steps:

1. Identification of the problem
2. Apply the code of ethics
3. Determine the nature and dimensions of the dilemmas
4. Generate potential courses of action.
5. Consider the potential consequences of all options, determine a course of action
6. Evaluate the selected course of action
7. Implement the course of action

References

1. Singh M. Oaths, codes, ethics and the essence of medicine: a time for resurrection. Natl Med J India. 1997;10(4):190–3.
2. Parsi RW. The international code of medical ethics of the world medical association. JAMA. 2022;328(20):37.
3. Varkey B. Principles of clinical ethics and their application to practice. Med Princ Pract. 2021;30:17–28. https://doi.org/10.1159/000509119.
4. Perrigault PF, Greco F. Ethical issues in neurocritical care. Rev Neurol (Paris). 2022;178(1–2):57–63.
5. Rosenfeld JV, et al. The clinical and ethical challenges of treating comatose patients following severe brain injury. Acta Neurochir. 2023;165:829–31. https://doi.org/10.1007/s00701-022-05376-7.
6. Hawley L, et al. Ethical considerations in chronic brain injury. J Head Trauma Rehabil. 2019;34(6):433–6.
7. Autonomy in Moral and Political Philosophy. The Stanford Encyclopedia of Philosophy (Fall 2020 Edition).
8. Beauchamp JF, Childress TL. Respect for autonomy. Principles of biomedical ethics. 4th ed. New York: Oxford University Press; 1994. p. 120–88.
9. Couillard P, Keith WA, Brownell. Ethical perspectives in neurology. Continuum Lifelong Learning Neurol. 2009;15(1):159–64.
10. Schreiner TG. Particular ethical issues in neurology and neuroscience research on human sub-

ject—a review article. Int J Med Rev Case Rep. 2020;4(11):5–10.
11. O'Brien J, Chantler C, J. Confidentiality and the duties of care. Med Ethics. 2003;29:36–40.
12. Galiatsatos P. Health equity and distributive justice considerations in critical care resource allocation. Lancet Respir Med. 2020;8(8):758–60.
13. Smith GP, Justice D, Care H. J Contemp Health Law Policy. 2002;18:421–30.
14. Fagerlin A, Schneider CE. Enough: the failure of the living will. Hastings Center Rep. 2004;34(2):30–42.
15. Council on Ethical and Judicial Affairs of the American Medical Association, Surrogate Decision Making E8.081. http://www.ama-assn.org.
16. Choudhary H. Analysis of the common cause judgment: would living wills become a practical reality? ILI Law Rev. 2019:II.
17. Adelman E, Darin BZ. Surrogate decision making in neurocritical care. Continuum Lifelong Learning Neurol. 2012;18(3):655–8.
18. Berger JT, et al. Surrogate decision making: reconciling ethical theory and clinical practice. Ann Intern Med. 2008;149:48–53.
19. Cai X, et al. Patient preferences and surrogate decision making in neuroscience intensive Care units. Neurocrit Care. 2015;23(1):131–41. https://doi.org/10.1007/s12028-015-0149-2.
20. Devnani R, et al. How surrogates decide: a secondary data analysis of decision-making principles used by the surrogates of hospitalized older adults. Gen Intern Med. 2017;32(12):1285–93.
21. Thompson T, et al. Adherence to advance directives in critical care decision making: vignette study. BMJ. 2003;327(7422):1011.
22. Shalowitz DI, Garrett-Mayer E, Wendler D. The accuracy of surrogate decision makers: a systematic review. Arch Intern Med. 2006;166(5):493–7.
23. Azoulay E, Pochard F, Kentish-Barnes N, et al. Risk of post-traumatic stress symptoms in family members of intensive care unit patients. Am J Respir Crit Care Med. 2005;171(9):987–94.
24. Wynn S. Decision by surrogates: an overview of surrogate consent laws in the United States. Bifocal. 2014;36(1)
25. Boyd EA, et al. It's not just what the doctor tells me: factors that influence surrogate decision-makers' perceptions of prognosis. Crit Care Med. 2010;38(5):1270–5.
26. Evans LR, et al. Surrogate decision-makers' perspectives on discussing prognosis in the face of uncertainty. Am J Respir Crit Care Med. 2009;179(1):48–53.
27. Bernat JL. Observations on ethical issues in the neuro-ICU. Neurocrit Care. 2015;23:1–320.
28. White B, et al. What does "futility" mean? An empirical study of doctors' perceptions. Med J Aust. 2016;204(8):318.
29. Huynh TN, et al. The opportunity cost of futile treatment in the ICU. Crit Care Med. 2014;42:1977–82.
30. Schneiderman LJ. Defining medical futility and improving medical care. J Bioeth Inq. 2011;8:123–31.
31. Swetz KM, et al. Ten common questions (and their answers) on medical futility. Mayo Clin Proc. 2014;89:943–59.
32. Australian Medical Association. Position statement on end of life care and advance care planning. Canberra: AMA; 2014. https://ama.com.au/position-statement/positionstatement-end-life-care-and-advancecare-planning-2014. Accessed Sept 2015.
33. Farsides B. Respecting wishes and avoiding conflict: understanding the ethical basis for organ donation and retrieval. Br J Anaesth. 2012;108(S1):i73–9.
34. Amanda M. The authority of next-of-kin in explicit and presumed consent systems for deceased organ donation: an analysis of 54 nations. Nephrol Dial Transplant. 2012;27:2533–46.
35. Prabhu. Is presumed consent an ethically acceptable way of obtaining organs for transplant? J Intensive Care Society. 2019;20(2):92–7.
36. Truog RD. Consent for organ donation–balancing conflicting ethical obligations. NEJM. 2008;358:1209–11.
37. Truog RD, et al. Recommendations for end-of-life care in the intensive care unit: a consensus statement by the American College of Critical Care Medicine. Crit Care Med. 2008;36(3):953–63.
38. White DB, et al. Are physicians' recommendations to limit life support beneficial or burdensome? Bringing empirical data to the debate. Am J Respir Crit Care Med. 2009;180(4):320–5.
39. Zahuranec DB, et al. Do-not-resuscitate orders and predictive models after intracerebral hemorrhage. Neurology. 2010;75(7):626.
40. Wiesen J, et al. Medical, ethical, and legal aspects of end-of-life dilemmas in the intensive care unit. Cleve Clin J Med. 2021;88(9):516–27.
41. Forester-Miller H, David T. A practitioner's guide to ethical decision making. American Counseling Association; 1996.
42. American Counseling Association. Code of ethics. Alexeandria, VA; 2005.

61 Diagnosing Brain Death

Pratheema Ramachandran

61.1 Introduction

As early as 1950s, the concept of death had been always woven around the loss of cardiorespiratory functions. Gradually, there was a lot of development in the field of medicine like mechanical ventilation, cardiopulmonary resuscitation, etc. which could sustain a person artificially and the concept of death changed gradually with the advent of these measures. In 1959, a patient who was apneic and comatose state void of brain stem activity was first described as "le coma depasse" by Goulon and Molaret [1]. More interest propped up and the description of death was redefined with neurological criteria. Death by Neurological Criteria (DNC) attracted a lot of interest and research from 1959.

61.2 Brain Death or Brain Stem Death?

As such, the term "brain death" has met more than one concept. First of all, the original Harvard criteria, which was officially formulated in the US, included [2] the injury to the major structures of the brain—cerebrum, diencephalon, and cerebellum, and for the declaration of brain death, the loss of activity in all these structures needed to be confirmed except the loss of neuroendocrine function [3]. The other concept, mostly accepted in the UK, is that brain stem damage was termed as "brain death" and was considered as death of the human. It is clearly described that a severe infratentorial injury was enough to declare brain death. But there was also a third concept, which made it specific to confirm the loss of higher brain function to diagnose brain death [4–6]. Whatever the concepts may be, irreversible damage and loss of brainstem functions make the human incompatible with life. The declaration of death by neurological criteria is the way forward to decide on organ transplantation [7], which is an entire separate entity by itself. So, the declaration puts a clinician into multifaceted responsibilities including ethical and social aspects. Hence, it is imperative to have clear concepts and understanding of the do's and don'ts of brain-dead declaration. The following sections of this chapter will describe and analyze each and every step of the process.

61.3 Determination of Brain Death

The recognition and diagnosis of death by neurological criteria [8, 9] is of utmost importance and involves various stages. A careful step-by-step approach with clear documentation with the use

P. Ramachandran (✉)
Apollo Specialty Hospitals, OMR, Chennai, Tamil Nadu, India

H. Prabhakar et al. (eds.), *Principles and Practice of Neurocritical Care*,
https://doi.org/10.1007/978-981-99-8059-8_61

of standardized checklists (published by the World Brain Death Project) can avoid confusion among the treating team.

The steps for declaration of brain death are as follows.

A. Ensure etiology of brain injury
B. Exclusion of confounders and confirming irreversibility
C. Clinical testing of brain stem reflexes
D. Clinical motor testing
E. Apnea testing

These steps should be done in a sequential order [10], and the flow of order must not be changed as each one is of paramount importance to ensure correct diagnosis.

A. Ensure etiology of brain injury

The first and most major step to start with is the confirmation of etiology of brain injury. For this, a detailed history, clinical examination [11], and review of neuroimaging (Figs. 61.1, 61.2, and 61.3) which had led to the catastrophe need to be looked into. There should be no assumptions or guesses when it comes to the declaration. An unbiased personal review of the imaging and other tests helps to confirm the gravity of the situation and gives a better perspective to reconfirm irreversible brainstem injury.

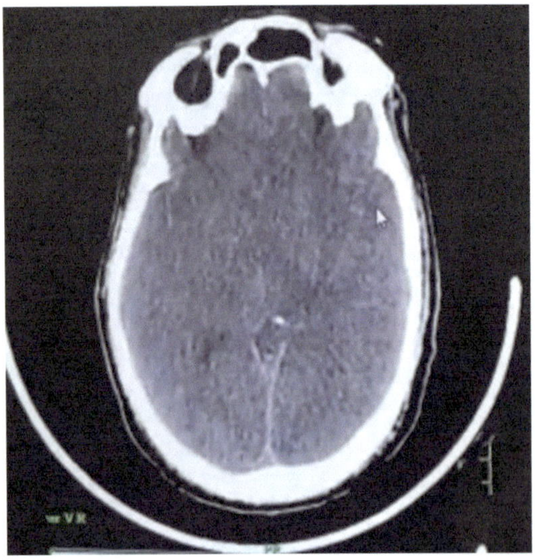

Fig. 61.1 CT scan showing features of severe cerebral edema (tight brain)

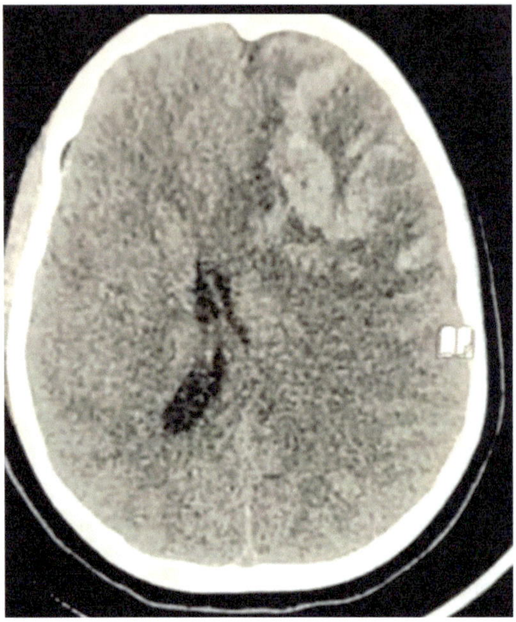

Fig. 61.2 CT scan showing left intraparenchymal bleed with midline shift

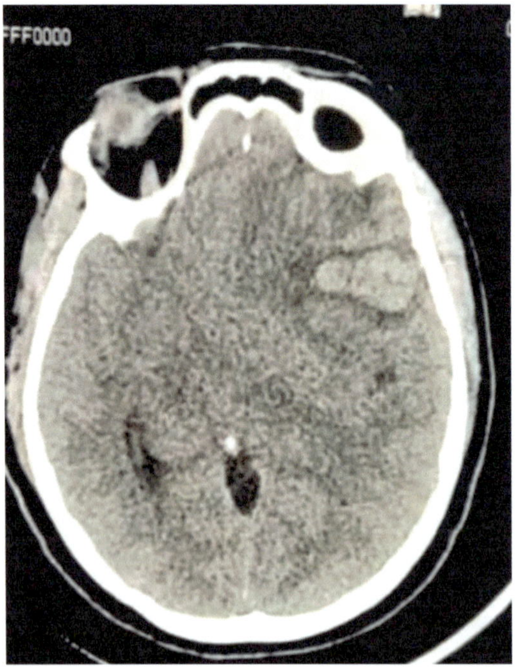

Fig. 61.3 CT scan showing left intraparenchymal bleed with midline shift and increased ICP

B. Exclusion of confounders and confirming irreversible damage

Testing for brain death should not be done if there is a normal neuroimaging, intact respiratory drive, or insufficient evaluation of the requirements for brain death. The confounding factors should be looked for and excluded before proceeding with the brain death testing. The confounders are drug overdose, hypothermia, and metabolic derangements like dyselectrolytemias.

Drug Overdose:

It can be difficult to determine brain death in a patient with a known overdose because brainstem reflexes are a crucial part of brain death [11, 12] and are known to occur with neuronal dysfunction from drug toxicity. There is a fear that xenobiotics with characteristics changing nerve transmission, producing apnea, or causing central nervous system depression may conceal intact brain activity and make the physical exam inaccurate, even while overdose and poisoning can truly be fatal. Also, an overdose indicates a strange circumstance in which a patient with a severe critical condition can recover without suffering long-term effects. It can be hard to rule out an overdose suspicion.

It is frequently uncertain what was ingested, when it was ingested, or what the history of the substances was. Even when poisoning is suspected, it may take hours or days to obtain xenobiotic drug concentrations, [13, 14] and toxicity frequently does not correlate with drug concentration in the blood compartment—a problem that was identified more than 40 years ago and is still present today. An overview of the instances and traits of xenobiotic poisoning (Table 61.1) that results in reversible loss of brainstem reflexes serves as a guide for medical professionals when attempting to diagnose brain death in these challenging patients.

CNS Depressants:

Before we start with the brain death testing, it is pertinent to exclude CNS depressants drug usage in the last 24 h. CNS depressants include benzodiazepines, opiates barbiturates, and ethanol.

Particularly, opioids are major confounders and mimic brain death in large doses. These drugs cause miosis which is a major distinguishing factor from the bilateral pupillary dilation found in cases of brain stem death. Paralytics agents, barbiturates, and benzodiazepines [12, 15–17] have prolonged action, particularly in cases of renal dysfunction. Train of four testing helps to detect muscle relaxants interference with the testing.

During most of the initial management of neuro cases, multiple CNS depressants are used in a desperate measure to manage the increasing intracranial pressure and reducing the cerebral metabolic rate [18–20], to an extent that some patients are put on induced barbiturate coma. Hence, declaring or testing for brain death requires a wait period from drug stoppage of the drug infusion allowing the drug to get excreted. It takes about [21–23] five half-lives for 97% of the drug to get eliminated from the body. Sometimes, even longer in cases of renal dysfunction. The

Table 61.1 Xenobiotics/drug overdoses mimicking brain death

S. no.	Xenobiotic	Mechanism	Treatment
	Snake envenomation	Neurotoxic effect, blockade of acetylcholine receptor or its release	Anti-snake venom
2	Baclofen	GABA agonist, blocks release of excitatory transmitters like glutamate, aspartate High doses cross the blood brain barrier	Supportive care
3.	Tricyclic antidepressants	Central and peripheral histamine antagonism	Bicarbonate infusion, urine alkalinisation, supportive care
4.	Bupropion	No clear mechanism	Supportive care
5.	Ethylene glycol	Alone or in combination with benzodiazepines cause severe axonal polyneuropathy	Multi organ support, treatment of renal failure

challenge is to balance the time to declare the patient brain dead and till then appropriate management of the prospective organ donor.

Temperature:

Hypothermia can be present because of the loss of thermostat/temperature control of the body or because of induced hypothermia. The measurement of core temperature should be done using central blood, rectal, esophageal, or gastric methods. Severe hypothermia can cause suspended animation, and it is important to ensure [24, 25] normothermia (37 °C) before declaration brain death. Hypothermia causes increased urine output mimicking diabetes inspidus, can also cause delayed elimination of the CNS depressant drugs from the body, can worsen shock, etc. Euthermia can be achieved by placing warmers and rewarming using warm IV fluids/fluid warmers, etc.

Dyselectrolytemia:

The most common electrolyte imbalances [19] that occur are hypernatremia, hypokalemia, hypophosphatemia, etc. The prime importance always goes to the high sodium levels. This can occur due to the increased free water loss due to posterior pitutary ischemia—ADH deficiency leading to diabetes insipidus. This can be managed by increasing free water input and avoiding sodium containing fluids along with desmopressin or vasopressin infusion.

Once the requirements have been met, it must be demonstrated that the brain injury is irreversible, which means that the loss of function is total and ongoing throughout time. The duration of "how long" is not well-established. Nonetheless, it is advised to wait at least 24 h after resuscitation following cardiac arrest, whether TTM is used or not, because brainstem function may not return right away. In general, additional observation is advised to dispel any doubts if there is any confusion about the condition's irreversibility before proceeding to testing of the brain stem reflexes.

C. Clinical Testing of Brain Stem Reflexes

The primary indications of brainstem function are reflexes mediated by the cranial nerves. Thus, establishing their absence is essential for the diagnosis of brain death. According to the intrinsic sensitivity [24, 26] of the cranial nerve networks and the impact of some ancillary factors in brain-dead patients, such as facial trauma, local edema, damage to tissues, and intracranial catheters affecting the assessment of reflexes, the testing and its individual significance varies and is challenging.

The assessment for the loss of brainstem reflexes is done after generating a comatose state with total nonresponse to maximal stimuli, as follows [27, 28]: absence of facial movement in response to noxious stimuli, loss of pupillary responsiveness, loss of corneal, oculocephalic, oculovestibular, gag, and cough reflexes, and absence of cerebrally mediated movement in response to noxious stimulation of the extremities.

Pupillary Reflex:

Elicited by flashing light over pupils.

Response: Pupillary constriction to light

Brain death: Mid position, Mid-sized pupils, No reaction to light

Remarks:

Quantitative pupilometry can be helpful to standardize response [28–30].

If pupils—small constricted—need to suspect and rule out opiate overdose/exclusive brain stem injury [31].

Corneal Reflex:

Elicited by touching near the iris with tip of gauze/drop of sterile saline.

Response—Blinking of eye

A unilateral or bilateral response of eyelid closure with upward deviation of the eye (Bell's phenomenon) indicates preserved brainstem functioning [32].

Oculocephalic Reflex:

Elicited by moving head horizontally from midline position.

Response—Movement of eyeball along with the head/in opposite direction

Challenge: This test is avoided in cervical spine/spinal cord injury

Oculovestibular Reflex:

Elicited by instilling cold saline into ear canal for 60 s.

Response—In comatose patients, eye deviation towards same side, nystagmus towards opposite side.

Patency of ear canal should be ensured/avoided in case of severe skull base or orbital trauma.

Cough/Gag Reflex:

Elicited by stimulating posterior pharyngeal wall with tongue depressor or trachea with suction catheter.

Response: gag/cough

Difficulty in severe facial trauma.

D. Clinical Motor Testing

To elicit motor response, deep pressure should be applied on the sternal notch, supraorbital notches, condyles at the level of the temporomandibular joints, and all four extremities proximally and distally. Differentiating spinal mediated from brain-mediated movements can be difficult and calls for a skilled clinician. An auxiliary test is necessary if results are still ambiguous. Triple flexion, decerebrate-like (extension) movements, the Babinski sign, and fasciculations are high-yield instances. An ancillary test is required if there is significant neuromuscular disease or facial trauma since these conditions may affect motor responses.

E. Apnea Testing

The purpose of apnea testing [33] is to let carbon dioxide gradually buildup which stimulates the medullary respiratory centers as much as possible. These centers are activated by the consequently acidic pH of the cerebrospinal fluid (CSF). Prior

Prerequisites: The following prerequisites must be satisfied before apnea testing can begin absence of clear spontaneous respirations; systolic blood pressure of at least 100 mmHg or mean arterial pressure of at least 60 in adults, normothermia (temperature of at least 36 °C); absence of hypoxia and eucapnia.

Preparation: An arterial line is placed for monitoring and sampling. The patient is preoxygenated with FiO_2 of 100% for about 10 min. The ventilator rate setting is adjusted to avoid carbon dioxide washout. Arterial blood gas (ABG) analysis is done.

Procedure: Chest and abdomen are exposed to observe for any movements. The ventilator is disconnected. The patient is oxygenated by passing a suction catheter into the endotracheal tube. Repeat ABG after 8–10 min, if PCO_2 is >20 mmHg above the baseline, then the apnea test is considered positive. If PCO_2 does not reach the expected value and the patient is stable, with no hypoxia or hypotension, the testing can be continued till the desired threshold is reached.

The apnea test is aborted and cannot be completely successful if hypotension, hypoxemia, or arrhythmias occur. There are instances of cardiac arrest reported during apnea testing.

The apnea test has been tried with various modifications too [33]. The use of CPAP over the endotracheal tube or AMBU bag with a PEEP valve etc. have been tried to avoid hypoxia during the conduct of the test.

Lazarus Sign:

Spinal reflexes [34, 35] like flexor plantar responses, flexor withdrawal responses, and deep-tendon reflexes can be noted after cerebral death. These can be explained by a spinal reflex arc, and they do not preclude brain death. The others reported were abdominal and cremasteric reflexes occurring several hours after brain death which was clinically and angiographically confirmed. The neck abdominal reflex (contraction of the abdominal muscles during passive flexion of the neck), flexion withdrawal reflex, and unilateral extension-pronation movements were described as early as 1973. These were named as "Lazarus Sign." It should be very clearly mentioned as spinally mediated reflexes, and this concerns anything to awareness or other higher functions [36].

61.4 Ancillary Testing

Ancillary testing is not required if a patient may be declared brain dead using clinical standards. Yet, a variety of conditions, such as the difficulty to finish a clinical test, the inability to rule out confounders, or the unclear interpretation of a specific test, may cause the provider to doubt the diagnosis. In this situation, ancillary testing is advised. Hence, ancillary testing is occasionally utilized in circumstances where a clinical examination is unlikely to provide a solution. Each examination has its limits, and these need to be considered when choosing the optimal test for a certain patient.

Financial aspects and equipment accessibility might also be considered. It is possible to think of an effective ancillary test as having the qualities of an ideal biomarker: it should be noninvasive, easily tested, affordable, generate data quickly, have high sensitivity and specificity, and should help prognosticate. Particularly, auxiliary tests must be free from confounding factors such sedative effects and false-positive results that could result in the incorrect diagnosis of brain death [37].

To date, no auxiliary test has met all these requirements, so it is necessary to weigh each test's risks and benefits individually, considering the particulars of each clinical situation.

The ancillary tests are based on the testing of two principles—electrophysiology and cerebral blood flow evaluation.

61.4.1 Tests Based on Electrophysiology of the Brain

Electrophysiology-based tests are EEG and evoke potential. These detect electrical signals and have their significance in neurocritical care. These tests are more helpful when the patient had undergone severe trauma to the brain and flow-based ancillary studies cannot be done due to practical difficulties.

Electroencephalogram (EEG): EEG detects cortical electrical activity and is more useful in ruling out residual cortical activity [38–40]. A major limitation is its inability to assess posterior fossa and brain stem electrical activity. Electrocerebral silence (Fig. 61.4) is seen in deeply comatose patients. Hence, it is not foolproof or a reliable ancillary test by itself.

Evoked Potentials: There are many types like Visual Evoked potentials (VEP), Somatosensory Evoked potentials (SSEP), and Auditory Evoked potentials (AEP). These tests [41–43] evaluate the entire pathway from cortical output to the peripheries, hence more informative than the EEG or along with EEG. Limitations are that

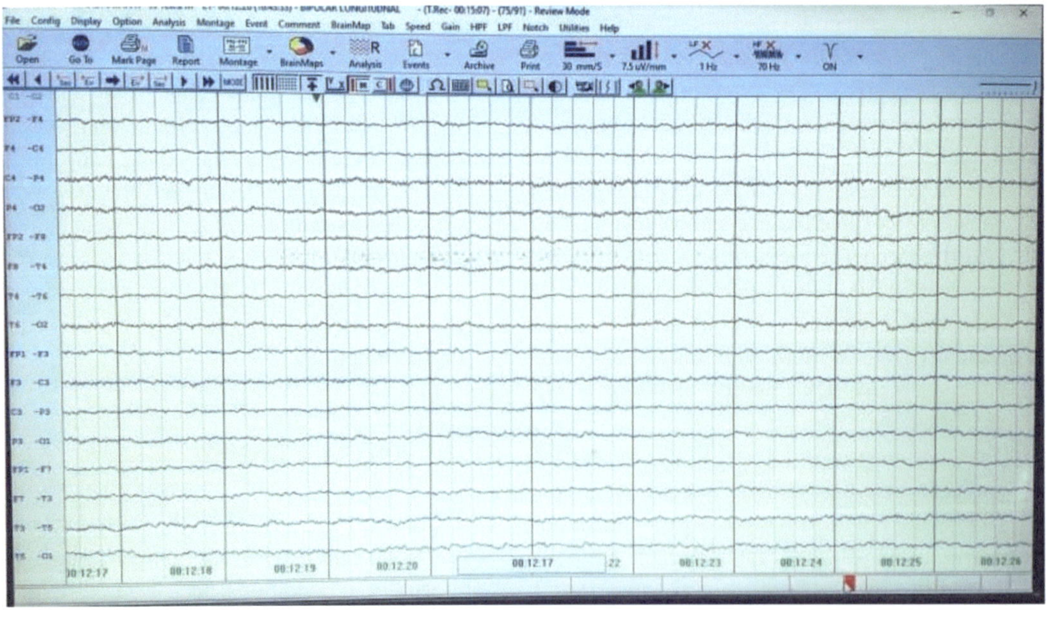

Fig. 61.4 Electrocerebral silence

these studies can study only specific pathways and general data cannot be elicited.

61.4.2 Tests Based on Blood Flow Evaluation of the Brain

These include tests which assess the circulation, perfusion, and the blood flow to the brain. These can be noninvasive like [44, 45] Magnetic Resonance imaging/Angiogram(MRA), Transcranial Doppler (TCD) [46–49] or minimally invasive involving injecting of a substance, either contrast as in [50, 51] CT angiogram (CTA), or a radionucleotide substance as in single photon emission computed tomography (SPECT) [52, 53] or invasive as [54, 55] digital subtraction angiography (DSA) (Table 61.2).

Despite so much research, evidence, and technologies worldwide, ancillary tests have their own challenges and limitations with respect to the data obtained and interpretation of the findings. Hence, no guidelines recommend brain death diagnosis exclusively only with the ancillary tests.

61.5 Special Situations

Brain death diagnosis in patients on extracorporeal membrane oxygenation (ECMO): In the past 2 to 3 decades [56], ECMO has been increasingly used and for distinct reasons like end stage heart failure, ARDS, post cardiac arrest status, etc. In the context of ECMO, oxygenation and carbon dioxide removal happen outside the body. They can have major neurological catastrophe, which can be from a bleed or malignant cerebral edema. In case a patient on ECMO becomes brain dead, the same principles are applied for testing and diagnosing brain death. Also, because venoarterial ECMO (V-A ECMO) bypasses the cardiac

Table 61.2 Ancillary tests based on blood flow

S. no	Procedure	Finding	Comments
1	Digital subtraction angiography (DSA)	Absence of flow of contrast at the entry of carotid and vertebral arteries into the skull correlates to absence of perfusion External carotid circulation will appear intact	Considered the gold standard. Limitations are available expertise, skill, cost, and transfer to an operating room/Cath lab
2.	Computed Tomogram Angiography (CTA)	Injection of iodinated contrast and evaluation of blood flow to the distal cerebral vasculature after a specific time period (usually 25–40 s), Absence of flow in the intracranial circulation with persistence in the extracranial carotid circulation is consistent with brain death	"Stasis filling"—contrast opacification of a vessel that is initially impeded by intracranial pressure, seen as absence of actual perfusion may be related to contrast timing and intracranial vessel length
3.	Single Positron emission Computed Tomography (SPECT)	Technetium-based compounds pass through the blood–brain barrier, circulate or are taken up by metabolically active parenchyma	Lipophobic compounds inadequately demonstrate flow through the posterior fossa, thus lipophilic preferred. Cannot be done at the bedside
4.	Magnetic Resonance Angiogram (MRA)	Greater resolution and detail regarding the extent of neurologic damage, and sheds lighter on plausible causes that may have been unclear	Subject to pitfalls of stasis filling disadvantage of increased time, expense, contraindications due to metallic implants, and concerns regarding nephrogenic systemic fibrosis
5.	Transcranial Doppler (TCD)	Measures dynamic changes of blood flow and confirms circulatory arrest when performed in the anterior and posterior circulations. Systolic spikes and oscillating flow appearance indicate obstruction to blood flow	Can be done at the bedside obtaining reliable measurements is tough with difficult bone windows and after decompressive procedures that may lower intracranial pressure

and pulmonary circuits, its use effectively prevents the arrest of cardiopulmonary function [57, 58] and requires death by neurological criteria as the main factor that determines death. The concept of apnea testing remains the same. The conduct is altered in which preoxygenation [59–61] is done by increasing the flow of gas to maintain FiO_2 100% and minimizing sweep gas to see if the CO_2 builds up gradually when there is no ventilation. There can be mixing of arterial blood [62, 63] and blood sampling should be done simultaneously at the arterial site and from near the membrane oxygenator. More studies are required for standardization and protocolisation of the methods.

61.5.1 Brain Death Diagnosis in Pediatric Population

All the steps of the procedure are the same as those with the adult population.

First is to ensure etiology of brain injury, then exclusion of confounders and confirming irreversibility. Then comes the clinical testing of brain stem reflexes, clinical motor testing, and apnea testing.

The minimum age in which brain death testing is done is 36–37 weeks of gestation [64, 65]. The number of examinations is two. The first examination is to check if the child has met the neurological criteria and the second test confirms if all the criteria are met. The observation period is 12 h if the age is more than 30 days, or 24 h if the age is less than 30 days. The examination is done by two different evaluators.

The apnea test is done as the same procedure as that of the adults. If not able to complete the apnea tests, ancillary tests are done.

61.5.2 Brain Death Diagnosis in Patients on Targeted Temperature Management

Previously, post cardiac patients were treated with therapeutic hypothermia in post cardiac arrest situations. It was a challenge to declare brain death in the setting of hypothermic patients. They were observed till they were rewarmed to euthermia [66–70] and sometimes the wait period was rough, and patients were unstable due to multiple factors like hypothermia induced diuresis, slow drug excretion, dyselectrolytemia, and hemodynamic instability. After many studies and after the recent TTM2 study, induced hypothermia has almost left the field of neurocritical care.

61.6 Conclusion

Neurocritical care is a fast growing and promising field, and the responsibility of the physicians in this field is immense. Brain death diagnosis and declaration is now gaining more importance and is practiced worldwide. The recognition, awareness, and appropriate training for the same is vital among the physicians. The need for organ donation too is gradually creeping up. The difference of the protocols in different countries is a concern which should be investigated, and it would be good if we could have standardized criteria and procedure worldwide.

References

1. Mollaret P, Goulon M. The depassed coma (preliminary memoir). Rev Neurol (Paris). 1959;101:3–15.
2. A definition of irreversible coma. Report of the Ad Hoc Committee of the Harvard Medical School to Examine the Definition of Brain Death. JAMA. 1968;205:337–40.
3. Lewis A, Bakkar A, Kreiger-Benson E, Kumpfbeck A, Liebman J, Shemie SD, et al. Determination of death by neurologic criteria around the world. Neurology. 2020;95:e299–309.
4. Diagnosis of brain death. Statement issued by the honorary secretary of the Conference of Medical Royal Colleges and their faculties in the United Kingdom on 11 October 1976. Br Med J. 1976;2:1187–8.
5. Fisher J. Re-examining death: against a higher brain criterion. J Med Ethics. 1999;25:473–6.
6. Jan MM. Brain death criteria the neurological determination of death. Neurosciences. 2008;13:350–5.
7. Shah SK, Truog RD, Miller FG. Death and legal fictions. J Med Ethics. 2011;37:719–22.
8. Claassen J, Doyle K, Matory A, Couch C, Burger KM, Velazquez A, et al. Detection of brain activation

in unresponsive patients with acute brain injury. N Engl J Med. 2019;380:2497–505.
9. Wijdicks EFM, Varelas PN, Gronseth GS, Greer DM, American Academy of Neurology. Evidence-based guideline update: determining brain. Death in adults: report of the quality standards Subcommittee of the American Academy of Neurology. Neurology. 2010;74:1911–8.
10. Greer DM, Shemie SD, Lewis A, Torrance S, Varelas P, Goldenberg FD, et al. Determination of brain death/death by neurologic criteria: the world brain death project. JAMA. 2020;324:1078–97.
11. Grzonka P, Tisljar K, Rüegg S, Marsch S, Sutter R. What to exclude when brain death is suspected. J Crit Care. 2019;53:212–7.
12. Neavyn MJ, Stolbach A, Greer DM, et al. ACMT position statement: determining brain death in adults after drug overdose. J Med Toxicol. 2017;13(3):271–3.
13. Wang A, Malik N, Shah O. Bupropion overdose mimicking brain death: a case report. Neurology. 2017;88(16 supp):6.058.
14. Stranges D, Lucerna A, Espinosa J, et al. A Lazarus effect: a case report of bupropion overdose mimicking brain death. World J Emerg Med. 2018;9(1):67–9.
15. Lasala GS, Sexton KJ, Okaneku J, Hand C, Vearrier D, Greenberg MI. Pentobarbital coma with loss of pupillary light refex. In: XXXV international congress of the European Association of Poisons Centres and Clinical Toxicologists (EAPCCT)—St Julian's, Malta. Clin Toxicol. 2015;53(4):302.
16. Druda DF, Gone S, Graudins A. Deliberate self-poisoning with a lethal dose of pentobarbital with confirmatory serum drug concentrations: survival after cardiac arrest with supportive care. J Med Toxicol. 2019;15(1):45–8.
17. Wijdicks EFM, Varelas PN, Gronseth GS, Greer DM. Evidence-based guideline update: determining brain death in adults. Neurology. 2010;74(23):1911–8.
18. Wijdicks EF. The diagnosis of brain death. N Engl J Med. 2001;344:1215–21.
19. Ostermann ME, Young B, Sibbald WJ, et al. Coma mimicking brain death following baclofen overdose. Intensive Care Med. 2000;26:1144–6.
20. Brenner RP. The interpretation of the EEG in stupor and coma. Neurologist. 2005;11:271–84.
21. Marrache F, Megarbane B, Pirnay S, et al. Difficulties in assessing brain death in a case of benzodiazepine poisoning with persistent cerebral blood flow. Hum Exp Toxicol. 2004;23:503–5.
22. Sztajnkrycer MD, Huang EE, Bond GR. Acute zonisamide overdose: a death revisited. Vet Hum Toxicol. 2003;45:154–6.
23. Caballero F, Lopez-Navidad A, Cotorruelo J, et al. Ecstasy-induced brain death and acute hepatocellular failure: multiorgan donor and liver transplantation. Transplantation. 2002;74:532–7.
24. Walker AE, Molinari GF. Criteria of cerebral death. Trans Am Neurol Assoc. 1975;100:29–35.
25. Roosen K, Klein M. Criteria, and diagnosis of brain death. Versicherungsmedizin. 1990;42:110–2.
26. Walker AE. Cerebral death. 3rd ed. Baltimore-Munich: Urban & Schwarzenberg; 1985. p. 1–198.
27. Wijdicks EFM. Brain death worldwide: accepted fact but no global consensus in diagnostic criteria. Neurology. 2002;58:20–5.
28. Shemie SD, Hornby L, Baker A, Teitelbaum J, Torrance S, Young K, et al. International guideline development for the determination of death. Intensive Care Med. 2014;40:788–97.
29. Phillips SS, Mueller CM, Nogueira RG, Khalifa YM. A systematic review assessing the current state of automated pupillometry in the NeuroICU. Neurocrit Care. 2019;31:142–61.
30. Solari D, Rossetti AO, Carteron L, Miroz J-P, Novy J, Eckert P, et al. Early prediction of coma recovery after cardiac arrest with blinded pupillometry. Ann Neurol. 2017;81:804–10.
31. Khandelwal A, Mishra RK, Singh S, Singh S, Rath GP. Dilated pupil as a diagnostic component of brain death-does it really matter? J Neurosurg Anesthesiol. 2019;31:356.
32. Pallis C. ABC of brain stem death. Diagnosis of brain stem death—II. Br Med J (Clin Res Edn). 1982;285:1641–4.
33. Busl KM, Lewis A, Varelas PN. Apnea testing for the determination of brain death: a systematic scoping review. Neurocrit Care. 2020;34:608. https://doi.org/10.1007/s12028-020-01015-0.
34. Jordan JE, Dyess E, Cliett J. Unusual spontaneous movements in brain-dead patients. Neurology 1985;35:1082 (Letter).
35. Jorgenson EO. Spinal man after brain death. The unilateral extension-pronation reflex of the upper limb as an indication of brain death. Aeta Neuroehir. 1973;28:259–73.
36. Mandel S, Arenas A, Scasta D. Spinal automatism in cerebral death. N Engl J Med. 1982;307:501.
37. Young GB, Shemie SD, Doig CJ, Teitelbaum J. Brief review: the role of ancillary tests in the neurological determination of death. Can J Anaesth. 2006;53:620–7.
38. Djurić S, Durić V, Milosević V, Stamenović J, Mihaljev-Martinov J. The role of neurophysiological methods in the conformation of brain death. Vojnosanit Pregl. 2013;70:309–14.
39. Knežević-Pogančev M, Pavlović M, Redžek-Mudrinić T. Isoelectric electroencephalogram cannot be equated with brain death. Clin Neurophysiol. 2010;4:e13.
40. Guérit JM. EEG and evoked potentials in the intensive care unit. Neurophysiol Clin/Clin Neurophysiol. 1999;29:301–17.
41. Facco E, Munari M, Gallo F, Volpin SM, Behr AU, Baratto F, et al. Role of short latency evoked potentials in the diagnosis of brain death. Clin Neurophysiol. 2002;113:1855–66.
42. Machado-Curbelo C, Roman-Murga JM. Usefulness of multimodal evoked potentials and the electroretinogram in the early diagnosis of brain death. Rev Neurol. 1998;27:809–17.

43. Sonoo M, Tsai-Shozawa Y, Aoki M, Nakatani T, Hatanaka Y, Mochizuki A, et al. N18 in median somatosensory evoked potentials: a new indicator of medullary function useful for the diagnosis of brain death. J Neurol Neurosurg Psychiatry. 1999;67:374–8.
44. Karantanas AH, Hadjigeorgiou GM, Paterakis K, Sfras D, Komnos A. Contribution of MRI, and MR angiography in early diagnosis of brain death. Eur Radiol. 2002;12:2710–6.
45. Sohn C-H, Lee H-P, Park JB, Chang HW, Kim E, Kim E, et al. Imaging findings of brain death on 3-tesla MRI. Korean J Radiol. 2012;13:54.
46. Ducrocq X, Braun M, Debouverie M, Junges C, Hummer M, Vespignani H. Brain death and transcranial Doppler: experience in 130 cases of brain-dead patients. J Neurol Sci. 1998;160:41–6.
47. Hassler W, Steinmetz H, Pirschel J. Transcranial Doppler study of intracranial circulatory arrest. J Neurosurg. 1989;71:195–201.
48. Conti A, Iacopino DG, Spada A, Cardali SM, Giusa M, La Torre D, et al. Transcranial Doppler ultrasonography in the assessment of cerebral circulation arrest: improving sensitivity by transcervical and transorbital carotid insonation and serial examinations. Neurocrit Care. 2009;10:326–35.
49. Lampl Y, Gilad R, Eschel Y, Boaz M, Rapoport A, Sadeh M. Diagnosing brain death using the transcranial Doppler with a transorbital approach. Arch Neurol. 2002;59:58–60.
50. Sawicki M, Sołek-Pastuszka J, Jurczyk K, Skrzywanek P, Guziński M, Czajkowski Z, et al. Original protocol using computed tomographic angiography for diagnosis of brain death: a better alternative to standard two-phase technique? Ann Transplant. 2015;20:449–60.
51. Dupas B, Gayet-Delacroix M, Villers D, Antonioli D, Veccherini MF, Soulillou JP. Diagnosis of brain death using two-phase spiral CT. AJNR Am J Neuroradiol. 1998;19:641–7.
52. Weckesser M, Schober O. Brain death revisited: utility confirmed for nuclear medicine. Eur J Nucl Med. 1999;26:1387–91.
53. Braum M, Ducrocq X, Huot JC, Audibert G, Anxionnat R, Picard L. Intravenous angiography in brain death: report of 140 patients. Neuroradiology. 1997;39:400–5.
54. Gomes AS, Hallinan JM. Intravenous digital subtraction angiography in the diagnosis of brain death. AJNR Am J Neuroradiol. 1983;4:21–4.
55. Flowers WM, Patel BR. Persistence of cerebral blood flow after brain death. South Med J. 2000;93:364–70.
56. Casadio MC, Coppo A, Vargiolu A, Villa J, Rota M, Avalli L, et al. Organ donation in cardiac arrest patients treated with extracorporeal CPR: a single centre observational study. Resuscitation. 2017;118:133–9.
57. Thiagarajan RR, Brogan TV, Scheurer MA, Laussen PC, Rycus PT, Bratton SL. Extracorporeal membrane oxygenation to support cardiopulmonary resuscitation in adults. Ann Thorac Surg. 2009;87:778–85.
58. Combes A, Hajage D, Capellier G, Demoule A, Lavoué S, Guervilly C, et al. Extracorporeal membrane oxygenation for severe acute respiratory distress syndrome. N Engl J Med. 2018;378:1965–7.
59. Hout MS, Hattler BG, Federspiel WJ. Validation of a model for flow-dependent carbon dioxide exchange in artificial lungs. Artif Organs. 2000;24:114–8.
60. Muralidharan R, Mateen FJ, Shinohara RT, Schears GJ, Wijdicks EFM. The challenges with brain death determination in adult patients on extracorporeal membrane oxygenation. Neurocrit Care. 2011;14:423–6.
61. Shah V, Lazaridis C. Apnea testing on extracorporeal membrane oxygenation: case report and literature review. J Crit Care. 2015;30:784–6.
62. Smilevitch P, Lonjaret L, Fourcade O, Geeraerts T. Apnea test for brain death determination in a patient on extracorporeal membrane oxygenation. Neurocrit Care. 2013;19:215–7.
63. Ihle J, Burrell A. Confirmation of brain death on VA-ECMO should mandate simultaneous distal arterial and post-oxygenator blood gas sampling. Intensive Care Med. 2019;45:1165–6.
64. Shemie SD, Doig C, Dickens B, Byrne P, Wheelock B, Rocker G, et al. Severe brain injury to neurological determination of death: Canadian forum recommendations. CMAJ. 2006;174:S1–13.
65. Committee on Fetus and Newborn, Papile L-A, Baley JE, Benitz W, Cummings J, Carlo WA, et al. Hypothermia and neonatal encephalopathy. Pediatrics. 2014;133:1146–50.
66. Dankiewicz J, Cronberg T, Lilja G, Jakobsen JC, Levin H, Ullén S, et al. Hypothermia versus normothermia after out-of-hospital cardiac arrest. N Engl J Med. 2021;384(2283–94):114.
67. Fernando SM, Di Santo P, Sadeghirad B, Lascarrou J-B, Rochwerg B, Mathew R, et al. Targeted temperature management following out-of-hospital cardiac arrest: a systematic review and network meta-analysis of temperature targets. Intensive Care Med. 2021;47(1078):115.
68. Lascarrou J-B, Merdji H, Le Gouge A, Colin G, Grillet G, Girardie P, et al. Targeted temperature management for cardiac arrest with nonshockable rhythm. N Engl J Med. 2019;381:2327–37.
69. Greer DM, Rosenthal ES, Wu O. Neuroprognostication of hypoxic-ischaemic coma in the therapeutic hypothermia era. Nat Rev Neurol. 2014;10:190–203.
70. Kurtek RW, Lai KK, Tauxe WN, Eidelman BH, Fung JJ. Tc-99m hexamethylpropylene amine oxime scintigraphy in the diagnosis of brain death and its implications for the harvesting of organs used for transplantation. Clin Nucl Med. 2000;25:7–10.

Brain Death and Organ Donation

62

Rahul Pandit

62.1 Introduction

The deceased organ donation rate of India is 0.52 per million population. Compared to some countries like the USA, it is 25.6 per million, the UK at 18.3 per million, and Spain at 32 per million [1].

There is an increasing organ demand [2], compared to the number of organs available for transplantation. A multi-disciplinary team approach is necessary for successful organ donation [3]. The physiology of all the available organs in the donor should be normalized and maintained till the time the organs are retrieved [2]. Intensivist plays a vital role in identification, declaration of brain death, and providing medical care to potential organ donors, thereby improving rates of graft survival, i.e., quality of organ donation [3–5].

R. Pandit (✉)
Sir HN Reliance Foundation Hospital and all Other Reliance Healthcare Initiatives,
Mumbai, Maharashtra, India

62.2 Potential Organ Donor [6]

A potential organ donor is defined by the presence of either brain death or a catastrophic injury to the brain which could progress beyond reversibility that may fulfil brain death criteria.

62.2.1 Historic Events [7–9]

Historically, death was defined by the presence of putrefaction or decapitation, failure to respond to painful stimuli, or the apparent loss of observable cardio respiratory action. But with the development in resuscitation measures and invention of mechanical ventilators, respiratory arrest was prevented. Vital functions can now be maintained artificially after the brain has ceased to function. Further increasing burden of medicolegal concepts necessitated definition of brain death.

In 1959, Mollaret and Goulon coined the term "le coma dèpassè" on brain death.

In 1968, an ad hoc committee at Harvard Medical School reexamined the definition of brain death.

Uniform Determination of Death Act (UDDA). The fundamental criterion is an individual who has sustained either (1) irreversible cessation of circulatory and respiratory functions, or (2) irreversible cessation of all functions of the entire brain, including the brain stem, is dead.

H. Prabhakar et al. (eds.), *Principles and Practice of Neurocritical Care*,
https://doi.org/10.1007/978-981-99-8059-8_62

1976 Conference of Medical Royal Colleges. It published the statement on diagnosis of brain death, and clinical diagnostic testing for brain death became more refined.

India follows the U.K Code. In India, the legal framework for organ donation is in place. According to the Transplantation of Human Organ Act **(THOA-1994)** legislation, deceased donation is a legal option (THOA 1994) [10, 11].

The Central Government has established a National Human Organs and Tissues Removal & Storage Network named NOTTO, which stands for National Organ and Tissue Transplant Organization. NOTTO has five regional networks ROTTO (Regional Organ & Tissue Transplant Organization) and each region of the country will develop SOTTO (State Organ and Tissue Transplant Organization) in every state/UT. This was based on the Transplantation of Human Organs and Tissues Rules, 2014.

Each hospital of the country related to transplant activity, either as retrieval or transplant center or both, has to link with NOTTO, through ROTTO/SOTTO as a part of National Networking.

62.2.2 What Does Brain Death Mean?

The Transplantation of Human Organs Act, 1994 (Central Act 42 of 1994) [10],—definition of death:

"Deceased person" means a person in whom permanent disappearance of all evidence of life occurs

1. By reason of brain-stem death
2. In a cardio-pulmonary sense at any time after live birth has taken place
3. **"Brain-stem death"** means the stage at which all functions of the **brain stem** have permanently and irreversibly ceased.

However, cause of irreversible coma has to be established, preconditions met, and confounding factors are to be ruled out [6–9, 12].

Brain death is commonly caused by, but not limited to causes below [7–9]

- Intracranial haemorrhage
- Ischaemic brain injury
- Head injury
- Cerebral anoxia/ischemic injury due to any cause
- Primary cerebral tumour

62.2.3 How Does Brain Death Occur [7, 8]

The following are caused in response to increased intracranial volume:

- Brain swelling
- Blood collections
- Obstruction to CSF flow (hydrocephalus)

The intracranial pressure (ICP) rises. As the skull is a fixed compartment, blood flow to the brain falls due to rising ICP and finally stops (Fig. 62.1).

The brain dies ⇒ Irreversible ⇒ Patient dies

Preconditions:

- Core temperature >32 °C,
- Metabolic parameters within acceptable range. [sodium >120–130 mEq and <150–160 mEq, Normo-glycaemia, Acid base status normal]
- No Endocrine disturbances, and
- Drug intoxication ruled out.

The criteria involved in the diagnosis and declaration of brain-death include:

- In the absence of conditions mimicking brain death
- Absence of brain-stem reflexes
- Apnea
- Irreversible coma

India follows the UK concept of brain-stem death, and the Transplantation of Human Organs (THO) Act was passed by the Indian parliament in

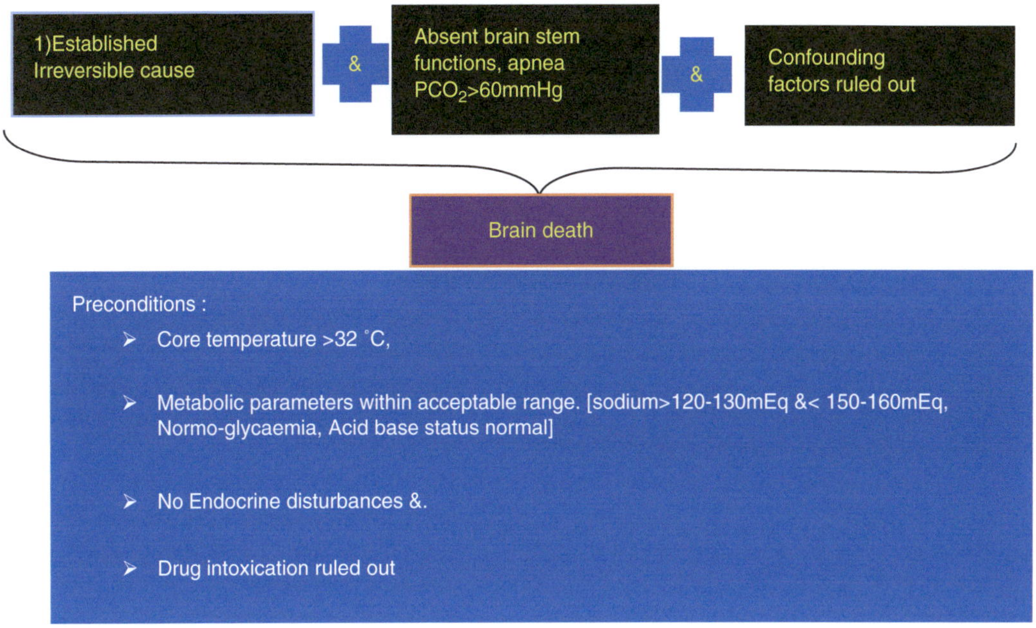

Fig. 62.1 Components of definition of brain death

1994 which legalized the brain-stem death [10]. In 1995, the THO rules were laid down which describe the brain-death certification procedure.

The state of Maharashtra has passed a resolution making it mandatory to declare and certify "brain-death." The Government Resolution underlines the responsibilities of hospitals registered under the THO Act 1994, that is, authorized transplant centers. As the large number of brain-death occurs in non-transplant hospitals, it makes for the appropriate authority (Director of Health Services) to register all hospitals in the state that have an operation theatre and ICU as Non-Transplant Organ Retrieval Centers (NTORCs). These hospitals are permitted to certify brain-death as per procedure and then conduct organ retrieval for therapeutic purposes but not permitted to perform actual transplantation. Thus, it is mandatory now for all NTORCs and authorized transplant centers in the state to certify and notify the brain-death cases to the Zonal Transplantation Co-ordination committee. This is a strong step to streamline the procedure for cadaveric organ retrieval and transplantation [8].

62.3 Determination of Brain Death/Tests for Brain Stem Death Certification [6–9, 12, 13]

Clinical examination is important for the determination of brain stem death.

History taking and physical examination findings that provide a clear etiology of brain dysfunction should be done, including the review of CT/MRI films.

The determination of brain death requires the identification of the proximate cause and irreversibility of coma. **The evaluation of a potentially irreversible coma should be established with appropriate clinical or neuro-imaging evidences.**

The exclusion of confounding factors that interfere in clinical diagnosis of brain death are as follows:

(a) Shock/hypotension—aim to have systolic BP $\geq$ 90–100 mmHg with vasopressors, if required

(b) Hypothermia—temperature <32 °C (core temperature)
(c) Exclude drugs known to alter neurologic, neuromuscular function like anesthetic agents, neuro-paralytic drugs, methaqualone, barbiturates, benzodiazepines, high-dose bretylium, amitriptyline, trichloroethylene, and alcohols

 Review medication and ICU observation chart for drugs given can wait for **at least 5 half-lives** with normal renal and liver function to exclude a drug effect. Use peripheral nerve stimulator for train of four **(TOF)** response to rule out muscle relaxant effect. This is particularly important where patients are referred from periphery to tertiary care center.
(d) Brain stem encephalitis. Review history and imaging
(e) Guillain–Barre syndrome. Review history and imaging
(f) Encephalopathy associated with hepatic failure, uremia, and hyperosmolar coma. Review history and imaging
(g) Severe hypophosphatemia. Check phosphate levels if in doubt

The following pre-requisites must be ruled out before carrying the test:

- Core temperature ≥36.5 °C or 97.7 °F
- Euvolemia or positive fluid balance in the previous 6 h
- Normal PCO_2 or arterial $PCO_2 \geq 40$ mmHg
- Normal PO_2. Pre-oxygenation for 15 min with 100% oxygen before carrying the apnea test, try to achieve an arterial $PO_2 \geq 200$ mmHg for safely conducting the test

Performance of a Complete Neurological Examination

I. Examination of the patient for the response to noxious stimuli is administered through a cranial nerve pathway. Spinal reflexes may be present. Suggested sites for **noxious stimuli are supraorbital grove bilaterally and trapezius squeeze bilaterally which have afferent and efferent from cranial nerve**
II. Absent pupillary reflex to direct and consensual light [**cranial nerve II and III**]; pupils need not be equal or dilated. Conditions and medications interfering in the pupillary reflex are orbital trauma, head injury, cataracts, and medications like high-dose dopamine, glutethimide, scopolamine, atropine, bretilium, or monoamine oxidase inhibitors.
III. Absent corneal reflex [**cranial nerve V and VII**], oculocephalic, cough, and gag reflexes [**cranial nerve IX and X**]. The corneal reflex may be altered as a result of facial weakness.
IV. Cold caloric test/absent oculovestibular reflex [**cranial nerve VIII, III and VI**]: The external auditory canal should be clear of cerumen. Elevate the patient's head by 30°. 20–50 mL of ice water irrigated into external auditory canal and over the tympanic membrane using a soft irrigation cannula. Labyrinthine injury or disease, anticholinergics, anticonvulsants, tricyclic antidepressants, and some sedatives may alter response. Tympanic membranes should be intact, allow 1 min after injection and at least 5 min between testing on each side.

62.4 Absent Respiratory Efforts in the Presence of Hypercarbia [12, 14] (Apnea Test)

62.4.1 Steps for Apnea Test

Pre-oxygenate patient with 100% O_2 for 15 min (to ensure denitrogenation of lungs) and do a base line ABG

- Connect a pulse oximetry and disconnect the ventilator.
- Deliver, 4–6 L/min of O_2, via endotracheal tube into the trachea using an soft catheter.
- Look closely for any respiratory movements (abdominal or chest excursions that produce adequate tidal volumes).

- Measure arterial PO_2, PCO_2, and pH after approximately 8–10 min and reconnect the ventilator (for every minute of apnea, $PaCO_2$ rises by approximately 3 mmHg).
- If respiratory movements are observed, the apnea test result is negative (i.e., it does not support the clinical diagnosis of brain death).
- Connect the ventilator if during testing:
  - The systolic blood pressure becomes <90 mmHg (or below age appropriate thresholds in children less than 18 years of age)
  - The pulse oximetry indicates significant oxygen desaturation
  - Cardiac arrhythmias develop

Immediately, draw an arterial blood sample and analyse arterial blood gas.

62.5 Interpretation [12, 14]

- **If respiratory movements are absent and arterial PCO_2 is ≥ 60 mmHg (*option:* In patients who are CO_2 retainers- 20 mmHg increase in PCO_2 over a baseline normal PCO_2), the apnea test result is positive (i.e., it supports the diagnosis of brain death).**
- If PCO_2 is <60 mmHg and PCO_2 increase is <20 mmHg (in CO2 Retainer) over baseline normal PCO_2, the result is indeterminate and a confirmatory test can be considered or apnea test is repeated.
- When appropriate 10 min apnea test can be repeated after pre-oxygenation for 15 min with an $Fi0_2$ of 1.0 and normalization of patients $PaCO_2$ to 40 mmHg.

62.6 Queries About Apnea Test [1, 14, 15]

(a) When should the Apnea test done?
(b) Who should do it?
(c) Is consent necessary of Apnea test?
(d) **Trouble shooting for Apnea test**

Table 62.1 Examples of observation periods in hours before testing for brain death. (Source: Pallis C Harley DH. ABC of Brainstem death BMJ publishing group: 1996)

Apneic coma after • Major neurosurgery • Confirmed aneurysm	>4 h
Head injury (no secondary brain damage from hematoma, shock, or brain hypoxia)	>6 h
Spontaneous intracerebral bleed	>6 h
Brain hypoxia (drowning and cardiac arrest)	>24 h
Any of the above (with suspicion of drug intoxication but no screening facilities)	50–100 h

(a) **When should the Apnea test done?**

The determination of brain death should be thorough and meticulous. Pallis and Harley stress the importance of appropriate duration of observation that must be provided to ensure irreversibility of the pathological processes. The suggested observation period is included in Table 62.1.

A formal evaluation of the brain stem reflexes is undertaken when the patient has fixed dilated pupils and absent cranial nerve reflexes for more than 4 h[1]. After the first clinical exam, the patient should be observed for a defined period of time for clinical manifestations that are inconsistent with the diagnosis of brain death. Most experts agree that a 6-h observation period is sufficient and reasonable in adults and children over the age of 2 years [13, 15].

62.7 Is Consent Necessary for Apnea Test?

- Consent is not necessary for carrying Apnea test (though an assent of family, informing them about the test been done).

62.8 Troubleshooting During Performance of Apnea Test [1, 12, 14]

1. Patient's systolic blood pressure (SBP) ≤100 mmHg: Vasopressors, inotropes, and fluid boluses need to be administered to keep the blood pressure (BP) above the target. The

apnoea test is aborted if systolic BP is ≤90 mmHg and the test needs to be repeated after stabilization.

2. Oxygen saturation not maintained during apnea testing:

   The apnea testing is terminated if the saturation is ≤85% for more than 30 s. The test can be retried with T-piece and continuous positive airway pressure of 10 cm H_2O and oxygen flow of 12.0 L/min. Reducing the positive end-expiratory pressure (PEEP) to 5 cm H_2O prior to disconnection from the ventilator for apnea testing can predict the tolerance to apnea.
3. Patient is hypothermic <35 °C: Guidelines for apnea testing are not valid and need to be repeated after correction of hypothermia.
4. The patient repeatedly desaturates or becomes hypotensive during apnea testing: One should consider ancillary tests for confirming brain death (electroencephalography, cerebral angiography, transcranial Doppler, and scintigraphy). **In India, the THOA act does not mandate about the use of ancillary tests (see the section 1.7**).
5. Baseline PaCO2 ≥ 40 mmHg or ≤35 mmHg: A rise of ≥20 mmHg above baseline can be considered a positive apnea test in patients with elevated baseline $PaCO_2$.

Reducing the frequency of ventilation to allow a $PaCO_2$ in the recommended range should be considered prior to the testing of Apnea.

62.8.1 Observations which Are Compatible and Incompatible with Brain Stem Death

Compatible:
- Spinal reflexes
- Sweating, blushing, and tachycardia
- Normotension without pharmacologic support
- Absence of diabetes insipidus

Incompatible:
- Decerebrate or decorticate posturing
- Extensor or flexor motor responses to painful stimuli
- Seizures

Reasons for spinal reflexes according to one hypothesis, the reflex movements represent hypoxia- and hypercapnia-induced activity of cervical cord neurons. Alternatively, they might be due to the disinhibition of movement generators of the spinal cord. Another hypothesis is that mechanical compression/decompression of the spinal root or cervical spinal cord by neck flexion/extension can generate movement [1, 12].

62.9 Ancillary Tests [1, 8, 13]

When the full clinical examination, including both assessments of brain stem reflexes and the apnoea test, is conclusively performed, **no additional testing is required to determine brain death.** Confirmatory tests like electroencephalography (EEG) cerebral angiography, transcranial Doppler, and radionuclide scan are not mandatory. **As per TOHA, the ancillary test is not mentioned at all; hence, its legal viability is challenging.**

Indications for ancillary tests are as follows:

1. Patients with skull or cervical injuries, cardiovascular instability [15]
2. Other factors like as severe facial trauma, otorrhagia, eye agenesis [15], which preclude the performance of a portion of the clinical examination
3. Reassure family members and medical staff [13]
4. Panel of doctors is in doubt or disagreement of the diagnosis [16]

62.10 Legal Aspects in India for Certification of Brain Death [1, 10, 13, 15, 16]

Who can certify?
How many doctors required?
How many times test needed?
What is the observation interval between the second set test?

62.10.1 Who Can Certify and How Many Doctors Required? [1, 10, 13, 16]

A Registered Medical Practitioner with appropriate authority should do Apnea test [10]. Diagnosis of brain death is established and recorded by two doctors, not belonging to the removal and transplantation teams. Out of the two doctors, one must be a specialist in neurology (Grade 1B). The order of examination is irrelevant, i.e., it does not matter whether the neurologist performs the first or the second examination [15].

Diagnosis of brainstem death requires a panel four doctors.

1. The doctor in charge of the patient
2. The doctor in charge of the hospital where the patient was treated
3. An independent specialist of unspecified specialty (physicians, surgeons, or intensivists) nominated from the panel of names approved by the appropriate authority
4. Neurologist or neurosurgeon or any other specialist from list above in point no 3

Amendments in the THO Act (2011) have allowed the selection of a surgeon/physician and an anesthetist/intensivist, in the event of the non-availability of neurosurgeon/neurologist.

Clinical examination and apnea test need to be done **two times** with an minimum **interval of 6 h.** After the second test, the team should start counselling the family regarding organ donation.

The time of death is the end of second apnea test.

62.11 Summary

Brain stem death is usually followed by an expected pattern of complex multiple organ failure; hence, an appropriate support to the donor before and after brain death can increase the number and quality of donor organs. The medical management of organ donor can be broadly divided into cardiovascular management, hormonal or management of metabolic derangement, management of temperature, respiration, hematological parameter, and nutritional support. The early identification of organs for donation helps to optimize the medical strategies. The guidance provided in this chapter though does not substitute proper clinical decision-making in particular case, but will help as the standard for intensivist for the management of brain death for organ and tissue donation.

References

1. Kumar L. Brain death and care of the organ donor. J Anaesthesiol Clin Pharmacol. 2016;32:146.
2. Kutsogiannis DJ, Pagliarello G, Doig C, Ross H, Shemie SD. Medical management to optimize donor organ potential: review of the literature. Can J Anaesth. 2006;53:820–30.
3. McKeown DW, Bonser RS, Kellum JA. Management of the heart beating brain-dead organ donor. Br J Anaesth. 2012;108(Suppl 1):i96–i107.
4. Bos EM, Leuvenink HGD, van Goor H, Ploeg RJ. Kidney grafts from brain dead donors: inferior quality or opportunity for improvement? Kidney Int. 2007;72:797–805.
5. de Lima Lopes Rodrigues S, de Escobar Ferraz Neto JB-H, da Costa Sardinha LA, Araujo S, Zambelli HJL, de Fátima Santana Ferreira Boin I, et al. Profile of effective donors from organ and tissue procurement services. Rev Bras Ter Intensiva. 2014;26(1):21–7.
6. Wood KE, Becker BN, McCartney JG, D'Alessandro AM, Coursin DB. Care of the Potential Organ Donor. N Engl J Med. 2004;351:2730–9.
7. de Groot YJ, Jansen NE, Bakker J, Kuiper MA, Aerdts S, Andrew IR. Maas imminent brain death: point of departure for potential heart-beating organ donor recognition. Intensive Care Med. 2010;36:1488–94.
8. Dhanwate AD. Brainstem death: a comprehensive review in Indian perspective. Indian J Crit Care Med. 2014;18(9):596–605.
9. National guidelines for organ and tissue donation Australasian Transplant Coordinators Association Incorporated. 4th Ed. 2008. http://www.atca.org.au/files/F.pdf. Accessed 10 Dec 2014.
10. Government of India. Transplantation of Human Organs Act, 1994. 1994. Central Act 42 of [cited 2007 Mar 9]. http://www.medindianet/tho/thobill1asp.
11. Shroff S. Legal and ethical aspects of organ donation and transplantation. Indian J Urol. 2009;25:348–55.
12. Wijdicks EFM. The diagnosis of brain-death. N Engl J Med. 2001;344:1215–21.
13. Goila AK, Pawar M. The diagnosis of brain death. Indian J Crit Care Med. 2009;13:7–11.
14. van der Jagt M, Lin M-S, Briegel J. Optimizing apnea test for determining brain death. Intensive

Care Med. 2016;42:117–8. https://doi.org/10.1007/s00134-015-4132-3.
15. Westphal GA, Garcia VD, de Souza RL, Franke CA, Vieira KD, Birckholz VRZ. Guidelines for the assessment and acceptance of potential brain-dead organ donors. Rev Bras Ter Intensiva. 2016;28(3):220–55.
16. Sethi NK, Sethi PK. Brainstem death: implications in India. JAPI. 2003;51:910–1.

Part X

Procedures in Neurocritical Care

63 External Ventricular Drain

Amit Goyal and Kumari Pallavi

63.1 Introduction

External ventricular drainage (EVD) is one of the most frequent neurosurgical procedures experienced in neurocritical care units [1]. It is a procedure consisting of placing a catheter into the ventricular system with the purpose of diverting the cerebrospinal fluid (CSF) flow extra-cranially or to monitor intracranial pressure (ICP). The most common indications include hemorrhagic strokes with intraventricular hemorrhage (IVH) or traumatic brain injury (TBI). Once in place, most frequent complications include catheter blockade or infection, necessitating the implementation of strict protocols for EVD maintenance [2]. This chapter discusses the indications, complications, and management of EVD in neurocritical care units.

63.2 Indications

EVD is generally an emergency procedure performed bedside. It is usually performed as a temporary measure to either drain CSF extra-cranially with an aim to reduce ICP or clear IVH, or to measure ICP in patients with intracranial hypertension [3–5]. Common indications of EVD insertion are listed in Table 63.1.

EVD in an open position functions as a conduit for extra-cranial CSF drainage. One of the most common indications is acute hydrocephalus (HCP) secondary to subarachnoid hemorrhage, malignant infarcts, posterior fossa tumors, and shunt failure [1, 4, 6–10]. It is also frequently used in patients with IVH for the purpose of clearing blood as well as reduction in ICP through continuous CSF drainage [1, 4, 11]. However, EVD placement does not result in the immediate clearance of intraventricular blood and has risk of getting blocked by blood clot. Continuous CSF drainage through EVD is also included in the brain trauma foundation (BTF) guidelines for reduction in the ICP burden after TBI [5]. EVD is also used as a mean to achieve intraoperative brain relaxation during brain tumor excision [12].

EVD is also considered the gold standard and more accurate mean for ICP monitoring [13, 14]. For this purpose, ventricular catheter is connected to an external strain-gauge transducer through a fluid filled catheter. Uninterrupted fluid column and leveling of transducer at the level of external auditory canal are pre-requisites for accurate ICP values [4]. BTF guidelines recommend ICP monitoring in TBI patients with Glasgow coma scale (GCS) <8, abnormal admission computed tomography (CT) scan or patients with normal CT scan with two or more of the following criteria: age >40 years, motor postur-

A. Goyal (✉) · K. Pallavi
Department of Neuronesthesia and Critical Care, Medanta—The Medicity, Gurgaon, Haryana, India

H. Prabhakar et al. (eds.), *Principles and Practice of Neurocritical Care*,
https://doi.org/10.1007/978-981-99-8059-8_63

Table 63.1 Indications of external ventricular drainage (EVD)

Extra-cranial CSF drainage
Acute HCP
• SAH
• Posterior circulation stroke with HCP
• Posterior cranial fossa tumor with HCP
• Malfunctioning of ventriculoperitoneal shunt
Clearance of ventricular blood
• SAH with IVH
• ICH with IVH
• Isolated IVH
Reduction in ICP
• TBI
• IVH
• ICH
• Intraoperative brain bulge
ICP monitoring
TBI
ICH
Acute subdural hematoma
AIS
Meningitis
Intraventricular administration of drugs
Antibiotic in CNS infections
rTPA in IVH
Vasospasm after SAH

CSF cerebrospinal fluid; *HCP* hydrocephalus; *SAH* subarachnoid hemorrhage; *IVH* intraventricular hemorrhage; *ICP* intracranial pressure; *TBI* traumatic brain injury; *ICH* intracerebral hemorrhage; *AIS* acute ischemic stroke; *CNS* central nervous system; *rTPA* recombinant tissue plasminogen activator

ing and systolic blood pressure < 90 mmHg [5]. Other indications for ICP monitoring may include patients with intracerebral hematoma (ICH), acute subdural hematoma (SDH), acute ischemic stroke (AIS), and meningitis [4, 13–15]. It may also be considered in patients with intracranial hypertension with associated factors such as, hypoxia, hypotension, anisocoria, midline shift >5 mm, and cerebral edema. Commercially available EVD systems have different units of ICP measurement (mmHg and cmH_2O) and clinician needs to be aware of it and apply appropriate conversion specifically while communicating to others [4]. Therefore, it is important for the hospitals to use uniform unit of measurement and reporting practices. Variability in ICP monitoring through EVD has also been reported by practices surveys and observational studies [16, 17].

EVD is also used as a conduit for therapeutic intraventricular drugs administration such as, recombinant tissue plasminogen activator (rTPA) for thrombolytic removal of IVH, intraventricular nicardipine for treatment of vasospasm after subarachnoid hemorrhage (SAH), and intraventricular antibiotics for the treatment of meningitis and ventriculitis [18–23]. However, efficacy and safety of this route for drugs administration is uncertain. Strict aseptic precautions must be followed while accessing the EVD system for drug administration. After the drug is administered, EVD should be clamped for 1 h, so that the drug does not drain out with CSF, as long as there is no neurological worsening or increase in ICP.

63.3 Insertion Procedure

Since EVD is frequently inserted after sudden neurological deterioration and the patient may not be stable for transport to the operating room, EVD insertion is commonly performed in neurocritical care units. Currently, there is no convincing evidence of significant increase in the risk of mechanical or infectious complications when EVD is placed bedside [10]. Prior to the procedure, coagulopathy and infection at the insertion site should be ruled out.

The ventricular system can be approached through four different surface landmark points, namely, Kocher's, Frazier's, Keen's and Dandy's points. Since the right frontal lobe is non-dominant in majority of population, right Kocher's point is usually the preferred site of entry into the right frontal horn of lateral ventricle (passing anterior to motor strip) [1, 2]. However in certain conditions such as right lateral ventricle hematoma, any vascular lesion in the trajectory of EVD or entry point infection, left Kocher's point is preferred for entry. After creating the burr hole, the catheter is directed towards medial canthus of the ipsilateral eye in coronal plane and ipsilateral external auditory meatus (EAM) in antero-posterior plane advancing towards foramen of monro. Once the CSF flow is conformed, the stylet is removed and the catheter is tunneled under the skin away from entry point and secured at the exit point before connecting to the external drainage system (Fig. 63.1). CSF samples are also collected for microbiology and biochemistry evaluation to rule out or trace the origin of any future ventriculostomy-associated infection. Following EVD insertion, a CT scan is commonly performed to confirm the catheter position (Fig. 63.2) and rule out any complication such as hemorrhage or extraventricular misplacement of catheter (Fig. 63.3) [24–26]. Technical advancement with guided ventriculostomy (CT guided, stereotactic guided) has increased the efficacy and accuracy of catheter placement [1, 26].

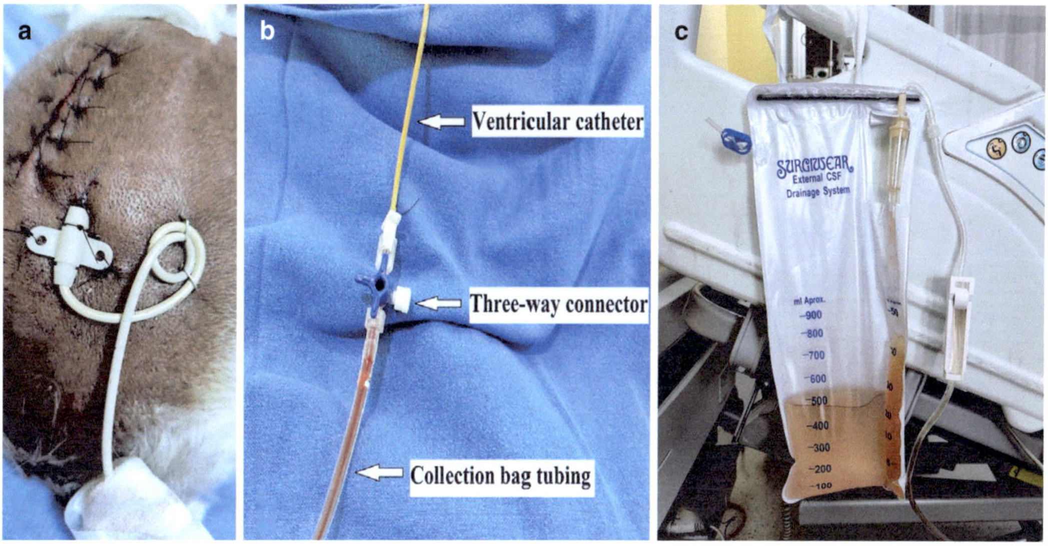

Fig. 63.1 (**a**) Image showing external ventricular drainage (EVD) tunneled under the skin away from entry point and secured at the exit point. (**b**) Ventricular catheter connected to the external drainage system through a three-way connector. (**c**) External CSF collection bag (with one small and one large chamber) fixed at the head end of patient's bed

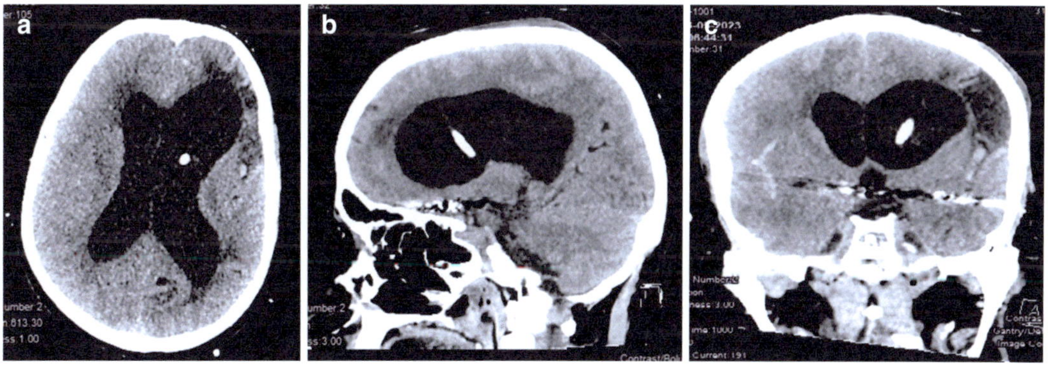

Fig. 63.2 Computed tomography (CT) image with axial section (**a**), sagittal section (**b**), and coronal section (**c**) showing position of ventricular catheter tip in the frontal horn of lateral ventricle

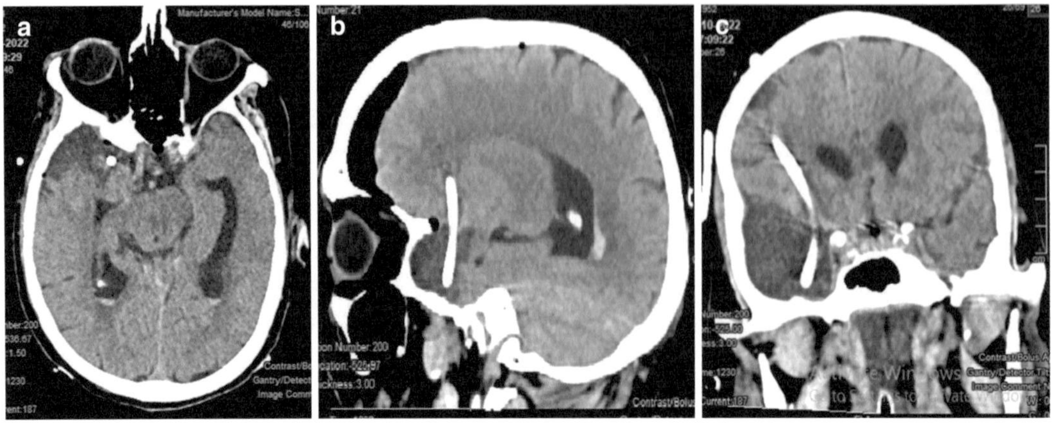

Fig. 63.3 Computed tomography (CT) image with axial section (**a**), sagittal section (**b**), and coronal section (**c**) showing extraventricular malposition of ventricular catheter

63.4 Management of EVD

After successful placement of EVD, most important aspects of EVD management are height of transducer (if purpose is ICP monitoring) or collecting system as well as rate of CSF drainage (i.e., mL/h). Manipulation of these factors is determined by the underlying pathology and opening pressure of CSF.

The height of the collecting system can be titrated as per the desired rate of CSF drainage to avoid under-/over-drainage. CSF drainage is generally not allowed >15–20 mL/h to avoid tear of bridging veins and subdural hemorrhage [3]. In a case of SAH with unsecured aneurysm, the initial height of the collecting system is set higher to avoid rapid drainage of CSF which can lead to re-bleeding [1]. The EVD height is lowered after aneurysm is secured. Titrated EVD drainage, including drainage at subatmospheric pressure may also be required to maintain CSF flow in certain conditions such as negative pressure hydrocephalus [27].

When purpose of EVD is ICP monitoring, the pressure transducer is kept at the level of foramen of monro, which corresponds to the level of EAM in the supine position and at the level of nasal bridge in the lateral position [28]. An incorrect level of transducer can produce erroneous ICP values (falsely low ICP above foramen of monro and falsely high ICP below foramen of monro). To avoid an erroneous value, the transducer must be re-leveled and zeroed after any change in position or disconnection of the system. During simultaneous CSF drainage, stopcock should turn "open" towards the transducer and "closed" towards the collecting system to acquire the ICP value [29].

CSF sampling should be performed only when infection is suspected [10, 30]. Sampling of CSF for laboratory evaluations should be performed under strict aseptic precautions to avoid any risk of infection. The sample port should be disinfected with 0.5% alcoholic chlorhexidine [31]. CSF should preferably be sampled through the proximal port (close to the ventricular catheter) rather than the distal port (close to the collection bag). Biochemistry parameters (sugars and protein) have shown high correlation between both the ports; however, white cell count and cultures have poor correlation [32, 33]. CSF should also not be sampled from the collection bag due to rapid degradation of cellular components [31]. Aspiration of CSF from either port should be very slow, not exceeding 1 mL/min.[2]

Regular inspection of the entire EVD system should be carried out to check for CSF leak, which may predispose to infection [29]. Color and clarity of CSF should also be monitored closely, which may reflect the intracranial pathology, such as blood in CSF may indicate SAH/IVH and cloudiness of CSF may indicate the presence of an infection [29, 31, 34]. Increase in CSF output should be noted as it may indicate rising ICP from edema or hemorrhage. Dressing should be performed with 0.9% saline and 0.5% alcoholic chlorhexidine every 24 h, or earlier if necessary, covering with sterile gauze and wrapping with bandages. When using an impermeable film, dressing change can be performed weekly [30, 31]. The drainage bag should be emptied when it reaches 2/3 or 3/4 of its volume capacity, as a full and heavy bag may alter or even stop the function of the system and the drainage of CSF [31].

Another important aspect of EVD management is the status of EVD during patient transport, change in position, and ambulation. Rapid and increased drainage during such maneuvers may increase the risk of intracranial hypotension, re-bleed of unsecured aneurysm, subdural hematomas, and reverse brain herniation. Therefore, it is a common practice to clamp the EVD during transport and change in position to avoid over drainage [3, 31, 35]. However, EVD clamping during transport has the associated risk of escalation of ICP specially in patients with pre-existing raised ICP and high hourly CSF output [3, 35]. EVD clamp trial prior to transport may help to identify patients at risk of developing intracranial hypertension. It is recommended to not routinely clamp the EVD during intra-hospital transport and decision should be based on hourly or daily CSF output, clamping trials in ICU and patient's tolerance to clamping [3]. ICP monitoring or closely monitored continuous CSF drainage may be considered during transport of patients who fail the pre-transport clamping trial. While clamping the EVD during transport, both proximal port (close to the ventricle catheter) and distal port (close to the collecting system) should be clamped [3].

63.4.1 Continuous Versus Intermittent EVD Drainage

There are two different strategies practiced for EVD drainage, "continuous and intermittent." Continuous drainage involves keeping the EVD "open" for continuous CSF drainage; whereas, intermittent drainage refers to "on demand" CSF drainage. It involves keeping the EVD "closed" and open only when required (increase in ICP or clinical deterioration). The choice between drainage strategies is commonly determined by the institutional practice. The main challenge with continuous drainage strategy is the decision regarding rate of drainage. This is generally decided based on pathology, clinical condition, neuroimaging, or ICP monitoring. Continuous strategy is generally preferred in patients with TBI and IVH, to achieve rapid reduction in ICP or clearance of blood [5, 36, 37]. But, it has associated higher rates of over drainage, ventriculostomy-associated infections (VAI) and non-functioning EVD [38–40]. On the other hand, intermittent drainage is safer with regards to EVD-related complications and is associated with shorter ICU and hospital length of stay and fewer EVD days (rapid weaning) [41].

63.4.2 EVD in SAH

EVD is frequently required in patients with SAH associated with acute hydrocephalus. Common practice in patients with unsecured aneurysm is to keep CSF drainage slow to avoid rapid reduction in ICP and increasing the risk of re-bleed due to increase in transmural pressure [1, 36]. It has been suggested that accelerated clearance of blood reduces the risk of vasospasm, delayed cerebral ischemia (DCI) and poor outcome, favoring continuous CSF drainage in SAH [42, 43]. In contrast, intermittent drainage may allow for the generation of pressure gradient necessary to re-establish the natural CSF pathway [4]. Current institutional practice favors the continuous drainage of CSF in SAH [36]. There is variability in the weaning approach of EVD in SAH. A pooled analysis showed that gradual weaning reduces the risk of shunt dependency but increases the risk of delayed ventriculoperitoneal (VP) shunt [44]. Another retrospective analysis showed reduction in the VP shunt rate with rapid weaning [41]. Number of EVD clamp trials have also shown association with VP shunt placement. More number of clamp trials is associated with fewer shunt insertion rate [45].

63.4.3 EVD in TBI

EVD has a dual role in TBI (monitoring & therapeutic). It is used for ICP monitoring as well as ICP control through CSF drainage. There is conflicting evidence for effectiveness of EVD in TBI outcome compared to intraparenchymal (IP) ICP monitoring [46–48]. The CENTRI-TBI study showed no difference in the outcome with IP monitor-guided or EVD-guided ICP management. But, a significant number of patients in IP group eventually required EVD for ICP control [48]. EVD has bigger advantage in the management of refractory intracranial hypertension [47, 48]. BTF also recommends the use of EVD for continuous CSF drainage to reduce the ICP burden in TBI [5]. Continuous CSF drainage may also reduce the need for additional ICP lowering measure such as hyperosmolar therapy. Other than cost effectiveness, early EVD may have additional advantage over IP monitor-guided ICP management in patients with refractory ICP.

63.4.4 EVD in ICH/IVH

ICH/IVH is frequently associated with acute HCP. EVD is indicated in large ICH/IVH for ICP management as well as clearance of intraventricular blood. EVD placement in ICH/IVH has shown good ICP control, lower mortality as well as IVH resolution [1, 4, 49–51], but it has not shown any significant improvement in outcome. It may also improve the CSF flow dynamics by clearance of ventricular blood and improving downstream resistance. Safety of intraventricular thrombolysis in IVH has been tested but CLEAR III trial did not show any significant improvement with intraventricular alteplase irrigation through EVD [18, 52].

63.4.5 Perioperative Management of EVD [3]

Pre-operative evaluation of the patient with EVD must include information regarding indication for EVD placement, ICP trends and waveform morphology (if ICP is monitored) and result of clamping trials if performed. Prior to shifting, integrity of the EVD system must be inspected and volume of CSF drained and drainage target must be communicated. If ICP is being monitored, the transducer must be leveled and zeroed at the level of EAM. Factors such as CSF output, clamping trials, and patient's response to clamping trials should be evaluated prior to decision for EVD status during transport [3]. If EVD is clamped during patient transport to OT or back to ICU, ICP may increase. Therefore, the transporting doctor should continuously monitor the patient for neurological worsening such as headache, reduced consciousness, anisocoria, neurological deficits, or raised ICP (if monitored) and manage the intracranial hypertension in a timely manner. Inside the operating room (OR), if feasible, EVD should be closed during change in patient position and it should be opened and re-leveled only after final patient's position. It is preferable to fix the transducer to OR table, so that changes in the table height does not affect the EVD functioning or ICP measurement. Since, positive pressure ventilation, anesthetic agents, and intraoperative hemodynamic changes may affect ICP, it is preferable to obtain frequent ICP values during intraoperative period. Documentation regarding intraoperative EVD management should include EVD status (open or clamped), collecting system's height relative to the reference level, color of CSF, amount of CSF drained, and ICP values.

63.5 EVD System and Troubleshooting

Since the EVD system has multiple connections, complex management system and remains in-situ for a considerably longer duration, it is prone to develop problems related to the EVD system (catheter, connectors, or tubing) and drainage volume despite appropriate maintenance and vigilance.

63.5.1 Accidental Disconnection

In case of inadvertent disconnection of the EVD system, the first response should be aimed at preventing leakage of CSF and maintaining the sterility of the ventricular catheter. A clamp should be applied immediately at the distal end of the catheter. To reduce the risk of contamination and infection, whole assembly distal to ventricular catheter must be replaced with a new and sterile kit. This should be followed by the verification of the patency of a new system to rule out catheter dislodgment and air bubbles in tubing [3, 52]. A CT scan can be performed to confirm the position of the ventricular catheter.

63.5.2 Drain Occlusion

Drain occlusion has an associated risk of increasing the ICP. If there is reduced/no CSF output or dampening of ICP waveform, the EVD system should be inspected for occlusion in a systemic manner, beginning from an insertion site to drainage bag distally. Mechanical factors such as a kink, debris or blood clot, air bubble and position of stopcocks should be ruled out first [2, 3, 53]. Patency may be restored by briefly lowering the collection bag to remove any air bubble or debris by CSF flow [2, 3, 34]. Otherwise, drainage tubing can be flushed towards a collecting bag to remove a clot or debris. Alternatively, the entire EVD kit can be replaced with a new one. If no flow is restored, the blockage of ventricular catheter proximally is suspected. Flushing the catheter upward can be considered though it has associated risk of increasing ICP, especially in patients with poor compliance. Sterile isotonic saline in a volume not exceeding 2 mL can be used to flush the catheter with close neuromonitoring for increase in ICP [3]. Flushing of tubing in either direction should be carried out under strict aseptic precautions. If CSF flow is still absent, a CT scan can be considered to rule out factors such as dislodged catheter or collapsed ventricles.

63.5.3 CSF Overdrainage

Rapid, large volume drainage of CSF can collapse the ventricles causing stretch and rupture of bridging veins resulting in subdural hemorrhage [3]. It can also increase the risk of re-bleed in patients with an unsecured aneurysm [1]. Overdrainage of CSF most commonly occur when the position of the patient or collecting system is changed with respect to each other (raising the head end or height of the bed, or lowering the height of collection bag) [3]. To avoid this, the collection bag can be fixed to the head end of the bed (Fig. 63.1c), or height of the collection bag should be changed immediately with respect to the patient. While changing the patient's position, the EVD system can be clamped though it can lead to increase in ICP. EVD should be unclamped as soon as possible as patients with critically elevated ICP may not tolerate even brief clamping of EVD. Overdrainage of CSF may also create pressure gradient between supratentorial and infratentorial compartment, increasing the risk of reverse herniation [53, 54]. To reverse the ventricle hypovolemia after overdrainage, lowering the patient's position (supine or trendelenburg position) with respect to collection bag can be considered [3].

63.5.4 CSF Leak

CSF leak from the catheter exit site is not an uncommon problem related to EVD. It is a major risk factor for EVD-related infection [55–57]. CSF leak at the catheter exit site >1 day is a major risk factor for infection [55]. CSF leak at the exit site indicates increase in the intraluminal resistance to CSF flow. Intraluminal resistance may increase when the catheter tip is lodged in IVH with its pores occluded by clot or when a clot enters inside the catheter lumen. Increasing the height of the collection bag or clamping of EVD during weaning may also increase the intraluminal resistance leading to CSF leak. IVH >10 mL has been found as a significant pre-disposing factor for CSF leak [55]. High intracranial pressures and poor wound healing may also contribute to the incidence of CSF leak. Placing a purse-string or vertical mattress suture at the exit site is the most common method of preventing CSF leak from the exit site [58, 59]. A CSF leak detection paper placed at the exit site has been used for easy detection of CSF leak [55]. Alternatively, a clear transparent dressing can be applied at the exit site with regular careful inspections. In case of suspected catheter occlusion, flushing of the catheter can be considered by the surgeon. EVD revision may also be required in some cases.

63.6 EVD and Infection

Since EVD is an invasive procedure and the EVD system has multiple connections, EVD-related infection is common with reported incidence of up to 32% [1, 2, 10]. Various factors associated with EVD infection have been identified and include systemic infection, previous craniotomy, depressed skull fracture, IVH, lack of tunneling of EVD catheter, CSF leak, catheter irrigation, frequent CSF sampling, and duration of EVD [1, 2, 10, 29, 34, 60, 61]. EVD management bundle suggested to prevent the EVD-related infection that includes aseptic insertion, tunneling of catheter away from insertion site, dressing of insertion site, peri-procedural prophylactic antibiotics, antimicrobial-impregnated catheters, limited manipulation of the closed system, and weaning to reduce EVD-related infection [1, 10, 62]. A single dose of prophylactic antimicrobial prior to EVD insertion is suggested against the use of antimicrobials for the duration of EVD due to the associated increased risk of resistant organisms and Clostridium difficile colitis [10, 63]. Antimicrobial-impregnated catheters have shown to reduce the risk of EVD-related infection and catheter colonization [10, 64–66]. Therefore, antimicrobial-impregnated catheters are recommended as part of comprehensive EVD management protocol. However, antimicrobial-impregnated catheters increase the risk of false-negative culture result when the CSF sample is drawn through it [67]. This may lead to potential delay in the detection of CSF infection or an inappropriately short duration of antibiotic therapy. Another important aspect of antimicrobial-impregnated catheters is economic consequence. The use of antimicrobial-impregnated catheter has shown to have significant impact on the cost savings due to decrease in the rate of infection [68]. The CSF collection system should be maintained in the upright position. If the collection system has to be placed flat, CSF from the small chamber should be emptied into the collection bag to prevent ascending infection from the collection chamber to drainage tubing.

The patient should be closely monitored for clinical signs of ventriculitis/meningitis for the duration EVD is in-situ. Fever, new or increasing headache, nuchal rigidity, and decreased level of consciousness indicate the need for CSF evaluation. In the setting of ventriculitis, intraventricular antimicrobials are recommended in patients who fail to respond to intravenous antimicrobials alone [10]. The infected ventricular catheter should be removed and replaced with a new catheter at different site if EVD requirement still persists [1].

63.7 Weaning and EVD Removal

EVD may be removed once the indication for EVD insertion (ICP monitoring or acute HCP) has been resolved. After the drainage of CSF or ventricular blood in acute HCP, CSF flow dynamics may return to normal allowing removal of EVD. However, CSF flow dynamics may not recover in some patients leading to chronic HCP requiring VP shunt for long-term CSF diversion. Once the clinical condition is stable, the decision of EVD removal or VP shunt placement depends upon the result of weaning or clamping trial. A conventional practice of EVD removal involves gradual weaning with stepwise increase in the drain height for several days prior to clamping of EVD. On the other hand, rapid weaning involves clamping of EVD as soon as weaning is started. During the weaning process, the patient is closely monitored for increase in ICP, neurological worsening and development of HCP. If patient fails the weaning trial, EVD is reopened followed by VP shunt placement. Compared to gradual weaning, rapid weaning is associated with fewer VP shunt placements, EVD-related infection and shorter length of ICU stay [41, 69, 70]. It is recommended that EVD weaning should be accomplished as quickly as it is clinically feasible, so as to minimize the total duration of EVD monitoring and EVD-related risks [10].

63.8 Ommaya Reservoir

Ommaya reservoir is a modification of conventional EVD. It is referred to a ventricular catheter connected to a reservoir which is placed under the scalp to provide long-term access to CSF or ventricle space. Various indications may include intraventricular administration of medication such as thrombolytics, antibiotics or chemotherapy, and aspiration or drainage of CSF [71–73]. Compared to conventional EVD, it is associated with a lower rate of infectious and non-infectious complications [74, 75]. It eliminates the conventional ventricular catheter-related complications such as catheter pull-outs, catheter blockage, and catheter breakage. Since it does not require long tunneling under the skin, it can be easily performed under local anesthesia.

For the external drainage of CSF, a scalp vein set is used. The needle is inserted percutaneously into the reservoir and the other end is connected to the collection bag with the help of a three-way connector (Fig. 63.4). The whole external assembly including the scalp vein set can be changed when the collection bag gets full. During patient transport or change in position, the conventional ventricular catheter may get dislodged or pulled out, necessitating re-insertion of a new catheter. However, with the combination of EVD & Ommaya reservoir, it is only the external assembly which gets disconnected during such accidents and ventricular catheter remains in place.

63.9 EVD and Thromboprophylaxis

Most patients requiring EVD have altered sensorium and are immobile with high risk of developing deep vein thrombosis. There is lack of strong evidence to guide the thromboprophylaxis practice and initiation timing in patients with EVD [10]. A sequential compression device or intermittent pneumatic compression device should be used from the first day of hospital admission. Chemoprophylaxis has been found to be safe with regards to ventriculostomy-associated hemorrhage and has shown to reduce the risk of venous thromboembolism [76]. Compared to late chemoprophylaxis, early chemoprophylaxis has not shown any significant increase in the risk of hemorrhagic complications after the placement of EVD [77]. The treating physician should weight the risks and benefits of chemoprophylaxis based on clinical profile of patient and stability of intracranial hemorrhage.

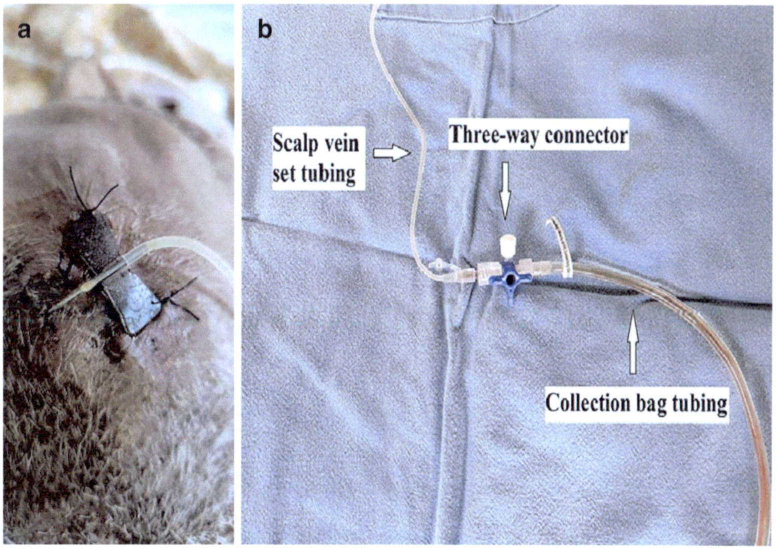

Fig. 63.4 (**a**) Scalp vein needle inserted percutaneously into Ommaya reservoir and fixed with stay sutures. (**b**) Scalp vein set connected to the collection bag with the help of a three-way connector

63.10 Conclusion

Patients in neurocritical care frequently require EVD for the purpose of draining CSF or ICP monitoring in various intracranial pathologies. Once in place, the EVD management approach differs for different indications and specific intracranial pathology. EVD is associated with several complications related to ventricular catheter, EVD system, drainage volume or infections. Compliance with the EVD management bundle reduces EVD-related infectious and non-infectious complications. The EVD management is generally a nursing responsibility; therefore, hospitals should adopt simple protocols for maintenance, troubleshooting, and monitoring for EVD making it technically less challenging.

References

1. Dey M, Jaffe J, Stadnik A, Awad IA. External ventricular drainage for intraventricular hemorrhage. Curr Neurol Neurosci Rep. 2012;12(1):24–33. https://doi.org/10.1007/s11910-011-0231-x.
2. Muralidharan R. External ventricular drains: management and complications. Surg Neurol Int. 2015;6(Suppl 6):S271–4. https://doi.org/10.4103/2152-7806.157620.
3. Lele AV, Hoefnagel AL, Schloemerkemper N, et al. Perioperative management of adult patients with external ventricular and lumbar drains: guidelines from the Society for Neuroscience in anesthesiology and critical care. J Neurosurg Anesthesiol. 2017;29(3):191–210. https://doi.org/10.1097/ANA.0000000000000407.
4. Chung DY, Olson DM, John S, Mohamed W, Kumar MA, Thompson BB, Rordorf GA. Evidence-based management of external ventricular drains. Curr Neurol Neurosci Rep. 2019;19(12):94. https://doi.org/10.1007/s11910-019-1009-9.
5. Carney N, Totten AM, O'Reilly C, et al. Guidelines for the management of severe traumatic brain injury, fourth edition. Neurosurgery. 2017;80(1):6–15. https://doi.org/10.1227/NEU.0000000000001432.
6. Wijdicks EF, Sheth KN, Carter BS, et al. Recommendations for the management of cerebral and cerebellar infarction with swelling: a statement for healthcare professionals from the American Heart Association/American Stroke Association. Stroke. 2014;45:1222–38.
7. Paldor I, Rosenthal G, Cohen JE, et al. Intracranial pressure monitoring following decompressive hemicraniectomy for malignant cerebral infarction. J Clin Neurosci. 2015;22:79–82.
8. Hedrich C, Gojo J, Azizi A, et al. Placement of EVD in pediatric posterior fossa tumors: safe and efficient or old-fashioned? The Vienna experience. Childs Nerv Syst. 2023;39:2079. https://doi.org/10.1007/s00381-023-05917-0.
9. Muthukumar N. Hydrocephalus associated with posterior fossa tumors: how to manage effectively? Neurol India. 2021;69, Suppl S2:342–9.
10. Fried HI, Nathan BR, Rowe AS, et al. The insertion and Management of External Ventricular Drains: an evidence-based consensus statement: a statement for healthcare professionals from the Neurocritical care society. Neurocrit Care. 2016;24(1):61–81. https://doi.org/10.1007/s12028-015-0224-8.
11. Ziai WC, Torbey MT, Naif NJ, et al. Frequency of sustained intracranial pressure elevation during treatment of severe intraventricular hemorrhage. Cerebrovasc Dis. 2009;27(4):403–10.
12. Gurjar HK, Mishra S, Garg K. Contralateral Ventriculostomy for intraoperative brain relaxation in supratentorial brain tumors. Neurol India. 2020;68(1):159–62.https://doi.org/10.4103/0028-3886.279710.
13. Le Roux P. Chapter 15. Intracranial pressure monitoring and management. In: Laskowitz D, Grant G, editors. Translational research in traumatic brain injury. Boca Raton, FL: CRC Press/Taylor and Francis Group; 2016.
14. Thamjamrassri T, Yuwapattanawong K, Chanthima P, Vavilala MS, Lele AV, EVDPoP Study Collaborators. A narrative review of the published literature, hospital practices, and policies related to external ventricular drains in the United States: the external ventricular drain publications, practices, and policies (EVDPoP) study. J Neurosurg Anesthesiol. 2022;34(1):21–8. https://doi.org/10.1097/ANA.0000000000000694.
15. Tariq A, Aguilar-Salinas P, Hanel RA, Naval N, Chmayssani M. The role of ICP monitoring in meningitis. Neurosurg Focus. 2017;43(5):E7. https://doi.org/10.3171/2017.8.FOCUS17419.
16. Olson DM, Batjer HH, Abdulkadir K, Hall CE. Measuring and monitoring ICP in neurocritical care: results from a national practice survey. Neurocrit Care. 2014;20(1):15–20.
17. Rogers M, Stutzman SE, Atem FD, Sengupta S, Welch B, Olson DM. Intracranial pressure values are highly variable after cerebral spinal fluid drainage. J Neurosci Nurs. 2017;49(2):85–9. https://doi.org/10.1097/JNN.0000000000000257.
18. Hanley DF, Lane K, McBee N, et al. Thrombolytic removal of intraventricular haemorrhage in treatment of severe stroke: results of the randomised, multicentre, multiregion, placebo-controlled CLEAR III trial. Lancet. 2017;389(10069):603–11. https://doi.org/10.1016/S0140-6736(16)32410-2.
19. Moradiya Y, Murthy SB, Newman-Toker DE, Hanley DF, Ziai WC. Intraventricular thrombolysis in intracerebral hemorrhage requiring ventriculostomy: a decade-long real-world experience. Stroke.

2014;45(9):2629–35. https://doi.org/10.1161/STROKEAHA.114.006067. Epub 2014 Jul 24.
20. Lu N, Jackson D, Luke S, et al. Intraventricular nicardipine for aneurysmal subarachnoid hemorrhage related vasospasm: assessment of 90 days outcome. Neurocrit Care. 2012;16:368–75.
21. Zahra K, Domingo RA, Turnbull MT, Santos CD, Peacock SH, Jackson DA, Tawk RG, Siegel JL, Freeman WD. Safety and tolerability of concentrated intraventricular Nicardipine for poor-grade aneurysmal subarachnoid hemorrhage-related vasospasm. J Pers Med. 2023;13(3):428. https://doi.org/10.3390/jpm13030428.
22. Lewin JJ 3rd, Cook AM, Gonzales C, et al. Current practices of intraventricular antibiotic therapy in the treatment of meningitis and ventriculitis: results from a multicenter retrospective cohort study. Neurocrit Care. 2019;30(3):609–16. https://doi.org/10.1007/s12028-018-0647-0.
23. Ng K, Mabasa VH, Chow I, Ensom MH. Systematic review of efficacy, pharmacokinetics, and administration of intraventricular vancomycin in adults. Neurocrit Care. 2014;20(1):158–71. https://doi.org/10.1007/s12028-012-9784-z.
24. Huyette DR, Turnbow BJ, Kaufman C, et al. Accuracy of the freehand pass technique for ventriculostomy catheter placement: retrospective assessment using computed tomography scans. J Neurosurg. 2008;108(1):88–91.
25. Kakarla UK, Kim LJ, Chang SW, et al. Safety and accuracy of bedside external ventricular drain placement. Neurosurgery. 2008;63(1 Suppl 1):ONS162–6. discussion ONS6–7.
26. Sarrafzadeh A, Smoll N, Schaller K. Guided (VENTRI-GUIDE) versus freehand ventriculostomy: study protocol for a randomized controlled trial. Trials. 2014;15:478.
27. Hunn BH, Mujic A, Sher I, Dubey AK, Peters-Willke J, Hunn AW. Successful treatment of negative pressure hydrocephalus using timely titrated external ventricular drainage: a case series. Clin Neurol Neurosurg. 2014;116:67–71. https://doi.org/10.1016/j.clineuro.2013.10.019.
28. Bisnaire D, Robinson L. Accuracy of levelling intraventricular collection drainage systems. J Neurosci Nurs. 1997;29:261–8.
29. Slazinski T, Anderson TA, Cattell E, Eigsti JE, Heimsoth S, Holleman J, et al. Care of the patient undergoing intracranial pressure monitoring/external ventricular drainage or lumbar drainage. Am Assoc Neurosci Nurs. 2011;43:1–37.
30. Hepburn-Smith M, Dynkevich I, Spektor M, Lord A, Czeisler B, Lewis A. Establishment of an external ventricular drain best practice guideline. J Neurosci Nurs. 2016;48:54–65. https://doi.org/10.1097/JNN.0000000000000174.
31. Vieira TW, Sakamoto VTM, Araujo BR, Pai DD, Blatt CR, Caregnato RCA. External ventricular drains: development and evaluation of a nursing clinical practice guideline. Nurs Rep. 2022;12(4):933–44. https://doi.org/10.3390/nursrep12040090.
32. Wong FW. Cerebrospinal fluid collection: a comparison of different collection sites on the external ventricular drain. Dynamics. 2011;22(3):19–24.
33. Kinast CB, Paal M, Liebchen U. Comparison of cerebrospinal fluid collection through the proximal and distal port below the overflow system from an external ventricular drain. Neurocrit Care. 2022;37(3):775–8. https://doi.org/10.1007/s12028-022-01615-y.
34. Woodward S, Addison C, Shah S, Brennan F, MacLeod A, Clements M. Benchmarking best practice for external ventricular drainage. Br J Nurs. 2002;11(1):47–53. https://doi.org/10.12968/bjon.2002.11.1.12217.
35. Chaikittisilpa N, Lele AV, Lyons VH, et al. Risks of routinely clamping external ventricular drains for intrahospital transport in neurocritically ill cerebrovascular patients. Neurocrit Care. 2017;26(2):196–204. https://doi.org/10.1007/s12028-016-0308-0.
36. Chung DY, Leslie-Mazwi TM, Patel AB, Rordorf GA. Management of External Ventricular Drains after Subarachnoid Hemorrhage: a multi-institutional survey. Neurocrit Care. 2017;26(3):356–61. https://doi.org/10.1007/s12028-016-0352-9.
37. Nwachuku EL, Puccio AM, Fetzick A, Scruggs B, Chang Y-F, Shutter LA, et al. Intermittent versus continuous cerebrospinal fluid drainage management in adult severe traumatic brain injury: assessment of intracranial pressure burden. Neurocrit Care. 2014;20(1):49–53.
38. Kim GS, Amato A, James ML, Britz GW, Zomorodi A, Graffagnino C, et al. Continuous and intermittent CSF diversion after subarachnoid hemorrhage: a pilot study. Neurocrit Care. 2011;14(1):68–72.
39. Kim JH, Desai NS, Ricci J, Stieg PE, Rosengart AJ, Hartl R, et al. Factors contributing to ventriculostomy infection. World Neurosurg. 2012;77(1):135–40. https://doi.org/10.1016/j.wneu.2011.04.017.
40. Olson DM, Zomorodi M, Britz GW, Zomorodi AR, Amato A, Graffagnino C. Continuous cerebral spinal fluid drainage associated with complications in patients admitted with subarachnoid hemorrhage. J Neurosurg. 2013;119(4):974–80. https://doi.org/10.3171/2013.6.JNS122403.
41. Rao SS, Chung DY, Wolcott Z, Sheriff F, Khawaja AM, Lee H, et al. Intermittent CSF drainage and rapid EVD weaning approach after subarachnoid hemorrhage: association with fewer VP shunts and shorter length of stay. J Neurosurg. 2019;132:1–6. https://doi.org/10.3171/2019.1.JNS182702.
42. Klimo P Jr, Kestle JR, MacDonald JD, Schmidt RH. Marked reduction of cerebral vasospasm with lumbar drainage of cerebrospinal fluid after subarachnoid hemorrhage. J Neurosurg. 2004;100(2):215–24. https://doi.org/10.3171/jns.2004.100.2.0215.
43. Kramer AH, Fletcher JJ. Locally-administered intrathecal thrombolytics following aneurysmal subarachnoid hemorrhage: a systematic review and meta-analysis. Neurocrit Care. 2011;14(3):489–99. https://doi.org/10.1007/s12028-010-9429-z.
44. Jabbarli R, Pierscianek D, Rölz R, et al. Gradual external ventricular drainage weaning reduces the

risk of shunt dependency after aneurysmal subarachnoid hemorrhage: a pooled analysis. Oper Neurosurg (Hagerstown). 2018;15(5):498–504. https://doi.org/10.1093/ons/opy009.
45. Ascanio LC, Gupta R, Adeeb N, et al. Relationship between external ventricular drain clamp trials and ventriculoperitoneal shunt insertion following non-traumatic subarachnoid hemorrhage: a single-center study. J Neurosurg. 2018;130(3):956–62. https://doi.org/10.3171/2017.10.JNS171644.
46. Bales JW, Bonow RH, Buckley RT, Barber J, Temkin N, Chesnut RM. Primary external ventricular drainage catheter versus intraparenchymal ICP monitoring: outcome analysis. Neurocrit Care. 2019;31(1):11–21. https://doi.org/10.1007/s12028-019-00712-9.
47. Liu H, Wang W, Cheng F, et al. External ventricular drains versus intraparenchymal intracranial pressure monitors in traumatic brain injury: a prospective observational study. World Neurosurg. 2015;83(5):794–800. https://doi.org/10.1016/j.wneu.2014.12.040.
48. Volovici V, Pisică D, Gravesteijn BY, et al. Comparative effectiveness of intracranial hypertension management guided by ventricular versus intraparenchymal pressure monitoring: a CENTER-TBI study. Acta Neurochir. 2022;164(7):1693–705. https://doi.org/10.1007/s00701-022-05257-z.
49. Hinson HE, Melnychuk E, Muschelli J, Hanley DF, Awad IA, Ziai WC. Drainage efficiency with dual versus single catheters in severe intraventricular hemorrhage. Neurocrit Care. 2012;16(3):399–405. https://doi.org/10.1007/s12028-011-9569-9.
50. Staykov D, Huttner HB, Lunkenheimer J, et al. Single versus bilateral external ventricular drainage for intraventricular fibrinolysis in severe ventricular haemorrhage. J Neurol Neurosurg Psychiatry. 2010;81(1):105–8. https://doi.org/10.1136/jnnp.2008.168427.
51. Warren AD, Li Q, Schwab K, et al. External ventricular drain placement is associated with lower mortality after intracerebral hemorrhage with intraventricular hemorrhage. Int J Emerg Med. 2022;15:51. https://doi.org/10.1186/s12245-022-00450-4.
52. Naff NJ, Hanley DF, Keyl PM, et al. Intraventricular thrombolysis speeds blood clot resolution: results of a pilot, prospective, randomized, double-blind, controlled trial. Neurosurgery. 2004;54(3):577–83.
53. Slazinski T, Anderson TA, Cattell E, et al. Care of the patient undergoing intracranial pressure monitoring/external ventricular drainage or lumbar drainage. Chicago, IL; 2011. p. 1–38. http://aann.org/publications/clinical-practice-guidelines. Accessed 25 Mar 2016.
54. Braksick SA, Himes BT, Snyder K, Van Gompel JJ, Fugate JE, Rabinstein AA. Ventriculostomy and risk of upward herniation in patients with obstructive hydrocephalus from posterior fossa mass lesions. Neurocrit Care. 2018;28(3):338–43. https://doi.org/10.1007/s12028-017-0487-3.
55. Korinek AM, Reina M, Boch AL, Rivera AO, De Bels D, Puybasset L. Prevention of external ventricular drain-related ventriculitis. Acta Neurochir. 2005;147:39–45.
56. Lyke KE, Obasanjo OO, Williams MA, O'Brien M, Chotani R, Perl TM. Ventriculitis complicating use of intraventricular catheters in adult neurosurgical patients. Clin Infect Dis. 2001;33:2028–33.
57. Park J, Choi YJ, Ohk B, Chang HH. Cerebrospinal fluid leak at percutaneous exit of ventricular catheter as a crucial risk factor for external ventricular drainage-related infection in adult neurosurgical patients. World Neurosurg. 2018;109:e398–403. https://doi.org/10.1016/j.wneu.2017.09.190.
58. Tailor JK, Kulkarni AV. Stopping CSF leaks at external ventricular drain exit sites: a technical note. Childs Nerv Syst. 2020;36(11):2841–4. https://doi.org/10.1007/s00381-020-04632-4.
59. Moscote-Salazar LR, Satyarthee GD. Multifaceted adjunct for prevention of cerebrospinal fluid leak following external ventricular drain placement to minimize incidence of infection. World Neurosurg. 2018;109:497–8. https://doi.org/10.1016/j.wneu.2017.10.124.
60. Hoefnagel D, Dammers R, Ter Laak-Poort MP, Avezaat CJ. Risk factors for infections related to external ventricular drainage. Acta Neurochir. 2008;150(3):209–14. https://doi.org/10.1007/s00701-007-1458-9.
61. Walek KW, Leary OP, Sastry R, et al. Risk factors and outcomes associated with external ventricular drain infections. Infect Control Hosp Epidemiol. 2022;43(12):1859–66. https://doi.org/10.1017/ice.2022.23.
62. Schade RP, Schinkel J, Visser LG, et al. Bacterial meningitis caused by the use of ventricular or lumbar cerebrospinal fluid catheters. J Neurosurg. 2005;102(2):229–34.
63. Ortiz R, Lee K. Nosocomial infections in neurocritical care. Curr Neurol Neurosci Rep. 2006;6(6):525–30.
64. Zabramski JM, Whiting D, Darouiche RO, et al. Efficacy of antimicrobial-impregnated external ventricular drain catheters: a prospective, randomized, controlled trial. J Neurosurg. 2003;98(4):725–30.
65. Abla AA, Zabramski JM, Jahnke HK, Fusco D, Nakaji P. Comparison of two antibiotic-impregnated ventricular catheters: a prospective sequential series trial. Neurosurgery. 2011;68(2):437–42. https://doi.org/10.1227/NEU.0b013e3182039a14.
66. Wang X, Dong Y, Qi XQ, Li YM, Huang CG, Hou LJ. Clinical review: efficacy of antimicrobial-impregnated catheters in external ventricular drainage—a systematic review and meta-analysis. Crit Care. 2013;17(4):234. https://doi.org/10.1186/cc12608.
67. Stevens EA, Palavecino E, Sherertz RJ, Shihabi Z, Couture DE. Effects of antibiotic-impregnated external ventricular drains on bacterial culture results: an in vitro analysis. J Neurosurg. 2010;113(1):86–92. https://doi.org/10.3171/2009.10.JNS09565.
68. Edwards NC, Engelhart L, Casamento EM, McGirt MJ. Cost-consequence analysis of antibiotic-impregnated shunts and external ventricular drains in hydrocephalus. J Neurosurg. 2015;122(1):139–47. https://doi.org/10.3171/2014.9.JNS131277.

69. Klopfenstein JD, Kim LJ, Feiz-Erfan I, et al. Comparison of rapid and gradual weaning from external ventricular drainage in patients with aneurysmal subarachnoid hemorrhage: a prospective randomized trial. J Neurosurg. 2004;100(2):225–9. https://doi.org/10.3171/jns.2004.100.2.0225.
70. Chung DY, Thompson BB, Kumar MA, et al. Association of external ventricular drain wean strategy with shunt placement and length of stay in subarachnoid hemorrhage: a prospective multicenter study. Neurocrit Care. 2022;36(2):536–45. https://doi.org/10.1007/s12028-021-01343-9.
71. Yang XT, Feng DF, Zhao L, Sun ZL, Zhao G. Application of the Ommaya reservoir in managing ventricular hemorrhage. World Neurosurg. 2016;89:93–100. https://doi.org/10.1016/j.wneu.2015.12.040.
72. Chen Y, Liu L, Zhu M. Intraventricular administration of antibiotics by Ommaya reservoir for patients with multidrug-resistant Acinetobacter baumannii central nervous system infection. Br J Neurosurg. 2021;35(2):170–3. https://doi.org/10.1080/02688697.2020.1777255.
73. de Oca M, Delgado M, Cacho Díaz B, Santos Zambrano J, et al. The comparative treatment of intraventricular chemotherapy by Ommaya reservoir vs. lumbar puncture in patients with leptomeningeal carcinomatosis. Front Oncologia. 2018;8:509. https://doi.org/10.3389/fonc.2018.00509.
74. Singh H, Patir R, Vaishya S, Miglani R, Kaur A. External ventricular drain related complications-whether continuous csf drainage via ommaya reservoir is the answer? Neurol India. 2020;68(2):458–61. https://doi.org/10.4103/0028-3886.284354.
75. Jha VC, Alam S. Role of Ommaya reservoir placement in hydrocephalus management following aneurysmal subarachnoid hemorrhage, an initial experience. Arq Bras Neurocir. 2022;41(3):e224–31.
76. Zachariah J, Snyder KA, Graffeo CS, et al. Risk of Ventriculostomy-associated hemorrhage in patients with aneurysmal subarachnoid hemorrhage treated with anticoagulant Thromboprophylaxis. Neurocrit Care. 2016;25(2):224–9. https://doi.org/10.1007/s12028-016-0262-x.
77. Tanweer O, Boah A, Huang PP. Risks for hemorrhagic complications after placement of external ventricular drains with early chemical prophylaxis against venous thromboembolisms. J Neurosurg. 2013;119(5):1309–13. https://doi.org/10.3171/2013.7.JNS13313.

Lumbar Drain

64

B. Nisha and Soniya Biswas

64.1 Introduction

Lumbar drains are used for temporary cerebrospinal fluid (CSF) diversion. A lumbar drain is a catheter that is inserted into the lumbar subarachnoid space to drain cerebrospinal fluid either continuously or intermittently. The lumbar drain catheter can be connected to a collection system which is used to collect and measure the collected CSF accurately. It is commonly inserted in neurosurgical patients and can be performed both at the bedside and in the operating room [1]. It is important to understand the indications, procedure, and complications of lumbar drain insertion to avoid any major disaster. This chapter will dwell into the considerations to be kept in mind while dealing with a lumbar drain.

64.2 Brief History

Continuous CSF drainage via spinal catheters was first performed by G Vorc'h in the 1960s [2]. He described its use for the reduction of intracranial pressure intraoperatively and for use in traumatic CSF leaks. McCullough et al. in 1988 proposed the use of CSF drainage as a modality to prevent spinal cord injury after the occlusion of thoracic aorta [3].

64.3 Relevant Anatomy

The choroid plexus of the ventricles in the brain produces the majority of CSF circulating within the central nervous system. CSF is replaced approximately three to four times a day with approximately 400–500 mL produced per day. In adults, the spinal cord is usually ends at the L1 or L2 vertebral levels as conus medullaris and the subarachnoid space continues up to the S2 vertebral level. Cauda equina floats freely in the subarachnoid space between the L2 and S2 level, and there is unlikely a chance of damage to the spinal cord or the nerve roots between these levels. Thus, L3/L4 and L4/L5 intervertebral spaces are the preferred level of lumbar drain insertion. This space can be identified by the intercristal/Toufier's/Jacoby's line which is a virtual horizontal line connecting the highest points of the iliac crest. To approach the subarachnoid space, the needle has to pierce the skin, subcutaneous tissue, supraspinous ligament, interspinous ligament, ligamentum flavum, dura mater, and the subarachnoid layer.

B. Nisha (✉)
Neuroanaesthesia and Critical Care, Apollo Speciality Hospitals, Madurai, Tamilnadu, India

S. Biswas
Rabindranath Tagore International Institute of Cardiac Sciences, Kolkata, West Bengal, India

H. Prabhakar et al. (eds.), *Principles and Practice of Neurocritical Care*,
https://doi.org/10.1007/978-981-99-8059-8_64

64.4 Indications

- Active CSF leak or those at risk for CSF leak, e.g., skull base procedures, prevention of CSF fistula
- To facilitate intraoperative brain relaxation and intraoperative exposure [4]
- In pituitary surgery to facilitate resection of suprasellar mass by injecting saline, detect CSF leak site by injecting fluorescein dye, and prevent and treat postoperative CSF leak [5, 6]
- Intrathecal antibiotics in bacterial/fungal meningitis, CSF sampling, evaluation of normal pressure hydrocephalus management [7, 8]
- Spinal cord protective strategy in open and endovascular thoracic aortic repair for patients at high risk of spinal cord injury [9]
- Malfunctioning or infected ventriculo-peritoneal shunts, and other neurological emergencies occurring due to infective, and neoplastic diseases

64.4.1 Craniotomy

Lumbar drains are used to facilitate brain relaxation to reduce retractor induced ischemic injury to brain. These cases include anterior skull base cases, retrosigmoid approaches, far lateral approaches, and suboccipital craniectomies [4].

64.4.2 Endoscopic Skull Base Surgery

Lumbar drains are commonly used in endoscopic skull base surgeries. It may be placed prior to or after an endoscopic endonasal approach to divert the CSF and allow for the skull base defect to heal without postoperative CSF leak [5].

64.4.3 CSF Leak

In cases of spontaneous or traumatic CSF leak, an LD can be placed prior to the attempted closure. It allows to identify the leak site by administering intrathecal fluorescein. Intrathecal injection of fluorescein dye through the lumbar drain intraoperatively during the repair of cerebrospinal fluid leaks is done to identify the location of defect and to confirm the watertight closure of the defect [6].

64.4.4 Thoracoabdominal Aortic Surgery

LD placement allows for CSF diversion and thereby reduce pressure in the intrathecal space. This may increase spinal cord perfusion pressure and result in the reduction of ischemic injury to the spinal cord. An LD can also be placed in cases of CSF leak following spine surgery [9].

64.5 Contraindications

The contraindications to the insertion of an LD include the following:

- Patient refusal
- Presence of significantly increased intracranial pressure
- Obstructive hydrocephalus
- Skin infection/spinal epidural abscess
- Coagulopathy/thrombocytopenia
- Anticoagulant therapy

64.6 Technique

64.6.1 Preprocedure Preparation

Detailed history—It is necessary to elicit the indication for the insertion of lumbar drain. Medication history should be taken in detail, especially intake of anticoagulants and antiplatelets. History suggestive of bleeding disorders or coagulopathy should be noted. Any history of previous spine surgery should be taken.

Examination—The spine, especially the lumbar region, should be examined. The presence of pre-existing neurological deficits should be noted.

Investigations—Complete blood count and coagulation profile should be done. A CT/MRI should be reviewed to rule out any contraindication for placing a lumbar drain like obstructive hydrocephalus.

64.6.2 Positioning and Equipment Setup

Lumbar drains are placed similar to a lumbar puncture, epidural, or intrathecal catheter placement.

The placement of an LD may be done prior to induction in an awake patient, or after the induction of anesthesia. The patient is placed in the lateral decubitus or sitting position. Using a strict aseptic technique, the lumbar catheter is typically inserted at the L3–4 or L4–5 level via a 14G Tuohy needle. It can be done via a median or paramedian approach. Figure 64.1 shows the equipment required for the procedure.

A kink resistant, flexible catheter with the guide wire is passed through the Tuohy needle into the intrathecal space. Secure the catheter firmly in place with the left hand and remove the guidewire from within the catheter. The catheter is secured approximately 5–8 cm past the needle into the intrathecal space. It should be stressed that the catheter should thread easily, similar to an epidural catheter. If resistance is felt, or the catheter is unable to proceed, both the needle and catheter should be removed as a single unit in order to prevent inadvertent shearing of the catheter [10].

The catheter can then be connected to the collection system with the catheter metal cap included in the kit. During cap placement, it is important to ensure that the end of catheter is not torn. A silk tie is generally used to secure the catheter tip to the cap (Fig. 64.2).

The catheter can then be connected to the collection system by a three-way stopcock. The catheter can be secured to the patient's skin with clear adhesive dressings.

The catheter can be flushed with sterile saline flush and connected to a sterile pressure monitoring kit and a closed collection system. The transducer should not be connected to any pressured flushing system [10].

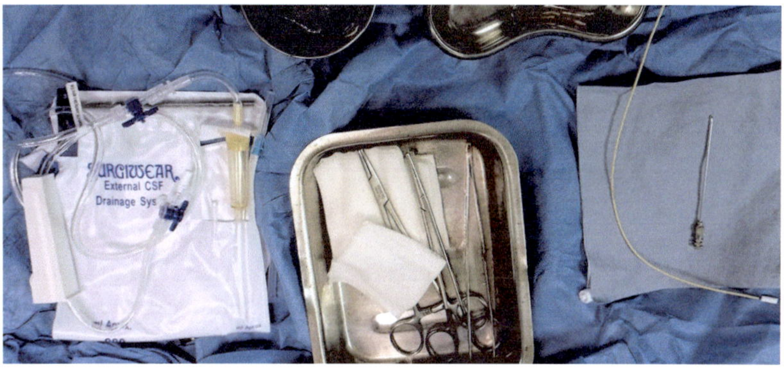

Fig. 64.1 Equipment required for insertion of lumbar drain

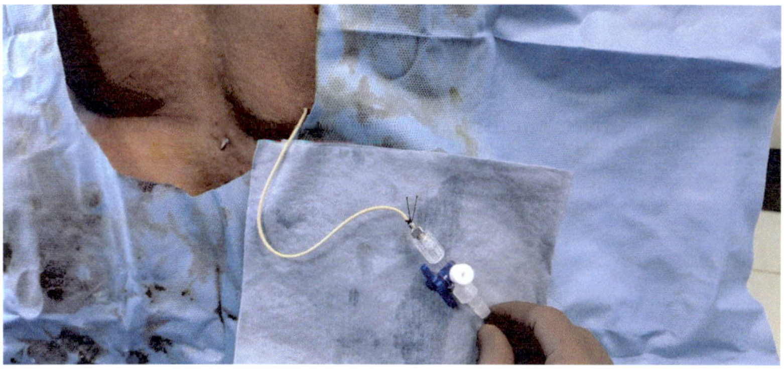

Fig. 64.2 Lumbar drain in situ

One can also opt for fluoroscopy-guided catheter placement. In this technique, the patient must be placed in a radiolucent table with the availability of C arm. Once CSF comes out, a contrast dye is injected. If the dye spreads diffusely, the space has been identified correctly. In the epidural space, the dye has an irregular pattern with multiple filling defects that is seen in the anteroposterior (AP) view and the dye is seen spreading along the spinolaminar line in the lateral view. In the subdural space, the "railroad track' appearance is seen in the AP view. Ultrasound and CT-guided placement can also be done [11].

64.6.3 CSF Drainage

CSF should be drained in a controlled and low resistive manner to avoid overdrainage and related complications like subdural bleed. As per the Society of Neuroanaesthesia and Critical Care guidelines, it should not exceed 10–20 mL/h.

64.6.4 Postprocedure Care

One should regularly check the lumbar drain dressing for soakage. The integrity of the whole system should be ensured. The drain rate should be kept in check. One should continuously look for any obstruction/underdrainage/overdrainage. Neurological examination should be done routinely to check for any damage to nerve roots or as a complication of CSF draining. Vitals including temperature should be checked at frequent intervals. The necessity to keep the lumbar drain in situ should be reviewed daily.

64.7 Complications

Intracerebral hemorrhage, tract hematoma or tract hemorrhages (0–41%)
Neural injury
Infection (0–50%)
Malposition
Occlusion and malfunction
Over drainage of CSF
Subdural or epidural hematoma
Re-bleeding from a ruptured cerebral aneurysm
Intracranial hypotension
Cerebellar tonsillar herniation
Pneumocephalus
Breakage of catheters with retained fragment of catheter
Postdural puncture headache

64.8 Management of Complications

64.8.1 Headache: Postdural Puncture Headache

CSF leak causes intrathecal hypotension resulting in traction on the meninges and cranial nerves. The amount of CSF drained can be reduced or drainage can be stopped to reduce headache. Good hydration and simple analgesics can be used.

64.8.2 Cerebral Herniation

Overdrainage of CSF can result in herniations, and the drainage must be stopped immediately.

64.8.3 Infection

Meningitis, cellulitis, and ventriculitis can be due to the following factors such as non-tunnelled catheters, non-sterile conditions, intraventricular haemorrhage, frequent sampling, irrigation of catheters, and longer in-situ duration. Cleansing the insertion site using an antimicrobial agent, institution of pre-LD-insertion antibiotics, avoiding routine CSF sampling, and limited manipulation of the CSF collecting system are the recommendations to decrease infection [12].

64.8.4 Catheter Shearing and Retained Catheter

This complication of LD placement can occur anywhere along the tract of the drain due to the shearing of the catheter from the needle. This is best avoided by not pulling the catheter while the catheter is still within the needle. It is also critical to remove the needle prior to the guidewire. The catheter can be snapped during removal as well. If the retained catheter is fully intradural, removal is not recommended unless the patient is symptomatic [13]. If the catheter is both intra- and extradural, the catheter must be removed. If the catheter is extradural, in most cases, removal is not needed.

64.8.5 Spinal Cord Injury/Paresthesia

The needle may penetrate the nerve roots leading to paresthesia, extremity weakness, or pain. If the patient reports these symptoms, an attempt can be made to place the drain at a different interspinous spaces. These symptoms are usually temporary as the damage to nerve roots is not usually permanent.

64.8.6 Severe Pre-existing CSF Leak

Insertion of an LD is particularly challenging in patients with CSF leak, resulting in low CSF volume within the thecal sac. It can be managed with the patient in reverse trendelenburg position or to utilize fluoroscopy. Occasionally, in such patients, it is possible to place the drain within the subarachnoid space with minimal cerebrospinal fluid or dry tap. When this is suspected, iodinated contrast can be administered through the drain to establish whether it is appropriately placed.

Prevention of Hemorrhagic and Infectious Complications Associated with External Ventricular and Lumbar Drains. *Class of Recommendation and Level of Evidence based on Guidelines From the Society for Neuroscience in Anaesthesiology and Critical Care* [1].

- Prior to the insertion of EVD and LD, prompt diagnosis and correction of coagulopathy utilizing institutional practice guidelines is recommended (Class I Recommendation; Level of Evidence E).
- Perioperative anticoagulation management with lumbar drain placement and removal should be performed within the framework of the current ASRA guidelines (Class I Recommendation; Level of Evidence E).
- Antibiotics should only be administered prior to the placement of a LD with the choice based on institutional practice (Class I Recommendation; Level of Evidence E).
- It is recommended to practice strict aseptic technique based on the national and institutional guidelines (Class I Recommendation; Level of Evidence E).

Perioperative Checklist for Patients with Lumbar Drain *based on Guidelines From the Society for Neuroscience in Anesthesiology and Critical Care*

- Obtain baseline neurological examination, Coagulation profile, use of antiplatelets and anticoagulants
- Review antibiotic plan for LD insertion in the operating room
- Review LD hourly CSF output to obtain baseline ICP if monitoring is done
- Review baseline CSF color and consistency
- Provide EVD and LD details during preoperative handoff between ICU and the anesthesia providers
- Transporting patients with LD with care & Confirm decision to travel with LD clamp vs. open
- Confirm availability of dedicated intravenous pole for LD mount
- Confirm leveling LD at phlebostatic axis or at lumbar catheter insertion site
- Ask the staff to inform in the following scenarios
  - Sudden decline in CSF drainage or no drainage from LD
  - Occlusion of LD
  - If the drain output is >15–20 mL at any time or in any given hour
  - Sudden change in CSF colour
  - Dampening or loss of ICP waveform

Management of EVD and LD in Special Clinical Scenarios. *Class of Recommendation and Level of Evidence based on Guidelines From the Society for Neuroscience in Anaesthesiology and Critical Care*

- LD tubing that is accidentally disconnected should be clamped immediately to prevent overdrainage of cerebrospinal fluid (Class I Recommendation; Level of Evidence C).
- If LD systems are contaminated by disconnection, all distal parts should be replaced with new sterile tubing (Class IIa Recommendation; Level of Evidence E).
- Routine flushing of the LD catheter should not be performed (Class III Recommendation; Level of Evidence E).
- In patients with ruptured cerebral aneurysm, sudden excessive drainage of cerebrospinal fluid prior to securing the aneurysm can provoke aneurysm re-rupture and should be avoided (Class III Recommendation: Level of Evidence C).
- Identification of LD tubing by appropriate labels and use of other visual aids is recommended to prevent confusion with intravenous ports (Class I Recommendation; Level of Evidence E).
- Accidental intrathecal injection should be recognized and reported to the neurosurgeon (Class IIa Recommendation; Level of Evidence E).
- Lavage of the intrathecal space after accidental injection is not recommended (Class III Recommendation; Level of Evidence C).
- Establish institutional standards to ensure safe intrathecal injection of fluorescein dye via lumbar drain in patients with suspected cerebrospinal fluid leak (Class I Level of Recommendation, Level of Evidence E).
- The ASRA guidelines on anticoagulation should be consulted to determine appropriateness of placement and removal of the LD.

References

1. Lele AV, Hoefnagel AL, Schloemerkemper N, Wyler DA, Chaikittisilpa N, Vavilala MS, et al. Perioperative management of adult patients with external ventricular and lumbar drains: guidelines from the society for neuroscience in anesthesiology and critical care. J Neurosurg Anesthesiol. 2017;29:191–210.
2. Livingston AJ, Laing B, Zwagerman NT, Harris MS. Lumbar drains: practical understanding and application for the otolaryngologist. Am J Otolaryngol. 2020;41:102740.
3. McCullough JL, Hollier LH, Nugent M. Paraplegia after thoracic aortic occlusion: influence of cerebrospinal fluid drainage. Experimental and early clinical results. J Vasc Surg. 1988;7(1):153–60.
4. Ackerman PD, Spencer DA, Prabhu VC. The efficacy and safety of preoperative lumbar drain placement in anterior skull base surgery. J Neurol Surg Rep. 2013;74(1):1–9.
5. Stokken J, Recinos PF, Woodard T, Sindwani R. The utility of lumbar drains in modern endoscopic skull base surgery. Curr Opin Otolaryngol Head Neck Surg. 2015;23(1):78–82.
6. Albu S, Florian IS, Bolboaca SD. The benefit of early lumbar drain insertion in reducing the length of CSF leak in traumatic rhinorrhea. Clin Neurol Neurosurg. 2016;142:43–7.
7. Woodworth GF, McGirt MJ, Williams MA, Rigamonti D. Cerebrospinal fluid drainage and dynamics in the diagnosis of normal pressure hydrocephalus. Neurosurgery. 2009;64(5):919–25, discussion 925–926.
8. Chotai S, Medel R, Herial NA, Medhkour A. External lumbar drain: a pragmatic test for prediction of shunt outcomes in idiopathic normal pressure hydrocephalus. Surg Neurol Int. 2014;5:12.
9. Fedorow CA, Moon MC, Mutch WA, Grocott HP. Lumbar cerebrospinal fluid drainage for thoracoabdominal aortic surgery: rationale and practical considerations for management. Anesth Analg. 2010;111(1):46–58.
10. Sladky JH, Piwinski SE. Lumbar puncture technique and lumbar drains. Atlas Oral Maxillofac Surg Clin North Am. 2015;23(2):169–76.
11. Chee CG, Lee GY, Lee JW, Lee E, Kang HS. Fluoroscopy-guided lumbar drainage of cerebrospinal fluid for patients in whom a blind beside approach is difficult. Korean J Radiol. 2015;16(4):860–5.
12. Coplin WM, Avellino AM, Kim DK, Winn HR, Grady MS. Bacterial meningitis associated with lumbar drains: a retrospective cohort study. J Neurol Neurosurg Psychiatry. 1999;67(4):468–73.
13. Hnenny L, Sabry HA, Raskin JS, Liu JJ, Roundy NE, Dogan A. Migrating lumbar intrathecal catheter fragment associated with intracranial subarachnoid hemorrhage. J Neurosurg Spine. 2015;22(1):47–51.

65 Percutaneous Tracheostomy

Kanwalpreet Sodhi, Navneh Samagh, Atul Phillips, and Manender Kumar

65.1 Introduction

Percutaneous dilatational tracheostomy (PDT) is one of the commonly performed bedside procedures in critically ill patients by intensivists. PDT has become the standard of care in modern intensive care unit (ICU) and is not only safe but also has resulted in sharp decline in use of surgical tracheostomy barring a few selected cases [1]. The foremost goal of PDT is to establish a safe airway in patients who cannot either protect their airway and/or require prolonged mechanical ventilation (MV). Other advantages include improved airway clearance and oral hygiene, efficient nursing care, better patient comfort and effective communication. Intended benefits of doing early tracheostomy in neurological patients entail reduced need for sedation, easier and faster weaning, and thereby shorter duration of MV, reduced ventilator associated pneumonia (VAP) rates, and reduced length of ICU stay contributing to better outcomes [2].

65.2 Indications

The classical indications of PDT in ICU (Table 65.1) are:

- Protect airway in patients who are at risk of aspiration.
- Prolonged mechanical ventilation.
- Facilitate weaning in difficult to wean patients.
- Improve broncho-pulmonary toileting.
- Minimize sedation requirement

Table 65.1 Indications of PDT

1. Prolonged MV > 7 days, in patients who are expected to have a meaningful recovery
2. Airway protection for neurologic disorders or traumatic brain injury
3. Upper airway obstruction due to stridor, foreign body, malignancy, trauma, infections
4. Bilateral vocal cord paralysis
5. Airway edema
6. Subglottic or tracheal stenosis
7. Intubation failure (cricothyrotomy is preferred)
8. Neuromuscular disorders for effective tracheobronchial toileting
9. As an adjunct to major head and neck surgery and airway or facial trauma management

K. Sodhi (✉)
Department of Critical Care, Deep Hospital, Ludhiana, Punjab, India

N. Samagh
Department of Anesthesiology, AIIMS, Bathinda, Punjab, India

A. Phillips
Fellow Neurocritical Care, Cummings School of Medicine University of Calgary, Alberta, Canada

M. Kumar
Department of Cardiac Anesthesia & Critical Care, Fortis Hospital, Ludhiana, Punjab, India

H. Prabhakar et al. (eds.), *Principles and Practice of Neurocritical Care*,
https://doi.org/10.1007/978-981-99-8059-8_65

Table 65.2 Contraindications to PDT

Absolute	Relative
Infants	Difficult anatomy (morbid obesity, enlarged thyroid gland, short neck, local malignancy, limited neck extension, tracheal deviation)
Lack of expertise	Pulsatile vessels in front of neck, high riding innominate artery
Local site infection	Close proximity to site of burns or surgical wound
Uncontrolled coagulopathy	Coagulopathy not corrected with reversal agents and blood products
Unstable cervical spine injuries	Previous cervical spine surgery/ tracheostomy
	High oxygen requirements: High PEEP >10 cm of H_2O or FiO_2 > 70%

65.3 Contraindications

There are few absolute contraindications for PDT and relative contraindications are now rarely considered contraindications due to procedural experience and availability of a wide range of procedural aids [1]. The absolute and relative contraindications are shown in Table 65.2.

65.4 Anatomy

Since the time PDT was first performed by Sheldon et al. in 1953, the technique has immensely metamorphosed and become advanced [3]. Anatomical mastery of the neck region therefore becomes obligatory as airway complications can be cataclysmic. The trachea is a tubular conduit extending in the subglottic space from the vocal cords to carina branching into bronchi. Adult trachea measures between 10 and 13 cm and tends to be shorter and narrower in females. The tracheal external diameter averages 2.3 cm with a standard wall thickness of 3 mm. The tracheal wall consists of 18–22 D-shaped incomplete tracheal "rings" with a cartilaginous anterolateral wall and a membranous posterior wall consisting of the trachealis muscle. Ageing leads to stiffening and narrowing of lateral lumen and increase in the anteroposterior diameter resulting in "saber-sheath" or scabbard trachea, which may be seen in chronic obstructive airway disease also [4].

65.4.1 Relationship with Surrounding Structures

The oesophagus runs along the posterior left border of the trachea, making the oesophagus prone to injury if the posterior tracheal wall is breached. The strap muscles (sternohyoid, sternothyroid, thyrohyoid, and omohyoid) overlie the trachea, protecting it. The thyroid gland typically overlies the second to fourth tracheal rings in the neck. Immediately lateral to the cervical trachea lies the recurrent laryngeal nerves and common carotid arteries, encased in the deep cervical fascia. The innominate artery originates at the right anterior aspect of the trachea and crosses over the distal and mid trachea as it arises from the aorta. The left common carotid artery runs superiorly from right-to-left over the left anterolateral trachea while the superior vena cava courses toward the right atrium along the right anterior aspect of the trachea. The cervical portion of the trachea lies anteriorly in the neck, dives posteriorly into the mediastinum with thymus. The anterior mediastinal contents overlie the thoracic trachea as it courses posterior to the heart. Paired anterior jugular veins are part of the superficial venous drainage system of the head and neck extending inferiorly to the left of the midline under the platysma. Common variants include a single anterior jugular vein formed in the midline and a plexus of smaller venous vessels found on the superior aspect replacing the anterior jugular veins [5].

65.4.2 Anatomic Landmarks for Tracheostomy

The ideal location for tracheostomy tube placement is between the second and third tracheal rings (Fig. 65.1). Always palpate the neck to identify key anatomical landmarks including the thyroid cartilage, cricoid cartilage and sternal notch. The thyroid notch identifies the superior aspect of the larynx in the midline. A palpable

Fig. 65.1 Anatomy of neck

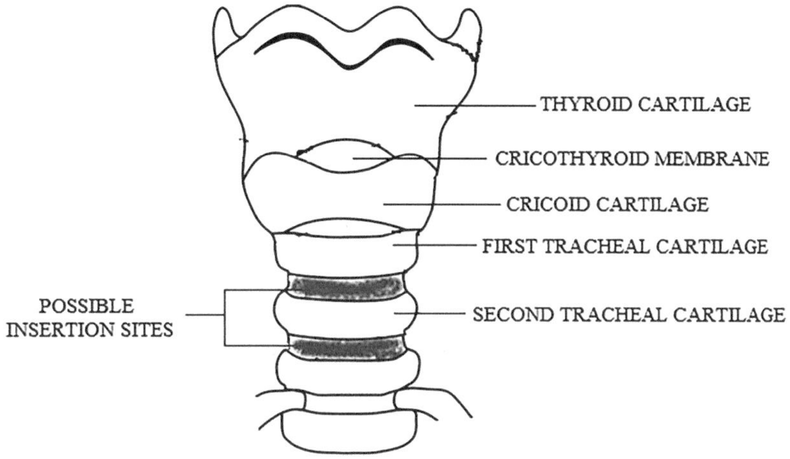

depression lying inferiorly between the cricoid and thyroid cartilages is the thickened cricothyroid membrane. Underlying the cricoid cartilage is the junction of the larynx and trachea. The skin incision is typically made 1–2 cm inferior to the cricoid. The sternal notch is an important landmark to identify a high-riding innominate artery by palpation. The trachea lies at a depth of 2–2.5 cm from the skin and follows the curvature of the cervical spine and it varies with age, increased pre-tracheal soft tissue, flexion-extension of the neck and diseases altering the curvature of spine [6]. The assessment of depth of trachea is imperative in patients in whom anatomical landmarks cannot be palpated and diagnostic ultrasound may be useful.

65.5 Techniques for Insertion of PDT

Since the initial PDT technique was described by Ciaglia et al [7] in mid 1980s, several modifications for insertion of PDT have been introduced in the last four decades. There is however not much evidence favoring one technique over the other [1]. The various techniques are as follows:

1. Ciaglia Serial Dilatational Technique

In this technique performed by Ciaglia et al. in 1985 [7], a cannula or needle is inserted into the trachea at the tracheostomy site. Guidewire is then inserted using the Seldinger technique and passed in the caudal direction. Next, a primary dilator is passed over the wire to start dilatation of the tract. A white plastic sheath is placed over the wire which acts as a guide for subsequent dilators. The dilator is inserted over the guide wire up to a safety ridge, to prevent damage to the curved dilator tip and prevent kinking of the guidewire. Multiple larger dilators are used sequentially till the tract is sufficiently dilated. A tracheostomy tube (TT) is loaded on the appropriately sized dilator which is passed over the guide wire and the plastic sheath into the trachea. Over time, this technique has undergone three major changes, i.e. site of insertion (moved caudal from cricoid cartilage by one or two tracheal interspaces), use of bronchoscopy and use of a single tapered dilator [1, 8].

2. Ciaglia Single Dilator Tracheostomy Technique

It is also known as Ciaglia Blue Rhino technique (Cook Critical Care, Bloomington, IN, USA). This technique introduced in 1999 is a modification of the Ciaglia technique and requires a simpler kit comprising a single-beveled curved hydrophilic dilator. This one-step dilatation is faster and associated with reduced loss of tidal volume during the procedure [1, 8].

3. Griggs Percutaneous Technique

This guidewire dilator forceps technique was described by Griggs et al. in 1990 and utilizes a specially designed dilating forceps (modified Howard Kelly forceps) for single-step dilatation of tissues in the pretracheal and tracheal space. And no special kit is required, it has potential to cause significant soft tissue damage [9].

4. Balloon Dilatational Tracheostomy (Ciaglia Blue Dolphin, Cook Medical)

This is the second generation of the Ciaglia technique with initial steps being same as the single dilator tracheostomy technique. However, a pressurized modified angioplasty balloon over a guidewire is used to dilate the trachea instead of a curved dilator. The balloon is inflated with saline to 11 atmospheric pressure for 15 s, resulting in the formation of a tracheal stoma. The balloon is then deflated and the TT is inserted in a single step. This technique is more useful in patients with cervical spine injury or recent spine surgery. Advantages of this technique are less pressure on tracheal wall as compared to other techniques, and reduced incidence of posterior tracheal wall injury as radial forces generated during insertion are less traumatic as compared to coaxial forces produced in other techniques [7, 10]. Disadvantages include longer duration of procedure and increased incidence of intra-tracheal bleeding [11].

5. Fantoni Translaryngeal Tracheostomy

It was first described by Fantoni and Ripamonti in 1997. This technique is not widely practiced as it is cumbersome and requires experience. This technique involves the insertion of the cannula or needle into the tracheal lumen with the guide wire directed in cranial and retrograde manner through the vocal cords into the mouth. The ETT is replaced by a narrower tube to maintain ventilation. A special tracheostomy device (combined dilator and tracheostomy tube) is attached to the guide wire and drawn back internally through the airway and out to the surface of the neck through the opening formed by the introducer needle. The tracheostomy tube is separated from the device and rotated 180°, so the open end faces down towards the carina [8, 12].

6. Frova's Percutaneous Tracheostomy

This technique was described in 2002, involves using a single-step screw-type dilator (PercuTwist kit; Rusch, Kernen, Germany). The dilator is rotated clockwise over the guidewire using a lifting motion and threaded into the tracheal stoma. It allows better control over the dilating manoeuvre throughout the procedure with the risk of injury to the posterior tracheal wall and tracheal ring fractures [8, 13].

65.5.1 Comparison of Different PDT Techniques

A systematic review was done by Cabrini et al. in 2012 including 13 studies comparing at least two PDT techniques. No major differences were observed between the techniques with the exception of the Fantoni technique which was associated with more serious complications [14]. Other studies found the Ciaglia Single Dilator Tracheostomy technique (aka Ciaglia Blue Rhino technique) to be better than other PDT techniques like PercuTwist, Blue Dolphin, and Griggs technique [11, 14–16].

65.6 Preparation and Steps of PDT

The preparation and procedure of PDT has been described in Table 65.3. Figure 65.2 gives a pictorial representation of steps of PDT.

Table 65.3 Preparation and steps of PDT [1, 8]

Initial checklist	Correct patient Correct equipment Written informed consent NPO status 6 h Check that coagulation profile is within normal limits Confirm withholding of anticoagulant drugs according to their half lives Availability of assistant to manage the airway
Monitoring	Heart rate, Blood pressure, SpO_2, Capnography Pre-procedure ultrasound of neck to identify the site of incision (not mandatory)
If bronchoscopy guided	Check the bronchoscope assembly Insert bronchoscope through the ET tube and orient the view for the operator to identify the desired entry point
Position	Properly position the patient to optimize the neck extension (a pillow may be placed underneath the shoulders to extend the neck)
Oxygenation	Keep FiO_2 100%. Do a thorough oral and endotracheal pre-procedural suctioning
Sedation	Adequately sedate and paralyze the patient with analgosedation and muscle relaxants
Repositioning of endotracheal tube	Deflate the ET cuff and withdraw ET under laryngoscopic/bronchoscopic vision until cuff is visualized just below cords, then reinflate the cuff
Sterile precautions	Clean skin with antiseptic solution and drape the patient
Skin infiltration	Infiltrate the skin at site of insertion with local anesthetic containing a vasoconstrictor (1-2% lignocaine with adrenaline)
Incision	Make a 2–2.5 cm transverse incision at insertion site Bluntly dissect subcutaneous fat and pretracheal tissue
Steps	1. Advance a 14-gauge sheathed introducer needle into trachea 2. Confirm tracheal placement of needle by aspiration of air into the saline filled syringe attached to the needle or direct visualization with bronchoscope 3. Withdraw the needle and insert guidewire using Seldinger technique through the plastic sheath 4. Dilate the insertion site with the help of dilators depending on the PDT technique 5. After adequate dilatation, dilator is removed and after adequate lubrication, tracheostomy tube with appropriate adapter is inserted into trachea over the guiding wire/catheter
Confirmation	Direct visualization of carina through the bronchoscope or by capnography

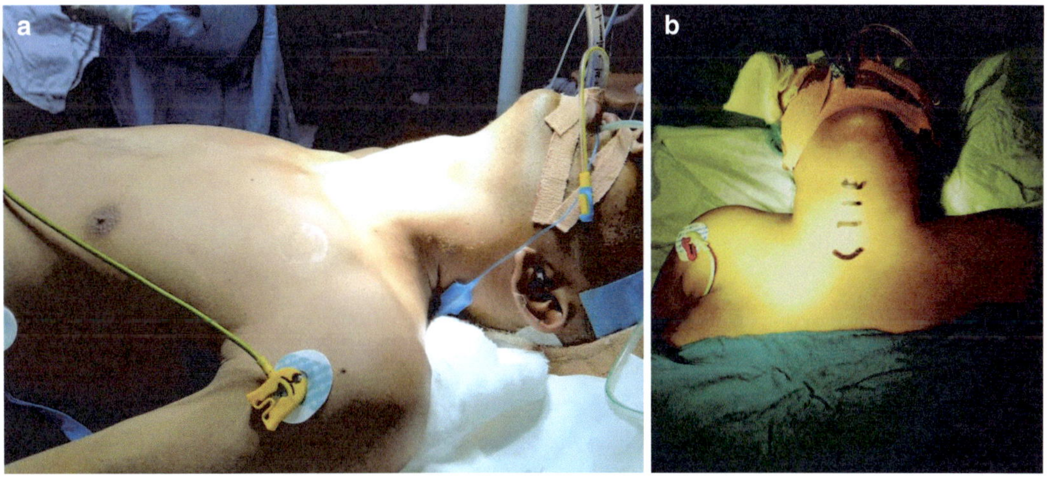

Fig. 65.2 Steps of PDT. (**a**) Patient position (**b**) Identificaiton of landmarks (**c**) Infiltartion of local anesthetic (**d**) Puncturing trachea (**e**) Aspiration of air (**f**) Guidewire insertion (**g-h**) Dilatation (**i**) Tracheostomy tube being inserted (**j**) Confirm placement

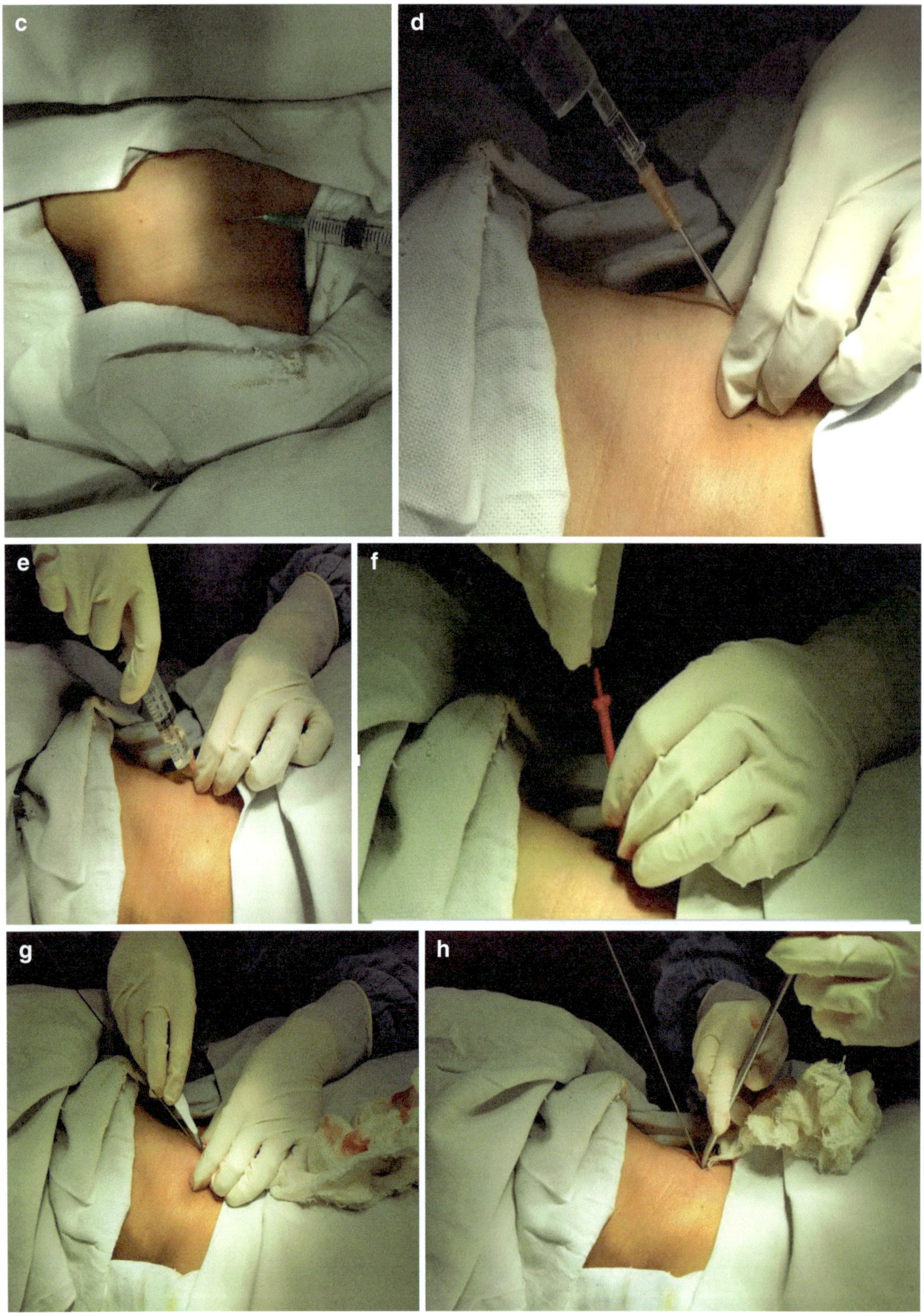

Fig. 65.2 (continued)

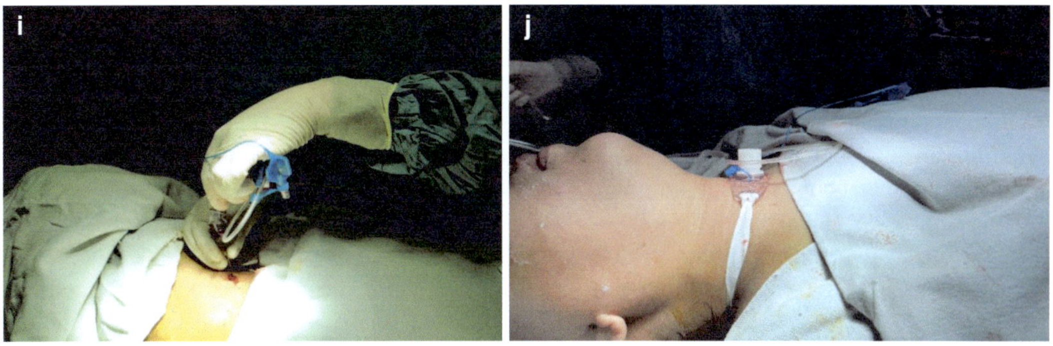

Fig. 65.2 (continued)

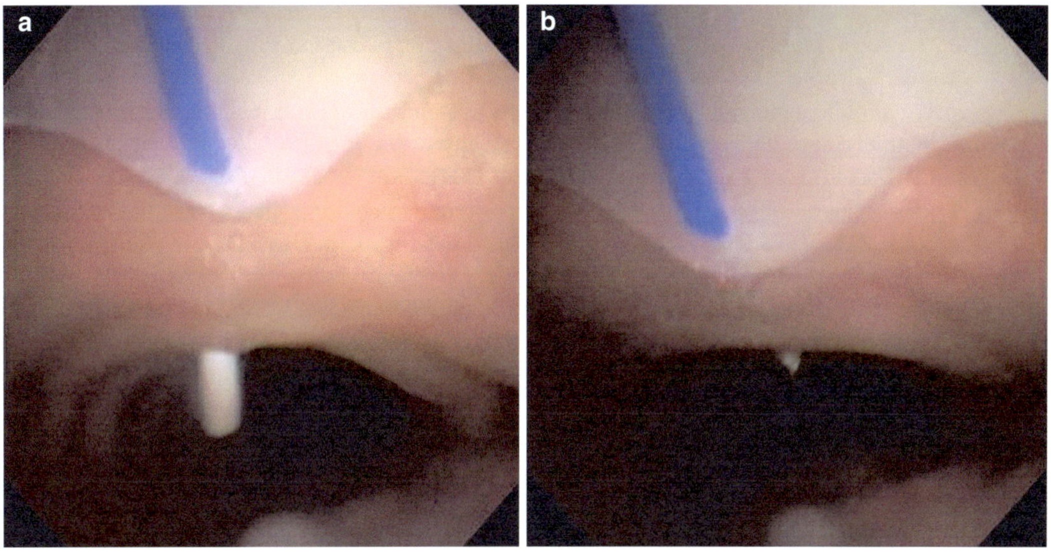

Fig. 65.3 Bronchoscopic View during PDT

65.7 Procedural Adjuncts

1. Bronchoscopy

Flexible bronchoscope during PDT is used for patients with difficult neck anatomy and can be a guide for the inexperienced operator [1]. Bronchoscope-assisted procedure is useful during PDT for the following reasons (Fig. 65.3):

(a) Real-time confirmation of needle placement into the trachea.
(b) Ensuring midline position of the needle.
(c) Confirmation of tube placement.

Avoiding injury to surrounding structures, posterior tracheal wall injury and preventing high placement of the tube are other benefits of using bronchoscope [17, 18]. However, there are certain concerns regarding the routine use of bronchoscope in neurological patients as it has been found to cause measurable increases in intracranial pressure (ICP) due to supine positioning for the procedure, increase in partial pressure of carbon dioxide (pCO2) and fall in oxygen saturation due to alveolar derecruitment [19]. Another concern is the requirement of specialized equipment and adequately trained manpower [20]. Due to insufficient data as of now, the routine use of bronchoscope is not currently recommended during PDT by most guidelines [1].

2. Preoperative Ultrasound [16]

Point-of-care ultrasonography (POCUS) in ICUs is increasingly being used as an adjunct to guide invasive procedures including PDT (Fig. 65.4). It is portable, noninvasive and readily available at the bedside in ICUs. Doing a pre-procedural POCUS of neck can help by:

(a) Estimation of distance from skin to the trachea.
(b) Accurate delineation of the position of the tracheal rings in patients without a clearly palpable tracheal anatomy to ensure midline punctures in patients such as morbidly obese, cervical spine injury patients where neck extension cannot be done or is not desired.
(c) Using POCUS to identify the puncture site allows for optimal site for TT insertion and was found to be different from puncture site identified by landmark technique in 24% cases [21].
(d) Ensures accurate placement of the introducer needle into the trachea.
(e) Identification of aberrant vessels—decreases risk of hemorrhage.
(f) Identification of enlarged thyroid isthmus.

Gobatto et al. in a retrospective study in 60 patients undergoing PDT observed that ultrasound-guided PDT (US-PDT) was safe, effective, with shorter procedure time and was comparable in clinical outcomes and complication rates to bronchoscopy-guided PDT procedures [22].

Similarly, in a prospective study among 74 patients, US-PDT was found to be more efficacious and a favorable alternative to bronchoscopy-guided PDT with a low complication rate in critically ill, obese patients [23].

In a meta-analysis (including three randomized and one nonrandomized controlled study) by Lin et al., in 474 patients, comparing the effectiveness of ultrasound-guided and anatomic landmark PDT, the authors concluded that real-time US-PDT resulted in increased first-pass success, decreased complications with no significant reduction in major bleeding or the total tracheostomy placement time [24]. Further randomized clinical trials are required before evidence-based recommendations for routine US-PDT are being made.

3. Laryngeal Mask Airway (LMA) [1, 21]

Some studies advocate the use of LMAs as an alternative to endotracheal tube (ETT) during PDT to prevent risks of accidental extubation and inadvertent puncture of ETT cuff [25]. However, in a study by Ambesh et al., a higher rate of potentially catastrophic complications (33%) in LMA group were seen as compared to the ETT group (3.3%) during PDT [26].

Another benefit of using LMA during fibre optically assisted PDT is better visualization of the trachea and larynx observed by Dosemeci et al. as compared to ETT [27]. On the other hand,

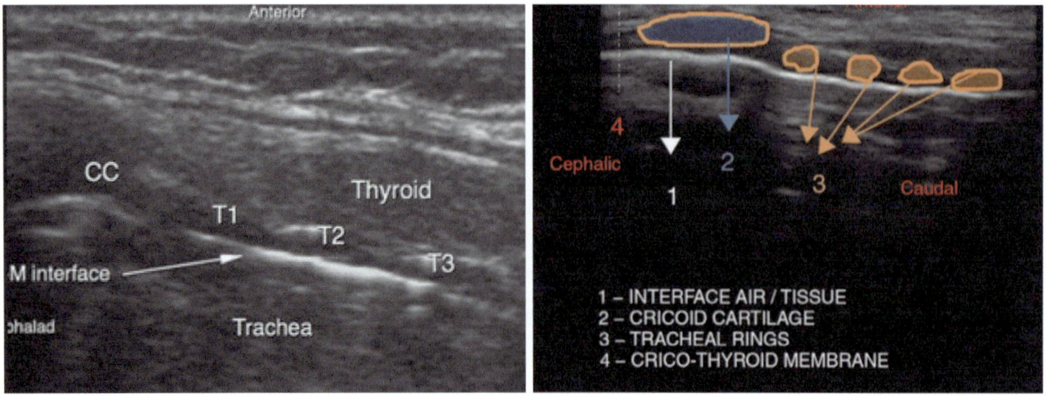

Fig. 65.4 Ultrasonography during PDT

its safety is questionable in critically ill patients requiring high degrees of ventilatory support. Hence, there is insufficient evidence to recommend the use of LMAs during PDT [25–28].

4. Capnography

Capnography can be used as a peri-procedure aid to monitor the adequacy of ventilation and for confirmation of the tracheal tube placement. Use of capnography is associated with the comparable success of confirmed needle placement, operating time, and complication rates as compared to bronchoscopy [29].

65.8 Special Considerations of PDT in Neurological Patients

Tracheostomy is an established technique for managing airway of critically ill patients with neurological problems including traumatic, non-traumatic brain injuries and stroke. Scales and colleagues, in a commentary on PDT, concluded that few special patient populations like those with underlying neurological problems may have different risk–benefit profiles than from general ICU patients [30]. If the primary brain injury is survivable and the patients have a reasonable prognosis, patients may have better prognosis by having earlier tracheostomy, but it may be prudent to wait longer otherwise.

The ultimate aim in any neurological patient is to avoid secondary insult to an already damaged brain, optimizing the most crucial parameters in neurointensive care medicine including ICP, cerebral perfusion pressure (CPP), and partial oxygen tension of brain tissue ($PBtO_2$). During PDT, fluctuations in ICP, CPP, and $PBtO_2$ are known to occur which should be avoided to prevent secondary brain insult [31–34].

In a retrospective study series of 289 tracheostomies in brain injury patients, severe complications were rare (1/289) with hypotension, transient hypoxia, and severe hypercapnia seen in in 3, 2, and 43 cases (15%), respectively. ICP rose temporarily in 24% of the cases but CPP remained unaffected. The authors found PDT to be a safe procedure for the most common neurosurgical diseases with short surgical time being the most important factor to avoid ICP increase [35].

TIP trial investigators recommend to use peri-procedural ICP and CPP monitoring in patients with severe cerebral dysfunction and those at risk of raised ICP [36]. Optic nerve sheath diameter (ONSD) monitoring using bedside ultrasound during PDT is a useful noninvasive monitor for clinicians in early recognition raised ICP but maybe cumbersome [37].

Thus, ICP surges during PDT should be safely managed with peri-procedural invasive or non-invasive ICP monitoring, appropriate sedation/analgesia, bolus of mannitol, or hypertonic saline or opening the ventriculostomy drain to lower ICP during the procedure [38].

65.9 Areas Requiring Special Considerations

1. Cervical spine injury

Patients with cervical spine injury are unable to extend their neck because of lack of cervical spine clearance and is a relative contraindication to PDT but studies report PDT to be safe, especially if done under ultrasound guidance. In a case series of 28 patients without cervical spine clearance, PDT was done with 96% success rate and low complication rate (7.1%) [39]. In another series comprising 16 patients with anterior cervical fusion following spinal cord injury, ultrasound-guided PDT was found to be much quicker and as safe as surgical tracheostomy [40].

2. Traumatic Brain Injury (TBI)

Patients with TBI can safely tolerate PDT with due intra-procedural considerations to mitigate the risks of raised ICP including use of sedation, appropriate ventilator settings, and avoiding bronchoscopy for procedure. If needed, it is better to shorten the time the bronchoscope is in the ETT, using a smaller diameter bronchoscope and minimizing suctioning during bronchoscopy. The procedure should be preferably performed in a controlled environment with close ICP and end-tidal CO_2 ($EtCO_2$) monitoring.

3. Pediatric Considerations

There have been concerns with the use of PDT in the airway management of children as the pediatric trachea is small and mobile and may compromise ventilation when performing bronchoscopic-guided PDT [41]. PDT is contraindicated in infants but has been safely performed in pediatric population. The technique standardized with some minor variations like vertical tracheal incision and use of pre- and/or post-operative bronchoscopy is safe with comparable complication rates as the surgical technique [42, 43]. A case series on PDT with 75% of study population below 2 years of age showed reduced cost and similar complication risk to operating room tracheostomies [44].

65.10 Decannulation

Decannulation is the process of removal of the tracheostomy tube once the need of the tracheostomy has resolved. There is no universally accepted protocol for decannulation and an individualized approach is needed [45]. Decannulation improves patient comfort, swallowing, and quality of life. The ideal set up to decannulate should be in an acute care setting and must be managed by a multi-disciplinary team.

1. Assessment for "Readiness" for Decannulation

The first step is to assess for the readiness for decannulation. The underlying cause for which the patient was tracheostomized should have been resolved. The patient should have adequate mentation, ability to obey commands, and maintain a patent airway. The patient should not be requiring ventilatory support (maintaining $SpO_2 > 95\%$ on room air) or should be manageable with noninvasive ventilation after decannulation [46].

2. Assessment of Cough [47, 48]

The ability to handle own's secretions and an effective cough reflex are important prerequisites before decannulation. Suctioning requirement should be less, and one study suggests it should be less than four times in previous 24 h or not more than two times in 8 h. The strength and adequacy of cough should be assessed by a speech therapist or physiotherapist and the patient must be able to generate an adequate peak expiratory flow rate (PEFR) (>160 L/min). The evaluation of upper airway patency and ruling out of any obstruction by endoscopy is prudent if the duration of mechanical ventilation is long. The lumen diameter should be more than 50% patent [49].

3. Assessment of Swallowing

The patient should be capable of taking liquids/semisolids without risk of aspiration. Airway patency can be assessed bedside by simply deflating the cuff and occluding the tracheostomy tube with a gloved finger for phonation. An objective assessment of bronchial micro-aspiration can be done by fibro-endoscopic examination or blue dye test [50]. A penetration-aspiration scale (PAS) is an 8-point scale used to characterize the depth and response to airway invasion during videofluoroscopy. A score of more than 5 confirms an aspiration event [51].

4. Decannulation Technique

The last step of the decannulation process is to give a trial of partially occluding the tracheostomy and allowing the patient to breathe. There are two techniques that have been mentioned viz. Corking technique and Blocking technique. In the former, the tube is deflated completely, then blocked and the patient is allowed to breathe around the tube and thereafter the tracheostomy tube can be removed; while in the latter, a smaller-sized tube or a fenestrated or cuff less tube is inserted as an intermediary step to decannulation [52].

5. Decannulation Failure [45, 53]

Reported incidence of decannulation failure is 2–5% which may become apparent sometimes by fourth day post decannulation. Some of the important causes for failure to decannulate are tracheal granuloma, tracheal stenosis, tracheomalacia, weak cough and vocal cord or laryngeal dysfunction. Inability to handle secretions, persistent neuro muscular weakness, poor lung capacity due to prolonged illness and ventilator dependency are

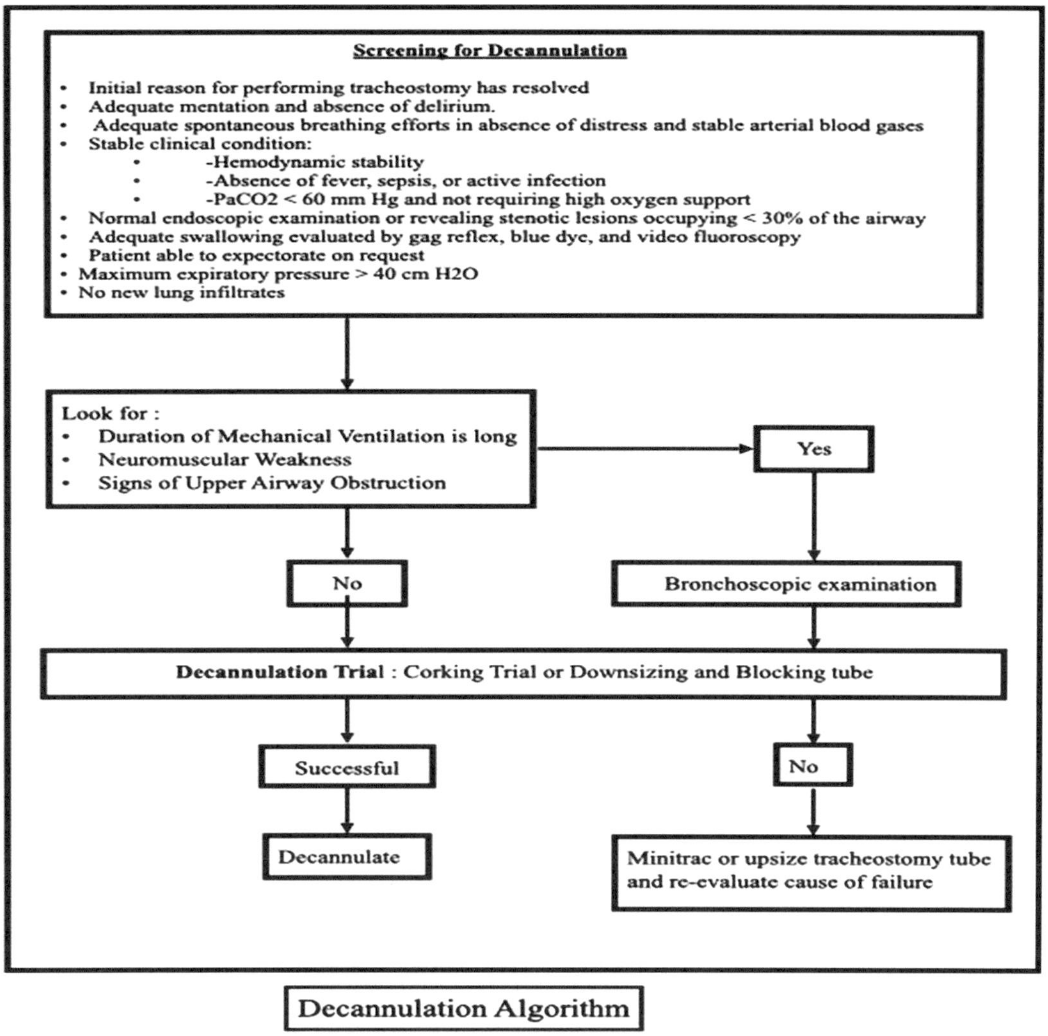

Fig. 65.5 Decannulation algorithm [54]

other causes in which patient may require long-term tracheotomy.

An algorithmic approach for decannulation is shown in Fig. 65.5.

65.11 Post Tracheostomy Care

Post tracheostomy care involves the following steps:

- Tube cuffs are typically low-pressure high-volume type and should be monitored to maintain cuff pressure in the range of 20–25 mmHg. Unmonitored overinflation can result in mucosal erosions and difficulty in feeding [52].
- Humidification of gases is important as this will aid in preventing formation of thick or dried up secretions, which are more prone to cause obstruction. [55]
- Head of the bed should be elevated to 30–45 degrees to minimize the risk of aspiration.
- Care should be taken while mobilizing and giving sides to patient and prevent accidental decannulation.
- Suctioning [56, 57]: The respiratory status of patients should be assessed at regular intervals to determine the need for suctioning as opposed to doing so at predetermined inter-

vals based on the consistency, quality of secretions and the patients ability to cough. The presence of noisy breathing, moist cough, dyspnea, restlessness, agitation, and increased inspiratory pressures on mechanical ventilation should alert the bedside nurse to need for urgent suction. Desaturation may be a late sign of need for suctioning. Masood et al. [58] studied the effect of implementing a standardized suctioning protocol and observed a reduction in tube obstruction. Suctioning should be done under strict aseptic precautions being mindful of the associated complications including hypoxia, arrhythmia, traumatic bleeding, and bronchospasm. Preoxygenation, monitoring of vitals during the procedure and maintenance of suction pressure around 120 mmHg can prevent inadvertent complications. Difficulty in passing the suction catheter should lead to suspicion of the tube being partially blocked or misplaced and requires immediate attention.

- Stoma care: Stoma should be cleaned daily with antiseptic solution and normal saline diluted in a 1:1 proportion. A small gauze must be placed under the flange of the tracheostomy as a cushion for skin. Dressing soiled with secretions should be changed, and any erythematous and infected stomal site should be treated with topical antiseptics.
- Tracheostomy tube change: The first tracheostomy tube change should not be done before 7 days post procedure. A person experienced to perform tracheostomy should be available at least while performing the first tube change. An algorithmic approach has been recommended for the tube change (Fig. 65.6).
- Multidisciplinary approach and Quality improvement programmes: Multidisciplinary tracheostomy teams are vital in improving

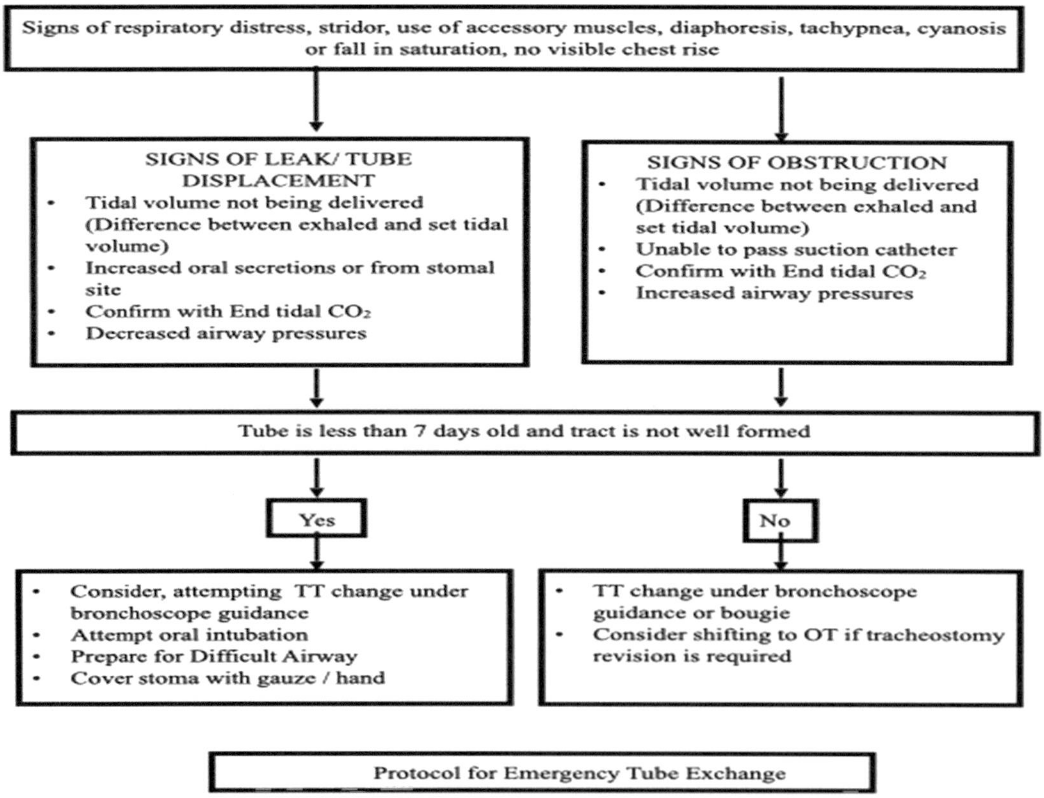

Fig. 65.6 Algorithm for tracheostomy tube change

outcomes in patients with tracheostomy. A study by Mah et al. [59], validates and addresses this vital service. In their study, an intensivist led multidisciplinary with a bundled approach not only improved patient satisfaction but also increased decannulation rates and tolerance of diet. The bundle included four measures: electronic set of post tracheostomy orders, tracking and follow-up of tracheostomized patients, decannulation protocol, and regular tracheostomy rounds. A single centre study by Sodhi et.al. showed that the support of a trained specialist tracheostomy nurse decreases the complication rates, re-admissions to ICU and reduces average length of ICU stay [60]. Trach trail [61] and Trach safe Initiatives [62] are quality-improvement programs based on patient centric pathways showing enhanced patients outcomes in terms of reduced ICU stay as well as in unanticipated mortalities at home, stressing the need to promote multidisciplinary approach to post tracheostomy patients.

65.12 Complications and Management

With increase in procedural experience, fewer complications are reported with the procedure [1]. The complications with PDT are almost similar as with the surgical technique [25]. As per the time of occurrence, they are divided into immediate (within few hours), early (0–7 days of procedure), and late (beyond day 7) (Table 65.4).

Most of the complications are preventable, and if at all they occur are self-limited or can be controlled with simple measures [1, 25]. The common complications of PDT along with the manifestation and treatment are included in Table 65.5.

65.13 Conclusion

PDT has become standard of care in modern ICUs worldwide and is safer to perform by use of POCUS in PDT which are available in most of the centres worldwide. However, evidence-based recommendations for routine POCUS in PDT require further validation. There are special considerations of PDT in neurocritical care patients including TBI, cervical spine injury, and pediatric neurological patients due to their underlying pathology which must be properly addressed.

Table 65.4 Complications of percutaneous tracheostomy

Immediate	Early	Late
Bleeding	Bleeding	Bleeding (tracheo-innominate artery bleed)
Hypoxia	Desaturation	Subglottic stenosis
Loss of airway	Tracheal tube obstruction	Tracheoesophageal fistula
False tract	Pneumothorax	Permanent voice changes due to vocal cord injury
Pneumothorax	Pneumomediastinum	Unplanned decannulation
Subcutaneous emphysema	Paratracheal placement	Infected stoma
Pneumomediastinum	Surgical emphysema	Difficulty in swallowing
Injury to posterior tracheal wall	Atelectasis	Difficult decannulation
Esophageal injury	Raised ICP	Scarring of the neck
Raised ICP	Accidental tube displacement	Delayed healing after decannulation

Table 65.5 Manifestations and management of complications of PDT

Timing	Complication	Manifestation	Management	Prevention
Immediate/ early	Bleeding	Venous oozing from stoma	• Usually self-limited • If not, then control with application of pressure • Use hemostatic agents • Purse-string suture can be applied • Frequent dressing changes • If persistent bleeding, chemical cauterization can be done with silver nitrate applied to the wound edge	Preoperative correction of coagulopathy Careful identification and control of bleeding points during the procedure Avoid overdilatation and creation of large stoma
	Hypoxia	Desaturation; drop in SpO_2 Can occur during suctioning	• 100% oxygen • Hand ventilation • Check for tube patency/ malpositioning	• Adequate preoxygenation • Precautions during suctioning: limit duration to <10 s, suction pressure < 120 mmHg
	Pneumothorax	Ventilation issues: high pressure alarms; CXR finding	• Immediate Intercostal drain placement • Needle thoracostomy as an emergency measure	Avoid coughing/bucking during procedure with adequate sedation
	Subcutaneous emphysema	Swelling around neck and chest; ventilation problems; high pressure alarms; CXR finding	• Confirm tube placement • No active intervention required • Typically disappears within 24 h	Avoid high airway pressures
	Paratracheal placement and posterior tracheal wall injury	Ventilation problems; excessive high pressure alarms	• Reposition the tube	Avoid excessive deep introduction of dilator into the airway, excessive downward force when advancing the tracheostomy-loaded dilator
	Bradycardia/asystole	Drop in heart rate Can occur during suctioning due to hypoxia or vagus nerve stimulation	• Immediately stop suctioning • Give 100% oxygen • May need atropine, if bradycardia persists	• Adequate preoxygenation before suctioning • Avoid deep suctioning • Restrict suction duration to <10 s
	Malpositioned tubes causing airway obstruction (may be indistinguishable from mucus plugging)	High-pressure alarms; ventilation problems or acute dyspnea	Exchanging the tube for another with a blunt tip opening	Rotation of the tube to bring the distal tip away from contact with the tracheal wall

Timing	Complication	Manifestation	Management	Prevention
Late	Subglottic stenosis	Usually manifest after decannulation with hoarseness, aphonia or abnormal cry	• Tracheal dilation is palliative • Definitive treatment: tracheal resection and reconstruction • Interventional bronchoscopic techniques (cryoprobe therapy, Nd:YAG and argon plasma coagulation)	• Maintain tracheostomy tube cuff pressure <30 mm Hg
	Bleeding (tracheoinnominate fistula)	Can be a catastrophic bleed	• Blood products • Immediate operative repair	• Avoid excessive cuff pressure (<30 mmHg)
	Tracheoesophageal fistula	Typically may present as foreign body in esophagus or feeds in tracheal suction	• Operative repair is indicated after the patient's critical illness has resolved	• Avoid excessive cuff pressure (<30 mmHg)
	Accidental decannulation	Tracheostomy tube out of the stoma	• Keep decannulated if patient conscious or • Replace the tube. • If unable to reinsert the tube, immediately perform translaryngeal intubation. • If there is no urgent need to secure the airway then the tracheostomy tube may be guided into the trachea bronchscopically	• Appropriate tube fixation • Careful patient mobilization
	Infections at stoma site	Redness, pain at stoma site Foul smelling pus at stoma	• Local site dressing • Systemic antibiotics	• Regular tracheostomy care • Limited disruption of tissue and minimal bleeding
	Atelectasis/lower respiratory tract infections	Fever Purulent tracheal secretions Increased O_2/ventilatory requirements	• Antibiotics	• Stringently following VAP bundle • Early tracheostomy when indicated

Acknowledgement The authors acknowledge Dr. Mandeep Kumar MD, DM, Assistant Professor, Santosh Medical College, Ghaziabad, for contributing the images (Figs. 65.2, 65.3, and 65.4).

References

1. Mehta C, Mehta Y. Percutaneous tracheostomy. Ann Card Anaesth. 2017;20:S19–25.
2. Astrachan DI, Kirchner JC, Goodwin WJ. Prolonged intubation vs. tracheotomy: complications, practical and psychological considerations. Laryngoscope. 1988;98:1165–9.
3. Sheldon CH, Pudenz RH, Freshwater DB, Cure BL. A new method for tracheostomy. J Neurosurg. 1955;12:428–31.
4. Muhammad JK, Major E, Patton DW. Evaluating the neck for percutaneous dilatational tracheostomy. J Craniomaxillofac Surg. 2000;28:336–42.
5. Epstein SK. Anatomy and physiology of tracheostomy. Respir Care. 2005;50(4):476–82.
6. Furlow PW, Mathisen DJ. Surgical anatomy of the trachea. Ann Cardiothorac Surg. 2018;7(2):255–60. https://doi.org/10.21037/acs.2018.03.01.
7. Ciaglia P, Firsching R, Syniec C. Elective percutaneous dilatational tracheostomy. A new and simple bedside procedure; preliminary report. Chest. 1985;87:715–9.
8. Batuwitage B, Webber S, Glossop A. Percutaneous tracheostomy. Contin Educ Anaesth Crit Care Pain. 2014;14:268–72.
9. Griggs WM, Myburgh J, Worthley L. A prospective comparison of a percutaneous tracheostomy technique with standard surgical tracheostomy. Intensive Care Med. 1991;17:261–3.
10. Zgoda MA, Berger R. Balloon facilitated percutaneous dilatational tracheostomy tube placement. Chest. 2005;128:3688–90.
11. Cianchi G, Zagli G, Bonizzoli M, Batacchi S, Camellia R, Biondi S, et al. Comparison between single-step and balloon dilatational tracheostomy in intensive care unit: a single-centre, randomized controlled study. Br J Anaesth. 2010;104:728–32.
12. Fantoni A, Ripamonti D. A non-derivative, non-surgical tracheostomy: the translaryngeal method. Intensive Care Med. 1997;23:386–92.
13. Frova G, Quintel M. A new simple method for percutaneous tracheostomy: controlled rotating dilation. A preliminary report. Intensive. Care Med. 2002;28:299–303.
14. Cabrini L, Monti G, Landoni G, Biondi-Zoccai G, Boroli F, Mamo D, et al. Percutaneous tracheostomy, a systematic review. Acta Anaesthesiol Scand. 2012;56:270–81.
15. Byhahn C, Wilke HJ, Halbig S, Lischke V, Westphal K. Percutaneous tracheostomy: Ciaglia blue rhino versus the basic Ciaglia technique of percutaneous dilational tracheostomy. Anesth Analg. 2000;91:882–6.
16. Van Heurn LW, Mastboom WB, Scheeren CI, Brink PR, Ramsay G. Comparative clinical trial of progressive dilatational and forceps dilatational tracheostomy. Intensive Care Med. 2001;27:292–5.
17. Marelli D, Paul A, Manolidis S, Walsh G, Odim JN, Burdon TA, et al. Endoscopic guided percutaneous tracheostomy: early results of a consecutive trial. J Trauma. 1990;30:433–5.
18. Barba CA, Angood PB, Kauder DR, Latenser B, Martin K, McGonigal MD, et al. Bronchoscopic guidance makes percutaneous tracheostomy a safe, cost-effective, and easy-to-teach procedure. Surgery. 1995;118:879–83.
19. Reilly PM, Anderson HL III, Sing RF, Schwab CW, Bartlett RH. Occult hypercarbia. An unrecognized phenomenon during percutaneous endoscopic tracheostomy. Chest. 1995;107:1760–3.
20. Rajajee V, Fletcher JJ, Rochlen LR, Jacobs TL. Real-time ultrasound-guided percutaneous dilatational tracheostomy: a feasibility study. Crit Care. 2011;15(1):R67.
21. Kollig E, Heydenreich U, Roetman B, Hopf F, Muhr G. Ultrasound and bronchoscopic controlled percutaneous tracheostomy on trauma ICU. Injury. 2000;31:663–8.
22. Gobatto AL, Besen BA, Tierno PF, Mendes PV, Cadamuro F, Joelsons D, et al. Comparison between ultrasound and bronchoscopy guided percutaneous dilatational tracheostomy in critically ill patients: a retrospective cohort study. J Crit Care. 2015;30(220):e13–7.
23. Ravi PR, Vijay MN. Real time ultrasound-guided percutaneous tracheostomy: is it a better option than bronchoscopic guided percutaneous tracheostomy? Med J Armed Forces India. 2015;71:158–64.
24. Lin K-T, Kao Y-S, Chiu C-W, Lin C-H, Chou C-C, Hsieh P-Y, et al. Comparative effectiveness of ultrasound-guided and anatomic landmark percutaneous dilatational tracheostomy: a systematic review and meta-analysis. PLoS One. 2021;16(10):e0258972.
25. Al-Ansari MA, Hijazi MH. Clinical review: percutaneous dilatational tracheostomy. Crit Care. 2005;10:202. https://doi.org/10.1186/cc3900.
26. Ambesh SP, Sinha PK, Tripathi M, Matreja P. Laryngeal mask airway vs endotracheal tube to facilitate bedside percutaneous tracheostomy in critically ill patients: a prospective comparative study. J Postgrad Med. 2002;48:11–5.
27. Dosemeci L, Yilmaz M, Gurpinar F, Ramazanoglu A. The use of the laryngeal mask airway as an alternative to the endotracheal tube during percutaneous dilatational tracheostomy. Intensive Care Med. 2002;28:63–7.
28. Raimondi N, Vidal MR, Calleja J, Quintero A, Cortés A, Celis E, et al. Evidence based guidelines for the use of tracheostomy in critically ill patients. J Crit Care. 2016;38:304–18. https://doi.org/10.1016/j.jcrc.2016.10.009.
29. Mallick A, Venkatanath D, Elliot SC, Hollins T, Nanda Kumar CG. A prospective randomized con-

trolled trial of capnography vs. bronchoscopy for blue rhino percutaneous tracheostomy. Anaesthesia. 2003;58:864–8.
30. Kuechler JN, Abusamha A, Ziemann S, Tronnier VM, Gliemroth J. Impact of percutaneous dilatational tracheostomy in brain injured patients. Clin Neurol Neurosurg. 2015;137:137–41. https://doi.org/10.1016/j.clineuro.2015.07.007.
31. Louh I, Freeman W. Safety and tolerability of percutaneous tracheostomy in neurocritical care patients with poor intracranial compliance. Crit Care Med. 2012;40:U230.
32. Stocchetti N, Parma A, Lamperti M, Songa V, Tognini L. Neurophysiological consequences of three tracheostomy techniques: a randomized study in neurosurgical patients. J Neurosurg Anesthesiol. 2000;12(4):307–13. https://doi.org/10.1097/00008506-200010000-00002.
33. Börm W, Gleixner M. Experience with two different techniques of percutaneous dilational tracheostomy in 54 neurosurgical patients. Neurosurg Rev. 2003;26:188–91. https://doi.org/10.1007/s10143-002-0248-3C.
34. Scales DC, Cuthbertson BH. Percutaneous dilatational tracheostomy: mostly safe, but do benefits outweigh risks? Crit Care. 2014;18:117.
35. Imperiale C, Magni G, Roberto F, Giovanni. Intracranial pressure monitoring during percutaneous tracheostomy "Percutwist" in critically ill neurosurgery patients. Anesth Analg. 2009;108(2):588–92. https://doi.org/10.1213/ane.0b013e31818f601b.
36. Kleffmann J, Pahl R, Deinsberger W, Ferbert A, Roth C. Effect of percutaneous tracheostomy on intracerebral pressure and perfusion pressure in patients with acute cerebral dysfunction (TIP trial): an observational study. Neurocrit Care. 2012;17(1):85–9. https://doi.org/10.1007/s12028-012-9709-x.
37. Kapoor I, Wanchoo J, Mahajan C, Singhal V, Roy H, Kumar S, et al. Effect of percutaneous tracheostomy on optic nerve sheath diameter [TONS trial]. Indian J Crit Care Med. 2021;25(4):382–7.
38. Louh IK, Freeman WD. Safety of percutaneous tracheostomy in neuro ICU patients with intracranial pressure monitoring. Crit Care. 2014;18:432.
39. Mayberry JC, Wu IC, Goldman RK, Chestnut RM. Cervical spine clearance and neck extension during percutaneous tracheostomy in trauma patients. Crit Care Med. 2000;28:3436–40.
40. Sustic A, Krstulovic B, Eskinja N, Zelic M, Ledic D, Turina D. Surgical tracheostomy versus percutaneous dilational tracheostomy in patients with anterior cervical spine fixation: preliminary report. Spine. 2002;27:1942–5.
41. Watters KF. Tracheostomy in infants and children. Respiratory Care Jun. 2017;62(6):799–825. https://doi.org/10.4187/respcare.05366.
42. Toursarkissian B, Fowler C, Zweng TN, Kearney PA. Percutaneous dilatational tracheostomy in children and teenagers. J Pediatr Surg. 1994;29:1421–4.
43. Raju A, Joseph DK, Diarra C, Ross SE. Percutaneous versus open tracheostomy in the pediatric trauma population. Am Surg. 2010;3:276–8.
44. Klotz DA, Hengerer AS. Safety of pediatric bedside tracheostomy in the intensive care unit. Arch Otolaryngol Head Neck Surg. 2001;127(8):950–5. https://doi.org/10.1001/archotol.127.8.950.
45. Connor HH, White AC. Tracheostomy decannulation. Respir Care. 2010;55(8):1076–81.
46. Kollef MH, Ahrens TS, Shannon W. Clinical predictors and outcomes for patients requiring tracheostomy in the intensive care unit. Crit Care Med. 1999;27(9):1714–20.
47. Hernández G, Ortiz R, Pedrosa A, Cuena R, Vaquero Collado C, Gonzalez Arenas P, et al. The indication of tracheotomy conditions the predictors of time to decannulation in critical patients. Med Intensiva. 2012;36(8):531–9.
48. Bach JR, Saporito LR. Indications and criteria for decannulation and transition from invasive to noninvasive long-term ventilatory support. Respir Care. 1994;39(5):515–28.
49. Rodrigues LB, Nunes TA. Importance of flexible bronchoscopy in decannulation of tracheostomy patients. Rev Col Bras Cir. 2015;42:2.
50. Béchet S, Hill F, Gilheaney Ó, Walshe M. Diagnostic accuracy of the modified Evan's blue dye test in detecting aspiration in subjects with tracheostomy: a systematic review of the evidence. Dysphagia. 2016;31(6):721–9.
51. Rosenbek JC, Robbins JA, Roecker EB, Coyle JL, Wood JL. A penetration-aspiration scale. Dysphagia. 1996;11(2):93–8.
52. Engels PT, Bagshaw SM, Meier M, Brindley PG. Tracheostomy: from insertion to decannulation. Can J Surg. 2009;52(5):427–33.
53. Law JH, Barnhart K, Rowlett W, de la Rocha O, Lowenberg S. Increased frequency of obstructive airway abnormalities with long-term tracheostomy. Chest. 1993;104(1):136–8.
54. Singh RK, Saran S, Baronia AK. The practice of tracheostomy decannulation-a systematic review. J Intensive Care. 2017;20(5):38. https://doi.org/10.1186/s40560-017-0234.
55. De Leyn P, Bedert L, Delcroix M, Depuydt P, Lauwers G, Sokolov Y, et al. Belgian Association of Pneumology and Belgian Association of Cardiothoracic Surgery. Tracheotomy: clinical review and guidelines. Eur J Cardiothorac Surg. 2007;32(3):412.
56. Petros S. Percutaneous tracheostomy. Crit Care. 1999;3(2):R5–R10. https://doi.org/10.1186/cc340.
57. Dunn PF, Goulet RL. Endotracheal tubes and airway appliances. Int Anesthesiol Clin. 2000;38(3):65–94. https://doi.org/10.1097/00004311-200007000-00006.
58. Masood MM, Farquhar DR, Biancaniello C, Hackman TG. Association of Standardized Tracheostomy Care Protocol Implementation and Reinforcement with the prevention of life-threatening respira-

tory events. JAMA Otolaryngol Head Neck Surg. 2018;144(6):527–32.
59. Mah JW, Staff II, Fisher SR, Butler KL. Improving decannulation and swallowing function: a comprehensive, multidisciplinary approach to post-tracheostomy care. Respir Care. 2017;62(2):137–43.
60. Sodhi K, Shrivastava A, Singla MK. Implications of dedicated tracheostomy care nurse program on outcomes. J Anesth. 2014;28(3):374–80. https://doi.org/10.1007/s00540-013-1718-1.
61. Ong T, Liu CC, Elder L, Hill L, Abts M, Dahl JP, et al. The trach safe initiative: a quality improvement initiative to reduce mortality among pediatric tracheostomy patients. Otolaryngol Head Neck Surg. 2020;163(2):221–31.
62. Cherney RL, Pandian V, Ninan A, Eastman D, Barnes B, King E, et al. The Trach Trail: a systems-based pathway to improve quality of tracheostomy care and interdisciplinary collaboration. Otolaryngol Head Neck Surg. 2020;163(2):232–43.

Bronchoscopy in Neuro ICU

66

Gunjan Chanchalani, Vivek Dave, and Anish Joshi

66.1 Introduction

Fibreoptic bronchoscopy (FOB) is one of the essential tools in critical care medicine, and it is being increasingly used for the diagnostic and therapeutic purpose in the intensive care units (ICUs). The safety, ease, and portability of bronchoscopy makes it one of the most popular and commonly requested invasive procedures in the ICU setting. The presence of round-the-clock trained critical care experts and the ready access of bronchoscope has broadened the diagnostic and therapeutic capabilities in the critically ill patients. But the procedure is not without complications and challenges, especially in a neuro ICU. The clinician must assess patient safety and perform procedures with utmost attention for better patient comfort [1].

The most common indications in diagnostic work-up are to visualize airway system, to examine and detect respiratory infections by means of bronchoalveolar lavage (BAL) and tissue sampling in specific situations. The main therapeutic indications are aspiration of bronchial secretions, mucus plug removal in cases of lobar atelectasis and diagnostic as well therapeutic in case of hemoptysis [2].

G. Chanchalani (✉)
KJ Somaiya Hospital, Mumbai, Maharashtra, India

V. Dave · A. Joshi
Critical Care Department, Narayana Multispeciality Hospital, Ahmedabad, Gujarat, India

66.2 Indications in Neuro ICU

There are a wide range of indications (Table 66.1) for FOB in neuro ICU like basic bronchoscopy with exploration, lavage, brushing, managing hemoptysis, and collecting samples as a primary techniques [3].

A. Infections

Neuro ICU patients often have a prolonged ICU stay, with prolonged periods of endotracheal intubations and tracheostomy, putting them at a greater risk of nosocomial pneumonia and ventilator associated events, often with resistant bugs. FOB is useful for collecting bronchoalveolar samples, thus increasing diagnostic accuracy of lower respiratory tract infections and thus facilitating targeted antimicrobial therapies. However, there is no clear cut evidence to support its routine use compared to standard practice, of administering antimicrobial therapies based on culture of endotracheal aspirates and clinical symptoms [4, 5].

B. Management of Airway Obstruction

Patients admitted with stroke, Parkinson's disease, motor neuron disease, meningoencephalitis, etc. often have a poor cough reflex,

H. Prabhakar et al. (eds.), *Principles and Practice of Neurocritical Care*,
https://doi.org/10.1007/978-981-99-8059-8_66

Table 66.1 Indications of bronchoscopy in a neuro ICU

Diagnostic	Therapeutic
Post trauma—identifying site of injury	Difficult intubation—especially in maxillofacial injuries
Pneumonia—non resolving	Percutaneous dilatational tracheostomy guidance
Hemoptysis—to identify source and site of bleeding	Foreign body removal
Failed extubation—to identify the cause	Secretion/atelectasis management—removal of mucus plugging
Unexplained infiltrates on X-ray or CT scan	Tumour—debridement of the tumor
Central airway obstruction whether benign or malignant	Tracheal stenosis—stent placement
Extent of tracheobronchial burn in patients with possible smoke inhalation/facial burns	Bleeding control using endobronchial blockers, cryotherapy, or argon laser therapy

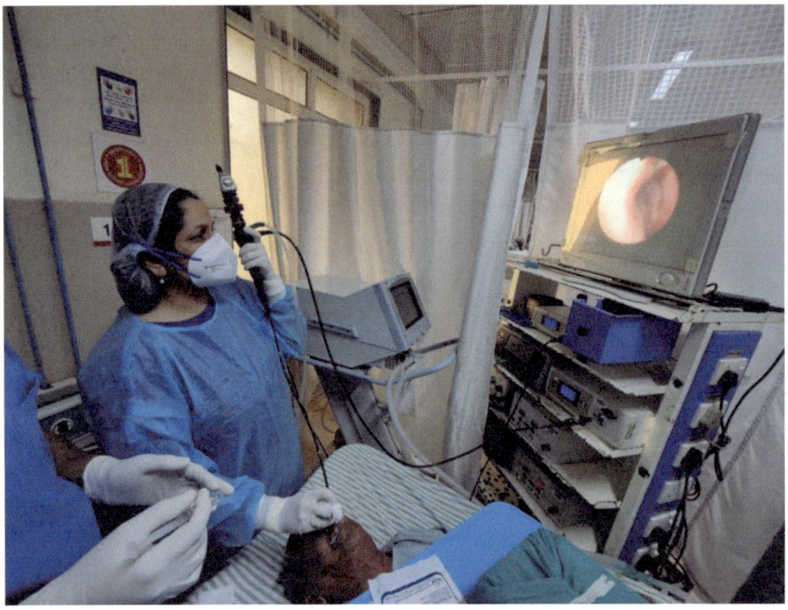

Fig. 66.1 FOB and airway examination

leading of secretion retention and aspiration. They are also at a higher risk of developing basal atelectasis. Thick secretions lead to mucus plugging in a bronchoalveolar tree which can give rise to lung collapse which can be confirmed by clinical parameters and chest radiography. Bedside FOB is helpful in clearing the bronchoalveolar tree and improving lung aeration, in situations where adequate chest physiotherapy and airway clearance techniques are unsuccessful. The bronchoscopic management of such cases includes the removal of thick endobronchial material by means of either suction or forceps. The overall success rate for the correction of acute atelectasis caused by airway obstruction due to mucus plugs is more than 70% in various reports [6, 7].

C. Bedside Tracheostomy in Neuro Patients

Early tracheostomy is a well-established procedure nowadays in patients with various neurological conditions, in whom there is anticipated prolong mechanical ventilatory requirement and also need to secure airways. FOB can be used as a guide while performing percutaneous dilatational tracheostomy in the ICU [8].

D. For Airway Evaluation

Inspection of the airway is required to localize the source of bleeding in cases of hemoptysis, with an intent to diagnose as well as control the bleeding source, and to clear the bronchus of the blood clots (Fig. 66.1).

FOB can also be performed to evaluate tracheomalacia or tracheal stenosis after tracheostomy. However, in certain selected and complicated cases, rigid bronchoscopy may be required [9].

66.3 The Procedure

An informed written consent should be taken by the patient or by the next of kin as often the critically ill neuro patients may not be in a position to give a consent.

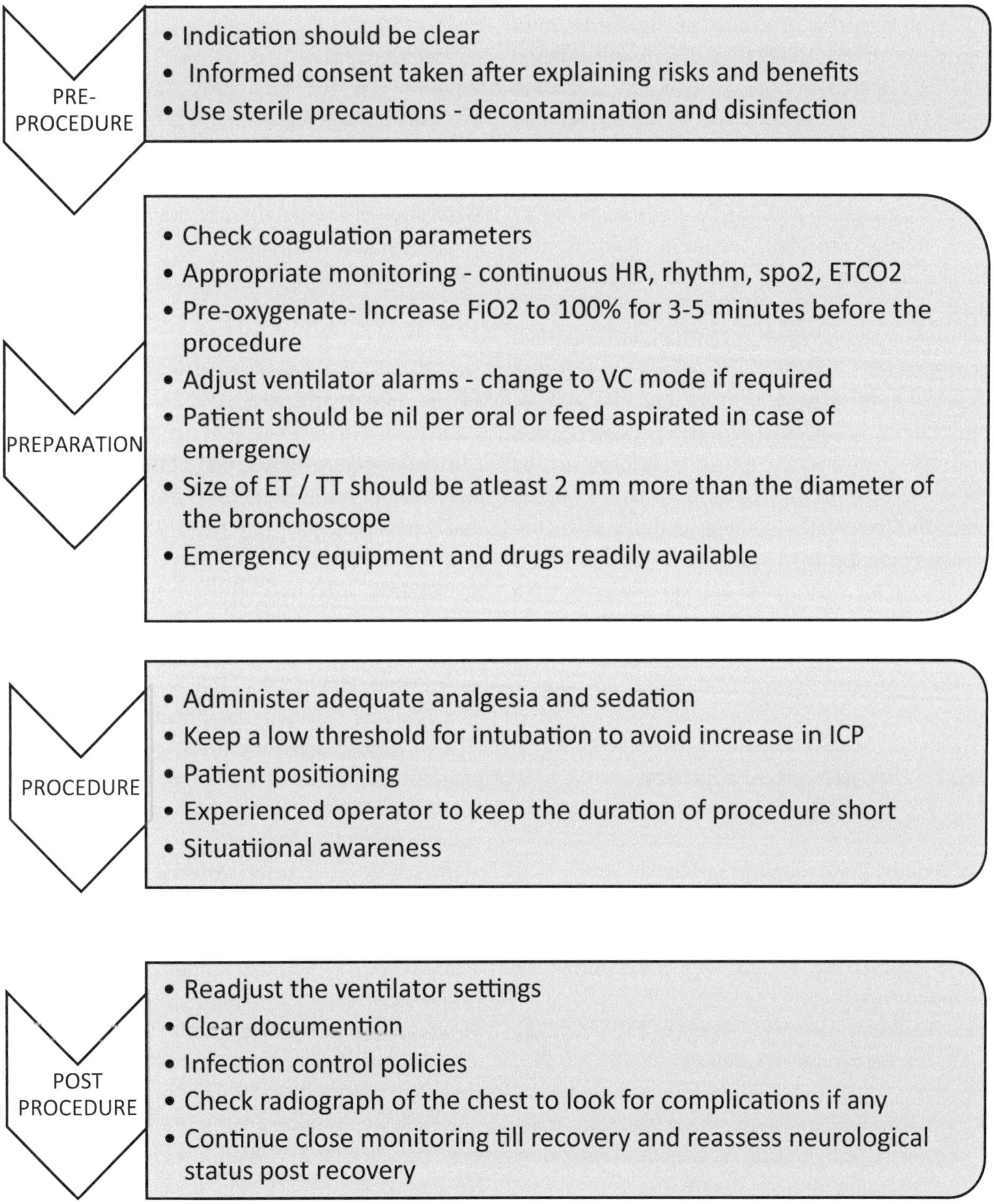

Flow Chart 61.1 Steps and precautions to be considered prior to, during, and after FOB in neuro ICU

In non-intubated patients, nil per oral of at least 8 h is recommended; however, in case of emergency and full stomach, it is better to intubate the patient for airway protection and the stomach contents aspirated via the nasogastric tube.

Topical anesthesia with 2% lidocaine is administered as a spray or via nebulisation. Obtunded patients or patients with poor cough reflex or high risk of aspiration should be intubated for airway protection. Adequate sedation may be required in order to facilitate a smooth procedure and to avoid a rise in the intracranial pressure (ICP).

In the ventilated patients, FOB can be performed through an endotracheal or tracheostomy tube, through specially adaptor attached, that allows bronchoscope to enter the circuit and airway, without disconnecting from mechanical ventilation and permitting ventilation throughout the procedure. However, this causes a significant increase in the airway pressure, and special caution should be exercised if the patient is on a pressure control mode. Close monitoring of the delivered tidal volume in order to avoid hypoxemia and hypercarbia should be done, also continuous monitoring of spo_2 and $ETCO_2$ is a must in all patients with neurological condition, CNS mass lesion or raised ICP [10]. It is recommended to have an ET/TT with inner diameter at least 2 mm larger than the size of the bronchoscope.

66.4 Bronchoscopy Safety Checklist

- Continuous SpO_2 monitoring
- Continuous $ETCO_2$ monitoring
- Continuous cardiac rate and rhythm monitoring
- NiBP monitoring—every 2–5 min/arterial BP monitoring
- In ventilated patients, increase FiO_2 to 1.0, 5–15 min prior to procedure
- Nursing support for sedation and monitoring
- Respiratory therapist support for ventilator management, monitoring of minute ventilation, and pressure limited volume loss
- Technical support to assist with procedure lavage, etc.

66.5 Contraindications

Contraindications to perform bronchoscopy in a critically ill neuro patient include the following:

- Respiratory rate > 30 bpm
- Impending respiratory failure in case of clinical use of accessory muscles
- PaO_2 < 70 mm Hg or SaO_2 < 90% with supplemental oxygen
- Requirement for minimally invasive BiPAP/CPAP ventilation
- Significantly altered mental status, without airway protection
- Acute ischemic heart disease or unstable angina
- Haemodynamic instability
- Critical cardiac dysrhythmias
- Known increased ICP

66.6 Complications

Currently, the use of bedside FOB has become a standard of care in examining and managing critical care patients. Improved knowledge and awareness regarding the procedure facilitates appropriate, safe, and effective use of bronchoscope. Overall, a FOB is a safe procedure with mortality is as low as 0.01% and in high risk, it varies from 0.08 to 2% (Table 66.2).

The most dreaded complication which can lead to further deterioration in patient's clinical condition is hypoxaemia. Hypoxaemia associated with FOB can lead to increase in cardiovascular workload and stress.

Increase in systolic arterial pressure and heart rate during FOB can lead to ECG changes in 10–15% of patients. Unexpected ST-T changes were reported in around 21% of patients [11]. In critically ill patients, there are chances of worsening of haemodynamic parameters and increase requirements of ionotropic agents. Bronchoscopy within 30 days of acute myocardial ischemia is associated with 5% mortality. It must be addressed with utmost caution in unstable angina patients. In the absence of ischemia with good clinical justification, FOB can be performed.

Table 66.2 Possible complications of performing FOB

Complications related to topical anaesthesia	Complications related to sedation and analgesia	Complications related to bronchoscopy	Complications related to sampling—Biopsy or brushing
Respiratory arrest	Hemodynamic instability	Airway obstruction	Pneumothorax
Cardiovascular collapse	Loss of airway reflexes and aspiration	Laryngospasm and bronchospasm	Haemorrhage
Convulsions		Hypoxaemia and/or hypercarbia	
Local anaesthetic toxicity		Cardiac arrhythmias/ hypotension	
		Vasovagal reaction	
		Haemorrhage	
		Pulmonary oedema	
		Pneumonia	

A potential complication of FOB is that it increases ICP while manipulating airway. The use of FOB increases the ICP with concomitant increase in mean arterial pressure; therefore, change in cerebral perfusion pressure is limited. But still, it can be performed in patients with reduced cranial compliance ensuring that sedation, analgesia, and relaxants are optimized.

Minor bleeding occurs in 0.19% and severe in 0.26% of bronchoscopies [12]. Bleeding risk is higher with the use of anticoagulation therapy, liver disease, or history of bleeding tendency. Haemoglobin, platelet count, and coagulation studies are supposed to be done when clinical risk factors suggest higher likelihood of coagulation abnormalities; however, abnormal results do not reliably predict the bleeding risk.

66.7 Bronchoscopy in Critically Ill Neuro Patient

It has been shown that FOB is relatively a safe procedure in neuro patients; however, it causes increase in the airway resistance with a drop in tidal volume and may increase the PEEP (positive end-expiratory pressure). These changes can cause an increase in the intracranial pressure, in the critically ill neuro patients.

Rise in the intra-thoracic pressure can reduce the venous return and thus reducing cardiac output. Frequent suctioning and lavage can also lead to alveolar collapse and often transient hypoxemia and rise in the $ETCO_2$ level, leading to an increase in the pulmonary vascular resistance. All these changes can contribute secondary brain injury.

Sustained increase in intracranial pressure leads to poor outcome in traumatic brain injury patients. Although no acute worsening in condition has been reported, secondary brain injury caused by localized cerebral ischemia is always a possibility [13]. The ICP returns to baseline levels after the procedure is completed. When performed with due care and precautions, FOB does not adversely affect neurologic status in patients with severe brain injury. Close monitoring with maintaining adequate oxygenation and carbon dioxide levels with adequate sedation and analgesia can make the procedure successful, without any bad consequences.

66.8 Conclusion

FOB is an integral part of critical care in ICU nowadays. The oxygenation strategy during FOB should be chosen according to the procedure, underlying cardiac function, oxygen requirement within the procedure, and the risk of worsening of respiratory and neurological status. It provides valuable diagnostic information and has therapeutic utility as well. It can be performed safely in neuro critically ill patients with appropriate clinical indications. Safety and benefits are the hallmark of its widespread use.

References

1. Ergan B, Nava S. The use of bronchoscopy in critically ill patients: considerations and complications. Expert Rev Respir Med. 2018;12(8):651–63. https://doi.org/10.1080/17476348.2018.1494576. Epub 2018 Jul 12
2. Kabadayi S, Bellamy MC. Bronchoscopy in critical care. BJA Educat. 2017;17:48–56. https://doi.org/10.1093/bjaed/mkw040.
3. Álvarez-Maldonado P, Redondo CN-P, Casillas-Enríquez JD, Navarro-Reynoso F, Cicero-Sabido R. Indications and efficacy of fiberoptic bronchoscopy in the ICU: have they changed since its introduction in clinical practice? Int Sch Res Notices. 2013;2013:217505. https://doi.org/10.5402/2013/217505.
4. Aridgides D, Dessaint J, Atkins G, Carroll J, Ashare A. Safety of research bronchoscopy with BAL in stable adult patients with cystic fibrosis. PLoS One. 2021;16(1):e0245696. https://doi.org/10.1371/journal.pone.0245696.
5. Jain K, Wainwright C, Smyth AR. Bronchoscopy-guided antimicrobial therapy for cystic fibrosis. Cochrane Database Syst Rev. 2013;(12):CD009530. https://doi.org/10.1002/14651858.CD009530.pub2. Update in: Cochrane Database Syst Rev. 2016;(1):CD009530.
6. Turner JS, Willcox PA, Hayhurst MD, Potgieter PD. Fiberoptic bronchoscopy in the intensive care unit—a prospective study of 147 procedures in 107 patients. Crit Care Med. 1994;22(2):259–64. https://doi.org/10.1097/00003246-199402000-00017.
7. Kreider ME, Lipson DA. Bronchoscopy for atelectasis in the ICU: a case report and review of the literature. Chest. 2003;124(1):344–50. https://doi.org/10.1378/chest.124.1.344.
8. Tsakiridis K, Darwiche K, Visouli AN, Zarogoulidis P, Machairiotis N, Christofis C, Stylianaki A, Katsikogiannis N, Mpakas A, Courcoutsakis N, Zarogoulidis K. Management of complex benign post-tracheostomy tracheal stenosis with bronchoscopic insertion of silicon tracheal stents, in patients with failed or contraindicated surgical reconstruction of trachea. J Thorac Dis. 2012;4 Suppl 1(Suppl 1):32–40. https://doi.org/10.3978/j.issn.2072-1439.2012.s002.
9. Noppen M, Stratakos G, Amjadi K, De Weerdt S, D'Haese J, Meysman M, Vincken W. Stenting allows weaning and extubation in ventilator- or tracheostomy dependency secondary to benign airway disease. Respir Med. 2007;101(1):139–45. https://doi.org/10.1016/j.rmed.2006.03.037. Epub 2006 May 18
10. Balwan A, Seder DB. Bronchoscopy in the NeuroICU. In: Lee K, editor. The NeuroICU book. 2nd ed. McGraw Hill; 2017. https://neurology.mhmedical.com/content.aspx?bookid=2155&sectionid=163967036. Accessed 16 Feb 2023.
11. Dweik RA, Mehta AC, Meeker DP, Arroliga AC. Analysis of the safety of bronchoscopy after recent acute myocardial infarction. Chest. 1996;110(3):825–8. https://doi.org/10.1378/chest.110.3.825.
12. Facciolongo N, Patelli M, Gasparini S, Lazzari Agli L, Salio M, Simonassi C, Del Prato B, Zanoni P. Incidence of complications in bronchoscopy. Multicentre prospective study of 20,986 bronchoscopies. Monaldi Arch Chest Dis. 2009;71(1):8–14. https://doi.org/10.4081/monaldi.2009.370.
13. Kerwin AJ, Croce MA, Timmons SD, Maxwell RA, Malhotra AK, Fabian TC. Effects of fiberoptic bronchoscopy on intracranial pressure in patients with brain injury: a prospective clinical study. J Trauma. 2000;48(5):878–82; discussion 882–3. https://doi.org/10.1097/00005373-200005000-00011.

MIX
Papier aus verantwortungsvollen Quellen
Paper from responsible sources
FSC® C105338

If you have any concerns about our products,
you can contact us on
ProductSafety@springernature.com

In case Publisher is established outside the EU,
the EU authorized representative is:
Springer Nature Customer Service Center GmbH
Europaplatz 3, 69115 Heidelberg, Germany

Printed by Libri Plureos GmbH
in Hamburg, Germany